Instructor Resources for Nursing Excellence

To aid in teaching your pharmacology course, use these resources designed to support your textbook.

Instructor's Resource Manual

Designed to help faculty plan and manage the pharmacology course, this manual includes:

- Detailed lecture notes with correlations to PowerPoint slides, organized by learning objectives
- Suggestions for classroom and clinical activities
- Comprehensive test questions with rationales, mapped to learning objectives
- Assignments using the **Companion Website** and the **Prentice Hall Nursing MediaLink DVD-ROM** that accompany the textbook

It also includes a **Strategies for Instructor Success** module for faculty that explains learning theories, planning for instruction, how to use effective pedagogies, assessing learning, and more! ISBN: 0-13-175676-1

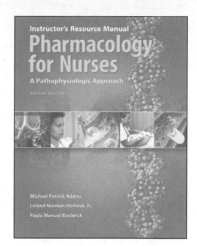

Instructor's Resource Manual
Pharmacology for Nurses
A Pathophysiologic Approach
SECOND EDITION

Michael Patrick Adams
Leland Norman Holland, Jr.
Paula Manuel Bostwick

Instructor's Resource DVD-ROM

This DVD-ROM includes all the textbook resources instructors need to teach pharmacology:

- Comprehensive **PowerPoint Presentation** that integrates lecture slides, images, animations, videos, and other resources
- **Classroom Response** questions set in PowerPoint slides *(Ask your Prentice Hall representative for more information about hardware to enhance your presentation.)*
- **First Day of Class** presentation to show your students how to use this textbook
- Complete **Image Gallery** in PowerPoint
- Additional **Media Resources**, such as videos and animations, to enhance your classroom presentations
- **TestGen** with questions in all NCLEX® formats, including questions mapped to the chapter learning objectives
- Link to the **Prentice Hall Instructors Resource Center** for additional resources (Internet connection required) ISBN: 0-13-175678-8

Alternate CD-ROM versions of this resource are also available from your Prentice Hall Representative.

Online Course Management

Prentice Hall OneKey is an integrated online resource that brings a variety of resources together in one convenient place for faculty and students using Blackboard and WebCT platforms. It provides you with the following:

FOR STUDENTS	FOR INSTRUCTORS
NCLEX-RN® Review Questions	Test Item Files
Case Studies	PowerPoint Presentations
Care Plan Activities	Media Gallery Resources
MediaLinks	Discussion Board
Email Communication	Class Announcements

For more information or to preview, go to:

http://cms.prenhall.com/webct/index.html

Bb
Blackboard
www.blackboard.com

http://cms.prenhall.com/blackboard/index.html

Dear Future Nurse,

When students are asked which subject in their nursing program is the most challenging, pharmacology always appears near the top of the list. The study of pharmacology demands that you apply knowledge from your past anatomy, physiology, and chemistry courses and integrate it with what you are learning in your current nursing courses. Lack of proper application of pharmacology can result in immediate and direct harm to the client. While pharmacology cannot be made easy, it can be made understandable if you make the proper connections to knowledge you learned in these courses. We wrote your textbook, **Pharmacology for Nurses,** to help you make these connections and to prepare you to provide safe, effective nursing care to your clients. How do we do this?

Learning pharmacology in context

When you learn drugs in association with diseases, you have an easier time connecting pharmacotherapy to therapeutic goals and client wellness. The approach of this textbook gives you a clearer picture of the importance of pharmacology to disease, and ultimately to nursing care. We focus on a holistic perspective to client care, which clearly shows the benefits and limitations of pharmacotherapy in curing or preventing illness.

Teaching through visuals

For nearly all students, learning is a highly visual process. Thus, we try to teach you the principles of drug action using different visual features. **Pharmacotherapy Illustrated** provides you with a visual overview of the drug therapy process and its impact on the disease, showing you specifically how the drug acts to counteract the effects of disease on the body. Also, to bring drug action to life, your DVD-ROM includes **Mechanism of Action** animations that clearly show drug action at the molecular, tissue, and system levels. These interactive animations correlate to the Prototype Drug boxes in the textbook chapters.

Providing a nursing focus

Once you understand how a drug works on the body—i.e., its actions, therapeutic effects, potential side effects and interactions, and more—you begin to understand the "why" of the interventions you will take as the nurse. For each drug class, **Nursing Considerations** sections discuss the major needs of the client, including general assessments, interventions, lifespan considerations, and client teaching for the entire classification. In addition, **Nursing Process Focus** charts identify clearly what nursing actions are most important for the most commonly prescribed drug classes and also address client education and discharge planning.

Putting it all together

At the end of each chapter, we added tools to help you test your understanding of the drugs and nursing care presented in that chapter:

- **Key Concepts** that provide a concise wrap-up of the essential ideas presented in each chapter, numbered to correspond to Key Concept sections within the chapter.
- **Review Questions** provide a way for you to test your knowledge; you can easily scan through the chapter to check your answers.
- **NCLEX® Review Questions** and **Critical Thinking Questions** help you apply essential components of nursing practice.
- **EXPLORE MediaLink** boxes refer you to additional resources, interactive exercises, and animations for that chapter on the **Prentice Hall MediaLink DVD-ROM** and **Companion Website.**

The following pages will show you how to make the most of your textbook and its resources to succeed in your pharmacology course. Although difficult and challenging, the study of pharmacology is truly a fascinating, lifelong journey. We hope that we have written a textbook that helps make that study easier and more understandable so that you will be able to provide safe, effective nursing care to clients undergoing drug therapy.

Regards,

Michael Patrick Adams   *Leland Norman Holland, Jr.*   *Paula Manuel Bostwick*

Learn how to use your textbook and its resources to help you learn pharmacology

Learning Pharmacology in Context

The vast majority of drugs are prescribed for specific diseases, yet many pharmacology textbooks fail to recognize the complex inter-relationships between pharmacology and disease. Learning drugs in the context of their associated diseases will make it easier for you to connect pharmacotherapy to therapeutic goals and client wellness. The pathophysiology approach of this textbook gives you a clearer picture of the importance of pharmacology to disease, and, ultimately to nursing care.

ANGINA PECTORIS

25.3 Pathogenesis of Angina Pectoris

Angina pectoris is acute chest pain caused by insufficient oxygen to a portion of the myocardium. More than 6 million Americans have angina pectoris, with over 350,000 new cases occurring each year. It is more prevalent in those over 55 years of age.

◀ **Disease and Body System Approach**

The organization by body systems (units) and diseases (chapters) clearly places the drugs in context with how they are used therapeutically. You can easily locate all relevant anatomy, physiology, pathophysiology, and pharmacology in the same chapter in which we present complete information for the drug classifications used to treat the disease(s) in each chapter. This organization builds the connection between pharmacology, pathophysiology, and the nursing care you learn in your clinical nursing courses.

Drugs at a Glance presents a quick way for you to see the classifications and prototypes that are covered in the chapter, organized by disorder drug class.

PharmFacts present pertinent facts and statistics related to the disease, providing you with a social and economic perspective of the disease.

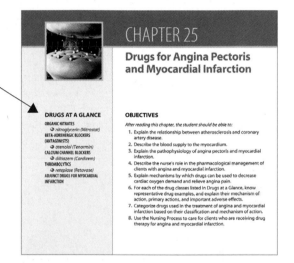

CHAPTER 25

Drugs for Angina Pectoris and Myocardial Infarction

DRUGS AT A GLANCE

ORGANIC NITRATES
  ⊘ *nitroglycerin (Nitrostat)*
BETA-ADRENERGIC BLOCKERS
(ANTAGONISTS)
  ⊘ *atenolol (Tenormin)*
CALCIUM CHANNEL BLOCKERS
  ⊘ *diltiazem (Cardizem)*
THROMBOLYTICS
  ⊘ *reteplase (Retavase)*
ADJUNCT DRUGS FOR MYOCARDIAL
INFARCTION

OBJECTIVES

After reading this chapter, the student should be able to:

1. Explain the relationship between atherosclerosis and coronary artery disease.
2. Describe the blood supply to the myocardium.
3. Explain the pathophysiology of angina pectoris and myocardial infarction.
4. Describe the nurse's role in the pharmacological management of clients with angina and myocardial infarction.
5. Explain mechanisms by which drugs can be used to decrease cardiac oxygen demand and relieve angina pain.
6. For each of the drug classes listed in Drugs at a Glance, know representative drug examples, and explain their mechanism of action, primary actions, and important adverse effects.
7. Categorize drugs used in the treatment of angina and myocardial infarction based on their classification and mechanism of action.
8. Use the Nursing Process to care for clients who are receiving drug therapy for angina and myocardial infarction.

℞ PROTOTYPE DRUG | Imipramine *(Tofranil)* | Tricyclic Antidepressant

ACTIONS AND USES

Imipramine blocks the reuptake of serotonin and norepinephrine into nerve terminals. It is used mainly for clinical depression, although it is occasionally used for the treatment of nocturnal enuresis in children. The nurse may find imipramine prescribed for a number of unlabeled uses including intractable pain, anxiety disorders, and withdrawal syndromes from alcohol and cocaine. Therapeutic effectiveness may not occur for 2 or more weeks.

ADMINISTRATION ALERTS

- Paroxismal diaphoresis can be a side effect of TCAs; therefore, diaphoresis may not be a reliable indicator of other disease states such as hypoglycemia.
- Imipramine causes anticholinergic effects and may potentiate effects of anticholinergic drugs administered during surgery.
- Do not discontinue abruptly, because rebound dysphoria, irritability, or sleeplessness may occur.
- Pregnancy category C.

PHARMACOKINETICS

Onset: < 1 h
Peak: 1–2 h PO; 30 min IV
Half-life: 8–16 h
Duration: Variable

ADVERSE EFFECTS

Side effects include sedation, drowsiness, blurred vision, dry mouth, and cardiovascular symptoms such as dysrhythmias, heart block, and extreme hypertension. Agents that mimic the action of norepinephrine or serotonin should be avoided because imipramine inhibits their metabolism and may produce toxicity. Some clients may experience photosensitivity and hypersensitivity to tricyclic drugs.

Contraindications: This drug should not be used in cases of acute recovery after MI, defects in bundle-branch conduction, and severe renal or hepatic impairment. Clients should not use this drug within 14 days of discontinuing MAOIs.

INTERACTIONS

Drug-Drug: Concurrent use of other CNS depressants, including alcohol, may cause sedation. Cimetidine (Tagamet) may inhibit the metabolism of imipramine, leading to increased serum levels and possible toxicity. Clonidine may decrease its antihypertensive effects, and increase risk for CNS depression. Use of oral contraceptives may increase or decrease imipramine levels. Disulfiram may lead to delirium and tachycardia. Antithyroid agents may produce agranulocytosis. Phenothiazines cause increased anticholinergic and sedative effects. Sympathomimetics may result in cardiac toxicity. Methylphenidate or cimetidine may increase the effects of imipramine and cause toxicity. Phenytoin is less effective when taken with imipramine. MAOIs may result in neuroleptic malignant syndrome.

Lab Tests: Imipramine produces altered blood glucose tests. Elevation of serum bilirubin and alkaline phosphatase is likely.

Herbal/Food: Herbal supplements such as evening primrose oil or ginkgo, which may lower the seizure threshold. St. John's wort used concurrently may cause serotonin syndrome.

Treatment of Overdose: There is no specific treatment for overdose. General supportive measures are recommended. Ensure an adequate airway, oxygenation, and ventilation. Monitor cardiac rhythm and vital signs. Gastric lavage may be indicated. Activated charcoal should be administered.

See the Companion Website for a Nursing Process Focus specific to this drug.

◀ **Prototype Approach and Prototype Drug Boxes**

The vast number of drugs available in clinical practice is staggering. To help you learn them, we use a prototype approach in which we introduce the one or two most representative drugs in each classification in detail. It can be less intimidating to focus your learning on one representative drug in each class. **Prototype Drug** boxes clearly summarize these important medications, presenting:

- Actions and Uses
- Administration Alerts
- Pharmacokinetics, including onset of action, duration, half-life, and peak effect, when known
- Adverse Effects and Contraindications
- Interactions with drugs, herbs, and food
- Treatment of Overdose and antidotes, where applicable

Teaching Through Visuals

For nearly all students, learning is a highly visual process. Thus, we use numerous visuals to help you review the anatomy and physiology of the body system as well as understand the principles of drug action on the body.

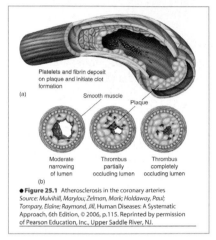

● **Figure 25.1** Atherosclerosis in the coronary arteries
Source: Mulvihill, Marylou; Zelman, Mark; Holdaway, Paul; Tompary, Elaine; Raymond, Jill, Human Diseases: A Systematic Approach, 6th Edition, © 2006, p.115. Reprinted by permission of Pearson Education, Inc., Upper Saddle River, NJ.

◀ **Vivid and Colorful Illustrations** help you review specific anatomy, physiology, and pathophysiology for a body system to help you better understand the impact of disease on that system.

Pharmacotherapy Illustrated boxes visually illustrate the drug therapy process and its impact on the disease, showing you specifically how the drug acts to counteract the effects of disease on the body. ▶

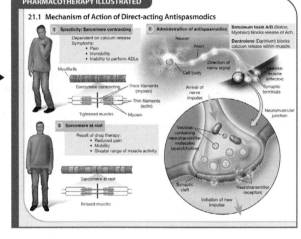

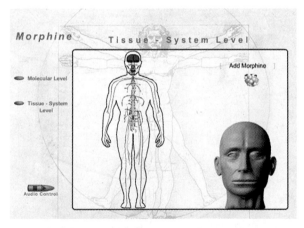

◀ **Mechanism of Action** animated tutorials on your **Prentice Hall Nursing MediaLink DVD-ROM** clearly show drug action at the molecular, tissue, organ, and system levels. These interactive animations—listed below—correlate to **Prototype Drug** and **Pharmacotherapy Illustrated** boxes in your book.

Mechanism of Action Animations

acetaminophen	Ch. 33	Doxazosin	Ch. 23	Lidocaine	Ch. 19	Ranitidine	Ch. 40
acyclovir	Ch. 36	epinephrine	Ch. 29	Lisinopril	Ch. 24	Reteplase	Ch. 25
Amiodarone	Ch. 26	epoietin alfa	Ch. 28	Methotrexate	Ch. 37	Salmeterol	Ch. 39
Atorvastatin	Ch. 22	escitalopram	Ch. 14	Methylphenidate	Ch. 16	saquinavir	Ch. 36
Calcitriol	Ch. 47	Estradiol	Ch. 45	Morphine	Ch. 18	Sildenafil	Ch. 46
ciprofloxacin	Ch. 34	Fluconazole	Ch. 35	Naproxen	Ch. 33	spironolactone	Ch. 30
Cyclobenzaprine	Ch. 21	Fluoxetine	Ch. 16	Nifedipine	Ch. 23	tegaserod	Ch. 41
cyclophosphamide	Ch. 37	Furosemide	Ch. 24	Omeprazole	Ch. 40	valproic acid	Ch. 15
Diazepam	Ch. 15	Glipizide	Ch. 44	Oxycodone	Ch. 18	venlafaxine	Ch. 16
Digoxin	Ch. 24	Heparin	Ch. 27	Penicillin	Ch. 34	Warfarin	Ch. 27
Diphenhydramine	Ch. 38	interferon alfa	Ch. 32	Pilocarpine	Ch. 49	Zidovudine	Ch. 36
Dopamine	Ch. 29	Levadopa	Ch. 20	Propranolol	Ch. 26	zolpidem	Ch. 14

Providing a Nursing Focus

Once you understand how a drug works on the body—i.e., its actions, therapeutic effects, potential side effects and interactions, and more—you begin to understand the "why" of the interventions you will take as the nurse. Each chapter guides you to the content that is essential for you to provide safe, effective drug therapy.

◀ **Nursing Considerations** appear within each drug class section and discuss the major needs of the client, including:
- General Assessments
- Interventions
- **Lifespan Considerations**
- **Client Teaching** for all the drugs in that classification, when applicable

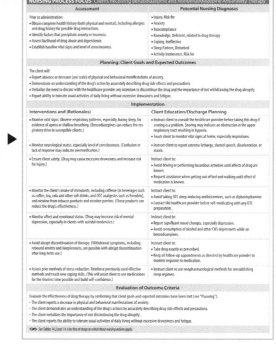

Nursing Process Focus charts present need-to-know nursing actions in the nursing process—assessment, nursing diagnoses, planning, implementation with interventions and rationales, evaluation—and include client teaching and discharge planning. Additional **Nursing Process Focus** charts are available on the Companion Website.

Avoiding Medication Errors are brief client-based scenarios that illustrate potential pitfalls that nurses encounter and can lead to medication errors. Each scenario ends with a question asking you to identify what went wrong, enabling you to watch for similar situations and deliver medications safely.

Natural Therapies boxes present popular herbal or dietary supplements clients may use along with conventional drugs. As a nurse, you need to assess clients to see if they are using any natural remedies that may have interactions with medications they are taking. ▶

◀ **Special Considerations** boxes present a variety of special issues related to culture, ethnicity, age, gender, and psychosocial concerns that nurses must consider during drug therapy.

Home & Community Considerations alert you to concerns and teaching implications for care settings outside the hospital. ▶

Putting It All Together

The tools at the end of each chapter and on the accompanying media resources help you test your understanding of the drugs and nursing care presented in that chapter. Using these tools will help you succeed in your pharmacology course, in the clinical setting, on the NCLEX-RN®, and ultimately in professional nursing practice.

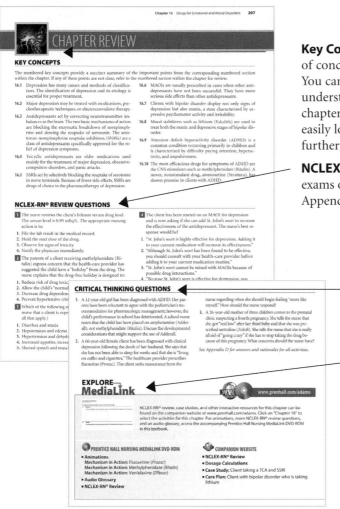

Key Concept Summary provides expanded summaries of concepts that correlate to sections within the chapter. You can use this succinct summary to ensure that you understand the concepts before moving on to the next chapter. The numbering of these concepts helps you easily locate that section within the chapter if you need further review.

NCLEX-RN® Review Questions prepare you for course exams on the chapter content using all NCLEX® formats. Appendix D provides answers and rationales.

Critical Thinking Questions help you apply the essential components of nursing care through case-based scenarios. Appendix D provides answers.

EXPLORE MediaLink directs you to resources for that chapter on the **Prentice Hall Nursing MediaLink DVD-ROM** and **Companion Website** that accompany your textbook.

 Prentice Hall Nursing MediaLink DVD-ROM

- **Audio Glossary** with pronunciations and definitions of every key term in the textbook
- **Drug Prototype Audio Pronunciations**
- **Drug Dosage Calculator**
- **Nursing in Action** video case studies for medication administration
- **NCLEX® Review** questions that emphasize the application of care and client education related to drug administration
- **Mechanism of Action** drug animation tutorials for prototype drugs, showing how drug action occurs at the tissue, organ, and system levels

CD-ROM versions of this resource can be purchased at www.MyPearsonStore.com using ISBN: 0-13-159712-4

Companion Website | www.prenhall.com/adams

- Additional **NCLEX® Review** questions with comprehensive rationales
- Pharmacology review activities that test your understanding of the drugs from each chapter: **Classification Reviews, Drug Reviews, Case Studies,** and **Care Plans**
- **Dosage Calculation** exercises
- **Nursing Process Focus** charts for drug prototypes
- **Preventing Medication Errors** review and activities
- **Student Success** module with advice and activities to help you be a successful nursing student
- And much more!

Student Assessment ... Real Nursing Skills ... Customized Study Plans ... The path to student success and nursing excellence in pharmacology!

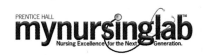

MyNursingLab is a user-friendly site that gives students the opportunity to test themselves on key concepts and skills in pharmacology. By using *MyNursingLab,* students can track their own progress through the course and use customized, media-rich, study plan activities to help them achieve success in the classroom, in clinical, and ultimately on the NCLEX-RN®. Students take a diagnostic pretest for each chapter, receive a customized study plan to work through based on the results, and conclude with a post test to assess competency. *MyNursingLab* can also help you, the instructor, to monitor class progress as students move through the curriculum.

To take a tour and see the power of **mynursinglab**, go to www.prenhall.com/nursing.

Ask your Prentice Hall Representative for more information and packaging options for including *MyNursingLab* and Prentice Hall OneKey in your curriculum.

BRIEF CONTENTS

UNIT 1 Core Concepts in Pharmacology 1

Chapter 1 Introduction to Pharmacology: Drug Regulation and Approval 2

Chapter 2 Drug Classes and Schedules 11

Chapter 3 Emergency Preparedness 18

Chapter 4 Principles of Drug Administration 27

Chapter 5 Pharmacokinetics 46

Chapter 6 Pharmacodynamics 56

UNIT 2 Pharmacology and the Nurse-Client Relationship 65

Chapter 7 The Nursing Process in Pharmacology 66

Chapter 8 Drug Administration Throughout the Lifespan 75

Chapter 9 Medication Errors and Risk Reduction 89

Chapter 10 Psychosocial, Gender, and Cultural Influences on Pharmacotherapy 99

Chapter 11 Herbal and Alternative Therapies 107

Chapter 12 Substance Abuse 117

UNIT 3 The Nervous System 129

Chapter 13 Drugs Affecting the Autonomic Nervous System 130

Chapter 14 Drugs for Anxiety and Insomnia 153

Chapter 15 Drugs for Seizures 169

Chapter 16 Drugs for Emotional and Mood Disorders 185

Chapter 17 Drugs for Psychoses 209

Chapter 18 Drugs for the Control of Pain 223

Chapter 19 Drugs for Local and General Anesthesia 244

Chapter 20 Drugs for Degenerative Diseases of the Nervous System 260

Chapter 21 Drugs for Neuromuscular Disorders 274

UNIT 4 The Cardiovascular and Urinary Systems 285

Chapter 22 Drugs for Lipid Disorders 286

Chapter 23 Drugs for Hypertension 301

Chapter 24 Drugs for Heart Failure 329

Chapter 25 Drugs for Angina Pectoris and Myocardial Infarction 345

Chapter 26 Drugs for Dysrhythmias 361

Chapter 27 Drugs for Coagulation Disorders 377

Chapter 28 Drugs for Hematopoietic Disorders 393

Chapter 29 Drugs for Shock 409

Chapter 30 Diuretic Therapy and Drugs for Renal Failure 423

Chapter 31 Drugs for Fluid Balance, Electrolyte, and Acid–Base Disorders 437

UNIT 5 The Immune System 453

Chapter 32 Drugs for Immune System Modulation 454

Chapter 33 Drugs for Inflammation and Fever 470

Chapter 34 Drugs for Bacterial Infections 483

Chapter 35 Drugs for Fungal, Protozoal, and Helminthic Infections 513

Chapter 36 Drugs for Viral Infections 532

Chapter 37 Drugs for Neoplasia 551

UNIT 6 The Respiratory System 577

Chapter 38 Drugs for Allergic Rhinitis and the Common Cold 578

Chapter 39 Drugs for Asthma and Other Pulmonary Disorders 593

UNIT 7 The Gastrointestinal System 609

Chapter 40 Drugs for Peptic Ulcer Disease 610

Chapter 41 Drugs for Bowel Disorders and Other Gastrointestinal Conditions 623

Chapter 42 Drugs for Nutritional Disorders 641

UNIT 8 The Endocrine System 659

Chapter 43 Drugs for Pituitary, Thyroid, and Adrenal Disorders 660

Chapter 44 Drugs for Diabetes Mellitus 681

Chapter 45 Drugs for Disorders and Conditions of the Female Reproductive System 696

Chapter 46 Drugs for Disorders and Conditions of the Male Reproductive System 717

UNIT 9 The Integumentary System and Eyes/Ears 731

Chapter 47 Drugs for Bone and Joint Disorders 732

Chapter 48 Drugs for Skin Disorders 752

Chapter 49 Drugs for Eye and Ear Disorders 770

Pharmacology for Nurses

A Pathophysiologic Approach

SECOND EDITION

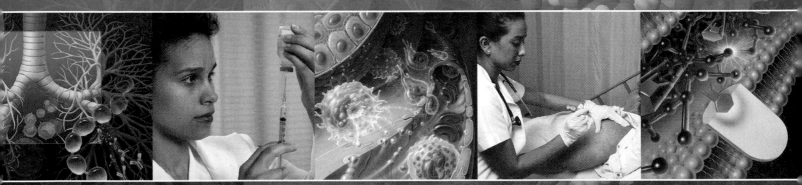

Michael Patrick Adams, PhD, RT(R)
Dean of Health Occupations
Pasco-Hernando Community College

Leland Norman Holland, Jr., PhD
Associate Academic Dean
Dean, College of Arts and Sciences
Southeastern University

Paula Manuel Bostwick, RN, MSN
Nursing Department Chair
Ivy Tech Community College

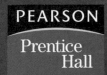

PEARSON
Prentice Hall

Upper Saddle River, New Jersey 07458

Library of Congress Cataloging-in-Publication Data

Adams, Michael
  Pharmacology for nurses : a pathophysiologic approach / Michael
Adams, Norman Holland, Paula Bostwick
    p. ; cm.
  ISBN 0-13-175665-6.
  1. Pharmacology. 2. Nurses.
    [DNLM: 1. Drug Therapy–nursing. 2. Pharmacology–Nurses'
Instruction. WB 330 A215p 2004] I. Holland, Norman (date). II.
Bostwick, Paula. III. Title.
  RM301.A32 2008
  615'. 1–dc22

                                                          2007020618

Publisher: Julie Levin Alexander
Publisher's Assistant: Regina Bruno
Editor-in-Chief: Maura Connor
Senior Managing Editor for Development: Marilyn Meserve
Development Editors: Elena M. Mauceri, Jennifer Maybin
Assistant Editor: Michael Giacobbe
Editorial Assistant: Mary Ellen Ruitenberg
Director of Marketing: Karen Allman
Senior Marketing Manager: Francisco Del Castillo
Marketing Specialist: Michael Sirinides
Managing Editor for Production: Patrick Walsh
Production Liaison: Faye Gemmellaro
Production Editor: Penny Walker, Aptara, Inc.
Media Product Manager: John J. Jordan
Media Development Editor: Dorothy Cook, Anita Castro
New Media Project Manager: Stephen J. Hartner
Manufacturing Manager: Ilene Sanford
Manufacturing Buyer: Pat Brown
Senior Design Coordinator: Maria Guglielmo Walsh
Interior Designer: Kenny Beck
Cover Designer: Pronk & Associates
Editorial Art Manager: Patrick Watson
Cover/Interior Art: Unit 1: Jim Dowdalls/Photo Researchers, Inc.;
Unit 2: © Jane Hurd/Phototake; Unit 3: Custom Medical Stock;
Unit 4: David Mack/Photo Researchers, Inc.; Unit 5: © Steve Oh,
M.S./Phototake; Unit 6: Phototake/Bodell Communications, Inc.;
Unit 7: © Steve Oh, M.S./Phototake; Unit 8: Michael Freeman/
Phototake; Unit 9: Custom Medical Stock
Interior Illustrations: Precision Graphics, Imagineering
Composition: Aptara, Inc.
Cover Printer: Lehigh Press
Printer/Binder: Courier/Kendallville

Notice: Care has been taken to confirm the accuracy of information presented in this textbook. The authors, editors, and the publisher, however, cannot accept responsibility for errors or omissions or for consequences from application of the information in this textbook and make no warranty, expressed or implied, with respect to its contents.

The authors and publisher have exerted every effort to ensure that drug selections and dosages set forth in this textbook are in accord with current recommendations and practices at the time of publication. However, in view of ongoing research, changes in government regulations, and the constant flow of information relating to drug therapy and drug reactions, the reader is urged to check the package inserts of all drugs for any change in indications of dosage and for added warnings and precautions. This is particularly important when the recommended agent is a new and/or infrequently employed drug.

Dedication

I dedicate this book to nursing educators, who contribute every day to making the world a better and more caring place.

—MPA

I would like to acknowledge the willful encouragement of Farrell and Norma Jean Stalcup. I dedicate this book to my beloved wife, Karen, and my three wonderful children, Alexandria Noelle, my double-deuce daughter, Caleb Jaymes, my number-one son, and Joshua Nathaniel, my number three "O."

—LNH

I dedicate the book to my husband Charles, the love of my life, my son C.J., and my daughter Bailey. Thank you for all of your love, support, and encouragement. I am so blessed to share my life with each of you.

—PMB

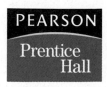

10 9 8 7 6 5 4 3 2 1
ISBN 10: 0-13-175665-6
EAN: 978-0-13-175665-6

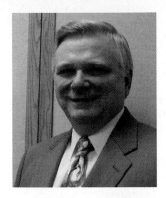

Michael Patrick Adams, PhD, RT(R), is the Dean of Health Occupations at Pasco-Hernando Community College. He is an accomplished and national speaker. The National Institute for Staff and Organizational Development in Austin, Texas, named Dr. Adams a Master Teacher. He has been registered by the American Registry of Radiologic Technologists for over 30 years. Dr. Adams obtained his Masters degree in Pharmacology from Michigan State University and his Doctorate in Education at the University of South Florida.

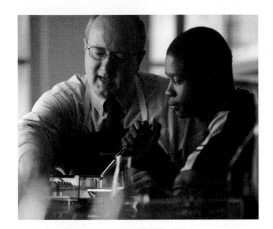

Leland Norman Holland, Jr., PhD (Norm) is the Associate Academic Dean and Dean of the College of Arts and Sciences at Southeastern University in Lakeland, Florida. He is actively involved in teaching and helping students prepare for service in medicine, nursing, dentistry, and allied health. He has taught pharmacology for 15 years at both the undergraduate and graduate levels. He is very much dedicated to the success of students preparing for work-life readiness. He comes to the teaching profession after spending several years doing basic science research at the VA Hospital in Augusta, Georgia, and the Medical College of Georgia, where he received his PhD in Pharmacology.

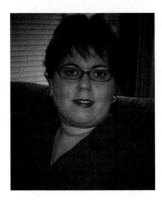

Paula Manuel Bostwick, RN, MSN is the Nursing Department Chair at Ivy Tech Community College in Fort Wayne, Indiana. She has been involved in nursing education for more than 15 years. She has clinical experience in medical-surgical and critical care nursing. Paula received her Masters of Science in Nursing from Ball State University.

CONTRIBUTORS

This textbook is a culmination of writing provided by many writers. The authors wish to extend their special thanks to the many nurse contributors who provided their unique knowledge and wisdom to this project. Their willingness to make such sacrifices to meet our deadlines is so appreciated. Their dedication to quality nursing education is very evident in this text.

Text Contributors

Marti Burton, RN, BS
Canadian Valley Technology Center
El Reno, Oklahoma
Chapter 15: Drugs for Seizures
Chapter 17: Drugs for Psychoses
Chapter 22: Drugs for Lipid Disorders
Chapter 23: Drugs for Hypertension

Margaret Gingrich, RN, MSN
Harrisburg Area Community College
Harrisburg, Pennsylvania
Chapter 35: Drugs for Fungal, Protozoal,
*   and Helminthic Infections*

Corinne C. Harmon, RN, MS, EdD, AOCN
Clemson University
Clemson, South Carolina
Chapter 18: Drugs for the Control of Pain
Chapter 26: Drugs for Dysrhythmias
Chapter 29: Drugs for Shock
Chapter 31: Drugs for Fluid Balance, Electrolyte, and Acid–Base
*   Disorders*
Chapter 34: Drugs for Bacterial Infections
Chapter 37: Drugs for Neoplasia

Helen W. Jones, RN, PhD, APN-C
Raritan Valley Community College
Somerville, New Jersey
Chapter 8: Drug Administration Throughout the Lifespan
Chapter 9: Medication Errors and Risk Reduction
Chapter 14: Drugs for Anxiety and Insomnia
Chapter 16: Drugs for Emotional and Mood Disorders

Darcus Kottwitz, RN, MSN
Fort Scott Community College
Fort Scott, Kansas
Chapter 19: Drugs for Local and General Anesthesia
Chapter 21: Drugs for Neuromuscular Disorders
Chapter 24: Drugs for Heart Failure
Chapter 27: Drugs for Coagulation Disorders
Chapter 41: Drugs for Bowel Disorders and Other
*   Gastrointestinal Conditions*
Chapter 44: Drugs for Diabetes Mellitus
Chapter 49: Drugs for Eye and Ear Disorders

Claudia R. Stoffel, RN, MSN
West Kentucky Community and Technical College
Paducah, Kentucky
Chapter 8: Drug Administration Throughout the Lifespan
Chapter 20: Drugs for Degenerative Diseases of the
*   Nervous System*
Chapter 36: Drugs for Viral Infections
Chapter 38: Drugs for Allergic Rhinitis and the Common Cold
Chapter 40: Drugs for Peptic Ulcer Disease
Chapter 42: Drugs for Nutritional Disorders
Chapter 46: Drugs for Disorders and Conditions of the Male
*   Reproductive System*

Frances M. Warrick, RN, MS
El Centro College
Dallas, Texas
Chapter 28: Drugs for Hematopoietic Disorders
Chapter 32: Drugs for Immune System Modulation
Chapter 45: Drugs for Disorders and Conditions of the Female
*   Reproductive System*

Jan Weust, RN, MSN
Ivy Tech Community College
Terre Haute, Indiana
Chapter 25: Drugs for Angina Pectoris and
*   Myocardial Infarction*
Chapter 43: Drugs for Pituitary, Thyroid, and
*   Adrenal Disorders*
Chapter 47: Drugs for Bone and Joint Disorders
Chapter 48: Drugs for Skin Disorders

Julie Will, RN, MSN
Ivy Tech Community College
Terre Haute, Indiana
Chapter 30: Diuretic Therapy and Drugs for Renal Failure
Chapter 33: Drugs for Inflammation and Fever
Chapter 39: Drugs for Asthma and Other Pulmonary
*   Disorders*

PRENTICE HALL NURSING MEDIALINK DVD-ROM

Peggy Pryzbycien, RN, MSN
Onondaga Community College
Syracuse, New York
Nursing In Action Cases

Margaret Gingrich, RN, MSN
Harrisburg Area Community College
Harrisburg, Pennsylvania
NCLEX Questions, Chapters 1–25

Patricia Teasley, RN, MSN, APRN, BC
Central Texas College
Killeen, Texas
NCLEX Questions, Chapters 26–49

COMPANION WEBSITE

Kelly L. Fisher, RN, PhD
Endicott College
Beverly, Massachusetts
Companion Website

Doris M. Marshalek, RN, MSN
Community College of Allegheny County
Pittsburgh, Pennsylvania
Case Studies, Care Plans

INSTRUCTOR RESOURCES

Rosanne C. Shinkle, RN, MN, ARNP
Florida Hospital College of Health Sciences
Orlando, Florida

Connie Dempsey, RN, MSN
Stark State College of Technology
North Canton, Ohio

Julie Traynor, RN, MS
Lake Region State College
Devils Lake, North Dakota

Terri L. Schwenk RN, MSN
Ivy Tech Community College
Terre Haute, Indiana

Kelly Gosnell, RN, MSN
Ivy Tech Community College
Terre Haute, Indiana

THANK YOU

W e are grateful to all the educators who reviewed the manuscript of this textbook. Their insights, suggestions, and eye for detail helped us to prepare a more relevant and useful book, one that focuses on the essential components of learning in the field of pharmacology.

Joy Ache-Reed, RN, MSN
Indiana Wesleyan University
Marion, Indiana

Mary Jane Araldi, RN, MSN
Fulton-Montgomery Community College
Johnstown, New York

Kathy Butcher, RN, BSN
Cuyahoga Community College
Cleveland, Ohio

Karen Stuart Champion, RN, MS
Indian River Community College
Fort Pierce, Florida

Darlene Clark, RN, MS
Pennsylvania State University
University Park, Pennsylvania

Kim Cooper, RN, MSN
Ivy Tech Community College
Terre Haute, Indiana

Pamela Covault, RN, MS
Neosho County Community College
Ottawa, Kansas

Nina Cuttler, APRN, MSN, BC
Central Carolina Technical College
Sumter, South Carolina

Karen D. Danielson, RN, MSN
North Central State College
Mansfield, Ohio

Barbara Duer, RN, 1MS
Rose State College
Midwest City, Oklahoma

Crystal Dunlevy, RRT, EdD
Cincinnati State Community & Technical College
Cincinnati, Ohio

Margaret Gingrich, RN, MSN
Harrisburg Area Community College
Harrisburg, Pennsylvania

Elizabeth Goodwin, RNC, MSN
Laramie County Community College
Cheyenne, Wyoming

Virginia Hallenbeck, RN, MS, CNS
Central Ohio Technical College
Newark, Ohio

Mark Hand, RN, MSN
Durham Technical Community College
Durham, North Carolina

Connie Heflin, RN, MSN
West Kentucky Community and Technical College
Paducah, Kentucky

Bobbie Hunt, RN, MSN
Davidson County Community College
Lexington, North Carolina

Helen W. Jones, RN, PhD, APN-C
Raritan Valley Community College
Somerville, New Jersey

Jack Keyes, PhD
Linfield College
Portland, Oregon

Kathleen N. Krov, RN, CNM, MSN, FLCCE-R
Raritan Valley Community College
Somerville, New Jersey

Bev Kubachka, RN, MS
Hocking College
Nelsonville, Ohio

Marina Martinez-Kratz, RN, MS
Jackson Community College
Jackson, Mississippi

Judy Maslowski, RN, MSN
University of Mary
Bismark, North Dakota

Mary Nifong, RN, MSN
Pikes Peak Community College
Colorado Springs, Colorado

Valerie M. O'Dell, RN, MSN
Youngstown State University
Youngstown, Ohio

Judith Pelletier, RN, MSN
Roxbury Community College
Roxbury Crossings, Massachusetts

Colleen Prunier, RN, MS, CARN, NP, CNS
Suffolk County Community College
Selden, New York

Janice Ramirez, RN, MSN
North Idaho College
Coeur d'Alene, Idaho

Susan Russell, RN
Columbia State Community College
Columbia, Tennessee

Phyl VonBargen-Sallee, RN, MS, CPNP
Oakland Community College
Waterford, Michigan

Jodene Scheller, RN, MSN
Lewis & Clark Community College
Godfrey, Illinois

Connie Schroeder, RN, MS
Danville Area Community College
Danville, Illinois

Cheryl Shaffer, RN, MS, ANP, PNP, PhD(c)
Suffolk County Community College
Selden, New York

Samantha Sinclair, RN, MSN, ANP-C
Suffolk County Community College
Selden, New York

Nancy Smith, RN, MS
Southern Maine Community College
South Portland, Maine

Diane Stewart, RN, MSN
Midwestern State University
Wichita Falls, Texas

Claudia R. Stoffel, RN, MSN
Paducah Community College
Paducah, Kentucky

Doris Stone, RN, MSN
Kentucky Community and Technical College System
Versailles, Kentucky

Prudence Twigg, APRN-BC, PhD(c)
Indiana University
Indianapolis, Indiana

Donna Van Houten, RN, MS
Gateway Community College
Phoenix, Arizona

Debra J. Walden, RN, MNSc
Arkansas State University
State University, Arkansas

Lori Warren, RN, MA, CPC, CCP, CLNC
Spencerian College
Jeffersonville, Indiana

Jan Weust, RN, MSN
Ivy Tech Community College
Terre Haute, Indiana

PREFACE

When students are asked which subject in their nursing program is the most challenging, pharmacology always appears near the top of the list. The study of pharmacology demands that students apply knowledge from a wide variety of the natural and applied sciences. To successfully predict drug action requires a thorough knowledge of anatomy, physiology, chemistry, and pathology as well as the social sciences of psychology and sociology. Lack of proper application of pharmacology can result in immediate and direct harm to the client; thus, the stakes in learning the subject are high.

Pharmacology cannot be made easy, but it can be made understandable, if the proper connections are made to knowledge learned in these other disciplines. The vast majority of drugs in clinical practice are prescribed for specific diseases, yet many pharmacology textbooks fail to recognize the complex interrelationships between pharmacology and pathophysiology. When drugs are learned in isolation from their associated diseases or conditions, students have difficulty connecting pharmacotherapy to therapeutic goals and client wellness. The pathophysiology approach of this textbook gives the student a clearer picture of the importance of pharmacology to disease, and ultimately to client care. The approach and rationale of this textbook focus on a holistic perspective to client care, which clearly shows the benefits and limitations of pharmacotherapy in curing or preventing illness. Although difficult and challenging, the study of pharmacology is truly a fascinating, lifelong journey.

Organization—A Body System and Disease Approach

Pharmacology for Nurses: A Pathophysiologic Approach is organized according to body systems (units) and diseases (chapters). Each chapter provides the complete information on the drug classifications used to treat the disease(s) classes. Specially designed headings cue students to each drug classification discussion.

The pathophysiology approach clearly places the drugs in context with how they are used therapeutically. The student is able to locate easily all relevant anatomy, physiology, pathology, and pharmacology in the same chapter in which the drugs are discussed. This approach provides the student with a clear view of the connection between pharmacology, pathophysiology, and the nursing care learned in other clinical courses. **PharmFacts** features, appearing in the disease chapters, present pertinent facts and statistics related to the disease, providing a social and economic perspective of the disease.

TEACHING DRUG PROTOTYPES

The vast number of drugs available in clinical practice is staggering. To facilitate learning, we use prototypes where the one or two most representative drugs in each classification are introduced in detail in the chapter. Students are less intimidated when they can focus their learning on one representative drug in each class. **Prototype Drug** boxes clearly describe these important medications. Within these boxes, the actions and uses of the drug are succinctly presented, including **Administration Alerts** that highlight vital information related to the administration of that drug and **Pharmacokinetic** information, such as onset of action, duration, half-life and peak effect, when known. The boxes also highlight contraindications, adverse effects, and drug-drug, herb-drug, and food-drug interactions, as well as **Treatment of Overdose** and antidotes, where applicable.

FOCUSED COVERAGE OF THE NURSING PROCESS

This textbook features a focused approach to the nursing process approach, which allows students to quickly find the content that is essential for them to know for safe, effective drug therapy. **Nursing Considerations** sections appear within each drug class discussion. These sections discuss the major needs of the client, including general assessments, interventions, lifespan considerations, and client teaching for the classification. **Client Education** is an important nursing intervention. Client education information in the Nursing Considerations sections and each Nursing Process Focus flowchart teaches students what essential information they need to convey to the client and caregiver. Integrated rationales for nursing actions provide the physiology of the drug action to answer the "why" of nursing interventions. This is key to developing critical thinking skills.

Nursing Process Focus charts provide a succinct, easy-to-read view of the most commonly prescribed drug class for the disease. The charts present need-to-know nursing actions in a format that reflects the "flow" of the Nursing Process: nursing assessment, potential nursing diagnoses, planning, interventions, client education and discharge planning, and evaluation. Rationales for interventions are included in parentheses. The Nursing Process Focus charts identify clearly what nursing actions are most important. Some prototype drugs have important nursing actions that are specific to that drug. In these instances, we provide a Nursing Process Focus chart in the text devoted solely to the prototype drug. Students can find Nursing Process Focus charts for every prototype drug on the Companion Website at **www.prenhall.com/adams**. The icon is provided at the bottom of each Prototype Drug box to remind the student that this content can be found on the Companion Website.

Teaching Pharmacology Through Visuals

For nearly all students, learning is a highly visual process. The textbook also incorporates generous use of artwork to illustrate and summarize key concepts. At the beginning of the system chapters, vivid and colorful illustrations help students review specific anatomy and physiology for a body system to help them better understand the impact of disease on that system. New to this edition is **Pharmacotherapy Illustrated,** a feature that provides students with a visual overview of the drug therapy related to the pathophysiology. Each of these boxes visually illustrates the drug therapy process and its impact on the disease, showing you specifically how the drug acts to counteract the effects of disease on the body.

Pharmacology for Nurses: A Pathophysiologic Approach is the first nursing pharmacology textbook to incorporate **Mechanism in Action** animations, which use computer simulations to clearly demonstrate drug action at the molecular, tissue, organ, and system levels. *MediaLink* tabs appear in the margin next to appropriate Prototype Drug boxes to direct the student to the full-color animation, including audio narrations that describe each step of the mechanism, on the included *Prentice Hall Nursing MediaLink DVD-ROM* that accompanies this book. Additional animations, which illustrate important pharmacological concepts such as agonists and antagonists, can also be found on the DVD-ROM.

Holistic Pharmacology

Pharmacology for Nurses: A Pathophysiologic Approach examines pharmacology from a holistic perspective. The **Special Considerations** features present pharmacology and nursing issues related to cultural, ethnic, age, gender, and psychosocial aspects. These features remind students that a drug's efficacy is affected as much by its pharmacokinetics as by the uniqueness of the individual. In addition, **Lifespan Considerations** are integrated throughout the textbook under the Nursing Considerations heading. This information alerts students to specific considerations for clients of various ages. **Natural Therapies** boxes present a popular herbal or dietary supplement that may be considered along with conventional drugs. Although the authors do not recommend the use of these alternative treatments in lieu of conventional medicines, the majority of clients use complementary and alternative therapies and the nurse must become familiar with how they affect client health. Herb-drug interactions are also included within the Prototype Drug boxes so nurses can monitor for any interactions that may result in clients using that medication. Nonpharmacological methods for controlling many diseases are also integrated into the chapters, and include lifestyle and dietary modifications.

A NOTE ABOUT TERMINOLOGY

The term "healthcare provider" is used to denote the physician, nurse practitioner, and any other health professional who is legally authorized to prescribe drugs.

Acknowledgments

When authoring a textbook such as this, a huge number of dedicated and talented professionals are needed to bring the initial vision to reality. Maura Connor, Editor-in-Chief, is responsible for helping us sculpt the vision for the text. Our Developmental Editors, Elena Mauceri and Jennifer Maybin, supplied the expert guidance and leadership to keep everyone on task and to be certain it reached its fruition on time. Providing the necessary expertise for our comprehensive supplement package was Michael Giacobbe, Associate Editor. Mary Ellen Ruitenberg, Editorial Assistant, did an outstanding job of managing the myriad office details. The work of Dorothy Cook and Anita Castro to coordinate the DVD-ROM and Companion Website development was invaluable.

The design staff at Prentice Hall, especially Maria Guglielmo Walsh, created magnificent text and cover designs. Patrick Watson, Art Coordinator, provided expertise on art, photography, and creation of the new Pharmacotherapy Illustrated features. Overseeing the production process with finesse was Faye Gemmellaro, Production Liaison at Prentice Hall. Penny Walker and the staff at Aptara provided expert and professional guidance in all aspects of the art and production process.

Although difficult and challenging, the study of pharmacology is truly a fascinating, lifelong journey. We hope that we have written a textbook that helps make that study easier and more understandable so that nursing students will be able to provide safe, effective nursing care to clients undergoing drug therapy. We hope students and faculty will share with us their experiences using this textbook and all its resources. Please contact us at NursingExcellence@prenhall.com.

Michael Adams

Norm Holland

Paula Bostwick

SPECIAL FEATURES

AVOIDING MEDICATION ERRORS

Chapter 16, p. 191
Chapter 22, p. 299
Chapter 26, p. 374
Chapter 27, p. 386
Chapter 31, p. 450
Chapter 32, p. 468
Chapter 34, p. 496
Chapter 38, p. 587
Chapter 43, p. 662
Chapter 47, p. 744

HOME & COMMUNITY CONSIDERATIONS

Accommodating Those With Bone and Joint Disorders, p. 738
Asthma Management in the Schools, p. 599
Aspirin for Cardiovascular Event Risk Reduction, p. 479
Caring for Loved Ones with Alzheimer's Disease, p. 268
Clients Taking Antidysrhythmics, p. 374
Clients Taking Anticoagulant Therapy, p. 380
CPR and Other Education for Heart Disease, p. 348
Educating Clients About OTC Medications for Bowel Disorders, Nausea, and Vomiting, p. 638
Educating Parents to Reduce Medication Errors in Children, p. 95
Helping Clients Manage Asthma, p. 605
Hepatotoxicity With Long-term Drug Therapies, p. 529
Hypernatremia in Athletes, p. 444
Impact of Diabetes on Community Resources, p. 694
Increasing Compliance in Heart Failure Treatment, p. 342
Muscle Relaxant Therapy in the Home Setting, p. 281
Nutritional Therapy for Clients Needing Diuretic Therapy, p. 433
Ophthalmic Drugs in the Home Setting, p. 778
OTC Drugs and Medication Errors, p. 96
Over-the-counter Medications for GI Disorders, p. 618
Postanesthesia Follow-up Care, p. 254
Preventing Medication Errors in the Home, p. 93
Promoting Safety With Medications that Affect the ANS, p. 150
Pseudoephedrine and Drug Abuse, p. 588
Recurrent Anaphylaxis, p. 421
Sample Packs of Medications for Erectile Dysfunction, p. 725
Serious Side Effects of Hormone Therapy, p. 702
Skin Disorders and Self-esteem, p. 765
Treating Clients With Hematopoietic Disorders, p. 396
Viral Infections, p. 545
Vitamin B$_9$ and Neural Tube Defects, p. 648

NATURAL THERAPIES

Acidophilus for Diarrhea, p. 629
Antibacterial Properties of Goldenseal, p. 509
Bilberry for Eye Health, p. 779
Black Cohosh for Menopause, p. 706
Burdock Root for Acne and Eczema, p. 765
Cayenne for Muscular Tension, p. 277
Chocolate and Grape Seed Extract for Hypertension, p. 308
Cloves and Anise as Natural Dental Remedies, p. 247
Coenzyme Q10 and Statins, p. 295
Complementary and Alternative Medicine for HIV, p. 548
Cranberry for Urinary Tract Infections, p. 433
Echinacea for Boosting the Immune System, p. 462
Feverfew for Migraines, p. 241
Fish Oil for COPD, p. 606
Fish Oils for Inflammation, p. 476
Garlic for Cardiovascular Health, p. 380
Ginger's Tonic Effects on the GI Tract, p. 621
Ginkgo Biloba and Garlic for Treatment of Dementia, p. 263
Ginseng and Myocardial Ischemia, p. 358
Glucosamine and Chondroitin for Osteoarthritis, p. 746
Hawthorn for Heart Failure, p. 342
The Ketogenic Diet, p. 173
Magnesium for Dysrhythmias, p. 374
Medication Errors and Supplements, p. 96
Melatonin, p. 157
Milk Thistle for Alcohol Liver Damage, p. 122
Saw Palmetto, p. 728
Sea Vegetables for Acidosis, p. 447
Selenium's Role in Cancer Prevention, p. 554
Stevia for Hyperglycemia, p. 691
St. John's Wort for Depression, p. 193
Tea Tree Oil for Fungal Infections, p. 529
Treatments for Thyroid Disease, p. 667
Valerian and Kava, p. 157
Vitamin C and the Common Cold, p. 647

NURSING PROCESS FOCUS

Clients Receiving
ACE-inhibitor Therapy, p. 318
Adrenergic-blocking Therapy, p. 142
Amphotericin B (Fungizone, Abelcet), p. 518
Androgen Therapy, p. 722
Antibacterial Therapy, p. 504
Anticholinergic Therapy, p. 148
Anticoagulant Therapy, p. 385
Antidepressant Therapy, p. 197
Antidiarrheal Therapy, p. 631
Antidysrhythmic Therapies, p. 370
Antihistamine Therapy, p. 584
Antineoplastic Therapy, p. 572

Antipyretic Therapy, p. 480
Antiretroviral Agents, p. 541
Antiseizure Drug Therapy, p. 182
Antithyroid Therapy, p. 671
Antituberculosis Agents, p. 509
Atypical Antipsychotic Therapy, p. 220
Benzodiazepine and Nonbenzodiazepine Antianxiety Therapy, p. 166
Beta-adrenergic Antagonist Therapy, p. 323
Bisphosphonates, p. 742
Bronchodilator Therapy, p. 602
Calcium Channel Blocker Therapy, p. 315
Calcium Supplements, p. 736
Cardiac Glycoside Therapy, p. 340
Colchicine, p. 749
Conventional Antipsychotic Therapy, p. 216
Direct Vasodilator Therapy, p. 326
Diuretic Therapy, pp. 312 and Inhibitor, p. 434
Drugs for Muscle Spasms or Spasticity, p. 280
Epoetin Alfa, p. 397
Ferrous Sulfate (Feosol, others), p. 405
Filgrastim (Neupogen), p. 400
Finasteride (Proscar), p. 728
Folic Acid, p. 649
General Anesthesia, p. 253
H_2-Receptor Antagonist Therapy, p. 616
HMG-CoA Reductase Inhibitor Therapy, p. 296
Hormone Replacement Therapy, p. 707
Immunostimulant Therapy, p. 464
Immunosuppressant Therapy, p. 467
Insulin Therapy, p. 687
Isotretinoin (Accutane), p. 763
IV Fluid Replacement Therapy for Shock, p. 416
Levodopa (Larodopa), p. 266
Lindane (Kwell), p. 759
Lithium (Eskalith), p. 201
Local Anesthesia, p. 250
Methylphenidate (Ritalin), p. 205
Nitroglycerin, p. 352
NSAID Therapy, p. 236
Ophthalmic Solutions for Glaucoma, p. 777
Opioid Therapy, p. 229
Oral Contraceptive Therapy, p. 703
Oral Hypoglycemic Therapy, p. 693
Oxytocin, p. 713
Parasympathomimetic Therapy, p. 145
Pharmacotherapy for Superficial Fungal Infections, p. 522
Sympathomimetic Therapy, p. 139
Systemic Glucocorticoid Therapy, p. 676
Thrombolytic Therapy, p. 389
Thyroid Hormone Replacement, p. 669
Total Parenteral Nutrition, p. 656
Triptan Therapy, p. 240

PHARMACOTHERAPY ILLUSTRATED

Mechanism of Action of Antihypertensive Drugs, p. 307
Mechanism of Action of Lipid-lowering Drugs, p. 294
Mechanism of Action of Local Anesthetics, p. 247
Mechanisms of Action of Alzheimer's Drugs, p. 270
Mechanisms of Action of Antiparkinsonism Drugs, p. 264
Mechanisms of Action of Antiprostatic Drugs, p. 726
Mechanisms of Action of Antiulcer Drugs, p. 614
Mechanisms of Action of Direct-acting Antispasmodics, p. 278
Mechanisms of Action of Diuretics, p. 427
Mechanisms of Action of Drugs for Anxiety, p. 155
Mechanisms of Action of Drugs Used for Heart Failure, p. 332
Mechanisms of Action of Drugs Used to Treat Angina, p. 349
Mechanisms of Active and Passive Immunity, p. 459
Model of the GABA Receptor–chloride Channel Molecule, p. 174

PHARMFACTS

Alternative Therapies in America, p. 109
Anesthesia and Anesthetics, p. 245
Angina Pectoris, p. 347
Anxiety Disorders, p. 156
Arthritis, p. 745
Asthma, p. 596
Attention Deficit–Hyperactivity Disorder, p. 202
Bacterial Infections, p. 484
Cancer, p. 553
Clients With Depressive Symptoms, p. 187
Clotting Disorders, p. 378
Community Health Statistics in the United States, p. 104
Consumer Spending on Prescription Drugs, p. 5
Degenerative Diseases of the Central Nervous System, p. 262
Diabetes Mellitus, p. 684
Dysrhythmias, p. 362
Epilepsy, p. 172
Extent of Drug Abuse, p. 15
Female Reproductive Conditions, p. 697
Fungal, Protozoal, and Helminthic Diseases, p. 514
Gastrointestinal Disorders, p. 624
Glaucoma, p. 773
Grapefruit Juice and Drug Interactions, p. 30
Headaches and Migraines, p. 237
Heart Failure, p. 330

SPECIAL FEATURES

Hematopoietic Disorders, p. 395
High Blood Cholesterol, p. 287
Inflammatory Disorders, p. 471
Insomnia, p. 157
Insomnia Linked to Insulin Resistance, p. 157
Male Reproductive Conditions and Disorders, p. 718
Marketing and Promotional Spending, p. 14
Minority Statistics and Healthcare Access, p. 102
Muscle Spasms, p. 275
Osteoporosis, p. 740
Pain, p. 224
Poisoning, p. 83
Possible Fetal Effects Caused by Specific Drug Use During Pregnancy, p. 80
Potential Chemical and Biological Agents for Terrorist Attacks, p. 19
Potentially Fatal Drug Reactions, p. 28
Psychoses, p. 210
Renal Disorders, p. 424
Shock, p. 410
Skin Disorders, p. 754
Statistics of Hypertension, p. 302
Substance Abuse in the United States, p. 119
Thyroid Disorders, p. 666
Time Length for New Drug Approvals, p. 8
Upper Gastrointestinal Tract Disorders, p. 611
Vaccines and Organ Transplants, p. 455
Viral Infections, p. 534
Vitamins, Minerals, and Nutritional Supplements, p. 642

PROTOTYPE DRUG

acetaminophen (Tylenol, others), p. 479
acyclovir (Zovirax), p. 545
alteplase (Activase), p. 388
aluminum hydroxide (Amphojel, others), p. 620
aminocaproic acid (Amicar), p. 390
amiodarone (Cordarone), p. 372
ammonium chloride, p. 449
amphotericin B (Fungizone), p. 517
aspirin (Acetylsalicylic Acid, ASA), p. 235
atenolol (Tenormin), p. 353
atorvastatin (Lipitor), p. 295
atropine (Atropair, Atropisol), p. 148
beclomethasone (Beclovent, Beconase, others), p. 604
benzocaine (Solarcaine, others), p. 760
benztropine (Cogentin), p. 268
bethanechol (Urecholine), p. 144
calcitriol (Calcijex, Rocaltrol), p. 739
calcium gluconate (Kalcinate), p. 736
cefotaxime (Claforan), p. 493
chloroquine (Aralen), p. 525
chlorothiazide (Diuril), p. 430
chlorpromazine (Thorazine), p. 213
cholestyramine (Questran), p. 297
ciprofloxacin (Cipro), p. 500
clopidogrel (Plavix), p. 387
clozapine (Clozaril), p. 219
colchicine, p. 749
cyanocobalamin (Crystamine, others), p. 403
cyclobenzaprine (Cycoflex, Flexeril), p. 277
cyclophosphamide (Cytoxan), p. 560
cyclosporine (Sandimmune, Neoral), p. 466
dantrolene sodium (Dantrium), p. 279
dextran 40 (Gentran 40, others), p. 441
dextromethorphan (Benylin, others), p. 590
diazepam (Valium), p. 177
digoxin (Lanoxin), p. 339
diltiazem (Cardizem), p. 354
diphenhydramine (Benadryl, others), p. 583
diphenoxylate with atropine (Lomotil), p. 629
donepezil (Aricept), p. 271
dopamine (Dopastat, Inotropin), p. 417
doxazosin (Cardura), p. 322
doxorubicin (Adriamycin), p. 564
enalapril (Vasotec), p. 318
epinephrine (Adrenalin), p. 420
epoetin alfa (Epogen, Procrit), p. 396
erythromycin (E-Mycin, Erythrocin), p. 497
escitalopram (Lexapro), p. 161
estrogen/progestin conjugated estrogens (Premarin) and conjugated estrogens with medroxyprogesterone (Prempro), p. 706
ethinyl estradiol with norethindrone (Ortho-Novum 1/35), p. 702
ethosuximide (Zarontin), p. 181
etidronate disodium (Didronel), p. 741
ferrous sulfate (Feosol, others), p. 404
fexofenadine (Allegra), p. 583
filgrastim (Neupogen), p. 399
finasteride (Proscar), p. 727
fluconazole (Diflucan), p. 519
fluticasone (Flonase, Flovent), p. 586
folic acid (Folacin, Folvite), p. 648
furosemide (Lasix), p. 336
gemfibrozil (Lopid), p. 298
gentamicin (Garamycin), p. 498
glipizide (Glucotrol, Glucotrol XL), p. 692
haloperidol (Haldol), p. 215
halothane (Fluothane), p. 252
heparin (Heplock), p. 383
hepatitis B vaccine (Recombivax HB, Engerix-B), p. 460
hydralazine (Apresoline), p. 325
hydrochlorothiazide (HydroDIURIL), p. 311

hydrocortisone (Cortef, Hydrocortone, others), p. 676
hydroxychloroquine sulfate (Plaquenil), p. 748
ibuprofen (Motrin, Advil), p. 475
imipramine (Tofranil), p. 191
interferon alfa-2A (Roferon-A), p. 463
ipratropium bromide (Atrovent, Combivent), p. 599
isoniazid (INH), p. 508
isosorbide dinitrate (Isordil, others), p. 338
isotretinoin (Accutane), p. 762
latanoprost (Xalatan), p. 775
levodopa (Larodopa), p. 265
levothyroxine (Synthroid), p. 669
lidocaine (Xylocaine), p. 249
lindane (Kwell), p. 757
lisinopril (Prinivil, Zestril), p. 334
lithium (Eskalith), p. 200
lorazepam (Ativan), p. 163
magnesium sulfate, p. 652
mebendazole (Vermox), p. 529
medroxyprogesterone acetate (Provera), p. 710
methotrexate (Folex, Mexate, others), p. 562
methylphenidate (Ritalin), p. 205
metoprolol (Lopressor), p. 337
metronidazole (Flagyl), p. 527
milrinone (Primacor), p. 341
morphine (Astramorph PF, Duramorph, others), p. 228
naloxone (Narcan), p. 231
nevirapine (Viramune), p. 539
nifedipine (Procardia), p. 314
nitroglycerin (Nitrostat, Nitro-Bid, Nitro-Dur, others), p. 351
nitrous oxide, p. 251
norepinephrine (Levarterenol, Levophed), p. 415
normal serum albumin (Albuminar, Albutein, Buminate, Plasbumin), p. 413
nystatin (Mycostatin), p. 521
omeprazole (Prilosec), p. 618
oxymetazoline (Afrin, others), p. 588
oxytocin (Pitocin, Syntocinon), p. 712
pancrelipase (Cotazym, Pancrease, others), p. 637
penicillin G (Pentids), p. 491
phenelzine (Nardil), p. 196
phenobarbital (Luminal), p. 176
phenylephrine (Neo-Synephrine), p. 138
phenytoin (Dilantin), p. 179
potassium chloride (KCl), p. 446
prazosin (Minipress), p. 141
prednisone (Meticorten, others), p. 477
procainamide (Procan, Procanbid, Pronestyl), p. 368
prochlorperazine (Compazine), p. 635
propranolol (Inderal), p. 369
propylthiouracil (PTU), p. 671
psyllium mucilloid (Metamucil, others), p. 627
raloxifene (Evista), p. 744

ranitidine HCl (Zantac), p. 615
regular insulin (Humulin R, Novolin R, and others), p. 686
reteplase (Retavase), p. 357
salmeterol (Serevent), p. 598
saquinavir (Fortovase, Invirase), p. 540
sertraline (Zoloft), p. 193
sibutramine (Meridia), p. 636
sildenafil (Viagra), p. 724
sodium bicarbonate, p. 448
sodium chloride (NaCl), p. 444
spironolactone (Aldactone), p. 432
succinylcholine (Anectine), p. 257
sumatriptan (Imitrex), p. 239
tamoxifen (Nolvadex), p. 569
tegaserod (Zelnorm), p. 632
testosterone base (Andro, others), p. 721
tetracycline (Achromycin, others), p. 495
thiopental (Pentothal), p. 255
timolol (Betimol, Timoptic, Timoptic XE), p. 776
trimethoprim-sulfamethoxazole (Bactrim, Septra), p. 502
valproic acid (Depakene), p. 180
vasopressin injection (Pitressin), p. 665
verapamil (Calan), p. 373
vincristine (Oncovin), p. 567
vitamin A (Aquasol A), p. 645
warfarin (Coumadin), p. 384
zafirlukast (Accolate), p. 605
zidovudine (Retrovir, AZT), p. 538
zolpidem (Ambien), p. 164

SPECIAL CONSIDERATIONS

Abuse of Volatile Inhalants by Children and Adolescents, p. 120
Adverse Drug Effects and Elderly Clients, p. 51
Age-related Issues in Drug Administration, p. 94
Alcoholism: Cultural and Environmental Influences, p. 101
Androgen Abuse by Athletes, p. 720
Asian Clients' Sensitivity to Propranolol, p. 371
The Challenges of Pediatric Drug Administration, p. 29
Chemotherapy in Elderly Patients, p. 570
Childhood Play Areas and Parasitic Infections, p. 527
Clients with Speaking, Visual, or Hearing Impairments, p. 69
Cultural Dietary Habits, p. 291
Cultural Effects on Immunizations, p. 461
Cultural Influences and the Treatment of Depression, p. 187
Cultural Influences on Pain Expression and Perception, p. 225
Cultural Remedies for Diarrhea, p. 630
Cultural Views and Treatments of Mental Illness, p. 212
Dietary Supplements and the Older Adult, p. 109
Enzyme Deficiency in Certain Ethnic Populations, p. 62
Estrogen Use and Psychosocial Issues, p. 708
Ethnic Considerations in Acetaminophen Metabolism, p. 480

SPECIAL FEATURES

Ethnic Groups and Smoking, p. 126

Ethnicity and ACE Inhibitor Action, p. 320

G6PD Deficiency and Antimalarials, p. 525

Hispanic Cultural Beliefs and Antibacterials, p. 488

HIV in the Pediatric and Geriatric Populations, p. 544

How Prescription Drug Costs Affect Senior Citizens, p. 8

H_2-Receptors and Vitamin B_{12} in Older Adults, p. 617

Impact of Anticholinergics on Male Sexual Function, p. 147

The Impact of Ethnicity and Lifestyle on Osteoporosis, p. 743

The Influence of Age on Pain Expression and Perception, p. 231

The Influence of Gender and Ethnicity on Angina, p. 348

Laxatives and Fluid–Electrolyte Balance, p. 445

Living With Alzheimer's and Parkinson's Diseases, p. 262

The New Fountain of Youth? p. 281

Non-English-Speaking and Culturally Diverse Clients, p. 71

Parasitic Infections in Children, p. 528

Pediatric Drug Research and Labeling, p. 83

Pediatric Dyslipidemias, p. 290

Psychosocial and Community Impact of Scabies and Pediculosis, p. 758

Psychosocial and Community Impacts of Alcohol-related Pancreatitis, p. 638

Psychosocial and Cultural Impacts of Young Diabetic Clients, p. 689

Psychosocial Issues and Compliance in Clients With Heart Failure, p. 341

Psychosocial Issues With Antiretroviral Drug Compliance, p. 538

Religious Affiliation and Disease Incidence, p. 102

Respiratory Distress Syndrome, p. 606

Seizure Etiologies Based on Genetics and Age-related Factors, p. 171

Shift Workers, Hypothyroidism, and Drug Compliance, p. 667

Vitamin Supplements and Client Communication, p. 645

Zero Tolerance in Schools, p. 204

DETAILED CONTENTS

About the Authors   xi
Contributors   xii
Thank You   xiv
Preface   xvi
Special Features   xviii

UNIT 1 Core Concepts in Pharmacology   1

Chapter 1   Introduction to Pharmacology: Drug Regulation and Approval   2

History of Pharmacology   3
Pharmacology: The Study of Medicines   4
Pharmacology and Therapeutics   4
Classification of Therapeutic Agents as Drugs, Biologics, and Alternative Therapies   4
Prescription and Over-the-Counter Drugs   4
Drug Regulations and Standards   5
The Role of the Food and Drug Administration   6
Stages of Approval for Therapeutic and Biological Drugs   7
Recent Changes to the Drug Approval Process   8
Canadian Drug Standards   9

Chapter 2   Drug Classes and Schedules   11

Therapeutic and Pharmacological Classification of Drugs   12
Chemical, Generic, and Trade Names for Drugs   13
Differences Between Brand-Name Drugs and Their Generic Equivalents   14
Controlled Substances and Drug Schedules   14
Canadian Regulations Restricting Drugs of Abuse   15

Chapter 3   Emergency Preparedness   18

The Nature of Bioterrorism   19
Role of the Nurse in Emergency Preparedness   20
Strategic National Stockpile   21
Anthrax   21
Viruses   22
Toxic Chemicals   23
Ionizing Radiation   23

Chapter 4   Principles of Drug Administration   27

Medication Knowledge, Understanding, and Responsibilities of the Nurse   28
The Rights of Drug Administration   29
Client Compliance and Successful Pharmacotherapy   29
Drug Orders and Time Schedules   30
Systems of Measurement   31
Enteral Drug Administration   32
Topical Drug Administration   34
Parenteral Drug Administration   38

Chapter 5   Pharmacokinetics   46

Pharmacokinetics: How the Body Handles Medications   47
The Passage of Drugs through Plasma Membranes   47
Absorption of Medications   48
Distribution of Medications   49
Metabolism of Medications   50
Excretion of Medications   51
Drug Plasma Concentration and Therapeutic Response   52
Plasma Half-life and Duration of Drug Action   53
Loading Doses and Maintenance Doses   53

Chapter 6   Pharmacodynamics   56

Pharmacodynamics and Interclient Variability   57
Therapeutic Index and Drug Safety   58
The Graded Dose–Response Relationship and Therapeutic Response   59
Potency and Efficacy   59
Cellular Receptors and Drug Action   60
Types of Drug–Receptor Interactions   61
Pharmacology of the Future: Customizing Drug Therapy   62

UNIT 2 Pharmacology and the Nurse-Client Relationship   65

Chapter 7   The Nursing Process in Pharmacology   66

Review of the Nursing Process   67
Assessment of the Client Related to Drug Administration   68
Nursing Diagnoses for the Client Receiving Medications   69
Setting Goals and Outcomes for Drug Administration   70

Key Interventions for Drug Administration 71

Evaluating the Effects of Drug Administration 72

Chapter 8 **Drug Administration Throughout the Lifespan** 75

Pharmacotherapy Across the Lifespan 76

Pharmacotherapy of the Pregnant Client 76

Pharmacotherapy of the Lactating Client 79

Client Teaching During Pregnancy and Lactation 80

Pharmacotherapy of Infants 81

Pharmacotherapy of Toddlers 82

Pharmacotherapy of Preschoolers and School-age Children 83

Pharmacotherapy of Adolescents 84

Pharmacotherapy of Young and Middle-aged Adults 84

Pharmacotherapy of Older Adults 85

Chapter 9 **Medication Errors and Risk Reduction** 89

Defining Medication Errors 90

Factors Contributing to Medication Errors 90

Nurse Practice Acts and Standards of Care 92

The Impact of Medication Errors 93

Reporting and Documenting Medication Errors 93

Strategies for Reducing Medication Errors 94

Providing Client Education for Medication Usage 95

How Healthcare Facilities Are Reducing Medication Errors 96

Governmental and Other Agencies That Track Medication Errors 96

Chapter 10 **Psychosocial, Gender, and Cultural Influences on Pharmacotherapy** 99

The Concept of Holistic Pharmacotherapy 100

Psychosocial Influences on Pharmacotherapy 101

Cultural and Ethnic Influences on Pharmacotherapy 101

Community and Environmental Influences on Pharmacotherapy 103

Genetic Influences on Pharmacotherapy 104

Gender Influences on Pharmacotherapy 104

Chapter 11 **Herbal and Alternative Therapies** 107

Alternative Therapies 108

Brief History of Therapeutic Natural Products 108

Herbal Product Formulations 109

Regulation of Herbal Products and Dietary Supplements 111

The Pharmacological Actions and Safety of Herbal Products 112

Specialty Supplements 114

Chapter 12 **Substance Abuse** 117

Overview of Substance Abuse 118

Neurobiological and Psychosocial Components of Substance Abuse 118

Physical and Psychological Dependence 119

Withdrawal Syndrome 119

Tolerance 120

Abused CNS Depressants 121

Cannabinoids 122

Hallucinogens 123

Abused CNS Stimulants 124

Nicotine 125

The Nurse's Role in Substance Abuse 126

UNIT 3 The Nervous System 129

Chapter 13 **Drugs Affecting the Autonomic Nervous System** 130

Autonomic Drugs 136

Adrenergic Agents (Sympathomimetics) 136

Nursing Process Focus Clients Receiving Sympathomimetic Therapy 138

Nursing Considerations 139

Adrenergic-blocking Agents 140

Nursing Considerations 141

Nursing Process Focus Clients Receiving Adrenergic-blocking Therapy 142

Cholinergic Agents (Parasympathomimetics) 143

Nursing Considerations 144

Nursing Process Focus Clients Receiving Parasympathomimetic Therapy 145

Cholinergic-blocking Agents (Anticholinergics) 146

Nursing Process Focus Clients Receiving Anticholinergic Therapy 148

Nursing Considerations 149

Chapter 14 **Drugs for Anxiety and Insomnia** 153

Anxiety Disorders 154

Insomnia 156

Central Nervous System Agents 158

Antidepressants 159

Benzodiazepines **160**

Nursing Considerations **161**

Barbiturates **163**

Nursing Process Focus Clients Receiving
Benzodiazepine and Nonbenzodiazepine
Antianxiety Therapy **166**

Chapter 15 **Drugs for Seizures** **169**

Seizures **170**

Drugs that Potentiate GABA **173**

*Barbiturates, Benzodiazepines, and Miscellaneous
GABA Agents* **173**

Nursing Considerations **174**

Benzodiazepines **176**

Nursing Considerations **176**

Drugs that Suppress Sodium Influx **178**

Hydantoin and Phenytoin-like Drugs **178**

Nursing Considerations **179**

Drugs that Suppress Calcium Influx **180**

Succinimides **180**

Nursing Considerations **181**

Nursing Process Focus Clients Receiving
Antiseizure Drug Therapy **182**

Chapter 16 **Drugs for Emotional and Mood
Disorders** **185**

Depression **186**

Antidepressants **188**

Tricyclic Antidepressants **188**

Nursing Considerations **190**

Selective Serotonin Reuptake Inhibitors **192**

Nursing Considerations **194**

Monoamine Oxidase Inhibitors **194**

Nursing Considerations **195**

Bipolar Disorder **196**

Nursing Process Focus Clients Receiving
Antidepressant Therapy **197**

Drugs for Bipolar Disorder **199**

Nursing Process Focus Clients Receiving Lithium
(Eskalith) **201**

Nursing Considerations **202**

**Attention Deficit–Hyperactivity
Disorder** **202**

**Drugs for Attention Deficit–Hyperactivity
Disorder** **203**

Nursing Considerations **204**

Nursing Process Focus Clients Receiving
Methylphenidate (Ritalin) **205**

Chapter 17 **Drugs for Psychoses** **209**

Schizophrenia **210**

**Conventional (Typical)
Antipsychotic Agents** **212**

Phenothiazines **212**

Nursing Considerations **214**

Nonphenothiazines **214**

Nursing Process Focus Clients Receiving
Conventional Antipsychotic Therapy **216**

Nursing Considerations **217**

Atypical Antipsychotic Agents **218**

Nursing Considerations **218**

Nursing Process Focus Clients Receiving
Atypical Antipsychotic Therapy **220**

Chapter 18 **Drugs for the Control of Pain** **223**

Opioid (Narcotic) Analgesics **226**

Nursing Process Focus Clients Receiving Opioid
Therapy **229**

Nursing Considerations **230**

Opioid Antagonists **231**

Nursing Considerations **231**

Nonopioid Analgesics **232**

*Nonsteroidal Anti-inflammatory Drugs
(NSAIDs)* **232**

Nursing Considerations **234**

Nursing Process Focus Clients Receiving NSAID
Therapy **236**

Tension Headaches and Migraines **237**

Nursing Considerations **239**

Nursing Process Focus Clients Receiving Triptan
Therapy **240**

Chapter 19 **Drugs for Local and General
Anesthesia** **244**

Local Anesthesia **245**

Local Anesthetics **245**

Nursing Considerations **248**

General Anesthesia **249**

Nursing Process Focus Clients Receiving Local
Anesthesia **250**

General Anesthetics **250**

Gaseous General Anesthetics **251**

Volatile Liquid General Anesthetics **252**

Nursing Process Focus Clients Receiving General
Anesthesia **253**

Nursing Considerations **254**

IV Anesthetics **254**

Nursing Considerations **255**

Nursing Considerations **258**

Chapter 20 **Drugs for Degenerative Diseases
of the Nervous System** **260**

Parkinson's Disease **261**

Parkinsonism Drugs **262**

Dopaminergics **262**

Nursing Considerations **264**

Anticholinergics **265**

Nursing Process Focus Clients Receiving
Levodopa (Larodopa) **266**

Nursing Considerations **267**

Alzheimer's Disease **268**

Drugs for Alzheimer's Disease **269**

*Acetylcholinesterase Inhibitors
(Parasympathomimetics)* **269**

Nursing Considerations **271**

**Chapter 21 Drugs for Neuromuscular
Disorders** **274**

Muscle Spasms **275**

Centrally Acting Skeletal Muscle Relaxants **276**

Spasticity **276**

Direct-acting Antispasmodics **278**

Nursing Considerations **279**

Nursing Process Focus Clients Receiving Drugs
for Muscle Spasms or Spasticity **280**

**UNIT 4 The Cardiovascular
and Urinary Systems** **285**

Chapter 22 Drugs for Lipid Disorders **286**

HMG-CoA Reductase Inhibitors/Statins **291**

Nursing Considerations **292**

Bile Acid Resins **293**

Nursing Considerations **294**

Nicotinic Acid (Niacin) **295**

Nursing Process Focus Clients Receiving
HMG-CoA Reductase Inhibitor Therapy **296**

Nursing Considerations **297**

Fibric Acid Agents **297**

Nursing Considerations **298**

Cholesterol Absorption Inhibitors **298**

Chapter 23 Drugs for Hypertension **301**

Diuretics **308**

Nursing Considerations **309**

Calcium Channel Blockers **311**

Nursing Process Focus Clients Receiving
Diuretic Therapy **312**

Nursing Considerations **314**

Nursing Process Focus Clients Receiving
Calcium Channel Blocker Therapy **315**

**Drugs Affecting the Renin–Angiotensin
System** **316**

Nursing Considerations **317**

Nursing Process Focus Clients Receiving
ACE-inhibitor Therapy **318**

Adrenergic Antagonists **320**

Nursing Considerations **322**

Nursing Process Focus Clients Receiving
Beta-adrenergic Antagonist Therapy **323**

Direct Vasodilators **324**

Nursing Considerations **324**

Nursing Process Focus Clients Receiving Direct
Vasodilator Therapy **326**

Chapter 24 Drugs for Heart Failure **329**

Pharmacotherapy of Heart Failure **332**

ACE Inhibitors **332**

Nursing Considerations **334**

Diuretics **335**

Nursing Considerations **335**

*Beta-adrenergic Blockers
(Antagonists)* **336**

Nursing Considerations **337**

Vasodilators **337**

Nursing Considerations **338**

Cardiac Glycosides **338**

Nursing Considerations **339**

Nursing Process Focus Clients Receiving Cardiac
Glycoside Therapy **340**

Phosphodiesterase Inhibitors **341**

Nursing Considerations **342**

**Chapter 25 Drugs for Angina Pectoris and
Myocardial Infarction** **345**

Angina Pectoris **346**

Organic Nitrates **349**

Nursing Considerations **350**

Beta-adrenergic Blockers (Antagonists) **351**

Nursing Considerations **352**

Nursing Process Focus Clients Receiving
Nitroglycerin **352**

Calcium Channel Blockers **353**

Nursing Considerations **354**

Myocardial Infarction **355**

Thrombolytics **355**

Nursing Considerations **357**

Antiplatelet and Anticoagulant Drugs **358**

Nitrates **358**

Beta-adrenergic Blockers **358**

*Angiotensin-converting Enzyme
(ACE) Inhibitors* **358**

Chapter 26 Drugs for Dysrhythmias **361**

Sodium Channel Blockers (Class I) **366**

Nursing Considerations **369**

Nursing Process Focus Clients Receiving
Antidysrhythmic Therapies **370**

*Beta-adrenergic Antagonists/Blockers
(Class II)* **371**

Nursing Considerations 371

Potassium Channel Blockers (Class III) 371

Nursing Considerations 372

Calcium Channel Blockers (Class IV) 373

Nursing Considerations 373

Chapter 27 **Drugs for Coagulation Disorders** 377

Anticoagulants 381

Nursing Considerations 382

Antiplatelet Agents 384

Nursing Process Focus Clients Receiving Anticoagulant Therapy 385

Nursing Considerations 386

Thrombolytics 387

Nursing Considerations 388

Nursing Process Focus Clients Receiving Thrombolytic Therapy 389

Hemostatics 389

Nursing Considerations 390

Chapter 28 **Drugs for Hematopoietic Disorders** 393

Hematopoietic Growth Factors 395

Human Erythropoietin and Related Drugs 395

Nursing Considerations 395

Nursing Process Focus Clients Receiving Epoetin Alfa 397

Colony-stimulating Factors 398

Nursing Considerations 398

Platelet Enhancers 399

Nursing Considerations 399

Nursing Process Focus Clients Receiving Filgrastim (Neupogen) 400

Anemias 401

Antianemic Agents 401

Vitamin B$_{12}$ and Folic Acid 401

Nursing Considerations 403

Iron 403

Nursing Considerations 404

Nursing Process Focus Clients Receiving Ferrous Sulfate (Feosol, others) 405

Chapter 29 **Drugs for Shock** 409

Fluid Replacement Agents 411

Nursing Considerations 413

Vasoconstrictors/Vasopressors 414

Nursing Considerations 415

Inotropic Agents 415

Nursing Process Focus Clients Receiving IV Fluid Replacement Therapy for Schock 416

Nursing Considerations 418

Anaphylaxis 418

Nursing Considerations 420

Chapter 30 **Diuretic Therapy and Drugs for Renal Failure** 423

Renal Failure 425

Diuretics 427

Nursing Considerations 428

Nursing Considerations 430

Nursing Considerations 431

Nursing Process Focus Clients Receiving Diuretic Therapy 434

Chapter 31 **Drugs for Fluid Balance, Electrolyte, and Acid–Base Disorders** 437

Fluid Balance 438

Fluid Replacement Agents 439

Nursing Considerations 441

Electrolytes 442

Nursing Considerations 444

Nursing Considerations 445

Acid–Base Balance 446

Nursing Considerations 447

Nursing Considerations 449

UNIT 5 **The Immune System** 453

Chapter 32 **Drugs for Immune System Modulation** 454

Vaccines 456

Nursing Considerations 458

Immunostimulants 461

Nursing Considerations 462

Immunosupressants 463

Nursing Process Focus Clients Receiving Immunostimulant Therapy 464

Nursing Process Focus Clients Receiving Immunosuppressant Therapy 467

Nursing Considerations 468

Chapter 33 **Drugs for Inflammation and Fever** 470

Inflammation 471

Nonsteroidal Anti-inflammatory Drugs 473

Nursing Considerations 475

Systemic Glucocorticoids (Corticosteroids) 476

Nursing Considerations 477

Fever 478

Nursing Considerations **478**

Nursing Process Focus Clients Receiving
Antipyretic Therapy **480**

Chapter 34   Drugs for Bacterial Infections 483

Antibacterial Agents 489
Penicillins 489

Nursing Considerations **490**

Cephalosporins 492

Nursing Considerations **493**

Tetracyclines 494

Nursing Considerations **494**

Macrolides 495

Nursing Considerations **496**

Aminoglycosides 497

Nursing Considerations **497**

Fluoroquinolones 499

Nursing Considerations **500**

Sulfonamides 501

Nursing Considerations **501**

Nursing Process Focus Clients Receiving
Antibacterial Therapy **504**

Tuberculosis 506

Nursing Considerations **508**

Nursing Process Focus Clients Receiving
Antituberculosis Agents **509**

**Chapter 35   Drugs for Fungal, Protozoal, and
Helminthic Infections 513**

**Drugs for Systemic Antifungal
Infections 515**

Nursing Considerations **516**

Azoles 517

Nursing Process Focus Clients Receiving
Amphotericin B *(Fungizone, Abelcet)* **518**

Nursing Considerations **520**

Drugs for Superficial Fungal Infections 520

Nursing Considerations **521**

Nursing Process Focus Clients Receiving
Pharmacotherapy for Superficial Fungal
Infections **522**

Protozoal Infections 522

Nursing Considerations **524**

Nursing Considerations **527**

Drugs for Helminthic Infections 528

Nursing Considerations **529**

Chapter 36   Drugs for Viral Infections 532

HIV-AIDS 534

*Reverse Transcriptase Inhibitors
(NRTIs, NNRTIs, and NtRTIs) 536*

Protease Inhibitors 538

Nursing Considerations **539**

Nursing Process Focus Clients Receiving
Antiretroviral Agents **541**

Herpesviruses 543

Nursing Considerations **545**

Influenza 546

Viral Hepatitis 547

Chapter 37   Drugs for Neoplasia 551

Alkylating Agents 557

Nursing Considerations **558**

Antimetabolites 560

Nursing Considerations **561**

Antitumor Antibiotics 563

Nursing Considerations **563**

**Natural Products (Plant Extracts
and Alkaloids) 565**

Nursing Considerations **566**

Hormones and Hormone Antagonists 567

Glucocorticoids 568

Gonadal Hormones 568

Antiestrogens 569

Androgen Antagonists 569

Nursing Considerations **569**

Biologic Response Modifiers 570

Nursing Process Focus Clients Receiving
Antineoplastic Therapy **572**

UNIT 6 The Respiratory System 577

**Chapter 38   Drugs for Allergic Rhinitis and the
Common Cold 578**

Allergic Rhinitis 580

*H_1-Receptor Antagonists/
Antihistamines 581*

Nursing Considerations **582**

Nursing Process Focus Clients Receiving
Antihistamine Therapy **584**

Intranasal Glucocorticoids 584

Nursing Considerations **586**

Decongestants 587

Nursing Considerations **588**

Common Cold 588

Antitussives 589

Nursing Considerations **590**

Expectorants and Mucolytics 591

**Chapter 39   Drugs for Asthma and Other
Pulmonary Disorders 593**

Asthma 595

Beta-adrenergic Agonists 596

Nursing Considerations **598**

Anticholinergics **598**

Nursing Considerations **599**

Methylxanthines **600**

Nursing Considerations **600**

Glucocorticoids **601**

Nursing Process Focus Clients Receiving Bronchodilator Therapy **602**

Nursing Considerations **603**

Leukotriene Modifiers **603**

Nursing Considerations **604**

Mast Cell Stabilizers **605**

Chronic Obstructive Pulmonary Disease **605**

UNIT 7 The Gastrointestinal System **609**

Chapter 40   Drugs for Peptic Ulcer Disease **610**

H_2-Receptor Antagonists **615**

Nursing Process Focus Clients Receiving H_2-Receptor Antagonist Therapy **616**

Nursing Considerations **616**

Proton Pump Inhibitors **617**

Nursing Considerations **617**

Antacids **618**

Nursing Considerations **619**

Antibiotics for H. Pylori **620**

Chapter 41   Drugs for Bowel Disorders and Other Gastrointestinal Conditions **623**

Constipation **625**

Laxatives **625**

Nursing Considerations **627**

Diarrhea **628**

Antidiarrheals **629**

Nursing Considerations **629**

Nursing Process Focus   Clients Receiving Antidiarrheal Therapy **631**

Nursing Considerations **631**

Nausea and Vomiting **632**

Antiemetics **633**

Antihistamines and Anticholinergic Agents **633**

Phenothiazines **633**

Glucocorticoids **633**

Selective Serotonin Reuptake Inhibitors (SSRIS) **633**

Other Antiemetics **633**

Nursing Considerations **633**

Hunger and Appetite **635**

Anorexiants **635**

Nursing Considerations **636**

Pancreatic Enzymes **637**

Nursing Considerations **638**

Chapter 42   Drugs for Nutritional Disorders **641**

Vitamins **642**

Lipid-soluble Vitamins **644**

Nursing Considerations **646**

Water-soluble Vitamins **646**

Nursing Considerations **648**

Nursing Process Focus Clients Receiving Folic Acid **649**

Minerals **649**

Nursing Considerations **652**

Nutritional Supplements **654**

Nursing Considerations **655**

Nursing Considerations **655**

Nursing Process Focus Clients Receiving Total Parenteral Nutrition **656**

UNIT 8 The Endocrine System **659**

Chapter 43   Drugs for Pituitary, Thyroid, and Adrenal Disorders **660**

Disorders of the Hypothalamus and the Pituitary Gland **662**

Growth Hormone (GH) **664**

Antidiuretic Hormone **665**

Nursing Considerations **666**

Thyroid Agents **667**

Nursing Considerations **668**

Nursing Process Focus Clients Receiving Thyroid Hormone Replacement **669**

Antithyroid Agents **670**

Nursing Process Focus Clients Receiving Antithyroid Therapy **671**

Nursing Considerations **672**

Adrenal Gland Disorders **673**

Glucocorticoids **674**

Nursing Considerations **675**

Nursing Process Focus Client Receiving Systemic Glucocorticoid Therapy **676**

Nursing Considerations **678**

Chapter 44   Drugs for Diabetes Mellitus **681**

Diabetes Mellitus **683**

Insulin **683**

Nursing Considerations **686**

Nursing Process Focus Clients Receiving Insulin Therapy **687**

Oral Hypoglycemics **689**

Nursing Considerations **691**

Nursing Process Focus Clients Receiving Oral Hypoglycemic Therapy **693**

Chapter 45 Drugs for Disorders and Conditions of the Female Reproductive System 696

Contraception 699
Oral Contraceptives 699

Nursing Considerations 701

Nursing Process Focus Clients Receiving Oral Contraceptive Therapy 703

Emergency Contraception and Pharmacological Abortion 704
Menopause 705

Nursing Process Focus Clients Receiving Hormone Replacement Therapy 707

Nursing Considerations 708

Uterine Abnormalities 708

Nursing Considerations 709

Labor and Breast-feeding 710
Oxytocics and Tocolytics 710

Nursing Considerations 712

Nursing Process Focus Clients Receiving Oxytocin 713

Female Infertility 714

Chapter 46 Drugs for Disorders and Conditions of the Male Reproductive System 717

Male Hypogonadism 718
Androgens 718

Nursing Considerations 720

Male Infertility 721
Erectile Dysfunction 721

Nursing Process Focus Clients Receiving Androgen Therapy 722

Nursing Considerations 723

Benign Prostatic Hyperplasia 725
Antiprostatic Agents 725

Nursing Considerations 728

Nursing Process Focus Clients Receiving Finasteride (Proscar) 728

UNIT 9 The Integumentary System and Eyes/Ears 731

Chapter 47 Drugs for Bone and Joint Disorders 732

Calcium-related Disorders 734

Nursing Considerations 735

Nursing Process Focus Clients Receiving Calcium Supplements 737

Nursing Considerations 738

Bisphosphonates 740

Nursing Process Focus Clients Receiving Bisphosphonates 742

Nursing Considerations 743

Selective Estrogen Receptor Modulators 743
Calcitonin 743
Hormone Replacement Therapy 743
Joint Disorders 745

Nursing Considerations 748

Nursing Process Focus Clients Receiving Colchicine Inhibitor 749

Chapter 48 Drugs for Skin Disorders 752

Skin Infections 754
Skin Parasites 756

Nursing Considerations 757

Sunburn and Minor Burns 758

Nursing Process Focus Clients Receiving Lindane (Kwell) 759

Nursing Considerations 760

Acne and Rosacea 761

Nursing Process Focus Clients Receiving Isotretinoin (Accutane) 763

Nursing Considerations 764

Dermatitis 765
Psoriasis 766
Topical Therapies 768
Systemic Therapies 768
Nonpharmacological Therapies 768

Chapter 49 Drugs for Eye and Ear Disorders 770

Glaucoma 772
Prostaglandins 773
Beta-adrenergic Blockers 773
Alpha$_2$-adrenergic Agonists 775
Carbonic Anhydrase Inhibitors 775
Cholinergic Agonists (Miotics) 775
Nonselective Sympathomimetics 775
Osmotic Diuretics 776

Nursing Considerations 776

Nursing Process Focus Clients Receiving Ophthalmic Solutions for Glaucoma 777

Ear Conditions 779
Otic Preparations 779

Nursing Considerations 780

Glossary 783
Appendix A 797
Appendix B 800
Appendix C 803
Appendix D 818
Appendix E 845
Index 847

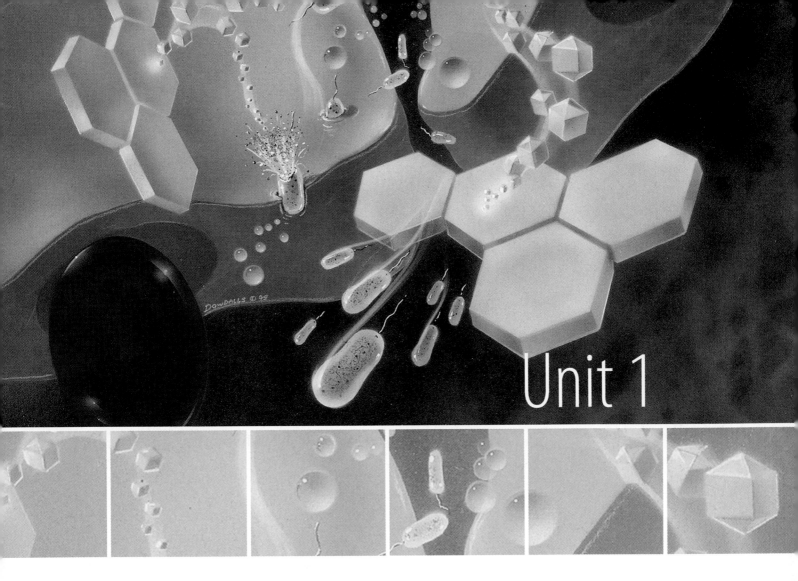

Unit 1

Core Concepts in Pharmacology

CHAPTER 1   Introduction to Pharmacology: Drug Regulation and Approval

CHAPTER 2   Drug Classes and Schedules

CHAPTER 3   Emergency Preparedness

CHAPTER 4   Principles of Drug Administration

CHAPTER 5   Pharmacokinetics

CHAPTER 6   Pharmacodynamics

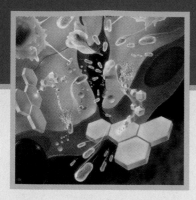

CHAPTER 1

Introduction to Pharmacology: Drug Regulation and Approval

OBJECTIVES

After reading this chapter, the student should be able to:

1. Identify key events in the history of pharmacology.
2. Explain the interdisciplinary nature of pharmacology, giving examples of subject areas needed to learn the discipline well.
3. Compare and contrast therapeutics and pharmacology.
4. Compare and contrast traditional drugs, biologics, and alternative therapies.
5. Identify the advantages and disadvantages of prescription and over-the-counter (OTC) drugs.
6. Identify key U.S. drug regulations that have ensured the safety and efficacy of medications.
7. Discuss the role of the U.S. Food and Drug Administration (FDA) in the drug approval process.
8. Explain the four stages of approval for therapeutic and biological drugs.
9. Discuss how the FDA has increased the speed with which new drugs reach consumers.
10. Describe the Canadian drug approval process and identify similarities between how drugs are approved in the United States.

MediaLink

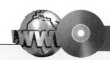

www.prenhall.com/adams

KEY TERMS

biologics *page 4*

clinical investigation *page 7*

clinical phase trials *page 7*

complementary and alternative therapies
  page 4

drug *page 4*

Food and Drug Administration (FDA) *page 6*

formulary *page 5*

medication *page 4*

NDA review *page 8*

pharmacology *page 4*

pharmacopoeia *page 5*

pharmacotherapy *page 4*

postmarketing surveillance *page 8*

preclinical investigation *page 7*

therapeutics *page 4*

More drugs are being administered to consumers than ever before. More than 3 billion prescriptions are dispensed each year in the United States. About half of all Americans take one prescription drug regularly, and at least one out of six persons takes at least three prescription drugs. The purpose of this chapter is to introduce the subject of pharmacology and to emphasize the role of government in ensuring that drugs, herbals, and other natural alternatives are safe and effective for public use.

1.1 History of Pharmacology

The story of pharmacology is rich and exciting, filled with accidental discoveries and landmark events. Its history likely began when a human first used a plant to relieve symptoms of disease. One of the oldest forms of health care, herbal medicine has been practiced in virtually every culture dating to antiquity. The Babylonians recorded the earliest surviving "prescriptions" on clay tablets in 3000 B.C. At about the same time, the Chinese recorded the *Pen Tsao* (Great Herbal), a 40-volume compendium of plant remedies dating to 2700 B.C. The Egyptians followed in 1500 B.C. by archiving their remedies on a document known as the Eber's Papyrus.

Little is known about pharmacology during the Dark Ages. Although it is likely that herbal medicine continued to be practiced, few historical events related to this topic were recorded. Pharmacology, and indeed medicine, could not advance until the discipline of science was eventually viewed as legitimate by the religious doctrines of the era.

The first recorded reference to the word *pharmacology* was found in a text entitled "Pharmacologia sen Manuductio and Materiam Medicum," by Samuel Dale, in 1693. Before this date, the study of herbal remedies was called "Materia Medica," a term that persisted into the early 20th century.

Although the exact starting date is obscure, modern pharmacology is thought to have begun in the early 1800s. At that time, chemists were making remarkable progress in isolating specific substances from complex mixtures. This enabled chemists to isolate the active agents morphine, colchicine, curare, cocaine, and other early pharmacological agents from their natural products. Pharmacologists could then study their effects in animals more precisely, using standardized amounts. Indeed, some of the early researchers used themselves as test subjects. Frederich Serturner, who first isolated morphine from opium in 1805, injected himself and three friends with a huge dose (100 mg) of his new product. He and his colleagues suffered acute morphine intoxication for several days afterward.

Pharmacology as a distinct discipline was officially recognized when the first department of pharmacology was established in Estonia in 1847. John Jacob Abel, who is considered the father of American pharmacology owing to his many contributions to the field, founded the first pharmacology department in the United States at the University of Michigan in 1890.

In the 20th century, the pace of change in all areas of medicine became exponential. Pharmacologists no longer needed to rely on the slow, laborious process of isolating active agents from scarce natural products; they could synthesize drugs in the laboratory. Hundreds of new drugs could be synthesized and tested in a relatively short time. More important, it became possible to understand how drugs produced their effects, down to their molecular mechanism of action.

The current practice of pharmacology is extremely complex and far advanced compared with its early, primitive history. The nurses and other health professionals who practice it, however, must never forget its early roots: the application of products to relieve human suffering. Whether a substance is extracted from the Pacific yew tree, isolated from a fungus, or created totally in a laboratory, the central purpose of pharmacology is to focus on the client and to improve the quality of life.

MediaLink ● Old-fashioned Remedies

1.2 Pharmacology: The Study of Medicines

The word **pharmacology** is derived from two Greek words, *pharmakon,* which means "medicine," and *logos,* which means "study." Thus, pharmacology is most simply defined as the study of medicines. Pharmacology is an expansive subject ranging from understanding how drugs are administered, to where they travel in the body, to the actual responses produced. To learn the discipline well, nursing students need a firm understanding of concepts from various foundation areas such as anatomy and physiology, chemistry, microbiology, and pathophysiology.

More than 10,000 brand-name drugs, generic drugs, and combination agents are currently available. Each has its own characteristic set of therapeutic applications, interactions, side effects, and mechanisms of action. Many drugs are prescribed for more than one disease, and most produce multiple effects on the body. Further complicating the study of pharmacology is the fact that drugs may elicit different responses depending on individual client factors such as age, sex, body mass, health status, and genetics. Indeed, learning the applications of existing medications and staying current with new drugs introduced every year is an enormous challenge for the nurse. The task, however, is a critical one for both the client and the healthcare practitioner. If applied properly, drugs can dramatically improve the quality of life. If applied improperly, can produce devastating consequences.

1.3 Pharmacology and Therapeutics

It is obvious that a thorough study of pharmacology is important to healthcare providers who prescribe drugs on a daily basis. Although state or provincial laws sometimes limit the kinds of drugs marketed and the methods used to dispense them, *all* nurses are directly involved with client care and are active in educating, managing, and monitoring the proper use of drugs. This applies not only to nurses in clinics, hospitals, and home healthcare settings but also to nurses who teach and to new students entering the nursing profession. In all these cases, it is necessary that individuals have a thorough knowledge of pharmacology to perform their duties. As nursing students progress toward their chosen specialty, pharmacology is at the core of client care and is integrated into every step of the nursing process. Learning pharmacology is a gradual, continuous process that does not end with graduation. Never does one completely master every facet of drug action and application. That is one of the motivating challenges of the nursing profession.

Another important area of study for the nurse, sometimes difficult to distinguish from pharmacology, is the study of therapeutics. Therapeutics is slightly different from the field of pharmacology, although the disciplines are closely connected. **Therapeutics** is the branch of medicine concerned with the prevention of disease and treatment of suffering. **Pharmacotherapy,** or *pharmacotherapeutics,* is

the application of drugs for the purpose of disease prevention and treatment of suffering. Drugs are just one of many tools available to the nurse for preventing or treating human suffering.

1.4 Classification of Therapeutic Agents as Drugs, Biologics, and Alternative Therapies

Substances applied for therapeutic purposes fall into one of the following three general categories.

- Drugs or medications
- Biologics
- Alternative therapies

A **drug** is a chemical agent capable of producing biological responses within the body. These responses may be desirable (therapeutic) or undesirable (adverse). After a drug is administered, it is called a **medication.** From a broad perspective, drugs and medications may be considered a part of the body's normal activities, from the essential gases that we breathe to the foods that we eat. Because drugs are defined so broadly, it is necessary to clearly separate them from other substances such as foods, household products, and cosmetics. Many agents such as antiperspirants, sunscreens, toothpaste, and shampoos might alter the body's normal activities, but they are not considered medically therapeutic, as are drugs.

Although most modern drugs are synthesized in a laboratory, **biologics** are agents naturally produced in animal cells, by microorganisms, or by the body itself. Examples of biologics include hormones, monoclonal antibodies, natural blood products and components, interferon, and vaccines. Biologics are used to treat a wide variety of illnesses and conditions.

Other therapeutic approaches include **complementary and alternative therapies.** These involve natural plant extracts, herbs, vitamins, minerals, dietary supplements, and many techniques considered by some to be unconventional. Such therapies include acupuncture, hypnosis, biofeedback, and massage. Because of their great popularity, herbal and alternative therapies are featured throughout this text wherever they show promise in treating a disease or condition. Herbal therapies are presented in Chapter 11∞.

1.5 Prescription and Over-the-Counter Drugs

Legal drugs are obtained either by a prescription or over the counter (OTC). There are major differences between the two methods of dispensing drugs. To obtain prescription drugs, an order must be given authorizing the client to receive the drug. The advantages to requiring an authorization are numerous. The healthcare provider has an opportunity to examine the client and determine a specific diagnosis. The practitioner can maximize therapy by ordering the proper drug for the client's condition, and by controlling the amount and frequency of drug to be dispensed. In addition, the healthcare provider has an opportunity to teach the client the proper use of the drug and what side effects to expect. In a few instances, a high margin of safety observed over many years can prompt a change in the status of a drug from prescription to OTC.

In contrast to prescription drugs, OTC drugs do not require a physician's order. In most cases, clients may treat themselves safely if they carefully follow instructions included with the medication. If clients do not follow these guidelines, OTC drugs can have serious adverse effects.

Clients prefer to take OTC drugs for many reasons. They may be obtained more easily than prescription drugs. No appointment with a physician is required, thus saving time and money. Without the assistance of a healthcare provider, however, choosing the proper drug for a specific problem can be challenging for a client. OTC drugs may react with foods, herbal products, prescription medications, or other OTC drugs. Clients may not be aware that some drugs can impair their ability to function safely. Self-treatment is sometimes ineffective, and the potential for harm may increase if the disease is allowed to progress.

1.6 Drug Regulations and Standards

Until the 19th century, there were few standards or guidelines to protect the public from drug misuse. The archives of drug regulatory agencies are filled with examples of early medicines, including rattlesnake oil for rheumatism; epilepsy treatment for spasms, hysteria, and alcoholism; and fat reducers for a slender, healthy figure. Many of these early concoctions proved ineffective, though harmless. At their worst, some contained hazardous levels of dangerous or addictive substances. It became quite clear that drug regulations were needed to protect the public.

The first standard commonly used by pharmacists was the **formulary,** or list of drugs and drug recipes. In the United States, the first comprehensive publication of drug

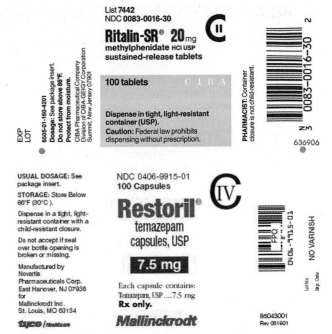

● **Figure 1.1** Examples of USP labels *Source: Courtesy of Novartis Pharmaceuticals Corporation and Mallinckrodt Pharmaceuticals.*

standards, called the *U.S. Pharmacopoeia* (*USP*), was established in 1820. A **pharmacopoeia** is a medical reference summarizing standards of drug purity, strength, and directions for synthesis. In 1852, a national professional society of pharmacists called the American Pharmaceutical Association (APhA) was founded. From 1852 to 1975, two major compendia maintained drug standards in the United States, the *U.S. Pharmacopoeia* and the *National Formulary* (*NF*) established by the APhA. All drug products were covered in the *USP*; pharmaceutical ingredients were the focus of the *NF*. In 1975, the two merged into a single publication, the *U.S. Pharmacopoeia–National Formulary* (*USP-NF*). The current document of about 2,400 pages contains 3,777 drug monographs in 164 chapters. Official monographs and interim revision announcements for the *USP-NF* are published regularly, with the full bound version printed every 5 years. Today, the USP label can be found on many medications verifying the purity and exact amounts of ingredients found within the container. Sample labels are illustrated in ● Figure 1.1.

In the early 1900s, the United States began to develop and enforce tougher drug legislation to protect the public. In 1902, the Biologics Control Act helped to standardize the quality of serums and other blood-related products. The Pure Food and Drug Act of 1906 gave the government power to control the labeling of medicines. In 1912, the Sherley Amendment prohibited the sale of drugs labeled with false therapeutic claims that were intended to defraud the consumer. In 1938, Congress passed the Food, Drug, and Cosmetic Act. This was the first law preventing the sale of drugs that had not been thoroughly tested before marketing. Later amendments to this law required drug companies to prove the safety and efficacy of any drug before it

PHARMFACTS

Consumer Spending on Prescription Drugs

- Spending on prescription drugs accounts for about 10% of national health spending.
- Between 1990 and 2000, prescription drug expenditures increased by more than 200%.
- The average number of prescription drugs taken per year increased from 7.9 prescriptions per person in 1994 to 12.0 prescriptions per person in 2004.
- The average cost of a prescription drug in 2004 was $63.59. This is an increase of 8.3% per year from 1994, when the average was $28.67 per prescription.
- Total pharmaceutical expenditures in the United States increased 11.4%, from $194 billion in 2002 to $216 billion in 2003.

MediaLink

Taking Medication

MediaLink

U.S. Pharmacopoeia

TIMELINE	REGULATORY ACTS, STANDARDS, AND ORGANIZATIONS
1820	A group of physicians established the first comprehensive publication of drug standards called the **U.S. Pharmacopeia (USP)**.
1852	A group of pharmacists founded a national professional society called the **American Pharmaceutical Association (APhA)**. The APhA then established the **National Formulary (NF)**, a standardized publication focusing on pharmaceutical ingredients. The *USP* continued to catalogue all drug related substances and products.
1862	This was the beginning of the **Federal Bureau of Chemistry**, established under the administration of President Lincoln. Over the years and with added duties, it gradually became the Food and Drug Administration (FDA).
1902	Congress passed the **Biologics Control Act** to control the quality of serums and other blood-related products.
1906	**The Pure Food and Drug Act** gave the government power to control the labeling of medicines.
1912	**The Sherley Amendment** made medicines safer by prohibiting the sale of drugs labeled with false therapeutic claims.
1938	Congress passed the **Food, Drug, and Cosmetic Act**. It was the first law preventing the marketing of drugs not thoroughly tested. This law now provides for the requirement that drug companies must submit a New Drug Application (NDA) to the FDA prior to marketing a new drug.
1944	Congress passed the **Public Health Service Act**, covering many health issues including biological products and the control of communicable diseases.
1975	The *U.S. Pharmacopeia* and *National Formulary* announced their union. The **USP-NF** became a single standardized publication.
1986	Congress passed the **Childhood Vaccine Act.** It authorized the FDA to acquire information about patients taking vaccines, to recall biologics, and to recommend civil penalties if guidelines regarding biologic use were not followed.
1988	The **FDA** was officially established as an agency of the **U.S. Department of Health and Human Services**.
1992	Congress passed the **Prescription Drug User Fee Act.** It required that nongeneric drug and biologic manufacturers pay fees to be used for improvements in the drug review process.
1994	Congress passed the **Dietary Supplement Health and Education Act** that requires clear labeling of dietary supplements. This act gives the FDA the power to remove supplements that cause a significant risk to the public.
1997	The **FDA Modernization Act** reauthorized the Prescription Drug User Fee Act. This act represents the largest reform effort of the drug review process since 1938.

● **Figure 1.2** A historical timeline of regulatory acts, standards, and organizations

could be sold within the United States. In reaction to the rising popularity of dietary supplements, Congress passed the Dietary Supplement Health and Education Act of 1994 in an attempt to control misleading industry claims. A brief timeline of major events in U.S. drug regulation is shown in ● Figure 1.2.

1.7 The Role of the Food and Drug Administration

Much has changed in the regulation of drugs in the past 100 years. In 1988, the **Food and Drug Administration (FDA)** was officially established as an agency of the U.S. Department of Health and Human Services. The Center for Drug Evaluation and Research (CDER), a branch of the FDA, exercises control over whether prescription drugs and OTC drugs may be used for therapy. The CDER states its mission as facilitating the availability of safe, effective drugs; keeping unsafe or ineffective drugs off the market; improving the health of Americans; and providing clear, easily understandable drug information for safe and effective use. Any pharmaceutical laboratory, whether private, public, or academic, must solicit FDA approval before marketing a drug.

Another branch of the FDA, the Center for Biologics Evaluation and Research (CBER), regulates the use of biologics including serums, vaccines, and blood products. One historical achievement involving biologics was the 1986 Childhood Vaccine Act. This act authorized the FDA to acquire information about clients taking vaccines, to recall biologics, and to recommend civil penalties if guidelines regarding biologics were not followed.

The FDA also oversees administration of herbal products and dietary supplements through the Center for Food Safety and Applied Nutrition (CFSAN). Herbal products and dietary supplements are regulated by the Dietary Supplement Health and Education Act of 1994. This act does not provide the same degree of protection for consumers as the Food, Drug, and Cosmetic Act of 1938. For example, herbal and dietary supplements may be marketed without prior approval from the FDA. This act is discussed in detail in Chapter 11∞.

1.8 Stages of Approval for Therapeutic and Biological Drugs

The amount of time spent by the FDA in the review and approval process for a particular drug depends on several checkpoints along a well-developed and organized plan. Therapeutic drugs and biologics are reviewed in four phases. These phases, summarized in ● Figure 1.3, are as follows:

1. Preclinical investigation
2. Clinical investigation
3. Review of the New Drug Application (NDA)
4. Postmarketing surveillance

Preclinical investigation involves extensive laboratory research. Scientists perform many tests on human and microbial cells cultured in the laboratory. Studies are performed in several species of animals to examine the drug's effectiveness at different doses, and to look for adverse effects. Extensive testing on cultured cells and in animals is essential because it allows the pharmacologist to predict whether the drug will cause harm to humans. Because laboratory tests do not always reflect the way a *human* responds, preclinical investigation results are always inconclusive. Animal testing may overestimate or underestimate the actual risk to humans.

Clinical investigation, the second stage of drug testing, takes place in three different stages termed **clinical phase trials.** Clinical phase trials are the longest part of the drug approval process. Clinical pharmacologists first perform tests on healthy volunteers to determine proper dosage and to assess for adverse effects. Large groups of selected clients with the particular disease are then given the medication. Clinical investigators from different medical specialties address concerns such as whether the drug is effective, worsens other medical conditions, interacts unsafely with existing medications, or affects one type of client more than others.

Clinical phase trials are an essential component of drug evaluations due to the variability of responses among clients. If a drug appears to be effective and without serious side effects, approval for marketing may be accelerated, or the drug may be used immediately in special cases with careful monitoring. If the drug shows promise but precautions are noted, the process is delayed until the pharmaceutical company remedies the concerns. In any case, an NDA must be submitted before a drug is allowed to proceed to the next stage of the approval process.

New Drug Development Timeline

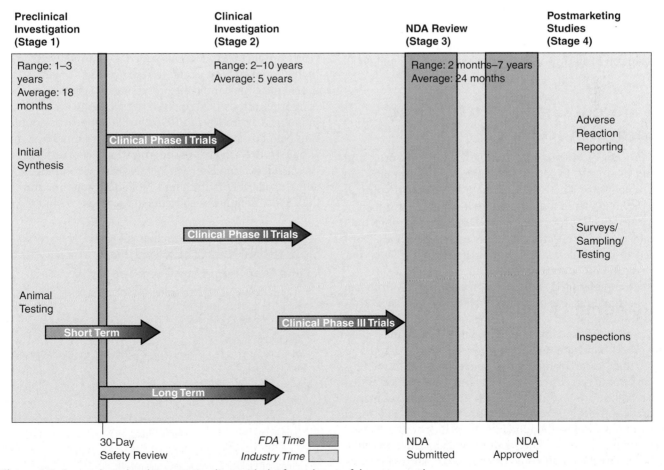

● **Figure 1.3** A new drug development timeline, with the four phases of drug approval

The **NDA review** is the third stage of the drug approval process. During this stage, clinical phase III trials and animal testing may continue depending on the results obtained from preclinical testing. By law, the FDA is permitted 6 months to initially review an NDA. If the NDA is approved, the process continues to the final stage. If the NDA is rejected, the process is suspended until noted concerns are addressed by the pharmaceutical company. The average NDA review time for new medications is approximately 17–24 months.

Postmarketing surveillance, the final stage of the drug approval process, begins after clinical trials and the NDA review have been completed. The purpose of this stage is to survey for harmful drug effects in a larger population. Some adverse effects take longer to appear and are not identified until a drug is circulated to large numbers of people. One example is the diabetes drug troglitazone (Rezulin), which was placed on the market in 1997. In 1998, Britain banned its use after discovering at least one death and several cases of liver failure in diabetic clients taking the medication. The FDA became aware of a number of cases in the United States in which Rezulin was linked with liver failure and heart failure. Rezulin was recalled in March 2000 after healthcare providers asked the FDA to reconsider its therapeutic benefits versus its identified risks.

The FDA holds public meetings annually to receive feedback from clients and professional and pharmaceutical organizations regarding the effectiveness and safety of new drug therapies. If the FDA discovers a serious problem, it will mandate that the drug be withdrawn from the market. The banning of Rezulin by the FDA is an ideal example of postmarketing surveillance in action. The FDA withdrew 11 prescription drugs from the market between 1997 and 2000.

1.9 Recent Changes to the Drug Approval Process

The process of isolating or synthesizing a new drug and testing it in cells, experimental animals, and humans can take many years. The NDA can include dozens of volumes of experimental and clinical data that must be examined in the drug review process. Some NDAs contain more than 100,000 pages. Even after all experiments have been concluded and clinical data have been gathered, the FDA review process can take several years.

Expenses associated with development of a new drug can cost pharmaceutical manufacturers millions of dollars. A recent study estimated the cost to bring a new drug to market at $802 million. These companies are often critical of the regulatory process and are anxious to get the drug marketed to recoup their research and development expenses. The public is also anxious to receive new drugs, particularly for diseases that have a high mortality rate. Although the criticisms of manufacturers and the public are certainly understandable—and sometimes justified—the fundamental priority of the FDA is to ensure that drugs are safe. Without an exhaustive review of scientific data the public could be exposed to dangerous medications, or those that are ineffective in treating disease.

MediaLink ● U.S. Drug Recalls

SPECIAL CONSIDERATIONS

How Prescription Drug Costs Affect Senior Citizens

Everyone complains about the high cost of prescription drugs, but senior citizens are particularly affected. The facts about senior citizens and prescription drugs are hard to ignore:

Americans older than age 65 constitute only 13% of the population but account for about 34% of all prescriptions dispensed and 40% of all OTC medications. More than 80% of all seniors take at least one prescribed medication each day. The average older person is taking more than four prescription medications at once, plus two OTC medications. Many of these medicines, such as those for hypertension and heart disease, are taken on a permanent basis.

Because seniors are usually retired, they are less likely than younger people to have insurance that covers the cost of prescription medications. On a fixed annual income, many seniors must choose between buying medications and purchasing adequate food or material necessities. The annual drug spending per senior grew from an average of $559 in 1992 to more than $1,200 in 2000. In 2005, the spending for prescription drugs among elderly clients was estimated to be at least 12% of total healthcare expenditures.

In the early 1990s, owing to pressures from organized consumer groups and various drug manufacturers, governmental officials began to plan how to speed up the drug review process. Reasons identified for the delay in the FDA drug approval process included outdated guidelines, poor communication, and insufficient staff to handle the workload.

In 1992, FDA officials, members of Congress, and representatives from pharmaceutical companies negotiated the Prescription Drug User Fee Act on a 5-year trial basis. This act required drug and biologic manufacturers to provide yearly product user fees. This added income allowed the FDA to hire more employees and to restructure its organization to more efficiently handle the processing of a greater number of drug applications. The result of restructuring was a resounding success. From 1992 to 1996, the FDA approved double the number of drugs while cutting some review times by as much as half. In 1997, the FDA Modernization Act reauthorized the Prescription Drug User Fee Act. Nearly 700 employees were added to the FDA's drug and biologics program, and more than $300 million was collected in user fees.

PHARMFACTS

Time Length for New Drug Approvals

- It takes about 11 years of research and development before a drug is submitted to the FDA for review.
- Phase I clinical trials take about 1 year and involve 20 to 80 normal, healthy volunteers.
- Phase II clinical trials last about 2 years and involve 100 to 300 volunteer clients with the disease.
- Phase III clinical trials take about 3 years and involve 1,000 to 3,000 clients in hospitals and clinic agencies.
- For every 5,000 chemicals that enter preclinical testing, only 5 make it to human testing. Of these 5 potential drugs, only 1 is finally approved.
- Since the 1992 Prescription Drug User Fee Act was passed, more than 700 drugs and biologics have come to the market.

TABLE 1.1	Steps of Approval for Drugs Marketed Within Canada
Step 1	Preclinical studies or experiments in culture, living tissue, and small animals are performed, followed by extensive clinical trials or testing done in humans.
Step 2	A drug company completes a *drug submission* to Health Canada. This report details important safety and effectiveness information including how the drug product will be produced and packaged, and expected therapeutic benefits and adverse reactions.
Step 3	A committee of drug experts including medical and drug scientists reviews the drug submission to identify potential benefits and drug risks.
Step 4	Health Canada reviews information about the drug product and passes on important details to health practitioners and consumers.
Step 5	Health Canada issues a Notice of Compliance (NOC) and Drug Identification Number (DIN). Both permit the manufacturer to market the drug product.
Step 6	Health Canada monitors the effectiveness and concerns of the drug after it has been marketed. This is done by regular inspection, notices, newsletters, and feedback from consumers and healthcare professionals.

1.10 Canadian Drug Standards

As in the United States, drug testing and risk assessment in Canada is a major priority. The Health Protection Branch (HPB) of the Canadian government serves under the auspices of the Department of Health and Welfare. The HPB's task is to protect Canadians from the potential health hazards of marketed products, imported goods, and environmental agents. The deputy minister enforces regulations concerned with consumer protection issues such as the Food and Drugs Act and the Tobacco Act.

Health Canada is the federal department working in partnership with provincial and territorial governments. It also coordinates its efforts with other federal departments to ensure proper management of health and safety issues.

The Health Products and Food Branch (HPFB) of Health Canada regulates the use of therapeutic substances through several national programs, the Therapeutic Products Programme (TPP), the Office of Natural Health Products, and the Food Directorate. The TPP covers such drugs as pharmaceuticals, narcotics, controlled and restricted drugs, and biologics. Some natural health products and food-based products called *nutraceuticals* are also regulated. The Office of Natural Products limits its focus to natural substances, for example, homeopathic and herbal remedies. The Food Directorate regulates nutraceuticals.

The Canadian Food and Drugs Act is an important regulatory document specifying that drugs cannot be marketed without a Notice of Compliance (NOC) and Drug Identification Number (DIN) from Health Canada. Amended guidelines date to 1953, stating that the use of foods, drugs, cosmetics, and therapeutic devices must follow established guidelines. Any drug that does not comply with standards established by recognized pharmacopoeias and formularies in the United States, Europe, Britain, or France cannot be labeled, packaged, sold, or advertised in Canada.

The drug approval process in Canada is illustrated in Table 1.1. Many similarities exist between drug regulation processes in Canada and the United States. These include the realization by both governments that they need to monitor natural products, dietary supplements and herbs, and newly developed traditional drug therapies.

MediaLink Canadian Drug Regulations

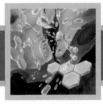

CHAPTER REVIEW

KEY CONCEPTS

The numbered key concepts provide a succinct summary of the important points from the corresponding numbered section within the chapter. If any of these points are not clear, refer to the numbered section within the chapter for review.

1.1 The history of pharmacology began thousands of years ago with the use of plant products to treat disease.

1.2 Pharmacology is the study of medicines. It includes the study of how drugs are administered and how the body responds.

1.3 The fields of pharmacology and therapeutics are closely connected. Pharmacotherapy is the application of drugs to prevent disease and ease suffering.

1.4 Therapeutic agents may be classified as traditional drugs, biologics, or alternative therapies.

1.5 Drugs are available by prescription or over the counter (OTC). Prescription drugs require an order from a healthcare provider.

1.6 Drug regulations were created to protect the public from drug misuse, and to assume continuous evaluation of safety and effectiveness.

1.7 The regulatory agency responsible for ensuring that drugs and medical devices are safe and effective is the Food and Drug Administration (FDA).

1.8 There are four stages of approval for therapeutic and biological drugs. These progress from cellular and animal testing to use of the experimental drug in clients with the disease.

1.9 Once criticized for being too slow, the FDA has streamlined the process to get new drugs to market more quickly.

1.10 Drug standards also ensure the effectiveness and safety of drugs for Canadian consumers.

CRITICAL THINKING QUESTIONS

1. Explain why a client might seek treatment from an OTC drug instead of a more effective prescription drug.

2. How does the FDA ensure the safety and effectiveness of drugs? How has this process changed in recent years?

3. In many respects, the role of the FDA continues long after the initial drug approval. Explain the continued involvement of the FDA.

See Appendix D for answers and rationales for all activities.

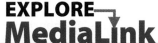 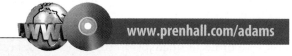

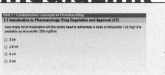 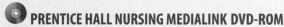 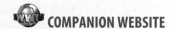

NCLEX-RN® review, case studies, and other interactive resources for this chapter can be found on the companion website at www.prenhall.com/adams. Click on "Chapter 1" to select the activities for this chapter. For animations, more NCLEX-RN® review questions, and an audio glossary, access the accompanying Prentice Hall Nursing MediaLink DVD-ROM in this textbook.

PRENTICE HALL NURSING MEDIALINK DVD-ROM
- Audio Glossary
- NCLEX-RN® Review

COMPANION WEBSITE
- NCLEX-RN® Review
- Case Study: Client with psoriasis
- Challenge Your Knowledge

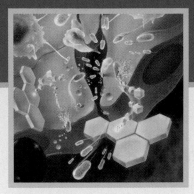

CHAPTER 2

Drug Classes and Schedules

OBJECTIVES

After reading this chapter, the student should be able to:

1. Explain the basis for placing drugs into therapeutic and pharmacological classes.
2. Discuss the prototype approach to drug classification.
3. Describe what is meant by a drug's mechanism of action.
4. Distinguish between a drug's chemical name, generic name, and trade name.
5. Explain why generic drug names are preferred to trade name drugs.
6. Discuss why drugs are sometimes placed on a restrictive list, and the controversy surrounding this issue.
7. Explain the meaning of a controlled substance.
8. Explain the U.S. Controlled Substance Act of 1970 and the role of the U.S. Drug Enforcement Agency in controlling drug abuse and misuse.
9. Identify the five drug schedules and give examples of drugs at each level.
10. Explain how drugs are scheduled according to the Canadian Controlled Drugs and Substances Act.

MediaLink 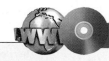 **www.prenhall.com/adams**

NCLEX-RN® review, case studies, and other interactive resources for this chapter can be found on the companion website at www.prenhall.com/adams. Click on "Chapter 2" to select the activities for this chapter. For animations, more NCLEX-RN® review questions, and an audio glossary, access the accompanying Prentice Hall Nursing MediaLink DVD-ROM in this textbook.

KEY TERMS

bioavailability *page 14*

chemical name *page 13*

combination drug *page 14*

controlled substance *page 15*

dependence *page 14*

generic name *page 13*

mechanism of action *page 12*

pharmacological classification *page 12*

prototype drug *page 12*

scheduled drugs *page 15*

therapeutic classification *page 12*

trade name *page 13*

withdrawal *page 15*

The student beginning the study of pharmacology is quickly confronted with hundreds of drugs having specific dosages, side effects, and mechanisms of action. Without a means of grouping or organizing this information, most students would be overwhelmed by the vast amounts of new data. Drugs can be classified by a number of different methods that provide logical systems for identifying drugs and determining the limitations of their use. This chapter presents methods of grouping drugs: by therapeutic or pharmacological classification, and by drug schedules.

2.1 Therapeutic and Pharmacological Classification of Drugs

One useful method of organizing drugs is based on their therapeutic usefulness in treating particular diseases. This is referred to as a **therapeutic classification.** Drugs may also be organized by **pharmacological classification.** A drug's pharmacological classification refers to the way an agent works at the molecular, tissue, and body system level. Both types of classification are widely used in categorizing the thousands of available drugs.

Table 2.1 shows the method of therapeutic classification, using cardiac care as an example. Many different types of drugs affect cardiovascular function. Some drugs influence blood clotting, whereas others lower blood cholesterol or prevent the onset of stroke. Drugs may be used to treat elevated blood pressure, heart failure, abnormal rhythm, chest pain, heart attack, or circulatory shock. Thus, drugs that treat cardiac disorders may be placed in several types of therapeutic classes, for example, anticoagulants, antihyperlipidemics, and antihypertensives.

A therapeutic classification need not be complicated. For example, it is appropriate to simply classify a medication as a "drug used for stroke" or a "drug used for shock." The key to therapeutic classification is to clearly state what a particular drug does clinically. Other examples of therapeutic classifications include antidepressants, antipsychotics, drugs for erectile dysfunction, and antineoplastics.

The pharmacological classification addresses a drug's **mechanism of action,** or *how* a drug produces its effect in the body. Table 2.2 shows a variety of pharmacological classifications using hypertension as an example. A diuretic treats hypertension by lowering plasma volume. Calcium channel blockers treat this disorder by decreasing cardiac contractility. Other drugs block intermediates of the renin–angiotensin pathway. Notice that each example describes *how* hypertension might be controlled. A drug's pharmacological classification is more specific than a therapeutic classification and requires an understanding of biochemistry and physiology. In addition, pharmacological classifications may be described with varying degrees of complexity, sometimes taking into account drugs' chemical names.

When classifying drugs, it is common practice to select a single drug from a class and compare all other medications with this representative drug. A **prototype drug**

TABLE 2.1 Organizing Drug Information by Therapeutic Classification	
Therapeutic Focus: Cardiac Care / Drugs Affecting Cardiovascular Function	
Therapeutic Usefulness	**Therapeutic Classification**
influence blood clotting	anticoagulants
lower blood cholesterol	antihyperlipidemics
lower blood pressure	antihypertensives
restore normal cardiac rhythm	antidysrhythmics
treat angina	antianginals

TABLE 2.2 Organizing Drug Information by Pharmacological Classification	
Focus on How a Therapy Is Applied: Pharmacotherapy for Hypertension May Be Achieved by:	
Mechanism of Action	**Pharmacological Classification**
lowers plasma volume	diuretic
blocks heart calcium channels	calcium channel blocker
blocks hormonal activity	angiotensin-converting enzyme inhibitor
blocks physiologic reactions to stress	adrenergic antagonist (or blocker)
dilates peripheral blood vessels	vasodilator

is the well-understood drug model with which other drugs in a pharmacological class are compared. By learning the prototype drug, students may predict the actions and adverse effects of other drugs in the same class. For example, by knowing the effects of penicillin V, students can extend this knowledge to the other drugs in the penicillin class of antibiotics. The original drug prototype is not always the most widely used drug in its class. Newer drugs in the same class may be more effective, have a more favorable safety profile, or have a longer duration of action. These factors may sway healthcare providers from using the original prototype drug. In addition, healthcare providers and pharmacology textbooks sometimes differ as to which drug should be the prototype. In any case, becoming familiar with the drug prototypes and keeping up with newer and more popular drugs is an essential part of mastering drugs and drug classes.

2.2 Chemical, Generic, and Trade Names for Drugs

A major challenge in studying pharmacology is learning thousands of drug names. Adding to this difficulty is the fact that most drugs have multiple names. The three basic types of drug names are chemical, generic, and trade names.

A **chemical name** is assigned using standard nomenclature established by the International Union of Pure and Applied Chemistry (IUPAC). A drug has only one chemical name, which is sometimes helpful in predicting a substance's physical and chemical properties. Although chemical names convey a clear and concise meaning about the nature of a drug, they are often complicated and difficult to remember or pronounce. For example, few nurses know the chemical name for diazepam: 7-chloro-1,3-dihydro-1-methyl-5-phenyl-2H-1,4-benzodiazepin-2-one. In only a

few cases, usually when the name is brief and easily remembered, will nurses use chemical names. Examples of useful chemical names include lithium carbonate, calcium gluconate, and sodium chloride.

More practically, drugs are sometimes classified by a *portion* of their chemical structure, known as the chemical group name. Examples are antibiotics such as fluoroquinolones and cephalosporins. Other common examples include phenothiazines, thiazides, and benzodiazepines. Although chemical group names may seem complicated when first encountered, knowing them will become invaluable as the nursing student begins to learn and understand major drug classes and actions.

The **generic name** of a drug is assigned by the U.S. Adopted Name Council. With few exceptions, generic names are less complicated and easier to remember than chemical names. Many organizations, including the Food and Drug Administration (FDA), the U.S. Pharmacopoeia, and the World Health Organization (WHO), routinely describe a medication by its generic name. Because there is only one generic name for each drug, healthcare providers often use this name, and students generally must memorize it.

A drug's **trade name** is assigned by the company marketing the drug. The name is usually selected to be short and easy to remember. The trade name is sometimes called the proprietary or product or brand name. The term *proprietary* suggests ownership. In the United States, a drug developer is given exclusive rights to name and market a drug for 17 years after a new drug application is submitted to the FDA. Because it takes several years for a drug to be approved, the amount of time spent in approval is usually subtracted from the 17 years. For example, if it takes 7 years for a drug to be approved, competing companies will not be allowed to market a generic equivalent drug for another 10 years. The

TABLE 2.3 Examples of Brand-name Products Containing Popular Generic Substances	
Generic Substance	**Brand Names**
aspirin	Acetylsalicylic Acid, Acuprin, Anacin, Aspergum, Bayer, Bufferin, Ecotrin, Empirin, Excedrin, Maprin, Norgesic, Salatin, Salocol, Salsprin, Supac, Talwin, Triaphen-10, Vanquish, Verin, ZORprin
diphenhydramine	Allerdryl, Benadryl, Benahist, Bendylate, Caladryl, Compoz, Diahist, Diphenadril, Eldadryl, Fenylhist, Fynex, Hydramine, Hydril, Insomnal, Noradryl, Nordryl, Nytol, Tusstat, Wehdryl
ibuprofen	Advil, Amersol, Apsifen, Brufen, Haltran, Medipren, Midol 200, Motrin, Neuvil, Novoprofen, Nuprin, Pamprin-IB, Rufen, Trendar

rationale is that the developing company should be allowed sufficient time to recoup the millions of dollars in research and development costs in designing the new drug. After 17 years, competing companies may sell a generic equivalent drug, sometimes using a different name, which the FDA must approve.

Trade names may be a challenge for students to learn because of the dozens of product names containing similar ingredients. In addition, a **combination drug** contains more than one active generic ingredient. This poses a problem in trying to match one generic name with one product name. As an example, refer to Table 2.3 and consider the drug diphenhydramine (generic name), also called Benadryl (one of many trade names). Diphenhydramine is an antihistamine. Low doses of diphenhydramine may be purchased over the counter (OTC); higher doses require a prescription. When looking for diphenhydramine, the nurse may find it listed under many trade names, such as Allerdryl and Compoz, provided alone or in combination with other active ingredients. Ibuprofen and aspirin are also examples of drugs with many different trade names. The rule of thumb is that the active ingredients in a drug are described by their generic name. The generic name of a drug is usually lowercased, whereas the trade name is capitalized.

2.3 Differences Between Brand-Name Drugs and Their Generic Equivalents

During its 17 years of exclusive rights to a new drug, the pharmaceutical company determines the price of the medication. Because there is no competition, the price is generally quite high. The developing company sometimes uses legal tactics to extend its exclusive rights, since this can mean hundreds of millions of dollars per year in profits for a popular medicine. Once the exclusive rights end, competing companies market the generic drug for less money, and consumer savings may be considerable. In some states, pharmacists may routinely substitute a generic drug when the prescription calls for a brand name. In other states, the pharmacist must dispense drugs directly as written by a healthcare provider or obtain approval before providing a generic substitute.

The companies marketing brand-name drugs often lobby aggressively against laws that might restrict the routine use of their brand-name products. The lobbyists claim that significant differences exist between a trade-name drug and its generic equivalent, and that switching to the generic drug may be harmful for the client. Consumer advocates, on the other hand, argue that generic substitutions should always be permitted because of the cost savings to clients.

Are there really differences between a brand-name drug and its generic equivalent? The answer is unclear. Despite the fact that the dosages may be identical, drug formulations are not always the same. The two drugs may have different inert ingredients. For example, if the drug is in tablet form, the active ingredients may be more tightly compressed in one of the preparations.

PHARMFACTS

Marketing and Promotional Spending

- When generic versions of paclitaxel (Taxol) became available, various legal tactics by Bristol-Myers Squibb delayed their entry to market. The estimated additional cost to consumers for 2 more years of patent extension was more than $1 billion.

- Promotional spending on prescription drugs rose to $27.7 billion in 2004, up from $16.6 billion in 2000 and $9.2 billion in 1996.

- Spending on consumer drug advertisements on television and in print media increased to $4.0 billion in 2004, up from $2.5 billion in 2000 and $791 million in 1996.

- Consumer advocates claim that promotional advertisements drive up demand for the newer, more expensive drugs over the older, less costly drugs that might be equally effective.

The key to comparing brand-name drugs and their generic equivalents lies in measuring the bioavailability of the two preparations. **Bioavailability** is the physiological ability of the drug to reach its target cells and produce its effect. Bioavailability may indeed be affected by inert ingredients and tablet compression. Anything that affects absorption of a drug, or its distribution to the target cells, can certainly affect drug action. Measuring how long a drug takes to exert its effect gives pharmacologists a crude measure of bioavailability. For example, if a client is in circulatory shock and it takes the generic-equivalent drug 5 minutes longer to produce its effect, that is indeed significant; however, if a generic medication for arthritis pain relief takes 45 minutes to act, compared with the brand-name drug, which takes 40 minutes, it probably does not matter which drug is prescribed.

To address this issue, some states (Florida, Kentucky, Minnesota, and Missouri, for example) have compiled a negative formulary list. A *negative formulary list* is a list of trade-name drugs that pharmacists may *not* dispense as generic drugs. These drugs must be dispensed exactly as written on the prescription, using the trade-name drug the physician prescribed. In some cases, pharmacists must inform or notify clients of substitutions. Pharmaceutical companies and some healthcare practitioners have supported this action, claiming that generic drugs—even those that have small differences in bioavailability and bioequivalence—could adversely affect client outcomes in those with critical conditions or illnesses. However, laws frequently change, in many instances, the efforts of consumer advocacy groups have led to changes in or elimination of negative formulary lists.

2.4 Controlled Substances and Drug Schedules

Some drugs are frequently abused or have a high potential for addiction. Technically, *addiction* refers to the overwhelming feeling that drives someone to use a drug repeatedly. **Dependence** is a related term, often defined as a

TABLE 2.4 U.S. Drug Schedules and Examples

Drug Schedule	Abuse Potential	Dependency Potential		Examples	Therapeutic Use
		Physical Dependence	Psychological Dependence		
I	highest	high	high	heroin, lysergic acid diethylamide (LSD), marijuana, and methaqualone	Limited or no therapeutic use
II	high	high	high	morphine, phencyclidine (PCP), cocaine, methadone, and methamphetamine	Used therapeutically with prescription; some drugs no longer used
III	moderate	moderate	high	anabolic steroids, codeine and hydrocodone with aspirin or Tylenol, and some barbiturates	Used therapeutically with prescription
IV	lower	lower	lower	dextropropoxyphene, pentazocine, meprobamate, diazepam, alprazolam	Used therapeutically with prescription
V	lowest	lowest	lowest	OTC cough medicines with codeine	Used therapeutically without prescription

physiological or psychological need for a substance. *Physical dependence* refers to an altered physical condition caused by the adaptation of the nervous system to repeated drug use. In this case, when the drug is no longer available, the individual expresses physical signs of discomfort known as **withdrawal.** In contrast, when an individual is *psychologically dependent,* there are few signs of physical discomfort when the drug is withdrawn; however, the individual feels an intense compelling desire to continue drug use. These concepts are discussed in detail in Chapter 12 ∞.

Drugs that cause dependency are restricted for use in situations of medical necessity, if at all allowed. According to law, drugs that have a significant potential for abuse are placed into five categories called schedules. These **scheduled drugs** are classified according to their potential for abuse: Schedule I drugs have the highest potential for abuse, and Schedule V drugs have the lowest potential for abuse. Schedule I drugs have little or no therapeutic value or are intended for research purposes only. Drugs in the other four schedules may be dispensed only in cases in which therapeutic value has been determined. Schedule V is the only category in which some drugs may be dispensed without a prescription because the quantities of the controlled drug are so low that the possibility of causing dependence is extremely remote. Table 2.4 gives the five drug schedules with examples. Not all drugs with an abuse potential are regulated or placed into schedules. Tobacco, alcohol, and caffeine are significant examples.

In the United States, a **controlled substance** is a drug whose use is restricted by the Controlled Substances Act of 1970 and later revisions. The Controlled Substances Act is also called the Comprehensive Drug Abuse Prevention and Control Act. Hospitals and pharmacies must register with the Drug Enforcement Administration (DEA) and then use their assigned registration numbers to purchase scheduled drugs. Hospitals and pharmacies must maintain complete records of all quantities purchased and sold. Drugs with higher abuse potential have more restrictions. For example, a special order form must be used to obtain Schedule II drugs, and orders must be written and signed by the healthcare provider. Telephone orders to a pharmacy are not permitted. Refills for Schedule II drugs are not permitted; clients must visit their healthcare provider first. Those convicted of unlawful manufacturing, distributing, or dispensing of controlled substances face severe penalties.

2.5 Canadian Regulations Restricting Drugs of Abuse

In Canada, until 1996 controlled substances were those drugs subject to guidelines outlined in Part III, Schedule G, of the Canadian Food and Drugs Act. According to these guidelines, a healthcare provider dispensed these medications only to clients suffering from specific diseases or illnesses. Regulated drugs included amphetamines, barbiturates, methaqualone, and anabolic steroids. Controlled drugs were labeled clearly with the letter *C* on the outside of the container.

PHARMFACTS

Extent of Drug Abuse

- In 2003, more than 10.9 million people reported driving under the influence of illegal drugs during the previous year.

- In 2003, 29.8% of the U.S. population 12 and older (70.8 million people) had smoked cigarettes during the past month. This figure includes 3.6 million young people aged 12 to 17. Although it is illegal in the United States to sell tobacco to underage youths, in most cases they are able to purchase them personally.

- From 1994 to 2003, emergency department records of abused substances such as gamma hydroxybutyric acid (GHB; street name *Fantasy*), ketamine (street names *jet, super acid, Special K,* among others), and MDMA (chemical name 3,4-methylenedioxymethamphetamine; street name *Ecstasy*) rose more than 2,000%.

- In 2003, more than 17 million Americans abused or were dependent on either alcohol or illicit drugs.

TABLE 2.5	Three-Schedule System for Drugs Sold in Canada
Drug Schedule	**Drug Type**
I	all prescription drugs
	drugs with no potential for abuse
	controlled drugs
	narcotic drugs
II	all nonprescription drugs monitored for sale by pharmacists
III	all nonprescription drugs not monitored for sale by pharmacists

Restricted drugs not intended for human use were covered in Part IV, Schedule H, of the Canadian Food and Drugs Act. These were drugs used in the course of a chemical or analytical procedure for medical, laboratory, industrial, educational, or research purposes. They included hallucinogens such as lysergic acid diethylamide (LSD), MDMA, and 2,5-dimethoxy-4-methylamphetamine (DOM; street name *STP*). Schedule F drugs were those drugs requiring a prescription for their sale. Examples were methylphenidate (Ritalin), diazepam (Valium), and chlordiazepoxide (Librium). Drugs such as morphine, heroin, cocaine, and cannabis were covered under the Canadian Narcotic Control Act and amended schedules. According to Canadian law, narcotic drugs were labeled clearly with the letter *N* on the outside of the container.

Today Canada's federal drug control statute is the Controlled Drugs and Substances Act. It repeals the Narcotic Control Act and Parts III and IV of the Food and Drug Act. It further establishes eight schedules of controlled substances; two classes of precursors are covered in one schedule. For a complete listing of drugs, see http://laws.justice.gc.ca/en/C-38.8/. The Controlled Drugs and Substances Act provides broad latitude to the Governor in Council to amend schedules as determined to be in the best interest of Canada's citizens. Drugs and substances covered in the Controlled Drugs and Substances Act correlate with agents named in three United Nations treaties: the Single Convention on Narcotic Drugs, the Convention on Psychotropic Substances, and United Nations Convention Against Illicit Traffic in Narcotic Drugs and Psychotropic Substances.

Throughout Canada, both prescription and nonprescription drugs must meet specific criteria for public distribution and use. Nonprescription drugs are provided according to guidelines and acts established by the respective Canadian provinces. One recent system establishes three general drug schedules (Table 2.5). Pharmacies must monitor those drugs used specifically to treat self-limiting discomforts such as cold, flu, and mild gastrointestinal or other symptoms. Other nonprescription drugs may be sold without monitoring.

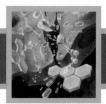

CHAPTER REVIEW

KEY CONCEPTS

The numbered key concepts provide a succinct summary of the important points from the corresponding numbered section within the chapter. If any of these points are not clear, refer to the numbered section within the chapter for review.

2.1 Drugs may be organized by their therapeutic or pharmacological classification.

2.2 Drugs have chemical, generic, and trade names. A drug has only one chemical or generic name but may have multiple trade names.

2.3 Generic drugs are less expensive than brand-name drugs, but they may differ in their bioavailability, that is, the ability of the drug to reach its target tissue and produce its action.

2.4 Drugs with a potential for abuse are restricted by the Controlled Substances Act and are categorized into schedules. Schedule I drugs are the most tightly controlled; Schedule V drugs have less potential for addiction and are less tightly controlled.

2.5 Canadian regulations restrict drugs as covered in its federal drug control statute: the Controlled Drugs and Substances Act.

CRITICAL THINKING QUESTIONS

1. What is the difference between therapeutic and pharmacological classifications? Identify the following classifications as therapeutic or pharmacological: beta-adrenergic blocker, oral contraceptive, laxative, folic acid antagonist, and antianginal agent.

2. What is a prototype drug, and how does it differ from other drugs in the same class?

3. A pharmacist decides to switch from a trade-name drug that was ordered by the physician to a generic-equivalent drug. What advantages does this substitution have for the client? What disadvantages might be caused by the switch?

4. Why are certain drugs placed in schedules? What extra precautions are healthcare providers required to take when prescribing scheduled drugs?

See Appendix D for answers and rationales for all activities.

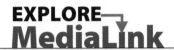
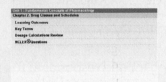
EXPLORE MediaLink

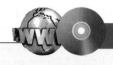
www.prenhall.com/adams

NCLEX-RN® review, case studies, and other interactive resources for this chapter can be found on the companion website at www.prenhall.com/adams. Click on "Chapter 2" to select the activities for this chapter. For animations, more NCLEX-RN® review questions, and an audio glossary, access the accompanying Prentice Hall Nursing MediaLink DVD-ROM in this textbook.

 PRENTICE HALL NURSING MEDIALINK DVD-ROM

- **Audio Glossary**
- **NCLEX-RN® Review**

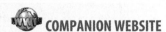 **COMPANION WEBSITE**

- **NCLEX-RN® Review**
- **Case Study:** Generic drugs
- **Challenge Your Knowledge**

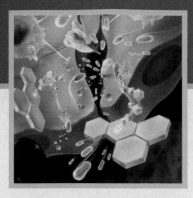

CHAPTER 3

Emergency Preparedness

OBJECTIVES

After reading this chapter, the student should be able to:

1. Explain why drugs are important in the context of emergency preparedness.
2. Discuss the role of the nurse in preparing for and responding to a bioterrorist act.
3. Identify the purpose and components of the Strategic National Stockpile (SNS).
4. Explain the threat of anthrax contamination and how it is transmitted.
5. Discuss the clinical manifestations and treatment of anthrax exposure.
6. Identify specific viruses that would most likely be used in a bioterrorist act.
7. Explain the advantages and disadvantages of vaccination as a means of preventing illness due to bioterrorist attacks.
8. Provide examples of chemical agents that might be used in a bioterrorism incident, and their treatments.
9. Describe the symptoms of acute radiation exposure and the role of potassium iodide (KI) in preventing thyroid cancer.

MediaLink

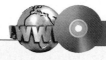

www.prenhall.com/adams

NCLEX-RN® review, case studies, and other interactive resources for this chapter can be found on the companion website at www.prenhall.com/adams. Click on "Chapter 3" to select the activities for this chapter. For animations, more NCLEX-RN® review questions, and an audio glossary, access the accompanying Prentice Hall Nursing MediaLink DVD-ROM in this textbook.

KEY TERMS

acute radiation syndrome *page 24*

anthrax *page 21*

bioterrorism *page 19*

ionizing radiation *page 23*

nerve agents *page 23*

Strategic National Stockpile (SNS) *page 21*

vaccine *page 22*

vendor-managed inventory (VMI) *page 21*

It is important that nursing students understand the role that drugs play in preventing or controlling global disease outbreaks. Drugs are the most powerful tools available to the medical community for countering worldwide epidemics and bioterrorist threats. If medical personnel could not identify, isolate, or treat the causes of global diseases, a major incident could easily overwhelm healthcare resources and produce a catastrophic loss of life. Drugs are a major component of emergency preparedness plans. This chapter discusses the role of pharmacology in the prevention and treatment of diseases or conditions that might develop in the context of a biological, chemical, or nuclear attack.

3.1 The Nature of Bioterrorism

Prior to the September 11, 2001, terrorist attacks on the United States, the attention of healthcare providers regarding disease outbreaks was focused mainly on the spread of traditional infectious diseases. These included possible epidemics caused by influenza, tuberculosis, cholera, and HIV. Table 3.1 lists the 10 most dangerous infectious diseases ranked according to which disorders caused the most deaths worldwide in the year 2000. Other infectious diseases such as food poisoning and sexually transmitted diseases were also common though considered less important, because they produced fewer fatalities.

The aftermath of the September 11, 2001, attacks prompted the healthcare community to expand its awareness of outbreaks and treatments to include bioterrorism and the health effects of biological and chemical weapons. **Bioterrorism** may be defined as the intentional use of infectious biological agents, chemical substances, or radiation to cause widespread harm or illness. The public has become more aware of the threat of bioterrorism because such federal agencies as the Centers for Disease Control and Prevention (CDC) and the U.S. Department of Defense have stepped up efforts to inform, educate, and prepare the public for disease outbreaks of a less traditional nature.

The goals of a bioterrorist are to create widespread public panic and to cause as many casualties as possible. There is no shortage of agents that can be used for this purpose. Indeed, some of these agents are easily obtainable and require little or no specialized knowledge to disseminate. Areas of greatest concern include acutely infectious diseases such as anthrax, smallpox, plague, and hemorrhagic

PHARMFACTS

Potential Chemical and Biological Agents for Terrorist Attacks

- Robert Stevens, the 63-year-old employee of American Media who died in Florida on October 5, 2001, was the first person to die from anthrax in the United States in 25 years.
- In 1979, accidental release of anthrax from a research lab in the Soviet Union killed 68 people. The problem was traced to a faulty air filter.
- The Ebola virus causes death by hemorrhagic fever in up to 90% of the clients who show clinical symptoms of infection.
- Ebola viruses are found in central Africa. Although the source of the viruses in nature remains unknown, monkeys (like humans) appear to be susceptible to infection and serve as sources of virus if infected.
- Widespread public smallpox vaccinations ceased in the United States in 1972.
- It is estimated that 7 million to 8 million doses of smallpox vaccine are in storage at the CDC. This stock cannot be easily replenished, since all vaccine production facilities were dismantled after 1980, and new vaccine production requires 24 to 36 months.
- Most nerve agents were originally produced in a search for insecticides, but because of their toxicity, they were evaluated for military use.
- Chemicals used in bioterrorist acts need not be sophisticated or difficult to obtain: Toxic industrial chemicals such as chlorine, phosgene, and hydrogen cyanide are used in commercial manufacturing and are readily available.

TABLE 3.1	The 10 Most Dangerous Infectious Diseases in the World, 2000		
Disease	**Causative Agent**	**Target**	**Deaths per Year (millions)**
influenza	*Haemophilus influenzae*	respiratory system	3.7
tuberculosis	*Mycobacterium tuberculosis*	lungs	2.9
cholera	*Vibrio cholerae*	digestive tract	2.5
AIDS	human immunodeficiency virus	immune response	2.3
malaria	*Plasmodium falciparum*	blood disorder	1.5
measles	rubeola virus	lungs and meninges	0.96
hepatitis B	hepatitis B virus (HBV)	liver	0.605
whooping cough	*Bordetella pertussis*	respiratory system	0.41
tetanus	*Clostridium tetani*	entire body (infections)	0.275
dengue fever	flavivirus	entire body (fever)	0.14

Source: July 2001 report by the WHO/Industry Drug Development Working Group—World Health Organization: http://www.who.int/en/

viruses; incapacitating chemicals such as nerve gas, cyanide, and chlorinated agents; and nuclear and radiation emergencies. The CDC has categorized the biological threats, based on their potential impact on public health, as shown in Table 3.2.

3.2 Role of the Nurse in Emergency Preparedness

Emergency preparedness is not a new concept. For more than 30 years, the Joint Commission on Accreditation of Healthcare Organizations (JCAHO) has required accredited hospitals to develop disaster plans and to conduct periodic emergency drills to determine readiness. Prior to the late 1990s, disaster plans and training focused on natural disasters such as tornadoes, hurricanes and floods, or accidents such as explosions that could cause multiple casualties. In the late 1990s, the JCAHO standards added the possibility of bioterrorism and virulent infectious organisms as rare, though possible, scenarios in disaster preparedness.

In 2001 JCAHO issued new standards that shifted the focus from disaster preparedness to emergency management. The newer standards included more than just responding to the immediate casualties caused by a disaster,

TABLE 3.2	Categories of Infectious Agents	
Category	**Description**	**Examples**
A	agents that can easily be disseminated or transmitted person to person; cause high mortality, with potential for major public health impact; might cause public panic and social disruption; require special action for public health preparedness	*Bacillus anthracis* (anthrax) *Clostridium botulinum* toxin (botulism) *Francisella tularensis* (tularemia) variola major (smallpox) viral hemorrhagic fevers such as Marburg and Ebola *Yersinia pestis* (plague)
B	moderately easy to disseminate; cause moderate morbidity and low mortality; require specific enhancements of CDC's diagnostic capacity and enhanced disease surveillance	*Brucella* species (brucellosis) *Burkholderia mallei* (glanders) *Burkholderia pseudomallei* (melioidosis) *Chlamydia psittaci* (psittacosis) *Coxiella burnetii* (Q fever) epsilon toxin of *Clostridium perfringens* food safety threats such as *Salmonella* and *E. coli* ricin toxin from *Ricinus communis* *Staphylococcus* enterotoxin B viral encephalitis water safety threats such as *Vibrio cholerae* and *Cryptosporidium parvum*
C	emerging pathogens that could be engineered for mass dissemination because of their availability, ease of production and dissemination, and potential for high morbidity and mortality rates and major health impacts	hantaviruses multidrug-resistant tuberculosis Nipah virus (NiV) tick-borne encephalitis viruses yellow fever

Source: http://www.bt.cdc.gov/agent/agentlist-category.asp

they also considered how an agency's healthcare delivery system might change during a crisis, and how it might return to normal operations following the incident. The expanded focus also included how the individual healthcare agency would coordinate its efforts with community resources, such as other hospitals and public health agencies. State and federal agencies revised their emergency preparedness guidelines in an attempt to plan more rationally for a range of disasters including possible bioterrorist acts.

Planning for bioterrorist acts requires close cooperation among all the different healthcare professionals. Nurses are central to the effort. Because a bioterrorist incident may occur in any community without warning, nurses must be prepared to respond immediately. The following elements underscore the key roles of nurses in meeting the challenges of a potential bioterrorist event:

- *Education* Nurses must maintain a current knowledge and understanding of emergency management relating to bioterrorist activities.

- *Resources* Nurses must maintain a current listing of health and law enforcement contacts and resources in their local communities who would assist in the event of bioterrorist activity.

- *Diagnosis and treatment* Nurses must be aware of the early signs and symptoms of chemical and biological agents, and their immediate treatment.

- *Planning* Nurses should be involved in developing emergency management plans.

3.3 Strategic National Stockpile

Should a chemical or biological attack occur, it would likely be rapid and unexpected, and would produce multiple casualties. Although planning for such an event is an important part of disaster preparedness, individual healthcare agencies and local communities could easily be overwhelmed by such a crisis. Shortages of needed drugs, medical equipment, and supplies would be expected.

The **Strategic National Stockpile (SNS),** formerly called the National Pharmaceutical Stockpile, is a program designed to ensure the immediate deployment of essential medical materials to a community in the event of a large-scale chemical or biological attack. Managed by the CDC, the stockpile consists of the following materials:

- Antibiotics
- Vaccines
- Medical, surgical, and client support supplies such as bandages, airway supplies, and IV equipment

The SNS has two components. The first is called a *push package,* which consists of a preassembled set of supplies and pharmaceuticals designed to meet the needs of an unknown biological or chemical threat. There are eight fully stocked 50-ton push packages stored in climate-controlled warehouses throughout the United States. They are in locations where they can reach any community in the

United States within 12 hours after an attack. The decision to deploy the push package is based on an assessment of the situation by federal government officials.

The second SNS component consists of a **vendor-managed inventory (VMI)** package. VMI packages are shipped, if necessary, after the chemical or biological threat has more clearly been identified. The materials consist of supplies and pharmaceuticals more specific to the chemical or biological agent used in the attack. VMI packages are designed to arrive within 24 to 36 hours.

The stockpiling of antibiotics and vaccines by local hospitals, clinics, or individuals for the purpose of preparing for a bioterrorist act is not recommended. Pharmaceuticals have a finite expiration date, and keeping large stores of drugs can be costly. Furthermore, stockpiling could cause drug shortages and prevent the delivery of these pharmaceuticals to communities where they may be needed most.

AGENTS USED IN BIOTERRORISM ACTS

Bioterrorists could potentially use any biological, chemical, or physical agent to cause widespread panic and serious illness. Knowing which agents are most likely to be used in an incident helps nurses plan and implement emergency preparedness policies.

3.4 Anthrax

One of the first threats following the terrorist attacks on the World Trade Center was **anthrax**. In the fall of 2001, five people died as a result of exposure to anthrax, presumably due to purposeful, bioterrorist actions. At least 13 U.S. citizens were infected, several governmental employees were threatened, and the U.S. Postal Service was interrupted for several weeks. There was initial concern that anthrax outbreaks might disrupt many other essential operations throughout the country.

Anthrax is caused by the bacterium *Bacillus anthracis,* which normally affects domestic and wild animals. A wide variety of hoofed animals are affected by the disease, including cattle, sheep, goats, horses, donkeys, pigs, American bison, antelopes, elephants, and lions. If transmitted to humans by exposure to an open wound, through contaminated food, or by inhalation, *B. anthracis* can cause serious damage to body tissues. Symptoms of anthrax infection usually appear 1 to 6 days after exposure. Depending on how the bacterium is transmitted, specific types of anthrax "poisoning" may be observed, each characterized by hallmark symptoms. Clinical manifestations of anthrax are summarized in Table 3.3.

B. anthracis causes disease by the emission of two types of toxins, edema toxin and lethal toxin. These toxins cause necrosis and accumulation of exudate, which produces pain, swelling, and restriction of activity, the general symptoms associated with almost every form of anthrax. Another component, the anthrax binding receptor, allows the

TABLE 3.3 Clinical Manifestations of Anthrax

Type	Description	Symptoms
cutaneous anthrax	most common but least complicated form of anthrax; almost always curable if treated within the first few weeks of exposure; results from direct contact of contaminated products with an open wound or cut	small skin lesions develop and turn into black scabs; inoculation takes less than 1 week; cannot be spread by person-to-person contact
gastrointestinal anthrax	rare form of anthrax; without treatment, can be lethal in up to 50% of cases; results from eating anthrax-contaminated food, usually meat	sore throat, difficulty swallowing, cramping, diarrhea, and abdominal swelling
inhalation anthrax	least common but the most dangerous form of anthrax; can be successfully treated if identified within the first few days after exposure; results from inhaling anthrax spores	initially, fatigue, and fever for several days, followed by persistent cough and shortness of breath; without treatment, death can result within 4–6 days

bacterium to bind to human cells and act as a "doorway" for both types of toxins to enter.

Further ensuring its chance for spreading, *B. anthracis* is spore forming. Anthrax spores can remain viable in soil for hundreds, and perhaps thousands, of years. Anthrax spores are resistant to drying, heat, and some harsh chemicals. These spores are the main cause for public health concern, because they are responsible for producing inhalation anthrax, the most dangerous form of the disease. After entry into the lungs, *B. anthracis* spores are ingested by macrophages and carried to lymphoid tissue, resulting in tissue necrosis, swelling, and hemorrhage. One of the main body areas affected is the mediastinum, which is a potential site for tissue injury and fluid accumulation. Meningitis is also a common pathology. If treatment is delayed, inhalation anthrax is lethal in almost every case.

B. anthracis is found in contaminated animal products such as wool, hair, dander, and bonemeal, but it can also be packaged in other forms, making it transmissible through the air or by direct contact. Terrorists have delivered it in the form of a fine powder, making it less obvious to detect. The powder can be inconspicuously spread on virtually any surface, making it a serious concern for public safety.

The antibiotic ciprofloxacin (Cipro) has traditionally been used for anthrax prophylaxis and treatment. For prophylaxis, the usual dosage is 500 mg PO (by mouth), every 12 hours for 60 days. If exposure has been confirmed, ciprofloxacin should immediately be administered at a usual dose of 400 mg IV (intravenously), every 12 hours. Other antibiotics are also effective against anthrax, including penicillin, vancomycin, ampicillin, erythromycin, tetracycline, and doxycycline. In the case of inhalation anthrax, the FDA has approved the use of ciprofloxacin and doxycycline in combination for treatment.

Many members of the public have become intensely concerned about bioterrorism threats and have asked their healthcare provider to provide them with ciprofloxacin. The public should be discouraged from seeking the prophylactic use of antibiotics in cases where anthrax exposure has not been confirmed. Indiscriminate, unnecessary use of antibiotics can be expensive, can cause significant side effects, and can promote the appearance of resistant bacterial strains. The student should refer to Chapter 34 ∞ to review the precautions and guidelines regarding the appropriate use of antibiotics.

Although anthrax immunization (vaccination) has been licensed by the FDA for 30 years, it has not been widely used because of the extremely low incidence of this disease in the United States prior to September 2001. The **vaccine** has been prepared from proteins from the anthrax bacteria, dubbed "protective antigens." Anthrax vaccine works the same way as other vaccines: by causing the body to make protective antibodies and thus preventing the onset of disease and symptoms. Immunization for anthrax consists of three subcutaneous injections given 2 weeks apart, followed by three additional subcutaneous injections given at 6, 12, and 18 months. Annual booster injections of the vaccine are recommended. At this time, the CDC recommends vaccination for only select populations: laboratory personnel who work with anthrax, military personnel deployed to high-risk areas, and those who deal with animal products imported from areas with a high incidence of the disease.

There is an ongoing controversy regarding the safety of the anthrax vaccine and whether it is truly effective in preventing the disease. Until these issues are resolved, the use of anthrax immunization will likely remain limited to select groups. Vaccines and the immune response are discussed in more detail in Chapter 32 ∞.

3.5 Viruses

In 2002, the public was astounded as researchers announced that they had "built" a poliovirus, a threat that U.S. health officials thought had essentially been eradicated in 1994. Although virtually eliminated in the Western Hemisphere, polio was reported in at least 27 countries as late as 1998. The infection persists among infants and children in areas with contaminated drinking water or food, mainly in underdeveloped regions of India, Pakistan, Afghanistan, western and central Africa, and the Dominican Republic. In the United States, polio remains a potential threat in 1 of

MediaLink Anthrax Vaccine Immunization Program (AVIP)

MediaLink Other Biological Threats

300,000 to 500,000 clients who are vaccinated with the oral poliovirus vaccine.

The current concern is that bioterrorists will culture the poliovirus and release it into regions where people have not been vaccinated. An even more dangerous threat is that a mutated strain, for which there is no effective vaccine, might be developed. Because the genetic code of the poliovirus is small (around 7,500 base pairs), it can be manufactured in a relatively simple laboratory. Once the virus is isolated, hundreds of different mutant strains could be produced in a very short time.

In addition to polio, smallpox is considered a potential biohazard. Once thought to have been eradicated from the planet in the 1970s, the variola virus that causes this disease has been harbored in research labs in several countries. Much of its genetic code (200,000 base pairs) has been sequenced and is public information. The disease is spread person to person as an aerosol or droplets or by contact with contaminated objects such as clothing or bedding. Only a few viral particles are needed to cause infection. If the virus is released into an unvaccinated population, as many as one in three could die.

There are no effective therapies for treating clients infected by most types of viruses that could be used in a bioterrorist attack. For some viruses, however, it is possible to create a vaccine that could stimulate the body's immune system in a manner that could be remembered at a later date. In the case of smallpox, a stockpile of the vaccine exists in enough quantity to administer to every person in the United States. The variola vaccine provides a high level of protection if given prior to exposure, or up to 3 days later. Protection may last from 3 to 5 years. The following are contraindications to receiving the smallpox vaccine, unless the individual has confirmed face-to-face contact with an infected client:

- Persons with (or a history of) atopic dermatitis or eczema
- Persons with acute, active, or exfoliative skin conditions
- Persons with altered immune states (e.g., HIV, AIDS, leukemia, lymphoma, immunosuppressive drugs)
- Pregnant and breast-feeding women
- Children younger than 1 year
- Persons who have a serious allergy to any component of the vaccine

It has been suggested that multiple vaccines be created, mass produced, and stockpiled to meet the challenges of a terrorist attack. Another suggestion has called for mass vaccination of the public, or at least those healthcare providers and law enforcement employees who might be exposed to infected clients.

Vaccines have side effects, some of which are quite serious. In the case of smallpox vaccination, for example, it is estimated that there might be as many as 250 deaths for every million people inoculated. If the smallpox vaccine was given to every person in the United States (approxi-

mately 300 million), possible deaths from vaccination could exceed 75,000. In addition, terrorists having some knowledge of genetic structure could create a modified strain of the virus that renders existing vaccines totally ineffective. It appears, then, that mass vaccination is not an appropriate solution until research can produce safer and more effective vaccines.

3.6 Toxic Chemicals

Although chemical warfare agents have been available since World War I, medicine has produced few drug antidotes. Many treatments provide minimal help other than to relieve some symptoms and provide comfort following exposure. Most chemical agents used in warfare were created to cause mass casualties; others were designed to cause so much discomfort that soldiers would be too weak to continue fighting. Potential chemicals that could be used in a terrorist act include nerve gases, blood agents, choking and vomiting agents, and those that cause severe blistering. Table 3.4 provides a summary of selected chemical agents and known antidotes and first-aid treatments.

The chemical category of main pharmacological significance is **nerve agents.** Exposure to these acutely toxic chemicals can cause convulsions and loss of consciousness within seconds, and respiratory failure within minutes. Almost all signs of exposure to nerve gas agents relate to overstimulation by the neurotransmitter acetylcholine (Ach) at both central and peripheral sites located throughout the body.

Acetylcholine is normally degraded by the enzyme acetylcholinesterase (AchE) in the synaptic space. Nerve agents block AchE, increasing the action of acetylcholine in the synaptic space; therefore, all symptoms of nerve gas exposure such as salivation, increased sweating, muscle twitching, involuntary urination and defecation, confusion, convulsions, and death are the direct result of Ach overstimulation. To remedy this condition, nerve agent antidote and Mark I injector kits that contain the anticholinergic drug atropine or a related medication are available in cases where nerve agent release is expected. Atropine blocks the attachment of Ach to receptor sites and prevents the overstimulation caused by the nerve agent. Neurotransmitters, synapses, and autonomic receptors are discussed in detail in Chapter 13 ∞.

3.7 Ionizing Radiation

In addition to releasing biological and chemical weapons, it is possible that bioterrorists could develop nuclear bombs capable of mass destruction. In such a scenario, the greatest number of casualties would be due to the physical blast itself. Survivors, however, could be exposed to high levels of **ionizing radiation** from hundreds of different radioisotopes created by the nuclear explosion. Some of these radioisotopes emit large amounts of radiation and persist in the environment for years. As was the case in the 1986 Chernobyl

TABLE 3.4	Chemical Warfare Agents and Treatments	
Category	**Signs of Discomfort/Fatality**	**Antidotes/First Aid**
Nerve Agents		
GA—Tabun (liquid) GB—Sarin (gaseous liquid) GD—Soman (liquid) VX (gaseous liquid)	Depending on the nerve agent, symptoms may be slower to appear and cumulative depending on exposure time: miosis, runny nose, difficulty breathing, excessive salivation, nausea, vomiting, cramping, involuntary urination and defecation, twitching and jerking of muscles, headaches, confusion, convulsion, coma, death.	Nerve agent antidote and Mark I injector kits with atropine are available. Flush eyes immediately with water. Apply sodium bicarbonate or 5% liquid bleach solution to the skin. Do not induce vomiting.
Blood Agents		
hydrogen cyanide (liquid)	Red eyes, flushing of the skin, nausea, headaches, weakness, hypoxic convulsions, death	Flush eyes and wash skin with water. For inhalation of mist, oxygen and amyl nitrate may be given. For ingestion of cyanide liquid, 1% sodium thiosulfate may be given to induce vomiting.
cyanogen chloride (gas)	Loss of appetite, irritation of the respiratory tract, pulmonary edema, death	Oxygen and amyl nitrate may be given. Give client milk or water. Do not induce vomiting.
Choking/Vomiting Agents		
phosgene (gas)	Dizziness, burning eyes, thirst, throat irritation, chills, respiratory and circulatory failure, cyanosis, frostbite-type lesions	Provide fresh air. Administer oxygen. Flush eyes with normal saline or water. Keep client warm and calm.
Adamsite—DM (crystalline dispensed in aerosol)	Irritation of the eyes and respiratory tract, tightness of the chest, nausea, and vomiting	Rinse nose and throat with saline, water, or 10% solution of sodium bicarbonate. Treat the skin with borated talcum powder.
Blister/Vesicant Agents		
phosgene oxime (crystalline or liquid) mustard—lewisite mixture—HL nitrogen mustard—HN-1, HN-2, HN-3 sulfur mustard agents	Destruction of mucous membranes, eye tissue, and skin (subcutaneous edema), followed by scab formation Irritation of the eyes, nasal membranes, and lungs; nausea and vomiting; formation of blisters on the skin; cytotoxic reactions in hematopoietic tissues including bone marrow, lymph nodes, spleen, and endocrine glands	Flush affected area with copious quantities of water. If ingested, do not induce vomiting. Flush affected area with water. Treat the skin with 5% solution of sodium hypochlorite or household bleach. Give milk to drink. Do not induce vomiting. Skin contact with lewisite may be treated with 10% solution of sodium carbonate.

Source: Chemical Fact Sheets at the U.S. Army Center for Health Promotion and Preventive Medicine website: http://chppm_www.apgea.army.mil/dts/dtchemfs.htm

nuclear accident in Ukraine, the resulting radioisotopes could travel through wind currents, to land thousands of miles away from the initial explosion. Smaller scale radiation exposure could occur through terrorist attacks on nuclear power plants or by the release of solid or liquid radioactive materials into public areas.

The acute effects of ionizing radiation have been well documented and depend primarily on the dose of radiation that the client receives. **Acute radiation syndrome,** sometimes called *radiation sickness,* can occur within hours or days after extreme doses. Immediate symptoms are nausea, vomiting, and diarrhea. Later symptoms in-

clude weight loss, anorexia, fatigue, and bone marrow suppression. Clients who survive the acute exposure are at high risk for developing various cancers, particularly leukemia.

Symptoms of nuclear and radiation exposure remain some of the most difficult to treat pharmacologically. Apart from the symptomatic treatment of radiation sickness, taking potassium iodide (KI) tablets after an incident or an attack is the only recognized therapy specifically designed for radiation exposure. One of the radioisotopes produced by a nuclear explosion is iodine-131. Because iodine is naturally concentrated in the thyroid gland, I-131 will immediately enter the thyroid and damage thyroid cells. For example, following the Chernobyl nuclear disaster, the incidence of thyroid cancer in Ukraine jumped from 4 to 6 cases per million people to 45 cases per million. If taken prior to, or immediately following, a nuclear incident, KI can prevent up to 100% of the radioactive iodine from entering the thyroid gland. It is effective even if taken 3 to 4 hours after radiation exposure. Generally, a single 130-mg dose is necessary.

Unfortunately, KI protects only the thyroid gland from I-131. It has no protective effects on other body tissues, and it offers no protection against the dozens of other harmful radioisotopes generated by a nuclear blast. As with vaccines and antibiotics, the stockpiling of KI by local healthcare agencies or individuals is not recommended. Interestingly, I-131 is also a medication used to shrink the size of an overactive thyroid gland. Thyroid medications are presented in Chapter 43 ∞.

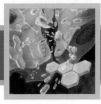

CHAPTER REVIEW

KEY CONCEPTS

The numbered key concepts provide a succinct summary of the important points from the corresponding numbered section within the chapter. If any of these points are not clear, refer to the numbered section within the chapter for review.

3.1 Bioterrorism is the deliberate use of a biological or physical agent to cause panic and mass casualties. The health aspects of biological and chemical agents have become important public issues.

3.2 Nurses play key roles in emergency preparedness, including providing education, resources, diagnosis and treatment, and planning.

3.3 The Strategic National Stockpile (SNS) is used to rapidly deploy medical necessities to communities experiencing a chemical or biological attack. The two components are the push package and the vendor-managed inventory.

3.4 Anthrax can enter the body through ingestion or inhalation, or by the cutaneous route. Antibiotic therapy can be successful if given prophylactically or shortly after exposure.

3.5 Viruses such as polio, smallpox, and those causing hemorrhagic fevers are potential biological weapons. If available, vaccines are the best treatments.

3.6 Chemicals and neurotoxins are potential bioterrorist threats for which there are no specific antidotes.

3.7 Potassium iodide (KI) may be used to block the effects of acute radiation exposure on the thyroid gland, but it is not effective for protecting other organs.

NCLEX-RN® REVIEW QUESTIONS

1 The nurse recognizes which of the following to be initial symptoms of inhaled anthrax? (Select all that apply.)

1. Cramping and diarrhea
2. Skin lesions that develop into black scabs
3. Fever
4. Headache
5. Cough and dyspnea

2 Potassium iodine (KI) taken immediately following a nuclear incident can prevent 100% of radioactive iodine from entering which body organ?

1. Brain
2. Thyroid
3. Kidney
4. Liver

3 Soldiers who may have been exposed to nerve gas agents can be expected to display which of these symptoms?

1. Convulsions and loss of consciousness
2. Memory loss and fatigue
3. Malaise and hemorrhaging
4. Fever and headaches

4 Which of these medications is primarily used for the treatment of anthrax?

1. Diphtheria vaccine
2. Amoxicillin (Amoxil)
3. Ciprofloxacin (Cipro)
4. Smallpox vaccine

5 The CDC categorized biological threats based on their:

1. Potential adverse effects.
2. Potential impact on public health.
3. Potential cost of treatment.
4. Potential loss of life.

CRITICAL THINKING QUESTIONS

1. Why is the medical community opposed to the mass vaccination of the general public for potential bioterrorist threats such as anthrax and smallpox?

2. Why does the protective effect of KI not extend to body tissues other than the thyroid gland?

3. Why do nurses play such a central role in emergency preparedness?

See Appendix D for answers and rationales for all activities.

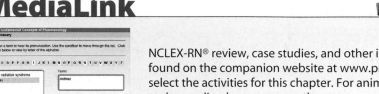

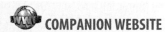
www.prenhall.com/adams

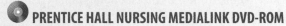

NCLEX-RN® review, case studies, and other interactive resources for this chapter can be found on the companion website at www.prenhall.com/adams. Click on "Chapter 3" to select the activities for this chapter. For animations, more NCLEX-RN® review questions, and an audio glossary, access the accompanying Prentice Hall Nursing MediaLink DVD-ROM in this textbook.

PRENTICE HALL NURSING MEDIALINK DVD-ROM
- Audio Glossary
- NCLEX-RN® Review

COMPANION WEBSITE
- NCLEX-RN® Review
- Case Study: Bioterrorism
- Challenge Your Knowledge

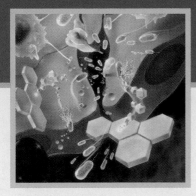

CHAPTER 4

Principles of Drug Administration

OBJECTIVES

After reading this chapter, the student should be able to:

1. Discuss drug administration as a component of safe, effective nursing care, utilizing the nursing process.
2. Describe the roles and responsibilities of the nurse regarding drug administration.
3. Explain how the five rights of drug administration affect client safety.
4. Give specific examples of how the nurse can increase client compliance in taking medications.
5. Interpret drug orders that contain abbreviations.
6. Compare and contrast the three systems of measurement used in pharmacology.
7. Explain the proper methods of administering enteral, topical, and parenteral drugs.
8. Compare and contrast the advantages and disadvantages of each route of drug administration.

MediaLink

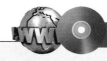 www.prenhall.com/adams

NCLEX-RN® review, case studies, and other interactive resources for this chapter can be found on the companion website at www.prenhall.com/adams. Click on "Chapter 4" to select the activities for this chapter. For animations, more NCLEX-RN® review questions, and an audio glossary, access the accompanying Prentice Hall Nursing MediaLink DVD-ROM in this textbook.

KEY TERMS

allergic reaction *page 29*

anaphylaxis *page 29*

apothecary system *page 31*

ASAP order *page 31*

astringent effect *page 37*

buccal route *page 33*

compliance *page 29*

enteral route *page 32*

enteric coated *page 32*

five rights of drug administration *page 29*

household system *page 31*

intradermal (ID) *page 38*

intramuscular (IM) *page 39*

intravenous (IV) *page 43*

metric system of measurement *page 31*

parenteral route *page 38*

PRN order *page 31*

routine orders *page 31*

single order *page 31*

standing order *page 31*

STAT order *page 30*

subcutaneous *page 38*

sublingual route *page 33*

sustained release *page 32*

three checks of drug administration *page 29*

The primary role of the nurse in drug administration is to ensure that prescribed medications are delivered in a safe manner. Drug administration is an important component of providing comprehensive nursing care that incorporates all aspects of the nursing process. In the course of drug administration, nurses will collaborate closely with physicians, pharmacists, and, of course, their clients. The purpose of this chapter is to introduce the roles and responsibilities of the nurse in delivering medications safely and effectively.

4.1 Medication Knowledge, Understanding, and Responsibilities of the Nurse

Whether administering drugs or supervising drug use, the nurse is expected to understand the pharmacotherapeutic principles for all medications given to each client. Given the large number of different drugs and the potential consequences of medication errors, this is indeed an enormous task. The nurse's responsibilities include knowledge and understanding of the following:

- What drug is ordered
  - Name (generic and trade) and drug classification
  - Intended or proposed use
  - Effects on the body
  - Contraindications
  - Special considerations, (e.g., how age, weight, body fat distribution, and individual pathophysiological states affect pharmacotherapeutic response)
  - Side effects
- Why the medication has been prescribed for this particular client
- How the medication is supplied by the pharmacy
- How the medication is to be administered, including dosage ranges
- What nursing process considerations related to the medication apply to this client

PHARMFACTS

Potentially Fatal Drug Reactions

Toxic Epidermal Necrolysis (TEN)

- Severe and deadly drug-induced allergic reaction
- Characterized by widespread epidermal sloughing, caused by massive disintegration of keratinocytes
- Severe epidermal detachment involving the top layer of the skin and mucous membranes
- Multisystem organ involvement and death if the reaction is not recognized and diagnosed
- Occurs when the liver fails to properly break down a drug, which then cannot be excreted normally
- Associated with use of some anticonvulsants (phenytoin [Dilantin], carbamazepine [Tegretol]), the antibiotic trimethoprim/sulfamethoxazole [Bactrim, Septra]), and other drugs, but can occur with the use of any prescription or OTC preparation, including ibuprofen (Advil, Motrin)
- Risk of death decreases if the offending drug is quickly withdrawn and supportive care is maintained
- Skin sloughing of 30% or more of the body

Stevens–Johnson Syndrome (SJS)

- Usually prompted by the same or similar drugs as TEN
- Begins within 1 to 14 days of pharmacotherapy
- Start of SJS usually signaled by nonspecific upper respiratory infection (URI) with chills, fever, and malaise
- Generalized blisterlike lesions follow within a few days
- Skin sloughing of 10% of the body

Before any drug is administered, the nurse must obtain and process pertinent information regarding the client's medical history, physical assessment, disease processes, and learning needs and capabilities. Growth and developmental factors must always be considered. It is important to remember that a large number of variables influence a client's response to medications. Having a firm understanding of these variables can increase the success of pharmacotherapy.

A major goal of studying pharmacology is to limit the number and severity of adverse drug events. Many adverse effects are preventable. Professional nurses can routinely avoid many serious adverse drug effects in their clients by applying their experience and knowledge of pharmacotherapeutics to clinical practice. Some adverse effects, however, are not preventable. It is vital that the nurse be prepared to recognize and respond to potential adverse effects of medications.

Allergic and anaphylactic reactions are particularly serious effects that must be carefully monitored and prevented, when possible. An **allergic reaction** is an acquired hyperresponse of body defenses to a foreign substance (allergen). Signs of allergic reactions vary in severity and include skin rash with or without itching, edema, runny nose, or reddened eyes with tearing. On discovering that the client is allergic to a product, it is the nurse's responsibility to alert all personnel by documenting the allergy in the medical record and by applying labels to the chart and medication administration record (MAR). An appropriate, agency-approved bracelet should be placed on the client to alert all caregivers to the specific drug allergy. Information related to drug allergy must be communicated to the physician and pharmacist so the medication regimen can be evaluated for cross-sensitivity among various pharmacologic products.

Anaphylaxis is a severe type of allergic reaction that involves the massive, systemic release of histamine and other chemical mediators of inflammation that can lead to life-threatening shock. Symptoms such as acute dyspnea and the sudden appearance of hypotension or tachycardia following drug administration are indicative of anaphylaxis, which must receive immediate treatment. The pharmacotherapy of allergic reactions and anaphylaxis is covered in Chapters 38 and 29 ∞, respectively.

4.2 The Rights of Drug Administration

The traditional **five rights of drug administration** form the operational basis for the safe delivery of medications. The five rights offer simple and practical guidance for nurses to use during drug preparation, delivery, and administration, and focus on individual performance. The five rights are as follows:

1. Right client
2. Right medication
3. Right dose
4. Right route of administration
5. Right time of delivery

Additional rights have been added over the years, depending on particular academic curricula or agency policies. Additions to the original five rights include considerations such as the right to refuse medication, the right to receive drug education, the right preparation, and the right documentation. Ethical and legal considerations regarding the five rights are discussed in Chapter 9 ∞.

The **three checks of drug administration** that nurses use in conjunction with the five rights help to ensure client safety and drug effectiveness. Traditionally these checks incorporate the following:

1. Checking the drug with the MAR or the medication information system when removing it from the medication drawer, refrigerator, or controlled substance locker
2. Checking the drug when preparing it, pouring it, taking it out of the unit-dose container, or connecting the IV tubing to the bag
3. Checking the drug before administering it to the client

Despite all attempts to provide safe drug delivery, errors continue to occur, some of which are fatal. Although the nurse is held accountable for preparing and administering medications, safe drug practices are a result of multidisciplinary endeavors. Responsibility for accurate drug administration lies with multiple individuals, including physicians, pharmacists, and other healthcare professionals. Factors contributing to medication errors are presented in Chapter 9 ∞.

4.3 Client Compliance and Successful Pharmacotherapy

Compliance is a major factor affecting pharmacotherapeutic success. As it relates to pharmacology, **compliance** is taking a medication in the manner prescribed by the practitioner, or in the case of OTC drugs, following the instructions on the label. Client noncompliance ranges from not taking the medication at all to taking it at the wrong time or in the wrong manner.

Although the nurse may be extremely conscientious in applying all the principles of effective drug administration, these strategies are of little value unless the client agrees that

---

SPECIAL CONSIDERATIONS

The Challenges of Pediatric Drug Administration
Administering medication to infants and young children requires special knowledge and techniques. The nurse must have knowledge of growth and development patterns. When possible, the child should be given a choice regarding the use of a spoon, dropper, or syringe. A matter-of-fact attitude should be presented in giving a child medications: Using threats or dishonesty is unacceptable. Oral medications that must be crushed for the child to swallow can be mixed with honey, flavored syrup, jelly, or fruit puree to avoid unpleasant tastes. Medications should not be mixed with certain dietary products, such as potatoes, milk, or fruit juices, to mask the taste, because the child may develop an unpleasant association with these items and refuse to consume them in the future. To prevent nausea, medications can be preceded and followed with sips of a carbonated beverage that is poured over crushed ice.

the prescribed drug regimen is personally worthwhile. Before administering the drug, the nurse should use the nursing process to formulate a personalized care plan that will best enable the client to become an active participant in his or her care (see Chapter 8 ∞). This allows the client to accept or reject the pharmacologic course of therapy, based on accurate information that is presented in a manner that addresses individual learning styles. It is imperative to remember that a responsible, well-informed adult always has the legal option to refuse to take any medication.

In the plan of care, it is important to address essential information that the client must know regarding the prescribed medications. This includes factors such as the name of the drug, why it has been ordered, expected drug actions, associated side effects, and potential interactions with other medications, foods, herbal supplements, or alcohol. Clients need to be reminded that they share an active role in ensuring their own medication effectiveness and safety.

Many factors can influence whether clients comply with pharmacotherapy. The drug may be too expensive or may not be approved by the client's health insurance plan. Clients sometimes forget doses of medications, especially when they must be taken three or four times per day. Clients often discontinue the use of drugs that have annoying side effects or those that impair major lifestyle choices. Adverse effects that often prompt noncompliance are headache, dizziness, nausea, diarrhea, or impotence.

Clients often take medications in an unexpected manner, sometimes self-adjusting their doses. Some clients believe that if one tablet is good, two must be better. Others believe they will become dependent on the medication if it is taken as prescribed; thus, they take only half the required dose. Clients are usually reluctant to admit or report noncompliance to the nurse for fear of being reprimanded or feeling embarrassed. Because the reasons for noncompliance are many and varied, the nurse must be vigilant in questioning clients about their medications. When

pharmacotherapy fails to produce the expected outcomes, noncompliance should be considered a possible explanation.

4.4 Drug Orders and Time Schedules

Healthcare providers use accepted abbreviations to communicate the directions and times for drug administration. Table 4.1 lists common abbreviations that relate to universally scheduled times.

A **STAT order** refers to any medication that is needed immediately, and is to be given only once. It is often associated with emergency medications that are needed for life-threatening situations. The term *STAT* comes from *statim*, the Latin word meaning "immediately." The physician normally notifies the nurse of any STAT order so it can be obtained from the pharmacy and administered immediately. The time between writing the order and administering the drug should be 5 minutes or less. Although not as urgent, an **ASAP** (as soon as

TABLE 4.1	Drug Administration Abbreviations
Abbreviation	**Meaning**
ac	before meals
ad lib	as desired/as directed
AM	morning
bid	twice per day
cap	capsule
gtt	drop
h or hr	hour
IM	intramuscular
IV	intravenous
no	number
pc	after meals; after eating
PO	by mouth
PM	afternoon
PRN	when needed/necessary
q	every
qh	every hour
qid	four times per day
q2h	every 2 hours (even)
q4h	every 4 hours (even)
q6h	every 6 hours (even)
q8h	every 8 hours (even)
q12h	every 12 hours
Rx	take
STAT	immediately; at once
tab	tablet
tid	three times per day

The Institute for Safe Medical Practices recommends that the following abbreviations be avoided because they can lead to medication errors: qd: instead use "daily" or "every day"; qhs: instead use "nightly"; qod: instead use "every other day."

possible) **order** should be available for administration to the client within 30 minutes of the written order.

The **single order** is for a drug that is to be given only once, and at a specific time, such as a preoperative order. A **PRN order** (Latin: *pro re nata*) is administered *as required* by the client's condition. The nurse makes the judgment, based on client assessment, as to when such a medication is to be administered. Orders not written as STAT, ASAP, NOW, or PRN are called **routine orders.** These are usually carried out within 2 hours of the time the order is written by the physician. A **standing order** is written in advance of a situation that is to be carried out under specific circumstances. An example of a standing order is a set of postoperative PRN prescriptions that are written for all clients who have undergone a specific surgical procedure. A common standing order for clients who have had a tonsillectomy is "Tylenol elixir 325 mg PO q6h PRN sore throat." Because of the legal implications of putting all clients into a single treatment category, standing orders are no longer permitted in some facilities.

Agency policies dictate that drug orders be reviewed by the attending physician within specific time frames, usually at least every 7 days. Prescriptions for narcotics and other scheduled drugs are often automatically discontinued after 72 hours, unless specifically reordered by the physician. Automatic stop orders do not generally apply when the number of doses or an exact period of time is specified.

Some medications must be taken at specific times. If a drug causes stomach upset, it is usually administered *with* meals to prevent epigastric pain, nausea, or vomiting. Other medications should be administered *between* meals because food interferes with absorption. Some CNS drugs and antihypertensives are best administered *at bedtime*, because they may cause drowsiness. Sildenafil (Viagra) is unique in that it should be taken 30 to 60 minutes prior to expected sexual intercourse, to achieve an effective erection. The nurse must pay careful attention to educating clients about

the timing of their medications, to enhance compliance and to increase the potential for therapeutic success.

Once medications are administered, the nurse must correctly document that they have been given to the client. It is necessary to include the drug name, dosage, time administered, any assessments, and the nurse's signature. If a medication is refused or omitted, this fact must be recorded on the appropriate form within the medical record. It is customary to document the reason, when possible. Should the client voice any concerns or complaints about the medication, these should also be included.

4.5 Systems of Measurement

Dosages are labeled and dispensed according to their weight or volume. Three systems of measurement are used in pharmacology: metric, apothecary, and household.

The most common system of drug measurement uses the **metric system.** The volume of a drug is expressed in terms of liters (L) or milliliters (ml). The cubic centimeter (cc) is a measurement of volume that is equivalent to 1 ml of fluid, but the *cc* abbreviation is no longer used because it can be mistaken for the abbreviation for unit (u) and cause medication errors. The metric weight of a drug is stated in kilograms (kg), grams (g), milligrams (mg), or micrograms (mcg). Note that the abbreviation μg should not be used for microgram, because it too can be confused with other abbreviations and cause a medication error.

The **apothecary** and **household systems** are older systems of measurement. Although most physicians and pharmacies use the metric system, these older systems are still encountered. Until the metric system totally replaces the other systems, the nurse must recognize dosages based on all three systems of measurement. Approximate equivalents between metric, apothecary, and household units of volume and weight are listed in Table 4.2.

TABLE 4.2 Metric, Apothecary, and Household Approximate Measurement Equivalents		
Metric	**Apothecary**	**Household**
1 ml	15–16 minims	15–16 drops
4–5 ml	1 fluid dram	1 teaspoon or 60 drops
15–16 ml	4 fluid drams	1 tablespoon or 3–4 teaspoons
30–32 ml	8 fluid drams or 1 fluid ounce	2 tablespoons
240–250 ml	8 fluid ounces (1/2 pint)	1 glass or cup
500 ml	1 pint	2 glasses or 2 cups
1 l	32 fluid ounces or 1 quart	4 glasses or 4 cups or 1 quart
1 mg	1/60 grain	————
60–64 mg	1 grain	————
300–325 mg	5 grains	————
1 g	15–16 grains	————
1 kg	————	2.2 pounds

To convert grains to grams: Divide grains by 15 or 16. To convert grams to grains: Multiply grams by 15 or 16. To convert minims to milliliters: Divide minims by 15 or 16.

Because Americans are very familiar with the teaspoon, tablespoon, and cup, it is important for the nurse to be able to convert between the household and metric systems of measurement. In the hospital, a glass of fluid is measured in milliliters—an 8-oz glass of water is recorded as 240 ml. If a client being discharged is ordered to drink 2,400 ml of fluid per day, the nurse may instruct the client to drink ten 8-oz glasses or 10 cups of fluid per day. Likewise, when a child is to be given a drug that is administered in elixir form, the nurse should explain that 5 ml of the drug is the same as 1 teaspoon. The nurse should encourage the use of accurate medical dosing devices at home, such as oral dosing syringes, oral droppers, cylindrical spoons, and medication cups. These are preferred over the traditional household measuring spoon because they are more accurate. Eating utensils that are commonly referred to as teaspoons or tablespoons often do not hold the volume that their names imply.

ROUTES OF DRUG ADMINISTRATION

The three broad categories of routes of drug administration are enteral, topical, and parenteral, and there are subsets within each of these. Each route has both advantages and disadvantages. Whereas some drugs are formulated to be given by several routes, others are specific to only one route. Pharmacokinetic considerations, such as how the route of administration affects drug absorption and distribution, are discussed in Chapter 5 ∞.

Certain protocols and techniques are common to all methods of drug administration. The student should review the drug administration guidelines in the following list before proceeding to subsequent sections that discuss specific routes of administration.

- Review the medication order and check for drug allergies.
- Wash your hands and apply gloves, if indicated.
- Use aseptic technique when preparing and administering parenteral medications.
- Identify the client by asking the person to state his or her full name (or by asking the parent or guardian), checking the identification band, and comparing this information with the MAR.
- Ask the client about known allergies.
- Inform the client of the drug's name and method of administration.
- Position the client for the appropriate route of administration.
- For enteral drugs, assist the client to a sitting position.
- If the drug is prepackaged (unit dose), remove it from the packaging at the bedside when possible.
- Unless specifically instructed to do so in the orders, do not leave drugs at the bedside.
- Document the medication administration and any pertinent client responses on the MAR.

Nursing in Action — Administering a Nasal Spray

4.6 Enteral Drug Administration

The **enteral route** includes drugs given orally and those administered through nasogastric or gastrostomy tubes. Oral drug administration is the most common, most convenient, and usually the least costly of all routes. It is also considered the safest route because the skin barrier is not compromised. In cases of overdose, medications remaining in the stomach can be retrieved by inducing vomiting. Oral preparations are available in tablet, capsule, and liquid forms. Medications administered by the enteral route take advantage of the vast absorptive surfaces of the oral mucosa, stomach, or small intestine.

TABLETS AND CAPSULES

Tablets and capsules are the most common forms of drugs. Clients prefer tablets or capsules over other routes and forms because of their ease of use. In some cases, tablets may be scored for more individualized dosing.

Some clients, particularly children, have difficulty swallowing tablets and capsules. Crushing tablets or opening capsules and sprinkling the drug over food or mixing it with juice will make it more palatable and easier to swallow. However, the nurse should not crush tablets or open capsules unless the manufacturer specifically states this is permissible. Some drugs are inactivated by crushing or opening, whereas others severely irritate the stomach mucosa and cause nausea or vomiting. Occasionally, drugs should not be crushed because they irritate the oral mucosa, are extremely bitter, or contain dyes that stain the teeth. Most drug guides provide lists of drugs that may not be crushed. Guidelines for administering tablets or capsules are given in Table 4.3A.

The strongly acidic contents within the stomach can present a destructive obstacle to the absorption of some medications. To overcome this barrier, tablets may have a hard, waxy coating that enables them to resist the acidity. These **enteric-coated** tablets are designed to dissolve in the alkaline environment of the small intestine. It is important that the nurse not crush enteric-coated tablets because the medication would then be directly exposed to the stomach environment.

Studies have clearly demonstrated that compliance declines as the number of doses per day increases. With this in mind, pharmacologists have attempted to design new drugs that may be administered only once or twice daily. **Sustained-release** tablets or capsules are designed to dissolve very slowly. This releases the medication over an extended time and results in a longer duration of action for the medication. Also called extended-release (XR), long-acting (LA), or slow-release (SR) medications, these forms allow for the convenience of once or twice a day dosing. Extended-release medications must not be crushed or opened.

Giving medications by the oral route has certain disadvantages. The client must be conscious and able to swallow properly. Certain types of drugs, including proteins, are inactivated by digestive enzymes in the stomach and small intestine. Medications absorbed from the stomach and small intestine first travel to the liver, where they may be inactivated before they ever reach their target organs. This

TABLE 4.3 Enteral Drug Administration

Drug Form	Administration Guidelines
A. tablet, capsule, or liquid	1. Assess that client is alert and has ability to swallow. 2. Place tablets or capsules into medication cup. 3. If liquid, shake the bottle to mix the agent, and measure the dose into the cup at eye level. 4. Hand the client the medication cup. 5. Offer a glass of water to facilitate swallowing the medication. Milk or juice may be offered if not contraindicated. 6. Remain with client until all medication is swallowed.
B. sublingual	1. Assess that client is alert and has ability to hold medication under tongue. 2. Place sublingual tablet under tongue. 3. Instruct client not to chew or swallow the tablet, or move the tablet around with tongue. 4. Instruct client to allow tablet to dissolve completely before swallowing saliva. 5. Remain with client to determine that all the medication has dissolved. 6. Offer a glass of water, if client desires.
C. buccal	1. Assess that client is alert and has ability to hold medication between the gums and the cheek. 2. Place buccal tablet between the gum line and the cheek. 3. Instruct client not to chew or swallow the tablet, or move the tablet around with tongue. 4. Instruct client to allow tablet to dissolve completely before swallowing saliva. 5. Remain with client to determine that all of the medication has dissolved. 6. Offer a glass of water, if client desires.
D. nasogastric and gastrostomy	1. Administer liquid forms when possible to avoid clogging the tube. 2. If solid, crush finely into powder and mix thoroughly with at least 30 ml of warm water until dissolved. 3. Assess and verify tube placement. 4. Turn off feeding, if applicable to client. 5. Aspirate stomach contents and measure the residual volume. If greater than 100 ml for an adult, check agency policy. 6. Return residual via gravity and flush with water. 7. Pour medication into syringe barrel and allow to flow into the tube by gravity. Give each medication separately, flushing between with water. 8. Keep head of bed elevated for 1 hour to prevent aspiration. 9. Reestablish continual feeding, as scheduled. Keep head of bed elevated 45° to prevent aspiration.

process, called *first-pass metabolism,* is discussed in Chapter 5 ∞. The significant variation in the motility of the GI tract and in its ability to absorb medications can create differences in bioavailability. In addition, children and some adults have an aversion to swallowing large tablets and capsules, or to taking oral medications that are distasteful.

SUBLINGUAL AND BUCCAL DRUG ADMINISTRATION

For sublingual and buccal administration, the tablet is not swallowed but kept in the mouth. The mucosa of the oral cavity contains a rich blood supply that provides an excellent absorptive surface for certain drugs. Medications given by this route are not subjected to destructive digestive enzymes, nor do they undergo hepatic first-pass metabolism.

For the **sublingual route,** the medication is placed under the tongue and allowed to dissolve slowly. Because of the rich blood supply in this region, the sublingual route results in a rapid onset of action. Sublingual dosage forms are most often formulated as rapidly disintegrating tablets or as soft gelatin capsules filled with liquid drug.

When multiple drugs have been ordered, the sublingual preparations should be administered after oral medications have been swallowed. The client should be instructed not to move the drug with the tongue, nor to eat or drink anything until the medication has completely dissolved. The sublingual mucosa is not suitable for extended-release formulations because it is a relatively small area and is constantly being bathed by a substantial amount of saliva. Table 4.3B and ● Figure 4.1a present important points regarding sublingual drug administration.

To administer by the **buccal route,** the tablet or capsule is placed in the oral cavity between the gum and the cheek. The client must be instructed not to manipulate the medication with the tongue; otherwise, it could get displaced to

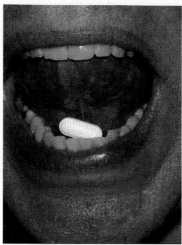

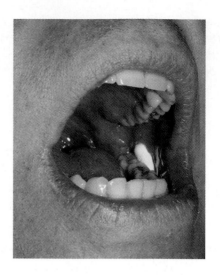

(a)   (b)

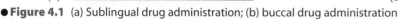

● **Figure 4.1** (a) Sublingual drug administration; (b) buccal drug administration

the sublingual area, where it would be more rapidly absorbed, or to the back of the throat, where it could be swallowed. The buccal mucosa is less permeable to most medications than the sublingual area, providing for slower absorption. The buccal route is preferred over the sublingual route for sustained-release delivery because of the greater mucosal surface area of the former. Drugs formulated for buccal administration generally do not cause irritation and are small enough to not cause discomfort to the client. As with the sublingual route, drugs administered by the buccal route avoid first-pass metabolism by the liver and the enzymatic processes of the stomach and small intestine. Table 4.3C and ● Figure 4.1b provide important guidelines for buccal drug administration.

NASOGASTRIC AND GASTROSTOMY DRUG ADMINISTRATION

Clients with a nasogastric tube or enteral feeding mechanism such as a gastrostomy tube may have their medications administered through these devices. A nasogastric (NG) tube is a soft, flexible tube inserted by way of the nasopharynx with the tip lying in the stomach. A gastrostomy (G) tube is surgically placed directly into the client's stomach. Generally, the NG tube is used for short-term treatment, whereas the G tube is inserted for clients requiring long-term care. Drugs administered through these tubes are usually in liquid form. Although solid drugs can be crushed or dissolved, they tend to cause clogging within the tubes. Sustained-release release drugs should not be crushed and administered through NG or G tubes. Drugs administered by this route are exposed to the same physiological processes as those given orally. Table 4.3D gives important guidelines for administering drugs through NG or G tubes.

4.7 Topical Drug Administration

Topical drugs are those applied locally to the skin or the membranous linings of the eye, ear, nose, respiratory tract,

urinary tract, vagina, and rectum. These applications include the following:

- *Dermatologic preparations* Drugs applied to the skin, the topical route most commonly used. Formulations include creams, lotions, gels, powders, and sprays.
- *Instillations and irrigations* Drugs applied into body cavities or orifices. These include the eyes, ears, nose, urinary bladder, rectum, and vagina.
- *Inhalations* Drugs applied to the respiratory tract by inhalers, nebulizers, or positive-pressure breathing apparatuses. The most common indication for inhaled drugs is bronchoconstriction due to bronchitis or asthma; however, a number of illegal, abused drugs are taken by this route because it provides a very rapid onset of drug action (see Chapter 12 ∞). Additional details on inhalation drug administration can be found in Chapter 39 ∞.

Many drugs are applied topically to produce a *local* effect. For example, antibiotics may be applied to the skin to treat skin infections. Antineoplastic agents may be instilled into the urinary bladder via catheter to treat tumors of the bladder mucosa. Corticosteroids are sprayed into the nostrils to reduce inflammation of the nasal mucosa due to allergic rhinitis. Local, topical delivery produces fewer side effects compared with oral or parenteral administration of the same drug. This is because topically applied drugs are absorbed very slowly, and amounts reaching the general circulation are minimal.

Some drugs are given topically to provide for slow release and absorption of the drug in the general circulation. These agents are administered for their *systemic* effects. For example, a nitroglycerin patch is applied to the skin not to treat a local skin condition but to treat a systemic condition, coronary artery disease. Likewise, prochlorperazine (Compazine) suppositories are inserted rectally not to treat a disease of the rectum but to alleviate nausea.

The distinction between topical drugs given for local effects and those given for systemic effects is an important one

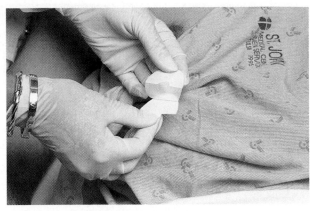

(a)

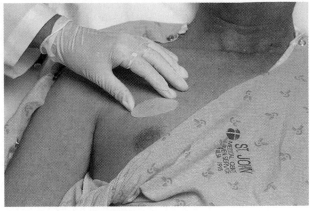

(b)

● **Figure 4.2** Transdermal patch administration: (a) protective coating removed from patch; (b) patch immediately applied to clean, dry, hairless skin and labeled with date, time, and initials *Source: Pearson Education/PH College.*

for the nurse. In the case of local drugs, absorption is undesirable and may cause side effects. For systemic drugs, absorption is essential for the therapeutic action of the drug. With either type of topical agent, drugs should not be applied to abraded or denuded skin, unless directed to do so.

TRANSDERMAL DELIVERY SYSTEM

The use of transdermal patches provides an effective means of delivering certain medications. Examples include nitroglycerin for angina pectoris and scopolamine (Transderm-Scop) for motion sickness. Although transdermal patches contain a specific amount of drug, the rate of delivery and the actual dose received may be variable. Patches are changed on a regular basis, using a site rotation routine, which should be documented in the MAR. Before apply-

ing a transdermal patch, the nurse should verify that the previous patch has been removed and disposed of appropriately. Drugs to be administered by this route avoid the first-pass effect in the liver and bypass digestive enzymes. Table 4.4A and ● Figure 4.2 illustrate the major points of transdermal drug delivery.

OPHTHALMIC ADMINISTRATION

The ophthalmic route is used to treat local conditions of the eye and surrounding structures. Common indications include excessive dryness, infections, glaucoma, and dilation of the pupil during eye examinations. Ophthalmic drugs are available in the form of eye irrigations, drops, ointments, and medicated disks. ● Figure 4.3 (a) and (b) and Table 4.4 give guidelines for adult administration.

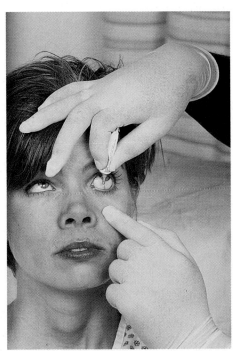

(a)

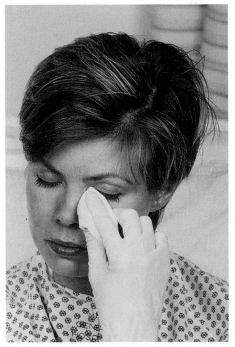

(b)

● **Figure 4.3** (a) Instilling an eye ointment into the lower conjunctival sac; (b) pressing on the nasolacrimal duct *Source: ©Jenny Thomas Photography.*

TABLE 4.4	Topical Drug Administration
Drug Form	**Administration Guidelines**
A. transdermal	1. Obtain transdermal patch, and read manufacturer's guidelines. Application site and frequency of changing differ according to medication.
	2. Apply gloves before handling, to avoid absorption of the agent by the nurse.
	3. Remove previous medication or patch, and cleanse area.
	4. If using a transdermal ointment, apply the ordered amount of medication in an even line directly on the premeasured paper that accompanies the medication tube.
	5. Press patch or apply medicated paper to clean, dry, and hairless skin.
	6. Rotate sites to prevent skin irritation.
	7. Label patch with date, time, and initials.
B. ophthalmic	1. Instruct client to lie supine or sit with head slightly tilted back.
	2. With nondominant hand, pull lower lid down gently to expose the conjunctival sac, creating a pocket.
	3. Ask client to look upward.
	4. Hold eyedropper 1/4–1/8 inch above the conjunctival sac. Do not hold dropper over eye, as this may stimulate the blink reflex.
	5. Instill prescribed number of drops into the center of the pocket. Avoid touching eye or conjunctival sac with tip of eyedropper.
	6. If applying ointment, apply a thin line of ointment evenly along inner edge of lower lid margin, from inner to outer canthus.
	7. Instruct the client to close eye gently. Apply gentle pressure with finger to the nasolacrimal duct at the inner canthus for 1–2 minutes, to avoid overflow drainage into nose and throat, thus minimizing risk of absorption into the systemic circulation.
	8. With tissue, remove excess medication around eye.
	9. Replace dropper. Do not rinse eyedropper.
C. otic	1. Instruct client to lie on side or to sit with head tilted so that affected ear is facing up.
	2. If necessary, clean the pinna of the ear and the meatus with a clean washcloth to prevent any discharge from being washed into the ear canal during the instillation of the drops.
	3. Hold dropper 1/4 inch above ear canal, and instill prescribed number of drops into the side of the ear canal, allowing the drops to flow downward. Avoid placing drops directly on the tympanic membrane.
	4. Gently apply intermittent pressure to the tragus of the ear three or four times.
	5. Instruct client to remain on side for up to 10 minutes to prevent loss of medication.
	6. If cotton ball is ordered, presoak with medication and insert it into the outermost part of ear canal.
	7. Wipe any solution that may have dripped from the ear canal with a tissue.
D. nasal drops	1. Ask the client to blow the nose to clear nasal passages.
	2. Draw up the correct volume of drug into dropper.
	3. Instruct the client to open and breathe through the mouth.
	4. Hold the tip of the dropper just above the nostril, and without touching the nose with the dropper, direct the solution laterally toward the midline of the superior concha of the ethmoid bone—not the base of the nasal cavity, where it will run down the throat and into the eustachian tube.
	5. Ask the client to remain in position for 5 minutes.
	6. Discard any remaining solution that is in the dropper.
E. vaginal	1. Instruct the client to assume a supine position with knees bent and separated.
	2. Place water-soluble lubricant into medicine cup.
	3. Apply gloves; open suppository and lubricate the rounded end.
	4. Expose the vaginal orifice by separating the labia with nondominant hand.
	5. Insert the rounded end of the suppository about 8–10 cm along the posterior wall of the vagina, or as far as it will pass.
	6. If using a cream, jelly, or foam, gently insert applicator 5 cm along the posterior vaginal wall and slowly push the plunger until empty. Remove the applicator and place on a paper towel.
	7. Ask the client to lower legs and remain lying in the supine or side-lying position for 5–10 minutes following insertion.

TABLE 4.4 Topical Drug Administration *(Continued)*	
Drug Form	**Administration Guidelines**
F. rectal suppositories	1. Instruct the client to lie on left side (Sims' position). 2. Apply gloves; open suppository and lubricate the rounded end. 3. Lubricate the gloved forefinger of the dominant hand with water-soluble lubricant. 4. Inform the client when the suppository is to be inserted; instruct the client to take slow, deep breaths and deeply exhale during insertion, to relax the anal sphincter. 5. Gently insert the lubricated end of suppository into the rectum, beyond the anal–rectal ridge to ensure retention. 6. Instruct the client to remain in the Sims' position or lie supine to prevent expulsion of the suppository. 7. Instruct the client to retain the suppository for at least 30 minutes to allow absorption to occur, unless the suppository is administered to stimulate defecation.

Although the procedure is the same with a child, it is advisable to enlist the help of an adult caregiver. In some cases, the infant or toddler may need to be immobilized with arms wrapped to prevent accidental injury to the eye during administration. For the young child, demonstrating the procedure using a doll facilitates cooperation and decreases anxiety.

OTIC ADMINISTRATION

The otic route is used to treat local conditions of the ear, including infections and soft blockages of the auditory canal. Otic medications include eardrops and irrigations, which are usually ordered for cleaning purposes. Administration to infants and young children must be performed carefully to avoid injury to sensitive structures of the ear. ● Figure 4.4 and Table 4.4C present key points in administering otic medications.

NASAL ADMINISTRATION

The nasal route is used for both local and systemic drug administration. The nasal mucosa provides an excellent absorptive surface for certain medications. Advantages of this route include ease of use and avoidance of the first-pass effect and digestive enzymes. Nasal spray formulations of corticosteroids have revolutionized the treatment of allergic rhinitis owing to their high safety margin when administered by this route.

Although the nasal mucosa provides an excellent surface for drug delivery, there is the potential for damage to the cilia within the nasal cavity, and mucosal irritation is common. In addition, unpredictable mucus secretion among some individuals may affect drug absorption from this site.

Drops or sprays are often used for their local **astringent effect;** that is, they shrink swollen mucous membranes or loosen secretions and facilitate drainage. This brings immediate relief from the nasal congestion caused by the common cold. The nose also provides the route to reach the nasal sinuses and the eustachian tube. Proper positioning of the client prior to instilling nose drops for sinus disorders depends on which sinuses are being treated. The same holds true for treatment of the eustachian tube. Table 4.4D and ● Figure 4.5 illustrate important facts related to nasal drug administration.

VAGINAL ADMINISTRATION

The vaginal route is used to deliver medications for treating local infections and to relieve vaginal pain and itching. Vaginal medications are inserted as suppositories, creams, jellies, or foams. It is important that the nurse explain the purpose of treatment and provide for privacy and client dignity. Before inserting vaginal drugs, the nurse should instruct the client to empty her bladder, to lessen both the discomfort during treatment and the possibility of irritating or injuring the vaginal lining. The client should be offered a perineal pad following administration. Table 4.4E and ● Figure 4.6 (a) and (b) provide guidelines regarding vaginal drug administration.

RECTAL ADMINISTRATION

The rectal route may be used for either local or systemic drug administration. It is a safe and effective means of delivering drugs to clients who are comatose or who are experiencing nausea and vomiting. Rectal drugs are normally in suppository form, although a few laxatives and

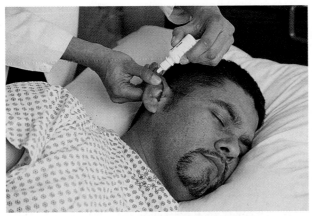

● **Figure 4.4** Instilling eardrops *Source: ©Elena Dorfman.*

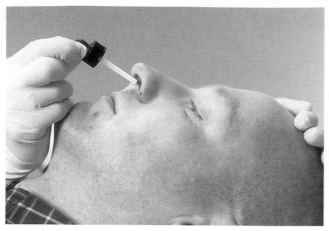

● **Figure 4.5** Nasal drug administration *Source: Pearson Education/PH College.*

diagnostic agents are given via enema. Although absorption is slower than by other routes, it is steady and reliable provided the medication can be retained by the client. Venous blood from the lower rectum is not transported by way of the liver; thus, the first-pass effect is avoided, as are the digestive enzymes of the upper GI tract. Table 4.4F gives selected details regarding rectal drug administration.

4.8 Parenteral Drug Administration

Parenteral administration refers to the dispensing of medications by routes other than oral or topical. The **parenteral route** delivers drugs via a needle into the skin layers, subcutaneous tissue, muscles, or veins. More advanced parenteral delivery includes administration into arteries, body cavities (such as intrathecal), and organs (such as intracardiac). Parenteral drug administration is much more invasive than topical or enteral. Because of the potential for introducing pathogenic microbes directly into the blood or body tissues, aseptic techniques must be strictly applied. The nurse is ex-

pected to identify and use appropriate materials for parenteral drug delivery, including specialized equipment and techniques involved in the preparation and administration of injectable products. The nurse must know the correct anatomical locations for parenteral administration, and safety procedures regarding hazardous equipment disposal.

INTRADERMAL AND SUBCUTANEOUS ADMINISTRATION

Injection into the skin delivers drugs to the blood vessels that supply the various layers of the skin. Drugs may be injected either intradermally or subcutaneously. The major difference between these methods is the depth of injection. An advantage of both methods is that they offer a means of administering drugs to clients who are unable to take them orally. Drugs administered by these routes avoid the hepatic first-pass effect and digestive enzymes. Disadvantages are that only small volumes can be administered, and injections can cause pain and swelling at the injection site.

An **intradermal (ID)** injection is administered into the dermis layer of the skin. Because the dermis contains more blood vessels than the deeper subcutaneous layer, drugs are more easily absorbed. Intradermal injection is usually employed for allergy and disease screening or for local anesthetic delivery prior to venous cannulation. Intradermal injections are limited to very small volumes of drug, usually only 0.1 to 0.2 ml. The usual sites for ID injections are the nonhairy skin surfaces of the upper back, over the scapulae, the high upper chest, and the inner forearm. Guidelines for intradermal injections are given in Table 4.5A (page 40) and ● Figure 4.7.

A **subcutaneous** injection is delivered to the deepest layers of the skin. Insulin, heparin, vitamins, some vaccines, and other medications are given in this area because the sites are easily accessible and provide rapid absorption. Body sites that are ideal for subcutaneous injections include the following:

• Outer aspect of the upper arms, in the area above the triceps muscle

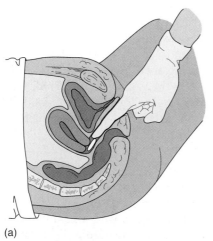

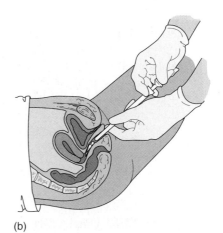

(a)   (b)

● **Figure 4.6** Vaginal drug administration: (a) instilling a vaginal suppository; (b) using an applicator to instill a vaginal cream
Source: Pearson Education/PH College.

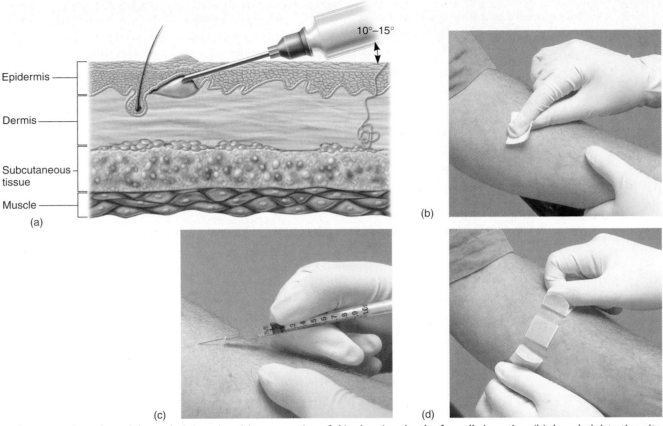

10°–15°

Epidermis

Dermis

Subcutaneous
tissue

Muscle

(a)

(b)

(c)

(d)

● **Figure 4.7** Intradermal drug administration: (a) cross section of skin showing depth of needle insertion; (b) the administration site is prepped; (c) the needle is inserted, bevel up at 10–15°; (d) the needle is removed and the puncture site is covered with an adhesive bandage *Source: Pearson Education/PH College.*

- Middle two-thirds of the anterior thigh area
- Subscapular areas of the upper back
- Upper dorsogluteal and ventrogluteal areas
- Abdominal areas, above the iliac crest and below the diaphragm, 1.5 to 2 inches out from the umbilicus

Subcutaneous doses are small in volume, usually ranging from 0.5 to 1 ml. The needle size varies with the client's quantity of body fat. The length is usually half the size of a pinched/bunched skinfold that can be grasped between the thumb and forefinger. It is important to rotate injection sites in an orderly and documented manner, to promote absorption, minimize tissue damage, and alleviate discomfort. For insulin, however, rotation should be within an anatomical area to promote reliable absorption and maintain consistent blood glucose levels. When performing subcutaneous injections, it is not necessary to aspirate prior to the injection. Note that tuberculin syringes and insulin syringes are not interchangeable, so the nurse should not substitute one for the other. Table 4.5B and ● Figure 4.8 include important information regarding subcutaneous drug administration.

INTRAMUSCULAR ADMINISTRATION

An **intramuscular (IM)** injection delivers medication into specific muscles. Because muscle tissue has a rich blood supply, medication moves quickly into blood vessels to produce a more rapid onset of action than with oral, ID, or subcutaneous administration. The anatomical structure of muscle permits this tissue to receive a larger volume of medication than the subcutaneous region. An adult with well-developed muscles can safely tolerate up to 4 ml of medication in a large muscle, although only 2 to 3 ml is recommended. The deltoid and triceps muscles should receive a maximum of 1 ml.

A major consideration for the nurse regarding IM drug administration is the selection of an appropriate injection site. Injection sites must be located away from bone, large blood vessels, and nerves. The size and length of needle are determined by body size and muscle mass, the type of drug to be administered, the amount of adipose tissue overlying the muscle, and the age of the client. Information regarding IM injections is given in Table 4.5 and ● Figure 4.9. The four common sites for intramuscular injections are as follows:

1. *Ventrogluteal site* The preferred site for IM injections. This area provides the greatest thickness of gluteal muscles, contains no large blood vessels or nerves, is sealed off by bone, and contains less fat than the buttock area, thus eliminating the need to determine the depth of subcutaneous fat. It is a suitable site for children and infants over 7 months of age.

TABLE 4.5 Parenteral Drug Administration	
Drug Form	**Administration Guidelines**
A. intradermal route	1. Prepare medication in a tuberculin or 1-ml syringe with a preattached 26- to 27-gauge, 3/8- to 5/8-inch needle.
	2. Apply gloves and cleanse injection site with antiseptic swab in a circular motion. Allow to air dry.
	3. With thumb and index finger of nondominant hand, spread skin taut.
	4. Insert needle, with bevel facing upward, at angle of 10–15°.
	5. Advance needle until entire bevel is under skin; do not aspirate.
	6. Slowly inject medication to form small wheal or bleb.
	7. Withdraw needle quickly, and pat site gently with sterile 2 × 2 gauze pad. Do not massage area.
	8. Instruct the client not to rub or scratch the area.
	9. Draw circle around perimeter of injection site. Read in 48 to 72 hours.
B. subcutaneous route	1. Prepare medication in a 1- to 3-ml syringe using a 23- to 25-gauge, 1/2- to 5/8-inch needle. For heparin, the recommended needle is 3/8 inch and 25–26 gauge.
	2. Choose site, avoiding areas of bony prominence, major nerves, and blood vessels. For heparin, check with agency policy for the preferred injection sites.
	3. Check previous rotation sites and select a new area for injection.
	4. Apply gloves and cleanse injection site with antiseptic swab in a circular motion.
	5. Allow to air dry.
	6. Bunch the skin between thumb and index finger of nondominant hand or spread taut if there is substantial subcutaneous tissue.
	7. Insert needle at 45° or 90° angle depending on body size: 90° if obese; 45° if average weight. If the client is very thin, gather skin at area of needle insertion and administer at 90° angle.
	8. For nonheparin injections, aspirate by pulling back on plunger. If blood appears, withdraw the needle, discard the syringe, and prepare a new injection. For heparin, do not aspirate, as this can damage surrounding tissues and cause bruising.
	9. Inject medication slowly.
	10. Remove needle quickly, and gently massage site with antiseptic swab. For heparin, do not massage the site, as this may cause bruising or bleeding.
C. intramuscular route: ventrogluteal, vastus lateralis, and deltoid muscle sites	1. Prepare medication using a 20- to 23-gauge, 1- to 1.5-inch needle.
	2. Apply gloves and cleanse injection site with antiseptic swab in a circular motion. Allow to air dry.
	3. Locate site by placing the hand with heel on the greater trochanter and thumb toward umbilicus. Point to the anterior iliac spine with the index finger, spreading the middle finger to point toward the iliac crest (forming a V). Inject medication within the V-shaped area of the index and third finger.
	4. Insert needle with smooth, dartlike movement at a 90° angle within V-shaped area.
	5. Aspirate, and observe for blood. If blood appears, withdraw the needle, discard the syringe, and prepare a new injection.
	6. Inject medication slowly and with smooth, even pressure on the plunger.
	7. Remove needle quickly.
	8. Apply pressure to site with a dry, sterile 2 × 2 gauze and massage vigorously to create warmth and promote absorption of the medication into the muscle.
D. intravenous route	1. To add drug to an IV fluid container:
	a. Verify order and compatibility of drug with IV fluid.
	b. Prepare medication in a 5- to 20-ml syringe using a 1- to 1.5-inch, 19- to 21-gauge needle. (Typically in an adult, a 22-gauge needle is used for fluid administration, but the size may vary with the client's body size and the reason for IV administration.)
	c. Apply gloves and assess injection site for signs and symptoms of inflammation or extravasation.
	d. Locate medication port on IV fluid container and cleanse with antiseptic swab.
	e. Carefully insert needle or access device into port and inject medication.
	f. Withdraw needle and mix solution by rotating container end to end.
	g. Hang container and check infusion rate.

TABLE 4.5	Parenteral Drug Administration (*Continued*)
Drug Form	**Administration Guidelines**
	2. To add drug to an IV bolus (IV push) using existing IV line or IV lock (reseal):
	a. Verify order and compatibility of drug with IV fluid.
	b. Determine the correct rate of infusion.
	c. Determine if IV fluids are infusing at proper rate (IV line) and that IV site is adequate.
	d. Prepare drug in a syringe.
	e. Apply gloves and assess injection site for signs and symptoms of inflammation or extravasation.
	f. Select injection port, on tubing, closest to insertion site (IV line).
	g. Cleanse tubing or lock port with antiseptic swab and insert needle into port.
	h. If administering medication through an existing IV line, occlude tubing by pinching just above the injection port.
	i. Slowly inject medication over designated time; usually not faster that 1 ml/min, unless specified.
	j. Withdraw syringe. Release tubing and ensure proper IV infusion if using an existing IV line.
	k. If using an IV lock, check agency policy for use of saline flush before and after injecting medications.

2. *Deltoid site* Used in well-developed teens and adults for volumes of medication not to exceed 1 ml. Because the radial nerve lies in close proximity, the deltoid is not generally used, except for small-volume vaccines, such as for hepatitis B in adults.

3. *Dorsogluteal site* Used for adults and for children who have been walking for at least 6 months. The site is safe as long as the nurse appropriately locates the injection landmarks to avoid puncture or irritation of the sciatic nerve and blood vessels.

4. *Vastus lateralis site* Usually thick and well developed in both adults and children, the middle third of the muscle is the site for IM injections.

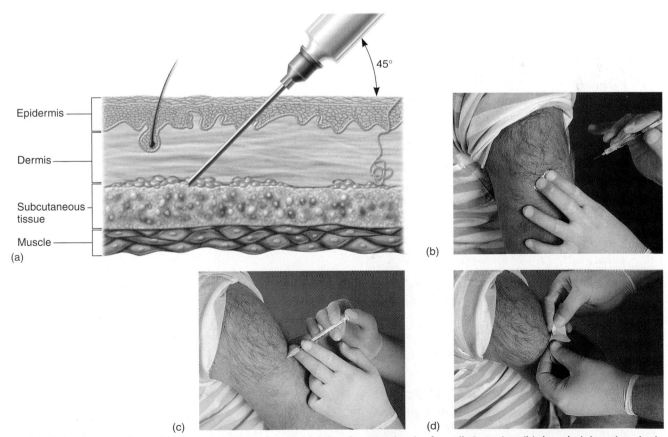

● **Figure 4.8** Subcutaneous drug administration: (a) cross section of skin showing depth of needle insertion; (b) the administration site is prepped; (c) the needle is inserted at a 45° angle; (d) the needle is removed and the puncture site is covered with an adhesive bandage *Source: Pearson Education/PH College.*

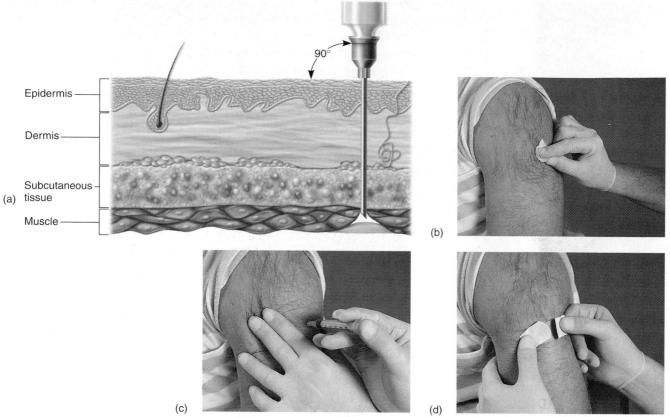

Epidermis

Dermis

Subcutaneous tissue

Muscle

(a)

90°

(b)

(c)

(d)

● **Figure 4.9** Intramuscular drug administration: (a) cross section of skin showing depth of needle insertion; (b) the administration site is prepped; (c) the needle is inserted at a 90° angle; (d) the needle is removed and the puncture site is covered with an adhesive bandage
Source: Pearson Education/PH College.

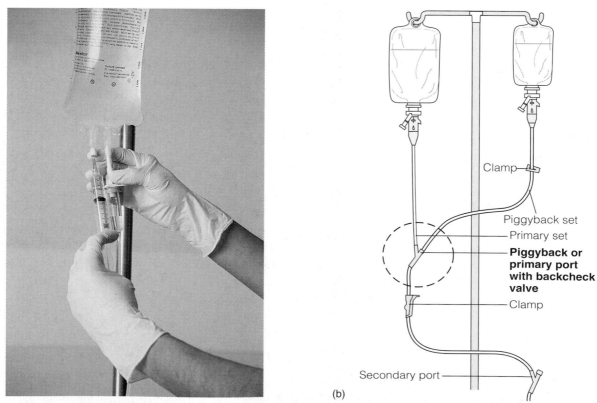

Clamp

Piggyback set

Primary set

Piggyback or primary port with backcheck valve

Clamp

Secondary port

(a)

(b)

● **Figure 4.10** Secondary intravenous lines: (a) a tandem intravenous alignment; (b) an intravenous piggyback (IVPB) alignment

Chapter 4 Principles of Drug Administration **43**

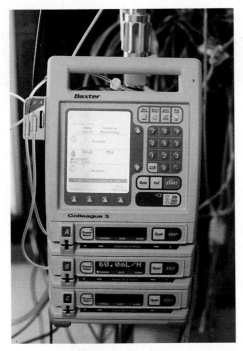

●**Figure 4.11** A Baxter infusion pump.

INTRAVENOUS ADMINISTRATION

Intravenous (IV) medications and fluids are administered directly into the bloodstream and are immediately available for use by the body. The IV route is used when a very rapid onset of action is desired. So with other parenteral routes, IV medications bypass the enzymatic process of the digestive system and the first-pass effect of the liver. The three basic types of IV administration are as follows:

1. *Large-volume infusion* For fluid maintenance, replacement, or supplementation. Compatible drugs may be mixed into a large-volume IV container with fluids such as normal saline or Ringer's lactate. Table 4.5D and ● Figure 4.10 illustrate this technique.

2. *Intermittent infusion* Small amount of IV solution that is arranged tandem with or piggybacked to the primary large-volume infusion. Used to instill adjunct medications, such as antibiotics or analgesics, over a short time period. ● Figure 4.11 shows a Baxter infusion pump.

3. *IV bolus (push) administration* Concentrated dose delivered directly to the circulation via syringe to administer single-dose medications. Bolus injections may be given through an intermittent injection port or by direct IV push. Details on the bolus administration technique are given in Table 4.5D and ● Figure 4.12.

Although the IV route offers the fastest onset of drug action, it is also the most dangerous. Once injected, the medication cannot be retrieved. If the drug solution or the needle is contaminated, pathogens have a direct route to the bloodstream and body tissues. Clients who are receiving IV injections must be closely monitored for adverse reactions. Some adverse reactions occur immediately after injection; others may take hours or days to appear. Antidotes for drugs that can cause potentially dangerous or fatal reactions must always be readily available.

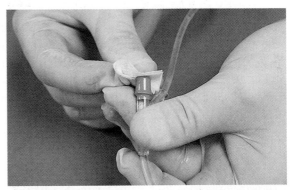

(a)

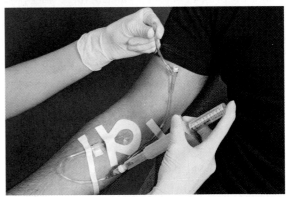

(b)

●**Figure 4.12** IV bolus administration. (a) The part is cleaned; (b) the drug is administered through the port using a needleless syringe.

Nursing in Action Administering Medications by IV Piggyback

Nursing in Action Administering Medications by IV Push

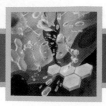

CHAPTER REVIEW

KEY CONCEPTS

The numbered key concepts provide a succinct summary of the important points from the corresponding numbered section within the chapter. If any of these points are not clear, refer to the numbered section within the chapter for review.

4.1 The nurse must have a comprehensive knowledge of the actions and side effects of drugs before they are administered to limit the number and severity of adverse drugs events.

4.2 The five rights and three checks are guidelines for safe drug administration, which is a collaborative effort among nurses, physicians, and other healthcare professionals.

4.3 For pharmacologic compliance, the client must understand and personally accept the value associated with the prescribed drug regimen. Understanding the reasons for noncompliance can help the nurse increase the success of pharmacotherapy.

4.4 There are established orders and time schedules by which medications are routinely administered. Documentation of drug administration and reporting of side effects are important responsibilities of the nurse.

4.5 Systems of measurement used in pharmacology include the metric, apothecary, and household systems. Although the metric system is most commonly used, the nurse must be able to convert dosages among the three systems of measurement.

4.6 The enteral route includes drugs given orally and those administered through nasogastric or gastrostomy tubes. This is the most common route of drug administration.

4.7 Topical drugs are applied locally to the skin or membranous linings of the eye, ear, nose, respiratory tract, urinary tract, vagina, and rectum.

4.8 Parenteral administration is the dispensing of medications via a needle, usually into the skin layers (ID), subcutaneous tissue, muscles (IM), or veins (IV).

NCLEX-RN® REVIEW QUESTIONS

1 What is the primary role of a nurse in medication administration?

1. Ensure medications are administered and delivered in a safe manner.
2. Be certain that physician orders are accurate.
3. Inform the client that prescribed medications need be taken only if the client agrees with the treatment plan.
4. Assure client compliance by watching the client swallow all prescribed medications.

2 Before administering drugs by the enteral route, the nurse should evaluate which of the following?

1. Ability of the client to lie supine
2. Compatibility of the drug with IV fluid
3. Ability of the client to swallow
4. Patency of the injection port

3 Which of the following is the highest nursing priority when a client has an allergic reaction to a newly prescribed medication?

1. Instruct the client to remain calm.
2. Document the allergy in the medical record.
3. Notify the physician of the allergic reaction.
4. Place an allergy bracelet on the client.

4 The order reads, "Lasix 40 mg IV STAT." Which of the following actions should the nurse take?

1. Administer the medication within 30 minutes of the order.
2. Administer the medication within 5 minutes of the order.
3. Administer the medication as required by the client's condition.
4. Assess the client's urinary output prior to administration and hold medication if output is less than 30 mL/h.

5 Which of the following medications would not be administered through a nasogastric tube? (Select all that apply.)

1. Liquids
2. Enteric-coated tablets
3. Sustained-release tablets
4. Tablets
5. IV medications

CRITICAL THINKING QUESTIONS

1. Why do errors continue to occur despite the fact that the nurse follows the five rights and three checks of drug administration?

2. What strategies can the nurse employ to ensure drug compliance for a patient who is refusing to take his or her - medication?

3. Compare the oral, topical, IM, subcutaneous, and IV routes. Which has the fastest onset of drug action? Which routes avoid the hepatic first-pass effect? Which require strict aseptic technique?

4. What are the advantages of the metric system of measurement over the household or apothecary systems?

See Appendix D for answers and rationales for all activities.

 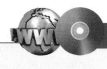

EXPLORE
MediaLink

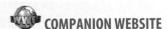
www.prenhall.com/adams

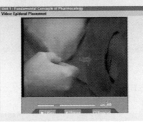

NCLEX-RN® review, case studies, and other interactive resources for this chapter can be found on the companion website at www.prenhall.com/adams. Click on "Chapter 4" to select the activities for this chapter. For animations, more NCLEX-RN® review questions, and an audio glossary, access the accompanying Prentice Hall Nursing MediaLink DVD-ROM in this textbook.

PRENTICE HALL NURSING MEDIALINK DVD-ROM

- **Audio Glossary**
- **NCLEX-RN® Review**
- **Nursing in Action**
  Administering Medications through a Nasogastric Tube
  Administering Dermatologic Medications
  Administering Eye Drops
  Administering Medications by IV Piggyback
  Administering Medications by IV Push
  Administering Subcutaneous Medications (Abdomen)
  Administering Subcutaneous Medications
  Administering a Z-track Medication
  Administering an IM Injection
  Administering Medication by Inhaler
  Administering a Nasal Spray
  Administering Ear Drops

COMPANION WEBSITE

- **NCLEX-RN® Review**
- **Case Study:** Client taking Glucotrol XL
- **Challenge Your Knowledge**

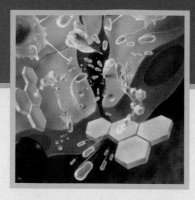

CHAPTER 5

Pharmacokinetics

OBJECTIVES

After reading this chapter, the student should be able to:

1. Explain the applications of pharmacokinetics to clinical practice.
2. Identify the four components of pharmacokinetics.
3. Explain how substances travel across plasma membranes.
4. Discuss factors affecting drug absorption.
5. Explain the metabolism of drugs and its applications to pharmacotherapy.
6. Discuss how drugs are distributed throughout the body.
7. Describe how plasma proteins affect drug distribution.
8. Identify major processes by which drugs are excreted.
9. Explain how enterohepatic recirculation might affect drug activity.
10. Explain the applications of a drug's plasma half-life ($t_{1/2}$) to pharmacotherapy.
11. Explain how a drug reaches and maintains its therapeutic range in the plasma.
12. Differentiate between loading and maintenance doses.

MediaLink

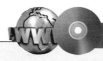

www.prenhall.com/adams

NCLEX-RN® review, case studies, and other interactive resources for this chapter can be found on the companion website at www.prenhall.com/adams. Click on "Chapter 5" to select the activities for this chapter. For animations, more NCLEX-RN® review questions, and an audio glossary, access the accompanying Prentice Hall Nursing MediaLink DVD-ROM in this textbook.

KEY TERMS

absorption   *page 48*

affinity   *page 49*

blood–brain barrier   *page 50*

conjugates   *page 50*

distribution   *page 49*

drug–protein complex   *page 49*

enterohepatic recirculation   *page 52*

enzyme induction   *page 50*

excretion   *page 51*

fetal–placental barrier   *page 50*

first-pass effect   *page 51*

hepatic microsomal enzyme system
   page 50

loading dose   *page 53*

maintenance dose   *page 54*

metabolism   *page 50*

minimum effective concentration   *page 53*

pharmacokinetics   *page 47*

plasma half-life (t½)   *page 53*

prodrug   *page 50*

therapeutic range   *page 53*

toxic concentration   *page 53*

Medications are given to achieve a desirable effect. To produce this therapeutic effect, the drug must reach its target cells. For some medications, such as topical agents used to treat superficial skin conditions, this is an easy task. For others, however, the process of reaching target cells in sufficient quantities to cause a physiological change may be challenging. Drugs are exposed to a myriad of different barriers and destructive processes after they enter the body. The purpose of this chapter is to examine factors that act on the drug as it attempts to reach its target cells.

5.1 Pharmacokinetics: How the Body Handles Medications

The term **pharmacokinetics** is derived from the root words *pharmaco*, which means "medicine" and *kinetics*, which means "movement or motion." Pharmacokinetics is thus the study of drug movement throughout the body. In practical terms, it describes how the body handles medications. Pharmacokinetics is a core subject in pharmacology, and a firm grasp of this topic allows nurses to better understand and predict the actions and side effects of medications in their patients.

Drugs face numerous obstacles in reaching their target cells. For most medications, the greatest barrier is crossing the many membranes that separate the drug from its target cells. A drug taken by mouth, for example, must cross the plasma membranes of the mucosal cells of the gastrointestinal tract and the capillary endothelial cells to enter the bloodstream. To leave the bloodstream, the drug must again cross capillary cells, travel through the interstitial fluid, and depending on the mechanism of action, the drug may also need to enter target cells and cellular organelles such as the nucleus, which are surrounded by additional membranes. These are just some of the membranes and barriers that a drug must successfully penetrate before it can elicit a response.

While seeking their target cells and attempting to pass through the various membranes drugs are subjected to numerous physiological processes. For medications given by the enteral route, stomach acid and digestive enzymes often act to break down the drug molecules. Enzymes in the liver and other organs may chemically change the drug molecule to make it less active. If the drug is seen as foreign by the body, phagocytes may attempt to remove it, or an immune response may be triggered. The kidneys, large intestine, and other organs attempt to excrete the medication from the body.

These examples illustrate pharmacokinetic processes: how the body handles medications. The many processes of pharmacokinetics are grouped into four categories: absorption, distribution, metabolism, and excretion, as illustrated in ● Figure 5.1.

5.2 The Passage of Drugs through Plasma Membranes

Pharmacokinetic variables depend on the ability of a drug to cross plasma membranes. With few exceptions, drugs must penetrate these membranes to produce their effects. Like other chemicals, drugs primarily use two processes to cross body membranes.

1. *Diffusion or passive transport* Movement of a chemical from an area of higher concentration to an area of lower concentration

2. *Active transport* Movement of a chemical against a concentration or electrochemical gradient

Plasma membranes consist of a lipid bilayer, with proteins and other molecules interspersed in the membrane. This lipophilic membrane is relatively impermeable

MediaLink Council on Family Health

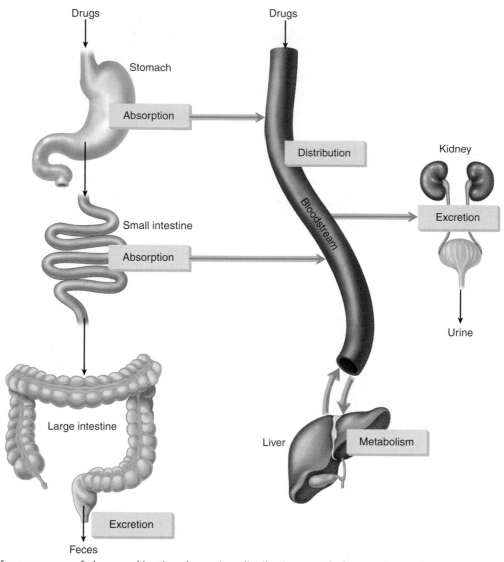

● **Figure 5.1** The four processes of pharmacokinetics: absorption, distribution, metabolism, and excretion

to large molecules, ions, and polar molecules. These physical characteristics have direct application to pharmacokinetics. For example, drug molecules that are small, nonionized, and lipid soluble will usually pass through plasma membranes by simple diffusion and more easily reach their target cells. Small water-soluble agents such as urea, alcohol, and water can enter through pores in the plasma membrane. Large molecules, ionized drugs, and water-soluble agents, however, will have more difficulty crossing plasma membranes. These agents may use other means to gain entry, such as carrier proteins or active transport. Drugs may not need to enter the cell to produce their effects. Once bound to receptors, located on the plasma membrane, some drugs activate a second messenger within the cell, which produces the physiological change (see Chapter 6 ∞).

5.3 Absorption of Medications

Absorption is a process involving the movement of a substance from its site of administration, across body mem-

branes, to circulating fluids. Drugs may be absorbed across the skin and associated mucous membranes, or they may move across membranes that line the GI or respiratory tract. Most drugs, with the exception of a few topical medications, intestinal anti-infectives, and some radiological contrast agents, must be absorbed to produce an effect.

Absorption is the primary pharmacokinetic factor determining the length of time it takes a drug to produce its effect. In general, the more rapid the absorption, the faster the onset of drug action. Drugs that are used in critical care are designed to be absorbed within seconds or minutes. At the other extreme are drugs such as the contraceptive Mirena (levonorgestrel–releasing intrauterine system), which is a polyethylene tube placed in the uterus. The drug is absorbed slowly and provides contraceptive protection for up to 5 years.

Absorption is conditional on many factors. Drugs administered IV have the most rapid onset of action. Drugs in elixir or syrup formulations are absorbed faster than tablets or capsules. Drugs administered in high doses are generally

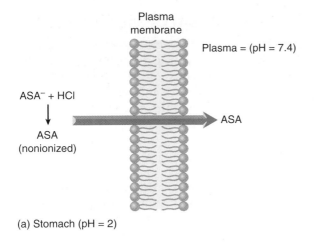

(a) Stomach (pH = 2)

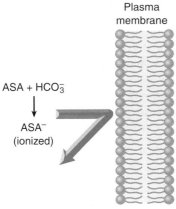

(b) Small intestine (pH = 8)

● **Figure 5.2** Effect of pH on drug absorption: (a) a weak acid such as aspirin (ASA) is in a nonionized form in an acidic environment and absorption occurs; (b) in a basic environment, aspirin is mostly in an ionized form and absorption is prevented

absorbed more quickly and have a more rapid onset of action than those given in low concentrations. Digestive motility, exposure to enzymes in the digestive tract, and blood flow to the site of drug administration also affect absorption.

The degree of ionization of a drug also affects its absorption. A drug's ability to become ionized depends on the surrounding pH. Aspirin provides an excellent example of the effects of ionization on absorption, as depicted in ● Figure 5.2. In the acid environment of the stomach, aspirin is in its *nonionized* form and thus readily absorbed and distributed by the bloodstream. As aspirin enters the alkaline environment of the small intestine, however, it becomes ionized. In its ionized form, aspirin is not as likely to be absorbed and distributed to target cells. Unlike acidic drugs, medications that are weakly basic are in their nonionized form in an *alkaline* environment; therefore, basic drugs are absorbed and distributed better in alkaline environments such as in the small intestine. The pH of the local environment directly influences drug absorption through its ability to ionize the drug. In simplest terms, it may help the student to remember that acids are absorbed in acids, and bases are absorbed in bases.

Drug–drug or food–drug interactions may influence absorption. Many examples of these interactions have been discovered. For example, administering tetracyclines with food or drugs containing calcium, iron, or magnesium can significantly delay absorption of the antibiotic. High-fat meals can slow stomach motility significantly and delay the absorption of oral medications taken with the meal. Dietary supplements may also affect absorption. Common ingredients in herbal weight-loss products such as aloe leaf, guar gum, senna, and yellow dock exert a laxative effect that may decrease intestinal transit time and reduce drug absorption (Scott & Elmer, 2002). The nurse must be aware of drug interactions and advise clients to avoid known combinations of foods and medications that significantly affect drug action.

5.4 Distribution of Medications

Distribution involves the transport of pharmacologic agents throughout the body. The simplest factor determining distribution is the amount of blood flow to body tissues. The heart, liver, kidneys, and brain receive the most blood supply. Skin, bone, and adipose tissue receive a lower blood flow; therefore, it is more difficult to deliver high concentrations of drugs to these areas.

The physical properties of the drug greatly influence how it moves throughout the body after administration. Lipid solubility is an important characteristic, because it determines how quickly a drug is absorbed, mixes within the bloodstream, crosses membranes, and becomes localized in body tissues. Lipid-soluble agents are not limited by the barriers that normally stop water-soluble drugs; thus, they are more completely distributed to body tissues.

Some tissues have the ability to accumulate and store drugs after absorption. The bone marrow, teeth, eyes, and adipose tissue have an especially high **affinity**, or attraction, for certain medications. Examples of agents that are attracted to adipose tissue are thiopental (Pentothal), diazepam (Valium), and lipid-soluble vitamins. Tetracycline binds to calcium salts and accumulates in the bones and teeth. Once stored in tissues, drugs may remain in the body for many months and are released very slowly back to the circulation.

Not all drug molecules in the plasma will reach their target cells, because many drugs bind reversibly to plasma proteins, particularly albumin, to form **drug–protein complexes**. Drug–protein complexes are too large to cross capillary membranes; thus, the drug is not available for distribution to body tissues. Drugs bound to proteins circulate in the plasma until they are released or displaced from the drug–protein complex. Only unbound (free) drugs can reach their target cells or be excreted by the kidneys. This concept is illustrated in ● Figure 5.3. Some drugs, such as the anticoagulant warfarin (Coumadin) are highly bound; 99% of the drug in the plasma exists in drug–protein complexes and is unavailable to reach target cells.

Drugs and other chemicals compete with one another for plasma protein–binding sites, and some agents have a

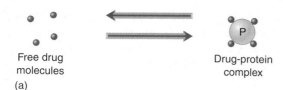

Free drug molecules

Drug-protein complex

(a)

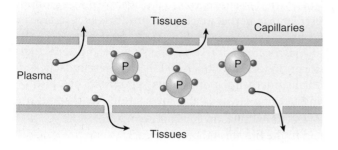

(b)

● **Figure 5.3** Plasma protein binding and drug availability: (a) drug exists in a free state or bound to plasma protein; (b) drug–protein complexes are too large to cross membranes

greater affinity for these binding sites than other agents. Drug–drug and drug–food interactions may occur when one agent displaces another from plasma proteins. The displaced medication can immediately reach high levels in the blood and produce adverse effects. An example is the drug warfarin (Coumadin). Drugs such as aspirin or cimetidine (Tagamet) displace warfarin from the drug–protein complex, thus raising blood levels of free warfarin and dramatically enhancing the risk of hemorrhage. Most drug guides give the percentage of medication bound to plasma proteins; when giving multiple drugs that are highly bound, the nurse should monitor the client closely for adverse effects.

The brain and placenta possess special anatomical barriers that inhibit many chemicals and medications from entering. These barriers are referred to as the **blood–brain barrier** and **fetal–placental barrier.** Some medications such as sedatives, antianxiety agents, and anticonvulsants readily cross the blood–brain barrier to produce their actions on the central nervous system. In contrast, most antitumor medications do not easily cross this barrier, making brain cancers difficult to treat.

The fetal–placental barrier serves an important protective function, because it prevents potentially harmful substances from passing from the mother's bloodstream to the fetus. Substances such as alcohol, cocaine, caffeine, and certain prescription medications, however, easily cross the placental barrier and can potentially harm the fetus. Consequently, no prescription medication, OTC drug, or herbal therapy should be taken by a clients who is pregnant without first consulting with a healthcare provider. The healthcare provider should always question female clients in the childbearing years regarding their pregnancy status before prescribing a drug. Chapter 7 ∞ presents a list of drug pregnancy categories for assessing fetal risk.

5.5 Metabolism of Medications

Metabolism, also called *biotransformation,* is the process of chemically converting a drug to a form that is usually more easily removed from the body. Metabolism involves complex biochemical pathways and reactions that alter drugs, nutrients, vitamins, and minerals. The liver is the primary site of drug metabolism, although the kidneys and cells of the intestinal tract also have high metabolic rates.

Medications undergo many types of biochemical reactions as they pass through the liver, including hydrolysis, oxidation, and reduction. During metabolism, the addition of side chains, known as **conjugates,** makes drugs more water soluble and more easily excreted by the kidneys.

Most metabolism in the liver is accomplished by the **hepatic microsomal enzyme system.** This enzyme complex is sometimes called the P-450 system, named after cytochrome P-450, which is a key component of the system. As they relate to pharmacotherapy, the primary actions of the hepatic microsomal enzymes are to inactivate drugs and accelerate their excretion. In some cases, however, metabolism can produce a chemical alteration that makes the resulting molecule *more* active than the original. For example, the narcotic analgesic codeine undergoes biotransformation to morphine, which has significantly greater ability to relieve pain. In fact, some agents, known as **prodrugs,** have no pharmacological activity unless they are first metabolized to their active form by the body. Examples of prodrugs include benazepril (Lotensin) and losartan (Cozaar).

Changes in the function of the hepatic microsomal enzymes can significantly affect drug metabolism. A few drugs have the ability to increase metabolic activity in the liver, a process called **enzyme induction.** For example, phenobarbital causes the liver to synthesize more microsomal enzymes. By doing so, phenobarbital increases the rate of its own metabolism, as well as that of other drugs metabolized in the liver. In these clients, higher doses of medication may be required to achieve the optimum therapeutic effect.

Certain clients have decreased hepatic metabolic activity, which may alter drug action. Hepatic enzyme activity is generally reduced in infants and elderly clients; therefore, pediatric and geriatric clients are more sensitive to drug therapy than middle-age clients. Clients with severe liver damage, such as that caused by cirrhosis, will require reductions in drug dosage because of the decreased metabolic activity. Certain genetic disorders have been recognized in which clients lack specific metabolic enzymes; drug dosages in these clients must be adjusted accordingly. The nurse should pay careful attention to laboratory values that may indicate liver disease so that doses may be adjusted accordingly.

Metabolism has a number of additional therapeutic consequences. As illustrated in ● Figure 5.4, drugs absorbed after oral administration cross directly into the hepatic portal circulation, which carries blood to the liver before it is distributed to other body tissues. Thus, blood passes through the liver circulation, some drugs can be completely metabolized to an inactive form before they ever reach the general

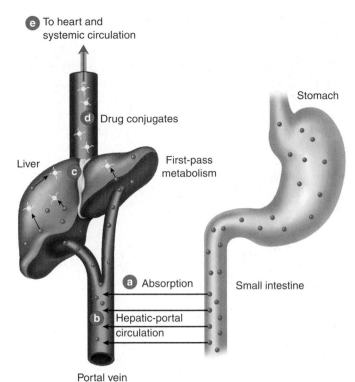

e To heart and systemic circulation

d Drug conjugates

Liver

c

First-pass metabolism

Stomach

a Absorption

b Hepatic-portal circulation

Small intestine

Portal vein

● **Figure 5.4** First-pass effect: (a) drugs are absorbed; (b) drugs enter hepatic portal circulation and go directly to liver; (c) hepatic microsomal enzymes metabolize drugs to inactive forms; (d) drug conjugates, leaving liver; (e) drug is distributed to general circulation

circulation. This **first-pass effect** is an important mechanism, since a large number of oral drugs are rendered inactive by hepatic metabolic reactions. Alternative routes of delivery that bypass the first-pass effect (e.g., sublingual, rectal, or parenteral routes) may need to be considered for these drugs.

5.6 Excretion of Medications

Drugs are removed from the body by the process of **excretion**. The rate at which medications are excreted determines their concentration in the bloodstream and tissues. This is important because the concentration of drugs in the bloodstream determines their duration of action. Pathological states, such as liver disease or renal failure, often increase the duration of drug action in the body because they interfere with natural excretion mechanisms. Dosing regimens must be carefully adjusted in these clients.

Although drugs are removed from the body by numerous organs and tissues, the primary site of excretion is the kidney. In an average-size person, approximately 180 L of blood is filtered by the kidneys each day. Free drugs, water-soluble agents, electrolytes, and small molecules are easily filtered at the glomerulus. Proteins, blood cells, conjugates, and drug–protein complexes are not filtered because of their large size.

On filtration at the renal corpuscle, chemicals and drugs are subjected to the process of reabsorption in the renal tubule. Mechanisms of reabsorption are the same as

absorption elsewhere in the body. Nonionized and lipid-soluble drugs cross renal tubular membranes easily and return to the circulation; ionized and water-soluble drugs generally remain in the filtrate for excretion.

Drug–protein complexes and substances too large to be filtered at the glomerulus are sometimes secreted into the distal tubule of the nephron. For example, only 10% of a dose of penicillin G is filtered at the glomerulus; 90% is secreted into the renal tubule. As with metabolic enzyme activity, secretion mechanisms are less active in infants and older adults.

Certain drugs may be excreted more quickly if the pH of the filtrate changes. Weak acids such as aspirin are excreted faster when the filtrate is slightly alkaline, because aspirin is ionized in an alkaline environment, and the drug will remain in the filtrate and be excreted in the urine. Weakly basic drugs such as diazepam (Valium) are excreted faster with a slightly acidic filtrate, because they are ionized in this environment. This relationship between pH and drug excretion can be used to advantage in critical care situations. To speed the renal excretion of acidic drugs such as aspirin in an overdosed client, nurses can administer sodium bicarbonate. Sodium bicarbonate will make the urine more basic, which ionizes more aspirin, causing it to be excreted more readily. The excretion of diazepam, on the other hand, can be enhanced by giving ammonium chloride. This will acidify the filtrate and increase the excretion of diazepam.

Impairment of kidney function can dramatically affect pharmacokinetics. Clients with renal failure will have diminished ability to excrete medications and may retain drugs for an extended time. Doses for these clients must be reduced, to avoid drug toxicity. Because small to moderate changes in renal status can cause rapid increases in serum drug levels, the nurse must constantly monitor kidney function in clients receiving drugs that may be nephrotoxic, or during pharmacotherapy with medications that have a narrow margin of safety. The pharmacotherapy of renal failure is presented in Chapter 30 ∞.

Organs other than the kidneys can serve as important sites of excretion. Drugs that can easily be changed into a gaseous form are especially suited for excretion by the respiratory system. The rate of respiratory excretion is

SPECIAL CONSIDERATIONS

Adverse Drug Effects and Elderly Clients

Adverse drug effects are more commonly recorded in elderly clients than in young adults or middle-age clients, because the geriatric population takes more drugs simultaneously (an average of seven) than other age groups. In addition, chronic diseases that affect pharmacokinetics are present more often in the elderly. One study (Doucet et al., 2002) of more than 2,800 inpatients older than age 70 found 500 adverse drug events at the time of admission. More than 60% of the adverse drug events were caused by drug–drug interactions. Of these, more than 46% were considered "preventable" because the drug–drug interaction was known. Excess doses were administered in almost 15% of the clients; healthcare providers often forgot to adjust doses for pharmacokinetic variables that change with aging.

dependent on factors that affect gas exchange, including diffusion, gas solubility, and pulmonary blood flow. The elimination of volatile anesthetics following surgery is primarily dependent on respiratory activity. The faster the breathing rate, the greater the excretion. Conversely, the respiratory removal of water-soluble agents such as alcohol is more dependent on blood flow to the lungs. The greater the blood flow into lung capillaries, the greater the excretion. In contrast with other methods of excretion, the lungs excrete most drugs in their original unmetabolized form.

Glandular activity is another elimination mechanism. Water-soluble drugs may be secreted into the saliva, sweat, or breast milk. The "funny taste" that clients sometimes experience when given IV drugs is an example of the secretion of agents into the saliva. Another example of glandular excretion is the garlic smell that can be detected when standing next to a perspiring person who has recently eaten garlic. Excretion into breast milk is of considerable importance for basic drugs such as morphine or codeine, as these can achieve high concentrations and potentially affect the nursing infant. Nursing mothers should always check with their healthcare provider before taking any prescription medication, OTC drug, or herbal supplement. Pharmacology of the pregnant or breast-feeding client is discussed in Chapter 7 ∞.

Some drugs are secreted in the bile, a process known as *biliary excretion*. In many cases, drugs secreted into bile will enter the duodenum and eventually leave the body in the feces. However, most bile is circulated back to the liver by **enterohepatic recirculation**, as illustrated in ● Figure 5.5. A percentage of the drug may be recirculated numerous times with the bile. Biliary reabsorption is extremely influential in prolonging the activity of cardiac glycosides, certain antibiotics, and phenothiazines. Recirculated drugs are ultimately metabolized by the liver and excreted by the kidneys. Recirculation and elimination of drugs through biliary excretion may continue for several weeks after therapy has been discontinued.

5.7 Drug Plasma Concentration and Therapeutic Response

The therapeutic response of most drugs is directly related to their level in the plasma. Although the concentration of the medication at its *target tissue* is more predictive of drug action, this quantity is impossible to measure in most cases. For example, it is possible to conduct a laboratory test that measures the serum level of the drug lithium carbonate (Eskalith) by taking a blood sample; it is a far different matter to measure the quantity of this drug in neurons within the

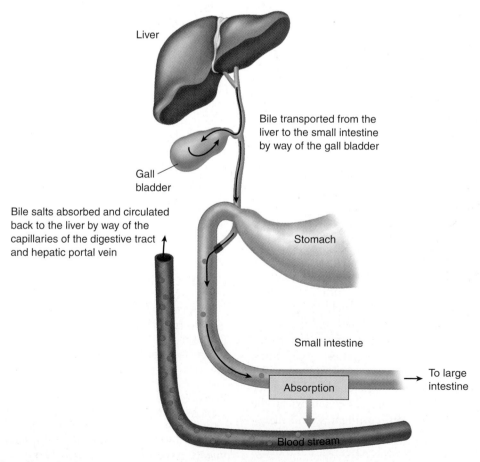

Liver

Bile transported from the liver to the small intestine by way of the gall bladder

Gall bladder

Bile salts absorbed and circulated back to the liver by way of the capillaries of the digestive tract and hepatic portal vein

Stomach

Small intestine

Absorption

To large intestine

Blood stream

● **Figure 5.5** Enterohepatic recirculation

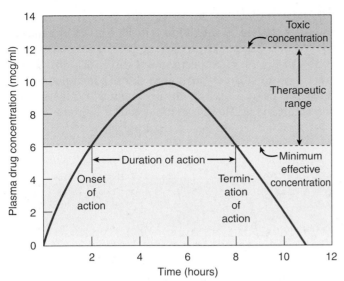

● **Figure 5.6** Single-dose drug administration: pharmacokinetic values for this drug are as follows: onset of action = 2 hours; duration of action = 6 hours; termination of action = 8 hours after administration; peak plasma concentration = 10 mcg/ml; time to peak drug effect = 5 hours; $t^{1/2}$ = 4 hours

CNS. Indeed, it is common practice for nurses to monitor the plasma levels of certain drugs that have a low safety profile.

Several important pharmacokinetic principles can be illustrated by measuring the serum level of a drug following a single-dose administration. These pharmacokinetic values are shown graphically in ● Figure 5.6. This figure demonstrates two plasma drug levels. First is the **minimum effective concentration,** the amount of drug required to produce a therapeutic effect. Second is the **toxic concentration,** the level of drug that will result in serious adverse effects. The plasma drug concentration *between* the minimum effective concentration and the toxic concentration is called the **therapeutic range** of the drug. These values have great clinical significance. For example, if the client has a severe headache and is given half of an aspirin tablet, the plasma level will remain below the minimum effective concentration, and the client will not experience pain relief. Two or three tablets will increase the plasma level of aspirin into the therapeutic range, and the pain will subside. Taking six or more tablets may result in adverse effects, such as GI bleeding or tinnitus. For each drug administered, the nurse's goal is to keep its plasma concentration in the therapeutic range. For some drugs, this therapeutic range is quite wide; for other medications, the difference between a minimum effective dose and a toxic dose can be dangerously narrow.

5.8 Plasma Half-life and Duration of Drug Action

The most common description of a drug's duration of action is its **plasma half-life ($t_{1/2}$),** defined as the length of time required for the plasma concentration of a medication to decrease by half after administration. Some drugs have a half-life

of only a few minutes, whereas others have a half-life of several hours or days. The greater the half-life, the longer it takes a medication to be excreted. For example, a drug with a $t_{1/2}$ of 10 hours would take longer to be excreted and thus produce a longer effect in the body than a drug with a $t_{1/2}$ of 5 hours.

The plasma half-life of a drug is an essential pharmacokinetic variable that has important clinical applications. Drugs with relatively short half-lives, such as aspirin ($t_{1/2}$ = 15 to 20 minutes) must be given every 3 to 4 hours. Drugs with longer half-lives, such as felodipine (Plendil) ($t_{1/2}$ = 10 hours), need be given only once a day. If a client has extensive renal or hepatic disease, the plasma half-life of a drug will increase, and the drug concentration may reach toxic levels. In these clients, medications must be given less frequently, or the dosages must be reduced.

5.9 Loading Doses and Maintenance Doses

Few drugs are administered as a single dose. Repeated doses result in an accumulation of drug in the bloodstream, as shown in ● Figure 5.7. Eventually, a plateau will be reached where the level of drug in the plasma is maintained continuously within the therapeutic range. At this level, the amount administered has reached equilibrium with the amount of drug being eliminated, resulting in the distribution of a continuous therapeutic level of drug to body tissues. Theoretically, it takes approximately four half-lives to reach this equilibrium. If the medication is given as a continuous infusion, the plateau can be reached quickly and be maintained with little or no fluctuation in drug plasma levels.

The plateau may be reached faster by administration of loading doses followed by regular maintenance doses. A **loading dose** is a higher amount of drug, often given only once or twice, that is administered to "prime" the

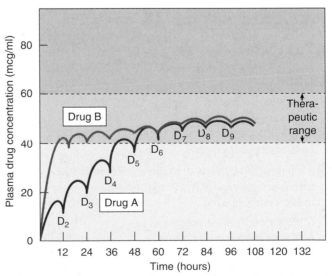

● **Figure 5.7** Multiple-dose drug administration: drug A (—) and drug B (—) are administered every 12 hours; drug B reaches the therapeutic range faster, because the first dose is a loading dose

bloodstream with a level sufficient to quickly induce a therapeutic response. Before plasma levels can drop back toward zero, intermittent **maintenance doses** are given to keep the plasma drug concentration in the therapeutic range. Although blood levels of the drug fluctuate with this approach, the equilibrium state can be reached almost as rapidly as with a continuous infusion. Loading doses are particularly important for drugs with prolonged half-lives and for situations in which it is critical to raise drug plasma levels quickly, as might be the case when administering an antibiotic for a severe infection. In Figure 5.7, notice that it takes almost five doses (48 hours) before a therapeutic level is reached using a routine dosing schedule. With a loading dose, a therapeutic level is reached within 12 hours.

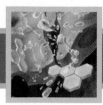

CHAPTER REVIEW

KEY CONCEPTS

The numbered key concepts provide a succinct summary of the important points from the corresponding numbered section within the chapter. If any of these points are not clear, refer to the numbered section within the chapter for review.

5.1 Pharmacokinetics focuses on the movement of drugs throughout the body after they are administered.

5.2 The physiological properties of plasma membranes determine movement of drugs throughout the body. The four components of pharmacokinetics are absorption, metabolism, distribution, and excretion.

5.3 Absorption is the process by which a drug moves from the site of administration to the bloodstream. Absorption depends on the size of the drug molecule, its lipid solubility, its degree of ionization, and interactions with food or other medications.

5.4 Distribution comprises the methods by which drugs are transported throughout the body. Distribution depends on the formation of drug–protein complexes and special barriers such as the placenta or brain barriers.

5.5 Metabolism is a process that changes a drug's activity and makes it more likely to be excreted. Changes in hepatic metabolism can significantly affect drug action.

5.6 Excretion processes remove drugs from the body. Drugs are primarily excreted by the kidneys but may be excreted into bile, by the lung, or by glandular secretions.

5.7 The therapeutic response of most drugs depends on their concentration in the plasma. The difference between the minimum effective concentration and the toxic concentration is called the therapeutic range.

5.8 Plasma half-life represents the duration of action for most drugs.

5.9 Repeated dosing allows a plateau drug plasma level to be reached. Loading doses allow a therapeutic drug level to be reached rapidly.

NCLEX-RN® REVIEW QUESTIONS

1 The client has a malignant brain tumor. What property of pharmacokinetics may cause difficulty in treating her tumor?

1. Blood–brain barrier
2. Drug–protein complexes
3. Affinity for neoplasms
4. Lack of active transport

2 A client with cirrhosis of the liver exhibits decreased metabolic activity. This will require what possible change in her drug regimen?

1. A reduction in the dosage of drugs.
2. A change in the timing of medication administration.
3. An increased dose of prescribed drugs.
4. All prescribed drugs must be given by intramuscular injection.

3 Some drugs may be completely metabolized by the liver circulation before ever reaching the general circulation. This effect is known as what?

1. Conjugation of drugs
2. Hepatic microsomal enzyme system
3. Blood–brain barrier
4. First-pass effect

4 A client who is in renal failure may have a diminished capacity to excrete medications. It is imperative that this client be assessed for what development?

1. Increased creatinine levels
2. Increased levels of blood urea nitrogen
3. Drug toxicity
4. Increased levels of potassium

5 The nurse understands that with glandular activity, water-soluble drugs may be secreted into (select all that apply):

1. Saliva
2. Sweat
3. Breast milk
4. Bile
5. Feces

CRITICAL THINKING QUESTIONS

1. Describe the types of obstacles drugs face from the time they are administered until they reach their target cells.

2. Why is the drug's plasma half-life important to the nurse?

3. How does the ionization of a drug affect its distribution in the body?

4. Explain why drugs that are metabolized through the first-pass effect may need to be administered by the parenteral route.

See Appendix D for answers and rationales for all activities.

EXPLORE MediaLink

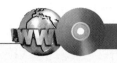

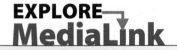

NCLEX-RN® review, case studies, and other interactive resources for this chapter can be found on the companion website at www.prenhall.com/adams. Click on "Chapter 5" to select the activities for this chapter. For animations, more NCLEX-RN® review questions, and an audio glossary, access the accompanying Prentice Hall Nursing MediaLink DVD-ROM in this textbook.

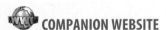
www.prenhall.com/adams

 PRENTICE HALL NURSING MEDIALINK DVD-ROM

- **Animation**
  Cytochrome
- **Audio Glossary**
- **NCLEX-RN® Review**

COMPANION WEBSITE

- **NCLEX-RN® Review**
- **Case Study:** Client using herbal supplements
- **Challenge Your Knowledge**

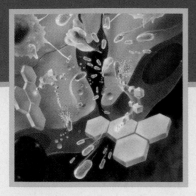

CHAPTER 6

Pharmacodynamics

OBJECTIVES

After reading this chapter, the student should be able to:

1. Apply principles of pharmacodynamics to clinical practice.
2. Discuss how frequency response curves may be used to explain how clients respond differently to medications.
3. Explain the importance of the median effective dose (ED_{50}) to clinical practice.
4. Compare and contrast median lethal dose (LD_{50}) and median toxicity dose (TD_{50}).
5. Discuss how a drug's therapeutic index is related to its margin of safety.
6. Identify the significance of the graded dose–response relationship to clinical practice.
7. Compare and contrast the terms *potency* and *efficacy*.
8. Distinguish between an agonist, a partial agonist, and an antagonist.
9. Explain the relationship between receptors and drug action.
10. Explain possible future developments in the field of pharmacogenetics.

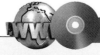

MediaLink

www.prenhall.com/adams

NCLEX-RN® review, case studies, and other interactive resources for this chapter can be found on the companion website at www.prenhall.com/adams. Click on "Chapter 6" to select the activities for this chapter. For animations, more NCLEX-RN® review questions, and an audio glossary, access the accompanying Prentice Hall Nursing MediaLink DVD-ROM in this textbook.

KEY TERMS

agonist *page 61*

antagonist *page 62*

efficacy *page 59*

frequency distribution curve
page 57

graded dose–response *page 59*

idiosyncratic response *page 62*

median effective dose (ED$_{50}$)
page 58

median lethal dose (LD$_{50}$) *page 58*

median toxicity dose (TD$_{50}$) *page 58*

nonspecific cellular responses
page 61

partial agonist *page 61*

pharmacodynamics *page 57*

pharmacogenetics *page 62*

potency *page 59*

receptor *page 60*

second messenger *page 61*

therapeutic index *page 58*

In clinical practice, nurses quickly learn that medications do not affect all clients in the same way: A dose that produces a dramatic response in one client may have no effect on another. In some cases, the differences among clients are predictable, based on the pharmacokinetic principles discussed in Chapter 5 ∞. In other cases, the differences in response are not easily explained. Despite this client variability, healthcare providers must choose optimal doses while avoiding unnecessary adverse effects. This is not an easy task given the wide variation of client responses within a population. This chapter examines the mechanisms by which drugs affect clients, and how the nurse can apply these principles to clinical practice.

6.1 Pharmacodynamics and Interclient Variability

The term **pharmacodynamics** comes from the root words *pharmaco*, which means "medicine," and *dynamics*, which means "change." In simplest terms, pharmacodynamics refers to how a medicine *changes* the body. A more complete definition explains pharmacodynamics as the branch of pharmacology concerned with the mechanisms of drug action and the relationships between drug concentration and responses in the body.

Pharmacodynamics has important clinical applications. Healthcare providers must be able to predict whether a drug will produce a significant change in clients. Although clinicians often begin therapy with average doses taken from a drug guide, intuitive experience often becomes the practical method for determining which doses of medications will be effective in a given client. Knowledge of therapeutic indexes, dose–response relationships, and drug–receptor interactions will help the nurse provide safe and effective treatment.

Interclient variability in responses to drugs can best be understood by examining a frequency distribution curve. A **frequency distribution curve,** shown in ● Figure 6.1, is a graphical representation of the number of clients responding to a drug action at different doses. Notice the wide range in doses that produced the client responses shown on the curve. A few clients responded to the drug at very

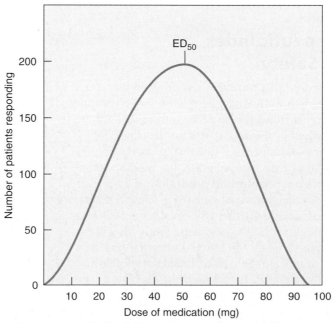

● **Figure 6.1** Frequency distribution curve: Interpatient variability in drug response

low doses. As the dose was increased, more and more clients responded. Some clients required very high doses to elicit the desired response. The peak of the curve indicates the largest number of clients responding to the drug. The curve does not show the *magnitude* of response, only whether a measurable response occurred among the clients. As an example, think of the given response to an antihypertensive drug as being a reduction of 20 mm Hg in systolic blood pressure. A few clients experienced the desired 20-mm reduction at a dose of only 10 mg of drug. A 50-mg dose gave the largest number of clients a 20-mm reduction in blood pressure; however, a few clients needed as much as 90 mg of drug to produce the same 20-mm reduction.

The dose in the middle of the frequency distribution curve represents the drug's **median effective dose (ED$_{50}$)**. The ED$_{50}$ is the dose required to produce a specific therapeutic response in 50% of a group of clients. Drug guides sometimes report the ED$_{50}$ as the average or standard dose.

The interclient variability shown in Figure 6.1 has important clinical implications. First, the nurse should realize that the standard or average dose predicts a satisfactory therapeutic response for only *half* the population. In other words, many clients will require more or less than the average dose for optimum pharmacotherapy. Using the systolic blood pressure example, assume that a large group of clients is given the average dose of 50 mg. Some of these clients will experience toxicity at this level because they needed only 10 mg to achieve blood pressure reduction. Other clients in this group will probably have no reduction in blood pressure. By observing the client, taking vital signs, and monitoring associated laboratory data, the nurse uses skills that are critical in determining whether the average dose is effective for the client. It is not enough to simply memorize an average dose for a drug; the nurse must know when and how to adjust this dose to obtain the optimum therapeutic response.

6.2 Therapeutic Index and Drug Safety

Administering a dose that produces an optimum therapeutic response for each individual client is only one component of effective pharmacotherapy. The nurse must also be able to predict whether the dose is safe for the client.

Frequency distribution curves can also be used to represent the safety of a drug. For example, the **median lethal dose (LD$_{50}$)** is often determined in preclinical trials, as part of the drug development process discussed in Chapter 1 ∞. The LD$_{50}$ is the dose of drug that will be lethal in 50% of a group of animals. As with ED$_{50}$, a group of animals will exhibit considerable variability in lethal dose; what may be a nontoxic dose for one animal may be lethal for another.

To examine the safety of a particular drug, the LD$_{50}$ can be compared with the ED$_{50}$, as shown in ● Figure 6.2a. In this example, 10 mg of drug X is the average *effective* dose, and 40 mg is the average *lethal* dose. The ED$_{50}$ and LD$_{50}$ are used to calculate an important value in pharmacology, a drug's **therapeutic index**, the ratio of a drug's LD$_{50}$ to its ED$_{50}$.

$$\text{Therapeutic index} = \frac{\text{median lethal dose LD}_{50}}{\text{median effective dose ED}_{50}}$$

The larger the difference between the two doses, the greater the therapeutic index. In Figure 6.2a, the therapeutic index is 4 (40 mg ÷ 10 mg). Essentially, this means that it would take an error in magnitude of *approximately* 4 times the average dose to be lethal to a client. Thus, the therapeutic index is a measure of a drug's safety margin: the higher the value, the safer the medication.

As another example, the therapeutic index of a second drug is shown in Figure 6.2b. Drug Z has the same ED$_{50}$ as drug X but shows a different LD$_{50}$. The therapeutic index for drug Z is only 2 (20 mg ÷ 10 mg). The difference between an effective dose and a lethal dose is very small for drug Z; thus, the drug has a narrow safety margin. The therapeutic index offers the nurse practical information on the safety of a drug, and a means to compare one drug with another.

Because the LD$_{50}$ cannot be experimentally determined in humans, the **median toxicity dose (TD$_{50}$)** is a more

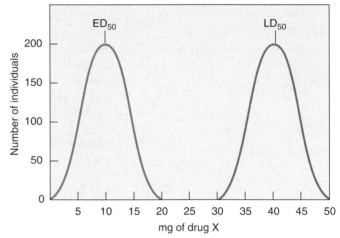

(a) Drug X : TI = $\dfrac{\text{LD}_{50}}{\text{ED}_{50}} = \dfrac{40}{10} = 4$

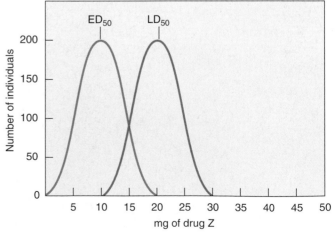

(b) Drug Z : TI = $\dfrac{\text{LD}_{50}}{\text{ED}_{50}} = \dfrac{20}{10} = 2$

● Figure 6.2 Therapeutic index: (a) drug X has a therapeutic index of 4; (b) drug Z has a therapeutic index of 2

practical value in a clinical setting. The TD_{50} is the dose that will produce a given toxicity in 50% of a group of clients. The TD_{50} value may be extrapolated from animal data or based on adverse effects recorded in client clinical trials.

6.3 The Graded Dose–Response Relationship and Therapeutic Response

In the previous examples, frequency distribution curves were used to graphically visualize client differences in responses to medications in a *population*. It is also useful to visualize the variability in responses observed within a *single client*.

The **graded dose–response** relationship is a fundamental concept in pharmacology. The graphical representation of this relationship is called a dose–response curve, as illustrated in ● Figure 6.3. By observing and measuring the client's response obtained at different doses of the drug, one can explain several important clinical relationships.

The three distinct phases of a dose–response curve indicate essential pharmacodynamic principles that have relevance to clinical practice. Phase 1 occurs at the lowest doses. The flatness of this portion of the curve indicates that few target cells have yet been affected by the drug. Phase 2 is the straight-line portion of the curve. This portion often shows a linear relationship between the amount of drug administered and the degree of response obtained from the client. For example, if the dose is doubled, twice as much response is obtained. This is the most desirable range of doses for pharmacotherapeutics, since giving more drug results in proportionately more effect; a lower drug dose gives less effect. In phase 3, a plateau is reached in which increasing the drug dose produces no additional therapeutic response. This may occur for a number of reasons. One explanation is that all the receptors for the drug are occupied. It could also mean that the drug has brought 100% relief, such as when a migraine headache has been terminated; giving higher doses produces no additional relief. In phase 3, although increasing the dose does not result in more therapeutic effect, the nurse should be mindful that increasing the dose may produce adverse effects.

6.4 Potency and Efficacy

Within a pharmacological class, not all drugs are equally effective at treating a disorder. For example, some antineoplastic drugs kill more cancer cells than others; some antihypertensive agents lower blood pressure to a greater degree than others; and some analgesics are more effective at relieving severe pain than others in the same class. Furthermore, drugs in the same class are effective at different doses; one antibiotic may be effective at a dose of 1 mg/kg, whereas another is most effective at 100 mg/kg. Nurses need a method to compare one drug with another so that they can administer treatment effectively.

There are two fundamental ways to compare medications within therapeutic and pharmacological classes. First is the concept of **potency.** A drug that is more potent will produce a therapeutic effect at a lower dose, compared with another drug in the same class. Consider two agents, drug X and drug Y, that both produce a 20-mm drop in blood pressure. If drug X produces this effect at a dose of 10 mg, and drug X at 60 mg, then drug X is said to be more potent. Thus, potency is a way to compare the doses of two independently administered drugs in terms of how much is needed to produce a particular response. A useful way to visualize the concept of potency is by examining dose–response curves. Compare the two drugs shown in ● Figure 6.4a. In this example, drug A is more potent because it requires a lower dose to produce the same response.

The second method used to compare drugs is called **efficacy**, which is the magnitude of maximal response that can be produced from a particular drug. In the example in Figure 6.4b, drug A is more efficacious because it produces a higher maximal response.

Which is more important to the success of pharmacotherapy, potency or efficacy? Perhaps the best way to understand these concepts is to use the specific example of headache pain. Two common OTC analgesics are ibuprofen (200 mg) and aspirin (650 mg). The fact that ibuprofen relieves pain at a lower dose indicates that this agent is *more potent* than aspirin. At recommended doses, however, both are equally effective at relieving headache pain; thus, they have the *same efficacy*. If the client is experiencing severe pain, however, neither aspirin nor ibuprofen has sufficient efficacy to bring relief. Narcotic analgesics such as morphine have a greater efficacy than aspirin or ibuprofen and can effectively treat this type of pain. From a pharmacotherapeutic perspective, efficacy is almost always more important than potency. In the previous example, the average dose is unimportant to the client, but

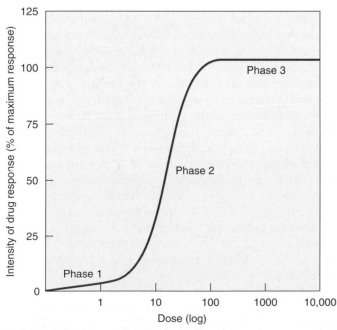

●**Figure 6.3** Dose–response relationship

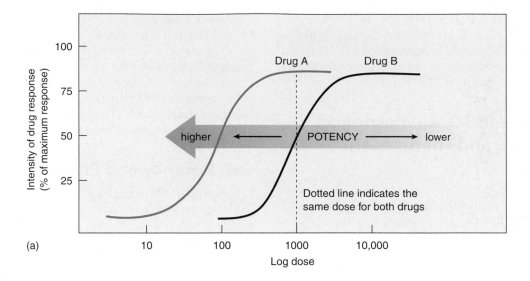

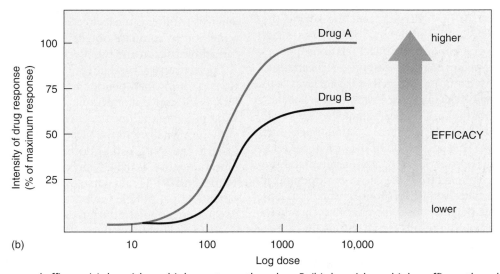

●**Figure 6.4** Potency and efficacy: (a) drug A has a higher potency than drug B; (b) drug A has a higher efficacy than drug B

headache relief is essential. As another comparison, the client with cancer is much more concerned about how many cancer cells have been killed (efficacy) than what dose the nurse administered (potency). Although the nurse will often hear claims that one drug is more potent than another, a more compelling concern is which drug is more efficacious.

6.5 Cellular Receptors and Drug Action

Drugs act by modulating or changing existing physiological and biochemical processes. To effect such changes requires that the drug interact with specific molecules and chemicals normally found in the body. A cellular macromolecule to which a medication binds to initiate its effects is called a **receptor**. The concept that a drug binds to a receptor to cause a change in body chemistry or physiology is a fundamental theory in pharmacology. Receptor theory explains the mechanisms by which most drugs produce their effects. It is important to understand, however, that these receptors do not exist in the body solely to bind drugs. Their normal function is to bind endogenous molecules such as hormones, neurotransmitters, and growth factors.

Although a drug receptor can be any type of macromolecule, the vast majority are proteins. As shown in ● Figure 6.5, a receptor may be depicted as a three-dimensional protein associated with a cellular plasma membrane. The extracellular structural component of a receptor often consists of several protein subunits arranged around a central canal or channel. Other receptors consist of many membrane-spanning segments inserted across the plasma membrane.

A drug attaches to its receptor in a specific manner, much like a lock and key. Small changes to the structure of a drug, or its receptor, may weaken or even eliminate

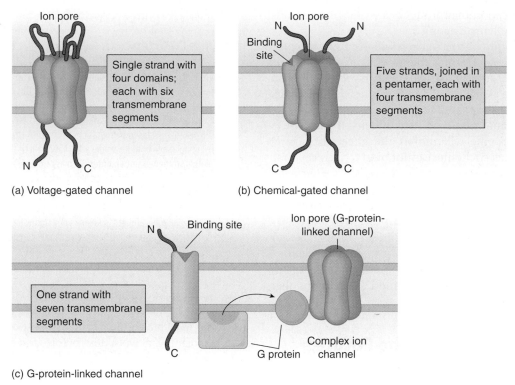

● Figure 6.5 Cellular receptors

binding between the two molecules. Once bound, drugs may trigger a series of **second messenger** events within the cell, such as the conversion of adenosine triphosphate (ATP) to cyclic adenosine monophosphate (cyclic AMP), the release of intracellular calcium, or the activation of specific G proteins and associated enzymes. These biochemical cascades initiate the drug's action by either stimulating or inhibiting a normal activity of the cell.

Not all receptors are bound to plasma membranes; some are intracellular molecules such as DNA or enzymes in the cytoplasm. By interacting with these types of receptors, medications are able to inhibit protein synthesis or regulate events such as cell replication and metabolism. Examples of agents that bind intracellular components include steroid medications, vitamins, and hormones.

Receptors and their associated drug mechanisms are extremely important in therapeutics. Receptor *subtypes* are being discovered and new medications are being developed at a faster rate than at any other time in history. These subtypes permit the "fine-tuning" of pharmacology. For example, the first medications affecting the autonomic nervous system affected all autonomic receptors. It was discovered that two basic receptor types existed in the body, alpha and beta, and drugs were then developed that affected only one type. The result was more specific drug action, with fewer adverse effects. Still later, several subtypes of alpha and beta receptors, including alpha-1, alpha-2, beta-1, and beta-2, were discovered that allowed even more specificity in pharmacotherapy. In recent years, researchers have further divided and refined these subtypes. It is likely that receptor research will continue to result in

the development of new medications that activate very specific receptors and thus direct drug action that avoids unnecessary adverse effects.

Some drugs act independently of cellular receptors. These agents are associated with other mechanisms, such as changing the permeability of cellular membranes, depressing membrane excitability, or altering the activity of cellular pumps. Actions such as these are often described as **nonspecific cellular responses**. Ethyl alcohol, general anesthetics, and osmotic diuretics are examples of agents that act by nonspecific mechanisms.

6.6 Types of Drug–Receptor Interactions

When a drug binds to a receptor, several therapeutic consequences can result. In simplest terms, a specific activity of the cell is either enhanced or inhibited. The actual biochemical mechanism underlying the therapeutic effect, however, may be extremely complex. In some cases, the mechanism of action is not known.

When a drug binds to its receptor, it may produce a response that *mimics* the effect of the endogenous regulatory molecule. For example, when the drug bethanechol (Urecholine) is administered, it binds to acetylcholine receptors in the autonomic nervous system and produces the same actions as acetylcholine. A drug that produces the same type of response as the endogenous substance is called an **agonist.** Agonists sometimes produce a greater maximal response than the endogenous chemical. The term **partial agonist** describes a medication that produces a weaker, or less efficacious, response than an agonist.

A second possibility is that a drug will occupy a receptor and *prevent* the endogenous chemical from acting. This drug is called an **antagonist**. Antagonists often compete with agonists for the receptor binding sites. For example, the drug atropine competes with acetylcholine for specific receptors in the autonomic nervous system. If the dose is high enough, atropine will inhibit the effects of acetylcholine, because acetylcholine cannot bind to its receptors.

Not all antagonism is associated with receptors. *Functional* antagonists inhibit the effects of an agonist not by competing for a receptor but by changing pharmacokinetic factors. For example, antagonists may slow the absorption of a drug. By speeding up metabolism or excretion, an antagonist can enhance the removal of a drug from the body. The relationships that occur between agonists and antagonists explain many of the drug–drug and drug–food interactions that occur in the body.

6.7 Pharmacology of the Future: Customizing Drug Therapy

Until recently, it was thought that single drugs should provide safe and effective treatment to every client in the same way. Unfortunately, a significant portion of the population either develops unacceptable side effects to certain drugs or is unresponsive to them. Many scientists and clinicians are now discarding the one-size-fits-all approach to drug therapy, which was designed to treat an entire population without addressing important inter-client variation.

With the advent of the Human Genome Project and other advances in medicine, pharmacologists are hopeful that

future drugs can be customized for clients with specific genetic similarities. In the past, unpredictable and unexplained drug reactions were labeled **idiosyncratic responses.** It is hoped that performing a DNA test before administering a drug may someday prevent these idiosyncratic side effects.

Pharmacogenetics is the area of pharmacology that examines the role of heredity in drug response. The greatest advances in pharmacogenetics have been the identification of subtle genetic differences in drug-metabolizing enzymes. Genetic differences in these enzymes are responsible for a significant portion of drug-induced toxicity. It is hoped that the use of pharmacogenetic information may someday allow for customized drug therapy. Although therapies based on a client's genetically based response may not be cost effective at this time, pharmacogenetics may radically change the way pharmacotherapy will be practiced in the future.

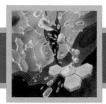

CHAPTER REVIEW

KEY CONCEPTS

The numbered key concepts provide a succinct summary of the important points from the corresponding numbered section within the chapter. If any of these points are not clear, refer to the numbered section within the chapter for review.

6.1 Pharmacodynamics is the area of pharmacology concerned with how drugs produce *change* in clients, and the differences in client responses to medications.

6.2 The therapeutic index, expressed mathematically as $TD_{50} \div ED_{50}$, is a value representing the margin of safety of a drug. The higher the therapeutic index, the safer the drug.

6.3 The graded dose–response relationship describes how the therapeutic response to a drug changes as the medication dose is increased.

6.4 Potency, the dose of medication required to produce a particular response, and efficacy, the magnitude of maximal response to a drug, are means of comparing medications.

6.5 Drug–receptor theory is used to explain the mechanism of action of many medications.

6.6 Agonists, partial agonists, and antagonists are substances that compete with drugs for receptor binding and can cause drug–drug and drug–food interactions.

6.7 In the future, pharmacotherapy will likely be customized to match the genetic makeup of each client.

NCLEX-RN® REVIEW QUESTIONS

1 Unpredictable and unexplained drug reactions are labeled what?

1. Adverse reactions
2. Idiosyncratic reactions
3. Enzyme-specific reactions
4. Unaltered reactions

2 A drug that occupies a receptor site and prevents endogenous chemicals from acting is termed what?

1. Antagonist
2. Partial agonist
3. Agonist
4. Protagonist

3 In considering the pharmacotherapeutic perspective, which property is considered to be of most importance?

1. Potency
2. Efficacy
3. Toxicity
4. Interaction with other drugs

4 The magnitude of maximal response that can be produced from a particular drug is considered to be what?

1. Efficacious
2. Toxic
3. Potent
4. Comparable

5 Morphine has a greater efficacy than (select all that apply):

1. Aspirin
2. Acetominophen
3. Inderal
4. Ibuprofen
5. Atenolol

CRITICAL THINKING QUESTIONS

1. If the ED_{50} is the dose required to produce an effective response in 50% of a group of patients, what happens in the "other" 50% of the patients after a dose has been administered?

2. Two drugs are competing for a receptor on a mast cell that will cause the release of histamine when activated. Compare the effects of an agonist versus an antagonist on this receptor. Which would likely be called an antihistamine, the agonist or the antagonist?

See Appendix D for answers and rationales for all activities.

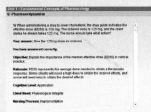

EXPLORE
MediaLink

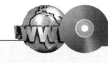

www.prenhall.com/adams

NCLEX-RN® review, case studies, and other interactive resources for this chapter can be found on the companion website at www.prenhall.com/adams. Click on "Chapter 6" to select the activities for this chapter. For animations, more NCLEX-RN® review questions, and an audio glossary, access the accompanying Prentice Hall Nursing MediaLink DVD-ROM in this textbook.

 PRENTICE HALL NURSING MEDIALINK DVD-ROM

- **Animation**
  Agonist
- **Audio Glossary**
- **NCLEX-RN® Review**

 COMPANION WEBSITE

- **NCLEX-RN® Review**
- **Case Study:** Potency and efficacy
- **Challenge Your Knowledge**

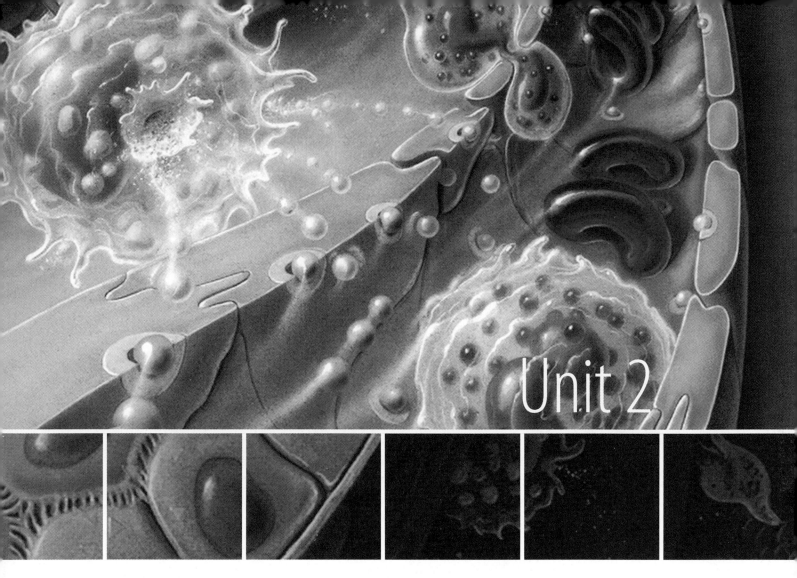

Unit 2

Pharmacology and the Nurse-Client Relationship

CHAPTER 7 The Nursing Process in Pharmacology

CHAPTER 8 Drug Administration Throughout the Lifespan

CHAPTER 9 Medication Errors and Risk Reduction

CHAPTER 10 Psychosocial, Gender, and Cultural Influences on Pharmacotherapy

CHAPTER 11 Herbal and Alternative Therapies

CHAPTER 12 Substance Abuse

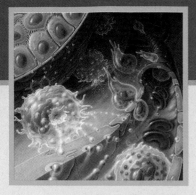

CHAPTER 7

The Nursing Process in Pharmacology

OBJECTIVES

After reading this chapter, the student should be able to:

1. Identify the steps of the Nursing Process.
2. Identify assessment data that is pertinent to medication administration.
3. Develop appropriate nursing diagnoses for clients receiving medications.
4. Identify realistic goals and outcomes during the planning stage for clients receiving medications.
5. Discuss key intervention strategies to be implemented for clients receiving medications.
6. Evaluate the outcomes of medication administration.
7. Apply the Nursing Process during medication administration utilizing the Nursing Process Focus flowcharts found in Chapters 13 through 49.

MediaLink 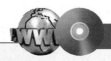 www.prenhall.com/adams

KEY TERMS

assessment   *page 67*
baseline data   *page 67*
evaluation   *page 68*
goal   *page 67*
interventions   *page 67*
nursing diagnoses   *page 67*
Nursing Process   *page 67*
objective data   *page 67*
outcome   *page 67*
planning   *page 67*
subjective data   *page 67*

The Nursing Process, a systematic method of problem solving, forms the foundation of all nursing practice. The use of the Nursing Process is particularly essential during medication administration. By using the steps of the Nursing Process, nurses can ensure that the interdisciplinary practice of pharmacology results in safe, effective, and individualized medication administration and outcomes for all clients under their care.

7.1 Review of the Nursing Process

Most nursing students enter a pharmacology course after taking a course on the fundamentals of nursing, during which the steps of the **Nursing Process** are discussed in detail. This section presents a brief review of those steps before discussing how they can be applied to pharmacology. Students who are unfamiliar with the Nursing Process are encouraged to consult one of the many excellent fundamentals of nursing textbooks for a more detailed explanation.

Assessment, the first step in the Nursing Process, is an ongoing process that begins with the nurse's initial contact with the client and continues with every interaction thereafter. During the initial assessment, **baseline data** are gathered that will be used to compare to information obtained during later interactions. Assessment consists of gathering **subjective data,** which include what the client says or perceives, and **objective data** gathered through physical assessment, laboratory tests, and other diagnostic sources.

Once the initial assessment data are gathered, the nurse makes clinical-based nursing judgments about the client and his or her responses to health and illness. **Nursing diagnoses** provide the basis for establishing goals and outcomes, planning interventions, and evaluating the effectiveness of the care given. Unlike medical diagnoses that focus on a disease or condition, nursing diagnoses focus on a client's response to actual or potential health and life processes. The North American Nursing Diagnosis Association (NANDA) defines nursing diagnoses as:

> A clinical judgment about individual, family, or community responses to actual or potential health/life processes. Per NANDA, nursing diagnoses provide the basis for selection of nursing interventions to achieve outcomes for which the nurse is accountable.

Nursing diagnoses are often the most challenging part of the Nursing Process. Sometimes the nurse identifies what is believed to be the client's problem, only to discover from further assessment that the planned goals, outcomes, and interventions have not "solved" the problem. A key point to remember is that nursing diagnoses focus on the *client's* needs, not the nurse's needs. A primary nursing role is to enable clients to become active participants in their own care. By including the client in identifying needs, the nurse encourages the client to take a more active role in working toward meeting the identified goals.

After a nursing diagnosis has been established, the nurse begins to plan ways to assist the client to return to, or maintain, an optimum level of wellness as defined by that diagnosis. Short- or long-term **goals** are established that focus on what the client will be able to do or achieve, not what the nurse will do. **Outcomes** are the objective measures of those goals. They specifically define what the client will do, under what circumstances, and within a specified time frame. Goals and outcomes are also discussed with the client or caregiver, and are prioritized to address immediate needs first.

Planning links strategies, or interventions, to the established goals and outcomes. Planning is the formal written process that communicates with all members of the healthcare team what the nurse will do to assist the client in meeting those goals. Each healthcare organization decides how this plan of care will be communicated, and it may be nurse centered or interdisciplinary.

Interventions are designed to meet the client's needs and ensure safe, effective care. As the nurse provides care, he or she makes ongoing reassessments and compares new data with the earlier data. The nurse compares the data with established nursing diagnoses, goals, and outcomes and begins the process of **evaluation.** Established nursing diagnoses are reviewed while taking into consideration the client's response to care. More assessment data are gathered as needed, and goals and outcomes are evaluated as to whether they were met, partially met, or not met at all. The process comes full circle as new or modified diagnoses are established, goals and outcomes redefined, and new interventions planned.

Nursing has not always relied on such an organized approach to nursing care, but has always been concerned with delivering safe and effective care. The administration of medications requires the use of the Nursing Process to ensure the best possible outcomes for the client. These steps will now be applied specifically to drug administration.

7.2 Assessment of the Client Related to Drug Administration

A health history and physical assessment are completed during the initial meeting between a nurse and client. Many pieces of data are gathered during this initial assessment that have specific implications for pharmacotherapy. Ongoing assessments after this time will provide additional data to help the nurse evaluate the outcomes of medication use. This section discusses pertinent assessment components and how they relate to drug administration.

The initial health history is tailored to the client's clinical condition. A complete history is the most detailed, but the appropriateness of this history must be considered given the client's condition. Often a problem-focused or "chief complaint" history is taken, focusing on the symptoms that led the client to seek care. In any history, key components must be assessed that may affect the successful outcome of drug administration. Essential questions to ask in the initial history relate to allergies; past medical history; medications used currently and in the recent past; personal and social history such as the use of alcohol, tobacco, or caffeine; health risks such as the use of street drugs or illicit substances; and reproductive health questions such as the pregnancy status of women of childbearing age. Table 7.1 provides pertinent questions that may be asked during an initial health history that provide baseline data before medications are administered. The health history is tailored to the client's condition,

TABLE 7.1 Health History Assessment Questions Pertinent to Drug Administration	
Health History Component Areas	**Pertinent Questions**
chief complaint	• How do you feel? (Describe) • Are you having any pain? (Describe) • Are you experiencing other symptoms? (Especially pertinent to medications are nausea, vomiting, headache, itching, dizziness, shortness of breath, nervousness or anxiousness, palpitations or heart "fluttering," weakness or fatigue)
allergies	• Are you allergic to any medications? • Are you allergic to any foods, environmental substances (e.g., pollen or "seasonal" allergies), tape, soaps, or cleansers? • What specifically happens when you experience an allergy?
past medical history	• Do you have a history of diabetes, heart or vascular conditions, respiratory conditions, neurological conditions? • Do you have any dermatologic conditions? • How have these been treated in the past? Currently?
family history	• Has anyone in your family experienced difficulties with any medications? (Describe) • Does anyone in your family have any significant medical problems?
drug history	• What prescription medications are you currently taking? (List drug name, dosage, frequency of administration) • What nonprescription/OTC medications are you taking? (List name, dosage, frequency) • What drugs, prescription or OTC, have you taken within the past month or two? • Have you ever experienced any side effects or unusual symptoms with any medications? (Describe) • What do you know, or have been taught, about these medications? • Do you use any herbal or homeopathic remedies? Any nutritional substances or vitamins?
health management	• Identify all the healthcare providers you have seen for health issues. • When was the last time you saw a healthcare provider? For what reason did you see this provider? • What is your normal diet? • Do you have any trouble sleeping?
reproductive history	• Is there any possibility you are pregnant? (Ask *every* woman of childbearing age) • Are you breast-feeding?
personal–social history	• Do you smoke? • What is your normal alcohol intake? • What is your normal caffeine intake? • Do you have any religious or cultural beliefs or practices concerning medications or your health that we should know about? • What is your occupation? What hours do you work? • Do you have any concerns regarding insurance or the ability to afford medications?
health risk history	• Do you have any history of depression or other mental illness? • Do you use any street drugs or illicit substances?

and all questions may not be appropriate during the initial assessment. Keep in mind that what is *not* being said may be as important as, or more important than, what *is* being said. For instance, a client may deny or downplay any symptoms of pain while grimacing or guarding a certain area from being touched. Nurses must use their observation skills during the history to gather such critical data.

Along with the health history, a physical assessment is completed to gather objective data on the client's condition. Vital signs, height and weight, a head-to-toe physical assessment, and lab specimens may be obtained. These values provide the baseline data to compare with future assessments and guide the healthcare provider in deciding which medications to prescribe. Many medications can affect the heart rate and blood pressure, and these especially should be noted. Baseline electrolyte values are important parameters to obtain, because many medications affect electrolyte balance. Renal and hepatic function tests are essential for many clients, particularly older adults and those who are critically ill, as these will be used to determine the proper drug dosage.

Once pharmacotherapy is initiated, ongoing assessments are conducted to determine the effects of the medications. Assessment should first focus on determining whether the client is experiencing the expected therapeutic benefits from the medications. For example, if a drug is given for symptoms of pain, has the pain subsided? If an antibiotic is given for an infection, have the signs of that infection—elevated temperature, redness or swelling, drainage from infected sites, etc.—improved over time? If a client is not experiencing the therapeutic effects of the medication, then further assessment must be done to determine the reason. Dosages and the scheduling of medications are reviewed, and serum drug levels may be obtained.

Assessment during pharmacotherapy also focuses on any side or adverse effects the client may be experiencing. Often, these effects are manifested in dermatologic, cardiovascular, gastrointestinal, or neurological symptoms. Here again, baseline data are compared with the current assessment to determine what changes have occurred since the initiation of pharmacotherapy. The Nursing Process Focus flowcharts provided in Chapters 13 through 49 ∞ illustrate key assessment data to be gathered associated with specific medications or classes of drugs.

Finally, an assessment of the ability of the client to assume responsibility for self-administration of medication is necessary. Will the client require assistance obtaining or affording the prescribed medications, or with taking them safely? What kind of medication storage facilities exist and are they adequate to protect the client, others in the home, and the efficacy of the medication? Does the client understand the uses and effects of this medication and how it is properly taken? Do assessment data suggest that the use of this medication might present a problem, such as difficulty swallowing large capsules or an inability to administer medication when home anticoagulant therapy has been ordered parenterally?

After analyzing the assessment data, the nurse determines client-specific nursing diagnoses appropriate for the drugs prescribed. These diagnoses will form the basis for the remaining steps of the Nursing Process.

7.3 Nursing Diagnoses for the Client Receiving Medications

Assessment data are used to develop a list of problems, or nursing diagnoses, that address the client's responses to health and life processes. These nursing diagnoses are used to set goals and plan care. They focus on the client's problems and are prioritized by importance to the client's clinical condition. Although the process of developing a nursing diagnosis is a challenging part of the Nursing Process, certain diagnoses often stand out as priorities. This section discusses common nursing diagnoses related to medication administration, and the development of appropriate nursing diagnosis statements.

Nursing diagnoses that focus on drug administration are the same as diagnoses written for other client condition–specific responses. They may address actual problems, such as the treatment of pain; focus on potential problems such as a risk for fluid volume deficit; or concentrate on maintaining the client's current level of wellness. The diagnosis is written as a one-, two-, or three-part statement depending on whether a wellness, risk, or actual problem has been identified. Actual and risk problems include the diagnostic statement and a related factor, or inferred cause. Actual diagnoses also contain a third part, the evidence gathered to support the chosen statement. There are many diagnoses appropriate to medication administration.

SPECIAL CONSIDERATIONS

Clients with Speaking, Visual, or Hearing Impairments

Verbal communication disorders may make obtaining responses from the client difficult. Communication may be facilitated by having the client write or draw responses. Clarify by paraphrasing the response back to the client. Use gestures, body language, and yes/no questions if writing or drawing is difficult. Allow adequate time for responses. Be especially aware of nonverbal clues, such as grimacing, when performing interventions that may cause discomfort or pain.

Provide adequate lighting for clients with visual impairments and be aware of how the phrasing of verbal communication affects the message conveyed. Remember that the nonverbal cues involved in communication may be missed by the client. Paraphrase responses back to clients to be sure they understood the message in the absence of nonverbal cues. Explain interventions in detail before implementing procedures or activities with the client.

Clients with hearing impairments benefit from communication that is spoken clearly and slowly in a low-pitched voice. Sit near the client and avoid speaking loudly or shouting, especially if hearing devices are used. Limit the amount of background noise when possible. Write or draw to clarify verbal communication, and use nonverbal gestures and body language to aid communication. Allow adequate time for communication and responses. Alert other members of the healthcare team that the client has a hearing impairment and may not hear a verbal answer to the nurse's call light given over an intercom system.

Some problems are nursing specific that the nurse can manage independently, whereas other problems are multidisciplinary and require collaboration with other members of the healthcare team. For any of the medications given to a client, there are often combinations of nursing-independent and collaborative diagnoses that can be established.

Two of the most common nursing diagnoses for medication administration are *Knowledge, Deficient* and *Noncompliance.* Knowledge deficit may be that the client has been given a new prescription and has no previous experience with the medication. This diagnosis may also be applicable when a client has not received adequate education about the drugs used in the treatment of his or her condition. When obtaining a medication history, the nurse should assess the client's knowledge regarding the drugs currently being taken and evaluate whether the drug education has been adequate. Sometimes a client refuses to take a drug that has been prescribed or refuses to follow the directions correctly. Noncompliance assumes that the client has been properly educated

about the medication and has made an informed decision not to take it. Because labeling a client's response as noncompliant may have a negative impact on the nurse–client relationship, it is vital that the nurse assess all possible factors leading to the noncompliance *before* establishing this diagnosis. Does the client understand why the medication has been prescribed? Has dosing and scheduling information been explained? Are side effects causing the client to refuse the medication? Do cultural, religious, social issues, or health beliefs have an impact on taking the medication? Is the noncompliance related to inadequate resources, either financial or social support? A thorough assessment of possible causes should be conducted before labeling the client's response as noncompliant.

Nursing diagnoses applicable to drug administration are often collaborative problems that require communication with other healthcare providers. For example, fluid volume deficit related to diuretic drugs may require additional interventions such as medical orders by the physician to ensure that electrolytes and intravascular fluid volume remain within normal limits. Nurses may assist the client with ambulation if weakness or postural hypotension occurs secondary to this fluid volume deficit independent of medical orders. Table 7.2 provides an abbreviated list of some of the common nursing diagnoses appropriate to drug administration. Although the list contains actual nursing diagnoses, these may also be identified as risk diagnoses. This is not an exhaustive list of all NANDA-approved diagnoses, and the establishment of new diagnoses is ongoing. The nurse is encouraged to consult books on nursing diagnoses for more information on establishing, writing, and researching other nursing diagnoses that may apply to drug administration.

TABLE 7.2 Common Nursing Diagnoses Applicable to Drug Administration

NANDA-Approved Nursing Diagnoses

Activity Intolerance	Knowledge, Deficient
Airway Clearance, Ineffective	Liver Function, Impaired, Risk for
Anxiety	Mobility: Physical, Impaired
Aspiration, Risk for	Nausea
Breathing Pattern, Ineffective	Noncompliance
Cardiac Output, Decreased	Nutrition, Imbalanced
Comfort, Enhanced, Readiness for	Oral Mucous Membrane, Impaired
Communication, Impaired Verbal	Pain
Constipation	Poisoning, Risk for
Contamination, Risk for	Self-Care Deficit
Coping, Ineffective	Sensory Perception, Disturbed
Diarrhea	Sexual Dysfunction
Distress, Moral	Skin Integrity, Impaired
Falls, Risk for	Sleep Pattern, Disturbed
Fatigue	Stress. Overload
Fluid Volume, Deficient	Suicide, Risk for
Fluid Volume, Excess	Swallowing, Impaired
Gas Exchange, Impaired	Therapeutic Regimen Management, Ineffective
Health Maintenance, Ineffective	
Human Dignity, Compromised, Risk for	Thermoregulation, Impaired
	Thought Processes, Disturbed
Hyperthermia	Tissue Perfusion, IneffectiveUrinary
Hypothermia	Incontinence
Infection, Risk for	Urinary Retention
Injury, Risk for	

Source: Adapted from North American Nursing Diagnosis Association, 2007–2008.

7.4 Setting Goals and Outcomes for Drug Administration

After the nurse has gathered client assessment data and formulated nursing diagnoses, goals and outcomes are developed and priorities established to assist in planning care, carrying out interventions, and evaluating the effectiveness of that care. Before administering and monitoring the effects of medications, nurses should establish clear, realistic goals and outcomes so that planned interventions ensure safe and effective use of these agents.

Goals are somewhat different from outcomes. Goals focus on what the client should be able to achieve and do, based on the nursing diagnosis established from the assessment data. Outcomes provide the specific, measurable criteria that will be used to evaluate the degree to which the goal was met. Both goals and outcomes are focused on what the client will achieve or do, are realistic, and are discussed with the client or caregiver. Priorities are established based on the assessment data and nursing diagnoses, with high-priority needs addressed before low-priority items. Safe and effective administration of medications, with the optimum therapeutic outcome possible, is the overall goal of any nursing plan of care.

Goals may be focused for the short term or long term, depending on the setting and situation. In the acute-care or ambulatory setting, short-term goals are most appropriate, whereas in the rehabilitation setting, long-term goals may be more commonly identified. For a client with a thrombus in the lower extremity who has been placed on anticoagulant therapy, a short-term goal may be that the client will not experience an increase in clot size, as evidenced by improving circulation to the lower extremity distal to the clot. A long-term goal might focus on teaching the client to effectively administer parenteral anticoagulant therapy at home. Like assessment data, goals should focus first on the therapeutic outcomes of medications, then on the treatment of side effects. For the client on pain medication, relief of pain is a priority established before treatment of the nausea, vomiting, or dizziness caused by the medication. The Nursing Process Focus flowcharts provided in Chapters 13 through 49 ∞ outline some of the common goals that might be developed with the client.

Outcomes are the specific criteria used to measure attainment of the selected goals. They are written to include the subject (the client in most cases), the actions required by that subject, under what circumstances, the expected performance, and the specific time frame in which the performance will be accomplished. In the example of the client who will be taught to self-administer anticoagulant therapy at home, an outcome may be written as: Client will demonstrate the injection of enoxaparin (Lovenox) using the preloaded syringe provided, given subcutaneously into the anterior abdominal areas, in 2 days (1 day prior to discharge). This outcome includes the subject (client), actions (demonstrate injection), circumstances (using a preloaded syringe), performance (SC injection into the abdomen), and time frame (2 days from now—1 day before discharge home). Writing specific outcomes also gives the nurse a concrete time frame to work toward assisting the client to meet the goals.

SPECIAL CONSIDERATIONS

Non-English-Speaking and Culturally Diverse Clients

Nurses should know, in advance, what translation services and interpreters are available in their healthcare facility to assist with communication. The nurse should use interpreter's services when available, validating with the interpreter that he or she is able to understand the client. Many dialects are similar but not the same, and knowing another language is not the same as understanding the culture. Can the interpreter understand the client's language and cultural expressions or nuances well enough for effective communication to occur? If a family member is interpreting, especially if a child is interpreting for a parent or relative, be sure that the interpreter first understands and repeats the information back to the nurse before explaining it in the client's own language. This is especially important if the translation is a summary of what has been said rather than a line-by-line translation. Before an interpreter is available, or if one is unavailable, use pictures, simple drawings, nonverbal cues, and body language to communicate with the client. Be aware of culturally based nonverbal communication behaviors (e.g., use of personal space, eye contact, or lack of eye contact). Gender sensitivities related to culture (e.g., male nurse or physician for female clients) and the use of touch are often sensitive issues. In the United States, an informal and personal style is often the norm. When working with clients of other cultures, adopting a more formal style may be more appropriate.

After goals and outcomes are identified based on the nursing diagnoses, a plan of care is written. Each agency determines whether this plan will be communicated as either nursing centered, interdisciplinary, or both. All plans should be client focused and include the client or caregiver in their development. The goals and outcomes identified in the plan of care will assist the nurse, and other healthcare providers, in implementing interventions and evaluating the effectiveness of that care.

7.5 Key Interventions for Drug Administration

After the plan of care has been written, making explicit any goals and outcomes based on established nursing diagnoses, the nurse implements this plan. Interventions are aimed at returning the client to an optimum level of wellness and limiting adverse effects related to the client's medical diagnosis or condition. Chapter 4 ∞ discusses interventions specific to drug administration, such as the five rights and the techniques of administering medications. This section focuses on other key intervention strategies that the nurse completes for a client receiving medications.

Monitoring drug effects is a primary intervention that nurses perform. A thorough knowledge of the actions of each medication is necessary to carry out this monitoring process. The nurse should first monitor for the identified therapeutic effect. A lack of sufficient therapeutic effect suggests the need to reassess pharmacotherapy. Monitoring may require a reassessment of the client's physical condition, vital signs, body weight, lab values, and/or serum drug levels. The client's statements about pain relief, as well as objective data, such as a change in blood pressure, are used to monitor the therapeutic outcomes of pharmacotherapy. The nurse also monitors for side and adverse effects and attempts to prevent or limit these effects when possible. Some side effects may be managed by the nurse independently of medical orders, whereas others require collaboration with physicians to alleviate client symptoms. For example, a client with nausea and vomiting after receiving a narcotic pain reliever may be comforted by the nurse who provides small frequent meals, sips of carbonated beverages, or frequent changes of linen. However, the physician or a nurse practitioner may need to prescribe an antiemetic drug to control the side effect of intense nausea.

Documentation of both therapeutic and adverse effects is completed during the intervention phase. This includes appropriate documentation of the administration of the medication, as well as the effects observed. Additional objective assessment data, such as vital signs, may be included in the documentation to provide more details about the specific drug effects. A client's statements can provide subjective detail to the documentation. Each healthcare facility determines where, when, and how to document the administration of medications and any follow-up assessment data that have been gathered.

Client teaching is a vital component of the nurse's interventions for a client receiving medications. Knowledge deficit, and even noncompliance, are directly related to the type and quality of medication education that a client receives. State nurse practice acts and regulating bodies such as JCAHO consider teaching to be a primary role for nurses, giving it the weight of law and key importance in accreditation standards. Because the goals of pharmcotherapy are the safe administration of medications, with the best therapeutic outcomes possible, teaching is aimed at providing the client with the information necessary to ensure this occurs. Every nurse–client interaction can present an opportunity for teaching. Small portions of education given over time are often more effective than large amounts of information given on only one occasion. Discussing medications each time they are administered is an effective way to increase the amount of education accomplished. Providing written material also assists the client to retain the information and review it later. Some medications come with a self-contained teaching program that includes videotapes. The client must be able to read and understand the material provided. Pharmacies may dispense client education pamphlets that detail all the effects of a mediation, but they are ineffective if the reading level is above what the client can understand, or is in a language unfamiliar to the client. Having the client summarize key points after the teaching has been provided may be used to verify that the client understands the information.

Elderly and pediatric clients often present special challenges to client teaching. Age-appropriate written or video materials and teaching that is repeated slowly and provided in small increments may assist the nurse in teaching these clients. It is often necessary to co-teach the client's caregiver. Parents of children must be included in the medication administration process. It is important that clients and their families understand the importance of consulting with their healthcare provider before taking any additional prescription or nonprescription medications. Table 7.3 summarizes key areas of teaching and provides sample questions the nurse might ask, or observations that can be made, to verify that teaching has been

effective. The Nursing Process Focus flowcharts in Chapters 13 through 49 ∞ also supply information on specific drugs and drug classes that is important to include in client teaching.

Medication administration in pediatric clients must be based on safe pediatric dosages, potential adverse drug reactions and medication predictability in this age group. Medication research often does not include children, so data are often unclear on safe pediatric doses potential adverse drug reactions and medication predictability. There is also great potential for medication errors, since drug administration in the pediatric population often requires drug calculations of smaller medication doses. The nurse must be vigilant to ensure the dosage is correct because small errors in drug doses have the potential to cause serious adverse effects in infants and children. The elderly population also presents the nurse with additional nursing considerations. Elderly clients often have chronic illnesses and age-related changes that may cause medication effects to be unpredictable. Because of chronic diseases, elderly clients often take multiple drugs that may cause many drug–drug interactions.

7.6 Evaluating the Effects of Drug Administration

Evaluation is the final step of the Nursing Process. It considers the effectiveness of the interventions in meeting established goals and outcomes. The process comes full circle as the nurse reassesses the client, reviews the nursing diagnoses, makes necessary changes, reviews and rewrites goals and outcomes, and carries out further interventions to meet the goals and outcomes. When evaluating the effectiveness of drug administration, the nurse assesses for optimum therapeutic effects and a minimal occurrence of side or adverse effects. The nurse also evaluates the effectiveness

TABLE 7.3 Important Areas of Teaching for a Client Receiving Medications	
Area of Teaching	**Important Questions and Observations**
therapeutic use and outcomes	• Can you tell me the name of your medicine and what the medicine is used for? • What will you look for to know that the medication is effective? (How will you know that the medicine is working?)
monitoring side and adverse effects	• Which side effects can you handle by yourself? (e.g., simple nausea, diarrhea) • Which side effects should you report to your healthcare provider? (e.g., extreme cases of nausea or vomiting, extreme dizziness, bleeding)
medication administration	• Can you tell me how much of the medication you are to take? (mg, number of tablets, ml of liquid, etc.) • Can you tell me how often you are to take it? • What special requirements are necessary when you take this medication? (e.g., take with a full glass of water; take on an empty stomach and remain upright for 30 minutes) • Is there a specific order in which you are to take your medications? (e.g., using a bronchodilator before using a corticosteroid inhaler) • Can you show me how you will give yourself the medication? (e.g., eye drops, subcutaneous injections) • What special monitoring is required before you take this medication? (e.g., pulse rate) Can you demonstrate this for me? Based on that monitoring, when should you *not* take the medication? • Do you know how, or where, to store this medication? • What should you do if you miss a dose?
other monitoring and special requirements	• Are there any special tests you are to have related to this medication? (e.g., finger-stick glucose levels, therapeutic drug levels) • How often should these tests be done? • What other medications should you *not* take with this medication? • Are there any foods or beverages you must not have while taking this medication?

of teaching provided and notes areas where further drug education is needed. Evaluation is not the end of the process but the beginning of another cycle as the nurse continues to work to ensure safe and effective medication use and active client involvement in his or her care. It is a check-point where the nurse considers the overall goal of safe and effective administration of medications and takes the steps necessary to ensure success of pharmacotherapy. The Nursing Process acts as the overall framework for working toward this success.

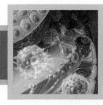

CHAPTER REVIEW

KEY CONCEPTS

The numbered key concepts provide a succinct summary of the important points from the corresponding numbered section within the chapter. If any of these points are not clear, refer to the numbered section within the chapter for review.

7.1 The Nursing Process is a systematic method of problem solving and consists of clearly defined steps: assessment, establishment of nursing diagnoses, planning care through the formulation of goals and outcomes, carrying out interventions, and evaluating the care provided.

7.2 Assessment of the client receiving medications includes health history information, physical assessment data, lab values and other measurable data, and an assessment of medication effects, both therapeutic and side effects.

7.3 Nursing diagnoses are written to address the client's responses related to drug administration. They are developed after an analysis of the assessment data, are focused on the client's problems, and are verified with the client or caregiver.

7.4 Goals and outcomes, developed from the nursing diagnoses, direct the interventions required by the plan of care. Goals focus on what the client should be able to achieve, and outcomes provide the specific, measurable criteria that will be used to measure goal attainment.

7.5 Interventions are aimed at returning the client to an optimum level of wellness through the safe and effective administration of medications. Key interventions required of the nurse include monitoring drug effects, documenting medications, and client teaching.

7.6 Evaluation begins a new cycle of care as new assessment data are gathered and analyzed, nursing diagnoses are reviewed or rewritten, goals and outcomes are refined, and new interventions are carried out.

NCLEX-RN® REVIEW QUESTIONS

1 Which of the following is an incorrect statement regarding nursing diagnosis?

1. It identifies the medical problem experienced by the client.
2. It is a clinical judgment made by the nurse.
3. It identifies the client's response to actual or potential health and life processes.
4. It determines nursing interventions for which the nurse is accountable.

2 An appropriately stated goal for a client with type 1 diabetes mellitus is:

1. The nurse will teach the client to recognize and respond to the signs and symptoms of hypoglycemia prior to discharge.
2. The client will demonstrate self-injection of insulin, using a preloaded syringe, into the subcutaneous tissue of the thigh prior to discharge.
3. The nurse will teach the client to accurately draw up the insulin dose in a syringe.
4. The client will be able to self-manage his diabetic diet and medications.

3 A 15-year-old adolescent with a history of type 1 diabetes presents to the emergency department in diabetic ketoacidosis. She has been successfully self-managing her diet and insulin therapy for the past 2 years. She confides in the nurse that she deliberately skipped some of her insulin doses because she didn't want to gain weight, and she is afraid of needle marks. Which of the following nursing diagnoses is most appropriate in this situation? (Select all that apply.)

1. Knowledge, Deficient
2. Self-Care Deficit
3. Noncompliance
4. Coping, Ineffective
5. Disbelief

4 Which factor is most important for the nurse to assess when evaluating the effectiveness of a client's drug therapy?

1. Client's promise to comply with drug therapy
2. Client's satisfaction with the drug
3. Cost of the medication
4. Evidence of therapeutic benefit

5 Which of the following is the part of the Nursing Process that has the nurse assess the effectiveness of the medication?

1. Assessment
2. Implementation
3. Diagnosis
4. Evaluation

CRITICAL THINKING QUESTIONS

1. A 13-year-old client from a rural community who is a cheer-leader has been diagnosed with type 1 diabetes. She is supported by a single mother who is frustrated with her daughter's eating habits. The client has lost weight since beginning her insulin regimen. The nurse notes that the client and her mother, who is very well dressed, are both extremely thin. Identify additional assessment data that the nurse would need to obtain before making the nursing diagnosis *Noncompliance*.

2. The drug regimen of the client in question 1 is evaluated, and the healthcare provider suggests a subcutaneous insulin pump to help control the client's fluctuating blood glucose levels. Write three nursing diagnoses related to this new therapy.

3. A nursing student is assigned to a licensed preceptor who is administering oral medications. The student notes that the preceptor administers the drugs safely but routinely fails to offer the client information about the drug being administered. Identify the information that the nurse should teach the client during medication administration.

See Appendix D for answers and rationales for all activities.

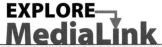
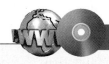

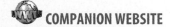
www.prenhall.com/adams

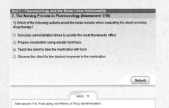

NCLEX-RN® review, case studies, and other interactive resources for this chapter can be found on the companion website at www.prenhall.com/adams. Click on "Chapter 7" to select the activities for this chapter. For animations, more NCLEX-RN® review questions, and an audio glossary, access the accompanying Prentice Hall Nursing MediaLink DVD-ROM in this textbook.

PRENTICE HALL NURSING MEDIALINK DVD-ROM

- **Audio Glossary**
- **NCLEX-RN® Review**

COMPANION WEBSITE

- **NCLEX-RN® Review**
- **Case Study:** Safe medication administration
- **Challenge Your Knowledge**

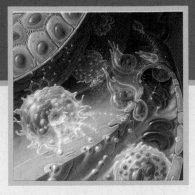

CHAPTER 8

Drug Administration Throughout the Lifespan

OBJECTIVES

After reading this chapter, the student should be able to:

1. Apply basic concepts of human growth and development to pharmacology.
2. Explain how physical, cognitive, and psychomotor development influence pharmacotherapeutics.
3. Describe physiological changes during pregnancy that may affect the absorption, distribution, metabolism, and excretion of drugs.
4. Describe how the sensitivity of the fetus to drugs changes with gestational age.
5. Match the five pregnancy categories with their definitions.
6. Identify techniques that the breastfeeding mother can use to reduce drug exposure to the newborn.
7. Describe physiological and biochemical changes that occur in the older adult, and how these affect pharmacotherapy.
8. Discuss the nursing and pharmacological implications associated with each of the following developmental age groups: prenatal, infancy, toddlerhood, preschool, school age, adolescence, young adulthood, middle adulthood, and older adulthood.

MediaLink

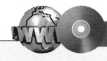 www.prenhall.com/adams

NCLEX-RN® review, case studies, and other interactive resources for this chapter can be found on the companion website at www.prenhall.com/adams. Click on "Chapter 8" to select the activities for this chapter. For animations, more NCLEX-RN® review questions, and an audio glossary, access the accompanying Prentice Hall Nursing MediaLink DVD-ROM in this textbook.

KEY TERMS

adolescence *page 84*

infancy *page 81*

middle adulthood *page 84*

older adulthood *page 84*

polypharmacy *page 85*

prenatal *page 77*

preschool child *page 83*

school-age child *page 83*

teratogen *page 77*

toddlerhood *page 82*

young adulthood *page 84*

Beginning with conception, and continuing throughout the lifespan, the organs and systems within the body undergo predictable physiological changes that influence the absorption, metabolism, distribution, and elimination of medications. Healthcare providers must recognize such changes to ensure that drugs are delivered in a safe and effective manner to clients of all ages. The purpose of this chapter is to examine how principles of developmental physiology and lifespan psychology apply to drug administration.

8.1 Pharmacotherapy Across the Lifespan

Growth is a term that characterizes the progressive increase in *physical* (bodily) size. *Development* is a related term that refers to the *functional* changes in the physical, psychomotor, and cognitive capabilities of a living being. Stages of growth and physical development usually go hand in hand, in a predictable sequence, whereas psychomotor and cognitive development have a tendency to be more variable in nature.

To provide optimum care, healthcare providers must understand *normal* growth and developmental patterns that occur throughout the lifespan. It is from this benchmark that *deviations* from the norm can be recognized, so that health-pattern impairments can be appropriately addressed. For pharmacotherapy to achieve its desired outcomes, such knowledge is essential.

The development of a person is a complex process that links the biophysical with the psychosocial, ethnocultural, and spiritual components to make each individual a unique human being. This whole-person view is essential to holistic care. The very nature of pharmacology requires that the nurse consider the individuality of each client and the specifics of age, growth, and development in relation to pharmacokinetics and pharmacodynamics.

DRUG ADMINISTRATION DURING PREGNANCY AND LACTATION

Healthcare providers exercise great caution when initiating pharmacotherapy during pregnancy or lactation. When possible, drug therapy is postponed until after pregnancy and lactation, or safer alternatives are attempted. There are some conditions, however, that are severe enough to require pharmacotherapy in such clients. These conditions include medications for treating preexisting illness, maternal illness unrelated to the pregnancy, or complications related to pregnancy. For example, if the client has epilepsy, hypertension, or a psychiatric disorder *prior to* the pregnancy, it would be unwise to discontinue therapy during pregnancy or lactation. Conditions such as gestational diabetes and gestational hypertension occur *during* pregnancy and must be treated for the safety of the growing fetus. In all cases, healthcare practitioners evaluate the therapeutic benefits of a given medication against its potential adverse effects.

8.2 Pharmacotherapy of the Pregnant Client

The pharmacotherapeutics of drug therapy in a pregnant client requires the healthcare provider to consider the effect both on the mother as well as on the growing fetus. The placenta is a semipermeable membrane: Some substances pass through to the fetus, whereas others are blocked. The fetal membranes contain enzymes that detoxify certain substances as they cross the membrane. For example, insulin from the mother is inactivated by placental enzymes during the early stages of pregnancy, preventing it from reaching the fetus (Chapter 44 ∞). In general, drugs that are water soluble, ionized, or bound to plasma proteins are less likely to cross the placenta.

PHYSIOLOGICAL CHANGES DURING PREGNANCY

During pregnancy, major physiological and anatomical changes occur in the endocrine, gastrointestinal (GI), cardiovascular, circulatory, and renal systems of clients. Some of these changes alter the pharmacodynamics of drugs administered to the client and may affect the success of pharmacotherapy.

ABSORPTION Hormonal changes as well as the pressure of the expanding uterus on the blood supply to abdominal organs affect the absorption of drugs given. Gastric emptying is delayed, and transit time for food and drugs in the GI tract is slowed by progesterone, which allows a longer time for absorption of oral drugs. Gastric acidity is also decreased, which can affect the absorption of certain drugs. Changes in the respiratory system during pregnancy—increased tidal volume and pulmonary vasodilation—may cause inhaled drugs to be absorbed more quickly.

DISTRIBUTION AND METABOLISM Hemodynamic changes in the pregnant client increase cardiac output, increase plasma volume, and change regional blood flow. The increased blood volume in the mother causes dilution of drugs and decreases plasma protein concentrations, affecting drug distribution. Blood flow to the uterus, kidneys, and skin is increased, whereas flow to the skeletal muscles is diminished. Alterations in lipid levels may alter drug transport and distribution, especially during the third trimester. Drug metabolism increases for certain drugs, most notably anticonvulsants such as carbamazepine, phenytoin, and valproic acid, which may require higher doses during pregnancy.

EXCRETION By the third trimester of pregnancy, blood flow through the kidneys increases 40% to 50%. This increase has a direct effect on renal plasma flow, glomerular filtration rate, and renal tubular absorption. Thus, drug excretion rates may be increased, affecting dosage timing and onset of action.

GESTATIONAL AGE AND DRUG THERAPY

The timing of drug therapy and the stage of fetal development critically affect the risk for possible fetal consequences. Because of the constant changes that occur during fetal development, the specific risk is dependent on when during gestation the drug is administered. Fetal consequences include intrauterine fetal death, physical malformations, growth impairment, behavioral abnormalities, and neonatal toxicity.

PRENATAL STAGE The **prenatal** stage is the time from conception to birth. This stage is subdivided into the embryonic period (conception to 8 weeks) and the fetal period (8 to 40 weeks or birth). In terms of pharmacotherapy, this is a strategic timeframe, because the nurse must take into consideration the health and welfare of both the pregnant client

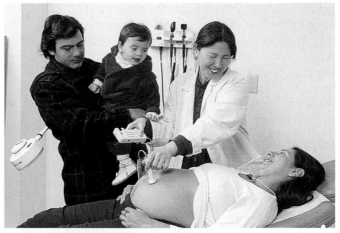

● **Figure 8.1** Treating the pregnant client
Source: © Jenny Thomas Photography.

as well as the child in utero (● Figure 8.1). Pharmacologically, the focus must be to eliminate potentially toxic agents that may harm the mother or unborn child. Agents that cause fetal malformations are termed **teratogens.** The baseline incidence of teratogenic events is approximately 3% of all pregnancies.

Before implantation, the developing ovum is usually unaffected by maternal use of drugs because there is not a vascular interchange between the mother and the baby. Thus, drugs are less likely to cause adverse fetal consequences. Drugs such as nicotine, however, can create a negative *environment* for the fetus and cause fetal damage, such as intrauterine growth retardation.

FIRST TRIMESTER After implantation, until days 58 to 60 postconception, when the skeleton and major fetal organs begin to form, the fetus is at greatest risk for developmental anomalies. If teratogenic drugs are used by the mother, major fetal malformations may occur, or the drug may even precipitate a spontaneous abortion. Unfortunately, accidental exposure may occur because the mother may take a medication before she knows she is pregnant. Whenever possible, drug therapy should be delayed until after the first trimester of pregnancy.

SECOND TRIMESTER During the second trimester (4 to 6 months) of pregnancy, development of the major organs has progressed considerably; however, exposure to certain substances taken by the mother can still cause considerable harm to the fetus. The nurse–client relationship is vital during this time, especially in terms of teaching. A woman who is pregnant can mistakenly believe that her unborn baby is safe from anything she consumes because the "baby is fully formed and just needs time to grow." During prenatal visits, the nurse must be vigilant in assessing and evaluating each client, so that any mistaken beliefs can be clarified.

THIRD TRIMESTER During the last trimester (7 to 9 months) of pregnancy, blood flow to the placenta increases and placental vascular membranes become thinner. Such alterations allow the transfer of more substances from the maternal circulation to the fetal blood. As a result, the fetus will receive larger doses of medications and other substances taken by the mother. Because the fetus lacks mature metabolic enzymes and efficient excretion mechanisms, medications will have a prolonged duration of action within the unborn child.

PREGNANCY DRUG CATEGORIES AND REGISTRIES

Fortunately, the number of prescription drugs strongly suspected or known to be teratogenic is small. In addition, in nearly every clinical situation requiring therapy with a known teratogen, there are alternative drugs that can be given with relative safety. New or infrequently used drugs for which there is inadequate safety information should be given to pregnant women only if the benefits clearly outweigh any theoretical risks.

The FDA has developed drug pregnancy categories that classify medications according to their risks during pregnancy. Table 8.1 lists the five pregnancy categories, which guide the healthcare team and the client in selecting drugs that are least hazardous for the fetus. Nurses who routinely work with women who are pregnant must memorize the drug pregnancy categories for medications commonly prescribed for their clients. Examples of category D or X drugs that have been associated with teratogenic effects include testosterone (Andro), estrogens (Premarin), ergotamine (Ergostat), all angiotensin-converting enzyme (ACE) inhibitors, methotrexate (Amethopterin), thalidomide (Thalomid), tetracycline (Achromycin), valproic acid (Depakote), and warfarin (Coumadin). In addition, alcohol, nicotine, and illicit drugs such as cocaine affect the unborn child.

It is impossible to experimentally test drugs for teratogenicity in human subjects during clinical trials. Although drugs are tested in pregnant laboratory animals, the structure of the human placenta is unique. Nonhuman primates such as monkeys and chimpanzees are most closely related genetically to human models but are rarely used because of the expense. Thus, the primary subjects used are rodents. This is problematic because rodents have different physiological, metabolic, and genetic characteristics. Most information about fetal malformations and abnormalities is extrapolated from these animal data and may be crude approximations of the actual risk to a human fetus. The actual risk to a human fetus may be much less, or magnitudes greater, than that predicted from animal data. The following statement bears repeating: *No prescription drug, over-the-counter (OTC) medication, herbal product, or dietary supplement should be taken during pregnancy unless the physician verifies that the therapeutic benefits to the mother clearly outweigh the potential risks for the unborn.*

The current A, B, C, D, and X pregnancy labeling system is simplistic and gives no *specific* clinical information to help guide nurses or their clients about a medication's true safety. The system does not indicate how the dose should be adjusted during pregnancy or lactation. Most drugs are category C because very high doses often produce teratogenic effects in animals. The FDA is in the process of updating these categories to provide more descriptive information about the risks and benefits of taking each medication. The new labels are expected to include pharmacokinetic and pharmacodynamic information that will suggest safe doses for the childbearing client. To gather this information, the FDA is encouraging all pregnant women who are taking medication to join a pregnancy registry that will survey drug effects on both the client and the fetus or newborn. Evaluation of a large number of pregnancies is needed to determine the effects of medicine on babies.

TABLE 8.1	FDA Pregnancy Categories
Category	**Definition**
A	Adequate, well-controlled studies in pregnant women have not shown an increased risk of fetal abnormalities.
B	Animal studies have revealed no evidence of harm to the fetus; however, there are no adequate, well-controlled studies in pregnant women.
	or
	Animal studies have shown an adverse effect, but adequate, well-controlled studies in pregnant women have failed to demonstrate a risk to the fetus.
C	Animal studies have shown an adverse effect, and there are no adequate, well-controlled studies in pregnant women.
	or
	No animal studies have been conducted, and there are no adequate, well-controlled studies in pregnant women.
D	Studies—either adequate and well controlled or observational—in pregnant women have demonstrated a risk to the fetus; however, the benefits of therapy may outweigh the potential risk.
X	Studies—either adequate and well controlled or observational—in animals or pregnant women have demonstrated positive evidence of fetal abnormalities. The use of the product is contraindicated in women who are or may become pregnant.

Source: U.S. Food and Drug Administration, 2001.

PREGNANCY REGISTRIES

Pregnancy registries help identify medications that are safe to be taken during pregnancy. These registries gather information from women who took medications during pregnancy. Information on babies born to women not taking the medication is then compared with data on babies born while medication was taken during pregnancy. The effects of the medication taken during pregnancy are then evaluated. Registries may be maintained by drug companies, governmental agencies or special-interest groups. Examples of pregnancy registries include the following:

- Antipsychotic medicines: http://www.motherisk.org/index.jsp
- Antiretroviral medicines: http://www.apregistry.com/
- Asthma medications: http://otispregnancy.org/otis_study_asthma.asp
- Epilepsy medications: http://www.massgeneral.org/aed/
- Rheumatoid arthritis medicines: http://otispregnancy.org/otis_study_ra.asp
- Immunosuppressant medicines: http://www.temple.edu/NTPR/

8.3 Pharmacotherapy of the Lactating Client

Breast-feeding is highly recommended as a means of providing nutrition, emotional bonding, and immune protection to the neonate. Many drugs, however, are able to enter breast milk, and a few have been shown to be harmful. As with the placenta, drugs that are ionized, water soluble, or bound to plasma proteins are less likely to enter breast milk. Central nervous system (CNS) medications are very lipid soluble and thus are more likely to be present in higher concentrations in milk and can be expected to have a greater effect on an infant. Although concentrations of CNS drugs in breast milk are found in higher amounts, they often remain at subclinical levels. Regarding the role of protein binding, drugs that remain in the maternal plasma bound to albumin are not able to penetrate the mother's milk supply. For example, warfarin is strongly bound to plasma proteins and thus has a reduced milk level because it is unable to transfer into the maternal milk.

The American Academy of Pediatrics (AAP) Committee on Drugs provides guidance on which drugs should be avoided during breast-feeding to protect the child's safety. Medications that pass into breast milk are indicated in drug guides. Nurses who work with women who are pregnant or breast-feeding should give careful attention to this information. Selected drugs that enter the breast milk and have been shown to produce adverse effects are listed in Table 8.2.

It is imperative that the nurse teach the lactating client that many prescription medications, OTC drugs, and herbal products are excreted in breast milk and have the potential to affect her child (● Figure 8.2). The same guidelines for drug use apply during the breast-feeding period as during pregnancy—drugs should be taken only if the benefits to the mother clearly outweigh the potential risks to the infant. The nurse should explore the possibility of postponing pharmacotherapy until the baby is weaned, or perhaps selecting a safer, nonpharmacological alternative therapy. If a drug is indicated, it is sometimes useful to administer it immediately after breast-feeding, or

TABLE 8.2	Selected Drugs Associated with Adverse Effects During Breast-feeding
Drug	**Reported Effect or Reasons for Concern**
amphetamine	irritability, poor sleeping pattern
cocaine	cocaine intoxication: irritability, vomiting, diarrhea, tremulousness, seizures
heroin	tremors, restlessness, vomiting, poor feeding
phencyclidine	potent hallucinogen
acebutolol (Sectral)	hypotension, bradycardia, tachypnea
atenolol (Tenormin)	cyanosis, bradycardia
bromocriptine (Parlodel)	suppresses lactation; may be hazardous to the mother
aspirin (salicylates)	metabolic acidosis
ergotamine (Ergostat)	vomiting, diarrhea, convulsions (doses used in migraine medications)
lithium (Eskalith)	one third to half the therapeutic blood concentration in infants
phenindione	anticoagulant: increased prothrombin and partial thromboplastin time
phenobarbital (Luminal)	sedation, infantile spasms after weaning from milk containing phenobarbital, methemoglobinemia
primidone (Mysoline)	sedation, feeding problems
sulfasalazine (Azulfidine)	bloody diarrhea

Source: From "The Transfer of Drugs and Other Chemicals into Human Breast Milk" by American Academy of Pediatrics, Committee on Drugs, 2001, *Pediatrics, 3*, pp. 776–782. Reprinted with permission.

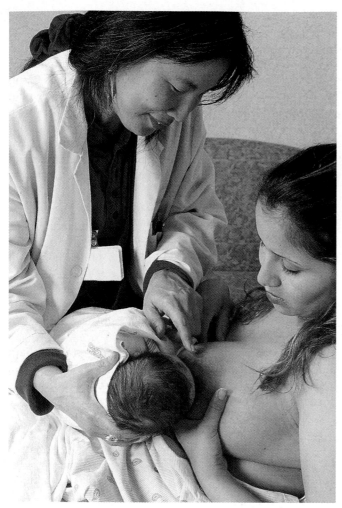

● **Figure 8.2** Treating the breast-feeding mother
Source: © *Jenny Thomas Photography.*

when the infant will be sleeping for an extended period, so that time elapses before the next feeding. This will reduce the amount of active drug products in the mother's milk when she does breast-feed her infant. The nurse can assist the mother in protecting the child's safety by teaching her to avoid illicit drugs, alcohol, and tobacco products during breast-feeding.

If a mother is receiving treatment with a radioactive drug (such as radioactive iodine, I-131), she should be advised to temporarily discontinue breast-feeding. During the time she is taking the radioactive substance, she should mechanically empty her breasts and discard the milk as directed. After she has concluded her treatment and her milk no longer contains radioactive substances, she can safely resume breast-feeding.

When considering the effects of drugs on the breast-feeding infant, the *amount* of drug that actually reaches the infant's tissues must be considered. Some medications are destroyed in the infant's GI system, are unable to be absorbed through the wall of the GI system, or are rapidly metabolized by the liver. Thus, although many drugs are found in breast milk, some are present in such small amounts that they cause no noticeable harm.

The last key factor in the effect of drugs on the infant relates to the infant's ability to metabolize small amounts of drugs. Premature, neonatal, and ill infants may be at greater risk for adverse effects because they lack drug metabolizing enzymes.

Some recommendations regarding medications given during lactation are as follows (Hale, 2004):

● Drugs with a shorter half-life are preferable. They generally peak rapidly and then are eliminated from the maternal plasma, which reduces the amount of drug exposure to the infant. The mother should not breast-feed while the drug is at its peak level.

● Drugs that have long half-lives (or active metabolites) should be avoided because they can accumulate in the infant's plasma. Examples include barbiturates, benzodiazepines, meperidine, and fluoxetine.

● Whenever possible, drugs with high protein-binding ability should be selected because they do not transfer as readily to the milk.

● Herbal products and dietary supplements should be avoided, unless specifically prescribed by the healthcare provider, because they may contain chemical ingredients that are harmful to the infant.

8.4 Client Teaching During Pregnancy and Lactation

Client education during pregnancy and lactation is critical to the success of pharmacotherapy and to the safety of the mother and baby. The nurse should perform an in-depth history and prenatal assessment to eliminate potentially hazardous substances, substitute alternative drugs, or adjust medication dosages. The client needs to be thoroughly

PHARMFACTS

Possible Fetal Effects Caused by Specific Drug Use During Pregnancy

■ Marijuana: low-birth-weight babies, increased risk of birth defects, increased risk of leukemia, increased behavioral problems, and decreased attention span

■ Cocaine: increased risk of miscarriage, premature delivery, malformations of fetal limbs and kidneys, later learning difficulties

■ Heroin: increased risk of miscarriage, low-birth-weight babies, babies born with neonatal abstinence syndrome (diarrhea, fever, sneezing, yawning, tremors, seizures, irregular breathing, and irritability)

■ Tobacco: increased risk of stillbirths, premature delivery, low-birth-weight babies, increased risk of sudden infant death syndrome (SIDS)

■ Alcohol: alcohol-related birth defects ranging from miscarriage and stillbirth to fetal alcohol syndrome (small stature; joint problems; and problems with attention, memory, intelligence, coordination, and problem solving)

Source: Data from Prevention Source, Vancouver, BC.

informed about the risks to both herself and her unborn child related to the use of drugs, alcohol, tobacco, alternative therapies, and OTC medications. Include the following points when teaching clients about drug therapy during pregnancy:

- Keep all scheduled physician appointments and laboratory visits for testing.

- Do not take other prescription drugs, OTC medications, herbal remedies, or dietary supplements without notifying your healthcare provider. Your healthcare provider may need to change a prescribed drug to another similar drug or change the drug dosage.

- Take iron, folic acid, and multivitamin supplements as prescribed during pregnancy.

- Eliminate alcohol and tobacco use.

- Join a pregnancy registry if you are taking prescription drugs.

- Understand that the adverse effects of drug treatment may be confused with common discomforts of pregnancy because they may be similar. These common discomforts include nausea, vomiting, heartburn, constipation, hypotension, heart palpitations, and fatigue.

- Use nonpharmacological alternatives such as massage for pain or calming music for anxiety, whenever possible, to minimize the need for drug therapy.

DRUG ADMINISTRATION DURING CHILDHOOD

As a child develops, physical growth and physiological changes mandate adjustments in the administration of medications. Although children may receive similar drugs via routes routes similar to those in adults, the nursing management for children is very different from that for adults. Factors for the nurse to consider include physiological variations, maturity of body systems, and greater fluid distribution in children. These factors can exaggerate or diminish the effectiveness of pediatric drug therapy. Drug dosages are vastly different in children. Almost all drug dosages are calculated on the basis of the infant's weight in kilograms. The following sections chronicle changes relevant to pharmacotherapy that occur in infancy, toddlerhood, preschool age, school age, and adolescence.

8.5 Pharmacotherapy of Infants

Infancy is the period from birth to 12 months of age. During this time, nursing care and pharmacotherapy are directed toward safety of the infant, proper dosing of prescribed drugs, and teaching parents how to administer medications properly.

When an infant is ill, it is sometimes traumatic for the parents. By having knowledge of growth and development, the nurse can assist the parents in caring for the baby (● Figure 8.3). The nurse should assess the infant's normal routines at home and attempt to follow these routines as closely as possible while the infant is hospitalized. Parents should be kept informed of specific orders for the infant such as fluid restrictions. Encourage the parents to participate in the care of the infant as much as they would like.

Medications administered at home to infants are often given via droppers into the eyes, ears, nose, or mouth. Infants with well-developed sucking reflexes may be willing to ingest oral drugs with a pleasant taste through a bottle nipple. Infant drops are given by placing the drops in the buccal pouch for the infant to swallow. Oral medications should be administered slowly to avoid aspiration. If rectal suppositories are administered, the buttocks should be held together for 5 to 10 minutes to prevent expulsion of the drug before absorption has occurred.

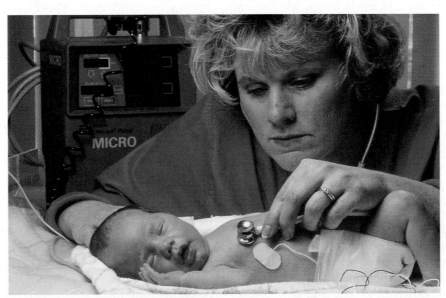

● **Figure 8.3** Treating the infant *Source: Pearson Education/PH College.*

Special considerations must be observed when administering IM or IV injections to infants. Unlike adults, infants lack well-developed muscle masses, so the smallest needle appropriate for the drug (preferably a 3/8-inch needle) should be used. The vastus lateralis is the preferred site for IM injections in infants and children younger than age 3, because this muscle has few nerves and is relatively well developed in infants. The gluteal site is usually contraindicated because of potential damage to the sciatic nerve, which may result in permanent disability. Because of the lack of choices for injection sites, the nurse must take care not to overuse a particular location, because inflammation and excessive pain may result. For IV sites, the feet and scalp often provide good venous access. After gaining IV access, it is important that the IV remain secured so the infant does not dislodge it. It is also important to check the IV site frequently and assess for signs of inflammation or infiltration.

Medications for infants are often prescribed in milligrams per kilogram per day (mg/kg/24h), rather than according to the baby's age in weeks or months. An alternative method of calculating doses is to use the infant's body surface area (BSA). The liver and kidneys of infants are immature; therefore, drugs will have a greater impact because of their prolonged duration of action. For these reasons, it is important to consider age and size in determining safe dosages of medications for infants.

From early infancy, the natural immunity a child receives from the mother in utero slowly begins to decline. The child's developing immune system must then take over. Childhood diseases that were once damaging or fatal can now be controlled through routine immunizations. The nurse plays a key role in educating parents about the importance of keeping their child's immunizations current. Vaccinations are discussed in Chapter 32 ∞.

8.6 Pharmacotherapy of Toddlers

Toddlerhood is the age period from 1 to 3 years. During this time, a toddler displays a tremendous sense of curiosity. The child begins to explore, wants to try new things, and tends to place everything in the mouth. This becomes a major concern for medication and household product safety. The nurse must be instrumental in teaching parents that poisons come in all shapes, sizes, and forms and include medicines, cosmetics, cleaning supplies, arts and crafts materials, plants, and food products that are improperly stored. Parents should be instructed to request child-resistant containers from the pharmacist and to stow all medications in secure cabinets.

Toddlers can swallow liquids and may be able to chew solid medications. When prescription drugs are supplied as flavored elixirs, it is important to stress that the child not be given access to the medications. Drugs must never be left at the bedside or within easy reach of the child. A child who has access to a bottle of cherry-flavored acetaminophen (Tylenol) may ingest a fatal overdose of the tasty liquid. Nurses should educate parents about the following means of protecting their children from poisoning:

* Read and carefully follow directions on the label before using drugs and household products.
* Store all drugs and harmful agents out of the reach of children and in locked cabinets.
* Keep all household products and drugs in their original containers. Never put chemicals in empty food or drink containers.
* Always ask for medication to be placed in child-resistant containers.
* Never tell children that medicine is candy.
* Keep the Poison Control Center number near phones, and call immediately when poisoning is suspected.
* Never leave medication unattended in a child's room or in areas where the child plays.

Administration of medications to toddlers can be challenging for the nurse. At this stage, the child is rapidly developing increased motor ability and learning to assert independence, but has extremely limited ability to reason or understand the relationship of medicines to health. Giving long, detailed explanations to the toddler will prolong the procedure and create additional anxiety. Short, concrete explanations followed by immediate drug administration are best for this age group. Physical comfort in the form of touching, hugging, or verbal praise following drug administration is important.

Oral medications that taste bad should be mixed with a vehicle such as jam, syrup, or fruit puree, if possible. Encourage parents to mix the medication in the smallest amount possible to ensure that the toddler receives all of it. The medication may be followed with a carbonated beverage or mint-flavored candy. Nurses should teach parents to avoid placing medicine in milk, orange juice, or cereals, because the child may associate these healthful foods with bad-tasting medications. Pharmaceutical companies often formulate pediatric medicines in sweet syrups to increase the ease of drug administration.

IM injections for toddlers should be given into the vastus lateralis muscle. IV injections may use scalp or feet veins; additional peripheral site options become available in late toddlerhood. The toddler presents additional safety issues to the nurse who is administering IV medications. The nurse must firmly secure the IV and then educate the parents about the dangers of the toddler's trying to pull away too quickly from the IV pump. It is often helpful to put longer tubing on a toddler's IV to give the child more play room. Suppositories may be difficult to administer because of the child's resistance. For any of these invasive administration procedures, having a parent in close proximity will usually reduce the toddler's anxiety and increase cooperation, but ask the parent prior to the procedure if he or she would like to assist. The nurse should take at least one helper into the room for assistance in restraining the toddler if necessary.

Pediatric Drug Research and Labeling

An estimated 75% of the medications prescribed for children contain no specific dosing information for pediatric clients. Without specific labeling information, healthcare providers have largely based their doses on the smaller weight of the child. Children, however, are not merely small adults; they have unique differences in physiology and biochemistry that may place them at risk in drug therapy.

Inclusion of children in clinical trials is an expensive and potentially risky process. Costs for testing drugs in large numbers of children in different age groups may reach as much as $35 million (Heinrich, 2001). Manufacturers have faced liability and malpractice issues associated with testing new medications in children. In 1997, Congress provided financial incentives for pharmaceutical manufacturers to test drugs in children. In return for comprehensive testing in children, the FDA granted the companies an additional 6 months of exclusive marketing rights for the drug. As a result of this effort, more than 28 drugs have been investigated in children, and 18 drug labels have been changed to incorporate the results of the research findings. Drugs that now have more specific pediatric labeling include ibuprofen (Motrin), ranitidine (Zantac), fluvoxamine (Luvox), etodolac (Lodine), and midazolam (Versed). The legislation was reauthorized until 2007, and extended to include the study of "off-patent" drugs in children and the establishment of an Office of Pediatric Therapeutics at the FDA.

8.7 Pharmacotherapy of Preschoolers and School-age Children

The **preschool child** ranges in age from 3 to 5 years. During this period, the child begins to refine gross and fine motor skills and develop language abilities. The child initiates new activities and becomes more socially involved with other children.

Preschoolers can sometimes comprehend the difference between health and illness and that medications are administered to help them feel better. Nonetheless, medications and other potentially dangerous products must still be safely stowed out of the child's reach.

In general, principles of medication administration that pertain to the toddler also apply to this age group. Preschoolers cooperate in taking oral medications if they are crushed or mixed with food or flavored beverages. After a child has been walking for about a year, the dorsogluteal site may be used for IM injections, because it causes less pain than the vastus lateralis site. The scalp veins can no longer be used for IV access; peripheral veins are used for IV injections.

Like toddlers, preschoolers often physically resist medication administration, and a long, detailed explanation of the procedure will promote additional anxiety. A brief explanation followed quickly by medication administration is usually the best method. Uncooperative children may need to be restrained, and clients older than 4 years may require two adults to administer the medication. Before and after medication procedures, the child may benefit from opportunities to play-act troubling experiences with dolls. When the child plays the role of doctor or nurse by giving a "sick" doll a pill or injection, comforting the doll, and explaining that the doll will now feel better, the little actor feels safer and more in control of the situation.

The **school-age child** is between 6 and 12 years of age. Some refer to this period as the *middle childhood* years. This is the time in a child's life when there is progression away from the family-centered environment to the larger peer-relationship environment. Rapid physical, mental, and social development occur, and early ethical–moral development begins to take shape. Thinking processes become progressively more logical and consistent.

During this time, most children remain relatively healthy, with immune system development well under way. Respiratory infections and GI upsets are the most common complaints. Because the child feels well most of the time, there is little concept of illness or the risks involved with ingesting a harmful substance offered to the child by a peer or older person.

The nurse is usually able to gain considerable cooperation from school-age children. Longer, more detailed explanations may be of value, because the child has developed some reasoning ability and can understand the relationship between the medicine and feeling better. When children are old enough to welcome choices, they can be offered limited dosing alternatives to provide a sense of control and to encourage cooperation. The option of taking one medication before another or the chance to choose which drink will follow a chewable tablet helps distract children from the issue of whether they will take the medication at all. It also makes an otherwise strange or unpleasant experience a little more enjoyable. Making children feel that they are willing participants in medication administration, rather than victims, is an important foundation for compliance. Praise for cooperation is appropriate for any pediatric client and sets the stage for successful medication administration in the future (● Figure 8.4).

School-age children can take chewable tablets and may swallow tablets or capsules. Many still resist injections and IV insertions. It is best to have help available for these procedures. The child should never be told that he or she is "too old" to cry and resist. The ventrogluteal site is preferred for IM injections, although the muscles of older children are developed enough for the nurse to use other sites.

Poisoning

According to the National Emergency Medical Association (NEMA):

- Each year, 2 million Americans are poisoned.
- Poisoning can be prevented through education and awareness.
- Many poisonings occur in children under 6 years of age.
- Adults can be poisoned by taking the wrong dose of medication, confusing different medications, or accidentally splashing a poison on the skin or in the eyes.

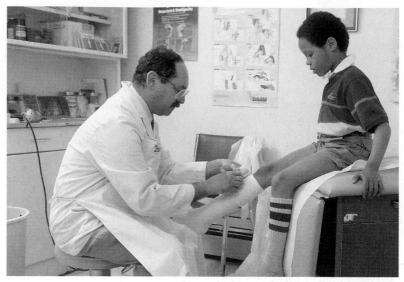

● Figure 8.4 Treating the younger school-age child *Source: Pearson Education/PH College.*

8.8 Pharmacotherapy of Adolescents

Adolescence is the time between ages 13 and 16 years. A person in this age group is able to think in abstract terms and come to logical conclusions based on a given set of observations. Rapid physical growth and psychological maturation have a great impact on personality development. The adolescent relates strongly to peers, wanting and needing their support, approval, and presence. Physical appearance and conformity with peers in terms of behavior, dress, and social interactions is important.

The most common needs for pharmacotherapy in this age group are for skin problems, headaches, menstrual symptoms, and sports-related injuries. There is an increased need for contraceptive information and counseling with sexually related health problems. This is also a time when weight becomes an issue for many teens, especially girls. Because anorexia nervosa and bulimia occur in this population, the nurse should carefully question adolescents about their eating habits and their use of OTC appetite suppressants or laxatives. Tobacco use and illicit drug experimentation may be prevalent in this population. Teenage athletes may use amphetamines to delay the onset of fatigue, and anabolic steroids to increase muscle strength and endurance. The nurse assumes a key role in educating adolescent clients about the hazards of tobacco use and illicit drugs.

The adolescent has a need for privacy and control in drug administration. The nurse should seek complete cooperation and communicate with the teen more in the manner of an adult than a child. Teens usually appreciate thorough explanations of their treatments, and ample time should be allowed for them to ask questions. Adolescents are often reluctant to admit their lack of knowledge, so the nurse should carefully explain important information regarding their medications and expected side effects, even if the client claims to understand. Teens are easily embarrassed, and the nurse should be sensitive to their needs for self-expression, privacy, and individuality, particularly when parents, siblings, or friends are present.

DRUG ADMINISTRATION DURING ADULTHOOD

When considering adult health, it is customary to divide this period of life into three stages: **young adulthood** (18 to 40 years), **middle adulthood** (40 to 65 years), and **older adulthood** (over 65 years). Within each of these divisions are similar biophysical, psychosocial, and spiritual characteristics that affect nursing and pharmacotherapy.

8.9 Pharmacotherapy of Young and Middle-aged Adults

The health status of younger adults is generally good; absorption, metabolic, and excretion mechanisms are at their peaks. There is minimal need for prescription drugs unless chronic diseases such as diabetes or immune-related conditions exist. The use of vitamins, minerals, and herbal remedies is prevalent in young adulthood. Prescription drugs are usually related to contraception or agents needed during pregnancy and delivery. Medication compliance is positive within this age range, because there is clear comprehension of benefit in terms of longevity and feeling well.

Substance abuse is a cause for concern in the 18 to 24 age group, with alcohol, tobacco products, amphetamines, and illicit drugs (marijuana and cocaine) a problem. For young adults who are sexually active, with multiple partners, prescription medications for the treatment of herpes, gonorrhea, syphilis, and HIV infections may be necessary.

The physical status of the middle-aged adult is on a par with that of the young adult until about 45 years of age. During this period of life, numerous transitions occur that often result in excessive stress. Middle-aged adults are sometimes

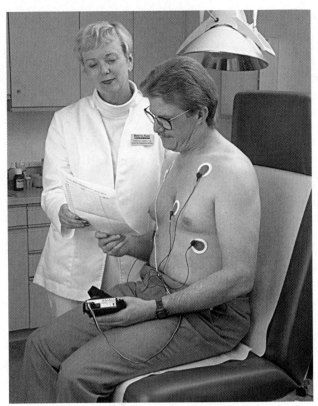

● **Figure 8.5** Treating the middle-aged adult *Source: Pearson Education/PH College.*

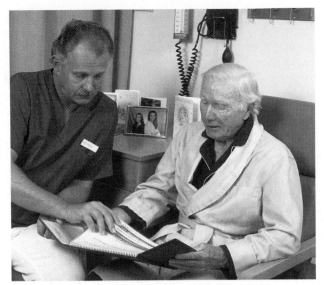

● **Figure 8.6** Treating the older adult *Source: Pearson Education/PH College.*

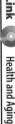

referred to as the "sandwich generation" because they are often caring for aging parents as well as children and grandchildren. Because of the pressures of work and family, middle-aged adults often take medication to control health alterations that could best be treated with positive lifestyle modifications. The nurse must emphasize the importance on overall health of lifestyle choices, such as limiting lipid intake, maintaining optimum weight, and exercising (● Figure 8.5).

Health impairments related to cardiovascular disease, hypertension, obesity, arthritis, cancer, and anxiety begin to surface in middle age. The use of drugs to treat hypertension, hyperlipidemia, digestive disorders, erectile dysfunction, and arthritis are becoming more common. Respiratory disorders related to lifelong tobacco use or exposure to secondhand smoke and environmental toxins may develop that require drug therapies. Adult-onset diabetes mellitus often emerges during this time of life. The use of antidepressants and antianxiety agents is prominent in the population older than 50.

8.10 Pharmacotherapy of Older Adults

During the 20th century, an improved quality of life and the ability to effectively treat many chronic diseases contributed to increased longevity. As individuals age, however, many physiological changes occur. The age-related changes in older adults influence the client's response to drugs, altering both the therapeutic and adverse effects, and creating special needs and risks. As a consequence of aging, clients experience an increasing number of chronic health disorders, and more drugs are prescribed to treat them. The taking of multiple drugs concurrently, known as **polypharmacy,** has become commonplace among older adults. Polypharmacy dramatically increases the risk for drug interactions and side effects.

Although predictable physiological and psychosocial changes occur with aging, significant variability exists among clients. For example, although cognitive decline and memory loss certainly occur along the aging continuum, there is a great variation in this population. Some individuals do not experience cognitive impairment at all. The nurse should avoid preconceived notions that elderly clients will have physical or cognitive impairment simply because they have reached a certain age. Careful assessment is always necessary (● Figure 8.6). The goal is to develop an individualized nursing care approach and to promote optimal quality of life because, for many clients, cure may not be a realistic goal.

When administering medications to older adults, the nurse should offer the client the same degree of independence and dignity that would be afforded middle-aged adults, unless otherwise indicated. Like their younger counterparts, older clients have a need to understand why they are receiving a drug and what outcomes are expected. Accommodations must be made for older adults who have certain impairments. Visual and auditory changes make it important for the nurse to provide drug instructions in large type and to obtain client feedback to be certain that medication instructions have been understood. Elderly clients with cognitive decline and memory loss can benefit from aids such as alarmed pill containers, medicine management boxes, and clearly written instructions. During assessment, the nurse should determine if the client is capable of self-administering medications or whether the assistance of a caregiver will be required. As long as small children are not present in the household, older clients with arthritis should be encouraged to ask the pharmacist for regular screw-cap medication bottles for ease of opening.

Older clients experience more adverse effects from drug therapy than does any other age group. Although some of these effects are due to polypharmacy, many of the adverse events are predictable, based on normal physiological and biochemical processes that occur during aging. The principal complications of drug therapy in the older adult population are degeneration of organ systems, multiple and severe illness, polypharmacy, and unreliable compliance. By understanding these changes, the nurse can avoid many adverse drug effects in older clients.

In older clients, the functioning ability of all major organ systems progressively declines. For this reason, all phases of pharmacokinetics are affected, and appropriate adjustments in therapy need to be implemented. Although most of the pharmacokinetic changes are due to reduced hepatic and renal drug elimination, other systems may also initiate a variety of changes. For example, immune system function diminishes with aging, so autoimmune diseases and infections occur more frequently in elderly clients. Thus, there is an increased need for influenza and pneumonia vaccinations. Normal physiological changes that affect pharmacotherapy of the older adult are summarized as follows:

ABSORPTION In general, absorption of drugs is slower in the older adult owing to diminished gastric motility and decreased blood flow to digestive organs. Increased gastric pH can delay absorption of medications that require high acidity to dissolve.

DISTRIBUTION Increased body fat in the older adult provides a larger storage compartment for lipid-soluble drugs and vitamins. Plasma levels are reduced, and the therapeutic response is diminished. Older adults have less body water, making the effects of dehydration more dramatic and increasing the risk for drug toxicity. For example, elderly clients who have reduced body fluid experience more orthostatic hypotension. The decline in lean body mass and total body water leads to an increased concentration of water-soluble drugs, because the drug is distributed in a smaller volume of water. The aging liver produces less albumin, resulting in decreased plasma protein-binding ability and increased levels of free drug in the bloodstream, thereby increasing the potential for drug–drug interactions. The aging cardiovascular system has decreased cardiac output and less efficient blood circulation, which slow drug distribution. This makes it important to initiate pharmacotherapy with smaller dosages and slowly increase the amount to a safe, effective level.

METABOLISM The liver's production of enzymes decreases, liver mass decreases, and the splanchnic blood flow is diminished, resulting in reduced hepatic drug metabolism. This change leads to an increase in the half-life of many drugs, which prolongs and intensifies drug response. The decline in hepatic function reduces first-pass metabolism. (Recall that first-pass metabolism relates to the amount of a drug that is removed from the bloodstream during the first circulation through the liver after the drug has been absorbed by the intestinal tract.) Thus, plasma levels are elevated, and tissue concentrations are increased for the particular drug. This change alters the standard dosage, the interval between doses, and the duration of side effects.

EXCRETION Older adults have reduced renal blood flow, glomerular filtration rate, active tubular secretion, and nephron function. This decreases drug excretion for drugs that are eliminated by the kidneys. When excretion is reduced, serum drug levels and the potential for toxicity markedly increase. Administration schedules and dosage amounts may need to be altered in many older adults owing to these changes in kidney function. Keep in mind that the most common etiology of adverse drug reactions in older adults is caused by the accumulation of toxic amounts of drugs secondary to impaired renal excretion.

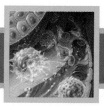

CHAPTER REVIEW

KEY CONCEPTS

The numbered key concepts provide a succinct summary of the important points from the corresponding numbered section within the chapter. If any of these points are not clear, refer to the numbered section within the chapter for review.

8.1 To contribute to safe and effective pharmacotherapy, it is essential for the nurse to understand and apply fundamental concepts of growth and development.

8.2 Pharmacotherapy during pregnancy should be conducted only when the benefits to the mother outweigh the potential risks to the unborn child. Pregnancy categories guide the healthcare provider in prescribing drugs for these clients.

8.3 Breast-feeding clients must be aware that drugs and other substances can appear in milk and cause adverse effects to the infant.

8.4 Client education is especially critical during pregnancy and lactation for the safety of the mother and baby and to ensure pharmacological outcomes.

8.5 During infancy, pharmacotherapy is directed toward the safety of the child and teaching the parents how to properly administer medications and care for the infant.

8.6 Drug administration to toddlers can be challenging; short, concrete explanations followed by immediate drug administration are usually best for the toddler.

8.7 Preschool and younger school-age children can begin to assist with medication administration.

8.8 Pharmacological compliance in the adolescent is dependent on an understanding and respect for the uniqueness of the person in this stage of growth and development.

8.9 Young adults constitute the healthiest age group and generally need few prescription medications. Middle-aged adults begin to suffer from stress-related illness such as hypertension.

8.10 Older adults take more medications and experience more adverse drug events than any other age group. For drug therapy to be successful, the nurse must make accommodations for age-related changes in physiological and biochemical functions.

NCLEX-RN® REVIEW QUESTIONS

1 A 16-year-old adolescent is 6 weeks' pregnant. Her acne has been exacerbated during the pregnancy. She asks the nurse if she can resume taking her isotretinoin (Accutane) prescription. The best response by the nurse is:

1. "Since you have a prescription for Accutane, it is safe to resume using it."
2. "You should check with your physician at your next visit."
3. "Accutane is known to cause birth defects and should never be taken during pregnancy."
4. "You should reduce the Accutane dosage by half during pregnancy."

2 To reduce the effect of a prescribed medication on the infant of a breast-feeding mother, the nurse should plan to administer the medication:

1. At night.
2. Immediately before the next feeding.
3. In divided doses at regular intervals around the clock.
4. Immediately after breast-feeding.

3 A client has arthritis in her hands. She takes several prescription drugs. Which statement by this client requires follow-up by the nurse?

1. "My pharmacist puts my pills in screw-top bottles to make it easier for me to take them."
2. "I fill my prescriptions once per month."
3. "I care for my 2-year-old grandson twice a week."
4. "My arthritis medicine helps my stiff hands."

4 A nurse is administering a liquid medication to a 15-month-old child. The most appropriate approach by the nurse is to:

1. Tell the child the medication is candy.
2. Mix the medication in 8 oz of orange juice.
3. Ask the child if she would like to take her medication now.
4. Sit her up, hold the medicine cup to her lips, and kindly instruct her to drink.

5 The nurse is preparing to give an injection to an infant. Using the image provided, select the preferred site for injections for newborns and infants.

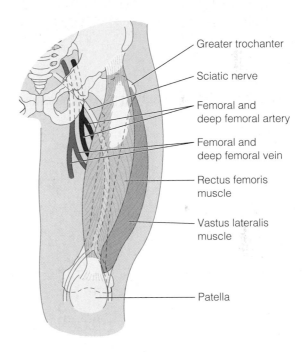

Greater trochanter

Sciatic nerve

Femoral and deep femoral artery

Femoral and deep femoral vein

Rectus femoris muscle

Vastus lateralis muscle

Patella

CRITICAL THINKING QUESTIONS

1. A 22-year-old pregnant client is diagnosed with pyelonephritis, and an antibiotic is prescribed. What information does the nurse need to safely administer the drug?

2. An 86-year-old male client is confused and anxious. His daughter wonders if "a small dose" of diazepam (Valium) might help her father to be less anxious. Prior to responding to the daughter or consulting the prescribing authority, the nurse should review age-related concerns. What are the nurse's concerns?

3. An 8-month-old child is prescribed acetaminophen (Tylenol) elixir for management of fever. She is recovering from gastroenteritis and is still having several loose stools per day. The child spits some of the elixir on her shirt. Does the nurse repeat the dose? What are the implications of this child's age and physical condition for oral drug administration?

See Appendix D for answers and rationales for all activities.

 EXPLORE MediaLink

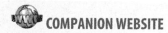 www.prenhall.com/adams

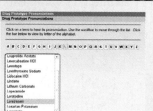

NCLEX-RN® review, case studies, and other interactive resources for this chapter can be found on the companion website at www.prenhall.com/adams. Click on "Chapter 8" to select the activities for this chapter. For animations, more NCLEX-RN® review questions, and an audio glossary, access the accompanying Prentice Hall Nursing MediaLink DVD-ROM in this textbook.

PRENTICE HALL NURSING MEDIALINK DVD-ROM

- **Audio Glossary**
- **NCLEX-RN® Review**

COMPANION WEBSITE

- **NCLEX-RN® Review**
- **Case Study:** Pharmacotherapy of toddlers
- **Challenge Your Knowledge**

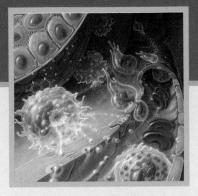

CHAPTER 9

Medication Errors and Risk Reduction

OBJECTIVES

After reading this chapter, the student should be able to:

1. Define a medication error.
2. Identify factors that contribute to medication errors.
3. Explain the relationship of standards of care to reducing medication errors.
4. Identify specific examples of the categories of medication errors.
5. Describe the severity of different categories of medication errors.
6. Explain how rules, policies, and procedures can help prevent medication errors.
7. Describe the impact of a medication error on all aspects of an agency or institution, including clients, staff nurses, administrative personnel, departments, and hospital or corporation.
8. Describe methods of reporting and documenting medication errors and incidents.
9. Describe strategies that the nurse may implement to reduce medication errors and incidents.
10. Identify client teaching information that can be used to reduce medication errors and incidents.
11. Identify efforts recommended by the FDA to monitor medication errors and incidents and provide information to healthcare providers.
12. Explain strategies used by healthcare organizations to reduce the number of medication errors and incidents.

MediaLink

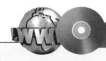

www.prenhall.com/adams

NCLEX-RN® review, case studies, and other interactive resources for this chapter can be found on the companion website at www.prenhall.com/adams. Click on "Chapter 9" to select the activities for this chapter. For animations, more NCLEX-RN® review questions, and an audio glossary, access the accompanying Prentice Hall Nursing MediaLink DVD-ROM in this textbook.

KEY TERMS

beneficence *page 90*

medication administration record (MAR)
  page 93

medication error *page 90*

medication error index *page 90*

nonmaleficence *page 90*

nurse practice act *page 92*

reasonable and prudent action *page 92*

risk management *page 96*

standards of care *page 92*

In their clinical practice, nurses are sensitive to the complexities of risk reduction and medication errors. They want to ensure client safety by striving to be 100% accurate when administering medications. Although nurses highly value proficiency and accuracy in giving medications, they may inadvertently commit an error that places their client at risk for injury. Doing harm to a client is every nurse's greatest fear. "To do no harm" is the ethical principle of **nonmaleficence,** and **beneficence** is the obligation to seek interventions that are beneficial for the client. These two principles guide nursing care in both theory and practice.

9.1 Defining Medication Errors

According to the National Coordinating Council for Medication Error Reporting and Prevention (NCC MERP), a **medication error** is "any preventable event that may cause or lead to inappropriate medication use or client harm while the medication is in the control of the healthcare professional, client, or consumer." NCC MERP also classifies medication errors and has developed the **medication error index**. This index categorizes medication errors by evaluating the extent of the harm an error can cause (● Figure 9.1).

Stated simply, a medication error is any error that occurs in the medication administration process whether or not it reaches the client. These errors may be related to misinterpretations, miscalculations, misadministrations, handwriting misinterpretation, and misunderstanding of verbal or phone orders.

9.2 Factors Contributing to Medication Errors

To be successful, proper medication administration involves a partnership between the healthcare provider and the client. This relationship is dependent on the competence of the healthcare provider, as well as the client's compliance with drug therapy. This dual responsibility provides a simple, though useful, way to conceptualize medication errors as resulting from healthcare provider error or client error. Clearly, the purpose of classifying and studying these errors is not to assess individual blame but to prevent future errors.

Factors contributing to medication errors by *healthcare providers* include, but are not limited to, the following:

- Omitting one of the rights of drug administration (see Chapter 4 ∞). Common errors include giving an incorrect dose, not giving an ordered dose, and giving an unordered drug.
- Failing to perform an agency system check. Both pharmacists and nurses must collaborate on checking the accuracy and appropriateness of drug orders prior to administering drugs to clients.
- Failing to account for client variables such as age, body size, and renal or hepatic function. Nurses should always review recent laboratory data and other information in the client's chart before administering medications, especially those drugs that have a narrow margin of safety.
- Giving medications based on verbal orders or phone orders, which may be misinterpreted or go undocumented. Nurses should remind the prescribing healthcare practitioner that medication orders must be in writing before the drug can be administered.
- Giving medications based on an incomplete order or an illegible order, when the nurse is unsure of the correct drug, dosage, or administration method. Incomplete orders should be clarified with the healthcare provider before the medication is administered. The NCC MERP

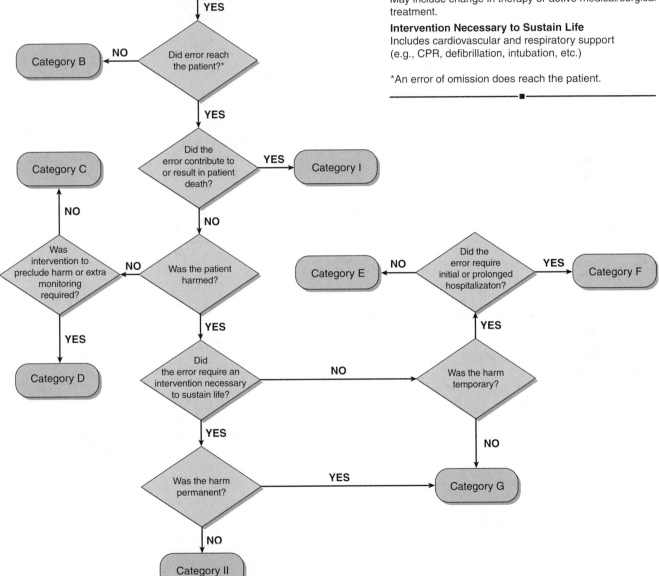

NCC MERP Index for Categorizing Medication Errors Algorithm

Harm
Impairment of the physical, emotional, or psychological function or structure of the body and/or pain resulting therefrom.

Monitoring
To observe or record relevant physiological or psychological signs.

Intervention
May include change in therapy or active medical/surgical treatment.

Intervention Necessary to Sustain Life
Includes cardiovascular and respiratory support (e.g., CPR, defibrillation, intubation, etc.)

*An error of omission does reach the patient.

MediaLink ● National Coordinating Council for Medication Error Reporting and Prevention (NCC MERP)

● **Figure 9.1** Index for Categorizing Medication Errors Algorithm © 2001 National Coordinating Council for Medication Error Reporting and prevention. All rights reserved. See also Figure 9.2, page 95 ∞.

recommends that written orders avoid certain abbreviations (Table 9.1) and include the following:

- A brief notation of purpose (for example, for pain)
- Metric system measurements except for therapies that use standard units such as insulin or vitamins

- Client age and, when appropriate, weight
- Drug name, exact metric weight or concentration, and dosage form
- A leading zero preceding a decimal number less than one (for example, 0.5 mg)

TABLE 9.1	Abbreviations to Avoid in Medication Administration	
Abbreviation	**Intended Meaning**	**Common Error**
U	units	Mistaken as a zero or a four (4) resulting in overdose. Also mistaken for "cc" (cubic centimeters) when poorly written.
μg	micrograms	Mistaken for "mg" (milligrams) resulting in an overdose.
q.d.	Latin abbreviation for every day	The period after the "Q" has sometimes been mistaken for an " I, " and the drug has been given "QID" (four times daily) rather than daily.
q.o.d.	Latin abbreviation for every other day	Misinterpreted as "QD" (daily) or "QID" (four times daily). If the "O" is poorly written, it looks like a period or "I."
SC or SQ	subcutaneous	Mistaken as "SL" (sublingual) when poorly written.
t i w	three times a week	Misinterpreted as "three times a day" or "twice a week."
D/C	discharge; also discontinue	Patient's medications have been prematurely discontinued when D/C, (intended to mean "discharge") was misinterpreted as "discontinue," because it was followed by a list of drugs.
hs	half strength	Misinterpreted as the Latin abbreviation "HS" (hour of sleep).
cc	cubic centimeters	Mistaken as "U" (units) when poorly written.
AU, AS, AD	Latin abbreviation for both ears, left ear, right ear	Misinterpreted as the Latin abbreviation "OU" (both eyes); "OS" (left eye); "OD" (right eye)
IU	international unit	Mistaken as IV (intravenous) or 10 (ten)
MS, MS04, MgS04	Confused for one another	Can mean morphine sulfate or magnesium sulfate

• Avoidance of abbreviations for drug names (for example, MOM, HCTZ) and Latin directions for use (NCC MERP, 2005).

• Practicing under stressful work conditions. Studies have correlated an increased number of errors with the stress level of nurses. Studies have also indicated that the rate of medication errors may increase when individual nurses are assigned to clients who are the most acutely ill.

Clients, or their home caregivers, may also contribute to medication errors by:

• Taking drugs prescribed by several practitioners without informing those healthcare providers about all prescribed medications.

• Getting their prescriptions filled at more than one pharmacy.

• Not filling or refilling their prescriptions.

• Taking medications incorrectly.

• Taking medications that may have been left over from a previous illness or prescribed for something else.

9.3 Nurse Practice Acts and Standards of Care

Each state has a **nurse practice act** that is designed to protect the public by defining the legal scope of practice. State boards of nursing or state nursing examiners ensure the enforcement of nurse practice acts. The nurse practice acts are important legislation, because they include the definition of professional nursing, part of which includes the safe delivery of medications. The professional nurse must be qualified to administer medications as defined in each nurse practice act.

All practicing nurses and student nurses should consult their state's nurse practice act prior to implementing care for clients. Because these acts are frequently amended and differ from state to state, practicing nurses should also periodically review their current nurse practice act for changes and updates.

Standards of care are the skills and learning commonly possessed by members of a profession. In nursing, standards of care are defined by nurse practice acts and the rule of **reasonable and prudent action**. This rule defines the standard of care as the actions that a reasonable and prudent nurse with equivalent preparation would perform under similar circumstances. What should the nurse do if the healthcare practitioner orders a dose of morphine that the nurse considers to be unsafe? If the nurse gives the medication and the client dies, who is responsible? If the nurse does not give the medication and the client suffers with pain or an adverse effect, who is responsible? Safeguarding the life and welfare of the client is the guiding principle. In cases of uncertainty, the nurse is legally judged by whether he or she acted within the jurisdiction of the state's nurse practice act and whether the actions were what a reasonable and prudent nurse would have done when faced with a similar dilemma.

Nurses who practice in clinical agencies need to understand and follow policies and procedures governing medication administration of the organization in which they practice. These policies and procedures establish the standards of care for that particular hospital or organization, and it is important that nurses adhere to those established policies and procedures. Common errors relate to failing to administer a medication at the prescribed time.

For example, an agency policy may identify that it is permissible to give a medication 30 minutes early or 30 minutes late for medications taken four times a day. The standards of care and the agency's policy manual are designed to help the nurse reduce medication errors and maintain client safety.

9.4 The Impact of Medication Errors

Medication errors are the most common cause of morbidity and preventable death within hospitals. When a medication error occurs, the repercussions can be emotionally devastating for the nurse and extend beyond the particular nurse and client involved. A medication error can increase the client's length of stay in the hospital, which increases costs and the time that a client is separated from his or her family. The nurse making the medication error may suffer self-doubt and embarrassment. If a high error rate occurs within a particular unit, the nursing unit may develop a poor reputation within the facility. If frequent medication errors or serious errors are publicized, the reputation of the facility may suffer, because it may be perceived as unsafe. Administrative personnel may also be penalized because of errors within their departments or the hospital as a whole

There are no acceptable incidence rates for medication errors. The goal of every healthcare organization should be to improve medication administration systems to prevent harm to clients due to medication errors. All errors, whether or not they affect the client, should be investigated with the goal of identifying ways to improve the medication administration process to prevent future errors. The investigation should occur in a nonpunitive manner that will encourage staff to report errors, thereby building a culture of safety within an organization. An error can alert nurses and healthcare administrators that a new policy or procedure needs to be implemented to reduce or eliminate medication errors.

9.5 Reporting and Documenting Medication Errors

When a nurse commits or observes an error, effects can be lasting and widespread. Although some errors go unreported, it is always the nurse's legal and ethical responsibility to report all occurrences. In severe cases, adverse reactions caused by medication errors may require the initiation of lifesaving interventions for the client. After such an incident, the client may require intense supervision and additional medical treatments.

The Food and Drug Administration (FDA) is concerned about medication errors at the federal level. Since 1992, the FDA has received about 20,000 reports of medication errors. Because these are voluntary reports, the actual number of errors is likely much higher. The FDA requires that nurses and other healthcare providers report medication errors for its database that is used to assist other professionals in avoiding similar mistakes. Medication errors, or situations that can lead to errors, may be reported in confidence directly to the FDA by telephone at 1-800-23-ERROR.

A second organization that has been established to provide assistance with medication errors is the National Coordinating Council for Medication Error Reporting and Prevention (NCC MERP). This organization was formed during the Pharmacopoeia Convention in 1995 to help standardize the medication error reporting system, examine interdisciplinary causes of medication errors, and promote medication safety. NCC MERP coordinates information on medication errors and provides medication error prevention education. The telephone number for NCC MERP is 1-800-822-8772.

DOCUMENTING IN THE CLIENT'S MEDICAL RECORD

Facility policies and procedures provide guidance on reporting medication errors. Documentation of the error should occur in a factual manner: The nurse should avoid blaming or making judgments. Documentation in the medical record must include specific nursing interventions that were implemented following the error to protect client safety, such as monitoring vital signs and assessing the client for possible complications. Documentation does not simply record that a medical error occurred. Failure to document nursing actions implies either negligence or failure to acknowledge that the incident occurred. The nurse should also document all individuals who were notified of the error. The **medication administration record (MAR)** is another source that should contain information about what medication was given or omitted.

WRITING AN INCIDENT REPORT

In addition to documenting in the client's medical record, the nurse making or observing the medication error should complete a written incident report. The specific details of the incident should be recorded, in a factual and objective manner. The incident report allows the nurse an opportunity to identify factors that contributed to the medication error. The incident report, however, is not included in the client's medical record.

Accurate documentation in the medical record and on the incident report is essential for legal reasons. These documents verify that the client's safety was protected and serve as a tool to improve medication administration processes.

HOME & COMMUNITY CONSIDERATIONS

Preventing Medication Errors in the Home

The U.S. Pharmacopeia's Safe Medication Use Expert Committee (Santell and Cousins, 2004) reports that medication errors occurring in the home are the result of communication problems (21%), knowledge deficit (19%), and inadequate or lacking monitoring (4%). Ten percent of errors are caused by lack of access to information. Warfarin is the drug most frequently (9%) associated with medication errors in the home; next in frequency are insulin (7%), morphine (4%), and vancomycin (4%). At the top of the list of error type are improper dose (36%) and omission errors (28%). In this study, the client, family, or caregiver is reported to be at fault in 39% of errors, the nurse in 36%, and the physician or pharmacist in 11%. This study points out the need for better client education, a role in which the nurse plays a large part.

Legal issues may worsen if there is an attempt to hide a mistake or delay corrective action, or if the nurse forgets to document interventions in the client's chart.

Hospitals and agencies monitor medication errors through quality improvement programs. The results of quality improvement programs alert staff and administrative personnel about trends within particular units and may serve as indicators of quality client care. Through data collection, specific solutions can be created to reduce the number of medication errors.

9.6 Strategies for Reducing Medication Errors

What can the nurse do in the clinical setting to avoid medication errors and promote safe administration? The nurse can begin by adhering to the four steps of the Nursing Process:

1. **Assessment:** Ask the client about allergies to food or medications, current health concerns, and use of over-the-counter (OTC) medications and herbal supplements. Ensure that the client is receiving the right dose, at the right time, and by the right route. Assess renal and liver functions, and determine if other body systems are impaired and could affect pharmacotherapy. Identify areas of needed client education with regard to medications.

2. **Planning:** Minimize factors that contribute to medication errors: Avoid using abbreviations that can be misunderstood, question unclear orders, do not accept verbal orders, and follow specific facility polices and procedures related to medication administration. Have the client restate dosing directions, including the correct dose of medication and the right time to take it. Ask the client to demonstrate an understanding of the goals of therapy.

3. **Implementation:** Be aware of potential distractions during medication administration and remove these distractions, if at all possible. When engaged in a medication-related task, focus entirely on the task. Noise, other events, and talking coworkers can distract the nurses' attention and result in a medication error. Practice the rights of medication administration: right client, right time and frequency of administration, right dose, right route of administration, right drug. Keep the following steps in mind as well:

   • Positively verify the identity of each client before administering the medication according to facility policy and procedures.

   • Use the correct procedures and techniques for all routes of administration. Use sterile materials and aseptic techniques when administering parenteral or eye medication.

   • Calculate medication doses correctly and measure liquid drugs carefully. Some medications, such as heparin, have a narrow safety margin for producing serious adverse effects. When giving these medications, ask a colleague or a pharmacist to check the calculations to make certain the dosage is correct.

   Always double-check pediatric calculations prior to administration.

   • Open medications immediately prior to administering the medication and in the presence of the client.

   • Record the medication on the MAR immediately after administration.

   • Always confirm that the client has swallowed the medication. Never leave the medication at the bedside unless there is a specific order that medications may be left there.

   • Be alert for long-acting oral dosage forms with indicators such as *LA*, *XL*, and *XR*. These tablets or capsules must remain intact for the extended-release feature to remain effective. Instruct the client not to crush, chew, or break the medication in half, because doing so could cause an overdose.

4. **Evaluation:** Assess the client for expected outcomes and determine if any adverse effects have occurred.

Nurses should know the most frequent types of drug errors and the severities of different categories of errors (● Figure 9.2). The FDA (Meadows, 2003) evaluated reports of fatal medication errors that it received from 1993 to 1998. The most common types of errors reported involved administering an improper dose (41%), giving the wrong drug (16%), and using the wrong route of administration (16%). Almost half of the fatal medication errors occurred in clients older than 60 years. There is an increase in the risk for errors in the elderly population because they often take multiple medications, have numerous healthcare providers, and are experiencing normal age-related changes in physiology. Children are another vulnerable population because they receive medication dosages based on weight (which increases the possibility of dosage miscalculations), and the therapeutic dosages are much smaller.

Nurses must be zealous in keeping up to date on pharmacotherapeutics and should never administer a medication until they are familiar with its uses and side effects. There are many venues by which the nurse can obtain updated medication knowledge. Each nursing unit should have current drug references available. Nurses can also call

SPECIAL CONSIDERATIONS

Age-related Issues in Drug Administration

The Pediatric Population

■ Always double-check calculations with another nurse for pediatric drug administration.

■ Medications may need to be crushed or administered in a liquid form.

■ Medications can have idiosyncratic effects on pediatric clients.

The Elderly Population

■ Remember that the frequency of adverse effects of medications is increased in elderly clients because of their slowed ability to absorb and metabolize medications.

■ Assess elderly clients for ability to swallow prior to administration of oral medications.

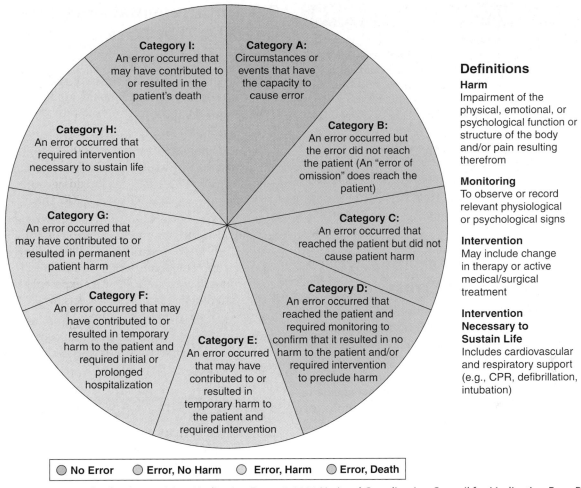

Definitions

Harm
Impairment of the physical, emotional, or psychological function or structure of the body and/or pain resulting therefrom

Monitoring
To observe or record relevant physiological or psychological signs

Intervention
May include change in therapy or active medical/surgical treatment

Intervention Necessary to Sustain Life
Includes cardiovascular and respiratory support (e.g., CPR, defibrillation, intubation)

Category I:
An error occurred that may have contributed to or resulted in the patient's death

Category A:
Circumstances or events that have the capacity to cause error

Category H:
An error occurred that required intervention necessary to sustain life

Category B:
An error occurred but the error did not reach the patient (An "error of omission" does reach the patient)

Category G:
An error occurred that may have contributed to or resulted in permanent patient harm

Category C:
An error occurred that reached the patient but did not cause patient harm

Category F:
An error occurred that may have contributed to or resulted in temporary harm to the patient and required initial or prolonged hospitalization

Category D:
An error occurred that reached the patient and required monitoring to confirm that it resulted in no harm to the patient and/or required intervention to preclude harm

Category E:
An error occurred that may have contributed to or resulted in temporary harm to the patient and required intervention

○ No Error   ○ Error, No Harm   ○ Error, Harm   ○ Error, Death

● **Figure 9.2** NCC MERP Index for Categorizing Medication Errors © 2001 National Coordinating Council for Medication Error Reporting and Prevention. All rights reserved.

the pharmacy to obtain information about the drug or, if available, look it up on the Internet using reliable sources. Many nurses are now relying on personal digital assistants (PDAs) to provide current information. These devices can be updated daily or weekly by downloading information so that the information is consistently current. Nurses need to familiarize themselves with research on preventing medical errors to maintain evidence-based practice skills.

9.7 Providing Client Education for Medication Usage

An essential strategy for avoiding medication errors is to educate the client by providing written age-appropriate handouts, audiovisual teaching aids about the medication, and contact information about whom to notify in the event of an adverse reaction.

Teach clients to:

• Know the names of all medications they are taking, the uses, when they should be taken, and the doses.

• Know what side effects need to be reported immediately.

• Read the label prior to each drug administration and use the medication device that comes with liquid

medications rather than household measuring spoons.

• Carry a list of all medications, including OTC drugs, as well as herbal and dietary supplements that are being taken. If possible, use one pharmacy for all prescriptions.

• Ask questions. Healthcare providers want to be partners in maintaining safe medication principles.

HOME & COMMUNITY CONSIDERATIONS

Educating Parents to Reduce Medication Errors in Children

Of the 105,603 errors documented by MEDMARX in a 2002 study (USP, 2003) 3,361 errors (3.2%) involved pediatric populations (birth to 16 years). Of these, 5.7% resulted in injury to the child. Many of these errors occur in the home or involve misinformation that can be corrected if parents or caregivers receive information on reducing such errors. Because medications for children are usually dosed by weight in kilograms, encourage parents to know their child's weight in kilograms and to reconfirm weight and dosage with the prescribing healthcare provider. Also advise parents to report their children's allergies to the healthcare provider and have children wear MedicAlert bracelets for any life-threatening allergies. Teach parents to identify their child's medication by size, shape, color, smell, and sight.

HOME & COMMUNITY CONSIDERATIONS

OTC Drugs and Medication Errors

Client use of OTC drugs and natural therapies is a common reason for adverse reactions and medication errors. For example, taking antibiotics can lower the effectiveness of oral contraceptives. OTC antihistamines can interact adversely with alcohol, sedatives, antidepressants, and antihypertensives. Encourage clients to

- Carry a list of all medications, including OTC drugs, dietary supplements, and medicinal herbs.
- Be sure family and various healthcare providers have a copy of this list. Include vitamins, laxatives, sleeping pills, and birth control pills.
- If possible, use one pharmacy for all prescriptions, because the pharmacist is an excellent resource for providing information about drug–drug and herbal/food interactions.

9.8 How Healthcare Facilities Are Reducing Medication Errors

There is a trend for healthcare agencies to use automated, computerized, locked cabinets for medication storage on client-care units. Each nurse on the unit has a code for accessing the cabinet and removing a medication dose. These automated systems also maintain an inventory of drug supplies.

Larger healthcare agencies often have **risk-management** departments to examine risks and minimize the number of medication errors. Risk-management personnel investigate incidents, track data, identify problems, and provide recommendations for improvement. Nurses collaborate with the risk-management committees to seek means of reducing medication errors by modifying policies and procedures within the institution. Examples of policies and procedures include:

- Correctly storing medication (light and temperature control).
- Reading the drug label to avoid using time-expired medications.
- Avoiding the transfer of doses from one container to another.
- Avoiding overstocking of medications.

9.9 Governmental and Other Agencies That Track Medication Errors

Several agencies, both governmental and private industry, track medication errors and provide updated reporting for consumers and healthcare professionals:

- The FDA's safety information and adverse-event reporting program is MedWatch. Its toll-free number is 1-800-332-1088, and its website is www.fda.gov/medwatch/how.htm
- The Institute for Safe Medication Practices (ISMP) accepts reports from consumers and healthcare professionals related to medication safety. It publishes *Safe Medicine*, a consumer newsletter about medication errors. The organization's number is 1-215-947-7797, and its website is www.ismp.org/pages/consumer.html
- MEDMARX is the U.S. Pharmacopeia's anonymous medication error reporting program used by hospitals. Its toll-free number is 1-800-822-8772, and its website is www.usp.org

NATURAL THERAPIES

Medication Errors and Supplements

Herbal, dietary, and vitamin supplements can have powerful actions and effects very similar to those of prescription drugs. Thus, when such supplements and drugs are taken together, the combined effect is much greater and may go beyond therapeutic to downright harmful. For example, many people with heart disease take garlic supplements in addition to warfarin (Coumadin) to prevent excessive clotting within blood vessels. Because garlic and warfarin are both strong anticoagulants, taking them together could result in abnormal bleeding.

Few studies have examined how concurrent use of a natural supplement affects the therapeutic effect of a prescription drug. There are exceptions (see "Hawthorne for Heart Failure" in Chapter 24), but the best way to avoid medication errors and potential harm is to encourage clients to report use of any herbal supplement to the healthcare provider.

(side margin, vertical) MediaLink MEDMARX MediaLink Institute for Safe Medication Practices (ISMP)

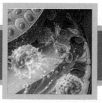

CHAPTER REVIEW

KEY CONCEPTS

The numbered key concepts provide a succinct summary of the important points from the corresponding numbered section within the chapter. If any of these points are not clear, refer to the numbered section within the chapter for review.

9.1 A medication error may be related to misinterpretations, miscalculations, misadministrations, handwriting misinterpretation, and misunderstanding of verbal or phone orders. Whether the client is injured or not, it is still a medication error.

9.2 Numerous factors contribute to medication errors, including ignoring the five rights of drug administration, failing to follow agency procedures or consider client variables, giving medications based on verbal orders, not confirming orders that are illegible or incomplete, and working under stressful conditions. Clients also contribute to errors by using more than one pharmacy, not informing healthcare providers of all medications they are taking, or not following instructions.

9.3 Nurse practice acts define professional nursing, including safe medication delivery. Standards of care are defined by nurse practice acts and the rule of reasonable and prudent action.

9.4 Medication errors affect client morbidity, mortality, and length of hospital stay. They also can damage the reputation of nurses, units, facility personnel, and the facility itself. There are no acceptable medication error incidence rates.

9.5 Nurses are legally and ethically responsible for reporting medication errors—whether or not they cause harm to a client—in the client's medical record and on an incident report. The FDA and NCC MERP are two agencies that track medication errors and provide data to help institute procedures to prevent them.

9.6 Nurses can reduce medication errors by adhering to the four steps of the Nursing Process—assessment, planning, implementation, and evaluation. Keeping up to date on pharmacotherapeutics and knowing common error types are instrumental to safe medication administration.

9.7 Client teaching includes providing age-appropriate medication handouts, and encouraging clients to keep a list of all prescribed medications, OTC drugs, herbal therapies, and vitamins they are taking and to report them to all healthcare providers.

9.8 Facilities use risk-management departments and agency policies and procedures to decrease the incidence of medication errors. Automated, computerized, locked cabinets for medication storage are a means of safekeeping of medications and keeping track of inventory at the unit level.

9.9 The FDA (MedWatch), the Institute of Safe Medication Practices (ISMP), and the U.S. Pharmacopeia (MEDMARX) are three agencies that track medication errors and provide databases of error incidence, error types, and levels of harm for healthcare professionals and/or consumers.

NCLEX-RN® REVIEW QUESTIONS

1 Each nurse is responsible for becoming familiar with the nurse practice acts of the state in which he or she practices because these acts:

1. Protect the nurse from malpractice suits.
2. Contain national standards and responsibilities.
3. Contain job descriptions for all nurses.
4. Define nursing practice and standards of care for the nurse practicing in a specific state.

2 The nurse administers a medication to the wrong client. The appropriate nursing action is to:

1. Monitor the client for adverse reaction before reporting the incident.
2. Document the error if the client has an adverse reaction.
3. Report the error to the physician, document the medication in the client record, and complete an incident report.
4. Notify the physician and document the error in the incident report only.

3 The client with liver dysfunction experiences toxicity to a drug following administration of several doses. This adverse reaction may have been prevented if the nurse had followed which phase of the nursing process?

1. Assessment
2. Planning
3. Implementation
4. Evaluation

4 Nurses have a legal and moral responsibility to report medication errors. The steps of reporting these errors include:

1. Punishing the nurse committing the error.
2. Monitoring unsafe medication orders.
3. Identifying potential unsafe medication facilities.
4. Examining interdisciplinary causes of errors and assisting professionals in ways to avoid mistakes.

5 The nurse has administered a medication to the wrong client. Which of the following is a correct action the nurse must take? (Select all that apply.)

1. Notify the physician.
2. Document that a medication error occurred in the nurses notes.
3. Assess vital signs.
4. Document medication on the medication administration record (MAR).
5. Complete a facility incident report.

CRITICAL THINKING QUESTIONS

1. A registered nurse is assigned to a team of eight clients. Six of these clients have medications scheduled for once-a-day dosing at 10 A.M. Explain how the nurse will be able to administer these drugs to the clients at the "right time."

2. A healthcare provider writes an order for Tylenol 3 PO q3–4 for mild pain. The nurse evaluates this order and is concerned that it is incomplete. Identify the probable concern and describe what the nurse should do prior to administering this medication.

3. A new nurse does not check an antibiotic dosage ordered by a healthcare provider for a pediatric client. The nurse subsequently overdoses a 2-year-old client, and an experienced nurse notices the error during the evening shift change. Identify each person who is responsible for the error and how each is responsible.

See Appendix D for answers and rationales for all activities.

EXPLORE MediaLink

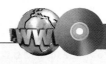 www.prenhall.com/adams

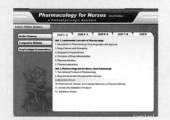

NCLEX-RN® review, case studies, and other interactive resources for this chapter can be found on the companion website at www.prenhall.com/adams. Click on "Chapter 9" to select the activities for this chapter. For animations, more NCLEX-RN® review questions, and an audio glossary, access the accompanying Prentice Hall Nursing MediaLink DVD-ROM in this textbook.

PRENTICE HALL NURSING MEDIALINK DVD-ROM

- **Audio Glossary**
- **NCLEX-RN® Review**

COMPANION WEBSITE

- **NCLEX-RN® Review**
- **Dosage Calculations**
- **Case Study:** Documentation of medication administration
- **Challenge Your Knowledge**

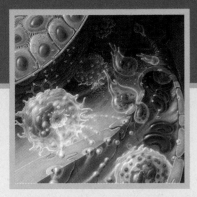

CHAPTER 10

Psychosocial, Gender, and Cultural Influences on Pharmacotherapy

OBJECTIVES

After reading this chapter, the student should be able to:

1. Describe fundamental concepts underlying a holistic approach to pharmacotherapy.
2. Describe the components of the human integration pyramid model.
3. Identify psychosocial and spiritual factors that can affect pharmacotherapeutics.
4. Explain how ethnicity can affect pharmacotherapeutic outcomes.
5. Identify examples of how cultural values and beliefs can influence pharmacotherapeutic outcomes.
6. Explain how community and environmental factors can affect healthcare outcomes.
7. Convey how genetic polymorphisms can influence pharmacotherapy.
8. Relate the implications of gender to the actions of certain drugs.

MediaLink

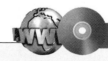 www.prenhall.com/adams

NCLEX-RN® review, case studies, and other interactive resources for this chapter can be found on the companion website at www.prenhall.com/adams. Click on "Chapter 10" to select the activities for this chapter. For animations, more NCLEX-RN® review questions, and an audio glossary, access the accompanying Prentice Hall Nursing MediaLink DVD-ROM in this textbook.

KEY TERMS

culture *page 102*
ethnic *page 102*
genetic polymorphism *page 104*
holistic *page 100*
psychology *page 101*
sociology *page 101*
spirituality *page 101*

It is convenient for a nurse to memorize an average drug dose, administer the medication, and expect all clients to achieve the same outcomes. Unfortunately, this is rarely the case. For pharmacotherapy to be successful, the needs of each individual client must be assessed and evaluated. In Chapter 5 ∞, variables such as absorption, metabolism, plasma protein binding, and excretion mechanisms were examined to help explain how these modify client responses to drugs. In Chapter 6 ∞, variability among client responses was explained in terms of differences in drug–receptor interactions. Chapter 8 ∞ examined how pharmacokinetic and pharmacodynamic factors change client responses to drugs throughout the lifespan. This chapter examines additional psychological, social, and biological variables that must be considered for optimum pharmacotherapy.

10.1 The Concept of Holistic Pharmacotherapy

To deliver the highest quality of care, the nurse must fully recognize the individuality and totality of the client. Each person must be viewed as an integrated biological, psychosocial, cultural, communicating whole, existing and functioning within the communal environment. Simply stated, the recipient of care must be regarded in a **holistic** context to better understand how established risk factors such as age, genetics, biological characteristics, personal habits, lifestyle, and environment increase a person's likelihood of acquiring specific diseases. Pharmacology has taken the study of these characteristics one step further—to examine and explain how they influence pharmacotherapeutic outcomes.

The *human integration pyramid*, shown in ● Figure 10.1, is a model of six categories that provides a basic framework of the functional environment and interrelationships in which human beings exist. This model provides a useful approach to addressing the nursing and pharmacological needs of clients within the collaborative practices of healthcare delivery. Where appropriate, concepts illustrated in the pyramid will be presented throughout this book as they relate to the various drug categories. All levels of the pyramid are important and interconnected: Some are specific to certain drug classes and nursing activities, whereas others apply more diversely across the pharmacotherapeutic spectrum.

By its very nature, modern (Western) medicine as it is practiced in the United States is seemingly incompatible with holistic medicine. Western medicine

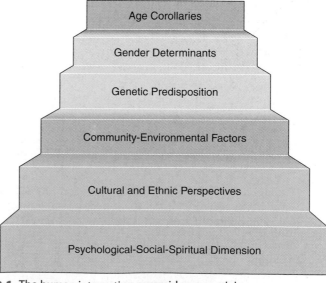

● **Figure 10.1** The human integration pyramid care model

focuses on specific diseases, their causes, and treatments. Disease is viewed as a malfunction of a specific organ or system. Sometimes, the disease is viewed even more specifically, and categorized as a change in DNA structure or a malfunction of one enzyme. Sophisticated technology is used to identify, image, and classify the specific structural or functional abnormality. Somehow, the total client is lost in this focus of categorizing disease. Too often, it does not matter how or why the client developed cancer, diabetes, or hypertension, or how he or she feels about it; the psychosocial and cultural dimensions are lost. Yet, these dimensions can have a profound impact on the success of pharmacotherapy. The nurse must consciously direct care toward a *holistic* treatment of each individual client, in his or her psychosocial, spiritual, and communal context.

10.2 Psychosocial Influences on Pharmacotherapy

Whereas science and medicine are founded on objective, logical, critical deliberation, psychology and sociology are based more on intuitive and subjective considerations. **Psychology** is the science that deals with normal and abnormal mental processes and their impact on behavior. **Sociology** studies human behavior within the context of groups and societies. **Spirituality** incorporates the capacity to love, to convey compassion and empathy, to give and forgive, to enjoy life, and to find peace of mind and fulfilment in living. The spiritual life overlaps with components of the emotional, mental, physical, and social aspects of living.

From a healthcare perspective, every human being should be considered as an integrated psychological, social, and spiritual being. Health impairments related to an individual's psychosocial situation often require a blending of individualized nursing care and therapeutic drugs, in conjunction with psychotherapeutic counselling. The term *psycho-social-spiritual* is appearing more frequently in nursing literature. It is now acknowledged that when clients have strong spiritual or religious beliefs, these may greatly influence their perceptions of illness and even affect the outcomes of pharmacotherapy. When illness imposes threats to health, the client commonly presents with psychological, social, and spiritual issues along with physical symptoms. Clients face concerns related to ill health, suffering, loneliness, despair, and death, and at the same time look for meaning, value, and hope in their situation. Such issues can have a great impact on wellness and preferred methods of medical treatment, nursing care, and pharmacotherapy.

The psychosocial history of the client is an essential component of the initial interview and assessment. This history delves into the personal life of the client, with inquiries directed toward lifestyle preferences, religious beliefs, sexual practices, alcohol intake, and tobacco and nonprescription drug use. The nurse must show extreme sensitivity when

gathering the data. If a trusting nurse–client relationship is not quickly established, the client will be reluctant to share important personal data that could affect nursing care.

The psychological dimension can exert a strong influence on pharmacotherapy. Clients who are convinced that their treatment is important and beneficial to their well-being will demonstrate better compliance with drug therapy. The nurse must ascertain the client's goals in seeking treatment, and determine whether drug therapy is compatible with those goals. Past experiences with health care may lead a client to distrust medications. Drugs may not be acceptable for the social environment of the client. For example, having to take drugs at school or in the workplace may cause embarrassment; clients may fear that they will be viewed as weak, unhealthy, or dependent. Some clients may believe that certain medications, such as antidepressants or seizure medications carry a social stigma, and therefore they will resist using them.

Clients who display positive attitudes toward their personal health and have high expectations regarding the results of their pharmacotherapy are more likely to achieve positive outcomes. The nurse plays a pivotal role in encouraging the client's positive expectations. The nurse must always be forthright in explaining drug actions and potential side effects. Trivializing the limitations of pharmacotherapy or minimizing potential adverse effects can cause the client to have unrealistic expectations regarding treatment. The nurse–client relationship may be jeopardized, and the client may acquire an attitude of distrust. As discussed in Chapter 9 ∞, the client has an ethical and legal right to receive accurate information regarding the benefits and effects of drug therapy.

10.3 Cultural and Ethnic Influences on Pharmacotherapy

Despite the apparent diverse cultural and ethnic differences among humans, we are, indeed, one species. It has been estimated that all humans share 99.8% of the same DNA sequences. The remaining 0.2% of the sequences that differ are shared among peoples with similar historical and geographic heritage.

MediaLink Healthy People 2010

SPECIAL CONSIDERATIONS

Religious Affiliation and Disease Incidence

Religious affiliation is correlated with a reduction in the incidence of some diseases such as cancer and coronary artery disease. Religious and spiritual factors often figure into important decisions for clients facing terminal illness and death, for example, the employment of advance directives such as the living will and the durable power of attorney for health care. Considerations of the meaning, purpose, and value of human life are used to make choices about the desirability of CPR and aggressive life support, or whether and when to forgo life support and accept death as appropriate and natural under the circumstances.

An **ethnic** group is a community of people having a common history and similar genetic heritage. Members of an ethnic group often share distinctive social and cultural traditions, which are maintained from generation to generation. These beliefs include a shared perception of health and illness.

Culture is a set of beliefs, values, religious rituals, and customs shared by a group of people. In some respects, culture and ethnicity are similar, and many people use the words interchangeably. Ethnicity more often is used to refer to *biological* and *genetic* similarities, whereas culture refers more to *social* similarities. For example, thousands of Africans were taken from their tribes and forcibly moved to America as part of the slave trade in the 1700s and 1800s.

PHARMFACTS

Minority Statistics and Healthcare Access

- In 2000, the majority ethnic group in the United States was non-Hispanic Whites, at 71%.
- By 2025, the population of non-Hispanic Whites is expected to decrease to 62%, and then fall to 55% by 2045.
- Sometime between 2050 and 2060, non-Hispanic White persons will themselves become a "minority," shrinking to less than half of all Americans.
- Whereas 89% of White non-Hispanics were covered by a health insurance plan, only 67% of Hispanics had such insurance in 2000. American Indians and Alaska Natives were less likely to have health insurance than other racial groups, with the exception of Hispanics.
- Eighty percent of Caucasians report having a regular doctor. This percentage is reduced to 57% for Hispanics, 68% for Asian Americans, and 70% for African Americans.
- African American (13%) and Hispanic (14%) adults are more than twice as likely as Caucasian (6%) adults to report no regular source of care, or that the emergency room is the usual source of care.
- Sixty-five percent of Caucasian Medicare beneficiaries reported that they were vaccinated against the flu in the past 12 months, versus only 43% of African Americans and 49% of Hispanics.
- Among part-time workers, 64% of Caucasians reported having employer-based insurance, whereas only 45% of African Americans and 40% of Hispanics did.
- Among workers earning more than $15 per hour, 79% of Caucasians reported that they were provided employer-based insurance, compared with 67% of African Americans and 54% of Hispanics.

Over several hundred years, many African Americans have adopted the cultural norms and lifestyles of European Americans. Others have kept some of their African cultural traditions and beliefs that have been passed on from generation to generation. As a group, however, all African Americans share genetic similarities to those living in Africa today and thus are considered as belonging to the same ethnic group.

Culture can be a dominant force influencing the relationship between client and nurse. The practitioner–client relationship is a cross-cultural encounter. The client brings religious and ideological beliefs that may challenge or conflict with what the healthcare provider believes to be in the best interests of the client. The client's definition of illness is, in fact, often based on his or her cultural beliefs and values. It is also important to remember that diversity exists not only *between* different cultures but also *within* individual cultures. Examples include differences between age groups or between genders within a given culture.

Cultural competence requires knowledge of the values, beliefs, and practices of various peoples, along with an attitude of awareness, openness, and sensitivity. Understanding and respecting the beliefs of the client are key to establishing and maintaining a positive therapeutic relationship that culminates in culturally sensitive nursing care. Therapeutic communication mandates that all healthcare providers bear in mind the cultural, racial, and social factors that make up each person, and how these affect behavior. Failure to take these beliefs seriously can undermine the client's ability to trust the nurse, and may even persuade some clients to avoid seeking medical care when it is needed.

Culture and ethnicity can affect pharmacotherapy in many ways. The nurse must keep in mind the following variables when treating clients in different ethnic groups.

- *Diet* Every culture has a unique set of foods and spices, which have the potential to affect pharmacotherapy. For example, Asian diets tend to be high in carbohydrates and low in protein and fat. African American diets are often higher in fat content.

- *Alternative therapies* Many cultural groups believe in using herbs and other alternative therapies either along with or in place of modern medicines. Some of these folk remedies and traditional treatments have existed for thousands of years and helped form the foundation for modern medical practice. Chinese clients may go to herbalists to treat their illnesses. Native Americans may take great care in collecting, storing, and using herbs to treat and prevent disease. Certain Hispanic cultures use spices and herbs to maintain a balance of hot and cold, which is thought to promote wellness. Therapeutic massage, heat, and tea infusions are used by many cultures. The nurse needs to interpret the effect of these herbal and alternative therapies on the desired pharmacotherapeutic outcomes.

- *Beliefs about health and disease* Each culture has distinct ways of viewing sickness and health. Some individuals seek the assistance of people in their community who they believe are blessed with healing powers. Native Americans may seek help from a tribal medicine man, or Hispanics from a *curandero* (folk healer). African Americans sometimes practice healing through the gifts of laying on of hands. The nurse must understand that clients may place great trust in these alternative healers, and should not demean their belief system.

- *Genetic differences* With the advent of DNA sequencing, hundreds of structural variants in metabolic enzymes have been discovered. Some of these appear more frequently in certain ethnic groups and have an impact on pharmacotherapeutics, as discussed in Section 10.5 ∞.

10.4 Community and Environmental Influences on Pharmacotherapy

A number of community and environmental factors have been identified that influence disease and its subsequent treatment. Population growth, complex technological advances, and evolving globalization patterns have all affected health care. Communities vary significantly in regard to urbanization levels, age distributions, socioeconomic levels, occupational patterns, and industrial growth. In much of the world, people live in areas lacking adequate sanitation and potable water supplies. All these community and environmental factors have the potential to affect health and access to pharmacotherapy.

Access to health care is perhaps the most obvious community-related influence on pharmacotherapy. There are many potential barriers to obtaining appropriate health care. Without an adequate health insurance plan, some people are reluctant to seek health care for fear of bankrupting the family unit. Older adults fear losing their retirement savings or being placed in a nursing home for the remainder of their lives. Families living in rural areas may have to travel great distances to obtain necessary treatment. Once treatment is rendered, the cost of prescription drugs may be far too high for clients on limited incomes. The nurse must be aware of these variables and have knowledge of social agencies in the local community that can assist in improving healthcare access.

Literacy is another community-related variable that can affect health care. Up to 48% of English-speaking clients do not have functional literacy—a basic ability to read, understand, and act on health information (Andrus & Roth, 2002). The functional illiteracy rate is even higher in certain populations, particularly non-English-speaking individuals and older clients. The nurse must be aware that these clients may not be able to read drug labels, understand written treatment instructions, or read brochures describing their disease or therapy. Functional illiteracy can result in a lack of understanding about the importance of pharmacotherapy and can lead to poor compliance. The nurse must attempt to identify these clients and provide them with brochures, instructions, and educational materials that can be understood. For non-English-speaking clients or those for whom English is their second language, the nurse should have proper materials in the client's primary language, or provide an interpreter who can help with accurate translations (● Figure 10.2). The nurse should ask the client to repeat

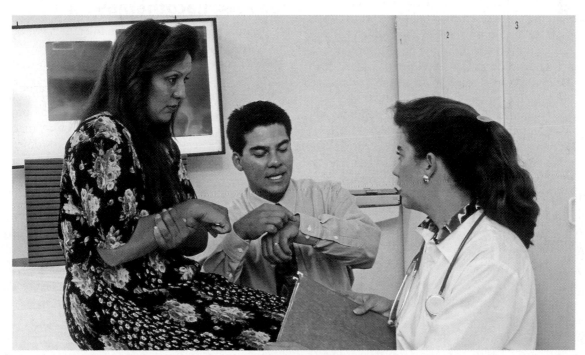

● **Figure 10.2** A nurse communicates with her non-English-speaking client through an interpreter
Source: Pearson Education/PH College.

important instructions, to ensure comprehension. The use of graphic-rich materials is appropriate for certain therapies.

10.5 Genetic Influences on Pharmacotherapy

Although 99.8% of human DNA sequences are like, the remaining 0.2% may result in significant differences in clients' ability to handle medications. Many of these differences are created when a mutation occurs in the portion of DNA responsible for encoding a certain metabolic enzyme. A single base mutation in DNA may result in an amino acid change in the enzyme, which alters its function. Hundreds of such mutations have been identified. These changes in enzyme structure and function are called **genetic polymorphisms**. The change may result in either increased or decreased drug metabolism, depending on the exact type of genetic polymorphism. The study of these polymorphisms is called *pharmacogenetics*.

Genetic polymorphisms are most often identified in specific ethnic groups, because people in an ethnic group have been located in the same geographic area and have married others within the same ethnic group for hundreds of generations. This causes the genetic polymorphism to be amplified and expressed within that population.

The relationship between client genetic factors and drug response has been documented for decades. The first polymorphism was discovered in the enzyme acetyltransferase, which metabolizes isoniazid (INH), a drug prescribed for tuberculosis. The metabolic process, known as *acetylation*, occurs abnormally slowly in certain Caucasians. The reduced hepatic metabolism and subsequent clearance by the kidney can cause the drug to build to toxic levels in these clients, who are known as *slow acetylators*. The opposite effect, fast acetylation, is found in many clients of Japanese descent.

In recent years, several other enzyme polymorphisms have been identified. Asian Americans are less able to metabolize codeine to morphine owing to an inherent absence of the enzyme debrisoquin, a defect that interferes with the analgesic properties of codeine. In another example, some persons of African American descent experience decreased effects from beta-adrenergic antagonist drugs such as propranolol (Inderal), because of genetically influenced variances in plasma renin levels. Another set of oxidation enzyme polymorphisms have been found that alter the response to warfarin (Coumadin), diazepam (Valium), and several other medications. Table 10.1 summarizes the three most common polymorphisms. Expanding knowledge about the physiological impact of heredity on pharmacotherapy may someday allow for personalization of the treatment process.

10.6 Gender Influences on Pharmacotherapy

A person's gender influences many aspects of health maintenance, promotion, and treatment, as well as drug response. For example, women tend to pay more attention to changes in health patterns and seek health care earlier than their male counterparts. Conversely, many women do not seek medical attention for potential cardiac problems, because heart disease is considered to be a "man's disease." Alzheimer's disease affects both men and women, but studies in various populations have shown that between 1.5 and 3 times as many women as men suffer from the disease. Alzheimer's disease is becoming recognized as a major

TABLE 10.1 Enzyme Polymorphisms of Importance to Pharmacotherapy		
Enzyme	**Result of Polymorphism**	**Drugs Using This Metabolic Enzyme/Pathway**
acetyltransferase	slow acetylation in Scandinavians, Jews, North African Caucasians; fast acetylation in Japanese	isoniazid, chlordiazepam, hydralazine, procainamide, caffeine
debrisoquin hydroxylase	poorly metabolized in Asians and African Americans	amitriptyline, imipramine, perphenazine, haloperidol, propranolol, metoprolol, codeine, morphine
mephenytoin hydroxylase	poorly metabolized in Asians and African Americans	diazepam, imipramine, barbiturates, warfarin

"women's health issue," comparable to osteoporosis, breast cancer, and fertility disorders.

Acceptance or rejection of the use of particular categories of medication may be gender based. Because of the side effects associated with certain medications, some clients do not take them appropriately—or take them at all. A common example is the use of certain antihypertensive agents in men. These may cause, as a common side effect, male impotence. In certain instances, male clients have suffered a stroke because they abruptly stopped taking the drug and did not communicate this fact to their healthcare provider. With open communication, dilemmas regarding drug problems and side effects can be brought into the open so alternative drug therapies can be considered. As with so many areas of health care, appropriate client teaching by the nurse is a key aspect in preventing or alleviating drug-related health problems.

Local and systemic responses to some medications can differ between genders. These response differences may be based on differences in body composition such as the fat-to-muscle ratio. In addition, cerebral blood flow variances between males and females may alter the response to certain analgesics. Some of the benzodiazepines used for anxiety have slower elimination rates in women, and this difference becomes even more significant if the woman is concurrently taking oral contraceptives. There are numerous gender-related situations that the nurse must understand to monitor drug actions and effects appropriately.

Until recently, the vast majority of drug research studies were conducted using only male subjects. It was wrongly assumed that the conclusions of these studies applied in the same manner to women. Since 1993, the FDA has formalized policies that require the inclusion of subjects of both genders during drug development. This includes analyses of clinical data by gender, assessment of potential pharmacokinetic and pharmacodynamic differences between genders, and, when appropriate, conducting additional studies specific to women's health.

Also of concern is gender inequity regarding prescription drug coverage. A common example is employer health plans that exclude women's contraceptive medications. It was not until a federal district court ruling in June 2001 that exclusion of prescription of female contraceptives by an employer's healthcare provider was deemed sex discrimination.

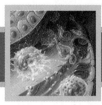

CHAPTER REVIEW

KEY CONCEPTS

The numbered key concepts provide a succinct summary of the important points from the corresponding numbered section within the chapter. If any of these points are not clear, refer to the numbered section within the chapter for review.

10.1 To deliver effective treatment, the nurse must consider the total client in a holistic context.

10.2 The psychosocial domain must be considered when delivering holistic care. Positive attitudes and high expectations toward therapeutic outcomes in the client may influence the success of pharmacotherapy.

10.3 Culture and ethnicity are two interconnected perspectives that can affect nursing care and pharmacotherapy. Differences in diet, use of alternative therapies, perceptions of wellness, and genetic makeup can influence client drug response.

10.4 Community and environmental factors affect health and the public's access to health care and pharmacotherapy. Inadequate access to healthcare resources and an inability to read or understand instructions may compromise treatment outcomes.

10.5 Genetic differences in metabolic enzymes that occur among different ethnic groups must be considered for effective pharmacotherapy. Small differences in the structure of enzymes can result in profound changes in drug response.

10.6 Gender can influence many aspects of health maintenance, promotion, and treatment, as well as medication response.

NCLEX-RN® REVIEW QUESTIONS

1 The client informs the nurse that he will use herbal compounds given by a family member to treat his hypertension. The appropriate action by the nurse is to:
1. Inform the client that the herbal treatments will be ineffective.
2. Obtain more information and determine whether the herbs are compatible with medications prescribed.
3. Notify the physician immediately.
4. Inform the client that the physician will not treat him if he does not accept the use of traditional medicine only.

2 The nurse provides teaching about a drug to an elderly couple. To ensure that the instructions are understood, the nurse should:
1. Provide detailed written material about the drug.
2. Provide labels and instructions in large print.
3. Assess the reading levels and have clients repeat instructions to determine understanding.
4. Provide instructions only when family members are present.

3 The nurse must understand gender issues related to drug therapy. Important considerations include:

1. Men seek health care earlier than women.
2. Women suffer from Alzheimer's disease in greater numbers than men.
3. Women are more likely to stop taking medications because of side effects.
4. All drug trials are conducted on male subjects.

4 The client informs the nurse that she will decide whether she will accept treatment after she prays with her family and minister. The nurse recognizes the role of spirituality in drug therapy as:

1. Irrelevant because medications act on scientific principles.
2. Important to the client's acceptance of medical treatment and response to treatment.
3. Harmless if it makes the client feel better.
4. Harmful, especially if treatment is delayed.

5 The client informs the nurse she is taking St. John's wort for depression. The nurse understands that St. John's wort, when mixed with medications, may (select all that apply):

1. Potentiate sedation.
2. Decrease cyclosporine levels.
3. Cause hyperglycemia.
4. Cause a hypertensive crisis.
5. Create euphoria.

CRITICAL THINKING QUESTIONS

1. A 72-year-old African American heart client, who has been treated for atrial flutter, is taking warfarin (Coumadin) 2.5 mg PO once a day. He comes to the clinic for his routine international normalized ratio (INR), which is no longer in the therapeutic range. The client lives in a rural area and has a large vegetable garden. What questions would a nurse need to ask to evaluate the cause of the decreased drug effectiveness?

2. An 82-year-old female client is admitted to the emergency department. She has been taking furosemide (Lasix) 40 mg PO daily as part of a regimen for congestive heart failure. She is confused and dehydrated. What gender-related considerations should the nurse make when assessing this client?

3. A 19-year-old male client of Mexican descent presents to a health clinic for migrant farm workers. In broken English, he describes severe pain in his lower jaw. An assessment reveals two abscessed molars and other oral health problems. Discuss the probable reasons for this client's condition.

See Appendix D for answers and rationales for all activities.

EXPLORE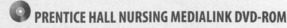
MediaLink

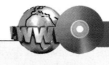
www.prenhall.com/adams

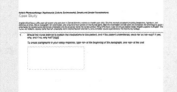

NCLEX-RN® review, case studies, and other interactive resources for this chapter can be found on the companion website at www.prenhall.com/adams. Click on "Chapter 10" to select the activities for this chapter. For animations, more NCLEX-RN® review questions, and an audio glossary, access the accompanying Prentice Hall Nursing MediaLink DVD-ROM in this textbook.

 PRENTICE HALL NURSING MEDIALINK DVD-ROM
- **Audio Glossary**
- **NCLEX-RN® Review**

COMPANION WEBSITE
- **NCLEX-RN® Review**
- **Case Study:** Cultural and ethnic influences
- **Challenge Your Knowledge**

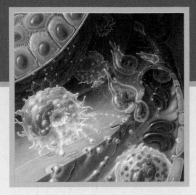

CHAPTER 11

Herbal and Alternative Therapies

OBJECTIVES

After reading this chapter, the student should be able to:

1. Explain the role of complementary and alternative medicine in client wellness.
2. Discuss reasons why herbal and dietary supplements have increased in popularity.
3. Identify the parts of an herb that may contain active ingredients and the types of formulations made from these parts.
4. Describe the strengths and weaknesses of the Dietary Supplement Health and Education Act (DSHEA) of 1994.
5. Describe some adverse effects that may be caused by herbal preparations.
6. Discuss the role of the nurse in teaching clients about complementary and alternative therapies.
7. Identify common drug–herbal interactions.
8. Explain how some herbal products are standardized based on specific active ingredients.

MediaLink 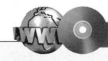 www.prenhall.com/adams

KEY TERMS

botanical *page 108*

complementary and alternative
  medicine (CAM) *page 108*

dietary supplement *page 111*

Dietary Supplement Health and Education
  Act (DSHEA) of 1994 *page 111*

herb *page 108*

specialty supplement *page 114*

Herbal supplements and alternative therapies represent a multibillion-dollar industry. Sales of dietary supplements alone exceed $17 billion annually, with more than 158 million consumers using them. Despite the fact that these therapies have not been subjected to the same scientific scrutiny as prescription medications, consumers turn to these treatments for a variety of reasons. Many people have the impression that natural substances have more healing power than synthetic medications. The ready availability of herbal supplements at a reasonable cost, combined with effective marketing strategies, has convinced many consumers to try them. This chapter examines the role of complementary and alternative therapies in the prevention and treatment of disease.

11.1 Alternative Therapies

Complementary and alternative medicine (CAM) comprises an extremely diverse set of therapies and healing systems that are considered to be outside mainstream health care. Although diverse, the major CAM systems have common characteristics. They:

- Focus on treating each person as an individual.
- Consider the health of the whole person.
- Emphasize the integration of mind and body.
- Promote disease prevention, self-care, and self-healing.
- Recognize the role of spirituality in health and healing.

Because of the popularity of CAM, considerable attention has recently focused on determining its effectiveness, or lack of effectiveness. Although research into these alternative systems is underway, few CAM therapies have been subjected to rigorous clinical and scientific study. It is likely that some of these therapies will be found ineffective, whereas others will become mainstream treatments. The line between what is defined as an alternative therapy and what is considered mainstream is constantly changing. Increasing numbers of healthcare providers are now accepting CAM therapies and recommending them to their clients. Table 11.1 describes some of these therapies.

Nurses have long known the value of CAM in preventing and treating disease. For example, prayer, meditation, massage, and yoga have been used for centuries to treat both body and mind. From a pharmacology perspective, much of the value of CAM therapies lies in their ability to reduce the need for medications. For instance, if a client can find anxiety relief through herbal products, massage, or biofeedback therapy, then the use of anxiolytic drugs may be reduced or eliminated. Reduction of drug dose leads to fewer adverse effects and improved compliance with drug therapy.

The nurse should be sensitive to the client's need for alternative treatment and not be judgmental. Both advantages and limitations must be presented to clients so they may make rational and informed decisions about their treatment. Pharmacotherapy and alternative therapies can serve complementary and essential roles in the healing of the total client.

11.2 Brief History of Therapeutic Natural Products

An **herb** is technically a **botanical** without any woody tissue such as stems or bark. Over time, the terms *botanical* and *herb* have come to be used interchangeably to refer to any plant product with some useful application either as a food enhancer, such as flavoring, or as a medicine.

The use of botanicals has been documented for thousands of years. One of the earliest recorded uses of plant products was a prescription for garlic in 3000 B.C.

TABLE 11.1   Complementary and Alternative Therapies

Healing Method	Examples
alternative healthcare systems	naturopathy
	homeopathy
	chiropractic
	Native American medicine (e.g., sweat lodges, medicine wheel)
	Chinese traditional medicine (e.g., acupuncture, Chinese herbs)
biological-based therapies	herbal therapies
	nutritional supplements
	special diets
manual healing	massage
	pressure-point therapies
	hand-mediated biofield therapies
mind–body interventions	yoga
	meditation
	hypnotherapy
	guided imagery
	biofeedback
	movement-oriented therapies (e.g., music, dance)
spiritual	shamans
	faith and prayer
others	bioelectromagnetics
	detoxifying therapies
	animal-assisted therapy

Eastern and Western medicine have recorded thousands of herbs and herb combinations reputed to have therapeutic value. Some of the most popular herbal supplements and their claimed applications are listed in Table 11.2.

With the birth of the pharmaceutical industry in the late 1800s, interest in herbal medicines began to wane. Synthetic drugs could be standardized, produced, and distributed more cheaply than natural herbal products. Regulatory agencies required that products be safe and effective, thus removing many products from the market. The focus of healthcare was on diagnosing and treating specific diseases, rather than on promoting wellness and holistic care. Most alternative therapies were no longer taught in medical or nursing schools; these healing techniques were criticized as being unscientific relics of the past.

Beginning in the 1970s and continuing to the present, alternative therapies and herbal medicine have experienced a remarkable resurgence, such that the majority of adult Americans are currently taking botanicals on a regular basis or have taken them in the past. This increase in popularity is due to factors such as increased availability of herbal products, aggressive marketing by the herbal industry, increased attention

to natural alternatives, and a renewed interest in preventive medicine. The gradual aging of the population has led to an increase in clients seeking therapeutic alternatives for chronic conditions such as pain, arthritis, hormone replacement therapy, and prostate difficulties. In addition, the high cost of prescription medicines has driven clients to seek less expensive alternatives. Nurses have been instrumental in promoting self-care and recommending CAM therapies for clients.

11.3 Herbal Product Formulations

The pharmacologically active chemicals in an herbal product may be present in only one specific part of the plant, or in all parts. For example, the active chemicals in chamomile are in the above-ground portion that includes the leaves, stems, and flowers. With other herbs, such as ginger, the underground rhizomes and roots are used for their healing properties. In collecting herbs for home use it is essential to know which portion of the plant contains the active chemicals.

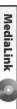

TABLE 11.2 Best-selling Herbal Supplements, in Rank Order

Rank	Herb	Medicinal Part	Primary Use(s)
1	garlic	bulbs	to reduce blood cholesterol, reduce blood pressure, provide anticoagulation
2	echinacea	entire plants	to enhance immune system, reduce inflammation
3	saw palmetto	ripe fruit/berries	to relieve urinary problems related to prostate enlargement
4	ginkgo	leaves and seeds	to improve memory, reduce dizziness
5	soy	beans	to provide source of protein, vitamins, and minerals; to relieve menopausal symptoms, prevent cardiovascular disease, prevent cancer
6	cranberry	berries/juices	to prevent urinary tract infection
7	ginseng	roots	to relieve stress, enhance immune system, decrease fatigue
8	black cohosh	roots	to relieve menopausal symptoms
9	St. John's wort	flowers, leaves, stems	to reduce depression, anxiety, and inflammation
10	milk thistle	seeds	to provide antitoxic therapy, protect against liver disease
11	evening primrose	seeds/oils	to provide source of essential fatty acids, relieve premenstrual or menopausal symptoms, relieve rheumatoid arthritis and other inflammatory symptoms
12	valerian	roots	to relieve stress, promote sleep
13	green tea		to provide antioxidant therapy; lower LDL cholesterol; prevent cancer; relieve stomach problems, nausea, vomiting
14	bilberry	berries/leaves	to terminate diarrhea, improve and protect vision, provide antioxidant therapy
15	grape seed	seeds/oils	to provide source of essential fatty acids, provide antioxidant therapy, restore microcirculation to tissues

Source: Data from Information Resources, Inc., Chicago, 2005

Most modern drugs contain only one active ingredient. This chemical is standardized, accurately measured, and delivered to the client in precise amounts. It is a common misconception that herbs also contain one active ingredient, which can be extracted and delivered to clients in precise doses, like drugs. Herbs actually may contain dozens of active chemicals, many of which have not yet been isolated, studied, or even identified. It is possible that some of these substances work together synergistically and may not have the same activity if isolated. Furthermore, the potency of an herbal preparation may vary depending on where it was grown and how it was collected and stored.

Recent attempts have been made to standardize herbal products, using a marker substance such as the percent flavones in ginkgo or the percent lactones in kava kava. Some of these standardizations are listed in Table 11.3. Until science can better characterize these substances, how-

TABLE 11.3 Standardization of Selected Herb Extracts

Herb	Standardization	Percent
black cohosh rhizome	triterpene glycosides	2.5
cascara sagrada bark	hydroxyanthracenic heterosides	20
echinacea purpurea herb	phenolics	4
ginger rhizome	pungent compounds	greater than 10
ginkgo leaf	flavoglycosides	24–25
	lactones	6
ginseng root	ginseosides	20–30
kava kava rhizome	kavalactones	40–45
milk thistle root	silymarin	80
saw palmetto fruit	fatty acids and sterols	80–90
St. John's wort	hypericins	0.3–0.5
	hyperforin	3–5

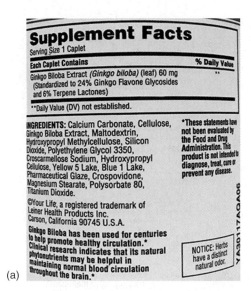

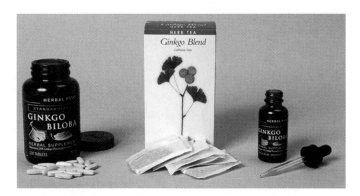

● **Figure 11.1** Two ginkgo biloba labels, note the lack of standardization in (a) 60 mg of extract, 24% ginkgo flavone glycosides and 6% terpenes and (b) 50:1 ginkgo leaf extract, 24% ginkgo flavone glycosides

ever, it is best to conceptualize the active ingredient of an herb as being the entire herb itself, and not just a single chemical. An example of the ingredients and standardization of ginkgo biloba is shown in ● Figure 11.1.

The two basic formulations of herbal products are solid and liquid. Solid products include pills, tablets, and capsules made from the dried herbs. Other solid products are salves and ointments that are administered topically. Liquid formulations are made by extracting the active chemicals from the plant using solvents such as water, alcohol, or glycerol. The liquids are then concentrated in various strengths and ingested. The various liquid formulations of herbal preparations are described in Table 11.4. ● Figure 11.2 illustrates different formulations of the popular herbal ginkgo biloba.

11.4 Regulation of Herbal Products and Dietary Supplements

Since the passage of the Food, Drug, and Cosmetic Act in 1936, Americans have come to expect that all approved prescription and OTC drugs have passed rigid standards of safety prior to being marketed. Furthermore, it is expected that these drugs have been tested for efficacy and that they

truly provide the medical benefits claimed by the manufacturer. Americans cannot and should not expect the same quality standards for herbal products. These products are regulated by a far less rigorous law, the **Dietary Supplement Health and Education Act (DSHEA) of 1994.**

According to the DSHEA, "dietary supplements" are specifically exempted from the Food, Drug, and Cosmetic Act. **Dietary supplements** are products intended to enhance or supplement the diet, such as botanicals, vitamins,

● **Figure 11.2** Three different ginkgo formulations: tablets, tea bags, and liquid extract

TABLE 11.4 Liquid Formulations of Herbal Products	
Product	**Description**
decoction	fresh or dried herbs are boiled in water for 30–60 minutes until much of the liquid has boiled off; very concentrated
extract	active ingredients are extracted using organic solvents to form a highly concentrated liquid or solid form; solvent may be removed or be part of the final product
infusion	fresh or dried herbs are soaked in hot water for long periods, at least 15 minutes; stronger than teas
tea	fresh or dried herbs are soaked in hot water for 5–10 minutes before ingestion; convenient
tincture	active ingredients are extracted using alcohol by soaking the herb; alcohol remains as part of the liquid

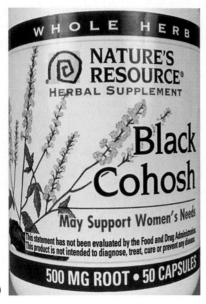

(a)

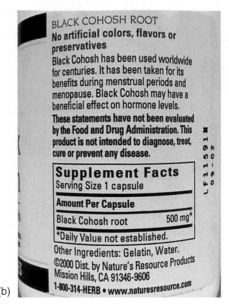

(b)

● **Figure 11.3** Labeling of black cohosh: (a) front label with general health claim and (b) back label with more health claims and FDA disclaimer

minerals, or other extracts or metabolites that are not already approved as drugs by the FDA. A major strength of the legislation is that it gives the FDA the power to remove from the market any product that poses a "significant or unreasonable" risk to the public. It also requires these products to be clearly labeled as "dietary supplements." An example of an herbal label for black cohosh is shown in ● Figure 11.3.

Unfortunately, the DSHEA has several significant flaws that have led to a lack of standardization in the dietary supplement industry, and to less protection for the consumer.

- Dietary supplements do not have to be tested prior to marketing.
- Efficacy does not have to be demonstrated by the manufacturer.
- The manufacturer does not have to prove the safety of the dietary supplement: To be removed from the market, the government has to prove that the dietary supplement is unsafe.
- Dietary supplements must state that the product is not intended to diagnose, treat, cure, or prevent any disease; however, the label may make claims about the product's effect on body structure and function, such as the following:
  - Helps promote healthy immune systems
  - Reduces anxiety and stress
  - Helps maintain cardiovascular function
  - May reduce pain and inflammation

The DSHEA does not regulate the accuracy of the label; the product may or may not contain the product listed, in the amounts claimed.

11.5 The Pharmacological Actions and Safety of Herbal Products

A key concept to remember when dealing with alternative therapies is that "natural" does not always mean "better" or "safe." There is no question that some botanicals contain active chemicals as powerful as, and perhaps more effective than, currently approved medications. Thousands of years of experience, combined with current scientific research, have shown that some herbal remedies have therapeutic actions. Because a substance comes from a natural product, however, does not make it safe or effective. For example, poison ivy is natural, but it certainly is not safe or therapeutic. Natural products may not offer an improvement over conventional therapy in treating certain disorders and, indeed, may be of no value whatsoever. Furthermore, a client who substitutes an unproven alternative therapy for an established, effective medical treatment may delay healing, suffer harmful effects, and endanger health.

Some herbal products contain ingredients that interact with prescription drugs. When obtaining medical histories, nurses should include questions on dietary supplements. Clients taking medications with potentially serious adverse effects such as insulin, warfarin (Coumadin), or digoxin (Lanoxin) should be warned never to take any herbal product or dietary supplement without first discussing their needs with a physician. Drug interactions with selected herbs are listed in Table 11.5. Herbal drug interactions are also noted, where applicable, in the prototype drug features throughout this text.

Another warning that must be heeded with natural products is to beware of allergic reactions. Most herbal products contain a mixture of ingredients, and it is not unusual to find dozens of different chemicals in teas and infusions

TABLE 11.5   Common Herb–Drug Interactions

Common (*Scientific*) Name	Interacts with	Comments
echinacea (*Echinacea purpurea*)	amiodarone anabolic steroids ketoconazole methotrexate	possible increased hepatotoxicity
feverfew (*Tanacetum parthenium*)	aspirin heparin NSAIDs warfarin	increased bleeding potential
garlic (*Allium sativum*)	aspirin insulin NSAIDs oral hypoglycemic agents warfarin	increased bleeding potential additive hypoglycemic effects increased bleeding potential additive hypoglycemic effects increased bleeding potential
ginger (*Zingiber officinalis*)	aspirin heparin NSAIDs warfarin	increased bleeding potential
ginkgo (*Ginkgo biloba*)	anticonvulsants aspirin heparin NSAIDs tricyclic antidepressants warfarin	possible decreased anticonvulsant effectiveness increased bleeding potential possible decreased seizure threshold increased bleeding potential
ginseng (*Panax quinquefolius/ Eleutherococcus senticosus*)	CNS depressants digoxin diuretics insulin oral hypoglycemic agents warfarin	potentiated sedation increased toxicity possible attenuated diuretic effects increased hypoglycemic effects increased hypoglycemic effects decreased anticoagulant effects
goldenseal (*Hydrastis canadensis*)	diuretics	possible attenuated diuretic effects
kava kava (*Piper methysticum*)	barbiturates benzodiazepines CNS depressants levodopa/carbidopa phenothiazines	potentiated sedation worsened Parkinson's symptoms increased risk and severity of dystonic reactions
St. John's wort (*Hypericum perforatum*)	CNS depressants cyclosporine efavirenz opiate analgesics protease inhibitors selective serotonin reuptake inhibitors theophylline tricyclic antidepressants warfarin	potentiated sedation possible decreased cyclosporine levels decreased antiretroviral activity increased sedation decreased antiretroviral activity of indinavir possible serotonin syndrome* decreased theophylline efficacy possible serotonin syndrome* decreased anticoagulant effects
valerian (*Valeriana officinalis*)	barbiturates benzodiazepines CNS depressants	potentiated sedation

*Serotonin syndrome: headache, dizziness, sweating, agitation
Source: Data modified from www.prenhall.com/drugguides

TABLE 11.6	Selected Specialty Supplements
Name	**Common Uses**
acidophilus	to maintain intestinal health
amino acids	to build protein, muscle strength, and endurance
coenzyme Q10	to prevent heart disease, provide antioxidant therapy
chondroitin	to alleviate arthritis and other joint problems
DHEA	to boost immune and memory functions
fish oil	to reduce cholesterol levels, enhance brain function, increase visual acuity due to presence of the omega-3 fatty acids
flaxseed oil	to reduce cholesterol levels, enhance brain function, increase visual acuity due to presence of the omega-3 fatty acids
glucosamine	to alleviate arthritis and other joint problems
methyl sulfonyl methane (MSM)	to reduce allergic reactions to pollen and foods, relieve pain and inflammation of arthritis and similar conditions
soy isoflavone	to reduce the risk of certain types of cancer

made from the flowers, leaves, or roots of a plant. Clients who have known allergies to certain foods or medicines should seek medical advice before taking a new herbal product. It is always wise to take the smallest amount possible when starting herbal therapy, even less than the recommended dose, to see if allergies or other adverse effects occur.

Nurses have an obligation to seek the latest medical information on herbal products, because there is a good possibility that their clients are using them to supplement traditional medicines. Clients should be advised to be skeptical of claims on the labels of dietary supplements and to seek health information from reputable sources. Nurses should never condemn a client's use of alternative medicines, but instead should be supportive and seek to understand the client's goals for taking the supplements. The healthcare provider will often need to educate clients on the role of CAM therapies in the treatment of their disorders and discuss which treatment or combination of treatments will best meet their health goals.

11.6 Specialty Supplements

Specialty supplements are nonherbal dietary products used to enhance a wide variety of body functions. These supplements form a diverse group of substances obtained from plant and animal sources. They are more specific in their action than herbal products and are generally targeted for one or a smaller number of conditions. The most popular specialty supplements are listed in Table 11.6.

In general, specialty supplements have a legitimate rationale for their use. For example, chondroitin and glucosamine are natural substances in the body necessary for cartilage growth and maintenance. Amino acids are natural building blocks of muscle protein. Flaxseed and fish oils contain omega fatty acids that have been shown to reduce the risk of heart disease in certain clients.

As with herbal products, the link between most specialty supplements and their claimed benefits is unclear. In some cases, the body already has sufficient quantities of the substance, taking additional amounts may be of no benefit. In other cases, the supplement is marketed for conditions for which the supplement has no proved effect. The good news is that these substances are generally not harmful, unless taken in large amounts. The bad news, however, is that they can give clients false hopes of an easy cure for chronic conditions such as heart disease or the pain of arthritis. As with herbal products, the health professional should advise clients to be skeptical about the health claims regarding the use of these supplements.

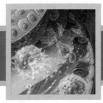

CHAPTER REVIEW

KEY CONCEPTS

The numbered key concepts provide a succinct summary of the important points from the corresponding numbered section within the chapter. If any of these points are not clear, refer to the numbered section within the chapter for review.

11.1 Complementary and alternative medicine is a set of diverse therapies and healing systems used by many people for disease prevention and self-healing.

11.2 Natural products obtained from plants have been used as medicines for thousands of years.

11.3 Herbal products are available in a variety of formulations, some contain standardized extracts, and others contain whole herbs.

11.4 Herbal products and dietary supplements are regulated by the Dietary Supplement Health and Education Act of

1994, which does not require safety or efficacy testing prior to marketing.

11.5 Natural products may have pharmacological actions and result in adverse effects, including significant interactions with prescription medications.

11.6 Specialty supplements are nonherbal dietary products used to enhance a wide variety of body functions. Like herbal products, most have not been subjected to controlled, scientific testing.

NCLEX-RN® REVIEW QUESTIONS

1 The nurse obtains information during the admission interview that the client is taking herbal supplements. What implications does this information have for the client's treatment?

1. This is not important, because herbal products are natural and pose no risk to the client.
2. These products are a welcome adjunct to conventional treatment.
3. The nurse must observe the client for allergic reactions.
4. The herbal products may interact with prescribed medications and affect drug action.

2 Appropriate teaching to provide safety for a client who is planning to use herbal products should include which of the following?

1. Take the smallest amount possible when starting herbal therapy, even less than the recommended dose, to see if allergies or other adverse effects occur.
2. Read the labels to determine composition of the product.
3. Research the clinical trials before using the products.
4. Read the labels to determine which diseases or disorders the product has been proved to treat or cure.

3 The client states he has been using the herbal product saw palmetto. The nurse recognizes that this supplement is often used to treat:

1. Insomnia.
2. Urinary problems associated with prostate enlargement.
3. Symptoms of menopause.
4. Urinary tract infection.

4 A client receiving warfarin (Coumadin) therapy reports use of the herb feverfew. The nurse observes the client for evidence of:

1. Liver toxicity.
2. Increased coagulation.
3. Renal dysfunction.
4. Increased bleeding potential.

5 The client has been taking sertraline hydrochloride (Zoloft), but just added St. John's wort for his depression. He now presents to the emergency department. The nurse recognizes the signs and symptoms of serotonin syndrome as (select all that apply):

1. Headache.
2. Dizziness.
3. Agitation.
4. Weight loss.
5. Sweating.

CRITICAL THINKING QUESTIONS

1. A 44-year-old breast cancer survivor is placed on tamoxifen (Nolvadex) 20 mg PO daily. Since receiving chemotherapy, the client has not had a menstrual cycle. She is concerned about being menopausal and wonders about the possibility of using a soy-based product as a form of natural hormone replacement. How should the nurse advise the client?

2. A 62-year-old male client is recuperating from a myocardial infarction. He is on the anticoagulant warfarin (Coumadin) and antidysrhythmic digoxin (Lanoxin). He talks to his wife about starting garlic to help lower his blood lipid levels, and ginseng because he has heard it helps in coronary artery disease. Discuss the potential concerns about the use of garlic and ginseng by this client.

3. The client has been taking St. John's wort for symptoms of depression. He is now scheduled for an elective surgery. What important preoperative teaching should be included?

See Appendix D for answers and rationales for all activities.

EXPLORE
MediaLink

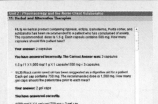

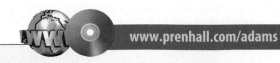

www.prenhall.com/adams

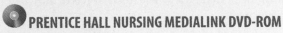

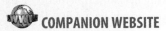

NCLEX-RN® review, case studies, and other interactive resources for this chapter can be found on the companion website at www.prenhall.com/adams. Click on "Chapter 11" to select the activities for this chapter. For animations, more NCLEX-RN® review questions, and an audio glossary, access the accompanying Prentice Hall Nursing MediaLink DVD-ROM in this textbook.

PRENTICE HALL NURSING MEDIALINK DVD-ROM

- **Audio Glossary**
- **NCLEX-RN® Review**

COMPANION WEBSITE

- **NCLEX-RN® Review**
- **Case Study:** Alternative therapies
- **Challenge Your Knowledge**

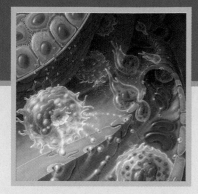

CHAPTER 12

Substance Abuse

DRUGS AT A GLANCE: ABUSED SUBSTANCES

CNS DEPRESSANTS
Sedatives and Sedative-Hypnotics
Barbiturates
Benzodiazepines
Opioids
Ethyl Alcohol
CANNABINOIDS
Marijuana
HALLUCINOGENS
LSD
Other Hallucinogens
CNS STIMULANTS
Amphetamines and Methylphenidate
Cocaine
Caffeine
NICOTINE

OBJECTIVES

After reading this chapter, the student should be able to:

1. Explain underlying causes of addiction.
2. Compare and contrast psychological and physical dependence.
3. Compare withdrawal syndromes for the various abused substance classes.
4. Discuss how nurses can recognize drug tolerance in clients.
5. Explain the major characteristics of abuse, dependence, and tolerance resulting from the following substances: alcohol, nicotine, marijuana, hallucinogens, CNS stimulants, sedatives, and opioids.
6. Describe the role of the nurse in delivering care to individuals who have substance abuse issues.

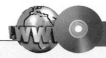

MediaLink   www.prenhall.com/adams

NCLEX-RN® review, case studies, and other interactive resources for this chapter can be found on the companion website at www.prenhall.com/adams. Click on "Chapter 12" to select the activities for this chapter. For animations, more NCLEX-RN® review questions, and an audio glossary, access the accompanying Prentice Hall Nursing MediaLink DVD-ROM in this textbook.

KEY TERMS

addiction   *page 118*

attention deficit–hyperactivity disorder
   (ADHD)   *page 125*

benzodiazepines   *page 121*

cross-tolerance   *page 120*

designer drugs   *page 118*

opioid   *page 121*

physical dependence   *page 119*

psychedelics   *page 123*

psychological dependence   *page 119*

reticular formation   *page 124*

sedative   *page 121*

substance abuse   *page 118*

tetrahydrocannabinol (THC)   *page 122*

tolerance   *page 120*

withdrawal syndrome   *page 119*

Substance abuse is the self-administration of a drug in a manner that does not conform to the norms within one's given culture or society. Throughout history, individuals have consumed both natural substances and prescription drugs to increase performance, assist with relaxation, alter psychological state, or to simply fit in with the crowd. Substance abuse has a tremendous economic, social, and public health impact on society. Although the terms *drug abuse* and *substance abuse* are sometimes used interchangeably, substance abuse is preferred, because many of these agents are not legal drugs or medications.

12.1 Overview of Substance Abuse

Abused substances belong to a number of diverse chemical classes. They have few structural similarities, but have in common an ability to affect the nervous system, particularly the brain. Some substances, such as opium, marijuana, cocaine, nicotine, caffeine, and alcohol, are obtained from natural sources. Others are synthetic or **designer drugs,** created in illegal laboratories for the express purpose of profiting from illicit drug trafficking.

Although the public often associates substance abuse with illegal drugs, this is not necessarily the case: Alcohol and nicotine are the two most commonly abused drugs. Legal, prescription medications such as methylphenidate (Ritalin) and meperidine (Demerol) are sometimes abused; ketamine and gamma hydrybutyrate (GHB) are examples of abused legal anesthetics. Anabolic steroids are legal medications commonly abused by athletes. Legal substances without prescription include volatile inhalants such as aerosols and paint thinners. Illegal substances that are frequently abused include marijuana, heroin (opioids), and hallucinogens such as lysergic acid diethylamide (LSD) and phencyclidine hydrochloride (PCP).

Several drugs once used therapeutically are now illegal owing to their high potential for abuse. Cocaine was once widely used as a local anesthetic, but today nearly all the cocaine acquired by users is obtained illegally. LSD is now illegal, although in the 1940s and 1950s, it was used in psychotherapy. Phencyclidine was popular in the early 1960s as an anesthetic, but was withdrawn from the market in 1965 because clients reported hallucinations, delusions, and anxiety after recovering from anesthesia. Many amphetamines once used for bronchodilation were discontinued in the 1980s after psychotic episodes were reported.

12.2 Neurobiological and Psychosocial Components of Substance Abuse

Addiction is an overwhelming compulsion that drives someone to repetitive drug-taking behavior, despite serious health and social consequences. It is impossible to accurately predict whether a person will become a substance abuser. Attempts to predict a person's addictive tendency using psychological profiles or genetic markers have largely been unsuccessful. Substance abuse depends on multiple complex, interacting variables. These variables focus on the following categories:

• *Agent or drug factors* Cost, availability, dose, mode of administration (e.g., oral, IV, inhalation), speed of onset/termination, and length of drug use

• *User factors* Genetic factors (e.g., metabolic enzymes, innate tolerance), propensity for risk-taking behavior, prior experiences with drugs, disease that may require a scheduled drug

• *Environmental factors* Social/community norms, role models, peer influences, educational opportunities

In the case of legal prescription drugs, addiction may begin with a legitimate need for pharmacotherapy. For example, narcotic analgesics may be indicated for pain relief, or sedatives for a sleep disorder. These drugs may result in a favorable experience,

PharmFacts

Substance Abuse in the United States

- Twenty-eight million Americans have used illicit drugs at least once.
- During the 2000–2001 school year, 25% of high school students used an illegal drug on a monthly or more frequent basis.
- An estimated 2.4 million Americans have used heroin during their lives.
- About one in five Americans has lived with an alcoholic while growing up. Children of alcoholic parents are four times more likely to become alcoholics than children of nonalcoholic parents.
- Alcohol is an important factor in 68% of manslaughters, 54% of murders, 48% of robberies, and 44% of burglaries.
- Among youth between the ages of 12 and 17, 7.2 million drank alcohol at least once in 2003. Girls were as likely as boys to drink alcohol.
- Barbiturate overdose is a factor in almost one third of all drug-related deaths.
- In 2003, 36% of 10th graders and 46% of 12th graders reported using marijuana and hashish.
- In 2003, 7.7% of high school seniors reported using cocaine, up from 5.9% in 1994.
- In 2002, 2 million Americans were currently using cocaine on a monthly basis; about 567,000 used crack cocaine.
- Approximately 70% of the cocaine entering the United States comes from Colombia and passes through south Florida.
- In 2003, 16% of 8th graders and 11% of 12th graders reported using volatile inhalants.
- In 2002, 30% of all Americans were cigarette smokers, including 25% of those between the ages of 12 and 25.
- In 2003, 43% of 10th graders and 54% of 12th graders reported they had tried smoking cigarettes. Eight percent of the 12th graders consumed more than half a pack or more each day.
- In 2003, 8% of 12th graders reported using Ecstasy (MDMA).
- LSD is one of the most potent drugs known, with only 25–150 mcg constituting a dose. In 2003, almost 9% of 12th graders reported using LSD.

such as pain relief or sleep, and clients will then want to repeat these positive experiences after the prescription has expired.

It is a common misunderstanding, even among some health professionals, that the therapeutic use of scheduled drugs creates large numbers of addicted clients. In fact, prescription drugs rarely cause addiction when used according to accepted medical protocols. The risk of addiction for prescription medications is primarily a function of the dose and the length of therapy. Because of this, medications having a potential for abuse are usually prescribed at the lowest effective dose and for the shortest time necessary to treat the medical problem. Nurses should administer these medications as prescribed for the relief of client symptoms, without undue fear of producing dependency. As mentioned in Chapters 1 and 2 ∞, numerous laws have been passed in an attempt to limit drug abuse and addiction.

12.3 Physical and Psychological Dependence

Whether a substance is addictive is related to how easily an individual can stop taking the agent on a repetitive basis. When a person has an overwhelming desire to take a drug and cannot stop, this condition is referred to as *substance dependence*. Substance dependence is classified into two categories, physical dependence and psychological dependence.

Physical dependence refers to an altered physical condition caused by the adaptation of the nervous system to repeated substance use. Over time, the body's cells become accustomed to the presence of the unnatural substance. With physical dependence, uncomfortable symptoms known as *withdrawal* result when the agent is discontinued. Opioids, such as morphine and heroin, may produce physical dependence rather quickly with repeated doses, particularly when taken intravenously. Alcohol, sedatives, some stimulants, and nicotine are other examples of substances that may easily produce physical dependence with extended use.

In contrast, **psychological dependence** produces no obvious signs of physical discomfort after the agent is discontinued. The user, however, has an overwhelming desire to continue substance use despite obvious negative economic, physical, or social consequences. This intense craving may be associated with the client's home environment or social contacts. Strong psychological craving for a substance may continue for months or even years and is often responsible for relapses during substance abuse therapy, and a return to drug-seeking behavior. Psychological dependence usually requires relatively high doses for a prolonged time, such as with marijuana and antianxiety drugs; however, psychological dependence may develop quickly, perhaps after only one use, for example with crack—a potent, inexpensive form of cocaine.

12.4 Withdrawal Syndrome

Once a person becomes physically dependent and the substance is discontinued, a **withdrawal syndrome** will occur. Symptoms of withdrawal syndrome may be particularly severe for those who are physically dependent on alcohol and sedatives. Because of the severity of the symptoms, the process of withdrawal from these agents is best accomplished in a substance abuse treatment facility. Examples of the types of withdrawal syndromes experienced with different abused substances are listed in Table 12.1.

Prescription drugs may be used to reduce the severity of withdrawal symptoms. For example, alcohol withdrawal can be treated with a short-acting benzodiazepine such as oxazepam (Serax), and opioid withdrawal can be treated with methadone. Symptoms of nicotine withdrawal may be relieved by replacement therapy in the form of nicotine patches or chewing gum. No specific pharmacological intervention is indicated for withdrawal from CNS stimulants, hallucinogens, marijuana, or inhalants.

With chronic substance abuse, people will often associate their conditions and surroundings, including social contacts with other users who are also taking the drug. Users tend to revert to drug-seeking behavior when they return to the company of other substance abusers. Counselors often encourage users to refrain from associating with past social contacts or having relationships with other substance abusers to lessen the possibility for relapse. The formation of new social contacts as a result of association with self-help

TABLE 12.1	Withdrawal Symptoms and Characteristics for Selected Drugs of Abuse		
Drug	Physiological and Psychological Effects	Toxicity Signs	Dependency Characteristics
alcohol	tremors, fatigue, anxiety, abdominal cramping, hallucinations, confusion, seizures, delirium	extreme somnolence, severe CNS depression, diminished reflexes, respiratory depression	moderate to high psychological dependence; moderate to extreme physical signs of withdrawal
barbiturates	insomnia, anxiety, weakness, abdominal cramps, tremor, anorexia, seizures, skin hypersenstivity reactions, hallucinations, delirium	severe CNS depression, tremor, diaphoresis, vomiting, cyanosis, tachycardia, Cheyne–Stokes respirations	moderate to high psychological dependence; moderate to extreme physical signs of withdrawal
benzodiazepines	insomnia, restlessness, abdominal pain, nausea, sensitivity to light and sound, headache, fatigue, muscle twitches	somnolence, confusion, diminished reflexes, coma	high psychological dependence; less severe physical signs
cocaine and amphetamines	mental depression, anxiety, extreme fatigue, hunger	dysrhythmias, lethargy, skin pallor, psychosis	high psychological dependence; less severe physical signs
hallucinogens	rarely observed; dependent on specific drug	panic reactions, confusion, blurred vision, increase in blood pressure, psychotic-like state	moderate to high psychological dependence; possible flashbacks
marijuana	irritability, restlessness, insomnia, tremor, chills, weight loss	euphoria, paranoia, panic reactions, hallucinations, psychotic-like state	high psychological dependence; little to no physical withdrawal signs
nicotine	irritability, anxiety, restlessness, headaches, increased appetite, insomnia, inability to concentrate, decrease in heart rate and blood pressure	heart palpitations, tachyarrythmias, confusion, depression, seizures	high psychological dependence; extreme physical signs of withdrawal
opioids	excessive sweating, restlessness, dilated pupils, agitation, goosebumps, tremor, violent yawning, increased heart rate and blood pressure, nausea/vomiting, abdominal cramps and pain, muscle spasms with kicking movements, weight loss	respiratory depression, cyanosis, extreme somnolence, coma	high psychological dependence; range of physical withdrawal signs

groups such as Alcoholics Anonymous helps some people transition to a drug-free lifestyle.

12.5 Tolerance

Tolerance is a biological condition that occurs when the body adapts to a substance after repeated administration. Over time, higher doses of the agent are required to produce the same initial effect. For example, at the start of pharmacotherapy, a client may find that 2 mg of a sedative is effective for inducing sleep. After taking the medication for several months, the client notices that it takes 4 mg or perhaps 6 mg to fall asleep. Development of drug tolerance is common for substances that affect the nervous system. *Tolerance should be thought of as a natural consequence of continued drug use and not be considered evidence of addiction or substance abuse.*

Tolerance does not develop at the same rate for all actions of a drug. For example, clients usually develop tolerance to the nausea and vomiting produced by narcotic analgesics after only a few doses. Tolerance to the mood-altering effects of these drugs and to their ability to reduce pain develops more slowly but eventually may be complete. On the other hand, tolerance never develops to the drug's ability to constrict the pupils. Clients will often endure annoying side effects of drugs, such as the sedation caused by antihistamines, if they know that tolerance will quickly develop to these effects.

Once tolerance develops to a substance, it often extends to closely related drugs. This phenomenon is known as

cross-tolerance. For example, a heroin addict will become tolerant to the analgesic effects of other opioids such as morphine or meperidine. Clients who have developed tolerance to alcohol will show tolerance to other CNS depressants such as barbiturates, benzodiazepines, and some general anesthetics. This has important clinical implications for the nurse, because doses of these related medications will need to be adjusted accordingly to obtain maximum therapeutic benefit.

SPECIAL CONSIDERATIONS

Abuse of Volatile Inhalants by Children and Adolescents

Many parents are concerned that their children will smoke tobacco or marijuana or become addicted to crack or amphetamines. Yet, few parents consider that the most common sources of abused substances are readily available in their own homes. Inhaling volatile chemicals, known as *huffing*, is most prevalent in the 10- to 12-year-old group and declines with age; one in five children has done this by the eighth grade. Virtually any organic compound can be huffed, including nail polish remover, spray paint, household glue, correction fluid, propane, gasoline, and even whipped cream propellants. These agents are available in the home, in stores, and in the workplace. They are inexpensive, legal, and can be used anytime and anywhere. Children can die after a single exposure or suffer brain damage, which may be manifested as slurred or slow speech, tremor, memory loss, or personality changes. Nurses who work with pediatric clients should be aware of the widespread nature of this type of abuse, and advise parents to keep a close watch on volatile substances.

MediaLink · The Temptation of Steroids

The terms *immunity* and *resistance* are often confused with tolerance. These terms more correctly refer to the immune system and infections and should not be used interchangeably with tolerance. For example, microorganisms become resistant to the effects of an antibiotic: They do not become tolerant. Clients become tolerant to the effects of pain relievers: They do not become resistant.

12.6 Abused CNS Depressants

CNS depressants are a group of drugs that cause clients to feel sedated or relaxed. Drugs in this group include barbiturates, nonbarbiturate sedative–hypnotics, benzodiazepines, alcohol, and opioids. Although the majority of these are legal substances, they are controlled owing to their abuse potential.

SEDATIVES AND SEDATIVE-HYPNOTICS

Sedatives, also known as *tranquilizers,* are prescribed for sleep disorders and certain forms of epilepsy. The two primary classes of sedatives are the barbiturates and the nonbarbiturate sedative–hypnotics. Their actions, indications, safety profiles, and addictive potential are roughly equivalent. Physical dependence, psychological dependence, and tolerance develop when these agents are taken for extended periods at high doses (Chapter 2 ∞). Clients sometimes abuse these drugs by faking prescriptions or by sharing their medication with friends. Sedatives are commonly combined with other drugs of abuse, such as CNS stimulants or alcohol. Addicts often alternate between amphetamines, which keep them awake for several days, and barbiturates, which are needed to help them relax and fall sleep.

Many sedatives have a long duration of action: Effects may last an entire day, depending on the specific drug. Users may appear dull or apathetic. Higher doses resemble alcohol intoxication, with slurred speech and motor incoordination. Four commonly abused barbiturates are pentobarbital (Nembutal), amobarbital (Amytal), secobarbital (Seconal), and a combination of secobarbital and amobarbital (Tuinal). The medical use of barbiturates and nonbarbiturate sedative–hypnotics has declined markedly over the past 20 years. The use of barbiturates in treating sleep disorders is discussed in Chapter 14 ∞, and their use in epilepsy is presented in Chapter 15 ∞.

Overdoses of barbiturates and nonbarbiturate sedative–hypnotics are extremely dangerous. The drugs suppress the respiratory centers in the brain, and the user may stop breathing or lapse into a coma. Death may result from barbiturate overdose. Withdrawal symptoms from these drugs resemble those of alcohol withdrawal and may be life threatening.

Benzodiazepines are another group of CNS depressants that have a potential for abuse. They are one of the most widely prescribed classes of drugs, and have largely replaced the barbiturates for certain disorders. Their primary indication is anxiety (Chapter 14 ∞), although they are also used to prevent seizures (Chapter 15 ∞) and as muscle relaxants (Chapter 21 ∞). Popular benzodiazepines include alprazolam (Xanax), diazepam (Valium), temazepam (Restoril), triazolam (Halcion), and midazolam (Versed).

Although they are a frequently prescribed drug class, benzodiazepine abuse is not common. Individuals abusing benzodiazepines may appear carefree, detached, sleepy, or disoriented. Death due to overdose is rare, even with high doses. Users may combine these agents with alcohol, cocaine, or heroin to augment their drug experience. If combined with these other agents, overdose may be lethal. The benzodiazepine withdrawal syndrome is less severe than that of barbiturates or alcohol.

OPIOIDS

Opioids, also known as *narcotic analgesics,* are prescribed for severe pain, persistent cough, and diarrhea. The opioid class includes natural substances obtained from the unripe seeds of the poppy plant such as opium, morphine, and codeine, and synthetic drugs such as propoxyphene (Darvon), meperidine (Demerol), oxycodone (OxyContin), fentanyl (Duragesic, Sublimaze), methadone (Dolophine), and heroin. The therapeutic effects of the opioids are discussed in detail in Chapter 18 ∞.

The effects of *oral* opioids begin within 30 minutes and may last over a day. *Parenteral* forms produce immediate effects, including the brief, intense rush of euphoria sought by heroin addicts. Individuals experience a range of CNS effects from extreme pleasure to slowed body activities and profound sedation. Signs include constricted pupils, an increase in the pain threshold, and respiratory depression.

Addiction to opioids can occur rapidly, and withdrawal can produce intense symptoms. Although extremely unpleasant, withdrawal from opioids is not life threatening, compared with barbiturate withdrawal. Methadone is a narcotic sometimes used to treat opioid addiction. Although methadone has addictive properties of its own, it does not produce the same degree of euphoria as other opioids, and its effects are longer lasting. Heroin addicts are switched to methadone to prevent unpleasant withdrawal symptoms. Since methadone is taken orally, clients are no longer exposed to serious risks associated with intravenous drug use, such as hepatitis and AIDS. Clients sometimes remain on methadone maintenance for a lifetime. Withdrawal from methadone is more prolonged than with heroin or morphine, but the symptoms are less intense.

ETHYL ALCOHOL

Ethyl alcohol, commonly known as *alcohol,* is one of the most commonly abused drugs. Alcohol is a legal substance for adults, and it is readily available as beer, wine, and liquor. The economic, social, and health consequences of alcohol abuse are staggering. Despite the enormous negative consequences associated with long-term use, small quantities of alcohol consumed on a daily basis have been found to reduce the risk of stroke and heart attack.

Alcohol is classified as a CNS depressant because it slows the region of the brain responsible for alertness and wakefulness. Alcohol easily crosses the blood–brain barrier, so its effects are observed within 5 to 30 minutes after consumption. Effects of alcohol are directly proportional to the amount consumed, and include relaxation, sedation, memory impairment, loss of motor coordination, reduced judgment, and decreased inhibition. Alcohol also imparts a characteristic odor to the breath and increases blood flow in certain areas of the skin, causing a flushed face, pink cheeks, or red nose. Although these symptoms are easily recognized, the nurse must be aware that other substances and disorders may cause similar effects. For example, many antianxiety agents, sedatives, and antidepressants can cause drowsiness, memory difficulties, and loss of motor coordination. Certain mouthwashes contain alcohol and cause the breath to smell alcoholic. During assessment, the skilled nurse must consider these factors before confirming alcohol use.

The presence of food in the stomach slows the absorption of alcohol, thus delaying the onset of drug action. *Metabolism,* or detoxification of alcohol by the liver, occurs at a slow, constant rate, which is not affected by the presence of food. The average rate is about 15 ml per hour—the practical equivalent of one alcoholic beverage per hour. If consumed at a higher rate, alcohol will accumulate in the blood and produce greater depressant effects on the brain. Acute overdoses of alcohol produce vomiting, severe hypotension, respiratory failure, and coma. Death due to alcohol poisoning is not uncommon. The nurse should teach clients to never combine alcohol consumption with other CNS depressants because their effects are cumulative, and profound sedation or coma may result.

Chronic alcohol consumption produces both psychological and physiological dependence and results in a large number of adverse health effects. The organ most affected by chronic alcohol abuse is the liver. Alcoholism is a common cause of *cirrhosis,* a debilitating and often fatal failure of the liver to perform its vital functions. Liver impairment causes in abnormalities in blood clotting and nutritional deficiencies, and sensitizes the client to the effects of all medications metabolized by the liver. For alcoholic clients, the nurse should begin therapy with reduced medication doses until the adverse effects of the medication can be assessed.

NATURAL THERAPIES

Milk Thistle for Alcohol Liver Damage

Excessive consumption of alcohol, as well as some psychotropic drugs, damages the liver. The active ingredient in the milk thistle plant (*Silybum marianum*), silymarin, has well-documented hepatoprotective qualities. Studies have shown that silymarin is able to neutralize the effects of alcohol, and actually stimulate liver regeneration. It acts as an antioxidant and free-radical scavenger. Anti-inflammatory and anticarcinogenic properties have also been documented (Song et al., 2006; Fraschini, Demartini, & Esposti 2002). Milk thistle may enhance the effectiveness of aspirin, increasing the risk of bleeding. Milk thistle also interacts with anticancer agents: It enhances the tumor-fighting effects of cisplatin and doxorubicin, and diminishes the effect of cisplatin and ifosfamide. Milk thistle may be found growing in North America, from Mexico to Canada.

The alcohol withdrawal syndrome is severe and may be life threatening. The use of anticonvulsants in the treatment of alcohol withdrawal is discussed in Chapter 15 ∞. Long-term treatment for alcohol abuse includes behavioral counseling and self-help groups such as Alcoholics Anonymous. Disulfiram (Antabuse) may be given to discourage relapses. Disulfiram inhibits acetaldehyde dehydrogenase, the enzyme that metabolizes alcohol. If a client consumes alcohol while taking disulfiram, he or she becomes violently ill within 5 to 10 minutes, with headache, shortness of breath, nausea/vomiting, and other unpleasant symptoms. Disulfiram is effective only in highly motivated clients, since the success of pharmacotherapy is entirely dependent on client compliance. Alcohol sensitivity continues for up to 2 weeks after disulfiram has been discontinued. As a pregnancy category X drug, disulfiram should never be taken during pregnancy.

In addition to disulfiram, acamprosate calcium (Campral, Forest) is an FDA-approved drug for maintaining alcohol abstinence in clients with alcohol dependence. Studies comparing the therapeutic benefit of disulfiram with acamprosate have not been fully demonstrated. The drug may benefit clients who are not candidates for naltrexone therapy. (Clients receiving naltrexone therapy or clients receiving methadone treatment are subject to withdrawal symptoms.) Acamprosate's mechanism of action involves the restoration of neuronal excitation—the alteration of gamma-aminobutyrate and glutamate activity in the CNS—and does not appear to have other central nervous system actions. Adverse reactions to acamprosate include diarrhea, flatulence, and nausea. The drug is contraindicated in clients with severe renal impairment but may be used in clients at increased risk for hepatoxicity.

12.7 Cannabinoids

Cannabinoids are substances obtained from the hemp plant *Cannabis sativa,* which thrives in tropical climates. Cannabinoid agents are usually smoked and include marijuana, hashish, and hash oil. Although more than 61 cannabinoid chemicals have been identified, the ingredient responsible for most of the psychoactive properties is delta-9-**tetrahydrocannabinol (THC).**

MARIJUANA

Marijuana, also known as *grass, pot, weed, reefer,* or *dope,* is a natural product obtained from *C. sativa.* It is the most commonly used illicit drug in the United States. Use of marijuana slows motor activity, decreases coordination, and causes disconnected thoughts, feelings of paranoia, and euphoria. It increases thirst and craving for food, particularly chocolate and other candies. One hallmark symptom of marijuana use is red or bloodshot eyes, caused by dilation of blood vessels. THC accumulates in the gonads.

When inhaled, marijuana produces effects that occur within minutes and last up to 24 hours. Because marijuana smoke is inhaled more deeply and held within the lungs for a longer time than cigarette smoke, marijuana smoke introduces four times more particulates (tar) into the lungs than tobacco smoke. Smoking marijuana on a daily basis may increase the risk of lung cancer and other respiratory disorders. Chronic use is associated with a lack of motivation in achieving or pursuing life goals.

Unlike many abused substances, marijuana produces little physical dependence or tolerance. Withdrawal symptoms are mild, if they are experienced at all. Metabolites of THC, however, remain in the body for months to years, allowing laboratory specialists to easily determine whether someone has taken marijuana. For several days after use, THC can also be detected in the urine. Despite numerous attempts to demonstrate therapeutic applications for marijuana, results have been controversial and the medical value of the drug remains to be proved.

12.8 Hallucinogens

Hallucinogens consist of a diverse class of chemicals that have in common the ability to produce an altered, dream-like state of consciousness. The prototype substance for this class, sometimes called **psychedelics,** is LSD. All hallucinogens are Schedule I drugs: They have no medical use.

LSD

For nearly all drugs of abuse, predictable symptoms occur in every user. Effects from hallucinogens, however, are highly variable and dependent on the mood and expectations of the user and the surrounding environment in which the substance is used. Two people taking the same agent will report completely different symptoms, and the same person may report different symptoms with each use. Users who take LSD or psilocybin (magic mushrooms, or shrooms) (● Figure 12.1) may experience symptoms such as laughter, visions, religious revelations, or deep personal insights. Common occurrences are hallucinations and afterimages projected onto people as they move. Users also report unusually bright lights and vivid colors. Some users hear voices; others report smells. Many experience a profound sense of truth and deep-directed thoughts. Unpleasant experiences can be terrifying and may include anxiety, panic attacks, confusion, severe depression, and paranoia.

LSD, also called *acid, the beast, blotter acid,* and *California sunshine,* is derived from a fungus that grows on rye and other grains. LSD is nearly always administered orally and can be manufactured in capsule, tablet, or liquid form. A common and inexpensive method for distributing LSD is to place drops of the drug on paper, often containing the images of cartoon characters or graphics related to drug culture. The paper is dried; users then ingest the paper containing the LSD to produce the drug's effects.

Psilocybin
(4-phosphoryl-DMT)

LSD

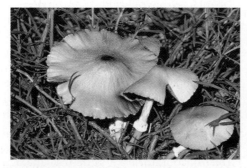
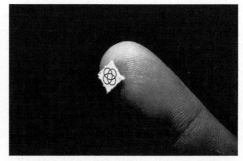

●**Figure 12.1** Comparison of the chemical structures of psilocybin and LSD. Psilocybin (left) is derived from a mushroom
Source: Pearson Education/PH College.

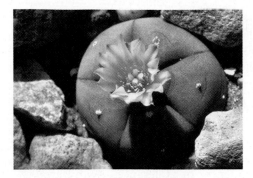

● **Figure 12.2** The chemical structure of mescaline, derived from the peyote cactus *Source: Pearson Education/PH College.*

LSD is distributed throughout the body immediately after use. Effects are experienced within an hour, and may last from 6 to 12 hours. LSD affects the central and autonomic nervous systems, increasing blood pressure, elevating body temperature, dilating pupils, and increasing the heart rate. Repeated use may cause impaired memory and inability to reason. In extreme cases, clients may develop psychoses. One unusual adverse effect is flashbacks, in which the user experiences the effects of the drug again, sometimes weeks, months, or years after the drug was initially taken. Although tolerance is observed, little or no dependence occurs with the hallucinogens.

OTHER HALLUCINOGENS

In addition to LSD, other hallucinogens that are abused include the following:

- *Mescaline* Found in the peyote cactus of Mexico and Central America (● Figure 12.2)

- *MDMA (3,4-methylenedioxymethamphetamine; XTC or Ecstasy)* An amphetamine originally synthesized for research purposes that has since become extremely popular among teens and young adults

- *DOM (2,5 dimethoxy-4-methylamphetamine)* A recreational drug often linked with rave parties as a drug of choice having the name STP

- *MDA (3,4-methylenedioxyamphetamine)* Called the love drug because it is believed to enhance sexual desires

- *Phenylcyclohexylpiperadine (PCP; angel dust or phencyclidine)* Produces a trancelike state that may last for days and results in severe brain damage

- *Ketamine (date rape drug or special coke)* produces unconsciousness and amnesia; primary legal use is as an anesthetic

12.9 Abused CNS Stimulants

Stimulants include a diverse family of drugs known for their ability to increase the activity of the CNS. Some are available by prescription for the treatment of narcolepsy, obesity, and attention deficit–hyperactivity disorder (ADHD).

As drugs of abuse, CNS stimulants are taken to produce a sense of exhilaration, improve mental and physical performance, reduce appetite, prolong wakefulness, or simply "get high." Stimulants include the amphetamines, cocaine, methylphenidate, and caffeine.

AMPHETAMINES AND METHYLPHENIDATE

CNS stimulants have effects similar to those of the neurotransmitter norepinephrine (Chapter 13 ∞). Norepinephrine affects awareness and wakefulness by activating neurons in a part of the brain called the **reticular formation.** High doses of amphetamines give the user a feeling of self-confidence, euphoria, alertness, and empowerment; but just as short-term use induces favorable feelings, long-term use often results in feelings of restlessness, anxiety, and fits of rage, especially when the user is coming down from a high induced by the drug.

Most CNS stimulants affect cardiovascular and respiratory activity, resulting in increased blood pressure and increased respiration rate. Other symptoms include dilated pupils, sweating, and tremors. Overdoses of some stimulants lead to seizures and cardiac arrest.

Amphetamines and dextroamphetamines were once widely prescribed for depression, obesity, drowsiness, and congestion. In the 1960s, it became recognized that the medical uses of amphetamines did not outweigh their risk for dependence. Owing to the development of safer medications, the current therapeutic uses of these drugs are extremely limited. Most substance abusers obtain these agents from illegal laboratories, which can easily produce amphetamines and make tremendous profits.

Dextroamphetamine (Dexedrine) may be prescribed for short-term weight loss when all other attempts to reduce weight have been exhausted, and to treat narcolepsy. Methamphetamine, commonly called *ice,* is often used as a recreational drug by users who like the rush that it gives them. It usually is administered in powder or crystal form, but it may also be smoked. Methamphetamine is a Schedule II drug marketed under the trade name Desoxyn, although most abusers obtain it from illegal methamphetamine (*meth*) laboratories. A structural analogue of methamphetamine, methcathinone (street name, *Cat*) is made illegally and snorted, taken orally, or injected IV. Methcathinone is a Schedule I agent.

Methylphenidate (Ritalin) is a CNS stimulant widely prescribed for children diagnosed with **attention deficit–hyperactivity disorder (ADHD).** Ritalin has a calming effect in children who are inattentive or hyperactive. By stimulating the alertness center in the brain, the child is able to focus on tasks for longer periods. This explains the paradoxical calming effects that this stimulant has on children, which is usually the opposite of that on adults. The therapeutic applications of methylphenidate are discussed in Chapter 16 ∞.

Ritalin is a Schedule II drug that has many of the same effects as cocaine and amphetamines. It is sometimes abused by adolescents and adults seeking euphoria. Tablets are crushed and used intranasally or dissolved in liquid and injected IV. Ritalin is sometimes mixed with heroin, a combination called a *speedball*.

COCAINE

Cocaine is a natural substance obtained from leaves of the coca plant, which grows in the Andes Mountains region of South America. Documentation suggests that the plant has been used by Andean cultures since 2500 B.C. Natives in this region chew the coca leaves, or make teas of the dried leaves. Because coca is taken orally, absorption is slow, and the leaves contain only 1% cocaine, so users do not suffer the ill effects caused by chemically pure extracts from the plant. In the Andean culture, use of coca leaves is not considered substance abuse because it is part of the social norms of that society.

Cocaine is a Schedule II drug that produces actions similar to those of the amphetamines, although its effects are usually more rapid and intense. It is the second most commonly abused illicit drug in the United States. Routes of administration include snorting, smoking, and injecting. In small doses, cocaine produces feelings of intense euphoria, a decrease in hunger, analgesia, illusions of physical strength, and increased sensory perception. Larger doses will magnify these effects and also cause rapid heartbeat, sweating, dilation of the pupils, and an elevated body temperature. After the feelings of euphoria diminish, the user is left with a sense of irritability, insomnia, depression, and extreme distrust. Some users report the sensation that insects are crawling under the skin. Users who snort cocaine develop a chronic runny nose, a crusty redness around the nostrils, and deterioration of the nasal cartilage. Overdose can result in dysrhythmias, convulsions, stroke, or death due to respiratory arrest. The withdrawal syndrome for amphetamines and cocaine is much less intense than that from alcohol or barbiturate abuse.

CAFFEINE

Caffeine is a natural substance found in the seeds, leaves, or fruits of more than 63 plant species throughout the world. Significant amounts of caffeine are consumed in chocolate, coffee, tea, soft drinks, and ice cream. Caffeine is sometimes added to OTC pain relievers because it has been shown to increase the effectiveness of these medications. Caffeine travels to almost all parts of the body after ingestion, and several hours are needed for the body to metabolize and eliminate the drug. Caffeine has a pronounced diuretic effect.

Caffeine is considered a CNS stimulant because it produces increased mental alertness, restlessness, nervousness, irritability, and insomnia. The physical effects of caffeine include bronchodilation, increased blood pressure, increased production of stomach acid, and changes in blood glucose levels. Repeated use of caffeine may result in physical dependence and tolerance. Withdrawal symptoms include headaches, fatigue, depression, and impaired performance of daily activities.

12.10 Nicotine

Nicotine is sometimes considered a CNS stimulant, and although it does increase alertness, its actions and long-term consequences place it in a class by itself. Nicotine is unique among abused substances in that it is legal, strongly addictive, and highly carcinogenic. Furthermore, use of tobacco can cause harmful effects to those in the immediate area who breathe secondhand smoke. Clients often do not consider tobacco use as substance abuse.

TOBACCO USE AND NICOTINE

The most common method by which nicotine enters the body is through the inhalation of cigarette, pipe, or cigar smoke. Tobacco smoke contains more than 1,000 chemicals, a significant number of which are carcinogens. The primary addictive substance present in cigarette smoke is nicotine. Effects of inhaled nicotine may last from 30 minutes to several hours.

Nicotine affects many body systems including the nervous, cardiovascular, and endocrine systems. Nicotine stimulates the CNS directly, causing increased alertness and ability to focus, feelings of relaxation, and light-headedness. The cardiovascular effects of nicotine include an accelerated heart rate and increased blood pressure, caused by activation of nicotinic receptors located throughout the autonomic nervous system (Chapter 13 ∞). These cardiovascular effects can be particularly serious in clients taking oral contraceptives: The risk of a fatal heart attack is 5 times greater in smokers than in nonsmokers. Muscular tremors may occur with moderate doses of nicotine, and convulsions may result from very high doses. Nicotine affects the endocrine system by increasing the basal metabolic rate, leading to weight loss. Nicotine also reduces appetite. Chronic use leads to bronchitis, emphysema, and lung cancer.

Both psychological and physical dependence occur relatively quickly with nicotine. Once started on tobacco, clients tend to continue their drug use for many years, despite overwhelming medical evidence that the quality of life will be adversely affected and their lifespan shortened. Discontinuation results in agitation, weight gain, anxiety, headache, and an extreme craving for the drug. Although nicotine replacement patches and gum assist clients in dealing with the unpleasant withdrawal symptoms, only 25% of clients who attempt to stop smoking remain tobacco-free a year later.

MediaLink   Cocaine Animation

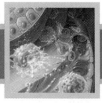

SPECIAL CONSIDERATIONS

Ethnic Groups and Smoking

The incidence of tobacco use varies among racial and ethnic groups. The highest rate is among American Indians and Alaska Natives. African Americans also have a high prevalence of smoking. The lowest prevalence is among Asian American and Hispanic women.

Smoking and other tobacco use are major contributors of the three leading causes of death in African Americans—heart disease, cancer, and stroke. African American men are at least 50% more likely to develop lung cancer than White men. Cerebrovascular disease is twice as high among African American men compared with White men. African American women do not fare any better: The incidence of strokes is twice as high among African American women as among White women. Nurses should educate their ethnic minority clients, particularly African Americans, about their increased risk of disease.

12.11 The Nurse's Role in Substance Abuse

The nurse serves a key role in the prevention, diagnosis, and treatment of substance abuse. A thorough medical history must include questions about substance abuse. In the case of IV drug users, the nurse must consider the possibility of HIV infection, hepatitis, tuberculosis, and associated diagnoses. Clients are often reluctant to report their drug use, for fear of embarrassment or being arrested. The nurse must be knowledgeable about the signs of substance abuse and withdrawal symptoms, and develop a keen sense of perception during the assessment stage. A trusting nurse–client relationship is essential to helping clients deal with their dependence. By using therapeutic communication skills and by demonstrating a nonjudgmental, empathetic attitude, the nurse can build a trusting relationship with clients.

It is often difficult for a healthcare provider not to condemn or stigmatize a client for his or her substance abuse. Nurses, especially those in large cities, are all too familiar with the devastating medical, economic, and social consequences of heroin and cocaine abuse. The nurse must be firm in disapproving of substance abuse, yet compassionate in trying to help the client receive treatment. A list of social agencies dealing with dependency should be readily available to provide clients. When possible, the nurse should attempt to involve family members and other close contacts in the treatment regimen. Educating the client and family members about the long-term consequences of substance abuse is essential.

CHAPTER REVIEW

KEY CONCEPTS

The numbered key concepts provide a succinct summary of the important points from the corresponding numbered section within the chapter. If any of these points are not clear, refer to the numbered section within the chapter for review.

12.1 A wide variety of substances may be abused by individuals, all of which share the common characteristic of altering brain physiology and/or perception.

12.2 Addiction is an overwhelming compulsion to continue repeated drug use that has both neurobiological and psychosocial components.

12.3 Certain substances can cause both physical and psychological dependence, which result in continued drug-seeking behavior despite negative health and social consequences.

12.4 The withdrawal syndrome is a set of uncomfortable symptoms that occur when an abused substance is no longer available. The severity of the withdrawal syndrome varies among the different drug classes.

12.5 Tolerance is a biological condition that occurs with repeated use of certain substances, and results in the necessity for higher doses to achieve the same initial response. Cross-tolerance occurs between closely related drugs.

12.6 CNS depressants, which include sedatives, opioids, and ethyl alcohol, decrease the activity of the brain, causing drowsiness, slowed speech, and diminished motor coordination.

12.7 Cannabinoids, which include marijuana, are the most frequently abused class of illegal substances. They cause less physical dependence and tolerance than the CNS depressants.

12.8 Hallucinogens, including LSD, cause an altered state of thought and perception similar to that found in dreams. Their effects are extremely variable and unpredictable.

12.9 CNS stimulants, including amphetamines, methylphenidate, caffeine, and cocaine, increase the activity of the CNS and produce increased wakefulness.

12.10 Nicotine is a powerful and highly addictive cardiovascular and CNS stimulant that has serious adverse effects with chronic use.

12.11 The nurse serves an important role in educating clients about the consequences of drug abuse and in recommending appropriate treatment.

NCLEX-RN® REVIEW QUESTIONS

1 Following a surgical procedure, the client states he does not want to take narcotic analgesics for pain because he is afraid he will become addicted to the drug. Response by the nurse is based on the knowledge that:

1. Dependence on narcotics is common among postoperative clients.
2. Addiction to prescription drugs is rare when used according to protocol.
3. Female clients are more likely to become addicted.
4. Addiction is rare if the client has a high pain threshold.

2 The client states she has been increasing the amount and frequency of the antianxiety drug she is using. The nurse understands that the client has most likely developed _____ to the drug.

1. Immunity
2. Tolerance
3. Resistance
4. Addiction

3 A 13-year-old boy has been showing signs of paranoia and anxiety and, according to his parents has been "acting very oddly," including recently being reclusive and locking himself in his room. On occasion, the young man has shown loss of coordination and an apparent distorted sense of time. The parents are very concerned, since they have been notified by the school nurse that their son has been implicated in drug activity. In the nurse's office, the young man asks if he can have a drink of water for "dry mouth." The nurse observes that his face is flushed and his eyes reddened. Which substance has the young man most likely used?

1. Heroin
2. Crack
3. Barbiturates
4. Marijuana

4 The client with a history of alcohol abuse is admitted to the hospital. The nursing care plan includes assessment of the client for which of the following symptoms indicative of alcohol withdrawal?

1. Mental depression, headaches, and hunger
2. Insomnia, nausea, and bradycardia
3. Tremors, hallucinations, and delirium
4. Weakness, hypotension, and violent yawning

5 The client states that she is going to quit smoking "cold turkey." The nurse teaches the client to expect which of the following symptoms during withdrawal from nicotine? (Select all that apply.)

1. Headaches and insomnia
2. Increased appetite
3. Tremors
4. Insomnia
5. Increased heart rate and blood pressure

CRITICAL THINKING QUESTIONS

1. A 16-year-old female client is hospitalized in the ICU following the ingestion of a high dose of MDMA (Ecstasy) at a street dance. Her mother cannot understand why her daughter could have such serious renal and cardiovascular complications after "just one dose." The nurse is concerned that the mother lacks sufficient knowledge to be helpful. What teaching does the nurse conduct?

2. The wife of a 24-year-old professional football player is admitted to the ER after being beaten and verbally abused by her husband. She says that he is under a great deal of stress and has been working hard to maintain peak athletic fitness. She says she has noticed that her husband becomes irritable easily. What assessments and interventions should the nurse perform?

3. A 44-year-old businessman travels weekly for his company and has had difficulty sleeping in "one hotel after another." He consulted his healthcare provider and has been taking secobarbital (Seconal) nightly to help him sleep. The client has called the nurse at the healthcare provider's office and has said, "I have just got to have something stronger." What does the nurse consider as part of the assessment?

See Appendix D for answers and rationales for all activities.

EXPLORE
MediaLink

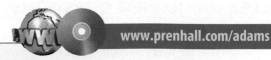

NCLEX-RN® review, case studies, and other interactive resources for this chapter can be found on the companion website at www.prenhall.com/adams. Click on "Chapter 12" to select the activities for this chapter. For animations, more NCLEX-RN® review questions, and an audio glossary, access the accompanying Prentice Hall Nursing MediaLink DVD-ROM in this textbook.

 PRENTICE HALL NURSING MEDIALINK DVD-ROM

- **Animation**
  Cocaine
- **Audio Glossary**
- **NCLEX-RN® Review**

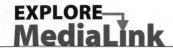 **COMPANION WEBSITE**

- **NCLEX-RN® Review**
- **Dosage Calculations**
- **Case Study:** CNS depressants
- **Challenge Your Knowledge**

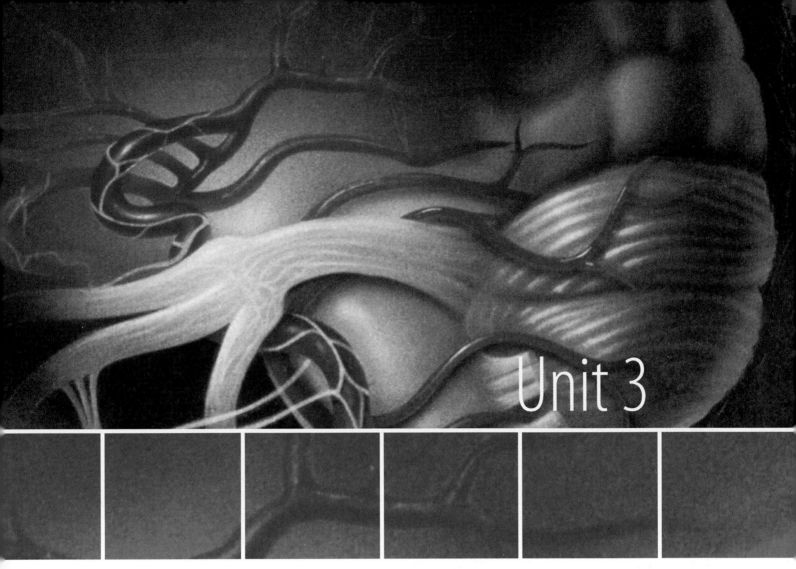

Unit 3

The Nervous System

CHAPTER 13   Drugs Affecting the Autonomic Nervous System

CHAPTER 14   Drugs for Anxiety and Insomnia

CHAPTER 15   Drugs for Seizures

CHAPTER 16   Drugs for Emotional and Mood Disorders

CHAPTER 17   Drugs for Psychoses

CHAPTER 18   Drugs for the Control of Pain

CHAPTER 19   Drugs for Local and General Anesthesia

CHAPTER 20   Drugs for Degenerative Diseases of the Nervous System

CHAPTER 21   Drugs for Neuromuscular Disorders

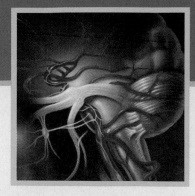

CHAPTER 13

Drugs Affecting the Autonomic Nervous System

DRUGS AT A GLANCE

ADRENERGIC AGENTS (SYMPATHOMIMETICS)
- *phenylephrine (Neo-Synephrine)*

ADRENERGIC BLOCKING AGENTS
- *prazosin (Minipress)*

CHOLINERGIC AGENTS (PARASYMPATHOMIMETICS)

Direct-acting Parasympathomimetics
- *bethanechol (Urecholine)*

Cholinesterase Inhibitors

CHOLINERGIC-BLOCKING AGENTS (ANTICHOLINERGICS)
- *atropine*

OBJECTIVES

After reading this chapter, the student should be able to:

1. Identify basic functions of the nervous system.
2. Identify important divisions of the peripheral nervous system.
3. Compare and contrast the actions of the sympathetic and parasympathetic divisions of the autonomic nervous system.
4. Explain the process of synaptic transmission and the neurotransmitters important to the autonomic nervous system.
5. Compare and contrast the types of responses that occur when drugs activate alpha$_1$-, alpha$_2$-, beta$_1$-, or beta$_2$-adrenergic receptors, and nicotinic or muscarinic receptors.
6. Discuss the classification and naming of autonomic drugs based on four possible actions.
7. Describe the nurse's role in the pharmacological management of clients receiving drugs affecting the autonomic nervous system.
8. For each of the drug classes listed in "Drugs at a Glance," explain the mechanism of drug action, primary actions, and important adverse effects.
9. Use the Nursing Process to care for clients receiving adrenergic agents, adrenergic-blocking agents, cholinergic agents, and cholinergic-blocking agents.

MediaLink 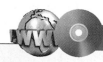 www.prenhall.com/adams

KEY TERMS

acetylcholine (Ach) *page 134*

acetylcholinesterase (AchE) *page 136*

adrenergic *page 134*

adrenergic antagonist *page 136*

alpha-receptor *page 134*

anticholinergic *page 136*

autonomic nervous system *page 131*

beta-receptor *page 134*

catecholamines *page 134*

central nervous system (CNS) *page 131*

cholinergic *page 135*

fight-or-flight response *page 131*

ganglionic synapse *page 132*

monoamine oxidase (MAO) *page 134*

muscarinic *page 136*

myasthenia gravis *page 143*

nicotinic *page 135*

norepinephrine (NE) *page 134*

parasympathetic nervous system *page 132*

parasympathomimetics *page 136*

peripheral nervous system *page 131*

postganglionic neuron *page 133*

preganglionic neuron *page 133*

rest-and-digest response *page 132*

somatic nervous system *page 131*

sympathetic nervous system *page 131*

sympathomimetic *page 136*

sympatholytic *page 136*

synapse *page 132*

synaptic transmission *page 133*

The study of nervous system pharmacology, or *neuropharmacology,* extends over the next eight chapters. Traditionally, neuropharmacology begins with a study of the autonomic nervous system. A firm grasp of autonomic physiology is necessary to understand cardiovascular, renal, respiratory, gastrointestinal, reproductive and ophthalmic function. Autonomic drugs are important because they mimic involuntary bodily functions. A thorough knowledge of autonomic drugs is essential to the treatment of disorders affecting many body systems, including abnormalities in heart rate and rhythm, hypertension, asthma, glaucoma, and even a runny nose. This chapter serves dual purposes. First, it is a concise review of autonomic nervous system physiology, a subject that is often covered superficially in anatomy and physiology classes. Second, it is an introduction to the four fundamental classes of autonomic drugs: adrenergic agents, cholinergic agents, adrenergic-blocking agents, and cholinergic-blocking agents.

13.1 The Peripheral Nervous System

The nervous system has two major divisions: the **central nervous system (CNS)** and the **peripheral nervous system.** The CNS consists of the brain and spinal cord. The peripheral nervous system consists of all nervous tissue outside the CNS, including sensory and motor neurons. The basic functions of the nervous system are as follows:

- Recognizing changes in the internal and external environments
- Processing and integrating the environmental changes that are perceived
- Reacting to the environmental changes by producing an action or response

● Figure 13.1 shows the functional divisions of the nervous system. In the peripheral nervous system, neurons either recognize changes to the environment (sensory division) or respond to these changes by moving muscles or secreting chemicals (motor division). The **somatic nervous system** consists of nerves that provide *voluntary* control over skeletal muscle. Nerves of the **autonomic nervous system,** on the other hand, exert *involuntary* control over the contraction of smooth muscle and cardiac muscle, and glandular activity. Organs and tissues regulated by neurons from the autonomic nervous system include the heart, digestive tract, respiratory tract, reproductive tracts, arteries, salivary glands, and portions of the eye.

13.2 The Autonomic Nervous System: Sympathetic and Parasympathetic Divisions

The autonomic nervous system has two divisions: the sympathetic and the parasympathetic nervous systems. With a few exceptions, organs and glands receive nerves from both branches of the autonomic nervous system. The major actions of the two divisions are shown in ● Figure 13.2. It is essential that the student learn these general actions early in the study of pharmacology, because knowledge of autonomic effects is used to predict the actions and side effects of many drugs.

The **sympathetic nervous system** is activated under conditions of stress, and produces a set of actions called the **fight-or-flight response.** Activation of this system will ready the body for an immediate response to a potential threat. The heart rate and blood pressure increase, and more blood is shunted to skeletal muscles. The liver immediately produces more glucose for energy. The bronchi dilate to allow more air into the lungs, and the pupils dilate for better vision.

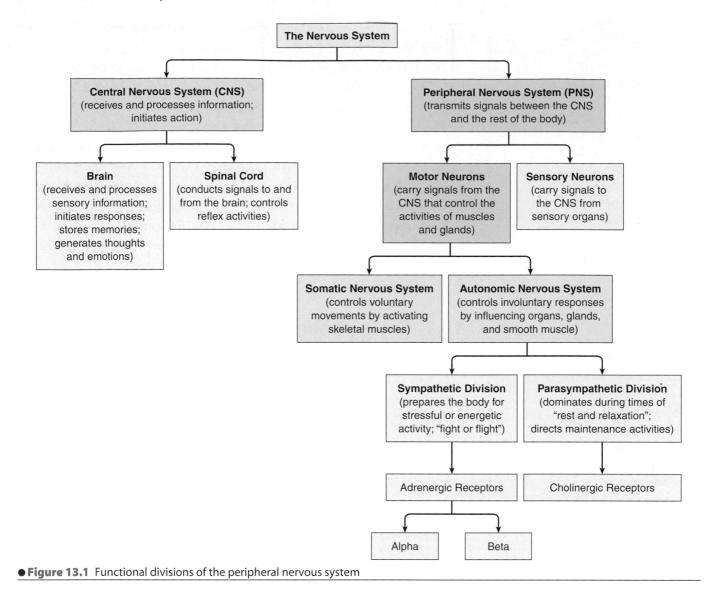

● **Figure 13.1** Functional divisions of the peripheral nervous system

Conversely, the **parasympathetic nervous system** is activated under nonstressful conditions and produces symptoms called the **rest-and-digest response.** Digestive processes are promoted, and heart rate and blood pressure decline. Not as much air is needed, so the bronchi constrict. Most of the actions of the parasympathetic division are the opposite of those of the sympathetic division.

A proper balance of the two autonomic branches is required for body homeostasis. Under most circumstances, the two branches cooperate to achieve a balance of readiness and relaxation. Because the branches produce mostly opposite effects, homeostasis may be achieved by changing one or both branches. For example, heart rate can be increased either by *increasing* the firing of sympathetic nerves or by *decreasing* the firing of parasympathetic nerves. This allows the body a means of fine-tuning its essential organ systems.

The sympathetic and parasympathetic divisions do not always produce opposite effects. For example, the constriction of arterioles is controlled entirely by the sympathetic branch.

Sympathetic stimulation causes constriction of arterioles, whereas lack of stimulation causes vasodilation. Sweat glands are controlled only by sympathetic nerves. In the male reproductive system, the roles are complementary. For example, erection of the penis is a function of the parasympathetic division, and ejaculation is controlled by the sympathetic branch.

13.3 Structure and Function of Autonomic Synapses

For information to be transmitted throughout the nervous system, neurons must communicate with one another, and with muscles and glands. In the autonomic nervous system this communication involves the connection of two neurons, in series. As the action potential travels along the first nerve, it encounters the first **synapse,** or juncture. Because this connection occurs outside the CNS, it is called the **ganglionic synapse.** The basic structure of a

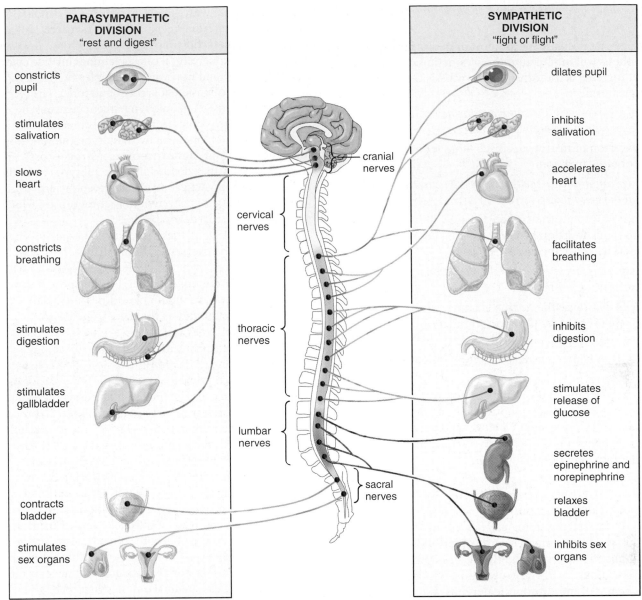

PARASYMPATHETIC DIVISION
"rest and digest"

constricts pupil

stimulates salivation

slows heart

constricts breathing

stimulates digestion

stimulates gallbladder

contracts bladder

stimulates sex organs

SYMPATHETIC DIVISION
"fight or flight"

dilates pupil

inhibits salivation

accelerates heart

facilitates breathing

inhibits digestion

stimulates release of glucose

secretes epinephrine and norepinephrine

relaxes bladder

inhibits sex organs

cranial nerves

cervical nerves

thoracic nerves

lumbar nerves

sacral nerves

● **Figure 13.2** Effects of the sympathetic and parasympathetic nervous systems *Source: Biology: A Guide to the Natural World, 2nd ed. (p. 558) by David Krogh, 2002, Upper Saddle River, NJ, Prentice Hall. Reprinted by permission.*

ganglionic synapse is shown in ● Figure 13.3. The nerve carrying the impulse exiting the spinal cord is called the **preganglionic neuron.** The nerve on the other side of the ganglionic synapse, waiting to receive the impulse, is the **postganglionic neuron.** Beyond the postganglionic neuron is the second synapse. The second synapse occurs at the target tissue.

A large number of drugs affect autonomic function by altering neurotransmitter activity at the second synapse. Some drugs are identical with endogenous neurotransmitters, or have a similar chemical structure, and are able to directly activate the gland or muscle. Others are used to block the activity of natural neurotransmitters. Following are the five general mechanisms by which drugs affect **synaptic transmission.**

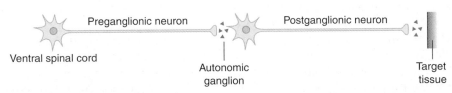

Preganglionic neuron   Postganglionic neuron

Ventral spinal cord

Autonomic ganglion

Target tissue

● **Figure 13.3** Basic structure of the autonomic pathway

• *Drugs may affect the synthesis of the neurotransmitter in the presynaptic nerve.*

Drugs that decrease the amount of neurotransmitter synthesis will inhibit autonomic function. Those drugs that increase neurotransmitter synthesis will have the opposite effect.

• *Drugs can prevent the storage of the neurotransmitter in vesicles within the presynaptic nerve.*

Prevention of neurotransmitter storage will inhibit autonomic function.

• *Drugs can influence the release of the neurotransmitter from the presynaptic nerve.*

Promoting neurotransmitter release will stimulate autonomic function, whereas slowing neurotransmitter release will have the opposite effect.

• *Drugs can prevent the normal destruction or reuptake of the neurotransmitter.*

Drugs that cause the neurotransmitter to remain in the synapse for a longer time will stimulate autonomic function.

• *Drugs can bind to the receptor site on the postsynaptic neuron.*

Drugs that bind to postsynaptic receptors and stimulate the nerve will increase autonomic function. Drugs that attach to the postsynaptic neuron and prevent the natural neurotransmitter from reaching its receptors will inhibit autonomic function.

The classic study of drugs affecting autonomic function centers around the last two mechanisms. It is important for the student to understand that autonomic drugs are not given to correct physiological defects in the autonomic nervous system. Compared with other body systems, the autonomic nervous system itself has remarkably little disease. Rather, drugs are used to stimulate or inhibit *target organs* of the autonomic nervous system, such as the heart, lungs, or digestive tract. With few exceptions, the disorder lies in the target organ, not the autonomic nervous system. Thus, when an "autonomic drug" such as norepinephrine (Levarterenol) is administered, it does not correct an autonomic disorder; it corrects dysfunction of that target organ naturally stimulated by the autonomic neurotransmnitter.

13.4 Norepinephrine and Acetylcholine

The two primary neurotransmitters of the autonomic nervous system are **norepinephrine (NE)** and **acetylcholine (Ach)**. A detailed knowledge of the underlying physiology of these neurotransmitters is required for proper understanding of drug action. When reading the following sections, the student should refer to the sites of acetylcholine and norepinephrine action shown in ● Figure 13.4.

In the sympathetic nervous system, norepinephrine is the neurotransmitter released at almost all postganglionic nerves.

The exception is sweat glands, in which acetylcholine is the neurotransmitter. Norepinephrine belongs to a class of agents called natural **catecholamines,** all of which are involved in neurotransmission. Natural catecholamines include epinephrine (adrenalin) and dopamine. Examples of synthetic catecholamines are isoproterenol and dobutamine. The receptors at the ends of postganglionic sympathetic neurons are called **adrenergic,** which comes from the word *adrenalin.*

Adrenergic receptors are of two basic types, **alpha-receptors (α-receptors)** and **beta-receptors (β-receptors)**. These receptors are further divided into the subtypes beta$_1$, beta$_2$, alpha$_1$, and alpha$_2$. Activation of each receptor subtype results in a characteristic set of physiological responses, which are generally summarized in Table 13.1.

The significance of these receptor subtypes to pharmacology cannot be overstated. Some drugs are selective and activate only one type of adrenergic receptor, whereas others affect all receptor subtypes. Furthermore, a drug may activate one type of receptor at low doses and begin to affect other receptor subtypes as the dose is increased. Committing the receptor types and their responses to memory is an essential step in learning autonomic pharmacology.

Norepinephrine (NE) is synthesized in the nerve terminal through a series of steps that require the amino acids phenylalanine and tyrosine. The final step of the synthesis involves the conversion of dopamine to norepinephrine. NE is stored in vesicles until an action potential triggers its release into the synaptic cleft. NE then diffuses across the cleft to alpha- or beta-receptors on the effector organ. The reuptake of NE back into the presynaptic neuron terminates its action. Once reuptake occurs, NE in the nerve terminal may be returned to vesicles for future use, or destroyed enzymatically by **monoamine oxidase (MAO)**. The enzyme catecholamine-*O*-methyl transferase (COMT) destroys NE at the synaptic cleft. The primary method for termination of NE action is through reuptake. Many drugs affect autonomic function by influencing the synthesis, storage, release, reuptake, or destruction of NE.

The adrenal medulla is a tissue closely associated with the sympathetic nervous system whose anatomical and physiological arrangement is much different from that of the rest of the sympathetic branch. Early in embryonic life, the adrenal medulla is part of the neural tissue destined to become the sympathetic nervous system. The primitive tissue splits, however, and the adrenal medulla becomes its own functional division. The preganglionic neuron from the spinal cord terminates in the adrenal medulla, and releases the neurotransmitter epinephrine directly into the blood. Once released, epinephrine travels to target organs, where it elicits the classic fight-or-flight symptoms. The action of epinephrine is terminated through hepatic metabolism, rather than reuptake.

Other types of adrenergic receptors exist. Although dopamine was once thought to function only as a chemical precursor to norepinephrine, research has determined that dopamine serves a larger role as a neurotransmitter. Five dopaminergic receptors (D$_1$ through D$_5$) have been discovered in the CNS. Dopaminergic receptors in the CNS are important to the action of certain antipsychotic medicines

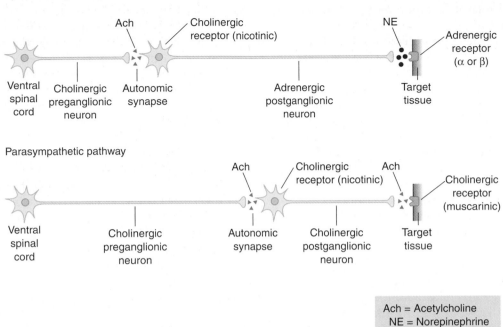

● **Figure 13.4** Receptors in the autonomic nervous system: (a) sympathetic division; (b) parasympathetic division

(Chapter 17 ∞) and in the treatment of Parkinson's disease (Chapter 20 ∞). Dopamine receptors in the peripheral nervous system are located in the arterioles of the kidney and other viscera. Although these receptors likely have a role in autonomic function, their therapeutic importance has yet to be discovered.

13.5 Acetylcholine and Cholinergic Transmission

Nerves releasing acetylcholine (Ach) are called **cholinergic** nerves. There are two types of cholinergic receptors that bind Ach, which are named after certain chemicals that bind to them (Table 13.1).

• *Nicotinic receptors*

At the ganglionic synapse in both the sympathetic and parasympathetic divisions of the autonomic nervous system

• *Muscarinic receptors*

Located on target tissues affected by postganglionic neurons in the parasympathetic nervous system

Early research on laboratory animals found that the actions of Ach at the *ganglia* resemble those of nicotine, the active agent found in tobacco products. Because of this similarity, receptors for Ach in the ganglia are called **nicotinic** receptors. Nicotinic receptors are also present in skeletal muscle, which is controlled by the somatic nervous system. Because these receptors are present in so many locations, drugs affecting nicotinic receptors produce profound effects on both the autonomic and somatic nervous systems. Activation of these cholinergic receptors causes tachycardia, hypertension, and increased tone and motility in the digestive tract. Although nicotinic receptor blockers were some of the first drugs used to treat hypertension, the only current therapeutic application of these agents, known as *ganglionic blockers*, is to produce muscle relaxation during surgical procedures (Chapter 19 ∞).

TABLE 13.1	Types of Autonomic Receptors		
Neurotransmitter	**Receptor**	**Primary Locations**	**Responses**
acetylcholine (cholinergic)	nicotinic	postganglionic neurons	stimulation of smooth muscle and gland secretions
	muscarinic	parasympathetic target: organs other than the heart	stimulation of smooth muscle and gland secretions
		heart	decreased heart rate and force of contraction
norepinephrine (adrenergic)	alpha$_1$	all sympathetic target organs except the heart	constriction of blood vessels, dilation of pupils
	alpha$_2$	presynaptic adrenergic nerve terminals	inhibition of release of norepinephrine
	beta$_1$	heart and kidneys	increased heart rate and force of contraction; release of renin
	beta$_2$	all sympathetic target organs except the heart	inhibition of smooth muscle

Nicotinic blocking agents have also been used in research to investigate the role of nicotinic receptors in learning and memory.

Activation of acetylcholine receptors affected by *postganglionic* nerve endings in the parasympathetic nervous system results in the classic symptoms of parasympathetic stimulation shown in Figure 13.2. Early research discovered that these actions closely resemble those produced when a client ingests the poisonous mushroom *Amanita muscaria*. Because of this similarity, these Ach receptors were named **muscarinic** receptors. Unlike the nicotinic receptors, which have few pharmacological applications, muscarinic receptors are affected by a number of medications, and these are discussed in subsequent sections of this chapter.

The physiology of acetylcholine affords several mechanisms by which drugs may act. Acetylcholine is synthesized in the presynaptic nerve terminal from choline and acetyl coenzyme A. Once synthesized, Ach is stored in vesicles in the presynaptic neuron. When an action potential reaches the nerve ending, Ach is released into the synaptic cleft, where it diffuses across to find nicotinic or muscarinic receptors. Ach in the synaptic cleft is rapidly destroyed by the enzyme **acetylcholinesterase (AchE),** and choline is reused. The choline is taken up by the presynaptic neuron to make more Ach, and the cycle is repeated. Drugs can affect the formation, release, receptor activation, or destruction of Ach.

AUTONOMIC DRUGS

13.6 Classification and Naming of Autonomic Drugs

Given the opposite actions of the sympathetic and parasympathetic nervous systems, autonomic drugs are classified based on one of four possible actions.

1. *Stimulation of the sympathetic nervous system*

   These drugs are called adrenergic agents or **sympathomimetics,** and they produce the classic symptoms of the fight-or-flight response. Natural or synthetic agents that produce a sympathomimetic response include the *catecholamines.*

2. *Inhibition of the sympathetic nervous system*

   These drugs are called adrenergic-blocking agents or **adrenergic antagonists,** and they produce actions *opposite* those of the sympathomimetics. The term **sympatholytics** is another name for adrenergic antagonists.

3. *Stimulation of the parasympathetic nervous system*

   These drugs are called cholinergic agents or **parasympathomimetics,** and they produce the characteristic symptoms of the rest-and-digest response.

4. *Inhibition of the parasympathetic nervous system*

   These drugs are called cholinergic-blocking agents, **anticholinergics,** parasympatholytics, or muscarinic blockers, and they produce actions *opposite* those of the cholinergic agents.

Students beginning their study of pharmacology often have difficulty understanding the terminology and actions of autonomic drugs. Examination of the four drug classes, however, makes it evident that only one group need be learned, because the others are logical extensions of the first. If the fight-or-flight actions of the sympathomimetics are learned, the other three groups can be deduced, because they are either the same or opposite. For example, both the sympathomimetics and the cholinergic-blocking agents increase heart rate and dilate the pupil. The other two groups, the cholinergic agents and the adrenergic-blocking agents, have the opposite effects—slowing heart rate and constricting the pupils. Although this is an oversimplification and exceptions do exist, it is a time-saving means of learning the basic actions and adverse effects of dozens of drugs affecting the autonomic nervous system. It should be emphasized again that mastering the actions and terminology of autonomic drugs early in the study of pharmacology will reap rewards later in the course when these drugs are applied to various systems.

ADRENERGIC AGENTS (SYMPATHOMIMETICS)

The adrenergic agents, also known as sympathomimetics, stimulate the sympathetic nervous system and induce symptoms characteristic of the fight-or-flight response. These drugs have clinical applications in the treatment of shock and hypotension.

13.7 Clinical Applications of Sympathomimetics

Sympathomimetics produce many of the same responses as the anticholinergics. However, because the sympathetic nervous system has alpha- and beta-subreceptors, the actions of many sympathomimetics are more specific and have wider therapeutic application (Table 13.2).

Sympathomimetics may be described chemically as catecholamines or noncatecholamines. The catecholamines have a chemical structure similar to norepinephrine and a short duration of action, and must be administered parenterally. The noncatecholamines can be taken orally and have longer durations of action, because they are not rapidly destroyed by monoamine oxidase.

Sympathomimetics act either directly or indirectly. Most sympathomimetics act directly by binding to and activating adrenergic receptors. Examples include the three endogenous catecholamines: epinephrine, norepinephrine, and dopamine. Other medications in this class act indirectly, by causing the release of norepinephrine from its vesicles on the presynaptic neuron or by inhibiting the reuptake or destruction of NE. Those that act by indirect mechanisms, such as amphetamine or cocaine, are used for their central effects on the brain rather than their autonomic effects. A few agents, such as ephedrine, act by both direct and indirect mechanisms.

Most effects of sympathomimetics are predictable based on their autonomic actions, dependent on which adrenergic receptor subtypes are stimulated. Because the receptor responses are so different, the student will need to memorize the specific subclass(es) of receptors activated by each

TABLE 13.2   Adrenergic Agents (Sympathomimetics)

Drug	Primary Receptor Subtype	Primary Use
albuterol (Proventil, Ventolin)	beta$_2$	asthma
clonidine (Catapres)	alpha$_2$ in CNS	hypertension
dexmedetomidine HCl (Precedex)	alpha$_2$ in CNS	sedation
dobutamine (Dobutrex)	beta$_1$	cardiac stimulant
dopamine (Intropin)	alpha$_1$ and beta$_1$	shock
epinephrine (Adrenalin, Primatene, others)	alpha and beta	cardiac arrest, asthma
formoterol (Foradil)	beta$_2$	asthma, COPD
isoproterenol (Isuprel)	beta$_1$ and beta$_2$	asthma, dysrhythmias, heart failure
metaproterenol (Alupent)	beta$_2$	asthma
metaraminol (Aramine)	alpha$_1$ and beta$_1$	shock
methyldopa (Aldomet)	alpha$_2$ in CNS	hypertension
norepinephrine (Levarterenol, Levophed)	alpha$_1$ and beta$_1$	shock
oxymetazoline (Afrin and others)	alpha	nasal congestion
phenylephrine (Neo-Synephrine)	alpha	nasal congestion
pseudoephedrine (Sudafed and others)	alpha and beta	nasal congestion
ritodrine (Yutopar)	beta$_2$	slowing of uterine contraction
salmeterol (Serevent)	beta$_2$	decongestant
terbutaline (Brethine and others)	beta$_2$	asthma

sympathomimetic. Specific subclasses of receptors and therapeutic applications are as follows:

- Alpha$_1$-receptor: treatment of nasal congestion or hypotension; cause mydriasis during ophthalmic examinations
- Alpha$_2$-receptor: treatment of hypertension through centrally-acting mechanism. (Autonomic alpha$_2$-receptors are also located on presynaptic membranes of postganglionic neurons and serve as autoreceptors for naturally occurring NE in the sympathetic nervous system. Activation of alpha$_2$-receptors reduces the release of NE.)
- Beta$_1$-receptor: treatment of cardiac arrest, heart failure, and shock
- Beta$_2$-receptor: treatment of asthma and premature labor contractions

Some sympathomimetics are nonselective, stimulating more than one type of adrenergic receptor. For example, epinephrine stimulates all four types of adrenergic receptors and is used for cardiac arrest and asthma. Pseudoephedrine (Sudafed and others) stimulates both alpha$_1$- and beta$_2$-receptors and is used as a nasal decongestant. Isoproterenol (Isuprel) stimulates both beta$_1$- and beta$_2$-receptors and is used to increase the rate, force, and conduction speed of the heart, and occasionally for asthma. The nonselective drugs generally cause more autonomic-related side effects than the selective agents.

The side effects of the sympathomimetics are mostly extensions of their autonomic actions. Cardiovascular effects such as tachycardia, hypertension, and dysrhythmias are particularly troublesome and may limit therapy. Large doses can induce CNS excitement and seizures. Other sympathomimetic responses that may occur are dry mouth, nausea, and vomiting. Some of these agents cause anorexia, which has led to their historical use as appetite suppressants. However, because of prominent cardiovascular side effects, sympathomimetics are now rarely used for this purpose.

Drugs in this class are found as prototypes in many other sections in this textbook. For additional prototypes of drugs in this class, see dopamine (Intropin), epinephrine (Adrenalin) and norepinephrine (Levophed) in Chapter 29 ∞, oxymetazoline (Afrin) in Chapter 38 ∞, and salmeterol (Serevent) in Chapter 39 ∞.

NURSING CONSIDERATIONS

The role of the nurse in sympathomimetic therapy involves careful monitoring of a client's condition and providing education as it relates to the prescribed drug treatment. Because adrenergic agents affect the heart, blood vessels, and the bronchi, they have a wide variety of uses, including the treatment of shock, hypotension, bronchial asthma, decreased cardiac output, cardiac arrest, and allergic reactions. Adverse effects are usually related to dosage and include hypertension, tachycardia, tremors, dizziness, dysrhythmias, urinary retention, and anorexia.

Because many of these medications are administered intravenously, carefully assess clients prior to and during

Pr PROTOTYPE DRUG | Phenylephrine *(Neo-Synephrine)* | Adrenergic Agent (Sympathomimetic)

ACTIONS AND USES

Phenylephrine is a selective alpha-adrenergic agonist that is available in several different formulations, including intranasal, ophthalmic, IM, subcutaneous, and IV. All its actions and indications are extensions of its sympathetic stimulation.

Intranasal administration—When applied intranasally by spray or drops, phenylephrine reduces nasal congestion by constricting small blood vessels in the nasal mucosa.

Topical administration—Applied topically to the eye during ophthalmic examinations, phenylephrine can dilate the pupil without causing significant cycloplegia.

Parental administration—The parenteral administration of phenylephrine can reverse acute hypotension caused by spinal anesthesia or vascular shock. Because phenylephrine lacks beta-adrenergic agonist activity, it produces relatively few cardiac side effects at therapeutic doses. Its longer duration of activity and lack of significant cardiac effects gives phenylephrine some advantages over epinephrine or norepinephrine in treating acute hypotension.

ADMINISTRATION ALERTS

- Parenteral administration can cause tissue injury with extravasation.
- Phenylephrine ophthalmic drops may damage soft contact lenses.
- Pregnancy category C.

PHARMACOKINETICS

Onset: Immediate IV; 10–15 min IM/subcutaneous

Peak: 5–10 min IV; 15–30 min IV/subcutaneous

Half-life: <15 min IV; 30–60 min IM/subcutaneous

Duration: 15–20 min IV; 30–120 min IM/subcutaneous; 3–6 h topical

ADVERSE EFFECTS

Topically and intranasally—When the drug is used topically or intranasally, side effects are uncommon. Intranasal use can cause burning of the mucosa and rebound congestion if used for prolonged periods (see Chapter 31 ∞). Ophthalmic preparations can cause narrow-angle glaucoma secondary to their mydriatic effect. High doses can cause reflex bradycardia owing to the elevation of blood pressure caused by stimulation of alpha$_1$-receptors.

Parenterally—When used parenterally, the drug should be used with caution in clients with advanced coronary artery disease or hypertension. Anxiety, restlessness, and tremor may occur owing to the drug's stimulation effect on the CNS. Clients with hyperthyroidism may experience a severe increase in basal metabolic rate, resulting in increased blood pressure and ventricular tachycardia.

Contraindications: This drug should not be used in clients with acute pancreatitis, heart disease, and hepatitis.

INTERACTIONS

Drug–Drug: Drug interactions may occur with MAO inhibitors, causing a hypertensive crisis. Increased effects may also occur with tricyclic antidepressants, ergot alkaloids, and oxytocin. Inhibitory effects occur with alpha-blockers and beta-blockers. This drug is incompatible with iron preparations (ferric salts).

Lab Tests: Unknown.

Herbal/Food: Unknown.

Treatment of Overdose: Overdose may cause tachycardia and hypertension. Treatment with an alpha-blocker such as phentolamine (Regitine) may be indicated to decrease blood pressure.

 See the Companion Website for a Nursing Process Focus specific to this drug.

---

administration. Frequently assess vital signs, skin color and integrity, capillary refill, and urine output while adrenergic agents are being administered. Inspect the IV site and surrounding tissues frequently for extravasation.

Be aware that severe hypertension is the primary manifestation of sympathomimetic toxicity. Assess for headache, confusion, seizures, and other related CNS changes.

Lifespan Considerations.   Use adrenergic agents carefully during pregnancy and lactation. Older adults are at increased risk for adverse reactions owing to chronic cardiovascular disease. Overdose in the elderly may include confusion, anxiety, restlessness, CNS depression, and death. Adrenergic agents should be used cautiously in children, as they are very sensitive to drug effects. Carefully calculate dosages in pediatric clients.

Client Teaching.   Client education as it relates to adrenergic agents should include the goals of therapy, the reasons for obtaining baseline data such as vital signs and the existence of underlying disorders, and possible drug side effects. Include the following points when teaching clients about adrenergic agonists:

- Do not take any other medications including herbal remedies and OTC drugs without notifying your health-care provider, because these may cause serious cardiovascular and CNS disturbances.
- If taking medication for asthma or other chronic lung diseases, follow the instructions on your inhaler. Adverse effects such as dizziness, palpitations, and tremors may occur with overuse.
- Adrenergic agents may elevate blood glucose levels. Monitor blood glucose levels carefully if you have diabetes.
- For severe allergies, always carry an epinephrine injection kit and notify your healthcare provider after usage.
- Use nasal decongestants for a short duration only, because rebound congestion may occur.
- Use proper medication self-administration techniques.
- Immediately report tremors, palpitations, changes in blood pressure, dizziness, urinary retention, or changes in skin integrity.

ADRENERGIC-BLOCKING AGENTS

Adrenergic blocking agents or antagonists inhibit the sympathetic nervous system and produce many of the same rest-and-digest symptoms as the parasympathomimetics. They have wide therapeutic application in the treatment of hypertension.

NURSING PROCESS FOCUS Clients Receiving Sympathomimetic Therapy

Assessment	Potential Nursing Diagnoses
Prior to administration: ■ Determine the reason for drug administration. ■ Monitor vital signs, urinary output, and cardiac output (initially and throughout therapy). ■ For treatment of nasal congestion, assess the nasal mucosa for changes such as excoriation or bleeding. ■ Obtain a complete health history including cautions and contraindications for drug use, allergies, drug history, and possible drug interactions. ■ Evaluate laboratory findings.	■ Knowledge, Deficient, related to drug therapy ■ Cardiac Output, Decreased ■ Tissue Perfusion, Ineffective ■ Injury, Risk for, related to side effect of drug therapy ■ Breathing Pattern, Ineffective, related to nasal congestion ■ Sleep Pattern, Disturbed ■ Pain

Planning: Client Goals and Expected Outcomes

The client will:
■ Exhibit a decrease in the symptoms for which the drug is being given.
■ Demonstrate an understanding of the drug's action by accurately describing drug side effects and precautions.
■ Demonstrate proper nasal or ophthalmic drug instillation technique.

Implementation

Interventions and (Rationales)	Client Education/Discharge Planning
■ IV: Frequently monitor IV insertion sites for extravasation. Use an infusion pump to deliver the medication. (An infusion pump will assure that medication is infused at the appropriate rate and will identify potential infiltration.) ■ Subcutaneous: Use a tuberculin syringe. (A tuberculin syringe permits extremely small dosages to be drawn up more exactly.) ■ Metered dose inhalation: Shake the container well and wait at least 2 minutes between doses of medication. (Waiting between doses allows for the maximum therapeutic effect.) ■ Ophthalmic: Instill only the prescribed number of drops when using ophthalmic solutions. (Deviating from the prescribed number of drops may either over- or underdose the medication.)	Instruct client to: ■ Use the drug strictly as prescribed, and do not "double up" on doses. ■ Take medication early in the day to prevent insomnia.
■ Monitor the client for side effects. (Side effects of sympathomimetics may be serious and may limit therapy.)	Instruct client to: ■ Immediately report shortness of breath, palpitations, dizziness, chest/arm pain or pressure, or other angina-like symptoms to the healthcare provider. ■ Consult the healthcare provider before attempting to use sympathomimetics to treat nasal congestion or eye irritation. ■ Monitor blood pressure, pulse, and temperature to ensure proper use of home equipment. ■ Consult the healthcare provider before taking any OTC drugs.
■ Monitor breathing patterns and observe for shortness of breath and/or audible wheezing. (Shortness of breath and audible wheezing may indicate that the client's asthma is worsening and additional interventions are needed.)	■ Instruct client to immediately report any difficulty breathing. Instruct clients with a history of asthma to consult their healthcare provider before using OTC drugs to treat nasal congestion.
■ Observe the client's responsiveness to light. (Some sympathomimetics cause photosensitivity by affecting the pupillary light accommodation/response.)	■ Instruct clients using ophthalmic sympathomimetics that transient stinging and blurred vision on instillation is normal. Headache and/or brow pain may also occur.
■ Provide eye comfort by reducing exposure to bright light in the environment; shield the eyes with a rolled washcloth or eye bandages. (This provides relief for severe photosensitivity.)	■ Instruct client to avoid driving and other activities requiring visual acuity until blurring subsides.
■ For clients receiving nasal sympathomimetics, observe the nasal cavity. Monitor for rhinorrhea and epistaxis. (Rhinorrhea and epistaxis may be a side effect of the medication.)	Instruct client to: ■ Observe nasal cavity for signs of excoriation or bleeding before instilling nasal spray or drops; review procedure for safe instillation of nasal sprays or eye drops. ■ Limit OTC usage of sympathomimetics; inform client about rebound nasal congestion.

(Continued)

13.8 Clinical Applications of Adrenergic Antagonists

Adrenergic antagonists act by directly blocking adrenergic receptors. The actions of these agents are specific to either alpha- or beta-blockade. Medications in this class have great therapeutic application and are the most widely prescribed class of autonomic drugs (see Table 13.3).

Alpha-adrenergic antagonists, or simply alpha-blockers, are used for their effects on vascular smooth muscle. By relaxing vascular smooth muscle in small arteries, alpha$_1$-blockers such as doxazosin (Cardura) cause vasodilation that results in decreased blood pressure. They may be used either alone or in combination with other agents in the treatment of hypertension (Chapter 23 ∞). A second use is in the treatment of benign prostatic hyperplasia (BPH), owing to their ability to increase urine flow (Chapter 46 ∞). The most common adverse effect of alpha-blockers is orthostatic hypotension, which occurs when a client abruptly changes from a recumbent to an upright position. Reflex tachycardia, nasal congestion, and impotence are other important side effects that may occur as a consequence of increased parasympathetic activity.

Beta-adrenergic antagonists may block beta$_1$-receptors, beta$_2$-receptors, or both types. Regardless of their receptor specificity, all beta-blockers are used therapeutically for their effects on the cardiovascular system. Beta-blockers decrease the rate and force of contraction of the heart, and slow electrical conduction through the atrioventricular node. Drugs that selectively block beta$_1$-receptors, such as atenolol (Tenormin), are called *cardioselective* agents. Because they have little effect on noncardiac tissue, they exert fewer side effects than nonselective agents such as propranolol (Inderal).

The primary use of beta-blockers is in the treatment of hypertension. Although the exact mechanism by which beta-blockers reduce blood pressure is not completely understood, it is thought that the reduction may be due to decreased cardiac output or to suppression of renin release by the kidneys. The student should refer to Chapter 23 ∞ for a more comprehensive description of the use of beta-blockers in hypertension management.

Beta-adrenergic antagonists have several other important therapeutic applications, discussions of which appear in many chapters in this textbook. By decreasing the cardiac workload, beta-blockers can ease the pain associated with angina pectoris (Chapter 25 ∞). By slowing electrical

TABLE 13.3   Adrenergic-blocking Agents (Antagonists)

Drug	Primary Receptor Subtype	Primary Use
acebutolol (Sectral)	beta$_1$	hypertension, dysrhythmias, angina
atenolol (Tenormin)	beta$_1$	hypertension, angina
carteolol (Cartrol)	beta$_1$ and beta$_2$	hypertension, glaucoma
carvedilol (Coreg)	alpha$_1$, beta$_1$, and beta$_2$	hypertension
doxazosin (Cardura)	alpha$_1$	hypertension
esmolol (Brevibloc)	beta$_1$	hypertension, dysrhythmias
metoprolol (Lopressor, Toprol)	beta$_1$	hypertension
nadolol (Corgard)	beta$_1$ and beta$_2$	hypertension
phentolamine (Regitine)	alpha	severe hypertension
℞ prazosin (Minipress)	alpha$_1$	hypertension
propranolol (Inderal)	beta$_1$ and beta$_2$	hypertension, dysrhythmias, heart failure
sotalol (Betapace)	beta$_1$ and beta$_2$	dysrhythmias
tamsulosin (Flomax)	alpha$_1$	benign prostatic hypertrophy
terazosin (Hytrin)	alpha$_1$	hypertension
timolol (Blocadren, Timoptic)	beta$_1$ and beta$_2$	hypertension, angina, glaucoma

conduction across the myocardium, beta-blockers are able to treat certain types of dysrhythmias (Chapter 26 ∞). Other therapeutic uses include the treatment of heart failure (Chapter 24 ∞), myocardial infarction (Chapter 25 ∞), and narrow-angle glaucoma (Chapter 49 ∞).

NURSING CONSIDERATIONS

The role of the nurse in adrenergic antagonist therapy involves careful monitoring of a client's condition and providing education as it relates to the prescribed drug treatment. Adrenergic antagonists work in one of two ways: (1) by blocking the effects of the adrenergic neurotransmitter receptors or (2) by inhibiting the release of norepinephrine and epinephrine. These drugs are used in the treatment of hypertension, dysrhythmias, angina, heart failure, BPH, and narrow-angle glaucoma.

Because adrenergic antagonists have a variety of effects on the heart and blood vessels, carefully assess the client's cardiovascular status prior to and during administration. Identify all medications, herbal remedies, and OTC drug contraindications for use with adrenergic antagonists.

Because many of these medications are metabolized by the liver, monitor hepatic function before and during therapy. Closely monitor clients with liver disease. Monitor renal function, because many of these drugs are eliminated mainly through the kidneys. The dose may need to be reduced if creatinine clearance is low.

If the client is receiving these medications for cardiac dysrhythmias, continuously monitor ECGs, heart rate, and blood pressure. Take apical heart rate and blood pressure readings prior to administration. If the heart rate is less that 60 beats per minute or if there is an irregularity, withhold the medication and notify the healthcare provider.

Assess the client for common side effects such as dizziness, drowsiness, headache, fatigue, palpitations, and dry mouth. Monitor for weight gain, edema, shortness of breath, or cough.

Lifespan Considerations.   Adrenergic antagonists should be used cautiously during pregnancy and lactation. With older adults, be aware of any chronic health conditions, and closely monitor these clients for adverse reactions.

Client Teaching.   Client education as it relates to adrenergic antagonists should include the goals of therapy, the reasons for obtaining baseline data such as vital signs and the existence of underlying disorders, and possible drug side effects. Include the following points when teaching clients about adrenergic antagonist therapy:

- Monitor your blood pressure daily.
- Ask for assistance before getting out of bed and walking, because dizziness may occur.
- Avoid driving for 12 to 24 hours after the first dose or when your dosage is increased.
- Immediately report dizziness or palpitations.
- Do not stop this medication abruptly. Discuss how to properly taper or discontinue your medication with your healthcare provider.

Pr PROTOTYPE DRUG | Prazosin *(Minipress)* | Adrenergic-blocking Agent

ACTIONS AND USES

Prazosin is a selective alpha$_1$-adrenergic antagonist that competes with norepinephrine at its receptors on vascular smooth muscle in arterioles and veins. Its major action is a rapid decrease in peripheral resistance that reduces blood pressure. It has little effect on cardiac output or heart rate, and it causes less reflex tachycardia than some other drugs in this class. Tolerance may occur to its antihypertensive effect. Its most common use is in combination with other agents, such as beta-blockers or diuretics, in the pharmacotherapy of hypertension. Prazosin has a short half-life and is often taken two or three times per day.

ADMINISTRATION ALERTS

- Give a low first dose to avoid severe hypotension.
- Safety during pregnancy (category C) or lactation is not established.

PHARMACOKINETICS

Onset: 2 h

Peak: 2–4 h

Half-life: 2–4 h

Duration: < 24 h

ADVERSE EFFECTS

Like other alpha-blockers, prazosin tends to cause orthostatic hypotension owing to alpha$_1$ inhibition in vascular smooth muscle. In rare cases, this hypotension can cause unconsciousness about 30 minutes after the first dose. To avoid this situation, the first dose should be very low and given at bedtime. Dizziness, drowsiness, or lightheadedness may occur. Reflex tachycardia may result from the rapid fall in blood pressure. Alpha blockade may cause nasal congestion or inhibition of ejaculation.

Contraindications: Safety during pregnancy and lactation is not established.

INTERACTIONS

Drug–Drug: Concurrent use of antihypertensives and diuretics results in extremely low blood pressure. Alcohol should be avoided.

Lab Tests: Increases urinary metabolites of vanillylmandelic acid (VMA) and norepinephrine, which are measured to screen for pheochromocytoma (adrenal tumor). Prazosin will cause false-positive results.

Herbal/Food: Do not use saw palmetto or nettle root products. Saw palmetto blocks alpha$_1$-receptors, resulting in the dilation of blood vessels and hypotensive response.

Treatment of Overdose: Overdose may cause hypotension. Blood pressure may be elevated by the administration of fluid expanders such as normal saline or vasopressors such as dopamine or dobutamine.

 See the Companion Website for a Nursing Process Focus specific to this drug.

NURSING PROCESS FOCUS Clients Receiving Adrenergic-blocking Therapy

Assessment	Potential Nursing Diagnoses
Prior to administration: • Assess vital signs, urinary output, and cardiac output (initially and throughout therapy). • Assess reason for drug administration. • Obtain complete health history, including cautions and contraindications for use, allergies, drug history, and possible drug interactions.	• Knowledge, Deficient, related to drug administration and effects • Sensory Perception, Disturbed • Injury, Risk for, related to dizziness, syncope • Urinary Elimination, Impaired • Sexual Dysfunction • Pain

Planning: Client Goals and Expected Outcomes

The client will:
• Exhibit a decrease in blood pressure with few adverse effects.
• Report a decrease in urinary symptoms such as hesitancy and difficulty voiding.
• Demonstrate an understanding of the drug's action by accurately describing drug side effects and precautions, and the importance of follow-up care.

Implementation

Interventions and (Rationales)	Client Education/Discharge Planning
• For prostatic hypertrophy, monitor for urinary hesitancy/feeling of incomplete bladder emptying, interrupted urinary stream. (These may be signs of decreased blood supply due to hypotension.)	• Instruct client to report increased difficulty with urinary voiding to healthcare provider.
• Monitor for syncope. (Alpha-adrenergic antagonists produce first-dose syncope phenomenon, and may cause loss of consciousness.)	Instruct client to: • Take this medication at bedtime, and to take the first dose *immediately* before getting into bed. Warn client about the first-dose phenomenon; reassure that this effect diminishes with continued therapy. • Avoid abrupt changes in position.
• Monitor vital signs, level of consciousness, and mood. (Adrenergic antagonists can exacerbate existing mental depression.)	• Instruct client to immediately report any feelings of dysphoria. • Interview client regarding suicide potential; obtain a "no-self-harm" verbal contract from the client.
• Monitor carefully for dizziness, drowsiness, or light-headedness. (These are signs of decreased blood flow to the brain due to the drug's hypotensive action.)	Instruct client: • To monitor vitals signs, especially blood pressure, ensuring proper use of home equipment. • Regarding the normotensive range of blood pressure; instruct client to consult the nurse regarding "reportable" blood pressure readings. • To report dizziness or syncope that persists beyond the first dose, as well as paresthesias and other neurological changes.
• Assess for blurred vision, tinnitus, epistaxis and edema. (These are potential side effects.)	Instruct client: • That nasal congestion may be a side effect. • To report any adverse reactions to the healthcare provider. • To avoid using OTC nasal decongestants with this medication.
• Monitor liver function. (These drugs may increase the risk of liver toxicity.)	Instruct client to: • Adhere to a regular schedule of laboratory testing for liver function as ordered by the healthcare provider. • Report signs and symptoms of liver toxicity: nausea, vomiting, diarrhea, rash, jaundice, abdominal pain, tenderness or distention, or change in color of stool. • Adhere to medication regimen.

Evaluation of Outcome Criteria

Evaluate the effectiveness of drug therapy by confirming that client goals and expected outcomes have been met (see "Planning").
• The client exhibits a decrease in blood pressure with minimal adverse effects.
• The client reports a decrease in urinary symptoms such as hesitancy and difficulty voiding.
• The client demonstrates an understanding of the drug's action by accurately describing drug side effects and precautions.

∞ *See Table 13.3 for a list of drugs to which these nursing actions apply.*

- Common side effects such as dizziness, drowsiness, headache, loss of energy and strength, palpitations, and dry mouth usually disappear after a few weeks of therapy.
- Follow your healthcare provider's suggestions for diet, exercise, stress reduction, and smoking cessation.

CHOLINERGIC AGENTS (PARASYMPATHOMIMETICS)

Parasympathomimetics are drugs that activate the parasympathetic nervous system. These cholinergic agents induce the rest-and-digest response.

13.9 Clinical Applications of Parasympathomimetics

The classic parasympathomimetic is acetylcholine, the endogenous neurotransmitter at cholinergic synapses in the autonomic nervous system. Acetylcholine, however, has almost no therapeutic use because it is rapidly destroyed after administration and produces many side effects. Recall that Ach is the neurotransmitter at the ganglia in both the parasympathetic and sympathetic divisions, and at the neuroeffector junctions in the parasympathetic nervous system, as well as in skeletal muscle. It is thus not surprising that administration of Ach or drugs that mimic Ach will have widespread and varied effects on the body.

Parasympathomimetics are divided into two subclasses, direct acting and indirect acting, based on their mechanism of action (Table 13.4). Direct-acting agents, such as bethanechol (Urecholine), bind to cholinergic receptors to produce the rest-and-digest response. Because direct-acting parasympathomimetics are relatively resistant to the destructive effects of the enzyme acetylcholinesterase, they have a longer duration of action than Ach. They are poorly absorbed across the GI tract and generally do not cross the blood–brain barrier. They have little effect on Ach receptors in ganglia. Because they are moderately selective to muscarinic receptors when used at therapeutic doses, direct-acting parasympathomimetics are sometimes called *muscarinic agonists.*

The indirect-acting parasympathomimetics, such as neostigmine (Prostigmin), inhibit the action of AchE. This inhibition allows endogenous Ach to avoid rapid destruction and remain on cholinergic receptors for a longer time, thus prolonging its action. These drugs are called *cholinesterase inhibitors.* Unlike the direct-acting agents, the cholinesterase inhibitors are nonselective and affect all Ach sites: autonomic ganglia, muscarinic receptors, skeletal muscle, and Ach sites in the CNS.

One of the first drugs discovered in this class, physostigmine (Antilirium), was obtained from the dried ripe seeds of *Physostigma venenosum,* a plant found in West Africa. The bean of this plant was used in tribal rituals. As research continued under secrecy during World War II, similar compounds were synthesized that produced potent neurological effects that could be used during chemical warfare. This class of agents now includes organophosphate insecticides such as malathion and parathion, and toxic nerve gases such as sarin. Nurses who work in agricultural areas may become quite familiar with the symptoms of acute poisoning with organophosphates. Poisoning results in intense stimulation of the parasympathetic nervous system, which may result in death, if untreated.

Because of their high potential for serious adverse effects, few parasympathomimetics are widely used in pharmacotherapy. Some have clinical applications in ophthalmology, because they reduce intraocular pressure in clients with glaucoma (Chapter 49 ∞). Others are used for their stimulatory effects on the smooth muscle of the bowel or urinary tract.

Several drugs in this class are used for their effects on acetylcholine receptors in skeletal muscle or in the CNS, rather than for their parasympathetic action. **Myasthenia gravis** is a disease characterized by destruction of nicotinic receptors on skeletal muscles. Administration of pyridostigmine (Mestinon) or neostigmine (Prostigmin) stimulates skeletal muscle contraction and helps reverse the severe muscle weakness characteristic of this disease. In addition, tacrine (Cognex) is useful in treating Alzheimer's disease

TABLE 13.4	Cholinergic Agents (Parasympathomimetics)	
Type	**Drug**	**Primary Use**
direct acting	ⓟ bethanechol (Urecholine)	to increase urination
	cevimeline HCl (Evoxac)	treatment of dry mouth
	pilocarpine (Isopto Carpine, Salagen)	glaucoma
cholinesterase inhibitors (indirect acting)	ambenonium (Mytelase)	myasthenia gravis
	donepezil (Aricept)	myasthenia gravis
	edrophonium (Tensilon)	diagnosis of myasthenia gravis
	galantamine hydrobromide (Razadyne)	glaucoma, treatment of anticholinergic overdose
	neostigmine (Prostigmin)	myasthenia gravis, to increase urination
	physostigmine (Antilirium)	Alzheimer's desease
	pyridostigmine (Mestinon)	Alzheimer's desease
	rivastigmine (Exelon)	Alzheimer's desease
	tacrine (Cognex)	Alzheimer's disease

because of its ability to increase the amount of acetylcholine in receptors in the CNS (Chapter 20 ∞).

NURSING CONSIDERATIONS

The role of the nurse in parasympathomimetic therapy involves careful monitoring of a client's condition and providing education as it relates to the prescribed drug treatment. These drugs are used in the treatment of urinary retention, myasthenia gravis, and Alzheimer's disease. Both direct- and indirect-acting parasympathomimetics are contraindicated for clients with hypersensitivity. Do not use in clients with obstruction of the gastrointestinal and urinary systems, because these drugs increase muscular tone and contraction. Additionally, do not use in clients with active asthma, bradycardia, hypotension, or Parkinson's disease.

Direct-acting Parasympathomimetics

Due to the stimulation of the CNS by these agents, several additional nursing actions are required. Take a careful assessment of past medical history for any of the following: angina pectoris, recent myocardial infarction, and dysrhythmias. Ask about possible use of lithium and adenosine, because both drugs are contraindicated owing to their interaction with nicotine. Lithium is a CNS agent that can produce significant muscarinic blockade to atropine. Adenosine is an antidysrhythmic agent, and its effect with nicotine can cause an increased risk of heart block.

Cholinesterase Inhibitors

The indirect-acting agents are contraindicated in clients with mechanical obstruction of either the intestine or urinary tract because of their ability to intensify smooth-muscle contractions. Smooth-muscle contractions can also occur in the bronchi, so use extreme caution when treating clients with asthma or chronic obstructive pulmonary disease (COPD).

Because these medications can inhibit acetylcholinesterase at many locations, Ach accumulates at the muscarinic and the neuromuscular junctions and causes side effects such as profuse salivation, increased muscle tone, urinary frequency, bronchoconstriction, and bradycardia. Keep atropine available to counteract the increased levels of Ach by providing selective blockage of muscarinic cholinergic receptors. Monitor the client for drug-induced insomnia.

Prior to administration, assess the client's condition for which parasympathomimetic therapy was ordered. Obtain baseline vital signs prior to any medication administration. Monitor the client's vital signs, because cholinergic agents may cause bradycardia and hypotension. Cholinergic agents may increase bronchial secretions and cause bronchoconstriction, so assess for dyspnea and auscultate the lungs and for evidence of rales or rhonchi. Administer with caution to clients with a recent history of asthma or COPD. Assess for bowel activity and discontinue the drug if bowel sounds are diminished or absent. Do not administer these drugs to clients with mechanical bowel obstruction.

Pr **PROTOTYPE DRUG** | Bethanechol *(Urecholine)* | Cholinergic Agent (Direct-acting Parasympathomimetic)

ACTIONS AND USES

Bethanechol is a direct-acting parasympathomimetic that interacts with muscarinic receptors to cause actions typical of parasympathetic stimulation. Its effects are most noted in the digestive and urinary tracts, where it stimulates smooth-muscle contraction. These actions are useful in increasing smooth-muscle tone and muscular contractions in the GI tract following general anesthesia. In addition, it is used to treat nonobstructive urinary retention in clients with atony of the bladder. Although poorly absorbed from the GI tract, it may be administered orally or by SC injection.

ADMINISTRATION ALERTS

- Never administer IM or IV.
- Oral and subcutaneous doses are *not* interchangeable.
- Monitor blood pressure, pulse, and respirations before administration and for at least 1 hour after subcutaneous administration.
- Pregnancy category C.

PHARMACOKINETICS

Onset: 30–90 min PO; 5–15 min subcutaneous

Peak: 60 min PO; 15–30 min subcutaneous

Half-life: 2–4 h PO; < 60 min subcutaneous

Duration: 6 h PO; 120 min subcutaneous

ADVERSE EFFECTS

The side effects of bethanechol are predicted from its parasympathetic actions. It should be used with extreme caution in clients with disorders that could be aggravated by increased contractions of the digestive tract, such as suspected obstruction, active ulcer, or inflammatory disease. The same caution should be exercised in clients with suspected urinary obstruction or COPD. Side effects include increased salivation, sweating, abdominal cramping, and hypotension that could lead to fainting.

Contraindications: Clients with asthma, epilepsy, or parkinsonism should not use this drug. Safety in pregnancy and lactation and in children younger than 8 years is not established.

INTERACTIONS

Drug–Drug: Drug interactions with bethanechol include increased cholinergic effects from cholinesterase inhibitors and decreased cholinergic effects from procainamide, quinidine, atropine, and epinephrine.

Lab Tests: May cause an increase in serum AST, amylase, and lipase.

Herbal/Food: Cholinergic effects caused by bethanechol may be antagonized by angel's trumpet, jimson weed, or scopalia.

Treatment of Overdose: Atropine sulfate is a specific antidote. Subcutaneous injection of atropine is preferred except in emergencies when the IV route may be used.

 See the Companion Website for a Nursing Process Focus specific to this drug.

NURSING PROCESS FOCUS Clients Receiving Parasympathomimetic Therapy

Assessment	Potential Nursing Diagnoses
Prior to administration: ■ Obtain complete health history including vital signs, allergies, and drug history for possible drug interactions. ■ Assess reason for drug administration. ■ Assess for contraindications of drug administration. ■ Assess for urinary retention, and urinary patterns initially and throughout therapy (direct acting). ■ Assess muscle strength, and neuromuscular status, ptosis, diplopia, and chewing.	■ Urinary Incontinence (direct acting) ■ Physical Mobility, Impaired (indirect acting) ■ Knowledge, Deficient, related to drug therapy ■ Injury, Risk for, related to side effects ■ Self-care, Deficient, related to disease process

Planning: Client Goals and Expected Outcomes

The client will:
■ Exhibit increased bowel/bladder function and tone by regaining normal pattern of elimination (direct acting).
■ Exhibit a decrease in myasthenia gravis symptoms such as muscle weakness, ptosis, and diplopia (indirect acting).
■ Demonstrate understanding of the drug's action by accurately describing drug indications, side effects, and precautions.
■ Exhibit an improvement in self-care activities.

Implementation

Interventions and (Rationales)	Client Education/Discharge Planning
All Parasympathomimetics	
■ Monitor for adverse effects such as abdominal cramping, diarrhea, excessive salivation, difficulty breathing, and muscle cramping. (These may indicate cholinergic crisis that requires atropine.)	■ Instruct client to report nausea, vomiting, diarrhea, rash, jaundice, or change in color of stool, or any other adverse reactions to the drug.
■ Monitor liver enzymes with initiation of therapy and weekly for 6 weeks. (Hepatotoxicity may occur.)	■ Instruct client to adhere to laboratory testing regimen for serum blood level tests of liver enzymes as directed.
■ Assess and monitor for appropriate self-care administration. (Possible complications related to inability to self-administer may occur.)	Instruct client to: ■ Take drug as directed on a regular schedule to maintain serum levels and control symptoms. ■ Not chew or crush sustained-release tablets. ■ Take oral parasympathomimetics on an empty stomach to lessen incidence of nausea and vomiting and to increase absorption.
Direct Acting	
■ Monitor intake and output ratio. Palpate abdomen for bladder distention. (These drugs have an onset of action of 60 minutes owing to binding of the drug to cholinergic receptors on the smooth muscle of the bladder, which relaxes the bladder to stimulate urination.)	■ Advise client to be near bathroom facilities after taking the drug.
■ Monitor for blurred vision. (This is a cholinergic effect.)	Advise client: ■ That blurred vision is a possible side effect and to take appropriate precautions. ■ Not to drive or perform hazardous activities until effects of the drugs are known.
■ Monitor for orthostatic hypotension. (This is a cholinergic effect.)	■ Instruct client to avoid abrupt changes in position. Avoid prolonged standing in one place.
Cholinesterase Inhibitors	
■ Monitor muscle strength, neuromuscular status, ptosis, diplopia, and chewing. (This determines if the therapeutic effect is achieved.)	■ Instruct client to report difficulty with vision or swallowing.
■ Schedule medication around meal times. (This will achieve therapeutic effect and aid in chewing and swallowing.)	■ Instruct client to take medication about 30 minutes before a meal.
■ Schedule activities to avoid fatigue. (Excess fatigue can lead to either a cholinergic or a myasthenic crisis.)	Instruct client to: ■ Plan activities according to muscle strength and fatigue. ■ Take frequent rest periods.

(Continued)

NURSING PROCESS FOCUS Clients Receiving Parasympathomimetic Therapy *(Continued)*	
Implementation	
Interventions and (Rationales)	**Client Education/Discharge Planning**
▪ Monitor for muscle weakness. (This symptom, depending on time of onset, indicates cholinergic crisis—overdose—or myasthenic crisis—underdose.)	Instruct client to: ▪ Report any severe muscle weakness that occurs 1 hour after administration of medication ▪ Report any muscle weakness that occurs 3 or more hours after medication administration, as this is a major symptom of myasthenic crisis

Evaluation of Outcome Criteria
Evaluate the effectiveness of drug therapy by confirming that the client goals and expected outcomes have been met (see "Planning"). ▪ The client exhibits normal patterns of elimination. ▪ The client exhibits a decrease in myasthenia gravis symptoms. ▪ The client demonstrates an understanding of the drug's action by accurately describing drug side effects and precautions. ▪ The client reports an increase in self-care abilities.
∞ *See Table 13.4 for a list of drugs to which these nursing applications apply.*

Record fluid intake and output and assess for urinary retention. Use with caution in clients with BPH, and do not administer to clients with mechanical obstruction of the urinary tract. Assess for fatigue and excessive salivation or sweating, because these may indicate overdosage.

For clients with myasthenia gravis, perform a baseline physical assessment of neuromuscular and respiratory function. Myasthenia gravis affects the muscles of the respiratory tract and other muscle groups owing to the destruction of nicotinic receptors on the skeletal muscles. Muscle weakness may be manifested as diplopia and ptosis of the upper eyelid. Other symptoms may include difficulty chewing, swallowing, and speaking; drooling; and inability to perform repetitive movements. Observe the client for difficult breathing that may occur because of decreased chest expansion and extreme fatigue.

In clients diagnosed with urinary retention, palpate the abdomen to identify urinary distention or discomfort. Ask the client about last fluid intake and time and amount of last urinary output. Continuously monitor vital signs, adverse drug reactions, and signs of cholinergic crisis.

Lifespan Considerations. For mothers who are breast-feeding, monitor the infant's respiratory patterns and any CNS changes prior to and after feedings. Monitor elderly clients for episodes of dizziness and sleep disturbances caused by CNS stimulation from the parasympathomimetic.

Client Teaching. Client education as it relates to cholinergic drugs should include the goals of therapy, the reasons for obtaining baseline data such as vital signs and the existence of underlying disorders, and the possible drug side effects. Include the following points when teaching clients about cholinergic drugs:

• Take the oral formulation of the drug on an empty stomach to decrease nausea and vomiting.

• Monitor your blood pressure and pulse daily. If pulse is less than 60, notify healthcare provider.

• Report decreased urine output.

• Take the drug as ordered and do not stop it abruptly.

• Report excessive sweating or perspiration, fatigue, and difficulty breathing.

CHOLINERGIC-BLOCKING AGENTS (ANTICHOLINERGICS)

Cholinergic-blocking agents are drugs that inhibit parasympathetic impulses. Suppressing the parasympathetic division induces symptoms of the fight-or-flight response.

13.10 Clinical Applications of Anticholinergics

Agents that block the action of acetylcholine are known by a number of names, including anticholinergics, cholinergic blockers, muscarinic antagonists, and parasympatholytics (see Table 13.5). Although the term *anticholinergic* is most commonly used, the most accurate term for this class of drugs is muscarinic antagonists, because at therapeutic doses, these drugs are selective for Ach muscarinic receptors, and thus have little effect on Ach nicotinic receptors.

Anticholinergics act by competing with acetylcholine for binding muscarinic receptors. When anticholinergics occupy these receptors, no response is generated at the neuroeffector organs. Suppressing the effects of Ach causes symptoms of sympathetic nervous system activation to predominate. Most therapeutic uses of the anticholinergics are predictable extensions of their parasympathetic-blocking actions: dilation of the pupils, increase in heart rate, drying of secretions, and relaxation of the bronchi. Note that these are also symptoms of sympathetic activation (fight or flight).

Historically, anticholinergics have been widely used for many different disorders. References to these agents, which are extracted from the deadly nightshade plant, *Atropa belladonna,* date to the ancient Hindus, the Roman Empire, and the Middle Ages. Because of plant's extreme toxicity, extracts of belladonna were sometimes used for intentional poisoning, including suicide, as well as in religious and

TABLE 13.5 Cholinergic-blocking Agents (Anticholinergics)

Drug	Primary Use
ⓟ atropine	to increase heart rate, dilate pupils
benztropine (Cogentin)	Parkinson's disease
cyclopentolate (Cyclogyl)	to dilate pupils
dicyclomine (Bentyl, others)	irritable bowel syndrome
glycopyrrolate (Robinul)	to produce a dry field prior to anesthesia, peptic ulcers
ipratropium (Atrovent)	asthma
oxybutynin (Ditropan)	incontinence
propantheline (Pro-Banthine)	irritable bowel syndrome, peptic ulcer
scopolamine (Hyoscine, Transderm-Scop)	motion sickness, irritable bowel syndrome, adjunct to anesthesia
tiotropium (spiriva)	asthma
trihexyphenidyl (Artane, others)	Parkinson's disease

beautification rituals. The name *belladonna* is Latin for "pretty woman." Roman women applied extracts of belladonna to the face to create the preferred female attributes of the time—pink cheeks and dilated, doelike eyes.

Therapeutic uses of anticholinergics include the following:

- *GI disorders* These agents decrease the secretion of gastric acid in peptic ulcer disease (Chapter 40 ∞). They also slow intestinal motility and may be useful for reducing the cramping and diarrhea associated with irritable bowel syndrome (Chapter 41 ∞).
- *Ophthalmic procedures* May be used to cause mydriasis or cycloplegia during eye procedures (Chapter 49 ∞).
- *Cardiac rhythm abnormalities* Can be used to accelerate the heart rate in clients experiencing bradycardia (Chapter 26 ∞).
- *Preanesthesia* Combined with other agents, anticholinergics can decrease excessive respiratory secretions and reverse the bradycardia caused by anesthetics (Chapter 19 ∞).
- *Asthma* A few agents, such as ipratropium (Atrovent), are useful in treating asthma, because of their ability to dilate the bronchi (Chapter 39 ∞).

The prototype drug, atropine, is used for several additional medical conditions owing to its effective muscarinic receptor blockade. These applications include reversal of adverse muscarinic effects and treatment of cholinergic agent poisoning, including that caused by overdose of bethanechol (Urecholine), cholinesterase inhibitors, or accidental ingestion of certain types of mushrooms or organophosphate pesticides.

Some of the anticholinergics are used for their effects on the CNS, rather than their autonomic actions. Scopolamine (Hyoscine, Transderm-Scop) is used to produce sedation and prevent motion sickness (Chapter 41 ∞); benztropine (Cogentin) is prescribed to reduce the muscular tremor and rigidity associated with Parkinson's disease; and donepezil (Aricept) has a slight memory enhancement effect in clients with Alzheimer's disease (Chapter 20 ∞).

Anticholinergics exhibit a relatively high incidence of side effects. Important adverse effects that limit their usefulness include tachycardia, CNS stimulation, and the tendency to cause urinary retention in men with prostate disorders. Adverse effects such as dry mouth and dry eyes occur owing to blockade of muscarinic receptors on salivary glands and lacrimal glands, respectively. Blockade of muscarinic receptors on sweat glands can inhibit sweating, which may lead to hyperthermia. Photophobia can occur because the pupil is unable to constrict in response to bright light. Symptoms of overdose (cholinergic crisis) include fever, visual changes, difficulty swallowing, psychomotor agitation, and/or hallucinations. (Use this simile to remember the signs of cholinergic crisis: "Hot as hades, blind as a bat, dry as a bone, mad as a hatter.") The development of safer and more effective drugs has greatly decreased the current use of anticholinergics. An exception is ipratropium (Atrovent), a relatively new anticholinergic used for clients with COPD. Because it is delivered via aerosol spray, this agent produces more localized action with fewer systemic side effects than atropine.

SPECIAL CONSIDERATIONS

Impact of Anticholinergics on Male Sexual Function

A functioning autonomic nervous system is essential for normal male sexual health. The parasympathetic nervous system is necessary for erections, whereas the sympathetic division is responsible for the process of ejaculation. Anticholinergic drugs block transmission of parasympathetic impulses and may interfere with normal erections. Adrenergic antagonists can interfere with the smooth-muscle contractions in the seminal vesicles and penis, resulting in an inability to ejaculate.

For male clients receiving autonomic medications, the nurse should include questions about sexual activity during the assessment process. For clients who are not sexually active, these side effects may be unimportant. For clients who are sexually active, however, drug-induced sexual dysfunction may be a major cause of noncompliance. The client should be informed to expect such side effects and to report them to the healthcare provider immediately. In most cases, alternative medications are available that do not affect sexual function. Inform the client that supportive counseling is available.

Pr PROTOTYPE DRUG | Atropine *(Atropair, Atropisol)* | Cholinergic-blocking Agent

ACTIONS AND USES

By occupying muscarinic receptors, atropine blocks the parasympathetic actions of Ach and induces symptoms of the fight-or-flight response. Most prominent are increased heart rate, bronchodilation, decreased motility in the GI tract, mydriasis, and decreased secretions from glands. At therapeutic doses, atropine has no effect on nicotinic receptors in ganglia or on skeletal muscle.

Although atropine has been used for centuries for a variety of purposes, its use has declined in recent decades because of the development of safer and more effective medications. Atropine may be used to treat hypermotility diseases of the GI tract such as irritable bowel syndrome, to suppress secretions during surgical procedures, to increase the heart rate in clients with bradycardia, and to dilate the pupil during eye examinations. Once widely used to cause bronchodilation in clients with asthma, atropine is now rarely prescribed for this disorder.

ADMINISTRATION ALERTS

- Never administer IM or IV.
- Oral and subcutaneous doses are *not* interchangeable.
- Monitor blood pressure, pulse, and respirations before administration and for at least 1 hour after subcutaneous administration.
- Pregnancy category C.

PHARMACOKINETICS

Onset: 30 min PO; 5–15 min subcutaneously

Peak: 60–90 min PO; 15–30 min subcutaneously

Half-life: 4 h PO; 120 min subcutaneously

Duration: 6 h PO; 4 h subcutaneously

ADVERSE EFFECTS

The side effects of atropine limit its therapeutic usefulness and are predictable extensions of its autonomic actions. Expected side effects include dry mouth, constipation, urinary retention, and an increased heart rate. Initial CNS excitement may progress to delirium and even coma.

Contraindications: Atropine is usually contraindicated in clients with glaucoma, because the drug may increase pressure within the eye. Atropine should not be administered to clients with obstructive disorders of the GI tract, paralytic ileus, bladder neck obstruction, benign prostatic hypertrophy, myasthenia gravis, cardiac insufficiency, or acute hemorrhage.

INTERACTIONS

Drug–Drug: Drug interactions with atropine include an increased effect with antihistamines, tricyclic antidepressants, quinidine, and procainamide, and decreased effects with levodopa.

Lab Tests: Unknown.

Herbal/Food: Use with caution with herbal supplements, such as aloe, sonna, buckthorn, and cascara sagrada, which may increase atropine's effect, particulary with chronic use of these herbs.

Treatment of Overdose: Accidental poisoning has occurred in children who eat the colorful, purple berries of the deadly nightshade, mistaking them for cherries. Symptoms of poisoning are those of intense parasympathetic stimulation. Overdose may cause CNS stimulation or depression. A short-acting barbiturate or diazepam (Valium) may be administered to control convulsions. Physostigmine is an antidote for atropine poisoning that quickly reverses the coma caused by large doses of atropine.

 See the Companion Website for a Nursing Process Focus specific to this drug.

NURSING PROCESS FOCUS   Clients Receiving Anticholinergic Therapy

Assessment	Potential Nursing Diagnoses
Prior to administration: - Obtain complete health history, including drug history, to determine possible drug interactions and allergies. - Assess reason for drug administration. - Assess for heart rate, blood pressure, temperature, and elimination patterns (initially and throughout therapy).	- Knowledge, Deficient, related to drug therapy - Cardiac Output, Decreased - Body Temperature, Imbalanced, Risk for - Oral Mucous Membrane, Impaired - Constipation - Urinary Retention - Injury, Risk for, related to effect of drug

Planning: Client Goals And Expected Outcomes

The client will:
- Exhibit a decrease in symptoms for which the medication is prescribed.
- Verbalize techniques to avoid hazardous side effects associated with anticholinergic therapy.
- Demonstrate an understanding of the drug's action by accurately describing drug side effects and precautions.

Implementation

Interventions and (Rationales)	Client Education/Discharge Planning
- Monitor for signs of anticholinergic crisis resulting from overdosage. (Fever, tachycardia, difficulty swallowing, ataxia, reduced urine output, psychomotor agitation, confusion, and hallucinations are signs of an anticholinergic crisis.)	- Instruct clients to report side effects related to therapy such as shortness of breath, cough, dysphagia, syncope, fever, anxiety, right upper quadrant pain, extreme lethargy, or dizziness.

NURSING PROCESS FOCUS Clients Receiving Anticholinergic Therapy *(Continued)*

Implementation

Interventions and (Rationales)	Client Education/Discharge Planning
▪ Report significant changes in heart rate, blood pressure, or the development of dysrhythmias. (Anticholinergics may cause increased heart rate and dysrhythmias owing to sympathetic nerve stimulation.)	▪ Instruct client to monitor vital signs, ensuring proper use of home equipment.
▪ Observe for side effects such as drowsiness, blurred vision, tachycardia, dry mouth, urinary hesitancy, and decreased sweating. (Sides effects are due to the blockade of muscarinic receptors.)	Instruct client to: ▪ Report side effects. ▪ Avoid driving and hazardous activities until effects of the drugs are known. ▪ Wear sunglasses to decrease the sensitivity to bright light.
▪ Provide comfort measures for dry mucous membranes such as applying lubricant to moisten lips and oral mucosa, assisting in rinsing mouth, and using artificial tears for dry eyes, as needed. (Dryness is due to anticholinergic effect.)	▪ Instruct client that oral rinses, sugarless gum or candy, and frequent oral hygiene may help relieve dry mouth. Avoid alcohol-containing mouthwashes, which can further dry oral tissue.
▪ Minimize exposure to heat or cold and strenuous exercise. (Anticholinergics can inhibit sweat gland secretions owing to direct blockade of the muscarinic receptors on the sweat glands. Sweating is necessary for clients to cool down, so the drug can increase their risk for hyperthermia.)	▪ Advise client to limit activity outside when the temperature is hot. Strenuous activity in a hot environment may cause heat stroke.
▪ Monitor intake and output ratio. Palpate abdomen for bladder distention. (Anticholinergics can block muscarinic receptors, which decreases tone and causes urinary retention.)	▪ Instruct client to notify healthcare provider if difficulty in voiding occurs.
▪ Monitor client for abdominal distention and auscultate for bowel sounds. (Anticholinergics block muscarinic receptors and may decreases tone and motility of intestinal smooth muscle.)	▪ Advise client to increase fluid and add bulk to the diet if constipation becomes a problem.

Evaluation of Outcome Criteria

Evaluate the effectivness of drug therapy by confirming that client goals and expected outcomes have been met (see "Planning").

- The client exhibits a decrease in symptoms for which the medication is prescribed.
- The client states techniques to avoid hazardous side effects associated with anticholinergic therapy.
- The client demonstrates an understanding of the drug's action by accurately describing drug side effects and precautions.

∞ *See Table 13.3 for a list of drugs to which these nursing actions apply.*

NURSING CONSIDERATIONS

The role of the nurse in anticholinergic therapy involves careful monitoring of a client's condition and providing education as it relates to the prescribed drug treatment. Perform a thorough medical history, including medications the client is currently taking that could cause drug–drug interactions. Antihistamines, in particular, can lead to excessive muscarinic blockade. Check for history of taking herbal supplements because some have atropinc-like actions that potentiate the effects of the cholinergic blockers and can be harmful to the client. For example, aloe, senna, buckthorn, and cascara sagrada may increase atropine's effect, particularly with chronic use of the herbs.

Do not use this class of drugs if the client has a history of acute-angle glaucoma. Anticholinergics block muscarinic receptors in the eye, creating paralysis of the iris sphincter, which can increase intraocular pressure.

Anticholinergics are contraindicated in clients with cardiopulmonary conditions such as COPD, asthma, heart disease, and hypertension, because blockade of cardiac muscarinic receptors prevents the parasympathetic nervous system from slowing the heart. The potential acceleration of heart rate may exacerbate these conditions. Clients with hyperthyroidism should not be given these medications, because in hyperthyroidism the heart rate is generally high, and administration of anticholinergics can cause dysrhythmias owing to norepinephrine release from sympathetic nerves that regulate heart rate.

Assess for baseline bowel and bladder function. Renal conditions are contraindications because of the effect of anticholinergics on bladder functioning. Gastrointestinal conditions such as ulcerative colitis and ileus are also contraindications, because blockade of muscarinic receptors in the intestine can decrease the tone and motility of intestinal smooth muscle, which can exacerbate intestinal conditions. Monitor clients with esophageal reflux and hiatal hernia, because anticholinergics reduce GI motility. Clients with gastroesophageal reflux disease (GERD) and hiatal hernia experience decreased muscle tone in the lower esophageal sphincter and delayed stomach emptying. Anticholinergics exacerbate these symptoms, increasing the risk of esophageal injury and aspiration. Clients with Down syndrome may be more sensitive to the effects of atropine owing to structural differences in the CNS caused by chromosomal abnormality (trisomy). Clients with Down syndrome also tend to have disorders such as GERD and heart disease, which may be adversely affected by anticholinergics.

Lifespan Considerations.   Anticholinergic drugs should be used cautiously in children, because adverse effects may be more severe. Safety has not been established during pregnancy and for lactating mothers. Anticholinergics may produce fetal tachycardia. When using these drugs in older adults, be alert for frequently seen adverse effects including mental confusion, hallucinations, urinary retention, constipation, and blurred vision.

Client Teaching.   Client education as it relates to anticholinergics should include the goals of therapy, the reasons for obtaining baseline data such as vital signs and the existence of underlying cardiac, renal, and other disorders, and possible drug side effects. Include the following points when teaching clients about anticholinergics:

- Avoid activities that may result in overheating, because the drug suppresses sweat glands and may lead to heat stroke.

- Avoid driving and other hazardous activities until effects of the drug are known, because drowsiness, dizziness, and blurred vision may occur.
- Increase fluids and fiber intake to prevent constipation.
- Use sugar-free hard candy, gum, or ice chips to minimize dry mouth, a common anticholinergic side effect.
- Report decreases in urine output or difficulty urinating.
- Administer ophthalmic preparations correctly.

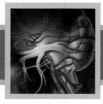

CHAPTER REVIEW

KEY CONCEPTS

The numbered key concepts provide a succinct summary of the important points from the corresponding numbered section within the chapter. If any of these points are not clear, refer to the numbered section within the chapter for review.

13.1 The peripheral nervous system is divided into a somatic portion, which is under voluntary control, and an autonomic portion, which is involuntary and controls smooth muscle, cardiac muscle, and glandular secretions.

13.2 Stimulation of the sympathetic division of the autonomic nervous system causes symptoms of the fight-or-flight response, whereas stimulation of the parasympathetic branch induces rest-and-digest responses.

13.3 Drugs can affect nervous transmission across a synapse by preventing the synthesis, storage, or release of the neurotransmitter; by preventing the destruction of the neurotransmitter; or by binding neurotransmitters to the receptors.

13.4 Norepinephrine is the primary neurotransmitter released at adrenergic receptors, which are divided into alpha and beta subtypes. Acetylcholine is the other primary neurotransmitter of the autonomic nervous system.

13.5 Acetylcholine is the primary neurotransmitter released at cholinergic receptors (nicotinic and muscarinic) in both the sympathetic and parasympathetic nervous systems. It is also the neurotransmitter at nicotinic receptors in skeletal muscle.

13.6 Autonomic drugs are classified by the receptors they stimulate or block: Sympathomimetics stimulate sympathetic nerves, and parasympathomimetics stimulate parasympathetic nerves; adrenergic antagonists inhibit the sympathetic division, whereas anticholinergics inhibit the parasympathetic branch.

13.7 Sympathomimetics act by directly activating adrenergic receptors, or indirectly by increasing the release of norepinephrine from nerve terminals. They are used primarily for their effects on the heart, bronchial tree, and nasal passages.

13.8 Adrenergic antagonists are used primarily for hypertension and are the most widely prescribed class of autonomic drugs.

13.9 Parasympathomimetics act directly by stimulating cholinergic receptors or indirectly by inhibiting acetylcholinesterase. They have few therapeutic uses because of their numerous side effects.

13.10 Anticholinergics act by blocking the effects of acetylcholine at muscarinic receptors, and are used to dry secretions, treat asthma, and prevent motion sickness.

NCLEX-RN® REVIEW QUESTIONS

1 Which of the following adverse drug effects would the nurse assess with the administration of adrenergic agents (sympathomimetics)?

1. Insomnia, nervousness, and anorexia
2. Nausea, vomiting, and hypotension
3. Nervousness, drowsiness, and hypertension
4. Bronchial dilation, hypotension, and bradycardia

2 Therapeutic uses for anticholinergics would include: (Select all that apply.)

1. Peptic ulcer disease.
2. Bradycardia.
3. Decreased sexual function.
4. Irritable bowel syndrome.
5. Urine retention.

3 Which of the following is not a potential adverse reaction of adrenergic antagonist medications?

1. Bronchodilation
2. Tachycardia
3. Edema
4. Heart failure

4 Elderly clients taking bethanechol (Urecholine) need to be assessed more frequently because of which of the following side effects?

1. Diaphoresis
2. Hypertension
3. Dizziness
4. Urinary retention

5 The client taking benztropine (Congentin) should be assessed for:

1. Heartburn.
2. Constipation.
3. Hypothermia.
4. Increased gastric motility.

CRITICAL THINKING QUESTIONS

1. A 24-year-old client (gravida 3, para 1) is admitted to the labor and delivery unit and states that she is having contractions. She is at 32 weeks gestation. The obstetrician initially begins tocolysis with magnesium sulfate and then switches the client to terbutaline (Brethine), 5 mg PO q4h around the clock. The nurse recognizes terbutaline as a beta$_2$-adrenergic agent. What nursing assessments should be made with a client receiving terbutaline therapy? What education does the client require in relation to terbutaline therapy? How will the nurse evaluate the medication's effectiveness?

2. A 74-year-old female client underwent a retropubic urethral suspension. She required a Foley catheter for 4 days postop and was still unable to void. She was recatheterized, and a bladder rehabilitation program was begun that included bethanechol (Urecholine). What nursing diagnosis should be considered as a part of this client's plan of care given this new drug regimen?

3. A 42-year-old male client was diagnosed with Parkinson's disease 4 years ago. He is being treated with a regimen of amantadine (Symmetrel), an indirect-acting dopaminergic agent, and benztropine mesylate (Cogentin). The nurse recognizes Cogentin as an anticholinergic agent. What should the nurse assess this client for? Discuss the potential side effects of benztropine that the nurse should assess for in this client.

See Appendix D for answers and rationales for all activities.

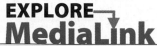

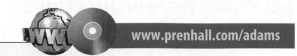

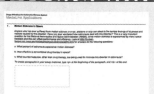

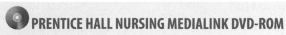

NCLEX-RN® review, case studies, and other interactive resources for this chapter can be found on the companion website at www.prenhall.com/adams. Click on "Chapter 13" to select the activities for this chapter. For animations, more NCLEX-RN® review questions, and an audio glossary, access the accompanying Prentice Hall Nursing MediaLink DVD-ROM in this textbook.

PRENTICE HALL NURSING MEDIALINK DVD-ROM

- **Audio Glossary**
- **NCLEX-RN® Review**

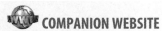

COMPANION WEBSITE

- **NCLEX-RN® Review**
- **Case Study:** Parasympathomimetics
- **Care Plan:** Client who receives atropine postoperatively
- **Dosage Calculations**
- **Nursing Process Focus**

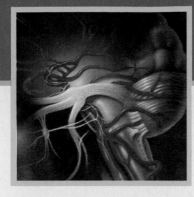

CHAPTER 14

Drugs for Anxiety and Insomnia

DRUGS AT A GLANCE

ANTIDEPRESSANTS
  📼 *escitalopram oxalate (Lexapro)*
BENZODIAZEPINES
  📼 *lorazepam (Ativan)*
BARBITURATES
NONBENZODIAZEPINE, NONBARBITURATE CNS DEPRESSANTS
  📼 *zolpidem (Ambien)*
Antiseizure Medication
Beta-blockers

OBJECTIVES

After reading this chapter, the student should be able to:

1. Identify the major types of anxiety disorders.
2. Discuss factors contributing to anxiety and explain some nonpharmacological therapies used to cope with this disorder.
3. Identify the regions of the brain associated with anxiety, sleep, and wakefulness.
4. Identify the three classes of medications used to treat anxiety and sleep disorders.
5. Explain the pharmacological management of anxiety and insomnia.
6. Describe the nurse's role in the pharmacological management of anxiety and insomnia.
7. Identify normal sleep patterns and explain how these might be affected by anxiety and stress.
8. Categorize drugs used for anxiety and insomnia based on their classification and mechanism of action.
9. For each of the classes listed in Drugs at a Glance, know representative drugs and explain their mechanisms of action, primary actions, and important adverse effects.
10. Use the Nursing Process to care for clients receiving drug therapy for anxiety and insomnia.

MediaLink

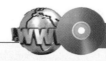

www.prenhall.com/adams

NCLEX-RN® review, case studies, and other interactive resources for this chapter can be found on the companion website at www.prenhall.com/adams. Click on "Chapter 14" to select the activities for this chapter. For animations, more NCLEX-RN® review questions, and an audio glossary, access the accompanying Prentice Hall Nursing MediaLink DVD-ROM in this textbook.

KEY TERMS

antidepressants *page 159*

anxiety *page 154*

anxiolytics *page 156*

electroencephalogram (EEG) *page 158*

generalized anxiety disorder (GAD) *page 154*

hypnotic *page 159*

insomnia *page 156*

limbic system *page 155*

long-term insomnia *page 157*

obsessive–compulsive disorder (OCD) *page 154*

panic disorder *page 154*

phobias *page 154*

post-traumatic stress disorder (PTSD) *page 155*

rebound insomnia *page 157*

REM sleep *page 158*

reticular activating system (RAS) *page 155*

reticular formation *page 155*

sedative *page 159*

sedative–hypnotic *page 159*

short-term or behavioral insomnia *page 157*

situational anxiety *page 154*

sleep debt *page 158*

social anxiety *page 154*

tranquilizer *page 159*

Clients experience nervousness and tension more often than any other symptoms. Seeking relief from these symptoms, they often turn to a variety of pharmacological and alternative therapies. Most healthcare providers agree that even though drugs do not cure the underlying problem, they can provide temporary help to calm clients who are experiencing acute anxiety, or who have simple sleep disorders. This chapter deals with drugs that treat anxiety, cause sedation, or help clients sleep.

ANXIETY DISORDERS

According to the *International Classification of Diseases*, 10th edition (ICD-10), **anxiety** is a state of "apprehension, tension, or uneasiness that stems from the anticipation of danger, the source of which is largely unknown or unrecognized." Anxious individuals can often identify at least some factors that bring on their symptoms. Most people state that their feelings of anxiety are disproportionate to any factual dangers.

14.1 Types of Anxiety Disorders

The anxiety experienced by people faced with a stressful environment is called **situational anxiety.** To a degree, situational anxiety is beneficial because it motivates people to accomplish tasks in a prompt manner—if for no other reason than to eliminate the source of nervousness. Situational stress may be intense, though clients often learn coping mechanisms to deal with the stress without seeking conventional medical intervention.

Generalized anxiety disorder (GAD) is a difficult-to-control, excessive anxiety that lasts 6 months or more. It focuses on a variety of life events or activities, and interferes with normal day-to-day functions. It is by far the most common type of stress disorder, and the one most frequently encountered by the nurse. Symptoms include restlessness, fatigue, muscle tension, nervousness, inability to focus or concentrate, an overwhelming sense of dread, and sleep disturbances. Autonomic signs of sympathetic nervous system activation that accompany anxiety include blood pressure elevation, heart palpitations, varying degrees of respiratory change, and dry mouth. Parasympathetic responses may consist of abdominal cramping, diarrhea, fatigue, and urinary urgency. Women are slightly more likely to experience GAD than men, and its prevalence is highest in the 20–35 age group.

A second category of anxiety, called **panic disorder,** is characterized by intense feelings of immediate apprehension, fearfulness, terror, or impending doom, accompanied by increased autonomic nervous system activity. Although panic attacks usually last less than 10 minutes, clients may describe them as seemingly endless. Up to 5% of the population will experience one or more panic attacks during their lifetime, with women being affected about twice as often as men.

Other categories of anxiety disorders include phobias, obsessive–compulsive disorder, and post-traumatic stress disorder. **Phobias** are fearful feelings attached to situations or objects. Common phobias include fear of snakes, spiders, crowds, or heights. A fear of crowds is termed **social anxiety.** Performers may experience feelings of dread, nervousness, or apprehension termed *performance anxiety.* Some anxiety is normal when a person faces a crowd or performs for a crowd, but extreme fear to the point of phobia is not normal. Phobias compel a client to avoid the fearful stimulus entirely to the point that his or her behavior is unnatural. Another unnatural behavior is **obsessive–compulsive disorder (OCD).** It involves recurrent, intrusive thoughts or repetitive behaviors that interfere with normal activities or relationships. Common examples include fear of exposure to germs and repetitive handwashing. **Post-traumatic stress disorder (PTSD)** is a type of situational anxiety that develops in response to reexperiencing a previous life event. Traumatic life events such as war, physical or sexual abuse, natural disasters, or murder may lead to a sense of helplessness and reexperiencing of the traumatic event. Hurricanes Katrina and Rita, as well as the terrorist attack on September 11, 2001, are examples of situations that may trigger PTSD. People who experience these types of traumatic life events are at risk for developing signs and symptoms of PTSD.

14.2 Specific Regions of the Brain Responsible for Anxiety and Wakefulness

Neural systems in the brain associated with anxiety and restlessness include the limbic system and the reticular activating system. These are illustrated in Pharmacotherapy Illustrated 14.1.

The **limbic system** is an area in the middle of the brain responsible for emotional expression, learning, and memory. Signals routed through the limbic system ultimately connect with the hypothalamus. Emotional states associated with this connection include anxiety, fear, anger, aggression, remorse, depression, sexual drive, and euphoria.

The hypothalamus is an important center responsible for unconscious responses to extreme stress such as high blood pressure, elevated breathing rate, and dilated pupils. These are responses associated with the fight-or-flight response of the autonomic nervous system, as presented in Chapter 13 ∞. The many endocrine functions of the hypothalamus are discussed in Chapter 43 ∞.

The hypothalamus connects with the **reticular formation,** a network of neurons found along the entire length of the brainstem, as shown in Pharmacotherapy Illustrated 14.1. Stimulation of the reticular formation causes heightened alertness and arousal; inhibition causes general drowsiness and the induction of sleep.

The larger area in which the reticular formation is found is called the **reticular activating system (RAS).** This structure

PHARMACOTHERAPY ILLUSTRATED

14.1 The reticular activating system and related regions in the brain are important areas of focus for drugs used to treat anxiety and anxiety-related symptoms.

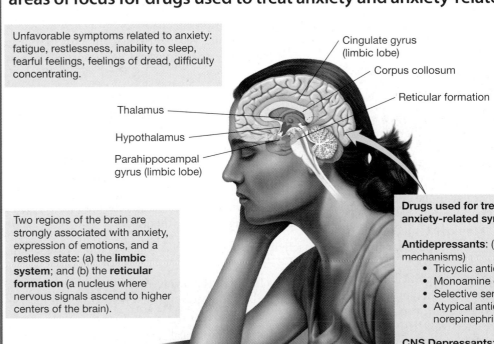

Unfavorable symptoms related to anxiety: fatigue, restlessness, inability to sleep, fearful feelings, feelings of dread, difficulty concentrating.

Cingulate gyrus (limbic lobe)

Corpus collosum

Reticular formation

Thalamus

Hypothalamus

Parahippocampal gyrus (limbic lobe)

Two regions of the brain are strongly associated with anxiety, expression of emotions, and a restless state: (a) the **limbic system**; and (b) the **reticular formation** (a nucleus where nervous signals ascend to higher centers of the brain).

Drugs used for treatment of anxiety and anxiety-related symptoms:

Antidepressants: (See Chapter 16 for specific mechanisms)
- Tricyclic antidepressants (TCAs)
- Monoamine oxidase inhibitors (MAOIs)
- Selective serotonin reuptake inhibitors (SSRIs)
- Atypical antidepressants including serotonin norepinephrine reuptake inhibitors (SNRIs)

CNS Depressants: (See Chapter 15 for specific mechanisms)
- Benzodiazepines
- Barbituates
- Other drugs

PHARMFACTS

Anxiety Disorders

- About 19 million Americans are diagnosed with anxiety every year.
- Other illnesses that commonly coexist with anxiety include depression, eating disorders, and substance abuse.
- The top five causes of anxiety (as listed in order) occur between the ages of 18 and 54.
  1. Phobia
  2. Post-traumatic stress
  3. Generalized anxiety
  4. Obsessive–compulsive feelings
  5. Panic

projects from the brainstem to the thalamus. The RAS is responsible for sleeping and wakefulness and performs an alerting function for the entire cerebral cortex. It helps a person focus attention on individual tasks by transmitting information to higher brain centers.

If signals are prevented from passing through the RAS, no emotion-related signals are sent to the brain, resulting in a reduction in general brain activity. If signals coming from the hypothalamus are allowed to proceed, then those signals are further routed through the RAS and on to higher brain centers. This is the neural mechanism thought to be responsible for feelings such as anxiety and fear. It is also the mechanism associated with restlessness and an interrupted sleeping pattern.

14.3 Anxiety Management Through Pharmacological and Nonpharmacological Strategies

Although stress itself may be incapacitating, it is often only a symptom of an underlying disorder. It is considered more productive to uncover and address the cause of the anxiety rather than to merely treat the symptoms with medications. Clients should be encouraged to explore and develop nonpharmacological coping strategies to deal with the underlying causes. Such strategies may include cognitive behavioral therapy, counseling, biofeedback techniques, meditation, and other complementary therapies. One model for stress management is shown in ● Figure 14.1.

When anxiety becomes severe enough to significantly interfere with daily activities of life, pharmacotherapy is indicated. In most types of stress, **anxiolytics,** or drugs having the ability to relieve anxiety, are quite effective. These include medications found within a number of therapeutic categories: central nervous system (CNS) agents such as antidepressants and CNS depressants; drugs for seizures (Chapter 15 ∞); emotional and mood disorder drugs (Chapter 16 ∞); antihypertensive agents (Chapter 23 ∞); and antidysrythmics (Chapter 26 ∞). Anxiolytics provide treatment for all the conditions mentioned in Section 14.1: phobias, post-traumatic stress disorder, generalized anxiety, obsessive–compulsive disorder, and panic attack.

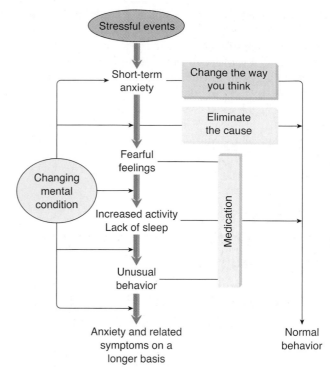

● **Figure 14.1** A model of anxiety in which stressful events or a changing mental condition can produce unfavorable symptoms, some of which may be controlled by medication

INSOMNIA

Insomnia is a condition characterized by a client's inability to fall asleep or remain asleep. Pharmacotherapy may be indicated if the sleeplessness interferes with normal daily activities.

14.4 Insomnia and Its Link to Anxiety

Why is it that we need sleep? During an average lifetime, about 33% of the time is spent sleeping, or trying to sleep. Although it is well established that sleep is essential for wellness, scientists are unsure of its function or how much is needed. Following are some theories:

- Inactivity during sleep gives the body time to repair itself.
- Sleep is a function that evolved as a protective mechanism. Throughout history, nighttime was the safest time of day.
- Sleep deals with "electrical" charging and discharging of the brain. The brain needs time for processing and filing new information collected throughout the day. When this is done without interference from the outside environment, these vast amounts of data can be retrieved through memory.

The acts of sleeping and waking are synchronized to many different bodily functions. Body temperature, blood pressure, hormone levels, and respiration all fluctuate on a

NATURAL THERAPIES

Melatonin

Melatonin is a natural hormone (*N*-acetyl-5-methoxytryptamine) produced especially at night by the pineal gland. Its secretion is stimulated by darkness and inhibited by light. Tryptophan is converted to serotonin and finally to melatonin. As melatonin production rises, alertness decreases, and body temperature starts to fall, both of which make sleep more inviting.

Melatonin production is also related to age. Children manufacture more melatonin than elderly clients; however, melatonin production begins to drop at puberty. Melatonin is one of only two hormones not regulated by the FDA and sold over the counter without a prescription (DHEA, or dehydroepiandrosterone, is the other). Supplemental melatonin, 0.5 to 3.0 mg at bedtime, is alleged to decrease the time required to fall asleep and to produce a deep and restful sleep. Melatonin should not be taken by pregnant or nursing clients, as there is a lack of studies to indicate its safety. Large doses of melatonin have been shown to inhibit ovulation, so women trying to conceive should reconsider taking melatonin.

People with severe allergies, autoimmune diseases, and immune system cancers such as lymphoma and leukemia should not take melatonin, because it could exacerbate such conditions by stimulating the immune system. Clients taking corticosteroids should be advised that melatonin may interfere with the efficacy of these hormones. Melatonin use in some children with seizure disorders may lead to increased seizure activity. Melatonin should not be given to healthy children, as they already produce it in abundance.

cyclic basis throughout the 24-hour day. When this cycle becomes impaired, pharmacological or other interventions may be needed to readjust it. Increased levels of the neurotransmitter serotonin help initiate the various processes of sleep.

Insomnia, or sleeplessness, is a disorder sometimes associated with anxiety. There are several major types of insomnia. **Short-term or behavioral insomnia** may be attributed to stress caused by a hectic lifestyle or the inability to resolve day-to-day conflicts within the home environment or the workplace. Worries about work, marriage, children, and health are common reasons for short-term loss of sleep. When stress interrupts normal sleeping patterns, clients cannot sleep because their minds are too active.

Foods or beverages containing stimulants such as caffeine may interrupt sleep. Clients may also find that the use

PHARMFACTS

Insomnia

- One third of the world's population has trouble sleeping during part of the year.
- Insomnia is more common in women than in men.
- Clients older than 65 sleep less than any other age group.
- Only about 70% of people with insomnia ever report this problem to their healthcare providers.
- People buy OTC sleep medications and combination drugs with sleep additives more often than any other drug category. Examples of trade-name products are Anacin PM, Excedrin PM, Nytol, Quiet World, Sleep-Eez, Sominex, Tylenol PM, and Unison.
- As a natural solution for sleep, some clients consider melatonin or herbal remedies such as valerian or kava (see Chapter 11 ∞).

PHARMFACTS

Insomnia Linked to Insulin Resistance

- Chronic lack of sleep may make people more prone to developing type 2 diabetes, or non-insulin-dependent diabetes mellitus (NIDDM).
- Chronic lack of sleep can provide the impetus for the body to develop a reduced sensitivity to insulin.
- In one study, healthy adults who averaged little more than 5 hours of sleep per night over 8 consecutive nights secreted 50% more insulin than those who averaged 8 hours of sleep per night for the same period. Those who slept less were 40% less sensitive to insulin than those who got more sleep.
- Sleep deprivation (6.5 hours or less per night) may explain why type 2 diabetes is becoming more prevalent.

of tobacco products makes them restless and edgy. Alcohol, although often enabling a person to fall asleep, may produce vivid dreams and frequent awakening that prevent restful sleep. Ingestion of a large meal, especially one high in protein and fat, consumed close to bedtime can interfere with sleep, owing to the increased metabolic rate needed to digest the food. Certain medications cause CNS stimulation, and these should not be taken immediately before bedtime. Stressful conditions such as too much light, uncomfortable room temperature (especially one that is too warm), snoring, sleep apnea, and recurring nightmares also interfere with sleep. **Long-term insomnia** is often caused by depression, manic disorders, and chronic pain.

Nonpharmacological means should be attempted prior to initiating drug therapy for sleep disorders. Long-term use of sleep medications is likely to worsen insomnia and may cause physical or psychological dependence. Some clients experience a phenomenon referred to as **rebound insomnia.** This condition occurs when a sedative drug is discontinued abruptly or after it has been taken for a long time; sleeplessness and symptoms of anxiety then become markedly worse.

Older clients are more likely to experience medication-related sleep problems. Drugs may seem to help the insomnia of an elderly client for a night or two, only to produce generalized brain dysfunction as the medication accumulates in the system. The agitated client may then be mistakenly

NATURAL THERAPIES

Valerian and Kava

Valerian (*Valeriana officinalis*) is a perennial plant native to Europe and North America. Kava (*Piper methysticum*) is a shrub native to the South Pacific islands. Both valerian and kava have active substances in their roots that affect the CNS. Valerian and kava are frequently used for anxiety and insomnia. Recent studies have shown that valerian may not be effective for insomnia, but this result may be dose dependent (Kennedy, Little, Haskell, & Scholey, 2006). High-quality research conducted on kava has proven its antianxiety effect (Ernst, 2006). These herbs are available as tinctures (alcohol mixture) or teas, or in capsule form. Valerian may increase the sedative effects of barbiturates. Kava may interact with a broad range of drugs, including barbiturates, benzodiazepines, and antiparkinsonism agents.

TABLE 14.1	Stages of Sleep
Stage	**Description**
NREM stage 1	At the onset of sleep, the client is in a stage of drowsiness for about 1 to 7 minutes. During this time, the client can be easily awakened. This stage lasts for about 4% to 5% of total sleep time.
NREM stage 2	The client can still be easily awakened. This stage constitutes the greatest amount of total sleep time, 45% to 55%.
NREM stage 3	The client may move into or out of a deeper sleep. Heart rate and blood pressure fall; gastrointestinal activity rises. This stage lasts for about 4% to 6% of total sleep time.
NREM stage 4	The deepest stage of sleep, this stage lasts a little longer than stage 1 or stage 3 sleep, about 12% to 15%. This is the stage during which nightmares occur in children. Sleepwalking is also a common behavior for this stage. Heart rate and blood pressure remain low; gastrointestinal activity remains high.
REM sleep	This stage is characterized by eye movement and a loss of muscle tone. Eye movement occurs in bursts of activity. Dreaming takes place in this stage. The mind is very active and resembles a normal waking state.

overdosed with further medication. Nurses, especially those who work in geriatric settings, are responsible for making accurate observations and reporting client responses to drugs so the healthcare provider can determine the lowest effective maintenance dose. When PRN medication is required for sleep, the nurse needs to conduct an individualized assessment of the individual, as well as follow-up evaluation and documentation of the medication's effect on the client.

14.5 Use of the Electroencephalogram to Diagnose Sleep and Seizure Disorders

The **electroencephalogram (EEG)** is a tool for diagnosing sleep disorders, seizure activity, depression, and dementia. Four types of brain waves—alpha, beta, delta, and theta—are identified by their shape, frequencies, and height on a graph. Brain waves give the healthcare provider an idea of how brain activity changes during various stages of sleep and consciousness. For example, alpha waves indicate an awake but drowsy client. Beta waves indicate an alert client whose mind is active.

Two distinct types of sleep can be identified with an EEG: nonrapid eye movement (NREM) sleep and rapid eye movement (REM) sleep. There are four progressive stages that advance into REM sleep. After NREM sleep has gone through the four stages, the sequence goes into reverse. Under normal circumstances, after returning from the depths of stage IV back to stage I of NREM, a person will still not awaken. Sleep quality begins to change; it is not as deep, and hormone levels and body temperature begin to rise. At that point, REM sleep occurs. **REM sleep** is often called paradoxical sleep, because the brain wave pattern of this stage is similar to that when persons are drowsy but awake. This is the stage during which dreaming occurs. People with normal sleep patterns move from NREM to REM sleep about every 90 minutes.

Clients who are deprived of stage IV NREM sleep experience depression and a feeling of apathy and fatigue. Stage IV NREM sleep appears to be linked to repair and restoration of the physical body, whereas REM sleep is as-

sociated with learning, memory, and the capacity to adjust to changes in the environment. The body requires the dream state associated with REM sleep to keep the psyche functioning normally. When test subjects are deprived of REM sleep, they experience a **sleep debt** and become frightened, irritable, paranoid, and even emotionally disturbed. Judgment is impaired, and reaction time is slowed. It is speculated that to make up for their lack of dreaming, these persons experience far more daydreaming and fantasizing throughout the day. The stages of sleep are shown in Table 14.1.

CENTRAL NERVOUS SYSTEM AGENTS

CNS agents are drugs that produce profound activity in the brain and spinal cord. CNS depressants are agents that slow neuronal activity in the brain. Clients experiencing anxiety or sleep disorders benefit from four general classes of medications: antidepressants, benzodiazepines, barbiturates, and nonbenzodiazepine/nonbarbiturate CNS depressants. Additional drug classes have anxiolytic activity and prevent stressful reactions in the body.

14.6 Treating Anxiety and Insomnia With CNS Agents

Antidepressants are frequently used to treat symptoms of anxiety. These drugs have an ability to reduce anxiety symptoms by altering levels of two important neurotransmitters in the brain, norepinephrine and serotonin. Restoration of neurotransmitter imbalances may reduce symptoms associated with depression, panic, obsessive–compulsive behavior and phobia. Typical antidepressants include tricyclic antidepressants (TCAs), selective serotonin reuptake inhibitors (SSRIs), and monoamine oxidase inhibitors (MAOIs). More detailed treatment of these drugs and their important mechanisms of action are covered in Chapter 16 ∞.

CNS depressants used for anxiety and sleep disorders are categorized into two major classes, the benzodiazepines and barbiturates. A third class consists of miscellaneous drugs that are chemically unrelated to the benzodiazepines or barbiturates but have similar therapeutic uses. Other CNS depressants that have a calming effect in the body include the opioids (Chapter 18 ∞) and ethyl alcohol (Chapter 12 ∞).

CNS depression should be viewed as a continuum ranging from relaxation, to sedation, to the induction of sleep and anesthesia. Coma and death are the end stages of CNS depression. Some drug classes are capable of producing the full range of CNS depression from calming to anesthesia, whereas others are less efficacious. Medications that depress the CNS are sometimes called **sedatives** because of their ability to sedate or relax a client. At higher doses, some of these drugs are called **hypnotics** because of their ability to induce sleep. Thus, the term **sedative–hypnotic** is often used to describe a drug with the ability to produce a calming effect at lower doses and the ability to induce sleep at higher doses. **Tranquilizer** is an older term, sometimes used to describe a drug that produces a calm or tranquil feeling.

Many CNS depressants can cause physical and psychological dependence, as discussed in Chapter 12 ∞. The withdrawal syndrome for some CNS depressants can cause life-threatening neurological reactions, including fever, psychosis, and seizures. Other withdrawal symptoms include increased heart rate and lowered blood pressure; loss of appetite; muscle cramps; impairment of memory, concentration, and orientation; abnormal sounds in the ears and blurred vision; and insomnia, agitation, anxiety, and panic. Obvious withdrawal symptoms typically last 2 to 4 weeks. Subtle ones can last months.

ANTIDEPRESSANTS

Starting in the 1960s, **antidepressants** were used mainly to treat depression or depression that accompanied anxiety. Today, antidepressants are used not only to treat major depression (Chapter 16 ∞), but also to treat anxiety conditions including general anxiety disorder, obsessive–compulsive disorder, panic, social phobia, and post-traumatic stress disorder. Given the effectiveness of antidepressants for these conditions, many believe that in the future, anxiolytics and antidepressants will no longer be treated as separate drug classes.

14.7 Antidepressants for Symptoms of Panic and Anxiety

For most clients, panic symptoms come in two stages. The first stage is termed *anticipatory anxiety,* in which the client begins to think about an upcoming challenge and starts to experience feelings of dread. The second stage is when physical symptoms such as shortness of breath, accelerated heart rate, and muscle tension start to emerge. Many of the stressful symptoms are associated with activation of the autonomic nervous system. For panic attacks, the most useful therapy is to help the client become motivated to face his or her fear and to suppress symptoms in one or more of these stages. If drugs can reduce the negative thoughts associated with the anticipatory component of panic, then there is less likelihood that the client will feel stressed. Drugs also reduce neuronal activity and actually suppress the autonomic nervous system, helping the client to remain calm. The client can then use self-help skills to control his or her behavior.

The primary medications used to reduce symptoms of panic and anxiety are the TCAs, MAOIs, and SSRIs. The medications with the longest track record for treating panic disorders are summarized in Table 14.2. The newer SSRIs treat not only panic symptoms but also symptoms of obsessive–compulsive disorder and phobias (Table 14.3). Popular SSRIs available for treatment of anxiety and

TABLE 14.2	**Antidepressants for Treatment of Panic Disorders**	
Drug	**Route and Adult Dose (max dose where indicated)**	**Adverse Effects**
TRICYCLIC ANTIDEPRESSANTS (TCAs)		
amitriptyline (Elavil)	PO, 75–100 mg/day, may gradually increase to 150–300 mg/day (use lower doses in nonhospitalized clients)	*Drowsiness, sedation, dizziness, orthostatic hypotension, dry mouth, constipation, urine retention, weight gain, tremor, dysrhythmias, blurred vision, slight mydriasis*
clomipramine (Anafranil)	PO; 75–300 mg/day in divided doses	
desipramine (Norpramin, Pertofrane and others)	PO, 75–100 mg/day at bedtime or in divided doses; may gradually increase to 150–300 mg/day (use lower doses in older adult clients)	<u>Heart block</u>
doxepin (Sinequan or Adapin)	PO; 30–150 mg/day at bedtime or in divided doses; may gradually increase to 300 mg/day (use lower doses in older adult clients)	
imipramine (Tofranil) (see page 191 for the Prototype Drug box ∞)	PO; 75–100 mg/day (max: 300 mg/day) in single or divided doses	
nortriptyline (Aventyl, Pamelor)	PO; 25 mg tid or qid, gradually increased to 100–150 mg/day	
MONOAMINE OXIDASE INHIBITORS (MAOIs)		
phenelzine (Nardil)	PO; 15 mg tid, rapidly increasing to at least 60 mg/day; may need up to 90 mg/day	*Orthostatic hypotension, constipation, dry mouth, nausea, anorexia*
tranylcypromine (Parnate)	PO; 30 mg/day in 2 divided doses (20 mg in AM, 10 mg in PM); may increase by 10 mg/day at 3-wk intervals (max: 60 mg/day)	

Italics indicate common adverse effects; <u>underlining</u> indicates serious adverse effects.

TABLE 14.3   Additional Antidepressants as Anxiolytics

Drug	Route and Adult Dose (max dose where indicated)	Adverse Effects
ATYPICAL ANTIDEPRESSANTS		
trazodone (Desyrel)	PO; 150 mg/day in divided doses; may increase by 50 mg/day over 3–4 days (max: 400–600 mg/day)	*Erratic heart rate and blood pressure, orthostatic hypotension, dry mouth, dizziness, somnolence, nausea, vomiting, sweating*
venlafaxine (Effexor) (classified as an SNRI; see Chapter 16 ∞)	PO; start with 37.5 mg/day sustained release and increase to 75–225 mg/day sustained release	Severe hostility, impulsivity, mental status changes that include extreme agitation progressing to delirium and coma, suicidality (especially in children)
SELECTIVE SEROTONIN REUPTAKE INHIBITORS (SSRIs)		
citalopram (Celexa)	PO; start at 20 mg/day; may increase to 40 mg/day if needed	*Nausea, vomiting, dry mouth, insomnia, somnolence, headache, nervousness, anxiety, GI disturbances, anorexia, agitation, dizziness, fatigue*
ⓟ escitalopram oxalate (Lexapro)	PO; 10 mg/day; may increase to 20 mg/day if needed after 1 wk	
fluoxetine (Prozac)	PO; 20 mg/day in AM; may increase by 20 mg/day at weekly intervals (max: 80 mg/day); when stable may switch to one 90-mg sustained-release capsule per week (max: 90 mg/wk)	Stevens-Johnson syndrome, extreme mania/hypomania, and suicidality (especially in children), abnormal bleeding, extreme psychomotor disturbances, seizures, autonomic instability with possible rapid fluctuations of vital signs, severe hyperthermia
fluvoxamine (Luvox)	PO; start with 50 mg/day; may increase slowly up to 300 mg/day given at bedtime or divided bid	
paroxetine (Paxil)	PO; 20–60 mg/day	
sertraline (Zoloft)	PO; begin with 50 mg/day; gradually increase every few weeks according to response (range: 50–200 mg)	

Italics indicate common adverse effects; underlining indicates serious adverse effects.

depression include citalopram (Celexa), escitalopram (Lexapro), fluoxetine (Prozac), paroxetine (Paxil), and sertraline (Zoloft). Escitalopram oxalate (Lexapro) is featured as a prototype drug for generalized anxiety disorder.

It is important to stress that the use of antidepressants must be monitored. In 2004, the Food and Drug Administration issued an advisory warning pointing out the potential warning signs of suicide in adults and children at the beginning of antidepressant treatment and when doses are changed. In addition, certain signs, which are the focus of anxiety therapy, might be expected with some antidepressant medications, for example, irritability, panic attacks, agitation, irritability, insomnia, and hostility. (See Chapter 16 ∞.)

As with all CNS agents, precautions must be taken to make sure medications are taken properly. See Chapter 16 ∞ for important primary actions and adverse effects of antidepressant drugs in general. Because of adverse reactions, some clients might find antidepressant treatment unacceptable.

Following is a brief summary of additional important considerations for each class of antidepressant.

- TCAs—Not recommended in clients with a history of heart attack, heart block, or arrhythmia; clients often have annoying anticholinergic effects such as dry mouth, blurred vision, urine retention, and hypertension (see Chapter 13 ∞); most TCAs are pregnancy category C or D; concurrent use with alcohol or other CNS depressants should be avoided; clients with asthma, gastrointestinal disorders, alcoholism, schizophrenia, or bipolar disorder should take TCAs extreme caution.

- SSRIs—Safer than other classes of antidepressants; less common sympathomimetic effects (increased heart rate and hypertension) and fever anticholinergic effects SSRIs can cause weight gain and sexual dysfunction; an overdose of this medication can cause confusion, anxiety, restlessness, hypertension, tremors, sweating, fever, and lack of muscle coordination.

- MAOIs—Clients should strictly avoid foods containing tyramine, a form of the amino acid tyrosine, to avoid a hypertensive crisis and should refrain from caffeine intake; MAOIs potentiate the effects of insulin and other diabetic drugs; common side effects include orthostatic hypotension, headache, and diarrhea; rarely used because of the potential for serious adverse effects.

- Atypical antidepressants including serotonin–norepinephrine reuptake inhibitors (SNRIs)—A number of side effects might be observed including insomnia, abnormal dreams, sweating, constipation, dry mouth, loss of appetite, weight loss, tremor, abnormal vision, headaches, nausea and vomiting, dizziness, and loss of sexual desire.

BENZODIAZEPINES

The benzodiazepines are one of the most widely prescribed drug classes. The root word *benzo* refers to an aromatic compound, one having a carbon ring structure attached to different atoms or to another carbon ring. Two nitrogen atoms incorporated into the second ring structure account for the diazepine (*di* = two; *azepine* = nitrogen) portion of the name.

Pr PROTOTYPE DRUG | Escitalopram *(Lexapro)* | Selective Serotonin Reuptake Inhibitor

ACTIONS AND USES

Escitalopram is a selective serotonin reuptake inhibitor (SSRI) that increases the availability of serotonin at specific postsynaptic receptor sites located within the CNS. Selective inhibition of serotonin reuptake results in antidepressant activity without production of symptoms of sympathomimetic or anticholinergic activity. This medication is indicated for conditions of generalized anxiety and depression. Unlabeled uses include the treatment of panic disorders.

ADMINISTRATION ALERTS

- You should not begin this medication until 14 days after administration of MAOI drugs.
- In cases of renal or hepatic impairment or in older adults, reduced doses are advised.
- Dose increments should be separated by at least 1 week.
- Pregnancy category C.

PHARMACOKINETICS

Onset: With once-daily dosing, steady-state plasma concentrations can be reached within 1 wk

Peak: 5 h

Half-life: 25–35 h

Duration: Variable

ADVERSE EFFECTS

Serious reactions include dizziness, nausea, insomnia, somnolennce, confusion, and seizures if taken in overdose.

Contraindications: This drug should not be used in clients who are breast-feeding or within 14 days of MAOI therapy.

INTERACTIONS

Drug–Drug: MAOIs should be avoided owing to serotonin syndrome, marked by autonomic hyperactivity, hyperthermia, rigidity, diaphoresis, and neuroleptic malignant syndrome. Combination with MAOIs could result in hypertensive crisis, hyperthermia, and autonomic instability.

Escitalopram will increase plasma levels of metoprolol and cimetidine. Concurrent use of alcohol and other CNS depressants may enhance CNS depressant effects; clients should avoid alcohol when taking this drug.

Lab Tests: Unknown.

Herbal/Food: Use caution with herbal supplements such as St. John's wort, which may cause serotonin syndrome and increase the effects of escitalopram.

Treatment of Overdose: There is no specific treatment for overdose. Treat symptoms, as indicated, including dizziness, confusion, nausea, vomiting, tremor, sweating, tachycardia, and seizures.

 See the Companion Website for a Nursing Process Focus specific to this drug.

See Chapter 16, page 197, for "Nursing Process Focus: Clients Receiving Antidepressant Therapy" ∞.

14.8 Treating Anxiety and Insomnia With Benzodiazepines

The benzodiazepines are drugs of choice for various anxiety disorders and for insomnia (see Table 14.4). Since the introduction of the first benzodiazepines—chlordiazepoxide (Librium) and diazepam (Valium)—in the 1960s, the class has become one of the most widely prescribed in medicine. Although about 15 benzodiazepines are available, all have the same actions and adverse effects, and differ primarily in their onset and duration of action. Some, such as midazolam (Versed), have a rapid onset time of 15 to 30 minutes; others, such as halazepam (Paxipam), take 1 to 3 hours to reach peak serum levels. The benzodiazepines are categorized as Schedule IV drugs, although they produce considerably less physical dependence and result in less tolerance than the barbiturates.

Benzodiazepines act by binding to the gamma-aminobutyric acid (GABA) receptor–chloride channel molecule. These drugs intensify the effect of GABA, which is a natural inhibitory neurotransmitter found throughout the brain. Most are metabolized in the liver to active metabolites and are excreted primarily in urine. One major advantage of the benzodiazepines is that they do not produce life-threatening respiratory depression or coma if taken in excessive amounts. Death is unlikely, unless the benzodiazepines are taken in large quantities in combination with other CNS depressants, or if the client suffers from sleep apnea.

Most benzodiazepines are given orally. Those that can be given parenterally, such as diazepam (Valium) and lorazepam (Ativan), should be monitored carefully owing to their rapid onset of CNS effects, and possible respiratory depression.

The benzodiazepines are drugs of choice for the short-term treatment of insomnia caused by anxiety, having replaced the barbiturates because of their greater margin of safety. Benzodiazepines shorten the length of time it takes to fall asleep and reduce the frequency of interrupted sleep. Although most benzodiazepines increase total sleep time, some reduce stage IV sleep, and some affect REM sleep. In general, the benzodiazepines used to treat short-term insomnia are different from those used to treat generalized anxiety disorder.

Benzodiazepines have a number of other important indications. Diazepam (Valium) is featured as a prototype drug in Chapter 15 ∞ for its use in treating seizure disorders. Other uses include treatment of alcohol withdrawal symptoms (Chapter 12 ∞), central muscle relaxation (Chapter 21 ∞), and as induction agents in general anesthesia (Chapter 19 ∞).

NURSING CONSIDERATIONS

The role of the nurse in benzodiazepine therapy involves careful monitoring of a client's condition and providing education as it relates to the prescribed drug treatment. Assess client needs for antianxiety drugs, including intensity and duration

TABLE 14.4 Benzodiazepines for Anxiety and Insomnia

Drug	Route and Adult Dose (max dose where indicated)	Adverse Effects
ANXIETY THERAPY		
alprazolam (Xanax)	For anxiety: PO; 0.25–0.5 mg tid For panic attacks: PO; 1–2 mg tid	*Drowsiness, sedation, lethargy, ataxia*
chlordiazepoxide (Librium)	Mild anxiety: PO, 5–10 mg tid or qid; IM/IV, 50–100 mg 1 h before a medical procedure Severe anxiety: PO, 20–25 mg tid or qid; IM/IV, 50–100 mg followed by 25–50 mg tid or qid	<u>Acute hyperexcited states, hallucinations, increased muscle spasticity, renal impairment, congenital defects among women who are pregnant, respiratory impairment due to hypersalivation.</u>
clonazepam (Klonopin)	PO; 1–2 mg/day in divided doses (max: 4 mg/day)	
clorazepate (Tranxene)	PO; 15 mg/day at bedtime (max: 60 mg/day in divided doses)	
diazepam (Valium) (see page 177 for the Prototype Drug box ∞)	PO, 2–10 mg bid; IM/IV, 2–10 mg: repeat if needed in 3–4 h	
halazepam (Paxipam)	PO; 20–40 mg tid or qid	
ⓟ lorazepam (Ativan)	PO; 2–6 mg/day in divided doses (max: 10 mg/day)	
oxazepam (Serax)	PO; 10–30 mg tid or qid	
INSOMNIA THERAPY		
estazolam (Prosom)	PO; 1 mg at bedtime; may increase to 2 mg if necessary	
flurazepam (Dalmane)	PO; 15–30 mg at bedtime	
quazepam (Doral)	PO; 7.5–15 mg at bedtime	
temazepam (Restoril)	PO; 7.5–30 mg at bedtime	
triazolam (Halcion)	PO; 0.125–0.25 mg at bedtime (max: 0.5 mg/day)	

Italics indicate common adverse effects; <u>underlining</u> indicates serious adverse effects.

of symptoms. Identify factors that precipitate anxiety or insomnia: physical symptoms, excessive CNS stimulation, excessive daytime sleep, or too little exercise or activity. Obtain a drug history, including hypersensitivity and the use of alcohol and other CNS depressants. Assess for the likelihood of drug abuse and dependence, and identify coping mechanisms used in managing previous episodes of stress, anxiety, and insomnia. Use cautiously in clients with a suicidal potential, because the risk of suicide may be increased. Assess for the existence of a primary sleep disorder, such as sleep apnea, because benzodiazepines depress respiratory drive.

Alterations in neurotransmitter activity produce changes in intraocular pressure; therefore, benzodiazepines are contraindicated in narrow-angle glaucoma. The presence of any organic brain disease is another contraindication, because these drugs alter the level of consciousness. Monitor liver and kidney function in long-term use. These drugs should be used cautiously in those clients with impaired renal or liver function. Consider the risk of respiratory depression when administering to clients with impaired respiratory function or in those taking other CNS depressants, and when giving intravenous doses. Assess for common side effects related to CNS depression such as drowsiness and dizziness, because these increase a client's risk of injury and may indicate a need for dose reduction. Should an overdose occur, flumazenil (Romazicon) is a specific benzodiazepine receptor antagonist that can be administered to reverse CNS depression.

Benzodiazepines are used illegally for recreation, most often by adolescents, young adults, and opioid or cocaine addicts. Therefore, help clients evaluate the social context of their environment, and take any precautions necessary to safeguard the medication supply.

Lifespan Considerations. Few studies of using benzodiazepines in the pediataric population have been done; therefore, it is recommended that they be used cautiously in this population. Because benzodiazepines cross the placenta and are excreted in breast milk, they are not recommended in pregnant or nursing women (pregnancy category D). Use cautiously in elderly clients, because metabolism and excretion are slowed, and there is a higher potenial for overdose. Assess elderly clients for oversedation, confusion, dizziness, and impaired mobility. Ensure that client safety is maintained.

Client Teaching. Client education as it relates to benzodiazepines should include the goals of therapy, the reasons for obtaining baseline data such as vital signs or the existence of underlying hepatic or renal disorders, and possible drug side effects. Include the following points when teaching clients about benzodiazepines:

- Use caution when driving or operating heavy machinery until the effect of the medication is known. Benzodiazepines can cause drowsiness and impair mental and physical functioning.
- Take the medication as directed. Do not exceed the ordered dosage.
- Avoid alcohol and other CNS depressants, because they may cause increased drowsiness.

Pr **PROTOTYPE DRUG** | Lorazepam *(Ativan)* | Benzodiazepine

ACTIONS AND USES

Lorazepam is a benzodiazepine that acts by potentiating the effects of GABA, an inhibitory neurotransmitter, in the thalamic, hypothalamic, and limbic levels of the CNS. It is one of the most potent benzodiazepines. It has an extended half-life of 10 to 20 hours, which allows for once or twice a day oral dosing. In addition to being used as an anxiolytic, lorazepam is used as a preanesthetic medication to provide sedation, and for the management of status epilepticus.

ADMINISTRATION ALERTS

- When administering IV, monitor respirations every 5 to 15 minutes. Have airway and resuscitative equipment accessible.
- Pregnancy category D.

PHARMACOKINETICS

Onset: 1–5 min IV; 15–30 min IM

Peak: 2 h PO; 90 min IM

Half-life: 10–20 h

Duration: Variable

ADVERSE EFFECTS

The most common side effects of lorazepam are drowsiness and sedation, which may decrease with time. When given in higher doses or by the IV route, more severe effects may be observed, such as amnesia, weakness, disorientation, ataxia, sleep disturbance, blood pressure changes, blurred vision, double vision, nausea, and vomiting.

Contraindications: This drug should not be used in clients with acute narrow-angle glaucoma, primary depressive disorders, or psychosis, and should be avoided for the management of severe uncontrolled pain

INTERACTIONS

Drug–Drug: Lorazepam interacts with multiple drugs. For example, concurrent use of CNS depressants, including alcohol, potentiates sedation effects and increases the risk of respiratory depression and death. Lorazepam may contribute to digoxin toxicity by increasing the serum digoxin level. Symptoms include visual changes, nausea, vomiting, dizziness, and confusion.

Lorazepam may decrease antiparkinsonism effects of levodopa and increase phenytoin levels.

Lab Tests: Unknown.

Herbal/Food: Use cautiously with herbal supplements. For example, sedation-producing herbs such as kava, valerian, chamomile, or hops may have an additive effect with medication. Stimulant herbs such as gotu-kola and ma huang may reduce the drug's effectiveness.

Treatment of Overdose: If overdose occurs, flumazenil (Romazicon), a specific benzodiazepine receptor antagonist, can be administered to reverse CNS depressant effects.

 See the Companion Website for a Nursing Process Focus specific to this drug.

- Do not stop taking medication suddenly, because withdrawal symptoms may occur.
- Store medication safely out of reach of children.

BARBITURATES

Barbiturates are drugs derived from barbituric acid. They are powerful CNS depressants prescribed for their sedative, hypnotic, and antiseizure effects that have been used in pharmacotherapy since the early 1900s.

14.9 Use of Barbiturates as Sedatives

Until the discovery of the benzodiazepines, barbiturates were the drugs of choice for treating anxiety and insomnia (see Table 14.5). Although barbiturates are still indicated for several conditions, they are rarely, if ever, prescribed for treating anxiety or insomnia because of significant side effects and the availability of more effective medications. The risk of psychological and physical dependence is high—several are Schedule II drugs. The withdrawal syndrome from barbiturates is extremely severe and can be fatal. Overdose results in profound respiratory depression, hypotension, and shock. Barbiturates have been used to commit suicide, and death due to overdose is not uncommon.

Barbiturates are capable of depressing CNS function at all levels. Like benzodiazepines, barbiturates act by binding to GABA receptor–chloride channel molecules, intensifying the effect of GABA throughout the brain. At low doses they reduce anxiety and cause drowsiness. At moderate doses they inhibit seizure activity (Chapter 15 ∞) and promote sleep, presumably by inhibiting brain impulses traveling through the limbic system and the reticular activating system. At higher doses, some barbiturates can induce anesthesia (Chapter 19 ∞).

When taken for prolonged periods, barbiturates stimulate the microsomal enzymes in the liver that metabolize medications. Thus, barbiturates can stimulate their own metabolism, as well as that of hundreds of other drugs that use these enzymes for their breakdown. With repeated use, tolerance develops to the sedative effects of the drug; this includes cross-tolerance to other CNS depressants such as the opioids. Tolerance does not develop, however, to the respiratory depressant effects. (See Chapter 15, page 182, for "Nursing Process Focus: Clients Receiving Antiseizure Drug Therapy." ∞)

TABLE 14.5 Barbiturates for Sedation and Insomnia

Drug	Route and Adult Dose (max dose where indicated)	Adverse Effects
SHORT ACTING		
pentobarbital sodium (Nembutal)	Sedative: PO; 20–30 mg bid or qid Hypnotic: PO, 120–200 mg; IM, 150–200 mg	<u>Respiratory depression, laryngospasm, apnea</u>
secobarbital (Seconal)	Sedative: PO; 100–300 mg/day in 3 divided doses Hypnotic: PO/IM; 100–200 mg	
INTERMEDIATE ACTING		
amobarbital (Amytal)	Sedative: PO; 30–50 mg bid or tid Hypnotic: PO/IM; 65–200 mg (max: 500 mg)	*Residual sedation*
aprobarbital (Alurate)	Sedative: PO; 40 mg tid Hypnotic: PO; 40–160 mg	<u>Agranulocytosis, angioedema, Stevens-Johnson syndrome, respiratory depression, circulatory collapse, apnea, respiratory depression, laryngospasm</u>
butabarbital sodium (Butisol)	Sedative: PO; 15–30 mg tid or qid Hypnotic: PO; 50–100 mg at bedtime	
LONG ACTING		
mephobarbital (Mebaral)	Sedative: PO; 32–100 mg tid or qid	*Drowsiness*
phenobarbital (Luminal) (see page 176 for the Prototype Drug box ∞)	Sedative: PO; 30–120 mg/day IV/IM; 100–200 mg/day	<u>Agranulocytosis, respiratory depression, Stevens–Johnson syndrome, exfoliative dermatitis (rare), CNS depression, coma, death</u>

Italics indicate common adverse effects; <u>underlining</u> indicates serious adverse effects.

14.10 Other CNS Depressants for Anxiety and Sleep Disorders

The final group of CNS depressants used for anxiety and sleep disorders consists of miscellaneous agents that are chemically unrelated to either benzodiazepines or barbiturates (see Table 14.6). In addition to nonbenzodiazepine, nonbarbiturate CNS depressants, other drugs used mainly for treatment of social anxiety symptoms include the antiseizure medication valproate (Depakote), and the beta blockers atenolol (Inderal) and propanolol (Tenormin). Drugs used mainly for insomnia therapy include the newest of all nonbenzodiazepine CNS depressants, zaleplon (Sonata), eszopiclone (Lunesta), and the relatively new drug zolpidem (Ambien). Older CNS depressants such as paraldehyde (Paracetaldehyde), chloral hydrate (Noctec), meprobamate

---

Pr **PROTOTYPE DRUG** | Zolpidem *(Ambien)* | Nonbenzodiazepine, Nonbarbiturate CNS Depressant

ACTIONS AND USES

Although a nonbenzodiazepine, zolpidem acts in a similar fashion to facilitate GABA-mediated CNS depression in the limbic, thalamic, and hypothalamic regions. It preserves stages III and IV of sleep and has only minor effects on REM sleep. The only indication for zolpidem is for short-term insomnia management (7 to 10 days).

ADMINISTRATION ALERTS

- Because of rapid onset, 7–27 minutes, give immediately before bedtime.
- Pregnancy category B.

PHARMACOKINETICS

Onset: 7–27 min

Peak: 0.5–2.3 h

Half-life: 1.7–2.5 h

Duration: 6–8 h

ADVERSE EFFECTS

Side effects include daytime sedation, confusion, amnesia, dizziness, depression, nausea, and vomiting.

Contraindications: Lactating women should not take this drug.

INTERACTIONS

Drug–Drug: Drug interactions with zolpidem include an increase in sedation when used concurrently with other CNS depressants, including alcohol. Phenothiazines augment CNS depression.

Lab Tests: Unknown.

Herbal/Food: When taken with food, absorption is slowed significantly, and the onset of action may be delayed.

Treatment of Overdose: Generalized symptomatic and supportive measures should be applied with immediate gastric lavage where appropriate. IV fluids should be administered as needed. Use of flumazenil (Romazicon) as a benzodiazepine receptor antagonist may be helpful.

See the Companion Website for a Nursing Process Focus specific to this drug.

MediaLink | Mechanism in Action: Zolpidem

TABLE 14.6   Miscellaneous Drugs for Anxiety and Insomnia

Drug	Route and Adult Dose (max dose where indicated)	Adverse Effects
NONBENZODIAZEPINE, NONBARBITURATE CNS DEPRESSANTS		
buspirone (BuSpar)	Sedative: PO; 7.5–15 mg in divided doses; may increase by 5 mg/day every 2–3 days if needed (max: 60 mg/day)	*Dizziness, headache, drowsiness, nausea, fatigue, ataxia vomiting, bitter metallic taste, dry mouth, diarrhea, hypotension*
chloral hydrate (Noctec)	Sedative: PO or by suppositories; 250 mg tid after meals Hypnotic: PO; 500 mg–1 g 15–30 min before bedtime	
dexmedetomidine HCl (Precedex)	Sedative: IV; loading dose 1 mcg/kg over 10 min; maintenance dose 0.2–0.7 mcg/kg/h	<u>Angioedema, cardiac arrest, exfoliative dermatitis (rare); Stevens-Johnson syndrome, anaphylaxis, respiratory failure, coma, sudden death</u>
eszopiclone (Lunesta)	Hypnotic: PO; 2 mg at bedtime; depending on the age, clinical response, and tolerance of the client, dose may be lowered to 1 mg PO	
ethchlorvynol (Placidyl)	Sedative: PO; 200 mg bid or tid Hypnotic: PO; 500 mg–1 g at bedtime	
glutethimide (Doriglute)	Hypnotic: PO 250–500 mg at bedtime	
meprobamate (Equanil)	Sedative: PO; 1.2–1.6 g/day in 3–4 divided doses (max: 2.4 g/day) Hypnotic: PO 400–800 mg	
paraldehyde (Paracetaldehyde)	Sedative: PO; 5–10 ml PRN Hypnotic: 10–30 ml PRN	
zaleplon (Sonata)	Hypnotic: PO 10 mg at bedtime (max: 20 mg/day)	
⊘ zolpidem (Ambien)	Hypnotic: PO; 5–10 mg at bedtime	
ANTISEIZURE MEDICATION		
valproic acid (Depakene) (see page 180 for the Prototype Drug box ∞)	Social anxiety symptoms: PO; 250 mg tid (max: 60 mg/kg/day)	*Sedation, drowsiness, nausea, vomiting, prolonged bleeding time* <u>Deep coma with overdose, liver failure, pancreatitis, prolonged bleeding time</u>
BETA BLOCKERS		
atenolol (Tenormin) (see page 353 for the Prototype Drug box ∞)	Social anxiety symptoms: PO; 25–100 mg/day	*Bradycardia, hypotension, confusion, fatigue, drowsiness*
propranolol (Inderal) (see page 369 for the Prototype Drug box ∞)	Social anxiety symptoms: PO; 40 mg bid (max: up to 320 mg/day)	<u>Anaphylactic reactions, Stevens–Johnson syndrome, toxic epidermal necrolysis, exfoliative dermatitis, agranulocytosis, aryngospasm, bronchospasm</u>

Italics indicate common adverse effects; <u>underlining</u> indicates serious adverse effects.

(Equanil), and glutethimide (Doriglute) have only historical interest, because they are so rarely prescribed owing to their potential for serious adverse effects. Buspirone (BuSpar) and zolpidem (Ambien) are commonly prescribed for their anxiolytic effects. Zolpidem (Ambien) and eszopiclone (Lunesta) are used for their hypnotic effects.

The mechanism of action for buspirone (BuSpar) is unclear but appears to be related to D_2 dopamine receptors in the brain. The drug has agonist effects on presynaptic dopamine receptors and a high affinity for serotonin receptors. Buspirone is less likely than benzodiazepines to affect cognitive and motor performance and rarely interacts with other CNS depressants. Common side effects include dizziness, headache, and drowsiness. Dependence and withdrawal problems are less of a concern with buspirone. Therapy may take several weeks to achieve optimal results.

Zolpidem (Ambien) is a Schedule IV controlled substance limited to the short-term treatment of insomnia. It is highly specific to the GABA receptor (Chapter 15 ∞) and produces muscle relaxation and anticonvulsant effects only at doses much higher than the hypnotic dose. As with other CNS depressants it should be used cautiously in clients with respiratory impairment, in the elderly, and when used concurrently with other CNS depressants. Lower dosages may be necessary. Also, because of the rapid onset of this drug (7 to 27 minutes), it should be taken just prior to expected sleep. Because zolpidem is metabolized in the liver and excreted by the kidneys, impaired liver or kidney function can increase serum drug levels. Zolpidem is in pregnancy category B. Zolpidem is used with caution in individuals with a high risk of suicide, because there is a potential for intentional overdose. Adverse reactions are usually minimal (mild nausea, dizziness, diarrhea, daytime drowsiness), but rebound insomnia may occur when the drug is discontinued. Other adverse effects are amnesia and sleepwalking.

Although structurally unrelated to other drugs used to treat insomnia, eszopiclone (Lunesta) has properties similar to those of zolpidem (Ambien). The effectiveness of eszopiclone

NURSING PROCESS FOCUS Clients Receiving Benzodiazepine and Nonbenzodiazepine Antianxiety Therapy

Assessment	Potential Nursing Diagnoses
Prior to administration: • Obtain complete health history (both physical and mental), including allergies and drug history for possible drug interactions. • Identify factors that precipitate anxiety or insomnia. • Assess likelihood of drug abuse and dependence. • Establish baseline vital signs and level of consciousness.	• Injury, Risk for • Anxiety • Noncompliance • Knowledge, Deficient, related to drug therapy • Coping, Ineffective • Sleep Pattern, Disturbed • Activity Intolerance, Risk for

Planning: Client Goals and Expected Outcomes

The client will:
• Report absence or decrease (use scale) of physical and behavioral manifestations of anxiety.
• Demonstrate an understanding of the drug's action by accurately describing drug side effects and precautions.
• Verbalize the need to discuss with the healthcare provider any intention to discontinue the drug and the importance of not withdrawing the drug abruptly.
• Report ability to tolerate usual activities of daily living without excessive drowsiness and fatigue.

Implementation

Interventions and (Rationales)	Client Education/Discharge Planning
• Monitor vital signs. Observe respiratory patterns, especially during sleep, for evidence of apnea or shallow breathing. (Benzodiazepines can reduce the respiratory drive in susceptible clients.)	• Instruct client to consult the healthcare provider before taking this drug if snoring is a problem. Snoring may indicate an obstruction in the upper respiratory tract resulting in hypoxia. • Teach client to monitor vital signs at home, especially respirations.
• Monitor neurological status, especially level of consciousness. (Confusion or lack of response may indicate overmedication.)	• Instruct client to report extreme lethargy, slurred speech, disorientation, or ataxia.
• Ensure client safety. (Drug may cause excessive drowsiness and increase risk for injury.)	Instruct client to: • Avoid driving or performing hazardous activities until effects of drug are known. • Request assistance when getting out of bed and walking until effect of medication is known.
• Monitor the client's intake of stimulants, including caffeine (in beverages such as coffee, tea, cola and other soft drinks, and OTC analgesics such as Excedrin), and nicotine from tobacco products and nicotine patches. (These products can reduce the drug's effectiveness.)	Instruct client to: • Avoid taking OTC sleep-inducing antihistamines, such as diphenhydramine. • Contact the healthcare provider before self-medicating with any OTC preparation.
• Monitor affect and emotional status. (Drug may increase risk of mental depression, especially in clients with suicidal tendencies.)	Instruct client to: • Report significant mood changes, especially depression. • Avoid consumption of alcohol and other CNS depressants while on benzodiazepines.
• Avoid abrupt discontinuation of therapy. (Withdrawal symptoms, including rebound anxiety and sleeplessness, are possible with abrupt discontinuation after long-term use.)	Instruct client to: • Take drug exactly as prescribed. • Keep all follow-up appointments as directed by healthcare provider to monitor response to medication.
• Assess prior methods of stress reduction. Reinforce previously used effective methods and teach new coping skills. (This will assist client to use medications for the shortest time possible and build self-confidence.)	• Instruct client to use nonpharmacological methods for reestablishing sleep regimen.

Evaluation of Outcome Criteria

Evaluate the effectiveness of drug therapy by confirming that client goals and expected outcomes have been met (see "Planning").
• The client reports a decrease in physical and behavioral manifestations of anxiety.
• The client demonstrates an understanding of the drug's actions by accurately describing drug side effects and precautions.
• The client verbalizes the importance of not discontinuing the drug abruptly.
• The client reports the ability to tolerate usual activities of daily living without excessive drowsiness and fatigue.

∞ *See Tables 14.2 and 14.4 for lists of drugs to which these nursing actions apply.*

has been shown in outpatient and sleep lab studies, but the drug has not directly been compared with zolpidem or other hypnotics. However, eszopiclone's longer elimination half-life, about twice as long as that of zolpidem, may give it an advantage in maintaining sleep and decreasing early-morning awakening. On the other hand, eszopiclone is more likely to cause daytime sedation.

Zaleplon (Sonata) may be useful for people who fall asleep but awake early in the morning, for example, 2:00 A.M. or 3:00

A.M. It is sometimes used for travel purposes and has been advertised by pharmaceutical companies for this purpose.

Two drugs not listed in Table 14.6 are diphenhydramine (Benadryl) and hydroxyzine (Vistaril). These are antihistamines that produce drowsiness and may be beneficial in calming clients. They offer the advantage of not causing dependence, although their use is often limited by anticholinergic side effects. Diphenhydramine is a common component of OTC sleep aids (Chapter 38 ∞).

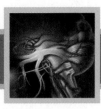

CHAPTER REVIEW

KEY CONCEPTS

The numbered key concepts provide a succinct summary of the important points from the corresponding numbered section within the chapter. If any of these points are not clear, refer to the numbered section within the chapter for review.

14.1 Generalized anxiety disorder is the most common type of anxiety; phobias, obsessive–compulsive disorder, panic attacks, and post-traumatic stress disorders are other important categories.

14.2 The limbic system and the reticular activating system are specific regions of the brain responsible for anxiety and wakefulness.

14.3 Anxiety can be managed through pharmacological and nonpharmacological strategies.

14.4 Insomnia is a sleep disorder that may be caused by anxiety. Nonpharmacological means should be attempted prior to initiating pharmacotherapy.

14.5 The electroencephalogram records brain waves and is used to diagnose sleep and seizure disorders.

14.6 CNS agents, including anxiolytics, sedatives, and hypnotics, are used to treat anxiety and insomnia.

14.7 When taken properly, antidepressants can reduce symptoms of panic and anxiety. Primary medications include tricyclic antidepressants (TCAs), monoamine oxidase inhibitors (MAOIs), and selective serotonin reuptake inhibitors (SSRIs).

14.8 Benzodiazepines are drugs of choice for generalized anxiety and insomnia.

14.9 Because of their side effects and high potential for dependency, barbiturates are arely used to treat insomnia.

14.10 Some commonly prescribed agents and CNS depressants not related to the benzodiazepines or barbiturates are used for the treatment of anxiety and sleeplessness.

NCLEX-RN® REVIEW QUESTIONS

1 The nurse should assess a client who is taking lorazepam (Ativan) for the development of which of these side effects?

1. Tachypnea
2. Astigmatism
3. Ataxia
4. Euphoria

2 A client is receiving temazepam (Restoril). Which of these responses should a nurse expect the client to have if the medication is achieving the desired affect?

1. The client sleeps in 3-hour intervals, awakes for a short time, and then falls back to sleep.
2. The client reports feeling less anxiety during activities of daily living.
3. The client reports having fewer episodes of panic attacks when stressed.
4. The client reports sleeping 7 hours without awakening.

3 A 32-year-old female client has been taking propranolol (Inderal) for her anxiety. On assessment, the nurse would identify which of the following symptoms as being related to Stevens–Johnson syndrome? (Select all that apply.)

1. Fever, chills, and malaise
2. Generalized blister-like lesions
3. Headache, nervousness, and insomnia
4. Skin sloughing
5. Edema

4 A client has been given instructions about the newly prescribed medication alprazolam (Xanax). Which of these statements, if made by the client, would indicate that the client needs further instruction?

1. "I will stop smoking by undergoing hypnosis."
2. "I will not drive immediately after I take this medication."
3. "I will stop the medicine when I feel less anxious."
4. "I will take my medication with food if my stomach feels upset."

5 A client has been taking diazepam (Valium) for 3 months. Which of these statements by the client would indicate that the outcome of medication therapy has been successful?

1. "I will need to take this medication for the rest of my life."
2. "I feel like I am able to cope with routine stress at my job."
3. "I like this medication. I know that I needed it to treat my anxiety, which is now better, but I think it just makes me feel good, so I am planning to stay on it for quite a while."
4. "I thought this medication would make me think clearly, but I don't feel any change in my feelings."

CRITICAL THINKING QUESTIONS

1. A 58-year-old male client underwent an emergency coronary artery bypass graft. He suffered complications while in the cardiac intensive care unit and spent 3 days on a ventilator. He is still experiencing a high degree of pain and also states that he cannot fall asleep. The client has been ordered secobarbital (Seconal) at night for sleep and also has a prescribed opioid analgesic. As the nurse, explain to the student nurse why both medications should be administered.

2. A 42-year-old female client with ovarian cancer suffered profound nausea and vomiting after her first round of chemotherapy. The oncologist has added lorazepam (Ativan)

2 mg per IV piggyback with ondansetron (Zofran) as part of the prechemotherapy regimen. Consult a drug handbook and discuss the purpose for adding this benzodiazepine.

3. An 82-year-old female client complains that she "just can't get good rest anymore." She says that she has come to her doctor to get something to help her sleep. What information can the nurse offer this client regarding the normal changes in sleep patterns associated with aging? What would you recommend for this client?

See Appendix D for answers and rationales for all activities.

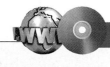

EXPLORE
MediaLink

www.prenhall.com/adams

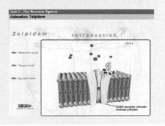

 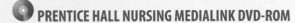

NCLEX-RN® review, case studies, and other interactive resources for this chapter can be found on the companion website at www.prenhall.com/adams. Click on "Chapter 14" to select the activities for this chapter. For animations, more NCLEX-RN® review questions, and an audio glossary, access the accompanying Prentice Hall Nursing MediaLink DVD-ROM in this textbook.

PRENTICE HALL NURSING MEDIALINK DVD-ROM

- **Animations**
  Mechanism in Action: Escitalopram (*Lexapro*)
  Mechanism in Action: Zolpidem (*Ambien*)
- **Audio Glossary**
- **NCLEX-RN® Review**

COMPANION WEBSITE

- **NCLEX-RN® Review**
- **Dosage Calculations**
- **Case Study:** Client taking lorazepam and digoxin
- **Care Plan:** Client experiencing severe anxiety attacks who is taking diazepam

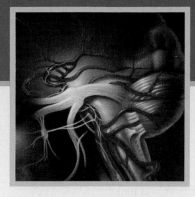

CHAPTER 15

Drugs for Seizures

DRUGS AT A GLANCE

DRUGS THAT POTENTIATE GABA ACTION
Barbiturates
　🖭 *phenobarbital (Luminal)*
Benzodiazepines
　🖭 *diazepam (Valium)*
Miscellaneous GABA Agents
HYDANTOINS AND
PHENYTOIN-LIKE DRUGS
　🖭 *phenytoin (Dilantin)*
　🖭 *valproic acid (Depakene)*
SUCCINIMIDES
　🖭 *ethosuximide (Zarontin)*

OBJECTIVES

After reading this chapter, the student should be able to:

1. Compare and contrast the terms epilepsy, seizures, and convulsions.
2. Recognize the causes of epilepsy.
3. Relate signs and symptoms to specific types of seizures.
4. Describe the nurse's role in the pharmacological management of epilepsy.
5. Explain the importance of client drug compliance in the pharmacotherapy of epilepsy.
6. For each of the drug classes listed in Drugs at a Glance, know representative drug examples and explain their mechanism of drug action, primary actions, and important adverse effects.
7. Categorize drugs used in the treatment of epilepsy based on their classification and mechanism of action.
8. Use the Nursing Process to care for clients receiving drug therapy for epilepsy.

MediaLink

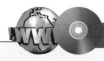 **www.prenhall.com/adams**

NCLEX-RN® review, case studies, and other interactive resources for this chapter can be found on the companion website at www.prenhall.com/adams. Click on "Chapter 15" to select the activities for this chapter. For animations, more NCLEX-RN® review questions, and an audio glossary, access the accompanying Prentice Hall Nursing MediaLink DVD-ROM in this textbook.

KEY TERMS

absence seizure   *page 176*

atonic seizure   *page 172*

convulsions   *page 170*

eclampsia   *page 171*

epilepsy   *page 170*

febrile seizure   *page 171*

gamma-aminobutyric acid (GABA)   *page 173*

generalized seizure   *page 171*

myoclonic seizure   *page 176*

partial (focal) seizure   *page 171*

seizure   *page 170*

status epilepticus   *page 174*

tonic–clonic seizure   *page 172*

E*pilepsy* may be defined as any disorder characterized by recurrent seizures. The symptoms of epilepsy depend on the type of seizure and may include blackout, fainting spells, sensory disturbances, jerking body movements, and temporary loss of memory. As the most common neurological disease, more than 2 million Americans have epilepsy. This chapter examines the pharmacotherapy of the different types of seizures.

SEIZURES

A **seizure** is a disturbance of electrical activity in the brain that may affect consciousness, motor activity, and sensation. The symptoms of seizure are caused by abnormal or uncontrollable neuronal discharges within the brain. These abnormal discharges can be measured using an electroencephalogram (EEG), a valuable tool in diagnosing seizure disorders. • Figure 15.1 compares normal and abnormal EEG recordings.

The terms *convulsion* and *seizure* are not synonymous. **Convulsions** specifically refer to involuntary, violent spasms of the large skeletal muscles of the face, neck, arms, and legs. Although some types of seizures do indeed involve convulsions, other seizures do not. Thus, it may be stated that all convulsions are seizures, but not all seizures are convulsions. Because of this difference, agents used to treat epilepsy will be described here as antiseizure medications, rather than anticonvulsants.

15.1 Causes of Seizures

A seizure is considered a symptom of an underlying disorder, rather than a disease in itself. There are many different etiologies of seizure activity. Seizures can result from acute situations or occur on a chronic basis, as with **epilepsy.** In some cases, the exact etiology may not be identified. The following are known causes of seizures.

- *Infectious diseases* Acute infections such as meningitis and encephalitis can cause inflammation in the brain.
- *Trauma* Physical trauma such as direct blows to the skull may increase intracranial pressure; chemical trauma such as the presence of toxic substances or the ingestion of poisons may cause brain injury.
- *Metabolic disorders* Changes in fluid and electrolytes such as hypoglycemia, hyponatremia, and water intoxication may cause seizures by altering electrical impulse transmission at the cellular level.
- *Vascular diseases* Changes in oxygenation such as those caused by respiratory hypoxia and carbon monoxide poisoning, and changes in perfusion such as those caused by hypotension, cerebral vascular accidents, shock, and cardiac dysrhythmias may be causes.

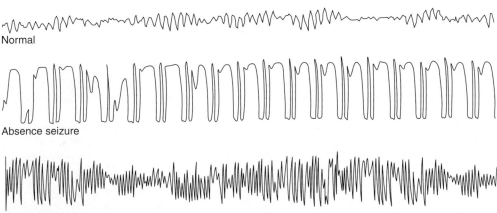

Normal

Absence seizure

Generalized tonic–clonic seizure

● **Figure 15.1** EEG recordings showing the differences between normal, absence seizure, and generalized tonic–clonic seizure tracings

- *Pediatric disorders* Rapid increase in body temperature may result in a **febrile seizure.**
- *Neoplastic disease* Tumors, especially rapidly growing ones, may occupy space, increase intracranial pressure, and damage brain tissue by disrupting blood flow.

Certain medications for mood disorders, psychoses, and local anesthesia when given in high doses may cause seizures because of increased levels of stimulatory neurotransmitters or toxicity. Seizures may also occur from drug abuse, as with cocaine, or during withdrawal syndromes from alcohol or sedative–hypnotic drugs.

Pregnancy is a major concern for clients with epilepsy. Additional barrier methods of birth control should be practiced to avoid unintended pregnancy, as some antiseizure medications decrease the effectiveness of oral contraceptives. Most antiseizure drugs are pregnancy category D. Clients should consult with their healthcare provider prior to pregnancy to determine the most appropriate plan of action for seizure control, given their seizure history. As some antiseizure drugs may cause folate deficiency, a condition correlated with increased risk of neural tube defects, vitamin supplements may be necessary. Pregnant women may experience seizures with **eclampsia,** a pregnancy-induced hypertensive disorder.

In some cases, the etiology of the seizures cannot be found. Clients may have a lower tolerance to environmental triggers, and seizures may occur when sleep deprived, exposed to strobe or flickering lights, or when small fluid and electrolyte imbalances occur. Seizures represent the most common serious neurological problem affecting children, with an overall incidence approaching 2% for febrile seizures and 1% for idiopathic epilepsy. Seizures that result from acute situations generally do not recur after the situation has been resolved. If a brain abnormality exists after the acute situation resolves, continuing seizures are likely.

Seizures can have a significant impact on the quality of life. They may cause serious injury if they occur while a person is driving a vehicle or performing a dangerous activity. Without pharmacotherapy, epilepsy can severely limit participation in school, employment, and social activities and can affect self-esteem. Chronic depression may accompany poorly controlled seizures. Proper treatment, however, can eliminate seizures completely in many clients. Important considerations in nursing care include identifying clients at risk for seizures, documenting the pattern and type of seizure activity, and implementing safety precautions. In collaboration with the client, healthcare provider, and pharmacist, the nurse is instrumental in achieving positive therapeutic outcomes. Through a combination of pharmacotherapy, client–family support, and education, effective seizure control can be achieved by the majority of clients.

15.2 Types of Seizures

The differing presentation of seizures relates to the areas of the brain affected by the abnormal electrical activity. Symptoms of a seizure can range from sudden, violent shaking and total loss of consciousness to muscle twitching or slight tremor of a limb. Staring into space, altered vision, and difficult speech are other behaviors a person may exhibit during a seizure. Determining the cause of recurrent seizures is important for planning appropriate treatment options.

Methods of classifying epilepsy have evolved over time. For example, the terms *grand mal* and *petit mal* epilepsy have, for the most part, been replaced by more descriptive and detailed categorization. Epilepsies are typically identified using the International Classification of Epileptic Seizures nomenclature, as partial (focal), generalized, and special epileptic syndromes (see Table 15.1). Types of **partial (focal)** or **generalized seizures** may be recognized based on symptoms observed during a seizure episode. Some symptoms are subtle and reflect the simple nature of neuronal misfiring in specific areas of the brain; others are more complex.

15.3 General Concepts of Epilepsy Pharmacotherapy

The choice of drug for epilepsy pharmacotherapy depends on the type of seizures the client is experiencing, the client's previous medical history, diagnostic studies, and the pathological processes causing the seizures. Once a medication is selected, the client is placed on a low initial dose. The amount is gradually increased until seizure control is achieved, or the side effects of the drug prevent additional increases in dose. Serum drug levels may be obtained to assist the healthcare provider in determining the most effective drug concentration. If seizure activity continues, a different medication is added in small-dose increments while the dose of the first drug is slowly reduced. Because seizures are likely to occur if antiseizure drugs are abruptly withdrawn, the medication is discontinued over a period of 6 to 12 weeks.

In most cases, effective seizure management can be obtained using a single drug. In some clients, two antiseizure medications may be necessary to control seizure activity, although additional side effects may become evident. Some antiseizure drug combinations may actually increase the incidence of seizures. The nurse should consult with current drug guides regarding compatibility before a second antiseizure agent is added to the regimen.

Once seizures have been controlled, clients are continued indefinitely on the antiseizure drug. After several years of being seizure free, clients may question the need for their medication. In general, withdrawal of antiseizure drugs should

---

SPECIAL CONSIDERATIONS

Seizure Etiologies Based on Genetics and Age-related Factors

- The etiologies that trigger the development of childhood epilepsy vary according to age.
- Congenital abnormalities of the CNS, perinatal brain injury, and metabolic imbalances are usually related to seizure activity in neonates, infants, and toddlers.
- Inherited epilepsies, CNS infections, and neurological degenerative disorders are linked to seizures that have their onset in later childhood.
- Cerebral trauma, cerebrovascular disorders, and neoplastic disease represent the most frequent causes of seizures in the adult population.

TABLE 15.1   Classification of Seizures and Symptoms

Classification	Type	Symptoms
partial	simple partial complex partial (psychomotor)	• olfacatory, auditory, and visual hallucinations • intense emotions • twitching of arms, legs, and face • aura (preceding) • brief period of confusion or sleepiness afterward with no memory of seizure • fumbling with or attempting to remove clothing • no response to verbal commands
general	absence (petit mal) **atonic** (drop attacks) **tonic–clonic** (grand mal)	• lasting a few seconds • seen most often in children (child stares into space, does not respond to verbal stimulation, may have fluttering eyelids or jerking) • misdiagnosed often (especially in child) as ADD or daydreaming • falling or stumbling for no reason • lasting a few seconds • aura (preceding) • intense muscle contraction (tonic phase) followed by alternating contraction and relaxation of muscles (clonic phase) • crying at beginning as air leaves lungs; loss of bowel/bladder control; shallow breathing with periods of apnea; usually lasting 1–2 minutes • disorientation and deep sleep after seizure (postictal state)
special syndromes	febrile seizure myoclonic seizure status epilepticus	• tonic–clonic activity lasting 1–2 minutes • rapid return to consciousness • most common in children between 3 months and 5 years of age • large jerking movements of a major muscle group, such as an arm • falling from a sitting position or dropping what is held • considered a medical emergency • continuous seizure activity possibly leading to coma and death

PHARMFACTS

Epilepsy

- The word *epilepsy* is derived from the Greek word *epilepsia*, meaning "to take hold of or to seize."
- About 2 million Americans have epilepsy.
- One of every 100 teenagers has epilepsy.
- Of the U.S. population, 10% will have a seizure within their lifetime.
- Most people with seizures are younger than 45 years of age.
- Contrary to popular belief, it is impossible to swallow the tongue during a seizure, and one should never force an object into the mouth of someone who is having a seizure.
- Epilepsy is not a mental illness; children with epilepsy have IQ scores equivalent to those of children without the disorder.
- Famous people who had epilepsy include Julius Caesar, Alexander the Great, Napoleon, Vincent van Gogh, Charles Dickens, Joan of Arc, and Socrates.
- Among 400,000 adult alcoholics going to the emergency department with withdrawal complaints, 60% of those clients have seizures within 6 hours after arriving at the hospital.

be attempted only after at least 3 years of being seizure free, and only under the close direction of the healthcare provider. Doses of medications are reduced slowly, one at a time, over a period of several months. If seizures recur during the withdrawal process, pharmacotherapy is resumed, usually with the same drug. The nurse must strongly urge clients to maintain compliance with pharmacotherapy and not attempt to discontinue antiseizure drug use without professional guidance. Table 15.2 lists antiseizure drugs, based on the type of seizure.

Holistic medicine, as a treatment philosophy considering the health and well-being of the whole person, does not differ from the standard treatment of epilepsy, according to the Epilepsy Foundation of America. Living a healthy, active life is good therapy for epilepsy, but only as an adjunct to medically prescribed antiseizure drug, not instead of it. With a valid diagnosis of epilepsy, there is no substitute for effective antiseizure pharmacotherapy. There are situations, however, in which the medicines cannot be tolerated. Sometimes another medical therapy, such as the ketogenic diet, is used, along with natural remedies.

Antiseizure pharmacotherapy is directed at controlling the movement of electrolytes across neuronal membranes

TABLE 15.2 Drugs Used in the Management of Specific Seizure Types

	PARTIAL SEIZURES	GENERALIZED SEIZURES		
		Absence, Atonic		Tonic–clonic
		SPECIAL EPILEPTIC SYNDROMES		
	Simple or Complex	Febrile seizures*	Myoclonic seizures	Status epilepticus
BARBITURATES AND BENZODIAZEPINES				
phenobarbital (Luminal)	✓		✓	✓
diazepam (Valium)		✓	✓	✓
lorazepam (Ativan)				✓
HYDANTOINS AND PHENYTOIN-LIKE AGENTS				
phenytoin (Dilantin)	✓			✓
carbamazepine (Tegretol)	✓			✓
valproic acid (Depakene)	✓	✓	✓	✓
SUCCINIMIDES				
ethosuximide (Zarontin)		✓		

* Preventing the onset of high fever is the best way to control febrile seizures.

or affecting neurotransmitter balance. In a resting state, neurons are normally surrounded by a higher concentration of sodium, calcium, and chloride ion. Potassium levels are higher inside the cell. An influx of sodium or calcium into the neuron *enhances* neuronal activity, whereas an influx of chloride ion *suppresses* neuronal activity.

The goal of antiseizure pharmacotherapy is to suppress neuronal activity just enough to prevent abnormal or repetitive firing. To this end, there are three general mechanisms by which antiseizure drugs act:

- Stimulating an influx of chloride ion, an effect associated with the neurotransmitter gamma-aminobutyric acid (GABA)

NATURAL THERAPIES

The Ketogenic Diet
The ketogenic diet is used when seizures cannot be controlled through pharmacotherapy or when there are unacceptable side effects to the medications. Before antiepileptic drugs were developed, this diet was a primary treatment for epilepsy. The ketogenic diet may be used for babies, children, or adults. With adults, however, it is harder to develop the ketones that are necessary for the diet.

The ketogenic diet is a stringently calculated diet that is high in fat and low in carbohydrates and protein. It limits water intake to avoid ketone dilution and carefully controls caloric intake. Each meal has the same ketogenic ratio of 4 g of fat to 1 g of protein and carbohydrate. Extra fat is usually given in the form of cream. Research suggests that the diet produces success rates similar to those of medication use, with one third of the children using it becoming seizure free, one third having their seizures reduced, and one third not responding. The diet appears to be equally effective for every seizure type, though those with drop attacks (atonic seizures) may be the most rapid responders. It also helps children with Lennox–Gastaut syndrome and shows promise in babies with infantile spasms. Side effects include hyperlipidemia, constipation, vitamin deficiencies, kidney stones, acidosis, and possibly slower growth rates. Those interested in trying the diet must consult with their healthcare provider; this is not a do-it-yourself diet and may be harmful if not carefully monitored by skilled professionals.

- Delaying an influx of sodium
- Delaying an influx of calcium

Within these three *pharmacological* classes are four major *chemical* classes: benzodiazepines, barbiturates, hydantoins, and succinimides. A fifth category consists of miscellaneous drug types not chemically related to the four major classes.

DRUGS THAT POTENTIATE GABA

Several important antiseizure drugs act by changing the action of **gamma-aminobutyric acid (GABA),** the primary inhibitory neurotransmitter in the brain. These agents mimic the effects of GABA by stimulating an influx of chloride ions that interact with the GABA receptor–chloride channel molecule. A model of this receptor is shown in Pharmacotherapy Illustrated 15.1. When the receptor is stimulated, chloride ions move into the cell, thus supressing the ability of neurons to fire.

BARBITURATES, BENZODIAZEPINES, AND MISCELLANEOUS GABA AGENTS

Barbiturates, benzodiazepines, and several miscellaneous drugs reduce seizure activity by intensifying GABA action. The major effect of enhancing GABA activity is CNS depression. These agents are listed in Table 15.3.

15.4 Treating Seizures With Barbiturates

The antiseizure properties of phenobarbital were discovered in 1912, and the drug is still one of the most commonly prescribed for epilepsy. As a class, barbiturates have a low margin for safety, cause profound CNS depression, and have a high potential for dependence. Phenobarbital,

PHARMACOTHERAPY ILLUSTRATED

15.1 Model of the GABA Receptor–Chloride Channel Molecules in Relationship to Epilepsy Pharmacotherapy

1 Seizure activity: Epilepsy

Uncontrolled neuronal discharge

Neuron

Abnormal EEG recording

2 Uncontrolled neuronal discharges

Na^+
Cl^-
Ca^{2+}

Cl^-

GABA

GABA receptor-chloride channel molecule

Benzodiazepines

Barbituates

3 Administration of antiseizure drugs

- Drugs that potentiate GABA actions:
  Benzodiazepines
  Barbituates
- Hydantoins and Phenytoin-like drugs
- Succinimides

4 Management of seizure activity

- Stimulating influx of Cl^-
- Delaying influx of Na^+ and Ca^{2+}

Normal EEG recording

Na^+
Cl^-
Ca^{2+}

however, is able to suppress abnormal neuronal discharges without causing sedation. It is inexpensive, long acting, and produces a low incidence of adverse effects. Phenobarbital is a drug of choice in the pharmacotherapy of neonatal seizures. When the drug is given orally, several weeks may be necessary to achieve optimum antiseizure activity.

Other barbiturates are occasionally used for epilepsy. Mephobarbital (Mebaral) is converted to phenobarbital in the liver, and offers no significant advantages over phenobarbital. Amobarbital (Amytal) is an intermediate-acting barbiturate that is given IM or IV to terminate **status epilepticus.** Unlike phenobarbital, which is a Schedule IV drug, amobarbital is a Schedule II drug and has a higher

risk for dependence; it is not given orally as an antiseizure drug.

NURSING CONSIDERATIONS

The role of the nurse in barbiturate therapy for seizures involves careful monitoring of a client's condition and providing education as it relates to the prescribed drug treatment. Barbiturates produce the most pronounced adverse effects of all antiseizure medications, so assess for sedation and respiratory depression. Because barbiturates are metabolized in the liver and excreted primarily in urine, monitor liver and kidney function regularly with long-term usage. Barbiturates cross the placenta and are excreted in breast milk; therefore,

TABLE 15.3   Antiseizure Drugs that Potentiate GABA Action

Drug	Route and Adult Dose (max dose where indicated)	Adverse Effects
BARBITURATES		
amobarbital (Amytal)	IV; 65–500 mg (max: 1 g)	*Somnolence*
pentobarbital (Nembutal)	PO/IM: 150–200 mg in 2 divided doses; IV: 100 mg, may increase to 500 mg if necessary	Agranulocytosis, Stevens–Johnson syndrome, angioedema, laryngospam, respiratory depression, CNS depression, coma, death
phenobarbital (Luminal)	For seizures: PO, 100–300 mg/day; IV/IM, 200–600 mg up to 20 mg/kg	
	For status epilepticus: IV, 15–18 mg/kg in single or divided doses (max: 20 mg/kg)	
secobarbital (Seconal)	IM/IV; 5.5 mg/kg repeated q3–4 h if necessary (IV infusion at less than 50 mg/15 sec)	
BENZODIAZEPINES		
clonazepam (Klonopin)	PO; 1.5 mg/day in 3 divided doses, increased by 0.5–1.0 mg every 3 days until seizures are controlled	*Drowsiness, sedation, ataxia*
clorazepate (Tranxene)	PO; 7.5 mg tid	Laryngospam, respiratory depression, cardiovascular collapse, coma
diazepam (Valium)	IM/IV: 5–10 mg (repeat as needed at 10–15 min intervals up to 30 mg; repeat again as needed every 2–4 h); IV push: administer emulsion at 5 mg/min	
lorazepam (Ativan) (see page 163 for the Prototype Drug box ∞)	IV: 4 mg injected slowly at 2 mg/min; if inadequate response after 10 min, may repeat once	
MISCELLANEOUS		
gabapentin (Neurontin)	For additional therapy: PO, start with 300 mg on Day 1; 300 mg bid on Day 2; 300 mg tid on day 3; continue to increase over 1 wk to a dose of 1,200 mg/day (400 mg tid); may increase to 1,800–2,400 mg/day	*Drowsiness, dizziness, fatigue, sedation, somnolence, vertigo, ataxia, confusion, asthenia, headache, tremor, nervousness, memory difficulty, difficulty concentrating, psychomotor slowing, nystagmus, paresthesia, nausea, vomiting, anorexia*
primidone (Mysoline)	PO; 250 mg/day, increased by 250 mg/wk up to max of 2 g in 2–4 divided doses	Serious disfiguring and debilitating rashes; sudden unexplained death in epilepsy (SUDEP); withdrawal seizures on discontinuation of drug
tiagabine (Gabitril)	PO; start with 4 mg/day; may increase by 4–8 mg/day every week up to 56 mg/day in 2–4 divided doses	
topiramate (Topamax)	PO; start with 50 mg/day, increased by 50 mg/wk to effectiveness (max: 1,600 mg/day)	

Italics indicate common adverse effects; underlining indicates serious adverse effects.

they are not recommended for pregnant or nursing women. Assess women of childbearing age for pregnancy or intent to become pregnant. There is an increased risk of congenital malformations when the drug is taken during the first trimester (pregnancy category D). These drugs may also produce folic acid deficiency, which is associated with an increased risk of neural tube birth defects, including spina bifida and hydrocephalus. Barbiturates may also decrease the effectiveness of oral contraceptives.

Barbiturates cause depletion of nutrients such as vitamins D and K, leading to reduced bone density (vitamin D deficiency) and impaired blood coagulability (vitamin K deficiency). Assess for bruising petechiae, epistaxis, GI bleeding, menorrhagia, and/or hematuria. The risk of respiratory depression must be considered when administering barbiturates to clients with impaired respiratory function or those taking other CNS depressants, and with intravenous doses. Monitor for common side effects such as drowsiness, dizziness, and postural hypotension, which increase a client's risk of injury.

Do not stop CNS depressants abruptly, as this can result in potentially life-threatening rebound seizure activity. Concurrent use of other antiseizure drugs may also decrease their anticonvulsant effect. Monitor clients taking gabapentin (Neurontin) and tiagabine (Gabitril) for dizziness and drowsiness.

Lifespan Considerations.   Elderly clients can be particularly at risk for significant vitamin deficiency caused by barbiturates owing to potential age-related nutritional imbalances. Assess for signs of diminished renal, hepatic, and respiratory function associated that would place elderly clients risk of CNS depression. GABA-enhancing drugs may produce an idiosyncratic response in children, resulting in restlessness and psychomotor agitation. Drugs with GABA-intensifying action are not recommended for pregnant or nursing women (pregnancy category D).

Client Teaching.   Client education as it relates to barbiturates should include the goals of therapy, the reasons for obtaining baseline data such as vital signs and the existence of underlying hepatic and renal disorders, and possible

Pr PROTOTYPE DRUG | Phenobarbital *(Luminal)* | Barbiturate

ACTIONS AND USES

Phenobarbital is a long-acting barbiturate, used for the management of a variety of seizures. It is also used for insomnia. Phenobarbital should not be used for pain relief, as it may increase a client's sensitivity to pain.

Phenobarbital acts biochemically in the brain by enhancing the action of the neurotransmitter GABA, which is responsible for suppressing abnormal neuronal discharges that can cause epilepsy.

ADMINISTRATION ALERTS

- Parenteral phenobarbital is a soft-tissue irritant. IM injections may produce local inflammatory reaction. IV administration is rarely used, because extravasation may produce tissue necrosis.
- Controlled substance: Schedule IV.
- Pregnancy category D.

PHARMACOKINETICS

Onset: 20–60 min PO; 5 min IV

Peak: 8–12 h PO; 30 min IV

Half-life: 2–6 days

Duration: 6–10 h PO; 4–10 h IV

ADVERSE EFFECTS

Phenobarbital is a Schedule IV drug that may cause dependence. Common side effects include drowsiness, vitamin deficiencies (vitamin D; folate, or B_9; and B_{12}), and laryngospasms. With overdose, phenobarbital may cause severe respiratory depression, CNS depression, coma, and death.

Contraindications: Administration of phenobarbital is inadvisable in cases of hypersensitivity to barbiturates; severe uncontrolled pain; preexisiting CNS depression; porphyrias; severe respiratory disease with dyspnea or obstruction; glaucoma or prostatic hypertrophy.

INTERACTIONS

Drug–Drug: Phenobarbital interacts with many other drugs. For example, it should not be taken with alcohol or other CNS depressants. These substances potentiate the action of barbiturates, increasing the risk of life-threatening respiratory depression or cardiac arrest. Phenobarbital increases the metabolism of many other drugs, reducing their effectiveness.

Lab Test: Barbiturates may affect bromsulphalein tests and increase serum phosphatase.

Herbal/Food: Kava and valerian may potentiate sedation.

Treatment of Overdose: There is no specific treatment for overdose. Drug removal may be accomplished by gastric lavage or use of activated charcoal. Hemodialysis may be effective in facilitating removal of phenobarbital from the body. Treatment is supportive and consists mainly of endotracheal intubation and mechanical ventilation. Treatment of bradycardia and hypotension may be necessary.

 See the Companion Website for a Nursing Process Focus specific to this drug.

---

drug side effects. Include the following points when teaching clients about barbiturates:

- Practice reliable contraception and notify your healthcare provider if pregnancy is planned or suspected because barbiturates can cause malformations during fetal development.
- Use another form of birth control in additon to oral contraceptives if you are taking barbiturates because they can decrease the effectiveness of oral contraceptives.
- Report signs and symtpoms of excessive bleeding such as nosebleeds, black stools, heavy periods, and/or blood in the urine.
- Immediately report severe drowsiness, signs of bleeding, or complaints of bone pain, especially in elderly clients.
- Avoid alcohol use.
- Avoid taking the herb ginkgo biloba because it can decrease the effects of barbiturates.

BENZODIAZEPINES

Like barbiturates, benzodiazepines intensify the effect of GABA in the brain. The benzodiazepines bind to the GABA receptor directly, suppressing abnormal neuronal foci.

15.5 Treating Seizures With Benzodiazepines

Benzodiazepines used in treating epilepsy include clonazepam (Klonopin), clorazepate (Tranxene), lorazepam (Ativan), and diazepam (Valium). Indications include **absence seizures** and **myoclonic seizures.** Parenteral diazepam is used to terminate status epilepticus. Because tolerance may begin to develop after only a few months of therapy with benzodiazepines, seizures may recur unless the dose is periodically adjusted. These agents are generally not used alone in seizure pharmacotherapy, but instead serve as adjuncts to other antiseizure drugs for short-term seizure control.

The benzodiazepines are one of the most widely prescribed classes of drugs, used not only to control seizures but also for anxiety, skeletal muscle spasms, and alcohol withdrawal symptoms.

NURSING CONSIDERATIONS

The role of the nurse in benzodiazepine therapy for seizures involves careful monitoring of a client's condition and providing education as it relates to the prescribed drug treatment. Assess the client's need for seizure medication by identifying frequency and symptoms of seizures and previous therapies used. Obtain a drug history including the use of

Pr PROTOTYPE DRUG | Diazepam *(Valium)* | Benzodiazepine

ACTIONS AND USES

Diazepam binds to the GABA receptor–chloride channels throughout the CNS. It produces its effects by suppressing neuronal activity in the limbic system and subsequent impulses that might be transmitted to the reticular activating system. Effects of this drug are suppression of abnormal neuronal foci that may cause seizures, calming without strong sedation, and skeletal muscle relaxation. When used orally, maximum therapeutic effects may take from 1 to 2 weeks. Tolerance may develop after about 4 weeks. When given IV, effects occur in minutes, and its anticonvulsant effects last about 20 minutes.

ADMINISTRATION ALERTS

- When administering IV, monitor respirations every 5 to 15 minutes. Have airway and resuscitative equipment accessible.
- Pregnancy category D.

PHARMACOKINETICS

Onset: 30–60 min PO; 15–30 min IV

Peak: 1–2 h PO; 15 min IV

Half-life: 20–50 h

Duration: 2–3 h PO; 15–60 min IV

ADVERSE EFFECTS

Because of tolerance and dependency, use of diazepam is reserved for short-term seizure control, or for status epilepticus. When given IV, hypotension, muscular weakness, tachycardia, and respiratory depression are common.

Contraindications: When administered in injectable form, this medication should be avoided under the following conditions: shock, coma, depressed vital signs, obstetrical patients, and infants less than 30 days of age. In tablet form, the medication should not be admnistered to infants less than 6 months of age, to patients with acute narrow-angle glaucoma or untreated open-angle glaucoma, or within 14 days of MAOI therapy.

INTERACTIONS

Drug–Drug: Diazepam should not be taken with alcohol or other CNS depressants because of combined sedation effects. Other drug interactions include cimetidine, oral contraceptives, valproic acid, and metoprolol, which potentiate diazepam's action; and levodopa and barbiturates, which decrease diazepam's action. Diazepam increases the levels of phenytoin in the bloodstream, and may cause phenytoin toxicity.

Lab Tests: Unknown.

Herbal/Food: Kava and chamomile may cause an increased effect.

Treatment of Overdose: If an overdose occurs, administer flumazenil (Romazicon), a specific benzodiazepine receptor antagonist to reverse CNS depression.

 See the Companion Website for a Nursing Process Focus specific to this drug.

CNS depressants and OTC drugs. Assess for the likelihood of drug abuse and dependence because benzodiazepines are Schedule IV drugs. Assess women of childbearing age for pregnancy, intent to become pregnant, or lactation status because these drugs are pregnancy category D and are secreted into breast milk. Benzodiazepines may also decrease the effectiveness of oral contraceptives.

Because benzodiazepines increase intraocular pressure, they should not be given to clients with narrow-angle glaucoma. Monitor liver and kidney function in long-term use These medications cause respiratory depression, so monitor respiratory function closely in clients with impaired respiratory function or who are taking other CNS depressants, and when administering IV doses. Assess for common side effects related to CNS depression such as drowsiness and dizziness. Should an overdose occur, administer flumazenil (Romazicon), a specific benzodiazepine receptor antagonist to reverse CNS depression.

Intravenous benzodiazepines such as diazepam (Valium) and lorazepam (Ativan) are used in the treatment of status epilepticus or continuous seizures. When administering these drugs IV, be sure to have supplemental oxygen and resuscitation equipment available. Monitor respiratory effort and oxygen saturation. Severe respiratory depression would be treated with intubation and ventilation rather than by reversing the benzodiazepine effects with flumazenil (Romazicon) beacuse of the need to terminate seizure activity. Because IV administration may cause hypotension, tachycar-

dia, and muscular weakness, monitor heart rhythm, heart rate, and blood pressure carefully. These drugs have a tendency to precipitate from solution and are irritating to veins, so do not mix them with other drugs or IV fluid additives and give them in as large a vein as possible. For more information on these drugs, see Chapter 14, page 166 ∞, "Nursing Process Focus: Clients Receiving Benzodiazepine and Nonbenzodiazepine Antianxiety Therapy."

Client Teaching. Client education as it relates to benzodiazepines should include the goals of therapy, the reasons for obtaining baseline data such as vital signs and the existence of underlying disorders, and possible drug side effects. Include the following points when teaching clients about benzodiazepines:

- Avoid alcohol use.
- Do not take any other prescription drugs (especially other CNS depressants or digoxin) and OTC medications, herbal remedies, or vitamins and minerals without notifying your healthcare provider.
- Limit tobacco use or the use of nicotine patches because they can decrease benzodiazepine effectiveness.
- Do not drive or perform hazardous activities until effects of the drug are known.
- Do not discontinue the drug abruptly because this may result in rebound seizure activity.
- Take the drug with food to prevent GI disturbances.

TABLE 15.4 Hydantoins and Phenytoin-like Drugs		
Drug	Route and Adult Dose (max dose where indicated)	Adverse Effects
HYDANTOINS		
fosphenytoin (Cerebyx)	IV; initial dose 15–20 mg PE*/kg at 100–150 mg PE/min followed by 4–6 mg PE/kg/day	*Somnolence, drowsiness, dissiness, nystagmus, gingival hyperplasia*
⊕ phenytoin (Dilantin)	PO; 15–18 mg/kg of 1-g initial dose; then 300 mg/day in 1–3 divided doses; may be gradually increased 100 mg/week	<u>Agranulocytosis, aplastic anemias; bullous, exfoliative, or purpuric dermatitis; Stevens–Johnson syndrome; toxic epidermal necrolysis; cardiovascular collapse; cardiac arrest</u>
PHENYTOIN-LIKE AGENTS		
carbamazepine (Tegretol)	PO; 200 mg bid, gradually increased to 800–1,200 mg/day in 3–4 divided doses	*Dizziness, ataxia, somnolence, headache, diplopia, blurred vision, transient indigestion, rhinitis, leukopenia, prolonged bleeding time, nausea, vomiting, anorexia*
felbamate (Felbatol)	Lennox–Gastaut syndrome: PO; start at 15 mg/kg/day in 3–4 divided doses; may increase 15 mg/kg at weekly intervals to max of 45 mg/kg/day	
	Partial seizures: PO; start with 1,200 mg/day in 3–4 divided doses; may increase by 600 mg/day every 2 wk (max: 3,600 mg/day)	<u>Agranulocytosis; aplastic anemias; bullous, exfoliative dermatitis; Stevens–Johnson syndrome; toxic epidermal necrolysis; bone marrow depression; acute liver failure; pancreatitis; heart block; respiratory depression</u>
lamotrigine (Lamictal)	PO; 50 mg/day for 2 wk, then 50 mg bid for 2 wk; may increase gradually up to 300–500 mg/day in 2 divided doses (max: 700 mg/day)	
⊕ valproic acid (Depakene, Depakote)**	PO/IV; 15 mg/kg/day in divided doses when total daily dose is greater than 250 mg; increase 5–10 mg every wk until seizures are controlled (max: 60 mg/kg/day)	
zonisamide (Zonegran)	PO; 100–400 mg/day	

* PE = phenytoin equivalents
**Other formulations of valproic acid include its salts, valproate and divalproex sodium.
Italics indicate common adverse effects; <u>underlining</u> indicates serious adverse effects.

• Take any precautions necessary to safeguard your medication supply because benzodiazepines are often used illegally for recreation.

DRUGS THAT SUPPRESS SODIUM INFLUX

This class of drugs dampens CNS activity by delaying an influx of sodium ions across neuronal membranes. Hydantoins and several other related antiseizure drugs act by this mechanism.

HYDANTOIN AND PHENYTOIN-LIKE DRUGS

Sodium channels guide the movement of sodium ions across neuronal membranes into the intracellular space. Sodium ion movement is the major factor that determines whether a neuron will undergo an action potential. If these channels are temporarily inactivated, neuronal activity will be suppressed. With hydantoin and phenytoin-like drugs, sodium channels are not blocked; they are just desensitized. If channels are blocked, neuronal activity completely stops, as occurs with local anesthetic drugs. These agents are listed in Table 15.4.

15.6 Treating Seizures With Hydantoins and Phenytoin-like Drugs

The oldest and most commonly prescribed hydantoin is phenytoin (Dilantin). Approved in the 1930s, phenytoin is a broad-spectrum drug that is useful in treating all types of epilepsy except absence seizures. It provides effective seizure suppression, without the abuse potential or CNS depression associated with barbiturates. Clients vary significantly in their ability to metabolize phenytoin; therefore, dosages are highly individualized. Because of the very narrow range between a therapeutic dose and a toxic dose, clients must be carefully monitored. The other hydantoins are used much less frequently than phenytoin. Phenytoin and fosphenytoin are first-line drugs in the treatment of status epilepticus.

Several widely used drugs share a mechanism of action similar to that of the hydantoins, including carbamazepine (Tegretol) and valproic acid (Depakene, Depakote), which is also available as valproate and divalproex sodium. Carbamazepine is a drug of choice for tonic-clonic and partial seizures, because it produces fewer adverse effects than phenytoin or phenobarbital. Valproic acid is a drug of choice for absence seizures and is used in combination with other drugs for partial seizures. Both carbamazepine and valproic acid are also used for bipolar disorder (Chapter 16 ∞). Newer antiseizure drugs having more limited uses include zonisamide (Zonegran), felbamate (Felbatol), and lamotrigine (Lamictal).

NURSING CONSIDERATIONS

The role of the nurse in hydantoin and phenytoin-like drug therapy for seizures involves careful monitoring of a client's condition and providing education as it relates to the prescribed drug treatment. Some hydantoin and phenytoin-like drugs are monitored via serum drug levels, so regular laboratory testing is required. Monitor the results, because if

Pr **PROTOTYPE DRUG** | Phenytoin *(Dilantin)* | Hydantoin

ACTIONS AND USES

Phenytoin acts by desensitizing sodium channels in the CNS responsible for neuronal responsivity. Desensitization prevents the spread of disruptive electrical charges in the brain that produce seizures. It is effective against most types of seizures except absence seizures. Phenytoin has antidysrhythmic activity similar to that of lidocaine (class IB). An unlabeled use is for digitalis-induced dysrhythmias.

ADMINISTRATION ALERTS

- When administering IV, mix with saline only, and infuse at the maximum rate of 50 mg/min. Mixing with other medications or dextrose solutions produces precipitate.
- Always prime or flush IV lines with saline before hanging phenytoin as a piggyback, since traces of dextrose solution in an existing main IV or piggyback line can cause microscopic precipitate formation, which become emboli if infused. Use an IV line with filter when infusing this drug.
- Phenytoin injectable is a soft-tissue irritant that causes local tissue damage following extravasation. To reduce the risk of soft-tissue damage, do not give IM; inject into a large vein or via central venous catheter.
- Avoid using hand veins to prevent serious local vasoconstrictive response (purple glove syndrome).
- Pregnancy category D.

PHARMACOKINETICS

Onset: Slowly and variably absorbed PO

Peak: 1.5–3 h prompt release; 4–12 h sustained release

Half-life: 22 h

Duration: 15 days

ADVERSE EFFECTS

Phenytoin may cause dysrhythmias, such as bradycardia or ventricular fibrillation, severe hypotension, and hyperglycemia. Severe CNS reactions include headache, nystagmus, ataxia, confusion and slurred speech, paradoxical nervousness, twitching, and insomnia. Peripheral neuropathy may occur with long-term use. Phenytoin can cause multiple blood dyscrasias, including agranulocytosis and aplastic anemia.

This medication may cause severe skin reactions, such as rashes, including exfoliative dermatitis, and Stevens–Johnson syndrome. Connective tissue reactions include lupus erythematosus, hypertrichosis, hirsutism, and gingival hypertrophy.

Contraindications: Clients with hypersensitivity to hydantoin products should be cautious. Rash, seizures due to hypoglycemia, sinus bradycardia, and heart block are contraindications.

INTERACTIONS

Drug–Drug: Phenytoin interacts with many other drugs, including oral anticoagulants, glucocorticoids, H_2 antagonists, antituberculin agents, and food supplements such as folic acid, calcium, and vitamin D. It impairs the efficacy of drugs such as digitoxin, doxycycline, furosemide, estrogens and oral contraceptives, and theophylline. Phenytoin when combined with tricyclic antidepressants can trigger seizures.

Lab Tests: Hydantoins may produce lower-than-normal values for dexamethasone or metapyrone tests. Phenytoin may increase serum levels of glucose, bromsulphalein, and alkaline phosphatase, and may decrease protein-bound iodine and urinary steroid levels.

Herbal/Food: Herbal laxatives (buckthorn, cascara sagrada, and senna) may increase potassium loss.

Treatment of Overdose: There is no specific treatment for overdose. Drug removal may be accomplished by gastric lavage, use of activated charcoal, or laxative. Treatment is supportive and consists mainly of maintaining the airway and breathing, monitoring phenytoin blood levels, and appropriately treating adverse symptoms.

 See the Companion Website for a Nursing Process Focus specific to this drug.

serum drugs levels stray outside the normal range, dosage adjustments must be made to avoid toxicity.

Assess for common signs of hydantoin toxicity, which include dizziness, ataxia, diplopia, and lethargy. These drugs affect vitamin K metabolism, so assess for signs of blood dyscrasias and bleeding by obtaining a CBC. Because hydantoins may also increase serum glucose levels, establish blood sugar levels using a finger-stick glucose test. Assess urine for hematuria and color changes such as pink, red, or brown, which may occur with phentoin therapy. Obtain a client history for hepatic or renal disease, because these drugs must be used cautiously with these conditions.

Several cases of fatal hepatotoxicity in clients taking valproic acid (Depakene, Depakote) have recently occurred. Assess the following types of clients extremely carefully before administering valproic acid because the risk for fatal hepatotoxicity is high: clients taking multiple antiseizure drugs, those with existing liver disease or organic brain disease, and those who are younger than 2 years of age. Obtain a careful health history

for heart block and seizures due to hypoglycemia because these medications are contraindicated for such conditions.

Lifespan Considerations. Obtain pregnancy tests on all women of childbearing age before beginning therapy because drugs in this class are pregnancy class D (phenytoin, carbamazepine, and valproic acid) or class C (felbamate and lamotrigine). Hydantoins may also decrease the effectiveness of oral contraceptives.

Client Teaching. Client education as it relates to hydantoin and phenytoin-like drugs should include the goals of therapy, the reasons for obtaining baseline data such as vital signs and any underlying disorders, and possible drug side effects. Include the following points when teaching clients about hydantoins and phenytoin-like drugs:

- Keep all scheduled physician appointments and laboratory visits for liver function tests.
- Immediately report signs of toxicity such as dizziness, difficulty walking, double vision, and fatigue.

Pr PROTOTYPE DRUG | Valproic Acid *(Depakene)* | Phenytoin-like Drugs

ACTIONS AND USES

The mechanism of action of valproic acid is the same as that of phenytoin, although effects on GABA and calcium channels may cause some additional actions. It is useful for a wide range of seizure types, including absence seizures and mixed types of seizures. Other uses include prevention of migraine headaches and treatment of bipolar disorder.

ADMINISTRATION ALERTS

- Valproic acid is a GI irritant. Advise clients not to chew extended-release tablets because mouth soreness will occur.
- Do not mix valproic acid syrup with carbonated beverages because they will trigger immediate release of the drug, which causes severe mouth and throat irritation.
- Open capsules and sprinkle on soft foods if client cannot swallow them.
- Pregnancy category D.

PHARMACOKINETICS

Onset: Readily absorbed from the GI tract

Peak: 1–4 h

Half-life: 5–20 h

Duration: Variable

ADVERSE EFFECTS

Side effects include sedation, drowsiness, GI upset, and prolonged bleeding time. Other effects include visual disturbances, muscle weakness, tremor, psychomotor agitation, bone marrow suppression, weight gain, abdominal cramps, rash, alopecia, pruritus, photosensitivity, erythema multiforme, and fatal hepatotoxicity.

Contraindications: Hypersensitivity may occur. This medication should not be administered to patients with liver disease, bleeding dysfunction, pancreatitis, and congenital metabolic disorders.

INTERACTIONS

Drug–Drug: Valproic acid interacts with many drugs. For example, aspirin, cimetidine, chlorpromazine, erythromycin, and felbamate may increase valproic acid toxicity. Concomitant warfarin, aspirin, or alcohol use can cause severe bleeding. Alcohol, benzodiazepines, and other CNS depressants potentiate CNS depressant action. Use of clonazepam concurrently with valproic acid may induce absence seizures. Valproic acid increases serum phenobarbital and phenytoin levels. Lamotrigine, phenytoin, and rifampin lower valproic acid levels.

Lab Tests: Unknown.

Herbal/Food: Unknown.

Treatment of Overdose: There is no specific treatment for overdose. Drug removal may be accomplished by gastric lavage, use of activated charcoal, or laxative. Treatment is supportive and consists mainly of maintaining the airway and breathing, monitoring phenytoin levels, and appropriately treating adverse symptoms.

 See the Companion Website for a Nursing Process Focus specific to this drug.

- Immediately report unsual bruising or bleeding from gums, nose, vagina, or rectum, or blood in the urine.
- Take only as prescribed.
- Imemdiately notify your healthcare provider if you have been diagnosed with liver or brain disease, heart block, or hypoglycemia.
- Immediately notify your healthcare provider if you suspect you are pregnant or are planning to become pregnant.

DRUGS THAT SUPPRESS CALCIUM INFLUX

Neurotransmitters, hormones, and some medications bind to neuronal membranes, stimulating the entry of calcium. Without calcium influx, neuronal transmission would not be possible. Succinimides delay entry of calcium into neurons by blocking calcium channels, increasing the electrical threshold and reducing the likelihood that an action potential will be generated. By raising the seizure threshold, succinimides keep neurons from firing too quickly, thus suppressing abnormal foci.

SUCCINIMIDES

Succinimides are medications that suppress seizures by delaying calcium influx into neurons. They are generally only effective against absence seizures. The succinimides are listed in Table 15.5.

15.7 Treating Seizures With Succinimides

Ethosuximide (Zarontin) is the most commonly prescribed drug in this class. It remains a drug of choice for absence seizures, although valproic acid is also effective for these

TABLE 15.5 **Succinimides**		
Drug	**Route and Adult Dose (max dose where indicated)**	**Adverse Effects**
Pr ethosuximide (Zarontin)	PO; 250 mg bid, increased every 4–7 days (max: 1.5 g/day)	*Drowsiness, dizzines, ataxia, epigastric distress, weight loss, anorexia, nausea, vomiting*
methsuximide (Celontin)	PO; 300 mg/day; may increase every 4–7 days (max: 1.2 g/day)	
phensuximide (Milontin)	PO; 0.5–1.0 g bid or tid	Agranulocytosis, pancytopenia, aplastic anemia, granulocytopenia

Italics indicate common adverse effects; underlining indicates serious adverse effects.

types of seizures. Some of the newer antiseizure agents, such as lamotrigine (Lamictal) and zonisamide (Zonegran), are being investigated for their roles in treating absence seizures. Lamotrigine has also been found to be effective in patients with partial seizures, usually in combination with other antiseizure medications.

NURSING CONSIDERATIONS

The role of the nurse in succinimide therapy for seizures involves careful monitoring of a client's condition and providing education as it relates to the prescribed drug treatment. Obtain a medical history regarding seizure activity and renal and hepatic function tests for baseline information. These drugs are metabolized by the liver and excreted by the kidneys. Succinimides should be used cautiously in clients with liver or renal insufficiency.

Review the client's current drug history to determine if any medications interact with succinimides, including other antiseizure drugs, phenothiazines, and antidepressants, because these medications lower the seizure threshold and can decrease the effectiveness of succinimides.

Observe for common adverse reactions during therapy, including drowsiness, headache, fatigue, dizziness, depression or euphoria, nausea and vomiting, diarrhea, weight loss, and abdominal pain. Monitor for life-threatening adverse reactions: severe mental depression with overt suicidal intent, Stevens–Johnson syndrome, and blood dyscrasias such as agranulocytosis, pancytopenia, and leukopenia.

Monitor seizure activity during therapy to determine the drug's efficacy. Assess for symptoms of overdose, which include CNS depression, stupor, ataxia, and coma. These symptoms may occur when ethosuximide (Zarontin) is given alone or in combination with other anticonvulsants. Monitor combined usage, and test regularly for serum levels of each drug.

Lifespan Considerations. Assess for pregnancy because succinimides are pregnancy category C.

Client Teaching. Client education as it relates to succinimide therapy should include the goals of therapy, the reasons for obtaining baseline data such as vital signs and the existence of underlying cardiac and hepatic disorders, and possible drug side effects. Include the following points when teaching clients about succinimides:

- Immediately report changes in mood, mental depression, or suicidal urges.
- Do not drive or perform hazardous activities until the drug's effects are known.
- Do not discontinue the drug abruptly because doing so may result in rebound seizure activity.
- Take with food to prevent GI disturbances.
- Immediately report symptoms that suggest infection such as fever, sore throat, or melancholy.
- Report weight loss and anorexia.

Pr **PROTOTYPE DRUG** | Ethosuximide *(Zarontin)* | Succinimide

ACTIONS AND USES

Ethosuximide is a drug of choice for absence (petit mal) seizures. It depresses the activity of neurons in the motor cortex by elevating the neuronal threshold. It is usually ineffective against psychomotor or clonic-tonic seizures; however, it may be given in combination with other medications that better treat these conditions. It is available in tablet and flavored-syrup formulations.

ADMINISTRATION ALERTS

- Do not abruptly withdrawal this medication because doing so may induce tonic-clonic seizures.
- Pregnancy category C.

PHARMACOKINETICS

Onset: Readily absorbed from the GI tract
Peak: 4 h
Half-life: 30 h in children; 60 h in adults
Duration: Variable

ADVERSE EFFECTS

Ethosuximide may impair mental and physical abilities. Psychosis or extreme mood swings, including depression with overt suicidal intent, can occur. Behavioral changes are more prominent in clients with a history of psychiatric illness. Central nervous system effects include dizziness, headache, lethargy, fatigue, ataxia, sleep pattern disturbances, attention difficulty, and hiccups. Bone marrow suppression and blood dyscrasias are possible, as is systemic lupus erythematosus.

Other reactions include gingival hypertrophy and tongue swelling. Common side effects are abdominal distress and weight loss.

Contraindications: Hypersensitivity may occur. Do not use this medication in cases of severe liver or kidney disease. Safety in children younger than 3 years of age has not been established.

INTERACTIONS

Drug–Drug: Ethosuximide increases phenytoin serum levels. Valproic acid causes ethosuximide serum levels to fluctuate (increase and decrease).

Lab Tests: Unknown.

Herbal/Food: Unknown.

Treatment of Overdose: There is no specific treatment for overdose. Drug removal may include emesis unless the client is dull, comatose, or convulsing. Treatment may be accomplished by gastric lavage, use of activated charcoal or cathartics, and general supportive measures. Hemodialysis may be effective in facilitating removal of ethosuximide from the body.

 See the Companion Website for a Nursing Process Focus specific to this drug.

NURSING PROCESS FOCUS Clients Receiving Antiseizure Drug Therapy

Assessment	Potential Nursing Diagnoses
Prior to administration: ■ Obtain a complete health history including allergies and drug history, to determine possible drug interactions. ■ Assess neurological status, including identification of recent seizure activity. ■ Assess growth and development.	■ Injury, Risk for, related to drug side effects ■ Knowledge, Deficient, related to drug therapy ■ Noncompliance, to medication regimen ■ Sleep pattern, Disturbed

Planning: Client Goals and Outcomes

The client will:

■ Experience the absence of, or a reduction in, the number or severity of seizures.

■ Avoid physical injury related to seizure activity or medication-induced sensory changes.

■ Demonstrate an understanding of the drug's action by accurately describing drug side effects and precautions.

Implementation

Interventions and (Rationales)	Client Education/Discharge Planning
■ Monitor neurological status, especially changes in level of consciousness and/or mental status. (Sedation may indicate impending toxicity.)	Instruct client to: ■ Report any significant change in sensorium, such as slurred speech, confusion, hallucinations, or lethargy. ■ Report any changes in seizure quality or unexpected involuntary muscle movement, such as twitching, tremor, or unusual eye movement. ■ Keep a seizure diary to chronicle seizures. ■ Be aware that some medications may cause initial drowsiness, which may decrease with continued treatment.
■ Monitor vital signs, especially blood pressure and depth and rate of respirations. (Barbiturates can cause severe respiratory depression.)	■ Instruct client to withold medication if any difficulty in breathing is experienced or if respirations are less than 12 breaths per minute.
■ Protect the client from injury during seizure events until therapeutic effects of drugs are achieved. (Barbiturates can cause drowsiness and dizziness.)	Instruct client to: ■ Avoid driving and other hazardous activities until effects of the drug are known. ■ Request assistance when getting out of bed and ambulating until effect of the drug is known.
■ Monitor effectiveness of drug therapy. Observe for developmental changes. (These may indicate a need for dose adjustment.)	Instruct client to: ■ Keep a seizure diary to chronicle symptoms phase, or during dose adjustment. ■ Take the medication exactly as ordered, including the same manufacturer's drug each time the prescription is refilled. (Switching brands may result in alterations in seizure control.) ■ Take a missed dose as soon as remembered, but do not take double doses. ■ Not discontinue barbiturates abruptly, since this can cause increased seizure activity.
■ Monitor children for paradoxical response to barbiturates. (Hyperactivity may occur.)	■ Instruct client/family members to notify the healthcare provider if the client exhibits hyperactive behavior.
■ Monitor for adverse effects. Observe for hypersensitivity, nephrotoxicity, and hepatotoxicity. (Most antiseizure medications are metabolized by the liver and excreted by the kidneys.)	Instruct client to: ■ Report side effects specific to drug regimen. ■ Report any signs of toxicity such as nausea, vomiting, rash, diarrhea, jaundice, abdominal pain, change in color of stool, flank pain, or blood in urine. ■ Adhere to a regular schedule of laboratory testing for liver and kidney function as ordered by the prescriber.
■ Monitor oral health. Observe for signs of gingival hypertrophy, bleeding, or inflammation. (These signs are phenytoin specific.)	Instruct client to: ■ Use a soft toothbrush and oral rinses as prescribed by the dentist. ■ Avoid mouthwashes containing alcohol. ■ Report changes in oral health such as excessive bleeding or inflammation of the gums. ■ Visit the dentist regularly.

NURSING PROCESS FOCUS Clients Receiving Antiseizure Drug Therapy *(Continued)*

Implementation

Interventions and (Rationales)	Client Education/Discharge Planning
▪ Monitor GI status. (Valproic acid is a GI irritant and anticoagulant.)	Instruct client to: ▪ Take the drug with food to reduce GI upset. ▪ Immediately report any severe or persistent heartburn, upper GI pain, nausea, or vomiting.
▪ Conduct guaiac stool testing for occult blood. (Phenytoin's CNS depressant effects decrease GI motility, producing constipation.)	▪ Instruct client to increase exercise, and fluid and fiber intake, to facilitate stool passage.
▪ Monitor nutritional status. (Phenytoin may cause decreased absorption of folic acid, vitamin D, magnesium, and calcium, leading to anemia and osteoporosis. Barbiturates may cause deficiencies in vitamin D, vitamin K, folate, and other B vitamins. Valproic acid may cause an increase in appetite and weight.)	Instruct client to: ▪ Immediately report signs of vitamin K deficiency: easy bleeding, tarry stools, bruising, and pallor. ▪ Immediately report signs of vitamin D deficiency: skin changes, dandruff, peripheral neuropathy, fatigue. ▪ Report significant changes in appetite or weight gain.

Evaluation of Outcome Criteria

Evaluate the effectiveness of drug therapy by confirming that client goals and expected outcomes have been met (see "Planning").

▪ The client reports having either no seizures or a reduction in seizure severity.

▪ The client is free of physical injury related to seizure activity or medication-induced sensory changes.

▪ The client demonstrates an understanding of the drug's action by accurately describing drug side effects and precautions.

∞ *See Tables 15.3 and 15.4 for lists of drugs to which these nursing actions apply.*

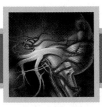

CHAPTER REVIEW

KEY CONCEPTS

The numbered key concepts provide a succinct summary of the important points from the corresponding numbered section within the chapter. If any of these points are not clear, refer to the numbered section within the chapter for review.

15.1 Seizures are associated with many causes, including head trauma, brain infection, fluid and electrolyte imbalance, hypoxia, stroke, brain tumors, and high fever in children.

15.2 The three broad categories of seizures are partial seizures, generalized seizures, and special epileptic syndromes. Each seizure type has a characteristic set of signs, and different drugs are used for different types.

15.3 Antiseizure drugs act by distinct mechanisms: potentiating GABA, and delaying the influx of sodium or calcium ions into neurons. Pharmacotherapy may continue for many years, and these agents must be withdrawn gradually to prevent seizure recurrence.

15.4 Barbiturates act by potentiating the effects of GABA. Phenobarbital is used for tonic-clonic and febrile seizures.

15.5 Benzodiazepines reduce seizure activity by intensifying GABA action. Their use is limited to being short-term adjuncts to other, more effective agents.

15.6 Hydantoin and phenytoin-like drugs act by delaying sodium influx into neurons. Phenytoin is a broad-spectrum drug used for all types of epilepsy except absence seizures.

15.7 Succinimides act by delaying calcium influx into neurons. Ethosuximide (Zarontin) is a drug of choice for absence seizures.

NCLEX-RN® REVIEW QUESTIONS

1 The nurse evaluates client teaching related to causes of seizures. Further teaching is needed if the client makes which of the following statements?

1. "Seizures can be caused by inflammation of the brain."

2. "Seizures can be caused by low blood sugar."

3. "My relative had seizures because of a large tumor growing in his muscles."

4. "Seizures may occur after a head injury."

2 The nursing student asks the nurse to explain the action of antiseizure medication. The nurse explains a mechanism of action as:

1. Suppression of the influx of chloride into the neuron.
2. Stimulation of the influx of calcium into the neuron.
3. Suppression of the influx of sodium into the neuron.
4. Stimulation of calcium and sodium needed to suppress seizure activity.

3 The nurse recognizes that several chemicals inhibit neurotransmitter function in the brain. The primary inhibitory transmitter in the brain is:

1. Sodium.
2. GABA.
3. Chloride.
4. Calcium.

4 The client, age 8, is prescribed valproic acid (Depokene) for treatment of a seizure disorder. The nurse should monitor the client closely for:

1. Hyperthermia.
2. Vitamin B deficiency.
3. Restlessness and agitation.
4. Respiratory distress.

5 Discharge teaching for a client receiving carbamazepine (Tegretol) should include:

1. Monitoring blood glucose and reporting decreased levels.
2. Expecting a discoloration of contact lenses.
3. Immediately reporting unusual bleeding or bruises to the healthcare provider.
4. Expecting a green discoloration of urine.

6 Which of the following medications may be used to treat partial seizures? (Select all that apply.)

1. Phenytoin (Dilantin)
2. Valproic acid (Depakene)
3. Diazepam (Valium)
4. Carbamazepine (Tegretol)
5. Ethosuximide (Zarontin)

CRITICAL THINKING QUESTIONS

1. The nurse practitioner reviews the laboratory results of a 16-year-old client who presents to the clinic with fatigue and pallor. The client's hematocrit is 26%, and the nurse notes multiple small petechiae and bruises over the arms and legs. This client has a generalized tonic-clonic seizure disorder that has been managed well on carbamazepine (Tegretol). Relate the drug regimen to this client's presentation.

2. A 24-year-old woman is brought to the emergency department by her husband. He tells the triage nurse that his wife has been treated for seizure disorder secondary to a head injury she received in an automobile accident. She takes Dilantin 100 mg q8h. He relates a history of increasing drowsiness and lethargy in his wife over the past 24 hours. A Dilantin level is performed, and the nurse notes that the results are 24 mcg/dl. Relate the drug regimen to this client's presentation.

3. The nurse is admitting a 17-year-old female client with a history of seizure disorder. The client has broken her leg in a car accident, in which she was the driver. The client states that she hates having to take Dilantin, and that she stopped the drug because she couldn't drive and it was making her ugly. Instead of reassuring the client, the nurse first considers the possible side effects of long-term phenytoin therapy. Explain possible long-term effects of phenytoin therapy and their impact on client compliance.

See Appendix D for answers and rationales for all activities.

EXPLORE
MediaLink

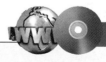 www.prenhall.com/adams

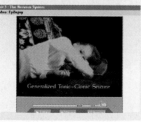

NCLEX-RN® review, case studies, and other interactive resources for this chapter can be found on the companion website at www.prenhall.com/adams. Click on "Chapter 15" to select the activities for this chapter. For animations, more NCLEX-RN® review questions, and an audio glossary, access the accompanying Prentice Hall Nursing MediaLink DVD-ROM in this textbook.

 PRENTICE HALL NURSING MEDIALINK DVD-ROM

- **Animations**
  Mechanism in Action: Diazepam (*Valium*)
  Mechanism in Action: Valproic Acid (*Depakene*)
- **Audio Glossary**
- **NCLEX-RN® Review**

COMPANION WEBSITE

- **NCLEX-RN® Review**
- **Dosage Calculations**
- **Case Study:** Client with seizures
- **Care Plan:** Client with a seizure disorder who is taking phenytoin

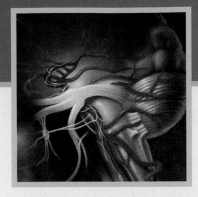

CHAPTER 16

Drugs for Emotional and Mood Disorders

DRUGS AT A GLANCE

ANTIDEPRESSANTS
Tricyclic Antidepressants (TCAs)
   🔊 *imipramine (Tofranil)*
Selective Serotonin Reuptake Inhibitors (SSRIs)
   🔊 *sertraline (Zoloft)*
MAO Inhibitors (MAOIs)
   🔊 *phenelzine (Nardil)*
Atypical Antidepressants
Serotonin–norepinephrine Reuptake Inhibitors (SNRIs)
DRUGS FOR BIPOLAR DISORDER
   🔊 *lithium (Eskalith)*
DRUGS FOR ATTENTION DEFICIT– HYPERACTIVITY DISORDER (ADHD)
CNS Stimulants
   🔊 *methylphenidate (Ritalin)*
Nonstimulant Drugs for ADHD

OBJECTIVES

After reading this chapter, the student should be able to:

1. Identify the two major categories of mood disorders and their symptoms.
2. Identify the symptoms of attention deficit–hyperactivity disorder.
3. Explain the etiology of clinical depression.
4. Discuss the nurse's role in the pharmacological management of clients with depression, bipolar disorder, or attention deficit–hyperactivity disorder.
5. For each of the drug classes listed in Drugs at a Glance, know representative drug examples, explain their mechanism of action, primary actions, and important adverse effects.
6. Categorize drugs used for mood and emotional disorders based on their classification and drug action.
7. Use the Nursing Process to care for clients receiving drug therapy for mood and emotional disorders.

MediaLink

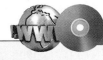

www.prenhall.com/adams

NCLEX-RN® review, case studies, and other interactive resources for this chapter can be found on the companion website at www.prenhall.com/adams. Click on "Chapter 16" to select the activities for this chapter. For animations, more NCLEX-RN® review questions, and an audio glossary, access the accompanying Prentice Hall Nursing MediaLink DVD-ROM in this textbook.

KEY TERMS

attention deficit–hyperactivity disorder
(ADHD)   *page 202*

bipolar disorder   *page 196*

depression   *page 186*

electroconvulsive therapy (ECT)   *page 187*

mania   *page 199*

monoamine oxidase inhibitor (MAOI)
page 194

mood disorder   *page 186*

mood stabilizer   *page 199*

selective serotonin reuptake inhibitor (SSRI)
page 192

serotonin–norepinephrine reuptake
inhibitor (SNRI)   *page 188*

serotonin syndrome (SES)   *page 193*

tricyclic antidepressant (TCA)   *page 188*

tyramine   *page 194*

nappropriate or unusually intense emotions are among the leading causes of mental health disorders. Although mood changes are a normal part of life, when those changes become severe and result in impaired functioning within the family, work environment, or interpersonal relationships, an individual may be diagnosed as having a **mood disorder**. The two major categories of mood disorders are depression and bipolar disorder. A third emotional disorder, attention deficit–hyperactivity disorder, is also included in this chapter.

DEPRESSION

Depression is a disorder characterized by a sad or despondent mood. Many symptoms are associated with depression, including lack of energy, sleep disturbances, abnormal eating patterns, and feelings of despair, guilt, and hopelessness. Depression is the most common mental health disorder of elderly adults, encompassing a variety of physical, emotional, cognitive, and social considerations.

16.1 Characteristics of Depression

Sometimes described as the most common mental illness, major depressive disorder is estimated to affect 5% to 10% of adults in the United States. The American Psychiatric Association's *Diagnostic and Statistical Manual of Mental Disorders,* 4th edition (DSM-IV), describes the following criteria for diagnosis of a major depressive disorder: a depressed mood plus at least five of the following symptoms lasting for a minimum of 2 weeks:

- Difficulty sleeping or sleeping too much
- Extremely tired; without energy
- Abnormal eating patterns (eating too much or not enough)
- Vague physical symptoms (GI pain, joint/muscle pain, or headaches)
- Inability to concentrate or make decisions
- Feelings of despair, lack of self-worth, guiltiness, and misery
- Obsessed with death (expressing a wish to die or to commit suicide)
- Avoiding psychosocial and interpersonal interactions
- Lack of interest in personal appearance or sex
- Delusions or hallucinations

The majority of depressed clients are not found in psychiatric hospitals but in mainstream everyday settings. For proper diagnosis and treatment to occur, the recognition of depression is a collaborative effort among healthcare providers. Because depressed clients are present in multiple settings and in all areas of practice, every nurse should possess proficiency in the assessment and nursing care of clients afflicted with this disorder. At times it is the pharmacist working in a neighborhood pharmacy or supermarket who may recognize that a person is depressed when the pharmacist observes him or her self-medicating with over-the-counter (OTC) remedies to enhance mood or to induce sleep.

Some women experience intense mood shifts associated with hormonal changes during the menstrual cycle, pregnancy, childbirth, and menopause. Up to 80% of women experience brief "baby blues" during the first 2 weeks after the birth of a baby. About 10% of new mothers will experience a major depressive disorder within the first 6 months postdelivery related to the dramatic hormonal shifts that occur during that period. Along with the hormonal changes, additional situational stresses such as responsibilities both at work and home, single parenthood, and caring for children and for aging parents, may contribute to the onset of symptoms. If mood is severely depressed and persists long enough, many women may benefit from medical treatment, including those with premenstrual

MediaLink ● The Geriatric Depression Scale (GDS)

SPECIAL CONSIDERATIONS

Cultural Influences and the Treatment of Depression

To fully understand any client who is suffering from depression, sociocultural factors must be fully considered.

- Depression (and other mental illness) is often ignored in many Asian communities because of the tremendous amount of stigma attached to it. Emotions are largely suppressed. Asian clients tend to come to the attention of mental health workers late in the course of their illness, and often have a feeling of hopelessness. It should be noted that Asians and African Americans generally metabolize antidepressants more slowly than other subgroups; therefore, initial doses should be reduced to avoid drug toxicity.

- Alternative therapies such as teas are often used to treat emotional illnesses within some Hispanic American groups; thus, medical help may not be sought for treatment of depression. There is often a stigma attached to mental health problems along with the belief that religious practices will solve mental health problems. Hispanics metabolize antidepressants about the same as other subgroups, although there are reports of greater susceptibility to anticholinergic effects.

- Some people of European origin deny that mental illness exists and therefore believe that depression will subside on its own. Higher doses of antidepressants are tolerated in this subgroup.

distress disorder, postpartum mood disorders, depression during pregnancy, or menopausal distress.

Because of the possible consequences of perinatal mood disorders, some states mandate that all new mothers receive information about these mood disorders prior to their discharge after giving birth. All levels of healthcare providers in obstetricians, offices, pediatric outclient settings, and family medicine centers are encouraged to conduct routine screening for symptoms of perinatal mood disorders.

During the dark winter months, some clients experience a type of depression known as *seasonal affective disorder (SAD)*. This type of depression is associated with a reduced release of the brain neurohormone melatonin. Exposing clients on a regular basis to specific wavelengths of light may relieve SAD depression and prevent future episodes.

16.2 Assessment and Treatment of Depression

The first step in implementing appropriate treatment for depression is a complete health examination. Certain drugs, such as glucocorticoids, levodopa, and oral contraceptives, can cause the same symptoms as depression, and the healthcare provider should rule out this possibility. Depression may be mimicked by a variety of medical and neurological disorders, ranging from B-vitamin deficiencies to thyroid gland problems to early Alzheimer's disease. If physical causes for the depression are ruled out, a psychological evaluation is often performed by a psychiatrist or psychologist to confirm the diagnosis.

During initial health examinations, inquiries should be made about alcohol and drug use, and any thoughts about death or suicide. This exam should include questions about any family history of depressive illness. If other family

members have been treated, the nurse should document what therapies they may have received and which were effective or helpful.

To determine a course of treatment, healthcare providers and nurses assess for well-accepted symptoms of depression. In general, severe depressive illness, particularly that which is recurrent, will require both medication and psychotherapy to achieve the best response. Counseling therapies help clients gain insight into and resolve their problems through verbal "give-and-take" with the therapist. Behavioral therapies help clients learn how to obtain more satisfaction and rewards through their own actions and how to unlearn the behavioral patterns that contribute to or result from their depression.

Short-term psychotherapies that are helpful for some forms of depression are *interpersonal* and *cognitive-behavioral therapies*. Interpersonal therapy focuses on the client's disturbed personal relationships that both cause and exacerbate the depression. Cognitive-behavioral therapies help clients change the negative styles of thought and behavior that are often associated with their depression.

Psychodynamic therapies focus on resolving the client's internal conflicts. These therapies are often postponed until the depressive symptoms are significantly improved.

In clients with serious and life-threatening mood disorders that are unresponsive to pharmacotherapy, **electroconvulsive therapy (ECT)** continues to be a useful treatment. Although ECT has been found to be safe, there are still deaths (1 in 10,000 clients) and other serious complications related to seizure activity and anesthesia caused by ECT (Janicak, 2002). Recent studies suggest that repetitive transcranial magnetic stimulation (rTMS) is an effective somatic treatment for major depression. This treatment requires surgical implant of the device, however. In contrast with ECT, rTMS has minimal effects on memory, does not require general anesthesia, and produces its effects without a generalized seizure.

Even with the best professional care, the client with depression may take a long time to recover. Many individuals with major depression have multiple bouts of the illness over the course of a lifetime. This can take its toll on the client's family, friends, and other caregivers who may sometimes feel burned out, frustrated, or even depressed themselves. They may experience episodes of anger toward the depressed loved one, only to subsequently suffer reactions

MediaLink ● Hamilton Rating Scale for Depression (HAM-D)

PHARMFACTS

Clients With Depressive Symptoms

- Major depression, manic depression, and situational depression are some of the most common mental health challenges worldwide.
- Clinical depression affects more than 19 million Americans each year.
- Fewer than half of those suffering from depression seek medical treatment.
- Most clients consider depression a weakness rather than an illness.
- There is no common age, sex, or ethnic factor related to depression—it can happen to anyone.

of guilt over being angry. Although such feelings are common, they can be distressing, and the caregiver may not know where to turn for help, support, or advice. It is often the nurse who is best able to assist the family members of a person suffering from emotional and mood disorders. Family members may need counseling themselves.

ANTIDEPRESSANTS

Drugs used to treat depression are categorized as antidepressants. Antidepressants treat major depression by enhancing mood. Over the years, *mood* has come to represent a broader term, encompassing feelings of phobia, obsessive compulsive behavior, panic, and anxiety. Thus, antidepressants are often prescibed for these disorders as well. Recent studies link depression and anxiety to similar neurotransmitter dysfunction, and both seem to respond to treatment with antidepressant medications (Chapter 14 ∞) Antidepressants are also beneficial in treating psychological and physical signs of pain (Chapter 18 ∞), especially in clients without major depressive disorder, for example, when mood problems are associated with debilitating conditions such as fibromylagia or muscle spasticity (see Chapter 21 ∞).

There is one important warning about antidepressants: In 2004, the U.S. Food and Drug Administration issued an advisory "black box warning" to be included at the beginning of drug package inserts and drug information sheets. The advisory was issued to clients, families, and health professioinals to closely monitor adults and children taking antidepressants for warning signs of suicide, espcially at the beginning of treatment and when doses are changed. The FDA further advised that certain signs might be expected among certain clients including anxiety, panic attacks, agitation, irritability, insomnia, impulsivity, hostility, and mania. The warning especially applies to children, who are at a greater risk for suicidal ideation.

16.3 Mechanism of Action of Antidepressants

Depression is associated with dysfunction of neurotransmitters in certain regions of the brain. Although medication does not completely restore normal chemical balance, it may help reduce depressive symptoms while the client develops effective means of coping.

It is theorized that antidepressants exert their effect through their action on certain neurotransmitters in the brain, including norepinephrine, dopamine, and serotonin. The two basic mechanisms of action are blocking the enzymatic breakdown of norepinephrine and slowing the reuptake of serotonin. The four primary classes of antidepressant drugs, also listed in Table 16.1, are as follows:

- Tricyclic antidepressants (TCAs)
- Selective serotonin reuptake inhibitors (SSRIs)
- Monoamine oxidase inhibitors (MAOIs)
- Atypical antidepressants including the serotonin–norepinephrine reuptake inhibitors (SNRIs) and other atypical antidepressants

The atypical antidepressants do not fit into the three major drug classes. Duloxetine (Cymbalta) and venlafaxine (Effexor), examples of atypical antidepressants, are **serotonin–norepinephrine reuptake inhibitors (SNRIs)**. They inhibit the reabsorption of serotonin and norepinephrine and elevate mood by increasing the levels of serotonin, norepinephrine, and dopamine in the central nervous system. In addition to treating major depression, duloxetine (Cymbalta) was approved by the Food and Drug Administration in 2004 for the treatment of neuropathic pain. Venlafaxine (Effexor), more recently used to relieve the symptoms of depression, is available in an intermediate-release form that requires two or three doses a day and an extended-release form that allows the client to take the medication just once a day.

Bupropion (Wellbutrin) not only inhibits the reuptake of serotonin but may also affect the activity of norepinephrine and dopamine. It should be used with caution in clients with seizure disorders because it lowers the seizure threshold. Wellbutrin is also marketed as Zyban for use in cessation of smoking. Maprotiline (Ludiomil) is similar to the TCAs in its therapeutic and adverse effects. Chemically, it is classified as a tetracyclic antidepressant and is used for the treatment of depression associated with anxiety and sleep disturbances. Trazodone (Desyrel) is most frequently used as a sleep aid, rather than as an antidepressant. The high levels of Desyrel needed for the amelioration of depression cause excessive sedation in many clients. Mirtazapine (Remerron) is used for depression and blocks presynaptic serotonin and norepinephrine receptors, thereby enhancing release of neurotransmitters from nerve terminals. Nefazodone (Serzone) is similar to Remeron. It was originally designed to treat depression causing minimal cardiovascular effects, fewer anticholinergic effects, less sedation, and less sexual dysfunction than the other antidepressants.

TRICYCLIC ANTIDEPRESSANTS

Named for their three-ring chemical structure, **tricyclic antidepressants (TCAs)** were the mainstay of depression pharmacotherapy from the early 1960s until the 1980s, and are still used today.

16.4 Treating Depression With Tricyclic Antidepressants

Tricyclic antidepressants act by inhibiting the reuptake of both norepinephrine and serotonin into presynaptic nerve terminals, as shown in ● Figure 16.1. TCAs are used mainly for major depression and occasionally for milder situational depression. Clomipramine (Anafranil) is approved for treatment of obsessive-compulsive disorder, and other TCAs are sometimes used as unlabeled treatments for panic attacks. One atypical use for TCAs, not related to psychopharmacology, is for the treatment of childhood enuresis (bed-wetting).

Shortly after their approval as antidepressants in the 1950s, it was found that the tricyclic antidepressants produced fewer side effects and were less dangerous than MAO inhibitors.

TABLE 16.1 Antidepressants

Drug	Route and Adult Dose (max dose where Indicated)	Adverse Effects
TRICYCLIC ANTIDEPRESSANTS (TCAs)		
amitriptyline (Elavil)	Adult: PO; 75–100 mg/day (may gradually increase to 150–300 mg/day); Geriatric: PO; 10–25 mg at bedtime (may gradually increase to 25–150 mg/day)	*Drowsiness, sedation, dizziness, orthostatic hypotension, dry mouth, constipation, urine retention, blurred vision, mydriasis*
amoxapine (Asendin)	Adult: PO; begin with 100 mg/day (may increase on day 3 to 300 mg/day); Geriatric: PO; 25 mg at bedtime; may increase every 3–7 days to 50–150 mg/day (max: 300 mg/day)	Bone marrow depression, seizures, heart block, MI, angioedema of face, tongue, or generalized
desipramine (Norpramin)	PO; 75–100 mg/day; may increase to 150–300 mg/day	
doxepin (Sinequan)	PO; 30–150 mg/day at bedtime; may gradually increase to 300 mg/day	
ⓟ imipramine (Tofranil)	PO; 75–100 mg/day (max: 300 mg/day)	
maprotiline (Ludiomil)	Mild to moderate depression: PO; start at 75 mg/day; gradually increase every 2 wk to 150 mg/day; Severe depression: PO; start at 100–150 mg/day; gradually increase to 300 mg/day	
nortriptyline (Aventyl, Pamelor)	PO; 25 mg tid or qid; may increase to 100–150 mg/day	
protriptyline (Vivactil)	PO; 15–40 mg/day in 3 to 4 divided doses (max: 60 mg/day)	
trimipramine (Surmontil)	PO; 75–100 mg/day (max: 300 mg/day)	
SELECTIVE SEROTONIN REUPTAKE INHIBITORS (SSRIs)		
citalopram (Celexa)	PO; start at 20 mg/day (max: 40 mg/day)	*Nausea, dry mouth, insomnia, somnolence, headache, nervousness, anxiety, insomnia, GI disturbances, dizziness, anorexia, fatigue*
escitalopram oxalate (Lexapro)	PO; 10 mg/day; may increase to 20 mg after 1 wk	
fluoxetine (Prozac)	PO; 20 mg/day in the AM, may increase by 20 mg/day at weekly intervals (max: 80 mg/day); when stable may switch to 90-mg sustained-release capsule once weekly (max: 90 mg/wk)	Stevens–Johnson syndrome
fluvoxamine (Luvox)	PO; start with 50 mg/day (max: 300 mg/day)	
paroxetine (Paxil)	Depression: PO; 10–50 mg/day (max: 80 mg/day); Obsessive-compulsive disorder: PO; 20–60 mg/day; Panic attacks: PO; 40 mg/day	
ⓟ sertraline (Zoloft)	Adult: PO; start with 50 mg/day; gradually increase every few weeks to a range of 50–200 mg; Geriatric: start with 25 mg/day	
ATYPICAL ANTIDEPRESSANTS		
duloxetine (Cymbalta) (SNRI)	PO; 40–60 mg/day in 1 or 2 divided doses	*Insomnia, nausea, dry mouth, constipation, increased blood pressure and heart rate, dizziness, somnolence, sweating, agitation, blurred vision, headache, dizziness, tremor, nausea, vomiting, drowsiness, increased appetite, orthostatic hypotension*
venlafaxine (Effexor) (SNRI)	PO; 25–125 mg tid	
bupropion (Wellbutrin; Zyban)	PO; 75–100 mg tid (greater than 450 mg/day increases risk for adverse reactions)	
mirtazapine (Remeron)	PO; 15 mg/day in a single dose at bedtime; may increase every 1–2 wk (max: 45 mg/day)	Stevens–Johnson syndrome, seizures
nefazodone (Serzone)	PO; 50–100 mg bid; may increase up to 300–600 mg/day	
trazodone (Desyrel)	PO; 150 mg/day; may increase by 50 mg/day every 3–4 days up to 400–600 mg/day	
MAO INHIBITORS (MAOIs)		
isocarboxazid (Marplan)	PO; 10–30 mg/day (max: 30 mg/day)	*Drowsiness, insomnia, orthostatic hypotension, blurred vision, nausea, constipation, anorexia, dry mouth, urine retention*
ⓟ phenelzine (Nardil)	PO; 15 mg tid (max: 90 mg/day)	
tranylcypromine (Parnate)	PO; 30 mg/day (give 20 mg in AM and 10 mg in PM); may increase by 10 mg/day at 3-wk intervals up to 60 mg/day	Respiratory collapse, hypertensive crisis, circulatory collapse

Italics indicate common adverse effects; <u>underlining</u> indicates serious adverse effects.

MediaLink • Mechanism in Action: Fluoxetine

MediaLink • Mechanism in Action: Venlafaxine

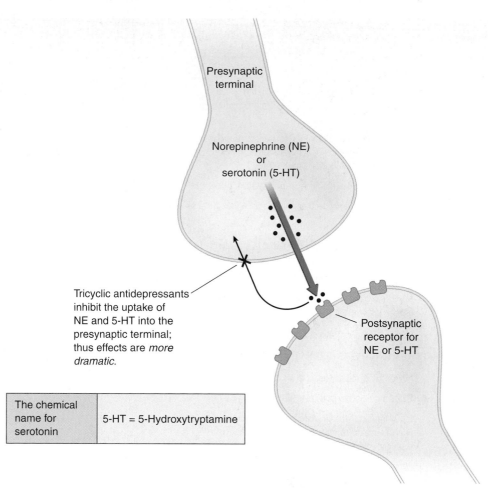

Presynaptic terminal

Norepinephrine (NE) or serotonin (5-HT)

Tricyclic antidepressants inhibit the uptake of NE and 5-HT into the presynaptic terminal; thus effects are *more dramatic.*

Postsynaptic receptor for NE or 5-HT

The chemical name for serotonin	5-HT = 5-Hydroxytryptamine

● **Figure 16.1** Tricyclic antidepressants produce their effects by inhibiting the reuptake of neurotransmitters into presynaptic nerve terminals. The neurotransmitters particularly affected are norepinephrine and serotonin.

However, TCAs have some unpleasant and serious side effects. The most common side effect is orthostatic hypotension, due to alpha₁ blockade on blood vessels. The most serious adverse effect occurs when TCAs accumulate in cardiac tissue. Although rare, cardiac dysrhythmias can occur.

Sedation is a frequently reported complaint at the initiation of therapy, though clients may become tolerant to this effect after several weeks of treatment. Most have a long half-life, which increases the risk of side effects for clients with delayed excretion. Anticholinergic effects, such as dry mouth, constipation, urinary retention, excessive perspiration, blurred vision, and tachycardia, are common. These effects are less severe if the drug is gradually increased to the therapeutic dose over 2 to 3 weeks. Significant drug interactions can occur with CNS depressants, sympathomimetics, anticholinergics, and MAO inhibitors. Since the advent of newer antidepressants that have fewer side effects, TCAs are less frequently used as first-line drugs in the treatment of depression and/or anxiety.

NURSING CONSIDERATIONS

The role of the nurse in TCA therapy involves careful monitoring of a client's condition and providing education as it relates to the prescribed drug treatment. The therapeutic effects of TCAs may take 2 to 6 weeks to occur. Suicide potential increases as blood levels of a TCA increase but have not yet reached their peak therapeutic levels. Monitor the client closely for symptoms of suicidal ideation throughout treatment. As clients begin to recover from both psychological and physical depression (psychological depression slows all body processes), their energy level rises.

Assessing previous health history is essential. TCAs are contraindicated in clients in the acute recovery phase of an MI, with heart block, or with a history of dysrhythmias, because of their effects on cardiac tissue. Because TCAs lower the seizure threshold, carefully monitor clients with epilepsy. Clients with urinary retention, narrow-angle glaucoma, or prostatic hypertrophy may not be good candidates for TCAs because of anticholinergic side effects. Annoying anticholinergic effects, coupled with the weight gain effect of TCAs, may lead to noncompliance. Tricyclics must be given with extreme caution to clients with asthma, cardiovascular disorders, gastrointestinal disorders, alcoholism, and other psychiatric disorders including schizophrenia and bipolar disorder. Most TCAs are pregnancy category C or D, so they are used during pregnancy or lactation only when medically necessary.

Significant drug interactions may occur with TCAs. Oral contraceptives may decrease the efficacy of tricyclics.

Pr PROTOTYPE DRUG │ Imipramine *(Tofranil)* │ Tricyclic Antidepressant

ACTIONS AND USES

Imipramine blocks the reuptake of serotonin and norepinephrine into nerve terminals. It is used mainly for clinical depression, although it is occasionally used for the treatment of nocturnal enuresis in children. The nurse may find imipramine prescribed for a number of unlabeled uses including intractable pain, anxiety disorders, and withdrawal syndromes from alcohol and cocaine. Therapeutic effectiveness may not occur for 2 or more weeks.

ADMINISTRATION ALERTS

- Paradoxical diaphoresis can be a side effect of TCAs; therefore, diaphoresis may not be a reliable indicator of other disease states such as hypoglycemia.
- Imipramine causes anticholinergic effects and may potentiate effects of anticholinergic drugs administered during surgery.
- Do not discontinue abruptly, because rebound dysphoria, irritability, or sleeplessness may occur.
- Pregnancy category C.

PHARMACOKINETICS

Onset: < 1 h

Peak: 1–2 h PO; 30 min IV

Half-life: 8–16 h

Duration: Variable

ADVERSE EFFECTS

Side effects include sedation, drowsiness, blurred vision, dry mouth, and cardiovascular symptoms such as dysrhythmias, heart block, and extreme hypertension. Agents that mimic the action of norepinephrine or serotonin should be avoided because imipramine inhibits their metabolism and may produce toxicity. Some clients may experience photosensitivity and hyper-sensitivity to tricyclic drugs.

Contraindications: This drug should not be used in cases of acute recovery after MI, defects in bundle-branch conduction, and severe renal or hepatic impairment. Clients should not use this drug within 14 days of discontinuing MAOIs.

INTERACTIONS

Drug-Drug: Concurrent use of other CNS depressants, including alcohol, may cause sedation. Cimetidine (Tagamet) may inhibit the metabolism of imipramine, leading to increased serum levels and possible toxicity. Clonidine may decrease its antihypertensive effects, and increase risk for CNS depression. Use of oral contraceptives may increase or decrease imipramine levels. Disulfiram may lead to delirium and tachycardia. Antithyroid agents may produce agranulocytosis. Phenothiazines cause increased anticholinergic and sedative effects. Sympathomimetics may result in cardiac toxicity. Methylphenidate or cimetidine may increase the effects of imipramine and cause toxicity. Phenytoin is less effective when taken with imipramine. MAOIs may result in neuroleptic malignant syndrome.

Lab Tests: Imipramine produces altered blood glucose tests. Elevation of serum bilirubin and alkaline phosphatase is likely.

Herbal/Food: Herbal supplements such as evening primrose oil or ginkgo, which may lower the seizure threshold. St. John's wort used concurrently may cause serotonin syndrome.

Treatment of Overdose: There is no specific treatment for overdose. General supportive measures are recommended. Ensure an adequate airway, oxygenation, and ventilation. Monitor cardiac rhythm and vital signs. Gastric lavage may be indicated. Activated charcoal should be administered.

 See the Companion Website for a Nursing Process Focus specific to this drug.

Cimetidine (Tagamet) interferes with their metabolism and excretion. Tricyclics affect the efficacy of clonidine (Catapres) and guanethidine (Ismelin). The nurse should observe clients for the effects of drugs that enhance the effects of TCAs, such as antidysrhythmics, antihistamines, antihypertensives, and CNS depressants. Clients who take cimetidine and atropine should also be monitored. Some drugs increase the rate of TCA metabolism and excretion from the body. These include carbamazepine (Tegretol), phenytoin (Dilantin), and rifampin (Rifadin), Cigarette smoking also diminishes the effect of TCAs.

Client Teaching.   Client education as it relates to tricyclic antidepressants should include the goals of therapy, the reasons for obtaining baseline data such as vital signs and the existence of underlying cardiac and renal disorders, and possible drug side effects. Include the following points when teaching clients about TCAs:

- Be aware that it may take several weeks or more to achieve the full therapeutic effect of the drug.
- Keep all scheduled follow-up appointments with your healthcare provider.
- Sweating, along with anticholinergic side effects, may occur.
- Take the medication exactly as prescribed and report side effects if they occur.
- Do not take other prescription drugs, OTC medications, or herbal remedies without notifying your healthcare provider.

AVOIDING MEDICATION ERRORS

A 23-year-old man was admitted this morning following a suicide attempt when his girlfriend broke up with him. When the nurse enters his room with his medications, he is talking on the telephone with his girlfriend. He makes eye contact with and motions for the nurse to leave his medications on the table so he can take them later. The nurse, not wanting to interrupt his conversation, puts the medications on the table, leaves the room, and charts the medications. What did the nurse do wrong?

See Appendix D for the suggested answer.

- Avoid using alcohol and other CNS depressants.
- Change positions slowly to avoid dizziness.
- Do not drive or engage in hazardous activities until the drug's sedative effect is known.
- Take the drug at bedtime if sedation occurs.
- Immediately discuss with your healthcare provider an intention or desire to become pregnant, because these drugs must be withdrawn over several weeks and not discontinued abruptly.

SELECTIVE SEROTONIN REUPTAKE INHIBITORS

Drugs that slow the reuptake of serotonin into presynaptic nerve terminals are called **selective serotonin reuptake inhibitors (SSRIs).** They have become drugs of choice in the treatment of depression because of their favorable side-effect profile.

16.5 Treating Depression With SSRIs

Serotonin is a natural neurotransmitter in the CNS, found in high concentrations in certain neurons in the hypothalamus, limbic system, medulla, and spinal cord. It is important to several body activities, including the cycling between NREM and REM sleep, pain perception, and emotional states. Lack of adequate serotonin in the CNS can lead to depression. Serotonin is metabolized to a less active substance by the enzyme monoamine oxidase (MAO). Serotonin is also known by its chemical name, 5-hydroxytryptamine (5-HT).

In the 1970s, it became increasingly clear that serotonin had a more substantial role in depression than once thought. Clinicians knew that the tricyclic antidepressants altered the sensitivity of serotonin to certain receptors in the brain, but they did not know how this change was connected with depression. Ongoing efforts to find antidepressants with fewer side effects led to the development of a third category of medications, the selective serotonin reuptake inhibitors (SSRIs).

Whereas the tricyclic class inhibit the reuptake of both norepinephrine and serotonin into presynaptic nerve terminals, the SSRIs selectively target for serotonin. Increased levels of serotonin in the synaptic gap induce complex neurotransmitter changes in presynaptic and postsynaptic neurons in the brain. Presynaptic receptors become less sensitive, and postsynaptic receptors become more sensitive. This mechanism is illustrated in ● Figure 16.2.

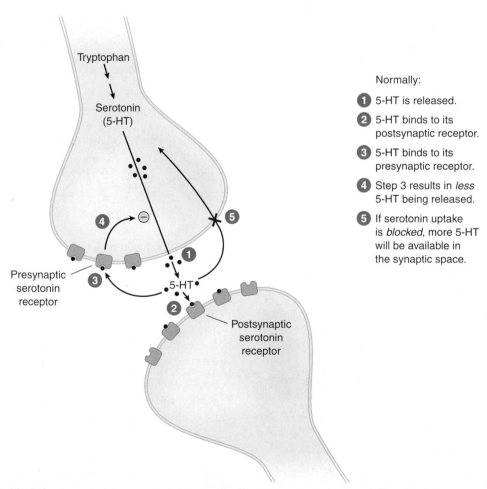

Normally:

1. 5-HT is released.
2. 5-HT binds to its postsynaptic receptor.
3. 5-HT binds to its presynaptic receptor.
4. Step 3 results in *less* 5-HT being released.
5. If serotonin uptake is *blocked*, more 5-HT will be available in the synaptic space.

● **Figure 16.2** SSRIs block the reuptake of serotonin into presynaptic nerve terminals. Increased levels of serotonin induce complex changes in presynaptic and postsynaptic neurons of the brain. Presynaptic receptors become less sensitive and postsynaptic receptors become more sensitive.

Pr PROTOTYPE DRUG | Sertraline *(Zoloft)* | Selective Serotonin Reuptake Inhibitor

ACTIONS AND USES

Sertraline is used for the treatment of depression, anxiety, obsessive-compulsive disorder, and panic. The antidepressant and anxiolytic properties of this drugs can be attributed to its ability to inhibit the reuptake of serotonin in the brain. Other uses include premenstrual dysphoric disorder, post-traumatic stress disorder, and social anxiety disorder. Therapeutic actions include enhancement of mood and improvement of affect with maximum effects observed after several weeks.

ADMINISTRATION ALERTS

- It is recommended that sertraline be given in the morning or evening.
- When administering sertraline as an oral liquid, mix with water, ginger ale, lemon/lime soda, lemonade, or orange juice. Follow manufacturer's instructions.
- Do not give concurrently with a MAO inhibitor or within 14 days of discontinuing MAOI medication.
- Pregnancy category C.

PHARMACOKINETICS

Onset: < 4 h

Peak: 5–8 h

Half-life: 2 h

Duration: Variable (extensive binding with serum proteins)

ADVERSE EFFECTS

Adverse effects include agitation, insomnia, headache, dizzines, somnolence, and fatigue. Take extreme precautions in clients with cardiac disease, hepatic impairment, seizure disorders, suicidal ideation, mania, or hypomania.

Contraindications: Concomitant use of sertraline and MAOIs or primozide is not advised. Antabuse should be avoided because of the alcohol content of the drug concentrate.

INTERACTIONS

Drug-Drug: Highly protein bound medications such as digoxin and warfarin should be avoided owing to risk of toxicity and increased blood concentrations leading to increased bleeding. MAOIs may cause neuroleptic malignant syndrome, extreme hypertension, and serotonin syndrome, characterized by headache, agitation, dizziness, fever, diarrhea, sweating, and shivering. Use cautiously with other centrally acting drugs to avoid adverse CNS effects.

Lab Tests: Sertraline results in asymptomatic liver function tests and a slight decrease in uric acid levels.

Herbal/Food: Clients should use precaution if taking St. John's wort or L-tryptophan to avoid serotonin syndrome.

Treatment of Overdose: There is no specific treatment for overdose. Emergency medical attention and general supportive measures may be necessary. Symptoms of overdose include nausea, vomiting, tremor, seizures, agitation, dizziness, hyperactivity, mydriasis, tachycardia, and coma.

 See the Companion Website for a Nursing Process Focus specific to this drug.

SSRIs have approximately the same efficacy at relieving depression as the MAO inhibitors and the tricyclics. The major advantage of the SSRIs, and the one that makes them drugs of choice, is their greater safety. Sympathomimetic effects (increased heart rate and hypertension) and anticholinergic effects (dry mouth, blurred vision, urinary retention, and constipation) are less common with this drug class. Sedation is also experienced less frequently, and cardiotoxicity is not observed. All drugs in the SSRI class have equal efficacy and similar side effects. In general, SSRIs elicit a therapeutic response more quickly than TCAs.

One of the most common side effects of SSRIs relates to sexual dysfunction. Up to 70% of both men and women can experience decreased libido and lack of ability to reach orgasm. In men, delayed ejaculation and impotence may occur. For clients who are sexually active, these side effects may result in noncompliance with pharmacotherapy. Other common side effects of SSRIs include nausea, headache, weight gain, anxiety, and insomnia. Weight gain may also lead to noncompliance.

Serotonin syndrome (SES) may occur when the client is taking another medication that affects the metabolism, synthesis, or reuptake of serotonin, causing serotonin to accumulate in the body. Symptoms can begin as early as 2 hours after taking the first dose or as late as several weeks after the initiating pharmacotherapy. SES can be produced by the concurrent administration of an SSRI with a MAOI, a tricyclic antidepressant, lithium, or a number of other medications. Symptoms of SES include mental status changes (confusion, anxiety, restlessness), hypertension, tremors, sweating, hyperpyrexia, or ataxia. Conservative treatment is to discontinue the SSRI and provide supportive care. In severe cases, mechanical ventilation and muscle relaxants may be necessary. If left untreated, death may occur.

NATURAL THERAPIES

St. John's Wort for Depression

St. John's wort (*Hypericum perforatum*) is an herb found throughout Great Britain, Asia, Europe, and North America commonly used as an antidepressant. It gets its name from a legend that red spots once appeared on its leaves on the anniversary of St. John's beheading. The word *wort* is a British term for "plant." Researchers once claimed that it produced its effects the same way MAO inhibitors do, by increasing the levels of serotonin, norepinephrine, and dopamine in the brain. More recent evidence suggests that it may selectively inhibit serotonin reuptake. Some claim that it is just as effective as fluoxetine (Prozac), paroxetine (Paxil), or sertraline (Zoloft) and with fewer side effects (Gastpar, Singer, & Zeller, 2006). St. John's wort has been reported to interact with several medications, including oral contraceptives, warfarin, digoxin, and cyclosporine (Fugh-Berman, 2000). It should not be taken concurrently with antidepressant medications.

An active ingredient in St. John's wort is a photoactive compound that when exposed to light, produces substances that can damage myelin. Clients have reported feeling stinging pain on the hands after sun exposure while taking the herbal remedy. Advise clients who take this herb to apply sunscreen or to wear protective clothing when outdoors.

NURSING CONSIDERATIONS

The role of the nurse in SSRI therapy involves careful monitoring of a client's condition and providing education as it relates to the prescribed drug treatment. Assess the client's needs for antidepressant therapy by noting the intensity and duration of symptoms and identifying factors that led to depression, such as life events and health changes. Obtain a careful drug history, including the use of CNS depressants, alcohol, and other antidepressants, especially MAOI therapy, because these may interact with SSRIs. Assess for hypersensitivity to SSRIs. Also ask the client about suicidal ideation, because the drugs may take several weeks before full therapeutic benefit is obtained. Obtain a history of any disorders of sexual function, because these drugs have a high incidence of side effects of this nature. Note any history of eating disorders, because SSRIs commonly cause weight gain, which may contribute to noncompliance in clients with distortions and concerns about body image.

Although the SSRIs are safer than other antidepressants, serious adverse effects can still occur. Obtain baseline liver function tests, because SSRIs are metabolized in the liver, and hepatic disease can result in higher serum levels. Obtain a baseline body weight to monitor weight gain.

Client Teaching. Client education as it relates to SSRIs should include the goals of therapy, the reasons for obtaining baseline data such as vital signs and the existence of underlying diorders or concurrent medication use, and possible drug side effects. Include the following points when teaching clients regarding SSRIs:

- SSRIs may take up to 5 weeks to reach their maximum therapeutic effectiveness.
- Do not take any prescription, OTC drugs, or herbal products without notifying your healthcare provider.
- Keep all follow-up appointments with your healthcare provider.
- Report side effects, including nausea, vomiting, diarrhea, sexual dysfunction, and fatigue.
- Do not drive or engage in hazardous activities until the drug's sedative effect is known
- Do not stop taking the drug suddenly after long-term use because withdrawal symptoms can occur. Although these symptoms are not lifethreatening, they are uncomfortable.
- Take most SSRIs in the morning with food to avoid GI upset and insomnia. Lexapro and Zoloft may be taken in the morning or evening. Take Remerron at bedtime because it usually causes excessive drowsiness, especially at lower doses.
- Exercise and restrict caloric intake to avoid weight gain.

MONOAMINE OXIDASE INHIBITORS

The group of drugs called **monoamine oxidase inhibitors (MAOIs)** inhibit monoamine oxidase, the enzyme that terminates the actions of neurotransmitters such as dopamine, norepinephrine, epinephrine, and serotonin. Because of their low safety margin, these drugs are reserved for clients who have not responded to TCAs or SSRIs.

16.6 Treating Depression With MAO Inhibitors

As discussed in Chapter 13, the action of norepinephrine at adrenergic synapses is terminated through two means: (1) reuptake into the presynaptic nerve and (2) enzymatic destruction by the enzyme monoamine oxidase. By decreasing the effectiveness of the enzyme monamine oxidase, the MAOIs limit the breakdown of norepinephrine, dopamine, and serotonin in CNS neurons. This creates higher levels of these neurotransmitters in the brain to facilitate neurotransmission and alleviate the symptoms of depression. MAO is located within presynaptic nerve terminals, as shown in ● Figure 16.3.

The monoamine oxidase inhibitors were the first drugs approved to treat depression, in the 1950s. They are as effective as TCAs and SSRIs in treating depression. However, because of drug–drug and food–drug interactions, hepatotoxicity, and the development of safer antidepressants, MAOIs are now reserved for clients who are not responsive to other antidepressant classes.

Common side effects of the MAOIs include orthostatic hypotension, headache, insomnia, and diarrhea. A primary concern is that these agents interact with a large number of foods and other medications, sometimes with serious effects. A hypertensive crisis can occur when a MAOI is used concurrently with other antidepressants or sympathomimetic drugs. Combining an MAOI with an SSRI can produce serotonin syndrome. If MAOIs are given with antihypertensives, the client can experience excessive hypotension. MAOIs also potentiate the hypoglycemic effects of insulin and oral antidiabetic drugs. Hyperpyrexia is known to occur in clients taking MAOIs with meperidine (Demerol), dextromethorphan (Pedia Care and others), and TCAs.

A hypertensive crisis can also result from an interaction between MAOIs and foods containing **tyramine,** a form of the amino acid tyrosine. Tyramine is usually degraded by MAO in the intestines. If a client is taking MAOIs, however, tyramine enters the bloodstream in high amounts and displaces norepinephrine in presynaptic nerve terminals. The result is a sudden release of norepinephrine, causing acute hypertension. Symptoms usually occur within minutes of ingesting the food and include occipital headache, stiff neck, flushing, palpitations, diaphoresis, and nausea. Myocardial infarctions and cerebral vascular accidents, though rare, are possible consequences as well. Calcium channel blockers may be given as an antidote. Because of their serious side effects when taken with foods and drugs, MAOIs are rarely used and are limited to clients with symptoms that are resistant to the more typical antidepressants and who are likely to comply with the restrictions regarding foods and drugs. Examples of foods containing tyramine are listed in Table 16.2.

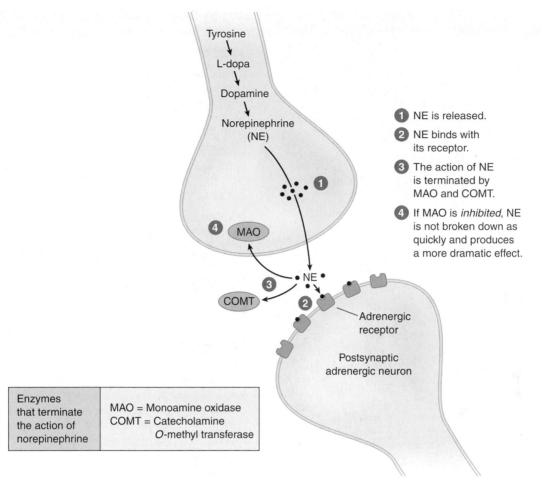

Tyrosine

L-dopa

Dopamine

Norepinephrine
(NE)

1 NE is released.

2 NE binds with
its receptor.

3 The action of NE
is terminated by
MAO and COMT.

4 If MAO is *inhibited*, NE
is not broken down as
quickly and produces
a more dramatic effect.

4 MAO

NE

3 COMT

2

Adrenergic
receptor

Postsynaptic
adrenergic neuron

Enzymes that terminate the action of norepinephrine	MAO = Monoamine oxidase COMT = Catecholamine O-methyl transferase

● **Figure 16.3** Termination of norepinephrine activity through enzyme activity in the synapse

NURSING CONSIDERATIONS

The role of the nurse in MAOI therapy involves careful monitoring of a client's condition and providing education as it relates to the prescribed drug treatment. A client taking an MAOI must refrain from foods that contain tyramine, which is found in many common foods. Assess cardiovascular status, because these agents may affect blood pressure. Phenelzine (Nardil) is contraindicated in cardiovascular disease, heart failure, CVA, hepatic or renal dysfunction, and paranoid schizophrenia. Obtain a CBC, because MAOIs can inhibit platelet function. Assess for the possibility of pregnancy, because these agents are pregnancy category C and enter breast milk. Use MAOIs with caution in epilepsy because they may lower the seizure threshold.

Take a careful drug history; common drugs that may interact with a MAOIs include other MAOIs, insulin,

TABLE 16.2	Foods Containing Tyramine		
Fruits	**Dairy Products**	**Alcohol**	**Meats**
avocados	cheese (cottage cheese is okay)	beer	beef or chicken liver
bananas	sour cream	wines (especially red wines)	paté
raisins	yogurt		meat extracts
papaya products, including meat tenderizers			pickled or kippered herring pepperoni
canned figs			salami
			sausage
			bologna/hot dogs
Vegetables	**Sauces**	**Yeast**	**Other Foods to Avoid**
pods of broad beans (fava beans)	soy sauce	all yeast or yeast extracts	chocolate

Pr **PROTOTYPE DRUG** | Phenelzine *(Nardil)* | Monoamine Oxidase Inhibitor

ACTIONS AND USES

Phenelzine produces its effects by irreversible inhibition of monoamine oxidase; therefore, it intensifies the effects of norepinephrine in adrenergic synapses. It is used to manage symptoms of depression not responsive to other types of pharmacotherapy, and is occasionally used for panic disorder. Drug effects may persist for 2 to 3 weeks after therapy is discontinued.

ADMINISTRATION ALERTS

- Washout periods of 2 to 3 weeks are required before introducing other drugs.
- Abrupt discontinuation of this drug may cause rebound hypertension.
- Pregnancy category C.

PHARMACOKINETICS

Onset: 30 min

Peak: 2–4 h

Half-life: 11 h

Duration: < 2 wk

ADVERSE EFFECTS

Common side effects are constipation, dry mouth, orthostatic hypotension, insomnia, nausea, and loss of appetite. It may increase heart rate and neural activity, leading to delirium, mania, anxiety, and convulsions. Severe hypertension may occur when ingesting foods containing tyramine. Seizures, respiratory depression, circulatory collapse, and coma may occur in cases of severe overdose.

Contraindications: Clients with cardiovascular or cerebrovascular disease, hepatic or renal impairment, and pheochromocytoma should not use this drug.

INTERACTIONS

Drug-Drug: Many other drugs affect the action of phenelzine. Concurrent use of tricyclic antidepressants and SSRIs should be avoided because the combination can cause temperature elevation and seizures. Opiates, including meperidine, should be avoided owing to increased risk of respiratory failure or hypertensive crisis. Sympathomimetics may precipitate a hypertensive crisis. Caffeine may result in cardiac dysrhythmias and hypertension.

Lab Tests: Phenelzine can produce a slightly false increase in serum bilirubin.

Herbal/Food: Ginseng may cause headache, tremors, mania, insomnia, irritability, and visual hallucinations. Concurrent use of ma huang or St. John's wort could result in hypertensive crisis.

Treatment of Overdose: Intensive symptomatic and supportive treatment may be required. Induction of emesis or gastric lavage with instillation of charcoal slurry may be helpful. Signs and symptoms of CNS stimulation, including seizures, should be treated with IV diazepam, given slowly. Hypertension should be treated appropriately with calcium channel blockers. Hypotension and vascular collapse should be treated with IV fluids and, if necessary, blood pressure titration with an IV infusion of dilute pressor agent. Body temperature should be monitored closely, and respiration should be supported with appropriate measures.

 See the Companion Website for a Nursing Process Focus specific to this drug.

---

caffeine-containing products, other antidepressants, meperidine (Demerol), and possibly opioids and methyldopa (Aldomet). There must be at least a 14-day interval between the use of MAOIs and these other drugs.

Some clients may not achieve the full therapeutic benefits of an MAOI for 4 to 8 weeks. Because depression continues during this time, clients may discontinue the drug if they believe it is not helping them. Symptoms of sleep disorder or anxiety are treated with short-term antianxiety agents and sleep aids until the therapeutic effects of the medication are achieved.

Because of the serious side effects possible with MAOIs, client education is vital. The client's ability to comprehend restrictions and be compliant with them may be impaired in a severely depressed state.

Client Teaching.   Client education as it relates to MAOIs should include the goals of therapy, the reasons for obtaining baseline data such as vital signs and the existence of underlying disorders, and possible drug side effects. Include the following points when teaching clients and their caregivers about MAOIs:

- Strictly observe dietary restrictions for foods containing tyramine.

- Do not take any prescription, OTC drugs, or herbal products without notifying your healthcare provider.
- Avoid caffeine.
- Wear a medic alert bracelet identifying the MAOI medication.
- Be aware that it may take several weeks or more to obtain the full therapeutic effect of drug.
- Keep all follow-up appointments with your healthcare provider.
- Do not drive or engage in hazardous activities until the drug's sedative effect is known; it may be taken at bedtime if sedation occurs.
- Observe for and report signs of impending stroke or myocardial infarction (MI).

BIPOLAR DISORDER

Once known as *manic depression,* **bipolar disorder** is characterized by extreme and opposite moods, episodes of depression that alternate with episodes of mania. Clients may oscillate rapidly between both extremes, or there may be

NURSING PROCESS FOCUS Clients Receiving Antidepressant Therapy

Assessment	Potential Nursing Diagnoses
Prior to administration: ■ Obtain a complete health history including allergies, family history of mood disorders, and possible drug interactions. ■ Establish baseline assessment of mood disorder. If possible, use a brief objective tool. ■ Frequency of assessment will relate to the severity of the mood disorder. ■ Obtain history of cardiac (including recent MI), renal, biliary, liver, and mental disorders including ECG and blood studies: CBC, platelets, glucose, blood urea nitrogen (BUN), creatinine, electrolytes, liver function tests and enzymes, and urinalysis. ■ Assess neurologic statusal, including seizure activity and identification of recent mood and behavior patterns.	■ Coping, Ineffective ■ Powerlessness ■ Thought Processes, Disturbed, related to side effects of drug, lack of positive coping skills ■ Knowledge, Deficient, related to drug therapy ■ Violence: Self-directed, Risk for ■ Urinary Retention, related to anticholinergic side effects of drug ■ Noncompliance, related to decreased sexual libido and/or weight gain ■ Risk for Injury, related to adverse side effects ■ Self-Care, Deficient, related to fatigue ■ Nutrition, Imbalanced, Less than body requirements, related to anorexia ■ Nutrition, Imbalanced, More than body requirements, related to side effects of medication or eating for comfort ■ Grieving, Dysfunctional, related to loss (such as loss of health, job, significant other, etc.)

Planning: Client Goals and Expected Outcomes

The client will:
- Report mood elevation (may use short objective tool, such as the Beck Depression Tool).
- Remain safe from self-harm or harm directed toward others.
- Actively engage in self-care activities.
- Report abilty to fall asleep and stay asleep as was able to do before depression.
- Demonstrate an understanding of the drug's action by accurately describing drug side effects and precautions.

Implementation

Interventions and (Rationales)	Client Teaching/Discharge Planning
■ Monitor vital signs, especially pulse and blood pressure, especially when initiating treatment. (Imipramine may cause orthostatic hypotension.)	Instruct client to: ■ Report any change in sensorium, particularly impending syncope. ■ Avoid abrupt changes in position. ■ Monitor vital signs (especially blood pressure) properly using home equipment ■ Consult the nurse regarding "reportable" blood pressure readings (e.g., lower than 80/50 mm Hg).
■ Administer accurately. Give TCAs at bedtime to aid in sleep and minimize daytime drowsiness. (Always practice safe techniques of medication administration. Giving medication at bedtime will minimize the side effect of drowsiness.)	■ Instruct client to take medication at bedtime to decrease daytime drowsines.
■ Observe for signs and symptoms of improved mood, keeping in mind that it may take 2 to 4 weeks to achieve therapeutic effectiveness. (The risk of suicide may increase as energy levels rise.)	Instruct client: ■ That it may take 2 to 4 weeks for mood to improve. ■ To report any feelings of suicide.
■ Observe for serotonin syndrome in SSRI use. (If suspected, discontinue drug and initiate supportive care. Respond according to ICU/emergency department protocols.)	■ Inform client that overdosage may result in serotonin syndrome, which can be life threatening.
■ Monitor for paradoxical diaphoresis. (This must be considered a significant sign, especially serious when coupled with nausea or vomiting or chest pain.)	■ Instruct client to seek immediate medical attention for dizziness, headache, tremor, nausea/vomiting, anxiety, disorientation, hyperreflexia, diaphoresis, and fever.
■ Monitor cardiovascular status. (Hypertension and stroke or MI and heart failure may be observed.)	■ Instruct client to immediately report severe headache, dizziness, paresthesias, bradycardia, chest pain, tachycardia, nausea or vomiting, or diaphoresis.
■ Monitor neurological status. Observe for somnolence and seizures. (TCAs may cause somnolence related to CNS depression. May reduce the seizure threshold.)	Instruct client to: ■ Report significant changes in neurological status, such as seizures, extreme lethargy, slurred speech, disorientation, or ataxia, and discontinue the drug. ■ Take dose at bedtime to avoid daytime sedation.

(Continued)

NURSING PROCESS FOCUS Clients Receiving Antidepressant Therapy *(Continued)*

Implementation

Interventions and (Rationales)	Client Teaching/Discharge Planning
■ Monitor mental and emotional status. Observe for suicidal ideation. (Therapeutic benefits may be delayed. If severely depressed, outclients should have no more than a 7-day medication supply.) Monitor for underlying or concomitant psychoses such as schizophrenia or bipolar disorders. (The drug may trigger manic states.) When used as antianxiety agents, client may need temporary antianxiety agent or sleep aid. (Therapeutic levels are not immediately reached.).	Instruct client: ■ To immediately report dysphoria or suicidal impulses ■ To commit to a "no-self-harm" verbal contract ■ That it may take 10 to 14 days before improvement is noticed, and about 1 month to achieve full therapeutic effect.
■ Observe for anticholinergic or antiadrenergic adverse effects. (Cardiovascular effects are most serious, but other unwanted effects include CNS symptoms, gastrointenstinal problems, blurred vision, urinary retention, sexual dysfunction, and weight gain).	■ Instruct client to report any changes bowel or bladder routines, blurred vision, weight gain, or sexual dysfunction.
■ Monitor sleep–wake cycle. Observe for insomnia and/or daytime somnolence. Establish baseline data on onset and duration of sleep disorder. (Baseline data provide information as to whether symptoms are improving.)	Instruct client to: ■ Take drug very early in the morning if insomnia occurs, to promote normal timing of sleep onset. ■ Avoid driving or performing hazardous activities until effects of drug are known. ■ Take at bedtime if daytime drowsiness persists. ■ Follow principles of sleep hygiene.
■ Monitor renal status and urinary output. (This drug may cause urine retention owing to muscle relaxation in urinary tract. Imipramine is excreted through the kidneys. Fluoxetine is slowly metabolized and excreted, increasing the risk of organ damage. Urinary retention may exacerbate existing symptoms of prostatic hypertrophy.)	Instruct client to: ■ Monitor fluid intake and output. ■ Notify the healthcare provider of edema, dysuria (hesitancy, pain, diminished stream), changes in urine quantity or quality (e.g., cloudy, with sediment). ■ Report fever or flank pain that may indicate a urinary tract infection related to urine retention
■ Use cautiously with elderly or young clients. (Diminished kidney and liver function related to aging can result in higher serum drug levels, and may require lower doses. Children, owing to an immature CNS, respond paradoxically to CNS drugs.)	Instruct client that: ■ The elderly may be more prone to side effects such as hypertension and dysrhythmias. ■ Children on imipramine for nocturnal enuresis may experience mood alterations.
■ Monitor gastrointestinal status. Observe for abdominal distention. (Muscarinic blockade reduces tone and motility of intestinal smooth muscle, and may cause paralytic ileus.)	Instruct client to: ■ Exercise, drink adequate amounts of fluid, and add dietary fiber to promote stool passage. ■ Consult the nurse regarding a bulk laxative or stool softener if constipation becomes a problem.
■ Monitor liver function and blood studies including CBC, differential, platelets, prothrombin time (PT), partial thromboplastin time (PTT), and liver enzymes. (These results determine signs and symptoms of hepatotoxicity.)	Instruct client to: ■ Report nausea, vomiting, diarrhea, rash, jaundice, epigastric or abdominal pain, tenderness, or change in color of stool. ■ Adhere to laboratory testing regimen for blood tests and urinalysis as directed.
■ Monitor hematologic status. Observe for signs of bleeding. (Imipramine may cause blood dyscrasias. Use with warfarin may increase bleeding time.)	Instruct client to: ■ Report excessive bruising, fatigue, pallor, shortness of breath, frank bleeding, and/or tarry stools. ■ Demonstrate guaiac testing on stool for occult blood.
■ Monitor immune/metabolic status. Use with caution in clients with diabetes mellitus or hyperthyroidism. (If given in hyperthyroidism, it can cause agranulocytosis. Imipramine may either increase or decrease serum glucose. Fluoxetine may cause initial anorexia and weight loss, but with prolonged therapy may result in weight gain of up to 20 lb.)	■ Instruct diabetic clients to monitor glucose level daily and consult nurse regarding reportable serum glucose levels (e.g., less than 70 and more than 140 mmol/L). ■ Instruct client that anorexia and weight loss will diminish with continued therapy.

NURSING PROCESS FOCUS Clients Receiving Antidepressant Therapy *(Continued)*

Implementation

Interventions and (Rationales)	Client Teaching/Discharge Planning
• Observe for extrapyramidal and anticholinergic effects. In overdosage, 12 hours of anticholinergic activity is followed by CNS depression. Do not treat overdosage with quinidine, procainamide, atropine, or barbiturates. (Quinidine and procainamide can increase the possibility of dysrhythmia, atropine can lead to severe anticholinergic effects, and barbiturates can lead to excess sedation.)	Instruct client to: • Immediately report involuntary muscle movement of the face or upper body (e.g., tongue spasms), fever, anuria, lower abdominal pain, anxiety, hallucinations, psychomotor agitation, visual changes, dry mouth, and difficulty swallowing. • Relieve dry mouth with (sugar-free) hard candies or chewing gum, and by drinking fluids. • Avoid alcohol-containing mouthwashes, which can further dry oral mucous membranes.
• Monitor visual acuity. Use with caution in narrow-angle glaucoma. (Imipramine may cause an increase in intraocular pressure. Anticholinergic effects may produce blurred vision.)	Instruct client to: • Report visual changes, headache, or eye pain. • Inform eye care professional of imipramine therapy.
• Ensure client safety. (Dizziness caused by postural hypotension increases the risk of fall injuries.)	Instruct client to: • Call for assistance before getting out of bed or attempting to ambulate alone. • Avoid driving or performing hazardous activities until blood pressure is stabilized and effects of the drug are known.

Evaluation of Outcome Criteria

Evaluate effectiveness of drug therapy by confirming that client goals and expected outcomes have been met (see "Planning").
• The client reports an elevation of mood.
• The client is free of self-harm and verbalizes no intent to harm others.
• The client initiates self-care activities.
• The client reports ability to fall asleep and stay asleep at night.
• The client demonstrates an understanding of the drug's action by accurately describing drug side effects and precautions.

∞ *See Table 16.1 for a list of drugs to which these nursing actions apply.*

prolonged periods when mood is normal. Depressive symptoms are the same collection of symptoms as were defined earlier in this chapter. Mania is characterized by excessive CNS stimulation that results in symptoms listed in section 16.7. To be diagnosed with bipolar disorder, these symptoms must be present for at least 1 week. Hypomania is characterized by the same symptoms, but they are less severe. Mania and hypomania may result from abnormal functioning of neurotransmitters or receptors in the brain. Hypomania may involve an excess of excitatory neurotransmitters (such as norepinephrine) or a deficiency of inhibitory neurotransmitters such as gamma-aminobutyric acid (GABA) (see Chapter 15 ∞). It is important to distiguish mania from the effects of drug use or abuse and also from schizophrenia.

16.7 Characteristics of Bipolar Disorder

During the depressive stages of bipolar disorder, clients exhibit the symptoms of major depression described earlier in this chapter. Clients with bipolar disorder also display signs of **mania,** an emotional state characterized by high psychomotor activity and irritability. Clients may shift from emotions of extreme depression to extreme rage and agitation. Symptoms of mania, as described in the following list, are generally the opposite of depressive symptoms:

• Inflated self-esteem or grandiosity
• Decreased need for sleep (e.g., feels rested after only 3 hours of sleep)
• Increased talkativeness or pressure to keep talking
• Flight of ideas or subjective feeling that thoughts are racing
• Distractibility (i.e., attention too easily drawn to unimportant or irrelevant external stimuli)
• Increased goal-directed activity (either socially, at work or school, or sexually) or psychomotor agitation
• Excessive involvement in pleasurable activities that have a high potential for painful consequences (e.g., unrestrained buying sprees, sexual indiscretions, or foolish business investments)

DRUGS FOR BIPOLAR DISORDER

Drugs for bipolar disorder are called **mood stabilizers,** because they have the ability to moderate extreme shifts in emotions between mania and depression. Some antiseizure drugs are also used for mood stabilization in bipolar clients.

TABLE 16.3 Drugs for Bipolar Disorder

Drug	Route and Adult Dose (max dose where indicated)	Adverse Effects
Pr lithium (Eskalith)	PO; initial: 600 mg tid; maintenance: 300 mg tid (max: 2.4 g/day)	*Headache, lethargy, fatigue, recent memory loss, nausea, vomiting, anorexia, abdominal pain, diarrhea, dry mouth, muscle weakness* Peripheral circulatory collapse
ANTISEIZURE DRUGS		
carbamazepine (Tegretol)	PO; 200 mg bid, gradually increased to 800–1200 mg/day in 3 to 4 divided doses	*Dizziness, ataxia, somnolence, headache, nausea, diplopia, blurred vision, sedation, drowsiness, nausea, vomiting, prolonged bleeding time*
lamotrigine (Lamictal)	PO; 50 mg/day for 2 weeks, then 50 mg bid for 2 weeks; may increase gradually up to 300–500 mg/day in 2 divided doses (max: 700 mg/day)	Heart block, aplastic anemia, respiratory depression, exfoliative dermatitis, Stevens–Johnson syndrome, toxic epidermal necrolysis, deep coma, death (with overdose), liver failure, pancreatitis
valproic acid (Depakene) (see page 180 for the Prototype Drug box ∞)	PO; 250 mg tid (max: 60 mg/kg/day)	

Italics indicate common adverse effects; underlining indicates serious adverse effects.

16.8 Pharmacotherapy of Bipolar Disorder

The traditional treatment of bipolar disorder is lithium (Eskalith), as monotherapy or in combination with other drugs. Lithium was approved in the United States in 1970. Before that time, its benefit in manic-depressive illness had been known; however, its therapeutic safety had not been proved. Antiseizure drugs (see Chapter 15 ∞), although not FDA approved, are used as unlabeled agents for mood stabilization. For example, carbamazepine (Tegretol) and valproic acid (Depakene) are antiseizure drugs that have adjunct uses in bipolar disease. Table 16.3 lists selected drugs used to treat bipolar disorder. Carbamazepine (Tegretol), valproic acid (Depakote), gabapentin (Neurontin), lamotrigine (Lamictal), topiramate (Topomax), and oxcarbazepine (Trileptal) all have some beneficial effects for mood stabilization.

Pr PROTOTYPE DRUG | Lithium *(Eskalith)* | Drugs for Bipolar Disorder

ACTIONS AND USES

Although the exact mechanism of action is not clear, lithium is thought to alter the activity of neurons containing dopamine, norepinephrine, and serotonin by influencing their release, synthesis, and reuptake. Therapeutic actions are stabilization of mood during periods of mania, and antidepressant effects during periods of depression. Lithium has neither antimanic nor antidepressant effects in individuals without bipolar disorder. After taking lithium for 2 to 3 weeks, clients are able to better concentrate and function in self-care.

ADMINISTRATION ALERTS

- Lithium has a narrow therapeutic/toxic ratio; risk of toxicity is high.
- Acute overdosage may be treated by hemodialysis.
- Pregnancy category D.

PHARMACOKINETICS

Onset:
 lithium carbonate: 30–60 min
 lithium citrate: 15–60 min

Peak: Variable

Half-life: 20–27 h

Duration: Variable

ADVERSE EFFECTS

Lithium may cause dizziness, fatigue, short-term memory loss, increased urination, nausea, vomiting, loss of appetite, abdominal pain, diarrhea, dry mouth, muscular weakness, and slight tremors. Clients should not have a salt-free diet when taking this drug, because it reduces lithium excretion.

Contraindications: This drug is contraindicated in debilitated clients and clients with severe cardiovascular disease, dehydration, or renal disease, and in cases of severe sodium depletion.

INTERACTIONS

Drug-Drug: Some drugs increase the rate at which the kidneys remove lithium from the bloodstream, including diuretics, sodium bicarbonate, and potassium citrate. Other drugs, such as methyldopa and probenecid, inhibit the rate of lithium excretion. Diuretics enhance excretion of sodium and increase the risk of lithium toxicity. Concurrent administration of anticholinergic drugs can cause urinary retention that, coupled with the polyuria effect of lithium, may cause a medical emergency. Alcohol can potentiate drug action.

Lab Tests: Unknown.

Herbal/Food: Unknown.

Treatment of Overdose: There is no specific treatment for overdose. Treatment is supportive, including gastric lavage, correction of fluid and electrolyte imbalance, and regulation of renal functioning. Hemodialysis is an effective and rapid means of removing the ion from the severely toxic client; however, recovery time may be prolonged.

Lithium has a narrow therapeutic index and is monitored via serum levels every 1 to 3 days when beginning therapy, and every 2 to 3 months thereafter. To ensure therapeutic action, concentrations of lithium in the blood must remain within the range of 0.6 to 1.5 mEq/L. Close monitoring encourages compliance and helps prevent toxicity. Lithium acts like sodium in the body, so conditions in which sodium is lost (e.g., excessive sweating or dehydration) can cause lithium toxicity. Lithium

overdose may be treated with hemodialysis and supportive care. Baseline studies of renal, cardiac, and thyroid status are indicated, as well as baseline electrolyte studies.

It is not unusual for other drugs to be used in combination with lithium for the control of bipolar disorder. During a client's depressed stage, a tricyclic antidepressant or bupropion (Wellbutrin) may be necessary. During the manic phases, a benzodiazepine will moderate manic symptoms. In cases of

NURSING PROCESS FOCUS Clients Receiving Lithium (Eskalith)

Assessment	Potential Nursing Diagnoses
Prior to administration: ▪ Obtain complete health history including allergies, drug history, and possible drug interactions. ▪ Assess mental and emotional status, including any recent suicidal ideation. ▪ Obtain cardiac history (including ECG and vital signs); renal and liver disorders, and blood studies: glucose, BUN, creatinine, electrolytes, and liver enzymes.	▪ Violence: Self-directed, Risk for ▪ Thought Processes, Disturbed ▪ Sleep Pattern, Disturbed ▪ Fluid Volume, Imbalanced, Risk for ▪ Self-Care Deficit: Dressing/Grooming

Planning: Client Goals and Expected Outcomes

The client will:
▪ Demonstrate stabilization of mood, including absence of mania and suicidal depression.
▪ Remain safe from self-harm or harm directed toward others.
▪ Engage in normal activities of daily living and report subjective improvement in mood.
▪ Report ability to fall and stay asleep.
▪ Demonstrate an understanding of the drugs' action by accurately describing drug side effects and precautions.

Implementation

Interventions and (Rationales)	Client Education/Discharge Planning
▪ Monitor mental and emotional status. Observe for mania and/or extreme depression. (Lithium should prevent mood swings.)	▪ Instruct client to keep a symptom log to document response to medication.
▪ Monitor electrolyte balance. (Lithium is a salt affected by dietary intake of other salts such as sodium chloride. Insufficient dietary salt intake causes the kidneys to conserve lithium, increasing serum lithium levels.)	Instruct client to: ▪ Monitor dietary salt intake; consume sufficient quantities, especially during illness or physical activity. ▪ Avoid activities that cause excessive perspiration.
▪ Monitor fluid balance. (Lithium causes polyuria by blocking effects of antidiuretic hormone.)	Instruct client to: ▪ Increase fluid intake to 1 to 1.5 L per day. ▪ Limit or eliminate caffeine consumption (caffeine has a diuretic effect, which can cause lithium sparing by the kidneys).
▪ Measure intake and output. Weigh client daily. (Short-term changes in weight are a good indicator of fluctuations in fluid volume. Excess fluid volume increases the risk of HF; pitting edema may signal HF.)	▪ Instruct client to notify healthcare provider of excessive weight gain or loss, or pitting edema.
▪ Monitor renal status, CBC, differential, BUN, creatinine, uric acid, and urinalysis. (Lithium may cause degenerative changes in the kidney, which increases drug toxicity.)	Instruct client to: ▪ Immediately report anuria, especially accompanied by lower abdominal tenderness, distention, headache, and diaphoresis. ▪ Inform healthcare provider of nausea, vomiting, diarrhea, flank pain or tenderness, and changes in urinary quantity and quality (e.g., sediment).
▪ Monitor cardiovascular status, vital signs including apical pulse, and status. (Lithium toxicity may cause muscular irritability resulting in cardiac dysrhythmias or angina. Use with caution in clients with a history of CAD or heart disease.)	Instruct client to: ▪ Immediately report palpitations, chest pain, or other symptoms suggestive of myocardial infarction. ▪ Monitor vital signs properly using home equipment.

(Continued)

NURSING PROCESS FOCUS Clients Receiving Lithium (Eskalith) (Continued)	
Implementation	
Interventions and (Rationales)	**Client Education/Discharge Planning**
▪ Monitor gastrointestinal status. (Lithium may cause dyspepsia, diarrhea, or metallic taste.)	▪ Instruct client to take drug with food to reduce stomach upset and report distressing GI symptoms.
▪ Monitor metabolic status. (Lithium may cause goiter with prolonged use and false-positive results on thyroid tests.)	▪ Instruct client to report symptoms of goiter or hypothyroidism: enlarged mass on neck, fatigue, dry skin, or edema.
Evaluation of Outcome Criteria	
Evaluate effectiveness of drug therapy by confirming that client goals and expected outcomes have been met (see "Planning"). ▪ The client demonstrates stabilization of mood, including absence of mania and suicidal depression. ▪ The client remains safe from self-harm or harm directed to others. ▪ The client initiates normal activities of daily living and reports an improvement in mood. ▪ The client reports being able to fall and stay asleep. ▪ The client demonstrates an understanding of the drug's action by accurately describing drug side effects and precautions.	

extreme agitation, delusions, or hallucinations, an antipsychotic agent may be indicated. Continued client compliance is essential to achieving successful pharmacotherapy, because some clients do not perceive their condition as abnormal.

NURSING CONSIDERATIONS

The role of the nurse in lithium therapy involves careful monitoring of a client's condition and providing education as it relates to prescribed drug treatment. Because lithium is a salt, clients with a history of cardiovascular and kidney disease should not take lithium. Clients frequently experience dehydration and sodium depletion; therefore, those on a low-salt diet should not be prescribed lithium. Assess for and identify signs and symptoms of lithium toxicity, which include diarrhea, lethargy, slurred speech, muscle weakness, ataxia, seizures, edema, hypotension, and circulatory collapse.

Lifespan Considerations. Lithium is contraindicated in pregnant and nursing women. It should also not be used by children younger than 12 years. It should be used with caution in older adults.

Client Teaching. Client education as it relates to lithium therapy should include the goals of therapy, the reasons for obtaining baseline data such as vital signs and the existence of cardiac and renal disorders, and possible drug side effects. Include the following points when teaching clients about lithium:

- Take medication as ordered, because compliance is the key to successful treatment.
- Keep all scheduled laboratory visits to monitor lithium levels.
- Do not change diet or decrease fluid intake, because any changes in diet and fluid status can affect therapeutic drug levels.
- Avoid alcohol use.
- Do not take other prescription medications, OTC drugs, or herbal products without notifying your healthcare provider.

- Do not stop taking this medication suddenly.
- Immediately report any increase in dilute urine, diarrhea, fever, or changes in mobility.
- Drink plenty of fluids to avoid dehydration.
- Practice reliable contraception and notify your healthcare provider if pregnancy is planned or suspected.

ATTENTION DEFICIT–HYPERACTIVITY DISORDER

A condition characterized by poor attention span, behavior control issues, and/or hyperactivity is called **attention deficit–hyperactivity disorder (ADHD)**. Although the condition is normally diagnosed in childhood, symptoms of ADHD may extend into adulthood.

16.9 Characteristics of ADHD

ADHD affects as many as 5% of all children. Most children diagnosed with this condition are between the ages of 3 and 7 years, and boys are 4 to 8 times more likely to be diagnosed than girls.

ADHD is characterized by developmentally inappropriate behaviors involving difficulty in paying attention or focusing on tasks. ADHD may be diagnosed when the child's hyperactive behaviors significantly interfere with normal play, sleep,

PHARMFACTS

Attention Deficit–Hyperactivity Disorder

- ADHD is the major reason why children are referred for mental health treatment.
- About half are also diagnosed with oppositional defiant or conduct disorder.
- About one fourth are also diagnosed with anxiety disorder.
- About one third are also diagnosed with depression.
- And about one fifth also have a learning disability.

or learning activities. Hyperactive children usually have increased motor activity that is manifested by a tendency to be fidgety and impulsive, and to interrupt and talk excessively during their developmental years; therefore, they may not be able to interact with others appropriately at home, school, or on the playground. In boys, the activity levels are usually more overt. Girls show less aggression and impulsiveness but more anxiety, mood swings, social withdrawal, and cognitive and language delays. Girls also tend to be older at the time of diagnosis, so problems and setbacks related to the disorder exist for a longer time before treatment interventions are undertaken. Symptoms of ADHD are described in the following list:

• Easy distractability

• Failure to receive or follow instructions properly

• Inability to focus on one task at a time and jumping from one activity to another

• Difficulty remembering

• Frequent loss or misplacement of personal items

• Excessive talking and interrupting other children in a group

• Inability to sit still when asked to do so repeatedly

• Impulsiveness

• Sleep disturbance

Most children with ADHD have associated challenges. Many find it difficult to concentrate on tasks assigned in school. Even if children are gifted, their grades may suffer because they have difficulty following a conventional routine; discipline may also be a problem. Teachers are often the first to suggest that a child be examined for ADHD and receive medication when behaviors in the classroom escalate to the point of interfering with learning. A diagnosis is based on psychological and medical evaluations.

The etiology of ADHD is not clear. For many years, scientists described this disorder as mental brain dysfunction and hyperkinetic syndrome, focusing on abnormal brain function and overactivity. A variety of physical and neurological disorders have been implicated; only a small percentage of those affected have a known cause. Known causes include contact with high levels of lead in childhood and prenatal exposure to alcohol and drugs. Genetic factors may also play a role, although a single gene has not been isolated and a specific mechanism of genetic transmission is not known. The interplay of genetics and environment may be a contributing dynamic. Recent evidence suggests that hyperactivity may be related to a deficit or dysfunction of dopamine, norepinephrine, and serotonin in the reticular activating system of the brain. Although once thought to be the culprits, sugars, chocolate, high-carbohydrate foods and beverages, and certain food additives have been disproved as causative or aggravating factors for ADHD.

The nurse is often involved in the screening and the mental health assessment of children with suspected ADHD. When a child is referred for testing, it is important to remember that both the child and family must be assessed. The family is screened with, or prior to, the child's evaluation. It is the nurse's responsibility to collect comprehensive data about the character and extent of the child's physical, psychological, and developmental health situation, to formulate the nursing diagnoses, and to create an individualized plan of care. A relevant nursing care plan can be created only if it is based on appropriate communication that fosters rapport and trust.

Once ADHD is diagnosed, the nurse is instrumental in educating the family regarding coping mechanisms that might be used to manage the demands of a child who is hyperactive. For the school-age child, the nurse often serves as the liaison to parents, teachers, and school administrators. The parents and child need to understand the importance of appropriate expectations and behavioral consequences. The child, from an early age and based on his or her developmental level, must be educated about the disorder and understand that there are consequences to inappropriate behavior. Self-esteem must be fostered in the child so that strengths in self-worth can develop. It is important for the child to develop a trusting relationship with healthcare providers and learn the importance of medication management and compliance.

One third to half of children diagnosed with ADHD also experience symptoms of attention dysfunction in their adult years. Symptoms of attention deficit disorder (ADD) in adults appear similar to mood disorders. Symptoms include anxiety, mania, restlessness, and depression, which can cause difficulties in interpersonal relationships. Some clients have difficulty holding jobs and may have increased risk for alcohol and drug abuse. Untreated ADD/ADHD has been linked to low self-esteem, diminished social success, and criminal or violent behaviors.

DRUGS FOR ATTENTION DEFICIT–HYPERACTIVITY DISORDER

The traditional drugs used to treat ADHD in children have been CNS stimulants. These drugs stimulate specific areas of the central nervous system that heighten alertness and increase focus. Recently, a non-CNS stimulant was approved to treat ADHD. Agents for treating ADHD are listed in Table 16.4.

16.10 Pharmacotherapy of ADHD

The main treatment for ADHD are CNS stimulants. Stimulants reverse many of the symptoms, helping clients focus on tasks. The most widely prescribed drug for ADHD is methylphenidate (Ritalin). Other CNS stimulants that are rarely prescribed include D- and L-amphetamine racemic mixture (Adderall), dextroamphetamine (Dexedrine), methamphetamine (Desoxyn), or pemoline (Cylert).

Clients taking CNS stimulants must be carefully monitored. CNS stimulants used to treat ADHD may create paradoxical hyperactivity. Adverse reactions include insomnia, nervousness, anorexia, and weight loss. Occasionally, a client may suffer from dizziness, depression, irritability, nausea, or abdominal pain. These are Schedule II controlled substances and pregnancy category C. Methylphenidate

TABLE 16.4	Drugs for Attention Deficit–Hyperactivity Disorder	
Drug	**Route and Adult Dose (max dose where indicated)**	**Adverse Effects**
CNS STIMULANTS		
D- and L-amphetamine racemic mixture (Adderall)	6 years old: PO; 5 mg one or two times/day; may increase by 5 mg at weekly intervals (max: 40 mg/day). 3–5 years old: PO; 2.5 mg 1 to 2 times/day; may increase by 2.5 mg at weekly intervals	*Irritability, nervousness, restlessness, insomnia, euphoria, palpitations*
dextroamphetamine (Dexedrine)	3–5 years old: PO; 2.5 mg 1 or 2 times/day; may increase by 2.5 mg at weekly intervals	Sudden death (reported in children with structural cardiac abnormalities), circulatory collapse, exfoliative dermatitis, anorexia, liver failure
	6 years old: PO; 5 mg 1 or 2 times/day; increase by 5 mg at weekly intervals (max: 40 mg/day)	
methamphetamine (Desoxyn)	6 years old: PO; 2.5–5 mg 1 or 2 times/day; may increase by 5 mg at weekly intervals (max: 20–25 mg/day)	
Ⓟ methylphenidate (Ritalin)	PO; 5–10 mg before breakfast and lunch, with gradual increase of 5–10 mg/week as needed (max: 60 mg/day)	
pemoline (Cylert)	6 years old: PO; 37.5 mg/day; may increase by 18.75 mg at weekly intervals (max: 112.5 mg/day)	
NONSTIMULANT FOR ADD/ADHD		
atomoxetine (Strattera)	PO; start with 40 mg in AM; may increase after 3 days to target dose of 80 mg/day given either once in the morning or divided morning and late afternoon/early evening; may increase to max of 100 mg/day if needed	*Headache, insomnia, upper abdominal pain, vomiting, decreased appetite* Severe liver injury (rare)

Italics indicate common adverse effects, underlining indicates serious adverse effects.

abuse has been increasing, especially among teens who take the drug to stay awake or as an appetite suppressant to lose weight.

Non-CNS stimulants have been tried for ADHD; however, they exhibit less efficacy. Clonidine (Catapres) is sometimes prescribed when clients are extremely aggressive, active, or have difficulty falling asleep. Atypical antidepressants such as bupropion (Wellbutrin) and tricyclics such as desipramine (Norpramine) and imipramine (Tofranil) are considered second-choice drugs, when CNS stimulants fail to work or are contraindicated.

A recent addition to the treatment of ADHD in children and adults is atomoxetine (Strattera). Although its exact mechanism is not known, it is classified as a norepinephrine reuptake inhibitor. Clients taking atomoxetine showed improved ability to focus on tasks and reduced hyperactivity. Efficacy appears to be equivalent to methylphenidate (Ritalin), although the drug is too new for long-term comparisons. Common side effects include headache, insomnia, upper abdominal pain, decreased appetite, and cough. Unlike methylphenidate, it is not a scheduled drug; thus, parents who are hesitant to place their child on stimulants now have a reasonable alternative. All children treated with atomexetine should be monitored closely for increased risk of suicide ideation.

SPECIAL CONSIDERATIONS

Zero Tolerance in Schools

Methylphenidate is an effective drug for treating ADHD and is often promoted by teachers and school counselors as an adjunct to improving academic performance and social adjustment. However, most schools have a "zero drug tolerance" policy, which creates a hostile environment for students who must take this drug. Zero tolerance policies generally prohibit the possession of *any* drug and define the school's right to search and seizure and the right to demand that students submit to random drug testing or screening as a condition of participating in sports and extracurricular activities. Schools maintain the right to suspend or expel students found in violation of such policies. In some districts, possession of scheduled drugs may also result in arrest and prosecution of the student.

Methylphenidate is a Schedule II controlled substance considered to have a high abuse potential. Students who take this drug should be made aware of the academic and social consequences of unauthorized possession of this medication. Most schools have strict guidelines regarding medication administration and require original prescriptions and containers of drug to be supplied to the school health office. Students should carry an official notice from the health-care provider regarding methylphenidate therapy that may be produced in the event of random drug testing.

NURSING CONSIDERATIONS

The role of the nurse in ADHD therapy involves careful monitoring of the client's condition and providing education as it relates to prescribed drug treatment. Take a thorough assessment prior to initiation of therapy. Methylphenidate (Ritalin) is contraindicated in clients with a history of cardiovascular disease, hypertension, hyperthyroidism, and seizure disorders. Review liver function tests, because clients receiving methylphenidate (Ritalin) can experience hepatotoxicity. Weight loss is common with all the ADHD medications, so weigh the client frequently. Offer clients high-calorie, nutritious meals and snacks.

Pr PROTOTYPE DRUG | Methylphenidate *(Ritalin)* | CNS Stimulant

ACTIONS AND USES

Methylphenidate activates the reticular activating system, causing heightened alertness in various regions of the brain, particularly those centers associated with focus and attention. Activation is partially achieved by the release of neurotransmitters such as norepinephrine, dopamine, and serotonin. Impulsiveness, hyperactivity, and disruptive behavior are usually reduced within a few weeks. These changes promote improved psychosocial interactions and academic performance.

ADMINISTRATION ALERTS

- Sustained-release tablets must be swallowed whole. Breaking or crushing SR tablets causes immediate release of the entire dose.
- Controlled substance: Schedule II drug.
- Pregnancy category C.

PHARMACOKINETICS

Onset: < 60 min

Peak: 2 h; 3–8 sustained release

Half-life: 2–4 h

Duration: 3–6 h; 8 h sustained release; 8–12 h extended release

ADVERSE EFFECTS

In a non-ADHD client, methylphenidate causes nervousness and insomnia. All clients are at risk for irregular heart beat, high blood pressure, and liver toxicity. Because methylphenidate is a Schedule II drug, it has the potential for causing dependence when used for extended periods. Periodic drug-free "holidays" are recommended to reduce drug dependence and to assess the client's condition.

Contraindications: Clients with a history of marked anxiety, agitation, psychosis, suicidal ideation, glaucoma, motor tics, or Tourette's disease should not use this drug.

INTERACTIONS

Drug–Drug: Methylphenidate interacts with many drugs. For example, it may decrease the effectiveness of anticonvulsants, anticoagulants, and guanethidine. Concurrent therapy with clonidine may increase adverse effects. Antihypertensives or other CNS stimulants could potentiate the vasoconstrictive action of methylphenidate. MAOIs may produce hypertensive crisis.

Lab Tests: Unknown.

Herbal/Food: Administration times relative to meals and meal composition may need individual titration.

Treatment of Overdose: There is no specific treatment for overdose. Signs and symptoms of acute overdose result principally from overstimulation of the CNS and from excessive sympathomimetic effects. Emergency medical attention and general supportive measures may be necessary.

MediaLink Mechanism in Action: Methylphenidate

Include families in the treatment of ADHD, because it affects the whole family. Family members should be taught to recognize signs of suicide ideation when atomoxetine is used.

Client Teaching. Client education as it relates to ADHD therapy should include the goals of therapy, the reasons for obtaining baseline data such as vital signs and the existence of other medical disorders, and possible drug side effects. Include the following points when teaching clients about ADHD therapy:

- Use caution when performing activities that require alertness.

- Take this medication as ordered or prescibed.
- Eat high-calorie, nutritious meals and weigh yourself weekly. Notify your healthcare provider of weight loss.
- Do not take other prescription medications, OTC drugs, or herbal products without notifying your healthcare provider.
- Keep all scheduled laboratory visits for testing.
- Do not discontinue medication suddenly.
- Keep medication in a secure location.

NURSING PROCESS FOCUS Clients Receiving Methylphenidate (Ritalin)

Assessment	Potential Nursing Diagnoses
Prior to administration: ■ Obtain a complete health history including allergies, drug history, and possible drug interactions. ■ Obtain history of neurological, cardiac, renal, biliary, and mental disorders including blood studies: CBC, platelets, liver enzymes. ■ Assess neurological status, including identification of recent behavioral patterns. ■ Assess growth and development.	■ Delayed Development, Risk for, related to growth retardation secondary to methylphenidate ■ Growth and Development, Delayed, related to increased motor activity, growth retardation secondary to methylphenidate, unsuccessful interpersonal relationships ■ Nutrition: Imbalanced, Less than Body Requirements ■ Knowledge, Deficient, related to drug therapy ■ Sleep Pattern, Disturbed

(Continued)

NURSING PROCESS FOCUS Clients Receiving Methylphenidate (Ritalin) *(Continued)*

Planning: Client Goals and Expected Outcomes

The client will:

- Experience subjective improvement in attention/concentration and reduction in impulsivity and/or psychomotor symptoms ("hyperactivity").
- Demonstrate an understanding of the drug's action by accurately describing drug side effects effects and precautions.

Implementation

Interventions and (Rationales)	Client Education/Discharge Planning
Monitor mental status and observe for changes in level of consciousness and adverse effects such as persistent drowsiness, psychomotor agitation or anxiety, dizziness, trembling or seizures. (These are adverse effects of CNS stimulants.)	Instruct client to report any significant increase in motor behavior, changes in sensorium, or feelings of dysphoria.
Use with caution in epilepsy. (Drug may lower the seizure threshold.)	Instruct client to discontinue drug immediately if seizures occur, and notify healthcare provider.
Monitor vital signs. (Stimulation of the CNS induces the release of catecholamines with a subsequent increase in heart rate and blood pressure.)	Instruct client to: - Immediately report rapid heartbeat, palpitations, or dizziness. - Monitor blood pressure and pulse properly using home equipment.
Monitor gastrointestinal and nutritional status. (CNS stimulation causes anorexia and elevates BMR, producing weight loss. Other GI side effects include nausea and vomiting and abdominal pain.)	Instruct client to: - Report any distressing GI side effects. - Take drug with meals to reduce GI upset and counteract anorexia; eat frequent, small nutrient-and calorie-dense snacks. - Weigh weekly and report significant losses over 1 lb.
Monitor laboratory tests such as CBC, differential, and platelet count. (Drug is metabolized in the liver and excreted by the kidneys; impaired organ function can increase serum drug levels. Drug may cause leukopenia and/or anemia.)	Instruct client to: - Report shortness of breath, profound fatigue, pallor, bleeding or excessive bruising (these are signs of blood disorder). - Report nausea, vomiting, diarrhea, rash, jaundice, abdominal pain, tenderness, distention, or change in color of stool (these are signs of liver disease). - Adhere to laboratory testing regimen for blood tests and urinalysis as directed.
Monitor effectiveness of drug therapy. (Dosage may be modified if symptoms continue.)	Instruct client to: - Schedule regular drug holidays - Not discontinue abruptly, as rebound hyperactivity or withdrawal symptoms may occur; taper the dose prior to starting a drug holiday. - Keep a behavior diary to chronicle symptoms and response to drug. - Safeguard medication supply owing to abuse potential.
Monitor growth and development. (Growth rate may stall in response to nutritional deficiency caused by anorexia.)	Instruct client that reductions in growth rate are associated with drug usage. Drug holidays may decrease this effect.
Monitor sleep–wake cycle. (CNS stimulation may disrupt normal sleep patterns.)	Instruct client that: - Insomnia may be adverse reaction. - Sleeplessness can sometimes be counteracted by taking the last dose no later than 4 PM. - Drug is not intended to treat fatigue; warn the client that fatigue may accompany washout period.

Evaluation of Outcome Criteria

Evaluate effectiveness of drug therapy by confirming that client goals and expected outcomes have been met (see "Planning").

- The client verbalizes improvement in attention and concentration and reduction in impulsivity and psychomotor symptoms ("hyperactivity").
- The client demonstrates an understanding of the drug's action by accurately describing drug side effects and precautions.

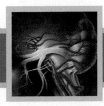

CHAPTER REVIEW

KEY CONCEPTS

The numbered key concepts provide a succinct summary of the important points from the corresponding numbered section within the chapter. If any of these points are not clear, refer to the numbered section within the chapter for review.

16.1 Depression has many causes and methods of classification. The identification of depression and its etiology is essential for proper treatment.

16.2 Major depression may be treated with medications, psychotherapeutic techniques, or electroconvulsive therapy.

16.3 Antidepressants act by correcting neurotransmitter imbalances in the brain. The two basic mechanisms of action are blocking the enzymatic breakdown of norepinephrine and slowing the reuptake of serotonin. The serotonin–norepinephrine reuptake inhibitors (SNRIs) are a class of antidepressants specifically approved for the relief of depression symptoms.

16.4 Tricyclic antidepressants are older medications used mainly for the treatment of major depression, obsessive-compulsive disorders, and panic attacks.

16.5 SSRIs act by selectively blocking the reuptake of serotonin in nerve terminals. Because of fewer side effects, SSRIs are drugs of choice in the pharmacotherapy of depression.

16.6 MAOIs are usually prescribed in cases when other antidepressants have not been successful. They have more serious side effects than other antidepressants.

16.7 Clients with bipolar disorder display not only signs of depression but also mania, a state characterized by expressive psychomotor activity and irritability.

16.8 Mood stabilizers such as lithium (Eskalith) are used to treat both the manic and depressive stages of bipolar disorder.

16.9 Attention deficit–hyperactivity disorder (ADHD) is a common condition occurring primarily in children and is characterized by difficulty paying attention, hyperactivity, and impulsiveness.

16.10 The most efficacious drugs for symptoms of ADHD are the CNS stimulants such as methylphenidate (Ritalin). A newer, nonstimulant drug, atomoxetine (Strattera), has shown promise in clients with ADHD.

NCLEX-RN® REVIEW QUESTIONS

1 The nurse reviews the client's lithium serum drug level. The serum level is 0.95 mEq/L. The appropriate nursing action is to:

1. File the lab result in the medical record.
2. Hold the next dose of the drug.
3. Observe for signs of toxicity.
4. Notify the physician immediately.

2 The parents of a client receiving methylphenidate (Ritalin) express concern that the health-care provider has suggested the child have a "holiday" from the drug. The nurse explains that the drug-free holiday is designed to:

1. Reduce risk of drug toxicity.
2. Allow the child's "normal" behavior to return.
3. Decrease drug dependence and assess status.
4. Prevent hypertensive crisis.

3 Which of the following symptoms would indicate to the nurse that a client is experiencing lithium toxicity? (Select all that apply.)

1. Diarrhea and ataxia
2. Hypotension and edema
3. Hypertension and dehydration
4. Increased appetite, increased energy, and memory loss
5. Slurred speech and muscle weakness

4 The client has been started on an MAOI for depression and is now asking if she can add St. John's wort to increase the effectiveness of the antidepressant. The nurse's best response would be?

1. "St. John's wort is highly effective for depression. Adding it to your current medication will increase its effectiveness."
2. "Although St. John's wort has been found to be effective, you should consult with your health-care provider before adding it to your current medication routine."
3. "St. John's wort cannot be mixed with MAOIs because of possible drug interactions."
4. "Because St. John's wort is effective for depression, you will not need your medication."

5 Which of the following would be a priority component of the teaching plan for a client prescribed phenelzine (Nardil) for treatment of depression?

1. Headache may occur.
2. Hyperglycemia may occur.
3. Read labels of food and over-the-counter drugs.
4. Monitor blood pressure for hypotension.

CRITICAL THINKING QUESTIONS

1. A 12-year-old girl has been diagnosed with ADHD. Her parents have been reluctant to agree with the pediatrician's recommendation for pharmacologic management; however, the child's performance in school has deteriorated. A school nurse notes that the child has been placed on amphetamine (Adderall), not methylphenidate (Ritalin). Discuss the developmental considerations that might support the use of Adderall.

2. A 66-year-old female client has been diagnosed with clinical depression following the death of her husband. She says that she has not been able to sleep for weeks and that she is "living on coffee and cigarettes." The healthcare provider prescribes fluoxetine (Prozac). The client seeks reassurance from the nurse regarding when she should begin feeling "more like myself." How should the nurse respond?

3. A 26-year-old mother of three children comes to the prenatal clinic suspecting a fourth pregnancy. She tells the nurse that she got "real low" after her third baby and that she was prescribed sertraline (Zoloft). She tells the nurse that she is really afraid of "going crazy" if she has to stop taking the drug because of this pregnancy. What concerns should the nurse have?

See Appendix D for answers and rationales for all activities.

EXPLORE MediaLink

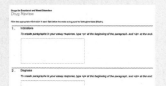

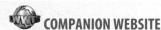

www.prenhall.com/adams

NCLEX-RN® review, case studies, and other interactive resources for this chapter can be found on the companion website at www.prenhall.com/adams. Click on "Chapter 16" to select the activities for this chapter. For animations, more NCLEX-RN® review questions, and an audio glossary, access the accompanying Prentice Hall Nursing MediaLink DVD-ROM in this textbook.

PRENTICE HALL NURSING MEDIALINK DVD-ROM

- **Animations**
  Mechanism in Action: Fluoxetine (*Prozac*)
  Mechanism in Action: Methylphenidate (*Ritalin*)
  Mechanism in Action: Venlafaxine (*Effexor*)
- **Audio Glossary**
- **NCLEX-RN® Review**

COMPANION WEBSITE

- **NCLEX-RN® Review**
- **Dosage Calculations**
- **Case Study:** Client taking a TCA and SSRI
- **Care Plan:** Client with bipolar disorder who is taking lithium

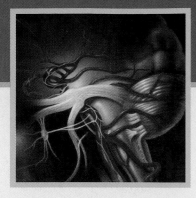

CHAPTER 17

Drugs for Psychoses

DRUGS AT A GLANCE

CONVENTIONAL (TYPICAL) ANTIPSYCHOTICS
Phenothiazines
    ☻ *chlorpromazine (Thorazine)*
Nonphenothiazines
    ☻ *haloperidol (Haldol)*
ATYPICAL ANTIPSYCHOTICS
    ☻ *clozapine (Clozaril)*
Dopamine System Stabilizers (DSSs)

OBJECTIVES

After reading this chapter, the student should be able to:

1. Explain theories for the etiology of schizophrenia.
2. Compare and contrast the positive and negative symptoms of schizophrenia.
3. Discuss the rationale for selecting a specific antipsychotic drug for the treatment of schizophrenia.
4. Explain the importance of client drug compliance in the pharmacotherapy of schizophrenia.
5. Describe the nurse's role in the pharmacological management of schizophrenia.
6. Explain the symptoms associated with extrapyramidal side effects of antipsychotic drugs.
7. For each of the drug classes listed in Drugs at a Glance, know representative drug examples, explain their mechanism of action, primary actions, and important adverse effects.
8. Categorize drugs used for psychoses based on their classification and drug action.
9. Use the Nursing Process to care for clients receiving drug therapy for psychoses.

MediaLink

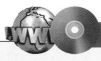

www.prenhall.com/adams

NCLEX-RN® review, case studies, and other interactive resources for this chapter can be found on the companion website at www.prenhall.com/adams. Click on "Chapter 17" to select the activities for this chapter. For animations, more NCLEX-RN® review questions, and an audio glossary, access the accompanying Prentice Hall Nursing MediaLink DVD-ROM in this textbook.

KEY TERMS

akathisia *page 214*

delusions *page 210*

dopamine type 2 (D$_2$) receptor *page 211*

dystonia *page 214*

extrapyramidal side effects (EPS) *page 214*

hallucinations *page 210*

illusions *page 210*

negative symptoms *page 211*

neuroleptic *page 212*

neuroleptic malignant syndrome *page 214*

paranoia *page 210*

Parkinsonism *page 214*

positive symptoms *page 211*

schizoaffective disorder *page 211*

schizophrenia *page 210*

tardive dyskinesia *page 214*

Severe mental illness can be incapacitating for the client and intensely frustrating for relatives and those dealing with the client on a regular basis. Before the 1950s, clients with acute mental dysfunction were institutionalized, often for their entire lives. The introduction of chlorpromazine (Thorazine) in the 1950s, and the development of newer agents, revolutionized the treatment of mental illness.

17.1 The Nature of Psychoses

A psychosis is a mental health condition characterized by **delusions** (firm ideas and beliefs not founded in reality), **hallucinations** (seeing, hearing, or feeling something that is not there), **illusions** (distorted perceptions of actual sensory stimuli), disorganized behavior, and a difficulty relating to others. Behavior may range from total inactivity to extreme agitation and combativeness. Some psychotic clients exhibit **paranoia,** an extreme suspicion and delusion that they are being followed, and that others are trying to harm them. Because they are unable to distinguish what is real from what is illusion, they are often viewed as insane.

Psychoses may be classified as *acute* or *chronic*. Acute psychotic episodes occur over hours or days, whereas chronic psychoses develop over months or years. Sometimes a cause may be attributed to the psychosis, such as brain damage, overdoses of certain medications, extreme depression, chronic alcoholism, and drug addiction. Genetic factors are known to play a role in some psychoses. Unfortunately, the vast majority of psychoses have no identifiable cause.

People with psychosis are usually unable to function normally in society without long-term drug therapy. Clients must see their healthcare provider periodically, and medication must be taken for life. Family members and social support groups are important sources of help for clients who cannot function without continuous drug therapy.

SCHIZOPHRENIA

Schizophrenia is a type of psychosis characterized by abnormal thoughts and thought processes, disordered communication, withdrawal from other people and the outside environment, and a high risk for suicide. Several subtypes of schizophrenic disorders are based on clinical presentation.

17.2 Signs and Symptoms of Schizophrenia

Schizophrenia is the most common psychotic disorder, affecting 1% to 2% of the population. Symptoms generally begin to appear in early adulthood, with a peak incidence in men 15 to 24 years of age, and women 25 to 34 years of age. Clients experience many different symptoms that may change over time. The following

PHARMFACTS

Psychoses

- Symptoms of psychosis are often associated with other mental health problems including substance abuse, depression, and dementia.
- Psychotic disorders are among the most misunderstood mental health disorders in North America.
- Approximately 3 million Americans have schizophrenia.
- Clients with psychosis often develop symptoms between the ages of 13 and the early 20s.
- As many as 50% of homeless people in America have schizophrenia.
- The probability of developing schizophrenia is 1 in 100 for the general population, 1 in 10 if one parent has the disorder, and 1 in 4 if both parents are schizophrenic.

symptoms may appear quickly or take several months or years to develop.

- Hallucinations, delusions, or paranoia
- Strange behavior, such as communicating in rambling statements or made-up words
- Rapid alternation between extreme hyperactivity and stupor
- Attitude of indifference or detachment toward life activities
- Strange or irrational actions
- Deterioration of personal hygiene, and job or academic performance
- Marked withdrawal from social interactions and inter-personal relationships

When observing clients with schizophrenia, nurses should look for both positive and negative symptoms. **Positive symptoms** are those that add on to normal behavior. These include hallucinations, delusions, and a disorganized thought or speech pattern. **Negative symptoms** are those that sub-tract from normal behavior. These symptoms include a lack of interest, motivation, responsiveness, or pleasure in daily activities. Negative symptoms are characteristic of the indif-ferent personality exhibited by many schizophrenics. Proper diagnosis of positive and negative symptoms is important for selection of the appropriate antipsychotic drug.

The cause of schizophrenia has not been determined, although several theories have been proposed. There appears to be a genetic component to schizophrenia, since many clients suffering from schizophrenia have family members who have been afflicted with the same disorder. Another theory suggests the disorder is caused by imbalances in neurotransmitters in specific areas of the brain. This theory suggests the possibility of overactive dopaminergic pathways in the basal nuclei, an area of the brain that controls motor activity. The basal ganglia (nuclei), shown in ● Figure 17.1, are responsible for starting and stopping synchronized mo-tor activity, such as leg and arm motions during walking.

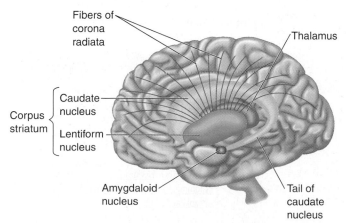

● **Figure 17.1** Basal ganglia: overactive dopamine D_2 receptors may be responsible for schizophrenia.

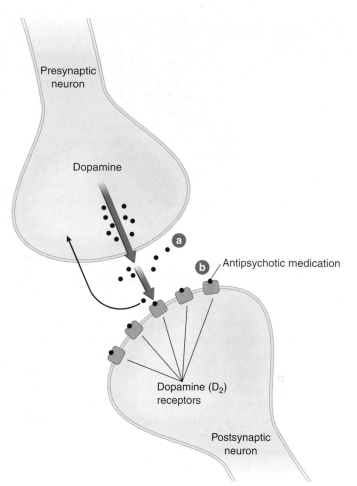

● **Figure 17.2** Mechanism of action of antipsychotic drugs: (a) overproduction of dopamine; (b) antipsychotic medication occupies D_2 receptor, preventing dopamine from stimulating the postsynaptic neuron.

Symptoms of schizophrenia seem to be associated with the **dopamine type 2 (D_2) receptor**. The basal nuclei are particularly rich in D_2 receptors, whereas the cerebrum contains very few. All antipsychotic drugs act by entering dopaminergic synapses and competing with dopamine. By blocking a majority of the D_2 receptors, antipsychotic drugs reduce the symptoms of schizophrenia. ● Figure 17.2 illustrates antipsychotic drug action at the dopaminergic receptor.

Schizoaffective disorder is a condition in which the client exhibits symptoms of both schizophrenia and mood disorder. For example, an acute schizoaffective reaction may include distorted perceptions, hallucinations, and delu-sions, followed by extreme depression. Over time, both pos-itive and negative psychotic symptoms will appear.

Many conditions can cause bizarre behavior, and these should be distinguished from schizophrenia. Chronic use of amphetamines or cocaine can create a paranoid syndrome. Certain complex partial seizures (see Chapter 15 ∞) can cause unusual symptoms that are sometimes mistaken for psychoses. Brain neoplasms, infections, or hemorrhage can also cause bizarre, psychotic-like symptoms.

SPECIAL CONSIDERATIONS

Cultural Views and Treatments of Mental Illness

Some cultures have very different perspectives on the cause of and treatment for mental illness. The foundation of many of these mental health treatments involves herbs and spiritual healing methods. American Indians may be treated by the community traditional "medicine man," who may treat mental symptoms with a sweat lodge and herbs. African Americans may go to a traditional voodoo priest or other healers for treatment, and they frequently use herbs to treat mental symptoms. Hispanics seek treatment from a folk healer, called a *curandero*; and they may use herbs such as chamomile, spearmint, and sweet basil for mental conditions. Members of some cultures may use amulets, or charms that are worn on a string or chain, to protect the wearer from evil spirits that are believed to cause mental illness.

17.3 Pharmacological Management of Psychoses

Management of severe mental illness is difficult. Many clients do not see their behavior as abnormal, and have difficulty understanding the need for medication. When that medication produces undesirable side effects, such as severe twitching or loss of sexual function, compliance diminishes and clients exhibit symptoms of their pretreatment illness. Agitation, distrust, and extreme frustration are common, as clients cannot comprehend why others are unable to think and see the same as them.

The primary goal of pharmacotherapy of schizophrenic clients is to reduce psychotic symptoms to a level that allows the client to maintain normal social relationships, including self-care and keeping a job. From a pharmacological perspective, therapy has both a positive and a negative side. Although many symptoms of psychosis can be controlled with current drugs, adverse effects are common and often severe. The antipsychotic agents do not cure mental illness, and symptoms remain in remission only as long as the client chooses to take the drug. The relapse rate for clients who discontinue their medication is 60% to 80%.

In terms of efficacy, there is little difference among the various antipsychotic drugs; there is no single drug of choice for schizophrenia. Selection of a specific drug is based on clinician experience, the occurrence of side effects, and the

needs of the client. For example, psychotic clients with Parkinson's disease need an antipsychotic with minimal extrapyramidal side effects. Those who operate machinery need a drug that does not cause sedation. Men who are sexually active may want a drug without negative effects on ejaculation. The experience and skills of the physician and mental health nurse are particularly valuable in achieving successful psychiatric pharmacotherapy.

CONVENTIONAL (TYPICAL) ANTIPSYCHOTIC AGENTS

Antipsychotic drugs are sometimes referred to as **neuroleptics.** The two basic categories of antipsychotic agents are conventional antipsychotics and atypical antipsychotics. The conventional drugs for psychoses include the phenothiazines and phenothiazine-like drugs.

PHENOTHIAZINES

The phenothiazines are most effective at treating the positive signs of schizophrenia, such as hallucinations and delusions, and have been the treatment of choice for psychoses for 50 years.

17.4 Treating Psychoses With Phenothiazines

The conventional antipsychotics, sometimes called first-generation or typical antipsychotics, include the phenothiazine and phenothiazine-like agents listed in Table 17.1. Within each category, agents are named by their chemical structure.

The first effective drug used to treat schizophrenia was the low-potency phenothiazine chlorpromazine (Thorazine), approved by the FDA for this use in 1954. Seven phenothiazines are now available to treat mental illness. All seven block the excitement associated with the positive symptoms of schizophrenia, although they differ in their potency and side-effect profiles. Hallucinations and delusions often begin to diminish within days. Other symptoms, however, may require as long as 7 to 8 weeks of pharmacotherapy to improve. Because of the high rate of recurrence of psychotic episodes, pharmacotherapy should be considered long term, often for the life of the client. Phenothiazines are thought to

TABLE 17.1 Conventional Antipsychotic Drugs: Phenothiazines		
Drug	**Route and Adult Dose (max dose where indicated)**	**Adverse Effects**
▶ chlorpromazine HCl (Thorazine)	PO; 25–100 mg tid or qid (max: 1000 mg/day) IM/IV; 25–50 mg (max: 600 mg q4–6h)	*Sedation, drowsiness, dizziness, extrapyramidal symptoms, constipation, photosensitivity, orthostatic hypotension*
fluphenazine HCl (Permitil, Prolixin)	PO; 0.5–10 mg/day (max: 20 mg/day)	
mesoridazine besylate (Serentil)	PO; 10–50 mg bid or tid (max: 400 mg/day)	<u>Agranulocytosis, pancytopenia, anaphylactoid reaction, tardive dyskinesia, neuroleptic malignant syndrome, hypothermia, adynamic ileus, sudden unexplained death</u>
perphenazine (Phenazine, Trilafon)	PO; 4–16 mg bid to qid (max: 64 mg/day)	
promazine HCl (Prozine, Sparine)	PO/IM; 10–200 mg q4–6 h (max: 1000 mg/day)	
thioridazine HCl (Mellaril)	PO; 50–100 mg tid (max: 800 mg/day)	
trifluoperazine HCl (Stelazine)	PO; 1–2 mg bid; (max: 20 mg/day)	

Italics indicate common adverse effects; <u>underlining</u> indicates serious adverse effects.

TABLE 17.2   Adverse Effects of Conventional Antipsychotic Agents

Effect	Description
acute dystonia	severe spasms, particularly the back muscles, tongue, and facial muscles; twitching movements
akathisia	constant pacing with repetitive, compulsive movements
anticholinergic effects	dry mouth, tachycardia, blurred vision
hypotension	particularly severe when client moves quickly from a recumbent to an upright position
neuroleptic malignant syndrome	high fever, confusion, muscle rigidity, and high serum creatine kinase; can be fatal
parkinsonism	tremor, muscle rigidity, stooped posture, and shuffling gait
sedation	usually diminishes with continued therapy
sexual dysfunction	impotence and diminished libido
tardive dyskinesia	bizarre tongue and face movements such as lip smacking and wormlike motions of the tongue; puffing of cheeks, uncontrolled chewing movements

act by preventing dopamine and serotonin from occupying their receptor sites in certain regions of the brain. This mechanism is illustrated in Figure 17.2

Although they revolutionized the treatment of severe mental illness, the phenothiazines exhibit numerous adverse effects that can limit pharmacotherapy. These are listed in Table 17.2. Anticholinergic effects such as dry mouth, postural hypotension, and urinary retention are common. Ejaculation disorders occur in a high percentage of clients taking phenothiazines; delay in achieving orgasm (in both men and women) is a common cause for noncompliance. Menstrual disorders are common. Each phenothiazine has

Pr PROTOTYPE DRUG | Chlorpromazine *(Thorazine)* | Phenothiazine

ACTIONS AND USES

Chlorpromazine provides symptomatic relief of positive symptoms of schizophrenia and controls manic symptoms in clients with schizoaffective disorder. Many clients must take chlorpromazine for 7 or 8 weeks before they experience improvement. Extreme agitation may be treated with IM or IV injections, which begin to act within minutes. Chlorpromazine can also control severe nausea and vomiting.

ADMINISTRATION ALERTS

- Do not crush or open sustained-release forms.
- When administered IM, give deep IM, only in the upper outer quadrant of the buttocks; client should remain supine for 30 to 60 minutes after injection, and then rise slowly.
- The drug must be gradually withdrawn over 2 to 3 weeks, and nausea/vomiting, dizziness, tremors, or dyskinesia may occur.
- IV forms should be used only during surgery or for severe hiccups.
- Pregnancy category C.

PHARMACOKINETICS

Onset: 30–60 mln

Peak: 2–4 h PO; 15–20 min IV

Half-life: 6 h

Duration: 30 h

ADVERSE EFFECTS

Strong blockade of alpha-adrenergic receptors and weak blockade of cholinergic receptors explain some of chlorpromazine's adverse effects. Common side effects are dizziness, drowsiness, and orthostatic hypotension.

Extrapyramidal side effects (EPS) occur more commonly in elderly, female, and pediatric clients who are dehydrated. Neuroleptic Malignant Syndrome (NMS) may also occur. Clients taking chlorpromazine who are exposed to warmer temperatures should be monitored more closely for symptoms of NMS.

Contraindications: Use is not advised during alcohol withdrawal or when the client is in a comatose state. Caution should be used with other conditions, including subcortical brain damage, bone marrow depression, and Reye's syndrome. Chlorpromazine is contraindicated in lactation.

INTERACTIONS

Drug–Drug: Chlorpromazine interacts with several drugs. For example, concurrent use with sedative medications such as phenobarbital should be avoided. Taking chlorpromazine with tricyclic antidepressants can elevate blood pressure. Concurrent use of chlorpromazine with antiseizure medication can lower the seizure threshold.

Lab Tests: Chlorpromazine may increase cephalin flocculation and possibly other liver function tests. False-positive results may occur for amylase, 5-hydroxyindole acetic acid, porphobilinogens, urobilinogen, and urine bilirubin. False-positive or false-negative pregnancy tests may result.

Herbal/Food: Kava and St. John's wort may increase the risk and severity of dystonia.

Treatment of Overdose: There is no specific treatment for overdose; clients are treated symptomatically. EPS may be treated with antiparkinsonism drugs, barbiturates, or diphenhydramine (Benadryl). Avoid producing respiratory depression with these treatments.

 See the Companion Website for a Nursing Process Focus specific to this drug.

a slightly different side-effect spectrum. For example, perphenazine (Phenazine, Trilafon) has a low incidence of anticholinergic effects, whereas mesoridazine (Serentil) has a high incidence of anticholinergic effects. Thioridazine (Mellaril) frequently causes sedation, whereas this side effect is less common with trifluoperazine (Stelazine).

Unlike many other drugs whose primary action is on the CNS (e.g., amphetamines, barbiturates, anxiolytics, alcohol), antipsychotic drugs do not cause physical or psychological dependence. They also have a wide safety margin between a therapeutic and a lethal dose; deaths due to overdoses of antipsychotic drugs are uncommon.

Extrapyramidal effects are a particularly serious set of adverse reactions to antipsychotic drugs. **Extrapyramidal side effects (EPS)** include acute dystonia, akathisia, Parkinsonism, and tardive dyskinesia. Acute **dystonias** occur early in the course of pharmacotherapy, and involve severe muscle spasms, particularly of the back, neck, tongue, and face. **Akathisia**, the most common EPS, is an inability to rest or relax. The client paces, has trouble sitting or remaining still, and has difficulty sleeping. Symptoms of phenothiazine-induced **Parkinsonism** include tremor, muscle rigidity, stooped posture, and a shuffling gait. Long-term use of phenothiazines may lead to **tardive dyskinesia,** which is characterized by unusual tongue and face movements such as lip smacking and wormlike motions of the tongue. If extrapyramidal effects are reported early and the drug is withdrawn or the dosage is reduced, the side effects can be reversible. With higher doses given for prolonged periods, the extrapyramidal symptoms may become permanent. The nurse must be vigilant in observing and reporting EPS, as prevention is the best treatment.

With the conventional antipsychotics, it is not always possible to control the disabling symptoms of schizophrenia without producing some degree of extrapyramidal effects. In these clients, drug therapy may be warranted to treat EPS symptoms. Concurrent pharmacotherapy with an anticholinergic drug may prevent some of the extrapyramidal signs (see Chapter 18 ∞). For acute dystonia, benztropine (Cogentin) may be given parenterally. Levodopa (Dopar, Larodopa) is usually avoided, since its ability to increase dopamine function antagonizes the action of the phenothiazines. Beta-adrenergic blockers and benzodiazepines are sometimes given to reduce signs of akathisia.

NURSING CONSIDERATIONS

The role of the nurse in phenothiazine therapy involves careful monitoring of a client's condition and providing education as it relates to the prescribed drug treatment. Because phenothiazines affect many body systems and can interact with drugs and alcohol, take a complete health history including any long-term physical problems (e.g., seizure disorders, cardiovascular disease), medication use, allergies, and lifestyle information such as the use of alcohol, illegal drugs, caffeine, smoking, or herbal preparations. This information allows the physician to individualize treatment and minimize the possibility of adverse reactions.

Assess for liver and kidney function, vision problems, and mental status to provide a baseline of the client's health status. Contraindications to the use of phenothiazine and phenothiazine-like drugs include CNS depression, bone marrow suppression, coma, alcohol withdrawal syndrome, lactation, age (children under age 6 months), and presence of Reye's syndrome. This class of drugs must be used with caution in clients with asthma, emphysema, respiratory infections, pregnancy (use only when benefits outweigh risks), and elderly persons or children.

Monitor clients for extrapyramidal symptoms. Symptoms include lip smacking; spasms of the face, tongue, or back muscles; facial grimacing; involuntary upward eye movements; jerking motions; extreme restlessness; stooped posture; shuffling gait; and tremors at rest. Report EPS symptoms to the physician immediately, because these symptoms may be reason to discontinue the drug.

A rare, though potentially life-threatening adverse effect is **neuroleptic malignant syndrome** (NMS), a toxic reaction to therapeutic doses of an antipsychotic drug. The onset of NMS varies from early in treatment to after several months of therapy. The client exhibits elevated temperature, unstable blood pressure, profuse sweating, dyspnea, muscle rigidity, and incontinence. Observe for these symptoms and report them immediately to the physician. This syndrome can lead to death if it is not recognized and treated.

In addition, assess the client for drowsiness and sedation, which are both common side effects of this type of medication owing to CNS depression. Evaluate the client's safety and ability to function.

Lifespan Considerations.   If the client is a child, assess for hyperexcitability, dehydration, or gastroenteritis as well as chickenpox or measles, because such conditions increase the potential for EPS. If possible, phenothiazines should not be given to children under 12 years of age. If the client is elderly, determine whether a lower dose may be indicated owing to the slower metabolism in older adults.

Client Teaching.   Client and family education is an especially important aspect of care for clients with mental illness. Client education as it relates to phenothiazines should include the goals of therapy, reasons for obtaining baseline data such as vital signs and the existense of underlying disorders, and possible drug side effects. Include the following points when teaching clients about phenothiazines:

- Immediately report signs and symptoms of EPS or NMS.
- Document on a calendar that each dose has been taken daily.
- Take the medication exactly as directed.
- Do not stop taking the drugs without the advice of the prescriber.

NONPHENOTHIAZINES

The nonphenothiazine antipsychotic medications have equal efficacy as the phenothiazines. Although the incidence of sedation and anticholinergic side effects is less, extrapyramidal effects may be common, particularly in elderly clients.

TABLE 17.3 Conventional Antipsychotic Drugs: Nonphenothiazines

Drug	Route and Adult Dose (max dose where indicated)	Adverse Effects
chlorprothixene (Taractan)	PO; 75–150 mg/day (max: 600 mg/day)	*Sedation, transient drowsiness, extrapyramidal symptoms, tremor, orthostatic hypotension*
haloperidol (Haldol)	PO; 0.2–5 mg bid or tid	
loxapine succinate (Loxitane)	PO; start with 20 mg/day and rapidly increase to 60–100 mg/day in divided doses (max: 250 mg/day)	<u>Tardive dyskinesia, neuroleptic malignant syndrome, laryngospasm, respiratory depression, hepatotoxicity, acute renal failure, sudden death</u>
molindone HCl (Moban)	PO; 50–75 mg/day in 3 to 4 divided doses; may increase to 100 mg/day in 3–4 days (max: 225 mg/day)	
pimozide (Orap)	PO; 1–2 mg/day in divided doses; gradually increase every other day to 7–16 mg/day (max: 10 mg/day)	
thiothixene HCl (Navane)	PO; 2 mg tid; may increase up to 15 mg/day (max: 60 mg/day)	

Italics indicate common adverse effects; <u>underlining</u> indicates serious adverse effects.

17.5 Treating Psychoses With Conventional Nonphenothiazines Antipsychotics

The conventional nonphenothiazine antipsychotic class consists of drugs whose chemical structures are dissimilar to the phenothiazines (Table 17.3). Introduced shortly after the phenothiazines, the nonphenothiazines were initially expected to produce fewer side effects. Unfortunately, this appears to not be the case. The spectrum of side effects for the nonphenothiazines is identical with that for the phenothiazines, although the degree to which a particular effect occurs depends on the specific drug. In general, the nonphenothiazine agents cause less sedation and fewer anticholinergic side effects than chlorpromazine (Thorazine) but exhibit an equal or even greater incidence of

Pr PROTOTYPE DRUG | Haloperidol *(Haldol)* | Nonphenothiazine

ACTIONS AND USES

Haloperidol is classified chemically as a butyrophenone. Its primary use is for the management of acute and chronic psychotic disorders. It may be used to treat clients with Tourette's syndrome and children with severe behavior problems such as unprovoked aggressiveness and explosive hyperexcitability. It is approximately 50 times more potent than chlorpromazine but has equal efficacy in relieving symptoms of schizophrenia. Haldol LA is a long-acting preparation that lasts for approximately 3 weeks following IM or subcutaneous administration. This is particularly beneficial for clients who are uncooperative or unable to take oral medications.

ADMINISTRATION ALERTS

- Do not abruptly discontinue, or severe adverse reactions may occur.
- The client must take medication as ordered for therapeutic results to occur.
- If the client does not comply with oral therapy, injectable extended-release haloperidol should be considered.
- Pregnancy category C.

PHARMACOKINETICS

Onset: 30–35 min
Peak: 2–6 h PO; 10–20 min IM
Half-life: 12–37 h PO; 10–19 h IV; 17–25 h IM
Duration: Variable

ADVERSE EFFECTS

Haloperidol produces less sedation and hypotension than chlorpromazine, but the incidence of EPS is high. Elderly clients are more likely to experience side effects and often are prescribed half the adult dose until the side effects of therapy can be determined. Although the incidence of NMS is rare, it can occur.

Contraindications: Pharmacotherapy with nonphenothiazines is not advised if the client is receiving medication for any of the following conditions: Parkinson's disease, seizure disorders, alcoholism, and severe mental depression.

INTERACTIONS

Drug–Drug: Haloperidol interacts with many drugs. For example, the following drugs decrease the effects/absorption of haloperidol: aluminum- and magnesium-containing antacids, levodopa (also increases chances of levodopa toxicity), lithium (increases chance of a severe neurological toxicity), phenobarbital, phenytoin (also increases chances of phenytoin toxicity), rifampin, and beta-blockers (may increase blood levels of haloperidol, thus leading to possible toxicity). Haloperidol inhibits the action of centrally acting antihypertensives.

Lab Tests: Unknown.

Herbal/Food: Kava may increase the effect of haloperidol.

Treatment of Overdose: In general, the symptoms of overdose are an exaggeration of known pharmacological effects and adverse reactions, the most prominent of which would be severe extrapyramidal reactions, hypotension, or sedation. With EPS, antiparkinsonism medication should be administered. Hypotension should be counteracted with IV fluids, plasma, or concentrated albumin, or vasopressor agents.

 See the Companion Website for a Nursing Process Focus specific to this drug.

NURSING PROCESS FOCUS Clients Receiving Conventional Antipsychotic Therapy

Assessment	Potential Nursing Diagnoses
Prior to administration: ■ Obtain a complete health history (medical and psychological) including allergies, drug history, and possible drug interactions. ■ Obtain baseline lab studies (electrolytes, CBC, BUN, creatinine, WBC, liver enzymes, and drug screens). ■ Assess for hallucinations, level of consciousness, and mental status. ■ Assess client support system(s).	■ Therapeutic Regimen Management, Ineffective, related to noncompliance with medication regimen, presence of side effects, and need for long-term medication use ■ Anxiety, related to symptoms of psychosis ■ Injury, Risk for, related to side effects of medication ■ Noncompliance, related to length of time before medication reaches therapeutic levels, desire to use alcohol or illegal drugs ■ Knowledge, Deficient, related to unfamiliarity with medications and their effects

Planning: Client Goals and Expected Outcomes

The client will:
■ Report a reduction of psychotic symptoms, including delusions, paranoia, irrational behavior, hallucinations.
■ Demonstrate an understanding of the drug's action by accurately describing drug side effects and precautions.
■ Immediately report side effects or adverse reactions.
■ Adhere to recommended treatment regimen.

Implementation

Interventions and (Rationales)	Client Education/Discharge Planning
■ Monitor for decrease of psychotic symptoms. (If client continues to exhibit symptoms of psychosis, the drug or dose may not be effective.)	Instruct client and caregiver to: ■ Notice increases or decreases of symptoms of psychosis, including hallucinations, abnormal sleep patterns, social withdrawal, delusions, or paranoia. ■ Contact physician if symptoms do not decrease over a 6-week period.
■ Monitor for side effects. (Problems with side effects may cause a decrease in compliance.)	Instruct client and caregiver: ■ About problems with drowsiness, dizziness, lethargy, headaches, blurred vision, skin rash, sweating, nausea/vomiting, lack of appetite, diarrhea, menstrual irregularities, depression, and blood pressure problems. ■ That impotence, gynecomastia, amenorrhea, and enuresis may occur.
■ Monitor for anticholinergic side effects such as orthostatic hypotension, constipation, anorexia, GU problems, respiratory changes, and visual disturbances. (These side effects may need to be treated so the client can continue with the medication.)	Instruct client to: ■ Avoid abrupt changes in position. ■ Avoid driving or performing hazardous activities until effects of the drug are known. ■ Report vision changes. ■ Increase dietary fiber, fluids, and exercise to prevent constipation. ■ Relieve symptoms of dry mouth with sugar-free hard candy or gum and frequent drinks of water. ■ Notify physician immediately if urinary retention occurs.
■ Monitor for EPS and NMS. (Presence of EPS may be sufficient reason for the client to discontinue the antipsychotic. NMS is life threatening and must be reported and treated immediately.)	Instruct client and caregiver to: ■ Recognize tardive dyskinesia, dystonia, akathisia, and pseudoparkinsonism. ■ Immediately seek treatment for elevated temperature, unstable blood pressure, profuse sweating, dyspnea, muscle rigidity, or incontinence.
■ Monitor for alcohol/illegal drug use. (Used concurrently, these cause an increased CNS depressant effect.)	■ Instruct client to avoid alcohol and illegal drug use. Refer client to community support groups such as AA or NA as appropriate.
■ Monitor caffeine use. (Use of caffeine-containing substances negates the effects of antipsychotics.)	Instruct client or caregiver about: ■ Common caffeine-containing products. ■ Acceptable substitutes, such as decaffeinated coffee and tea, and caffeine-free colas.
■ Monitor for cardiovascular changes, including hypotension, tachycardia, and ECG changes. (Haloperidol has fewer cardiotoxic effects than other antipsychotics, and may be preferred for clients with existing CV problems.)	■ Instruct client and caregiver that dizziness and falls, especially with sudden position changes, may indicate cardiovascular changes. Teach safety measures.

NURSING PROCESS FOCUS Clients Receiving Conventional Antipsychotic Therapy *(Continued)*

Implementation

Interventions and (Rationales)	Client Education/Discharge Planning
▪ Monitor for smoking. (Heavy smoking may decrease metabolism of haloperidol, leading to decreased efficacy.)	▪ Instruct client to stop or decrease smoking. Refer client to smoking cessation programs, if indicated.
▪ Monitor elderly clients closely. (Elderly clients may need lower doses and a more gradual dosage increase. Elderly women are at greater risk for developing tardive dyskinesia.)	▪ Instruct caregiver to observe for and immediately report unusual reactions such as confusion, depression, and hallucinations, and for symptoms of tardive dyskinesia. ▪ Instruct elderly clients or caregivers how to counteract anticholinergic effects of medication while taking into account any other existing medical problems.
▪ Monitor lab results, including RBC and WBC counts, and drug levels. (Use of some medications may cause changes in blood counts. Some medications can cause toxicity.)	▪ Instruct client and caregiver to keep appointments for laboratory testing.
▪ Monitor for use of medication. (All antipsychotics must be taken as ordered for therapeutic results to occur.)	▪ Instruct client and caregiver to take medication as prescribed, even if no therapeutic benefits are felt, because it may take several months for full therapeutic benefits to occur.
▪ Monitor for seizures. (This drug may lower the seizure threshold.)	▪ Instruct client and caregiver that seizures may occur and review appropriate safety precautions.
▪ Monitor client's environment. (The drug may cause the client to perceive a brownish discoloration of objects or photophobia. It may also interfere with the ability to regulate body temperature.)	Instruct client and caregiver to: ▪ Wear dark glasses to avoid discomfort from photophobia. ▪ Avoid temperature extremes. ▪ Be aware that perception of brownish discoloration of objects may appear, but it is not harmful.

Evaluation of Outcome Criteria

Evaluate the effectiveness of drug therapy by confirming that client goals and expected goals have been met (see "Planning").
▪ The client and family report a decrease in symptoms of psychosis including delusions, paranoia, and irrational behavior.
▪ The client demonstrates an understanding of the drug's action by accurately describing side effects and precautions.
▪ The client immediately reports adverse reactions.
▪ The client adheres to the recommended treatment regimen.

∞ *See Tables 17.1 and 17.3 for lists of drugs to which these nursing actions apply.*

extrapyramidal signs. Concurrent therapy with other CNS depressants must be carefully monitored, because of the potential additive effects.

Drugs in the nonphenothiazine class have the same therapeutic effects and efficacy as the phenothiazines. They are also believed to act by the same mechanism as the phenothiazines, that is, by blocking postsynaptic D_2 dopamine receptors. As a class, they offer no significant advantages over the phenothiazines in the treatment of schizophrenia.

NURSING CONSIDERATIONS

The role of the nurse in conventional nonphenothiazine therapy involves careful monitoring of a client's condition and providing education as it relates to the prescribed drug treatment. Because nonphenothiazines can also interact with many drugs, assess the client's drug use history, including current and past medications, to establish any previous allergic reactions or adverse effects from these medications. Assess elderly clients more carefully

than younger clients for unusual adverse reactions such as confusion, depression, and hallucinations that are drug induced.

Perform a complete baseline assessment, including physical assessment, mental status (orientation, affect, cognition), vital signs, lab studies (CBC, liver and renal function tests), preexisting medical conditions (especially cardiac, kidney, and liver function), and vision screening. Assess the available support system, because many psychiatric clients are unable to self-manage their drug regimen. Contraindications for this class of drugs include Parkinson's disease, CNS depression, alcoholism, seizure disorders, and age younger than 3 years.

Inform the client and caregivers that sedation is a less severe side effect than with phenothiazines, but there is a greater incidence of EPS with nonphenothiazine antipsychotics. A possible life-threatening adverse effect of antipsychotic drugs is NMS.

Because of the anticholinergic side effects of these drugs, monitor for dry mouth, urinary retention, constipation, and hypotension with resultant tachycardia. Compliance with this classification of drug is equally as important as with the phenothiazines. Assess for alcohol and illegal drug use, which causes an increased depressant effect when used with antipsychotic drugs. Caution the client that any form of caffeine used with these drugs will likely increase anxiety.

Lifespan Considerations. When assessing older clients, check for unusual reactions to haloperidol (Haldol). Older adults need smaller doses and more frequent monitoring with a gradual dose increase. There is an increased incidence of tardive dyskinesia in elderly women. This category of drugs is not safe for use with children younger than 2 years.

Client Teaching. Client education as it relates to conventional nonphenothiazines should include the goals of therapy, the reasons for obtaining baseline data, and possible drug side effects. Include the following points when teaching clients about nonphenothiazines:

- Immediately report signs and symptoms of EPS or NMS.
- Report continued or increased symptoms of psychosis.
- Avoid alcohol or illegal drug use.
- Avoid caffeine-containing beverages and foods.
- Report any complaints of dizziness, loss of consciousness, or falls.
- Immediately report any type of seizure activity.

ATYPICAL ANTIPSYCHOTIC AGENTS

Atypical antipsychotics treat both positive and negative symptoms of schizophrenia. They have become drugs of choice for treating psychoses.

17.6 Treating Psychoses With Atypical Antipsychotics

The approval of clozapine (Clozaril), the first atypical antipsychotic, marked the first major advance in the pharmacotherapy of psychoses since the discovery of chlorpromazine decades earlier. Clozapine, and the other drugs in this class, are called second generation, or atypical, because they have a broader spectrum of action than the conventional antipsychotics, controlling both the positive and negative symptoms of schizophrenia (Table 17.4). Furthermore, at therapeutic doses they exhibit their antipsychotic actions without producing the EPS effects of the conventional agents. Some drugs, such as clozapine, are especially useful for clients in whom other drugs have proved unsuccessful.

The mechanism of action of the atypical agents is largely unknown, but they are thought to act by blocking several different receptor types in the brain. Like the phenothiazines, the atypical agents block dopamine D_2 receptors. However, the atypicals also block serotonin (5-HT) and alpha-adrenergic receptors, which is thought to account for some of their properties. Because the atypical agents are only loosely bound to D_2 receptors, they produce fewer extrapyramidal side effects than the conventional antipsychotics.

Although there are fewer side effects with atypical antipsychotics, adverse effects are still significant, and clients must be carefully monitored. Although most antipsychotics cause weight gain, the atypical agents are associated with obesity and its risk factors. Risperidone (risperdal) and some of the other antipsychotic drugs increase prolactin levels, which can lead to menstrual disorders, decreased libido, and osteoporosis in women. in men, high prolactin levels can cause lack of libido and impotence. There is also concern that some atypical agents alter glucose metabolism, which can lead to type 2 diabetes.

NURSING CONSIDERATIONS

The role of the nurse in atypical antipsychotic therapy involves careful monitoring of a client's condition and providing education as it relates to the prescribed drug treatment. Take a complete health history, including

TABLE 17.4	Atypical Antipsychotic Drugs	
Drug	**Route and Adult Dose (max dose where indicated)**	**Adverse Effects**
aripiprazole (Abilify)	PO; 10–15 mg/day (max: 30 mg/day)	*Tachycardia, transient fever, sedation, dizziness, headache, light-headedness, somnolence, anxiety, nervousness, hostility, insomnia, nausea, vomiting, constipation, parkinsonism, akathisia*
ⓟ clozapine (Clozaril)	PO; start at 25–50 mg/day and titrate to a target dose of 50–450 mg/day in 3 days; may increase further (max: 900 mg/day)	
olanzapine (Zyprexa)	Adult: PO; start with 5–10 mg/day; may increase by 2.5–5 mg every week (range 10–15 mg/day; max: 20 mg/day). Geriatric: PO; start with 5 mg/day	Agranulocytosis, neuroleptic malignant syndrome (rare)
quetiapine fumarate (Seroquel)	PO; start with 25 mg bid; may increase to a target dose of 300–400 mg/day in divided doses	
risperidone (Risperdal)	PO; 1–6 mg bid; increase by 2 mg daily to an initial target dose of 6 mg/day	
ziprasidone (Geodon)	PO; 20 mg bid (max: 80 mg bid)	

Italics indicate common adverse effects; <u>underlining</u> indicates serious adverse effects.

Pr **PROTOTYPE DRUG** | Clozapine *(Clozaril)* | Atypical Antipsychotic

ACTIONS AND USES

Therapeutic effects of clozapine include remission of a range of psychotic symptoms including delusions, paranoia, and irrational behavior. Of severely ill clients, 25% show improvement within 6 weeks of starting clozapine; 60% show improvement within 6 months. Clozapine acts by interfering with the binding of dopamine to its receptors in the limbic system. Clozapine also binds to alpha-adrenergic, serotonergic, and cholinergic sites throughout the brain.

ADMINISTRATION ALERTS

- Give the client only a 1-week supply of clozapine at a time, to ensure return for weekly lab studies.
- Dose must be increased gradually.
- Pregnancy category B.

PHARMACOKINETICS

Onset: 2–4 wk

Peak: 2.5 h

Half-life: 8–12 h

Duration: Variable

ADVERSE EFFECTS

Because seizures and agranulocytosis are associated with clozapine use, a course of therapy with conventional antipsychotics is recommended before starting clozapine therapy. Common side effects are dizziness, drowsiness, headache, constipation, transient fever, salivation, flulike symptoms, and tachycardia. As with the conventional agents, elderly clients exhibit a higher incidence of orthostatic hypotension and anticholinergic side effects. Clozapine may also cause bone marrow suppression, which has proved fatal in some cases.

Contraindications: This drug should not be given to clients with myeloproliferative disorders or in cases of severe CNS depression.

INTERACTIONS

Drug–Drug: Clozapine interacts with many drugs. For example, it should not be taken with alcohol, other CNS depressants, or with drugs that suppress bone marrow function, such as anticancer drugs.

Concurrent use with antihypertensives may lead to hypotension. benzodiazepines taken with clozapine may lead to severe hypotension and a risk for respiratory arrest. Concurrent use of digoxin or warfarin may cause increased levels of those drugs, which could lead to increased cardiac problems or hemorrhage, respectively. If phenytoin is taken concurrently with clozapine, seizure threshold will be decreased.

Lab Tests: When treatment with clozapine is discontinued, white blood cell (WBC) count and absolute neutrophil count (ANC) should be monitored weekly for at least 4 weeks or until the WBC count is $\leq 3{,}500/mm^3$ and the ANC is $\leq 2{,}000/mm^3$.

Herbal/Food: Use with caution with herbal supplements, such as kava, which may increase CNS depression.

Treatment of Overdose: Activated charcoal, which may be used with sorbitol, may be as or more effective than emesis or gastric lavage, and should be considered in treating overdosage. Establish and maintain an airway; ensure adequate oxygenation and ventilation.

 See the Companion Website for a Nursing Process Focus specific to this drug.

---

seizure activity, cardiovascular status, psychological disorders, and neurological and blood diseases. Obtain baseline lab tests, including CBC, WBC with differential, electrolytes, BUN, creatinine, and liver enzymes. Continue to monitor the WBC with differential every week for the first 6 months, then every 2 weeks for the next 6 months, then every 4 weeks until the drug is discontinued, because these drugs can cause agranulocytosis and leukopenia. Assess for hallucinations, mental status, dementia, and bipolar disorder, initially and throughout therapy. Obtain the client's drug history to determine possible drug interactions and allergies.

Clozapine (Clozaril) is contraindicated in coma or severe CNS depression, uncontrolled epilepsy, history of clozapine-induced agranulocytosis, and leukopenia (WBC count <3,500). When atypical antipsychotics are given to clients with cardiovascular disorders and conditions that predispose the client to hypotension, monitor blood pressure closely for severe hypotension. Closely monitor for adverse effects in clients who are using other CNS depressants, including alcohol; those with renal or hepatic impairment; those who are exposed to extreme heat; elderly or young clients; and those with prostatic hypertrophy, glaucoma, or a history of paralytic ileus.

Lifespan Considerations. Atypical antipsychotics are contraindicated during pregnancy and lactation because they can cause harm to the developing fetus or to the infant. Instruct female clients to have a pregnancy test within 6 weeks of beginning therapy (be sure the test is negative), to use reliable birth control during treatment, and to notify their healthcare provider if they plan to become pregnant.

Client Teaching. Client education as it relates to atypical antipsychotic drugs should include the goals of therapy, reasons for obtaining baseline data such as vital signs and the existence of underlying disorders, and possible drug side effects. Include the following points when teaching clients and their families about atypical antipsychotic medications:

NURSING PROCESS FOCUS   Clients Receiving Atypical Antipsychotic Therapy

Assessment	Potential Nursing Diagnoses
Prior to administration: ■ Obtain a complete health history (medical and psychological) including allergies, drug history, and possible drug interactions. ■ Obtain baseline lab studies, especially RBC and WBC counts. ■ Assess for hallucinations, mental status, and level of consciousness. ■ Assess client support system(s).	■ Anxiety, related to symptoms of psychosis, side effects of medication ■ Injury, Risk for, related to side effects of medication, psychosis ■ Noncompliance, related to lack of understanding or knowledge, desire to use alcohol and caffeine-containing products.

Planning: Client Goals And Expected Outcomes

The client will:
■ Adhere to recommended treatment regimen.
■ Report a reduction of psychotic symptoms, including delusions, paranoia, irrational behavior, and hallucinations.
■ Demonstrate an understanding of the drug's actions by accurately describing drug side effects and precautions.

Implementation

Interventions and (Rationales)	Client Education/Discharge Planning
■ Monitor RBC and WBC counts. (Agranulocytosis [WBC below 3500] can be a life-threatening side effect of these medications, which may also suppress bone marrow and lower infection-fighting ability.)	■ Advise client and caregiver to keep appointments for laboratory testing. ■ Instruct client to immediately report any sore throat, signs of infection, fatigue without apparent cause, or bruising.
■ Observe for adverse effects. (These drugs may affect blood pressure, heart rate, and other autonomic functions.)	■ Instruct client and caregiver to report side effects, such as drowsiness, dizziness, depression, anxiety, tachycardia, hypotension, nausea/vomiting, excessive salivation, urinary frequency or urgency, incontinence, weight gain, muscle pain or weakness, rash, and fever.
■ Monitor for anticholinergic side effects. (These medications may cause mouth dryness, constipation, or urine retention.)	Instruct client and caregiver to: ■ Increase dietary fiber, fluids, and exercise to prevent constipation. ■ Relieve symptoms of dry mouth with sugar-free hard candy or chewing gum, and frequent drinks of water. ■ Immediately notify healthcare provider if urinary retention occurs. Possible catheter placement may be necessary.
■ Monitor for decrease of psychotic symptoms. (Decreased symptoms indicate an effective dose and type of medication.)	Instruct client and caregiver to: ■ Notice increases or decreases of symptoms of psychosis, including hallucinations, abnormal sleep patterns, social withdrawal, delusions, or paranoia. ■ Contact healthcare provider if symptoms do not decrease over a 6-week period.
■ Monitor for alcohol or illegal drug use. (Used concurrently, these will cause increased CNS depression. The client may decide to use alcohol or illegal drugs as a means of coping with symptoms of psychosis, so may stop taking the drug.)	■ Instruct client to avoid alcohol or illegal drug use. Refer client to AA, NA, or other support group as appropriate.
■ Monitor caffeine use. (Use of caffeine-containing substances inhibits the effects of antipsychotics.)	Instruct client and caregiver about: ■ Common caffeine-containing products. ■ Acceptable substitutes, including decaffeinated coffee and tea, and caffeine-free soda.
■ Monitor for smoking. (Heavy smoking may decrease blood levels of the drug.)	■ Instruct client to stop or decrease smoking. Refer to smoking cessation programs if indicated.
■ Monitor elderly clients closely. (Older clients may be more sensitive to anticholinergic side effects.)	■ Instruct elderly clients on ways to counteract anticholinergic effects of medication while taking into account any other existing medical problems.

Evaluation of Outcome Criteria

Evaluate the effectiveness of drug therapy by confirming that client goals and expected outcomes have been met (see "Planning").
■ The client adheres to recommended treatment regimen.
■ The client reports reduced symptoms of psychosis including delusions, paranoia, and irrational behavior.
■ The client demonstrates an understanding of the drug's action by accurately describing drug side effects and precautions.

∞ *See Table 17.4 for a list of drugs to which these nursing actions apply.*

- Change positions slowly to avoid dizziness and postural hypotension.
- Take the drug exactly as prescribed; do not make any dosage changes or stop taking the medication without the approval of your healthcare provider. Medication may take a minimum of 6 weeks before any therapeutic effects are noted.
- Keep all scheduled laboratory visits for tests.
- Notify your healthcare provider if no improvement in behavior is noted after 6 weeks of therapy.
- Avoid alcohol, illegal drug, caffeine, and tobacco use.
- Immediately report significant side effects, but continue taking the medication.
- Increase your intake of fruits, vegetables, and fluids if constipation occurs.

17.7 Treating Psychoses With Dopamine System Stabilizers

Owing to side effects caused by conventional and atypical antipsychotic medications, a new drug class was developed to better meet the needs of clients with psychoses (Bailey, 2003). The new class is called *dopamine system stabilizers (DSSs)* or dopamine partial agonists. Aripiprazole (Abilify) received FDA approval in November 2002 for the treatment of schizophrenia and schizoaffective disorder. Because aripiprazole controls both the positive and negative symptoms of schizophrenia, it is grouped in Table 17.4 with the atypical antipsychotic drugs.

Aripiprazole-treated clients appear to exhibit fewer EPS than clients treated with haloperidol (Haldol). Side effects include headache, nausea/vomiting, fever, constipation, and anxiety.

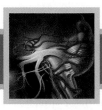

CHAPTER REVIEW

KEY CONCEPTS

The numbered key concepts provide a succinct summary of the important points from the corresponding numbered section within the chapter. If any of these points are not clear, refer to the numbered section within the chapter for review.

17.1 Psychoses are severe mental and behavioral disorders characterized by disorganized mental capacity and an inability to recognize reality.

17.2 Schizophrenia is a type of psychosis characterized by abnormal thoughts and thought processes, disordered communication, withdrawal from other people and the outside environment, and a high risk for suicide.

17.3 Pharmacological management of psychoses is difficult because the adverse effects of the drugs may be severe, and clients often do not understand the need for medication.

17.4 The phenothiazines have been effectively used for the treatment of psychoses for more than 50 years; however,

they have a high incidence of side effects. Extrapyramidal side effects (EPS) and neuroleptic malignant syndrome (NMS) are two particularly serious conditions.

17.5 The nonphenothiazine conventional antipsychotics have the same therapeutic applications and side effects as the phenothiazines.

17.6 Atypical antipsychotics are often preferred because they address both positive and negative symptoms of schizophrenia, and produce less dramatic side effects.

17.7 Dopamine system stabilizers are the newest antipsychotic class. It is hoped that this new class will have the same efficacy as other antipsychotic classes, with fewer serious side effects.

NCLEX-RN® REVIEW QUESTIONS

1 The client states he has not taken his antipsychotic drug for the past 2 weeks because it was causing sexual dysfunction. The name *antipsychotic* explains that continuing the medication as prescribed is important because:
1. Hypertensive crisis may occur with abrupt withdrawal.
2. Muscle twitching may occur.
3. Parkinson-like symptoms will occur.
4. Symptoms of psychosis are likely to return.

2 Prior to discharge, the nurse provides teaching related to side effects of phenothiazines to the client and caregivers. Which of the following should be included?
1. The client may experience withdrawal and slowed activity.
2. Severe muscle spasms may occur early in therapy.
3. Tardive dyskinesia is likely early in therapy.
4. Medications should be takes as prescribed to prevent side effects.

3 The client experiences EPS during therapy with phenothiazines. The nurse expects which of the following drugs to be prescribed?

1. Benztropine (Cogentin)
2. Diazepam (Valium)
3. Haloperidol (Haldol)
4. Lorazepam (Ativan)

4 Nursing implications of the administration of haloperidol (Haldol) to a client exhibiting psychotic behavior include which of the following? (Select all that apply.)

1. Take 1 hour before or 2 hours after antacids.
2. The incidence of EPS is high.
3. It is therapeutic if ordered on a PRN basis.
4. Haldol is contraindicated in Parkinson's disease, seizure disorders, alcoholism, and severe mental depression.
5. Crush the sustained-release form for easier swallowing.

5 Which of the following data collected by the nurse during the history and physical is a contraindication for a client to receive fluphenazine (Prolixin)?

1. Diabetes mellitus
2. Age older than 70
3. Bone marrow depression
4. Hypertension

CRITICAL THINKING QUESTIONS

1. A 22-year-old male client has been on haloperidol (Haldol LA) for 2 weeks for the treatment of schizophrenia. During a follow-up assessment, the nurse notices that the client keeps rubbing his neck and is complaining of neck spasms. What is the nurse's initial action? What is the potential cause of the sore neck and what would be the potential treatment? What teaching is appropriate for this client?

2. A 68-year-old client has been put on olanzapine (Zyprexa) for treatment of acute psychoses. What is a priority of care for this client? What teaching is important for this client?

3. A 20-year-old, newly diagnosed schizophrenic client has been on chlorpromazine (Thorazine) and is doing well. Today the nurse notices that the client appears more anxious and is demonstrating increased paranoia. What is the nurse's initial action? What is the potential problem? What client teaching is important?

See Appendix D for answers and rationales for all activities.

EXPLORE
MediaLink

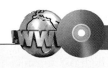 www.prenhall.com/adams

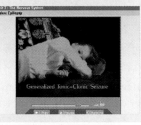
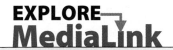

NCLEX-RN® review, case studies, and other interactive resources for this chapter can be found on the companion website at www.prenhall.com/adams. Click on "Chapter 17" to select the activities for this chapter. For animations, more NCLEX-RN® review questions, and an audio glossary, access the accompanying Prentice Hall Nursing MediaLink DVD-ROM in this textbook.

PRENTICE HALL NURSING MEDIALINK DVD-ROM
- **Animation**
  Mechanism in Action: Extrapyramidal Side Effects
- **Audio Glossary**
- **NCLEX-RN® Review**

COMPANION WEBSITE
- **NCLEX-RN® Review**
- **Dosage Calculations**
- **Case Study:** Client taking antipsychotics
- **Care Plan:** Client with schizophrenia taking chlorpromazine

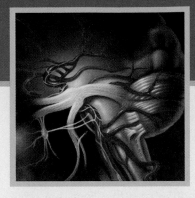

CHAPTER 18

Drugs for the Control of Pain

DRUGS AT A GLANCE

OPIOID (NARCOTIC) ANALGESICS
Opioid Agonists
  ⊙ *morphine (Astramorph PF, Duramorph, others)*
Opioid Antagonists
  ⊙ *naloxone (Narcan)*
Opioids with Mixed Agonist–Antagonist Activity
NONOPIOID ANALGESICS
Acetaminophen
Nonsteroidal Anti-inflammatory Drugs (NSAIDs)
  ⊙ *aspirin (acetylsalicylic acid, ASA)*
Centrally Acting Agents
ANTIMIGRAINE AGENTS
Ergot Alkaloids
Triptans
  ⊙ *sumatriptan (Imitrex)*

OBJECTIVES

After reading this chapter, the student should be able to:

1. Relate the importance of pain assessment to effective pharmacotherapy.
2. Explain the neural mechanism for pain at the level of the spinal cord.
3. Explain how pain can be controlled by inhibiting the release of spinal neurotransmitters.
4. Describe the role of nonpharmacological thera pies in pain management.
5. Compare and contrast the types of opioid receptors and their importance to pharmacology.
6. Explain the role of opioid antagonists in the diagnosis and treatment of acute opioid toxicity.
7. Describe the long-term treatment of opioid dependence.
8. Compare the pharmacotherapeutic approaches of preventing migraines with those of aborting migraines.
9. Describe the nurse's role in the pharmacological management of clients receiving analgesics and antimigraine drugs.
10. For each of the drug classes listed in Drugs at a Glance, know representative drug examples, and explain the mechanisms of drug action, primary actions, and important adverse effects.
11. Categorize drugs used in the treatment of pain based on their classification and mechanism of action.
12. Use the Nursing Process to care for clients receiving drug therapy for pain.

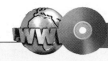

MediaLink   www.prenhall.com/adams

KEY TERMS

Aδ fibers   *page 225*

analgesic   *page 226*

aura   *page 237*

C fibers   *page 225*

cyclooxygenase   *page 233*

endogenous opioids   *page 225*

kappa receptor   *page 226*

methadone maintenance   *page 232*

migraine   *page 237*

mu receptor   *page 226*

narcotic   *page 226*

neuropathic pain   *page 224*

nociceptor   *page 225*

nociceptor pain   *page 224*

opiate   *page 226*

opioid   *page 226*

substance P   *page 225*

tension headache   *page 237*

Pain is a physiological and emotional experience characterized by unpleasant feelings, usually associated with trauma or disease. On a simple level, pain may be viewed as a defense mechanism that helps people avoid potentially damaging situations and encourages them to seek medical help. Although the neural and chemical mechanisms for pain are fairly straightforward, many psychological and emotional processes can modify this sensation. Anxiety, fatigue, and depression can increase the perception of pain. Positive attitudes and support from caregivers may reduce the perception of pain. Clients are more likely to tolerate their pain if they know the source of the sensation and the medical course of treatment designed to manage the pain. For example, if clients know that the pain is temporary, such as during labor or after surgery, they are more likely to accept the pain.

18.1 Assessment and Classification of Pain

The psychological reaction to pain is a subjective experience. The same degree and type of pain may be described as excruciating and unbearable by one client while not mentioned during physical assessment by another. Several numerical scales and survey instruments are available to help healthcare providers standardize the assessment of pain and measure the progress of subsequent drug therapy. Successful pain management depends on an accurate assessment of both the degree of pain experienced by the client and the potential underlying disorders that may be causing the pain. Selection of the correct therapy is dependent on the nature and character of the pain.

Pain can be classified as either acute or chronic. *Acute pain* is an intense pain occurring over a defined time, usually from injury to recovery. *Chronic pain* persists longer than 6 months, can interfere with daily activities, and is associated with feelings of helplessness or hopelessness.

Pain can also be classified as to its source. Injury to *tissues* produces **nociceptor pain.** This type of pain may be further subdivided into *somatic pain,* which produces sharp, localized sensations, or *visceral pain,* which is described as a generalized dull, throbbing, or aching pain. In contrast, **neuropathic pain** is caused by injury to *nerves* and typically is described as burning, shooting, or numb pain. Whereas nociceptor pain responds quite well to conventional pain-relief medications, neuropathic pain has less therapeutic success.

18.2 Nonpharmacological Techniques for Pain Management

Although drugs are quite effective at relieving pain in most clients, they can have significant side effects. For example, at high doses, aspirin causes gastrointestinal (GI) bleeding, and the opioids cause significant drowsiness and have the potential

PHARMFACTS

Pain

Pain is a common symptom:

- Approximately 16 million people experience chronic arthritic pain.
- More than 31 million adults report low back pain, with 19 million people experiencing this pain on a chronic basis.0
- At least 50 million people are fully or partially disabled as a result of pain.
- More than 50% of adults experience muscle pain each year.
- Up to 40% of people with cancer report moderate to severe pain.

MediaLink

The American Holistic Nurses Association

SPECIAL CONSIDERATIONS

Cultural Influences on Pain Expression and Perception

How a person responds to pain and chooses the type of pain management may be culturally determined. Establishment of a therapeutic relationship is of the utmost importance in helping a client attain pain relief. The nurse should respect the client's attitudes and beliefs about pain as well as choice of preferred treatment. Assessing the client's needs, beliefs, and customs by listening, showing respect, and allowing the client to help develop and choose treatment options to attain pain relief is the most culturally sensitive approach.

When assessing pain, the nurse must remember that some clients may openly express their feelings about and need for pain relief, whereas others may believe that the expression of pain symptoms, such as crying, is a sign of weakness. Pain management also varies according to cultural or religious beliefs. Traditional pain medications may or may not be preferred for pain control. Asians and Native Americans may prefer to use alternative therapies such as herbs, thermal therapies, acupuncture, massage, and meditation. Prayer plays an important role within African American and Hispanic cultures.

for dependence. Nonpharmacological techniques may be used in place of drugs, or as an adjunct to pharmacotherapy, to assist clients in obtaining adequate pain relief. When used concurrently with medication, nonpharmacological techniques may allow for lower doses and possibly fewer drug-related adverse effects. Some techniques used for reducing pain are as follows:

- Acupuncture
- Biofeedback therapy
- Massage
- Heat or cold packs
- Meditation or prayer
- Relaxation therapy
- Art or music therapy
- Imagery
- Chiropractic manipulation
- Hypnosis
- Therapeutic or physical touch
- Transcutaneous electrical nerve stimulation (TENS)
- Energy therapies such as Reiki and Qi gong

Clients with intractable cancer pain sometimes require more invasive techniques as rapidly growing tumors press on vital tissues and nerves. Furthermore, chemotherapy and surgical treatments for cancer can cause severe pain. Radiation therapy may provide pain relief by shrinking solid tumors that may be pressing on nerves. Surgery may be used to reduce pain by removing part of or the entire tumor. Injection of alcohol or another neurotoxic substance into neurons is occasionally performed to cause nerve blocks. Nerve blocks irreversibly stop impulse transmission along the treated nerves, and have the potential to provide total pain relief.

18.3 The Neural Mechanisms of Pain

The process of pain transmission begins when pain receptors are stimulated. These receptors, called **nociceptors,** are free nerve endings strategically located throughout the body. The nerve impulse signaling the pain is sent to the spinal cord along two types of sensory neurons, called Aδ and C fibers. **Aδ fibers** are wrapped in myelin, a lipid substance that speeds nerve transmission. **C fibers** are unmyelinated; thus, they carry information more slowly. The Aδ fibers signal sharp, well-defined pain, whereas the C fibers conduct dull, poorly localized pain.

Once pain impulses reach the spinal cord, neurotransmitters are responsible for passing the message along to the next neuron. Here, a neurotransmitter called **substance P** is thought to be responsible for continuing the pain message, although other neurotransmitter candidates have been proposed. Spinal substance P is critical because it controls whether pain signals will continue to the brain. The activity of substance P may be affected by other neurotransmitters released from neurons in the CNS. One group of neurotransmitters called **endogenous opioids** includes endorphins, dynorphins, and enkephalins. ● Figure 18.1 shows one point of contact where endogenous opioids modify sensory information at the level of the spinal cord. If the pain impulse reaches the brain, it may respond to the sensation with many possible actions, ranging from signaling the skeletal muscles to jerk away from a sharp object, to mental

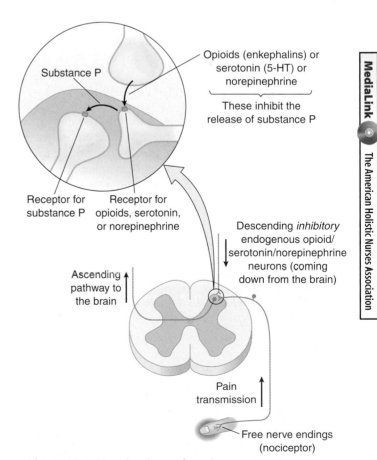

●**Figure 18.1** Neural pathways for pain

depression caused by thoughts of death or disability in those suffering from chronic pain.

The fact that the pain signal begins at nociceptors located within peripheral tissues and proceeds through the CNS allows several targets for the pharmacological intervention of pain transmission. In general, the two main classes of pain medications act at different locations: The nonsteroidal anti-inflammatory drugs (NSAIDs) act at the peripheral level, whereas the opioids act in the CNS.

OPIOID (NARCOTIC) ANALGESICS

Analgesics are medications used to relieve pain. The two basic categories of analgesics are the opioids and the nonopioids. An opioid analgesic is a natural or synthetic morphinelike substance responsible for reducing severe pain. Opioids are **narcotic** substances, meaning that they produce numbness or stuporlike symptoms.

18.4 Classification of Opioids

Terminology associated with the narcotic analgesic medications is often confusing. Several of these drugs are obtained from opium, a milky extract from the unripe seeds of the poppy plant, which contains more than 20 different chemicals having pharmacological activity. Opium consists of 9% to 14% morphine and 0.8% to 2.5% codeine. These natural substances are called **opiates.** In a search for safer analgesics, chemists have created several dozen synthetic drugs with activity similar to that of the opiates. **Opioid** is a general term referring to any of these substances, natural or synthetic, and is often used interchangeably with the term *opiate.*

Narcotic is a general term used to describe morphinelike drugs that produce analgesia and CNS depression. Narcotics may be natural, such as morphine, or synthetic such as meperidine (Demerol). In common usage, a narcotic analgesic is the same as an opioid, and the terms are often used interchangeably. In the context of drug enforcement, however, the term *narcotic* is often used to describe a much broader range of abused illegal drugs such as hallucinogens, heroin, amphetamines, and marijuana. In medical environments, the nurse should restrict use of the term narcotic to specifically refer to opioid substances.

Opioids exert their actions by interacting with at least six types of receptors: mu (types one and two), kappa, sigma,

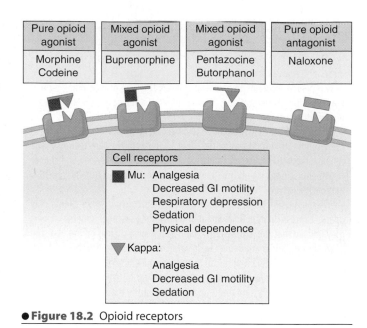

● **Figure 18.2** Opioid receptors

delta, and epsilon. From the perspective of pain management, the **mu** and **kappa receptors** are the most important. Drugs that stimulate a particular receptor are called *opioid agonists;* those that block a receptor are called *opioid antagonists.* The types of actions produced by activating mu and kappa receptors are listed in Table 18.1.

Some opioid agonists, such as morphine, activate both mu and kappa receptors. Other opioids, such as pentazocine (Talwin), exert mixed opioid agonist–antagonist effects by activating the kappa receptors but blocking the mu receptors. Opioid blockers such as naloxone (Narcan) inhibit both the mu and kappa receptors. This is the body's natural way of providing the mechanism for a diverse set of body responses from one substance. ● Figure 18.2 illustrates opioid actions on the mu and kappa receptors.

18.5 Pharmacotherapy With Opioids

Opioids are drugs of choice for moderate to severe pain that cannot be controlled with other classes of analgesics. More than 20 different opioids are available as medications, which may be classified by similarities in their chemical structures, by their mechanisms of action, or by their

TABLE 18.1	Responses Produced by Activation of Specific Opioid Receptors		
Response	Mu Receptor		Kappa Receptor
analgesia	✓		✓
decreased GI motility	✓		✓
euphoria	✓		
miosis			✓
physical dependence	✓		
respiratory depression	✓		
sedation	✓		✓

TABLE 18.2 Opioids for Pain Management

Drug	Route and Adult Dose (max dose where indicated)	Adverse Effects
OPIOID AGONISTS WITH MODERATE EFFICACY		
codeine	PO; 15–60 mg qid	*Sedation, nausea, constipation, dizziness*
hydrocodone bitartrate (Hycodan)	PO; 5–10 mg q4–6h PRN (max: 15 mg/dose)	
oxycodone hydrochloride (OxyContin); oxycodone terephthalate (Percocet-5, Roxicet, others)	PO; 5–10 mg qid PRN	Hepatotoxicity, respiratory depression, circulatory collapse, coma
propoxyphene hydrochloride (Darvon)	PO; 65 mg (HCl form) or 100 mg (napsylate form) q4h	
propoxyphene napsylate (Darvon-N)	PRN (max: 390 mg/day HCl; max : 600 mg/day napsylate)	
OPIOID AGONISTS WITH HIGH EFFICACY		
hydromorphone hydrochloride (Dilaudid)	PO; 1–4 mg q4–6h PRN	*Pruritis, constipation, nausea, sedation, drowsiness*
levorphanol tartrate (Levo-Dromoran)	PO; 2–3 mg tid—qid PRN	
meperidine hydrochloride (Demerol)	PO; 50–150 mg q3–4h PRN	Anaphylactoid reaction, cardiac arrest, severe respiratory depression or arrest
methadone hydrochloride (Dolophine)	PO; 2.5–10 mg q3–4h PRN	
⊕ morphine sulfate (Astramorph PF, Duramorph, others)	PO; 10–30 mg q4h PRN	
oxymorphone hydrochloride (Numorphan)	Subcutaneous/IM; 1–1.5 mg q4–6h PRN; 5 mg q4–6h PRN	
OPIOID ANTAGONISTS		
nalmefene hydrochloride (Revex)	Subcutaneous/IM/IV; use 1 mg/ml concentration Nonopioid dependent: 0.5 mg/70 kg Opioid dependent: 0.1 mg/70 kg	*Muscle and joint pains, difficulty sleeping, anxiety, headache, nervousness, vomiting*
⊕ naloxone hydrochloride (Narcan)	IV; 0.4–2 mg; may be repeated every 2–3 min up to 10 mg if necessary	Hepatotoxicity
naltrexone hydrochloride (Trexan, ReVia)	PO; 25 mg followed by another 25 mg in 1h if no withdrawal response (max: 800 mg/day)	
OPIOIDS WITH MIXED AGONIST–ANTAGONIST EFFECTS		
buprenorphine hydrochloride (Buprenex)	IM/IV; 0.3 mg q6h (max: 0.6 mg q4h)	*Drowsiness, dizziness, light-headedness, euphoria, nausea, clammy skin, sweating*
butorphanol tartrate (Stadol)	IM; 1–4 mg q3–4h PRN (max: 4 mg/dose)	
dezocine (Dalgan)	IV; 2.5–10 mg (usually 5 mg) q2–4h IM; 5–10 mg (usually 10 mg) q3–4h	Respiratory depression
nalbuphine hydrochloride (Nubain)	Subcutaneous/IM/IV; 10–20 mg q3–6h PRN (max: 160 mg/day)	
pentazocine hydrochloride (Talwin)	PO; 50–100 mg q3–4h (max: 600 mg/day) Subcutaneous/IM/IV; 30 mg q3–4h (max: 360 mg/day)	

Italics indicate common adverse effects; <u>underlining</u> indicates serious adverse effects.

efficacy (Table 18.2). The most clinically useful method is by efficacy, which places opiates into categories of strong or moderate narcotic activity. Morphine is the prototype drug for severe pain, and the drug against which all other opiates are compared.

Opiates produce many important effects other than analgesia. They are effective at suppressing the cough reflex and at slowing the motility of the GI tract for cases of severe diarrhea. As powerful CNS depressants, opioids can cause sedation, which may be either a therapeutic effect or a side effect, depending on the client's disease state. Some clients experience euphoria and intense relaxation, which are reasons why opiates are sometimes abused. There are many adverse effects, including respiratory depression, sedation, nausea, and vomiting.

All the narcotic analgesics have the potential to cause physical and psychological dependence, as discussed in Chapter 12 ∞. Dependence is more likely to occur when high doses are taken for extended periods. Many healthcare providers and nurses are hesitant to administer the proper amount of opioid analgesics for fear of causing client dependence or of producing serious adverse effects such as sedation or respiratory depression. Because of this undermedication, clients may not receive complete pain relief. When used according to accepted medical practice, clients can, and indeed should, receive the pain relief they need without fear of addiction or adverse effects.

It is common practice to combine opioids and nonnarcotic analgesics into a single tablet or capsule. The two classes of analgesics work synergistically to relieve pain, and

Pr PROTOTYPE DRUG | Morphine *(Astramorph PF, Duramorph, others)* | Opioid Agonist

ACTIONS AND USES

Morphine binds with both mu and kappa receptor sites to produce profound analgesia. It causes euphoria, constriction of the pupils, and stimulation of cardiac muscle. It is used for symptomatic relief of serious acute and chronic pain after nonnarcotic analgesics have failed, as preanesthetic medication, to relieve shortness of breath associated with heart failure and pulmonary edema, and for acute chest pain connected with MI.

ADMINISTRATION ALERTS

- Oral solution may be given sublingually.
- Oral solution comes in multiple strengths; carefully observe drug orders and labels before administering.
- Morphine causes peripheral vasodilation, which results in orthostatic hypotension.
- Pregnancy category D in long-term use or with high doses.

PHARMACOKINETICS

Onset: < 60 min

Peak: 60 min PO; 20–60 min rectally; 50–90 min subcutaneously; 30–60 min IM; 20 min IV

Half-life: 2–3h

Duration: Up to 7h

ADVERSE EFFECTS

Morphine may cause dysphoria (restlessness, depression, and anxiety), hallucinations, nausea, constipation, dizziness, and an itching sensation. Overdose may result in severe respiratory depression or cardiac arrest. Tolerance develops to the analgesic, sedative, and euphoric effects of the drug. Cross-tolerance also develops between morphine and other opioids such as heroin, methadone, and meperidine. Physical and psychological dependence develops when high doses are taken for prolonged periods.

Contraindications: Morphine may intensify or mask the pain of gallbladder disease, owing to biliary tract spasms. Morphine should also be avoided in cases of acute or severe asthma, GI obstruction, and severe hepatic or renal impairment.

INTERACTIONS

Drug–Drug: Morphine interacts with several drugs. For example, concurrent use of CNS depressants, such as alcohol, other opioids, general anesthetics, sedatives, and antidepressants such as MAO inhibitors and tricyclics, potentiates the action of opiates, increasing the risk of severe respiratory depression and death.

Lab Tests: Unknown.

Herbal/Food: Yohimbe, kava kava, valerian, and St. John's wort may potentiate the effect of morphine.

Treatment of Overdose: IV administration of naloxone is the specific treatment. Other treatments include activated charcoal, a laxative and a counter acting narcotic antagonist. Multiple doses may be needed.

 See the Companion Website for a Nursing Process Focus specific to this drug.

---

the dose of narcotic can be kept small to avoid dependence and opioid-related side effects. Five common combination analgesics are as follows:

- Vicodin (hydrocodone, 5 mg; acetaminophen, 500 mg)
- Percocet (oxycodone hydrochloride, 5 mg; acetaminophen, 325 mg)
- Percodan (oxycodone hydrochloride, 4.5 mg; oxycodone terephthalate, 0.38 mg; aspirin, 325 mg)
- Darvocet-N 50 (propoxyphene napsylate, 50 mg; acetaminophen, 325 mg)
- Empirin with Codeine No. 2 (codeine phosphate, 15 mg; aspirin, 325 mg)

Some opioids are used primarily for conditions other than pain. For example, alfentanil (Alfenta), fentanyl (Sublimaze), remifentanil (Ultiva), and sufentanil (Sufenta) are used for general anesthesia; these are discussed in Chapter 19. Codeine is most often prescribed as a cough suppressant and is covered in Chapter 38. Opiates used in treating diarrhea are presented in Chapter 41 ∞.

NURSING CONSIDERATIONS

The role of the nurse in opioid therapy for pain involves careful monitoring of a client's condition and providing education as it relates to the prescribed drug treatment. Perform an initial assessment to determine the presence or history of severe respiratory disorders, increased intracranial pressure (ICP), seizures, and liver or renal disease. Obtain an allergy history before administering these drugs. Obtain a complete blood count (CBC), and liver and renal function laboratory results including aspartate aminotransferase (AST), alanine aminotransferase (ALT), amylase, and bilirubin to rule out the presence of disease. Determine the character, duration, location, and intensity of pain before administering these agents. Obtain a history of current medication usage, especially alcohol and other CNS depressants, because these drugs will increase respiratory depression and sedation. Contraindications include hypersensitivity and conditions precluding IV opioid administration such as acute asthma or upper airway obstruction.

By activating primarily mu receptors, opioids may cause profound respiratory depression. Therefore, obtain vital signs, especially respirations, prior to and throughout the treatment regimen. Do not administer if respirations are below 12 breaths per minute. Narcotic antagonists such as naloxone (Narcan) should be readily available if respirations fall below 10 breaths per minute. Watch for decreasing level of consciousness, and ensure safety by keeping the bed in a low position with side rails raised. Assistance may be needed with ambulation and activities of daily living (ADLs).

NURSING PROCESS FOCUS Clients Receiving Opioid Therapy

Assessment	Potential Nursing Diagnoses
▪ Obtain a complete health history including allergies, drug history, and possible drug interactions. ▪ Assess pain (quality, intensity, location, duration) and effect on sleep pattern. ▪ Assess respiratory function. ▪ Assess level of consciousness before and after administration. ▪ Obtain vital signs.	▪ Knowledge, Deficient , related to drug therapy ▪ Pain, Acute, related to injury, disease, or surgical procedure ▪ Breathing Pattern, Ineffective, related to action of medication ▪ Constipation, related to action of medication ▪ Sleep Pattern, Disturbed, related to surgical pain

Planning: Client Goals and Expected Outcomes

The client will:
- Report pain relief or a reduction in pain intensity.
- Demonstrate an understanding of the drug's action by accurately describing drug side effects and precautions.
- Immediately report rebound pain, restlessness, anxiety, depression, hallucination, nausea, dizziness, constipation, or itching.
- Be free of preventable adverse drug effects.

Implementation

Interventions and (Rationales)	Client Education/Discharge Planning
▪ Opioids may be administered PO, subcutaneously, IM, IV, or rectally. (Ensure that correct route is administered.)	Instruct client: ▪ That oral *capsules* may be opened and mixed with cool foods; extended-release *tablets*, however, may not be chewed, crushed, or broken. ▪ That oral solution given sublingually may be in a higher concentration than solution for swallowing.
▪ Opioids are Schedule II controlled substances. (Opioids produce both physical and psychological dependence.)	Instruct client to: ▪ Take necessary steps to safeguard drug supply. ▪ Avoid sharing medications with others.
▪ Monitor liver function tests. (Opioids are metabolized in the liver. Hepatic disease can increase blood levels of opioids to toxic levels.)	Instruct client to: ▪ Report nausea, vomiting, diarrhea, rash, jaundice, abdominal pain, tenderness or distention, or change in color of stool. ▪ Keep scheduled laboratory appointments for liver function tests as ordered by the healthcare provider.
▪ Monitor vital signs, especially depth and rate of respirations/pulse oximetry. (Opioids can cause respiratory depression.) ▪ Withhold the drug if the client's respiratory rate is below 10, and notify the healthcare provider. (Opioids can cause respiratory depression.)	Instruct client or caregiver to: ▪ Monitor vital signs regularly, particularly respirations. ▪ Withhold medication for any difficulty in breathing or respirations below 10 breaths per minute; report symptoms to the healthcare provider.
▪ Monitor neurological status; perform neurochecks regularly. (Opioids can cause changes in sensorium, sluggish papillary response, and seizures.)	Instruct client to: ▪ Report headache or any significant change in sensorium, such as an aura or other visual affects that may indicate an impending seizure. ▪ Recognize seizures and methods to ensure personal safety during a seizure. ▪ Report any seizure activity immediately.
▪ If ordered PRN, administer medication on client request or when nursing observations indicate client expressions of pain. (Administering pain medication promptly helps prevent pain from becoming severe.)	▪ Instruct client to immediately alert the healthcare provider when pain returns or increases.
▪ Monitor renal status and urine output. (These drugs may cause urinary retention, which may exacerbate existing symptoms of benign prostatic hyperplasia or cause urinary tract infection.)	Instruct client or caregiver to: ▪ Measure and monitor fluid intake and output. ▪ Report symptoms of dysuria (hesitancy, pain, diminished stream), changes in urine quality or scanty urine output, fever or flank pain.

(Continued)

NURSING PROCESS FOCUS Clients Receiving Opioid Therapy *(Continued)*

Implementation

Interventions and (Rationales)	Client Education/Discharge Planning
▪ Monitor for other side effects such as restlessness, dizziness, anxiety, depression, hallucinations, nausea, and vomiting. (Hives or itching may indicate an allergic reaction due to the production of histamine.)	Instruct client or caregiver to: ▪ Recognize side effects and symptoms of an allergic or anaphylactic reaction. ▪ Immediately report any shortness of breath, tight feeling in the throat, itching, hives or other rash, feelings of dysphoria, nausea, or vomiting. ▪ Avoid the use of sleep-inducing OTC antihistamines without first consulting the healthcare provider.
▪ Monitor for constipation. (Opioids slow peristalsis.)	Instruct client to: ▪ Maintain an adequate fluid and fiber intake to facilitate stool passage. ▪ Use a stool softener or laxative as recommended by the healthcare provider.
▪ Ensure client safety. (Opioids can cause changes in sensorium, which may lead to falls.)	Instruct client to: ▪ Request assistance when getting out of bed. ▪ Avoid driving until effects of drug are known.
▪ Monitor frequency of requests and stated effectiveness of narcotic administered. (Opioids cause tolerance and dependence.)	Instruct client and caregiver: ▪ Regarding cross-tolerance issues. ▪ To monitor medication supply to observe for hoarding, which may signal an impending suicide attempt. ▪ That drug dependence in terminal illness must be viewed from the perspective of reduced life expectancy.

Evaluation of Outcome Criteria

Evaluate effectiveness of drug therapy by confirming that client goals and expected outcomes have been met (see "Planning").
▪ The client reports pain relief or a reduction in pain intensity.
▪ The client demonstrates an understanding of the drugs action by accurately describing side effects and precautions.
▪ The client immediately reports rebound pain, restlessness, anxiety, depression, hallucination, nausea, dizziness, constipation, or itching.
▪ The client is free of preventable adverse drug effects.

∞ *See Table 18.2 for a list of drugs to which these nursing actions apply.*

Another severe adverse reaction, increased ICP, occurs as an indirect result of respiratory depression. When respiration is suppressed, the CO_2 content of blood is increased, which dilates the cerebral blood vessels and causes ICP to rise. Similarly, orthostatic hypotension may also occur because of the blunting of the baroreceptor reflex and dilation of the peripheral arterioles and veins.

Continually monitor urine output for urinary retention, which may occur owing to increasing tone in the bladder sphincter, and through suppression of the bladder stimuli.

Side effects such as constipation, nausea, and vomiting occur owing to a combination of actions on the GI tract. Suppression of intestinal contractions, increase in tone of the anal sphincter, and inhibition of secretion of fluids into the intestine may result in constipation. Nausea or vomiting may occur secondary to the direct stimulation of the chemoreceptor trigger zone of the medulla, and an antiemetic may be indicated. Opioids may be contraindicated for clients suffering from diarrhea caused by infections, especially following antibiotic therapy (pseudomembranous colitis). Pathogens in the GI tract produce toxins that are shed during diarrhea; constipation causes toxins to build up in the body.

Client Teaching. Client education as it relates to opioids should include the goals of therapy, the reasons for obtaining baseline data such as vital signs and the existence of underlying renal or respiratory disorders, and possible drug side effects. Include the following points when teaching clients about opioids:

- Take medications exactly as prescribed.
- Do not take other prescription drugs, OTC medications, herbal remedies, or vitamins or minerals without notifying the healthcare provider.
- Keep all scheduled laboratory visits for liver function tests.
- Immediately report nausea and vomiting; diarrhea; rash; yellowing of the skin; abdominal pain, tenderness, or distention; or change in color of stool.
- Report any seizure activity immediately.
- Notify the healthcare provider if pain relief is not effective.
- Do not take medication if you experience excess drowsiness, confusion, or respiratory status.

The Influence of Age on Pain Expression and Perception

Pain control in both children and elderly clients can be challenging. Knowledge of developmental theories, the aging process, behavioral cues, subtle signs of discomfort, and verbal and nonverbal responses to pain are a must when it comes to effective pain management. Older clients may have a decreased perception of pain or may simply ignore pain as a "natural" consequence of aging. Because these clients frequently go undermedicated, a thorough assessment is needed. As with adults, belief in self-report when assessing for pain in children is important. Developmentally appropriate pain-rating tools are available and should be used on a consistent basis. Comfort measures should also be used.

When administering opioids for pain relief, always monitor clients closely. Smaller doses are usually indicated, and side effects may be heightened. Closely monitor decreased respirations, LOC, and dizziness. Take body weight prior to starting opioid administration and calculate doses accordingly. Keep bed and crib rails raised and the bed in low position at all times to prevent injury from falls. Some opioids, such as meperidine (Demerol), should be used cautiously in children. Many elderly clients take multiple drugs (polypharmacy), so it is important to obtain a complete list of all medications taken and check for interactions.

OPIOID ANTAGONISTS

Opioid antagonists are blockers of opioid activity. They are often used to reverse the symptoms of opioid toxicity or overdose, such as sedation or respiratory depression.

18.6 Pharmacotherapy With Opioid Antagonists

Opioid overdose can occur as a result of overly aggressive pain therapy or as a result of substance abuse. Any opioid may be abused for its psychoactive effects; however, morphine, meperidine, and heroin are preferred because of their potency. Although heroin is currently available as a legal analgesic in many countries, it is deemed too dangerous for therapeutic use by the FDA and is a major drug of abuse. Once injected or inhaled, heroin rapidly crosses the blood–brain barrier to enter the brain, where it is metabolized to morphine. Thus, the effects and symptoms of heroin administration are actually caused by the activation of mu and kappa receptors by morphine. The initial effect is an intense euphoria, called a *rush*, followed by several hours of deep relaxation.

Acute opioid intoxication is a medical emergency, with respiratory depression being the most serious problem. Infusion with the opioid antagonist naloxone (Narcan) may be used to reverse respiratory depression and other acute symptoms. In cases in which the client is unconscious and it is unclear which drug has been taken, opioid antagonists may be given to diagnose the overdose. If the opioid antagonist fails to quickly reverse the acute symptoms, the overdose was likely due to a nonopioid substance.

NURSING CONSIDERATIONS

The role of the nurse in opioid antagonist therapy involves careful monitoring of a client's condition and providing education as it relates to the prescribed drug treatment. Assess the client's respiratory status and administer the opioid antagonist if respirations are below 10 breaths per minute. Resuscitative equipment should be immediately accessible. Obtaining key medical information is a priority; include the presence or history of cardiovascular disease. Opioids increase cardiac workload, so they must be used with caution in clients with cardiovascular disease. Assess the social

---

Pr PROTOTYPE DRUG | Naloxone *(Narcan)* | Opioid Antagonist

ACTIONS AND USES

Naloxone is a pure opioid antagonist, blocking both mu and kappa receptors. It is used for complete or partial reversal of opioid effects in emergency situations when acute opioid overdose is suspected. Given intravenously, it begins to reverse opioid-initiated CNS and respiratory depression within minutes. It will immediately cause opioid withdrawal symptoms in clients physically dependent on opioids. It is also used to treat postoperative opioid depression. It is occasionally given as adjunctive therapy to reverse hypotension caused by septic shock.

ADMINISTRATION ALERTS

- Administer for respiratory rate of fewer than 10 breaths/minute. Keep resuscitative equipment accessible.
- Pregnancy category B.

PHARMACOKINETICS

Onset: 1–2 min IV; 2–5 min IM; 2–5 min subcutaneously

Peak: < 60 min

Half-life: 20–60 min

Duration: 60–100 min

ADVERSE EFFECTS

Naloxone itself has minimal toxicity. However, reversal of the effects of opioids may result in rapid loss of analgesia, increased blood pressure, tremors, hyperventilation, nausea and vomiting, and drowsiness.

Contraindications: Naloxone should not be used for respiratory depression caused by nonopioid medications.

INTERACTIONS

Drug–Drug: Drug interactions include a reversal of the analgesic effects of narcotic agonists and antagonists.

Lab Tests: Unknown.

Herbal/Food: Echinacea may increase the risk of hepatotoxicity.

Treatment of Overdose: Naloxone overdose requires the use of oxygen, IV fluids, vasopressors, and other supportive measures as indicated. These treatments may be useful in combination drug overdose (for example, pentazocine with naloxone [Talwin NX]).

 See the Companion Website for a Nursing Process Focus specific to this drug.

context of the client's environment for the potential for opioid dependency. Use opioid antagonists cautiously in clients who are physically dependent on opioids, because drug-induced withdrawal may be more severe than spontaneous opioid withdrawal. Caution is also advised for pregnant or lactating women, and in children.

Assess the client's pain level before administering these drugs and during therapy. During and immediately after the administration of opioid antagonists, check vital signs every 3 to 5 minutes (especially respiratory function and blood pressure), obtain air blood gas (ABG) levels and ECG, and monitor for drowsiness, tremors, hyperventilation, ventricular tachycardia, and loss of analgesia. If giving these drugs to drug-dependent clients, monitor for signs of opioid withdrawal such as cramping, vomiting, hypertension, and anxiety.

Opioid antagonists such as naltrexone (Depade, ReVia, and Trexan) are also used for the treatment of opioid addiction. Monitor for side effects during treatment, many of which reflect the opioid withdrawal syndromes. Symptoms include increased thirst, chills, fever, joint/muscle pain, CNS stimulation, drowsiness, dizziness, confusion, seizures, headache, nausea, vomiting, diarrhea, rash, rapid pulse and respirations, pulmonary edema, and wheezing. Check vital signs every 3 to 5 minutes. Continually assess respiratory function and cardiac status for tachycardia and hypertension. As with naloxone (Narcan), resuscitative equipment should be readily available.

Client Teaching. Client education as it relates to opioid antagonists should include the goals of therapy, the reasons for obtaining baseline data such as vital signs and the existence of underlying cardiovascular disorders, and possible drug side effects. Include the following points when teaching clients about opioid antagonists:

- Immediately report chills, nausea, vomiting, headache, CNS stimulation, or wheezing.
- Notify the healthcare provider of any pain or discomfort.
- Inform the healthcare provider if you are pregnant or lactating.

18.7 Treatment for Opioid Dependence

Although effective at relieving pain, the opioids have a greater risk for dependence than almost any other class of medications. Tolerance develops relatively quickly to the euphoric effects of opioids, causing abusers to escalate their doses and take the drugs more frequently. The higher and more frequent doses rapidly cause physical dependence in opioid abusers.

When physically dependent clients attempt to discontinue drug use, they experience extremely uncomfortable symptoms that convince many to continue their drug-taking behavior to avoid the suffering. As long as the drug is continued, they feel "normal," and many can continue work or social activities. In cases when the drug is abruptly discontinued, the

client experiences about 7 days of withdrawal symptoms before overcoming the physical dependence.

The intense craving characteristic of psychological dependence may occur for many months, and even years, following discontinuation of opioids. This often results in a return to drug-seeking behavior unless significant support groups are established.

One common method of treating opioid dependence is to switch the client from IV and inhalation forms of illegal drugs to methadone (Dolophine). Although an opioid, oral methadone does not cause the euphoria of the injectable opioids. Methadone does not cure the dependence, however, and the client must continue taking the drug to avoid withdrawal symptoms. This therapy, called **methadone maintenance,** may continue for many months or years, until the client decides to enter a total withdrawal treatment program. Methadone maintenance allows clients to return to productive work and social relationships without the physical, emotional, and criminal risks of illegal drug use.

A newer treatment option is to administer buprenorphine (Subutex), a mixed opioid agonist–antagonist, by the sublingual route. Buprenorphine is used early in opioid abuse therapy to prevent opioid withdrawal symptoms. Another combination agent, Suboxone, contains both buprenorphine and naloxone, and is used later in the maintenance of opioid addiction.

NONOPIOID ANALGESICS

The nonopioid analgesics include acetaminophen, NSAIDs, and a few centrally acting agents.

NONSTEROIDAL ANTI-INFLAMMATORY DRUGS (NSAIDS)

The NSAIDs inhibit cyclooxygenase, an enzyme responsible for the formation of prostaglandins. When cyclooxygenase is inhibited, inflammation and pain are reduced.

18.8 Pharmacotherapy With NSAIDs

NSAIDs are the drugs of choice for mild to moderate pain, especially for pain associated with inflammation. These drugs have many advantages over the opioids. Aspirin and ibuprofen are available OTC and are inexpensive. They are available in many different formulations, including those designed for children. They are safe and produce adverse effects only at high doses. The NSAIDs have antipyretic and anti-inflammatory activity, as well as analgesic properties. Some of the NSAIDs, such as the selective COX-2 inhibitors, are used primarily for their anti-inflammatory properties. The role of the NSAIDs in the treatment of inflammation and fever is discussed in Chapter 33 ∞. Table 18.3 highlights the common nonopioid analgesics.

The NSAIDs act by inhibiting pain mediators at the nociceptor level. When tissue is damaged, chemical mediators

TABLE 18.3   Nonopioid Analgesics

Drug	Route and Adult Dose (max dose where indicated)	Adverse Effects
acetaminophen (Tylenol) (see page 479 for the Prototype Drug box ∞)	PO; 325–650 mg q4–6h	*Hepatotoxicity in alcoholics* Hepatotoxicity, hepatic coma, acute renal failure
NSAIDS: Selective COX-2 Inhibitors		
celecoxib (Celebrex)	PO; 100–200 mg bid or 200 mg qid	*Abdominal pain, dizziness, headache, sinusitis, hypersensitivity* Cautious use due to FDA review
NSAIDS: Ibuprofen and Ibuprofen-type Drugs		
diclofenac (Cataflam, Voltaren)	PO; 50 mg bid–qid (max: 200 mg/day)	*Indigestion, nausea, occult blood loss, anorexia, headache, drowsiness, dizziness* Aplastic anemia, drug-induced peptic ulcer, GI bleeding, agranulocytosis, laryngospasm, laryngeal edema
diflunisal (Dolobid)	PO; 1,000 mg followed by 500 mg bid–tid	
etodolac (Lodine)	PO; 200–400 mg tid–qid	
fenoprofen calcium (Nalfon)	PO; 200 mg tid–qid	
flurbiprofen (Ansaid)	PO; 50–100 mg tid–qid (max: 300 mg/day)	
ibuprofen (Advil, Motrin)	PO; 400 mg tid–qid (max: 1,200 mg/day)	
indomethacin (Indocin)	PO; 25–50 mg bid–tid (max: 200 mg/day), or 75 mg sustained release 1–2 times/day	
ketoprofen (Actron, Orudis)	PO; 12.5–50 mg tid–qid	
ketorolac tromethamine (Toradol)	PO; 10 mg qid PRN (max: 40 mg/day)	
mefenamic acid (Ponstel)	PO; Loading dose: 500 mg; Maintenance dose: 250 mg q6h PRN	
meloxicam (Mobic)	PO; 7.5 mg/day (max: 15 mg/day)	
nabumetone (Relafen)	PO; 1,000 mg/day (max: 2,000 mg/day)	
naproxen (Naprosyn, Naprelen)	PO; 500 mg followed by 200–250 mg tid–qid (max: 1,000 mg/day)	
naproxen sodium (Aleve, Anaprox, others)	PO; 250–500 mg bid (max: 1,000 mg/day naproxen)	
ozaprozin (Daypro)	PO; 600–1,200 mg/day (max: 1,800 mg/day)	
piroxicam (Feldene)	PO; 10–20 mg 1–2 times/day (max: 20 mg/day)	
sulindac (Clinoril)	PO; 150–200 mg bid (max: 400 mg/day)	
tolmetin (Tolectin)	PO; 400 mg tid (max: 2 g/day)	
NSAIDS: Salicylates		
aspirin (acetylsalicylic acid, ASA)	PO; 350–650 mg q4h (max: 4 g/day)	*Heartburn, stomach pains, ulceration* Bronchospasm, anaphylactic shock, hemolytic anemia
choline salicylate (Arthropan)	PO; 435–870 mg (2.5–5 ml) q4h	
salsalate (Disalcid)	PO; 325–3,000 mg/day in divided doses (max: 4 g/day)	
CENTRALLY ACTING AGENTS		
clonidine (Catapres)	PO; 0.1 mg bid–tid (max: 0.8 mg/day)	*Hypotension, dry mouth, constipation, drowsiness, sedation, dizziness, vertigo, fatigue, headache* Anaphylactic reaction
tramadol (Ultram)	PO; 50–100 mg q4–6h PRN (max: 400 mg/day); may start with 25 mg/day, and increase by 25 mg q3days up to 200 mg/day	

Italics indicate common adverse effects; underlining indicates serious adverse effects.

are released locally, including histamine, potassium ion, hydrogen ion, bradykinin, and prostaglandins. Bradykinin is associated with the sensory impulse of pain. Prostaglandins can induce pain through the formation of free radicals.

Prostaglandins are formed with the help of two enzymes called **cyclooxygenase** type 1 (COX-1) and cyclooxygenase type 2 (COX-2). Aspirin inhibits both COX-1

and COX-2. Because the COX-2 enzyme is more specific for the synthesis of those prostaglandins that cause pain and inflammation, the selective COX-2 inhibitors provide more specific pain relief and are used primarily for their anti-inflammatory properties. Celecoxib (Celebrex) and rofecoxib (Vioxx), once top-selling arthritis medications have been linked to the risk of heart attack and stroke. Vioxx was removed from the market on September 30, 2004,

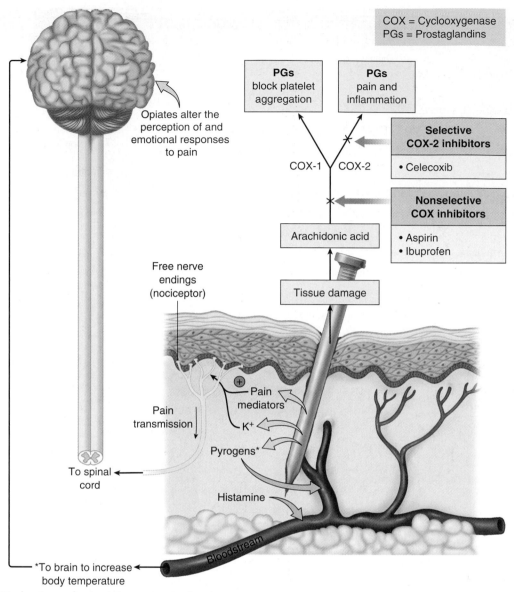

COX = Cyclooxygenase
PGs = Prostaglandins

PGs
block platelet
aggregation

PGs
pain and
inflammation

COX-1 COX-2

**Selective
COX-2 inhibitors**

• Celecoxib

**Nonselective
COX inhibitors**

• Aspirin
• Ibuprofen

Arachidonic acid

Tissue damage

Opiates alter the
perception of and
emotional responses
to pain

Free nerve
endings
(nociceptor)

⊕ Pain
mediators

K⁺

Pyrogens*

Pain
transmission

Histamine

To spinal
cord

Bloodstream

*To brain to increase
body temperature

● **Figure 18.3** Mechanisms of pain at the nociceptor level

after a study revealed that this drug was linked to heart attacks. Strokes, blood clots, and cardiovascular injuries. ● Figure 18.3 illustrates the mechanisms involved in pain at the nociceptor level.

Several important nonopioid analgesics are not classified as NSAIDs. Acetaminophen is a nonopioid analgesic that is equally as effective as aspirin and ibuprofen in relieving pain. Acetaminophen is featured as a prototype antipyretic on page 479 in Chapter 33 ∞. Clonidine (Catapres) and tramadol (Ultram) are centrally acting analgesics. Tramadol has weak opioid activity, though it is not thought to relieve pain by this mechanism.

NURSING CONSIDERATIONS

The role of the nurse in NSAID therapy involves careful monitoring of a client's condition and providing education as it relates to the prescribed drug treatment. Because

NSAIDs are readily available, inexpensive, and taken orally, clients sometimes forget that these medications can have serious side effects. The inhibition of COX-1 by aspirin makes it more likely to cause peptic ulcers and GI bleeding and acute renal failure. Ibuprofen exerts less of an effect on COX-1 inhibition, so it produces less gastric bleeding than aspirin.

When caring for clients taking high doses of these drugs, complete a thorough assessment for the presence or history of hypersensitivity, bleeding disorders, peptic ulcers, severe renal/hepatic disease, and pregnancy. NSAIDs are not recommended for clients with these conditions. Perform renal and liver function studies (blood urea nitrogen [BUN], creatinine, AST, ALT, and hemoglobin) before and during pharmacotherapy. Assess the location, character, and intensity of pain initially for baseline data and throughout treatment to determine effectiveness. Aspirin has many drug interactions; therefore, obtain a

Pr **PROTOTYPE DRUG** | Aspirin *(Acetylsalicylic Acid, ASA)* | NSAID, Salicylate

ACTIONS AND USES

Aspirin inhibits prostaglandin synthesis involved in the processes of pain and inflammation and produces mild to moderate relief of fever. It has limited effects on peripheral blood vessels, causing vasodilation and sweating. Aspirin has significant anticoagulant activity, and this property is responsible for its ability to reduce the risk of mortality following MI, and to reduce the incidence of strokes. Aspirin has also been found to reduce the risk of colorectal cancer, although the mechanism by which it affords this protective effect is unknown.

ADMINISTRATION ALERTS

- Platelet aggregation inhibition caused by aspirin is irreversible. Aspirin should be discontinued 1 week prior to elective surgery.
- Aspirin is excreted in the urine and affects urine testing for glucose and other metabolites, such as vanillylmandelic acid (VMA).
- Pregnancy category D.

PHARMACOKINETICS

Onset: 1 h

Peak: 2–4 h

Half-life: 15–20 min (aspirin); 2–3 h (salicylate at low dose); more than 20 h (salicylate at high dose)

Duration: 24 h

ADVERSE EFFECTS

At high doses, such as those used to treat severe inflammatory disorders, aspirin may cause gastric discomfort and bleeding because of its antiplatelet effects. Enteric-coated tablets and buffered preparations are available for clients who experience GI side effects.

Contraindications: Because aspirin increases bleeding time, it should not be given to clients receiving anticoagulant therapy such as warfarin, heparin, and plicamycin.

INTERACTIONS

Drug–Drug: Concurrent use of phenobarbital, antacids, and glucocorticoids may decrease aspirin's effects. Aspirin may potentiate the action of oral hypoglycemic agents. Effects of NSAIDs, uricosuric agents such as probenecid, beta-blockers, spironolactone, and sulfa drugs may be decreased when combined with aspirin. Insulin, methotrexate, phenytoin, sulfonamides, and penicillin may increase effects. When aspirin is taken with alcohol, pyrazolone derivatives, steroids, or other NSAIDs, there is an increased risk for gastric ulcers.

Lab Tests: Aspirin may cause prolonged prothrombin time by decreasing prothrombin production. Aspirin may also interfere with pregnancy tests, and decrease serum levels of cholesterol, potassium, PBI, T_3, and T_4. High salicylate levels may cause abnormalities in liver function tests.

Herbal/Food: Feverfew, garlic, ginger, and gingko may increase the risk of bleeding.

Treatment of Overdose: Treatment may include any of the following: activated charcoal, gastric lavage, laxative, or drug therapy for overdose symptoms such as dizziness, drowsiness, abdominal pain, or seizures.

 See the Companion Website for a Nursing Process Focus specific to this drug.

complete inventory of drugs taken by the client list. Contraindications include hypersensitivity to aspirin or other NSAIDs; bleeding disorders such as hemophilia, von Willebrand's disease, and telangiectasia; and favism (genetic G6PD enzyme deficiency). When clients are taking high doses of these medications, it is important to monitor them for nephrotoxicity (dysuria, hematuria, and oliguria), blood dyscrasias, hepatitis, and allergic responses (rash and urticaria). Also monitor clients for nausea, abdominal pain, anorexia, dizziness, and drowsiness. To decrease GI upset, give the medication with food and plenty of fluids. Do not crush enteric-coated tablets.

Lifespan Consideration. Exercise extreme caution in administering aspirin to children and teenagers. Aspirin has been implicated in the development of Reye's syndrome when given to children with flulike illnesses. Febrile, dehydrated children can rapidly develop aspirin toxicity. Use aspirin with caution in clients who are pregnant or lactating. Pregnancy category C (D in third trimester) denotes potential harm to the fetus.

Client Teaching. Client education as it relates to nonopioid analgesic therapy should include the goals of therapy; the reasons for obtaining baseline data such as

vital signs and the existence of underlying bleeding, renal, hepatic, or pregnancy disorders; and possible drug side effects. Include the following points when teaching clients about nonopioid analgesics:

- Do not administer aspirin to children and teenagers.
- Take medications with food and plenty of fluids to prevent GI upset.
- Immediately report nausea, blood in stools or urine, abdominal pain, anorexia, dizziness, rash, or itching.
- Keep all scheduled laboratory visits for renal and liver function tests.
- Report a history of bleeding disorders.

TENSION HEADACHES AND MIGRAINES

Headaches are some of the most common complaints of clients. Living with headaches can interfere with ADLs, thus causing great distress. The pain and inability to focus and concentrate result in work-related absences and difficulties

NURSING PROCESS FOCUS   Clients Receiving NSAID Therapy

Assessment	Potential Nursing Diagnoses
Prior to administration: ■ Obtain a complete health history including allergies, drug history, and possible drug interactions. ■ Determine pain and analgesic usage patterns. ■ Identify infectious agents or other factors responsible for inflammation or pain.	■ Pain, Acute, related to injury or surgical procedure ■ Pain, Chronic, related to back injury ■ Knowledge, Deficient, related to drug therapy ■ Health Maintenance, Ineffective, related to chronic pain

Planning: Client Goals and Expected Outcomes

The client will:
■ Report pain relief or a reduction in pain intensity.
■ Demonstrate an understanding of the drug's action by accurately describing drug side effects and precautions.
■ Report ability to manage activities of daily living.
■ Immediately report unresolved, untoward, or rebound pain; persistent fever; blurred vision; tinnitus; bleeding; changes in color of stool or urine.

Implementation

Interventions and (Rationales)	Client Education/Discharge Planning
■ NSAIDs may be administered PO or PR. When suppositories are used, monitor integrity of rectum. (Rectal bleeding may occur.)	Instruct client to: ■ Not cut or crush enteric-coated tablets. Regular tablets may be broken or pulverized and mixed with food. ■ Administer liquid aspirin immediately after mixing because it breaks down rapidly. ■ Not take ibuprofen and naproxen concurrently. ■ Consult the healthcare provider regarding appropriate OTC analgesics for specific types of pain. ■ Consult the nurse regarding aspirin therapy following surgery. ■ Advise laboratory personnel of aspirin therapy when providing urine samples.
■ Monitor vital signs, especially temperature. (Increased pulse and blood pressure may indicate discomfort; when accompanied by pallor and/or dizziness may indicate bleeding.)	Instruct client to: ■ Report rapid heartbeat, palpitations, dizziness, or pallor. ■ Properly monitor blood pressure and temperature using home equipment.
■ Monitor for signs of GI bleeding or hepatic toxicity. (NSAIDs can be a local irritant to the GI tract with anticoagulant action that is metabolized in the liver.)	Instruct client to: ■ Report any bleeding, abdominal pain, anorexia, heartburn, nausea, vomiting, jaundice, or a change in the color or character of stools. ■ Use the proper method of obtaining stool samples and home testing for occult blood.
■ Monitor complete blood count (CBC) for signs of anemia related to blood loss. (Nonopioids may cause GI bleeding.)	Instruct client to: ■ Keep scheduled laboratory appointments for testing as ordered by the healthcare provider. ■ Take NSAIDs with food to reduce stomach upset.
■ Assess for character, duration, location, and intensity of pain and the presence of inflammation. (Pain assessment may indicate need for additional therapies.)	Instruct client to: ■ Notify the healthcare provider if pain or inflammation remains unresolved. ■ Take only the prescribed amount to decrease the potential for adverse effects.
■ Monitor for hypersensitivity reaction. (Hypersensitivity reactions may be a medical emergency.)	■ Instruct client to immediately report shortness of breath, wheezing, throat tightness, itching, or hives. If these occur, stop taking aspirin immediately and inform the healthcare provider.
■ Monitor urine output and edema in feet/ankles. (Medication is excreted through the kidneys. Long-term use may lead to renal dysfunction.)	■ Instruct client to immediately report changes in urination, flank pain, or pitting edema.

NURSING PROCESS FOCUS Clients Receiving NSAID Therapy *(Continued)*

Implementation

Interventions and (Rationales)	Client Education/Discharge Planning
■ Monitor for sensory changes such as tinnitus or blurred vision. (Tinnitus and blurred vision may be signs of toxicity.)	Instruct client to: ■ Immediately report any sensory changes in sight or hearing, especially blurred vision or ringing in the ears. ■ Keep scheduled appointments with the healthcare provider.

Evaluation of Outcome Criteria

Evaluate effectiveness of drug therapy by confirming that client goals and expected outcomes have been met (see "Planning").

■ The client reports pain relief or reduction in pain intensity.

■ The client demonstrates an understanding of the drug's actions by accurately describing drug side effects and precautions.

■ The client manages activities of daily living.

■ The client reports unresolved, untoward, or rebound pain; persistent fever; blurred vision; tinnitus; bleeding; changes in color of stool or urine.

∞ *See Table 18.3 under "NSAIDS" for a list of drugs to which these nursing actions apply.*

caring for home and family. When the headaches are persistent, or occur as migraines, drug therapy is warranted.

18.9 Classification of Headaches

Of the several varieties of headaches, the most common type is the **tension headache.** This condition occurs when muscles of the head and neck become very tight because of stress, causing a steady and lingering pain. Although quite painful, tension headaches are self-limiting and generally considered an annoyance rather than a medical emergency. Tension headaches can usually be effectively treated with OTC analgesics such as aspirin, acetaminophen, or ibuprofen.

The most painful type of headache is the **migraine,** which is characterized by throbbing or pulsating pain, sometimes preceded by an aura. **Auras** are sensory cues that let the client know that a migraine attack is coming soon. Examples of sensory cues are jagged lines or flashing lights, or special smells, tastes, or sounds. Most migraines are accompanied by nausea and vomiting. Triggers for migraines include nitrates, monosodium glutamate (MSG)—found in many Asian foods, red wine, perfumes, food additives, caffeine, chocolate, and aspartame. By avoiding foods containing these substances, some clients can prevent the onset of a migraine attack.

18.10 Drug Therapy for Migraine Headaches

There are two primary goals for the pharmacological therapy of migraines (Table 18.4). The first is to stop migraines in progress, and the second is to prevent migraines from occurring. For the most part, the drugs used to abort migraines are different from those used for prophylaxis. Drug therapy is most effective if begun before a migraine has reached a severe level.

The two major drug classes used as antimigraine agents, the triptans and the ergot alkaloids, are both serotonin (5-HT) agonists. Serotonergic receptors are found throughout the CNS, and in the cardiovascular and GI systems. At least five receptor subtypes have been identified. In addition to the triptans, other drugs acting at serotonergic receptors include the popular antianxiety agents fluoxetine (Prozac) and buspirone (BuSpar).

Pharmacotherapy of migraine termination generally begins with acetaminophen or NSAIDs. If OTC analgesics are unable to abort the migraine, the drugs of choice are often the triptans. The first of the triptans, sumatriptan (Imitrex), was marketed in the United States in 1993. These agents are selective for the 5-HT$_1$-receptor subtype, and they are thought to act by constricting certain intracranial vessels. They are effective in aborting migraines with or without auras. Although oral forms of the triptans are most convenient, clients who experience nausea and vomiting during the migraine may require an alternative dosage form. Intranasal formulations and prefilled syringes of triptans are available for clients who are able to self-administer the medication.

For clients who are unresponsive to triptans, the ergot alkaloids may be used to abort migraines. The first purified

MediaLink

Tension Headaches and Migraines

PHARMFACTS

Headaches and Migraines

■ About 28 million Americans suffer from headaches and migraines.

■ Of all migraines, 95% are controlled by drug therapy and other measures.

■ Before puberty, more boys have migraines than girls.

■ After puberty, women have four to eight times more migraines than men have.

■ Headaches and migraines appear mostly among people in their 20s and 30s.

■ Persons with a family history of headache or migraine have a higher chance of developing these disorders.

TABLE 18.4   Antimigraine Drugs

Drug	Route and Adult Dose (max dose where indicated)	Adverse Effects
ERGOT ALKALOIDS*		
dihydroergotamine mesylate (D.H.E. 45, Migranal)	IM; 1 mg; may be repeated at 1-h intervals to a total of 3 mg (max: 6 mg/wk)	*Weakness, nausea, vomiting, abnormal pulse*
ergotamine tartrate (Ergostat) ergotamine with caffeine (Cafergot, Ercaf, others)	PO; 1–2 mg followed by 1–2 mg q30min until headache stops (max: 6 mg/day or 10 mg/wk)	<u>Delirium, convulsive seizures, intermittent claudication</u>
TRIPTANS		
almotriptan (Axert)	PO; 6.25–12.5 mg; may repeat in 2 h if necessary (max: 2 tabs/day)	*Asthenia, tingling , warming sensation, dizziness, vertigo*
eletriptan (Relpax)	PO; 20–40 mg; may repeat in 2 if necessary (max: 80 mg/day)	
frovatriptan (Frova)	PO; 2.5 mg; may repeat in 2 if necessary (max: 7.5 mg/day)	<u>Coronary artery vasospasm, MI, cardiac arrest</u>
naratriptan (Amerge)	PO; 1–2.5 mg; may repeat in 4 h if necessary (max: 5 mg/day)	
rizatriptan (Maxalt)	PO; 5–10 mg; may repeat in 2 h if necessary (max: 30 mg/day); 5 mg with concurrent propranolol (max: 15 mg/day)	
℗ sumatriptan (Imitrex)	PO; 25 mg for 1 dose (max: 100 mg)	
zolmitriptan (Zomig)	PO; 2.5–5 mg; may repeat in 2 h if necessary (max: 10 mg/day)	
BETA-ADRENERGIC BLOCKERS*		
atenolol (Tenormin) (see page 353 for the Prototype Drug box ∞)	PO; 25–50 mg/day (max: 100 mg/day)	*Bradycardia, hypotension, CHF*
metoprolol (Lopressor)	PO; 50–100 mg 1–2 times/day (max: 450 mg/day)	<u>Bronchospasm, exfoliative dermatitis, agranulocytosis, membrane irritation, rash</u>
propranolol hydrochloride (Inderal) (see page 369 for the Prototype Drug box ∞)	PO; 80–240 mg/day in divided doses; may need 160–240 mg/day	
timolol (Blocadren)	PO; 10 mg bid; may increase to 60 mg/day in 2 divided doses	
CALCIUM CHANNEL BLOCKERS**		
nifedipine (Procardia) (see page 314 for the Prototype Drug box ∞)	PO; 10–20 mg tid (max: 180 mg/day)	*Dizziness, light-headedness, facial flushing, heat sensitivity, diarrhea*
nimodipine (Nimotop)	PO; 60 mg q4h for 21 days; start therapy within 96 hours of subarachnoid hemorrhage	<u>MI, hepatotoxicity</u>
verapamil hydrochloride (Isoptin) (see page 373 for the Prototype Drug box ∞)	PO; 40–80 mg tid (max: 360 mg/day)	
TRICYCLIC ANTIDEPRESSANTS**		
amitryptyline hydrochloride (Elavil)	PO; 75–100 mg/day	*Sedation, drowsiness, orthostatic hypotension, blurred vision, slight mydriasis, dry mouth, urinary retention*
imipramine (Tofranil) (see page 191 for the Prototype Drug box ∞)	PO; 75–100 mg/day (max: 300 mg/day)	<u>MI, arrythmias, heart block, agranulocytosis, angioedema</u>
MISCELLANEOUS AGENTS**		
valproic acid (Depakene, Depakote) (see page 180 for the Prototype Drug box ∞)	PO; 250 mg bid (max: 1,000 mg/day)	*Nausea, vomiting, sedation, drowsiness, discoloration of urine (for vitamin B_2)*
methysergide (Sansert)	PO; 4–8 mg/day in divided doses	<u>Deep coma with overdose, liver failure, bone marrow depression</u>
riboflavin (vitamin B_2)	As a supplement: PO; 5–10 mg/day For deficiency: PO; 5–30 mg/day in divided doses	

Italics Indicate common adverse effects; <u>underlining</u> indicates serious adverse effects.
*For terminating migraines; **for preventing migraines.

Pr PROTOTYPE DRUG | Sumatriptan (*Imitrex*) | Antimigraine Agent, Triptan

ACTIONS AND USES

Sumatriptan belongs to a relatively new group of antimigraine drugs known as the triptans. The triptans act by causing vasoconstriction of cranial arteries; this vasoconstriction is moderately selective and does not usually affect overall blood pressure. This medication is available in oral, intranasal, and subcutaneous forms. Subcutaneous administration terminates migraine attacks in 10 to 20 minutes; the dose may be repeated 60 minutes after the first injection, to a maximum of two doses per day. If taken orally, sumatriptan should be administered as soon as possible after the migraine is suspected or has begun.

ADMINISTRATION ALERTS

- Sumatriptan may produce cardiac ischemia in susceptible persons with no previous cardiac events. Healthcare providers may opt to administer the initial dose of sumatriptan in the healthcare setting.
- Sumatriptan's systemic vasoconstrictor activity may cause hypertension and may result in dysrhythmias or myocardial infarction. Keep resuscitative equipment accessible.
- Sumatriptan selectively reduces carotid arterial blood flow. Monitor changes in level of consciousness and observe for seizures.
- Pregnancy category C.

PHARMACOKINETICS

Onset: 15 min nasal; 30 min PO; 10 min subcutaneous

Peak: 2 h PO; 1 h subcutaneous

Half-life: 2 h

Duration: 24–48 h

ADVERSE EFFECTS

Some dizziness, drowsiness, or a warming sensation may be experienced after taking sumatriptan; however, these effects are not normally severe enough to warrant discontinuation of therapy.

Contraindications: Because of its vasoconstricting action, the drug should be used cautiously, if at all, in clients with recent myocardial infarction, or with a history of angina pectoris, hypertension, or diabetes.

INTERACTIONS

Drug–Drug: Sumatriptan interacts with several drugs. For example, an increased effect may occur when taken with monoamine oxidase inhibitors (MAOIs) and selective serotonin reuptake inhibitors (SSRIs). Further vasoconstriction can occur when taken with ergot alkaloids and other triptans.

Lab Tests: Unknown.

Herbal/Food: Ginkgo, ginseng, echinacea, and St. John's wort may increase triptan toxicity.

Treatment of Overdose: Treatment may include drug therapy for the following symptoms: weakness, lack of coordination, watery eyes and mouth, tremors, seizures, or breathing problems.

 See the Companion Website for a Nursing Process Focus specific to this drug.

---

alkaloid, ergotamine (Ergostat), was isolated from the ergot fungus in 1920, although the actions of the ergot alkaloids had been known for thousands of years. Ergotamine is an inexpensive drug that is available in oral, sublingual, and suppository forms. Modifications of the original molecule have produced a number of other pharmacologically useful drugs, such as dihydroergotamine (Migranal). Dihydroergotamine is given parenterally and as a nasal spray. Because the ergot alkaloids interact with adrenergic and dopaminergic receptors as well as serotonergic receptors, they produce multiple actions and side effects. Many ergot alkaloids are pregnancy category X drugs.

Drugs for migraine prophylaxis include various classes of drugs that are discussed in other chapters of this textbook. These include beta-adrenergic blockers, calcium channel blockers, antidepressants, and antiseizure drugs. Because all these drugs have the potential to produce side effects, prophylaxis is initiated only if the incidence of migraines is high and the client is unresponsive to the drugs used to abort migraines. Of the various drugs, the beta-blocker propranolol (Inderal) is one of the most commonly prescribed. Amitriptyline (Elavil), an antidepressant, is preferred for clients who may have a mood disorder or suffer from insomnia in addition to their migraines.

NURSING CONSIDERATIONS

The role of the nurse in antimigraine therapy involves careful monitoring of a client's condition and providing education as it relates to the prescribed drug treatment. Before starting clients on antimigraine medications, gather information about the frequency and intensity of the migraine headaches and the presence or history of myocardial infarction (MI), angina, and hypertension. Also, gather information about the presence or history of renal and liver disease, diabetes, and pregnancy. Obtain the results of lab tests to assess for underlying renal and liver disease.

Assess apical pulse, respirations, and blood pressure. Because migraines may be stress related, investigate a client's stress level and coping mechanisms. Always assess for hypersensitivity and the use of other medications such as monoamine oxidase inhibitors (MAOIs) or selective serotonin reuptake inhibitors (SSRIs), both of which can cause an increased effect of triptans.

Assess the client's neurological status, including level of consciousness (LOC), blurred vision, nausea and vomiting, and tingling in extremities. These signs or symptoms may indicate a migraine is beginning. Provide a quiet, calm environment with decreased noise and subdued lighting, and

NURSING PROCESS FOCUS Clients Receiving Triptan Therapy

Assessment	Potential Nursing Diagnoses
Prior to administration: • Obtain a complete health history including allergies, drug history, and possible drug interactions. • Determine pain and analgesic usage patterns. • Identify infectious agents or other factors responsible for inflammation or pain. • Assess level of consciousness before and after administration.	• Pain, Acute, related to severe headache • Knowledge, Deficient, related to drug therapy • Coping, Ineffective, related to chronic pain • Health Maintenance, Ineffective, related to inability to manage activities of daily living

Planning: Client Goals and Expected Outcomes

The client will:
• Report pain relief or a reduction in pain intensity.
• Demonstrate an understanding of the drug's action by accurately describing drug side effects and precautions.
• Immediately report shortness of breath, chest tightness or pressure, jaw pain, untoward or worsened rebound headache, seizures, or other neurological changes.
• Be able to adequately perform activities of daily living.

Implementation

Interventions and (Rationales)	Client Education/Discharge Planning
• Administer the first dose of the medication under supervision. (Cardiac assessments may occur during this time.)	• Instruct client that the first dose may need to be given under medical supervision, in the event of cardiac side effects. Reassure client that this is merely a precautionary measure.
• Monitor vital signs, especially blood pressure and pulse. (Triptans have vasoconstrictor action.)	• Instruct client to properly monitor vital signs, especially blood pressure and pulse, using home equipment.
• Observe for changes in severity, character, or duration of headache. (Sudden severe headaches of "thunderclap" quality can signal subarachnoid hemorrhage. Headaches that differ in quality and are accompanied by such signs as fever, rash, or stiff neck may herald meningitis.)	Instruct client: • That changes in the character of migraines could signal other, potentially more serious, disorders. • About warning signs of stroke and discuss other conditions such as meningitis that may cause headache.
• Monitor neurological status; perform neurochecks regularly. (Dizziness or light-headedness may be a result of coronary ischemia.)	Instruct client: • That feeling dizzy or light-headed can be the result of the drug's action on the CNS, or coronary ischemia. • To report episodes of severe dizziness or impending syncope immediately. • To review emergency response and safety measures in the event of a seizure.
• Monitor for possible side effects, including dizziness, drowsiness, warming sensation, tingling, light-headedness, weakness, or neck stiffness due to vasoconstriction. (Such symptoms can result from decreased blood flow to the brain related to reduced carotid arterial blood supply.)	Instruct client: • To immediately report side effects to the healthcare provider. • Regarding symptoms suggestive of stroke or MI that may require immediate emergency intervention and transport to a hospital.
• Monitor dietary intake of foods that contain tyramine. (These foods may trigger an acute migraine.)	• Instruct client to avoid or limit foods containing tyramine, such as pickled foods, beer, wine, and aged cheeses.
• Monitor kidney and liver function via laboratory tests. (Assesses liver and renal function with regard to medication administration.)	Instruct client to: • Report nausea, vomiting, diarrhea, rash, jaundice, abdominal pain, tenderness, distention, or change in color of stool. • Keep scheduled laboratory appointments for liver function testing as ordered by the healthcare provider.

Evaluation of Outcome Criteria

Evaluate effectiveness of drug therapy by confirming that client goals and expected outcomes have been met (see "Planning").
• The client reports a reduction in pain intensity.
• The client demonstrates an understanding of the drug's actions by accurately describing the drug side effects and precautions.
• The client reports shortness of breath, chest tightness or pressure, jaw pain, untoward or worsening rebound headache, seizures, or other neurological changes.
• The client demonstrates improved ability to manage activities of daily living.

∞ *See Table 18.4 under "Triptans" for a list of drugs to which these nursing actions apply.*

organize care to limit disruptions and decrease neural stimulation. Apply cold packs to help lessen the uncomfortable effects of the migraine.

Monitor for possible side effects, including dizziness, drowsiness, vasoconstriction, warming sensations, tingling, light-headedness, weakness, and neck stiffness. Use with caution during pregnancy or lactation. Sumatriptan (Imitrex) is excreted in breast milk. Advise the client that the drug could be harmful to the fetus or infant. Contraindications include hypertension, myocardial ischemia, coronary artery disease (CAD), history of MI, dysrhythmia or heart failure, high-risk CAD profile, and diabetes, because the vasoconstriction action of the drugs used for these disorders may worsen migraine pain.

The ergot alkaloids promote vasoconstriction, which terminates ongoing migraines. Side effects may include nausea, vomiting, weakness in the legs, myalgia, numbness and tingling in fingers and toes, angina-like pain, and tachycardia. Toxicity may be evidenced by constriction of peripheral arteries, resulting in cold, pale, numb extremities and muscle pain. Sumatriptan (Imitrex) is metabolized in the liver and excreted by the kidneys; impaired organ function can increase serum drug levels. Monitor the client for long-term use of these medications, because they can cause physical dependence.

Client Teaching.   Client education as it relates to drug therapy for migraines should include the goals of therapy, the reasons for obtaining baseline data such as vital signs and the existence of underlying cardiovascular disorders, and possible drug side effects. Include the following points when teaching clients regarding the ergot alkaloids:

- Take medication immediately after onset of symptoms.
- Control, avoid, or eliminate factors that trigger a headache or migraine, such as fatigue, anxiety, and alcohol.
- Report muscle pain, numbness, and cold extremities.
- Do not overuse any of these drugs, because physical dependence may result.

NATURAL THERAPIES

Feverfew for Migraines

Feverfew (*Tanacetum parthenium*) is an herb that originated in southeastern Europe and is now found all over Europe, Australia, and North America. The common name feverfew is derived from its antipyretic properties. The leaves contain the active ingredients, the most prevalent of which is a lactone known as parthenolide. Standardization of this herb is based on the percent parthenolide in the product.

Feverfew has an overall spectrum of action resembling that of aspirin. The herb has been shown to exert anti-inflammatory and antispasmodic effects, as well as to inhibit platelet aggregation. Feverfew extract has also been shown to contain a novel type of mast cell inhibitor that inhibits anti-IgE-induced histamine release. In clinical trials, feverfew was associated with a reduction in number and severity of migraine attacks, as well as a reduction in vomiting (Evans and Taylor, 2006). The most common adverse effect is mouth ulceration, which occurs in about 10% of feverfew users.

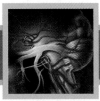

CHAPTER REVIEW

KEY CONCEPTS

The numbered key concepts provide a succinct summary of the important points from the corresponding numbered section within the chapter. If any of these points are not clear, refer to the numbered section within the chapter for review.

18.1   Pain is assessed and classified as acute or chronic, nociceptor land or neuropathic.

18.2   Nonpharmacological techniques such as massage, biofeedback therapy, and meditation are often important adjuncts to effective pain management.

18.3   Neural mechanisms include pain transmission via Aδ or C fibers and the release of substance P.

18.4   Opioids are natural or synthetic substances extracted from the poppy plant that exert their effects through interaction with mu and kappa receptors.

18.5   Opioids are the drugs of choice for severe pain. They also have other important therapeutic effects including dampening of the cough reflex and slowing of the motility of the GI tract.

18.6   Opioid antagonists may be used to reverse the symptoms of opioid toxicity or overdose, such as sedation and respiratory depression.

18.7   Opioid withdrawal can result in severe symptoms, and dependence is often treated with methadone maintenance.

18.8   Nonopioid analgesics, such as aspirin, acetaminophen, and the selective COX-2 inhibitors, are effective in treating mild to moderate pain, inflammation, and fever.

18.9   Headaches are classified as tension headaches or migraines. Migraines may be preceded by auras, and symptoms include nausea and vomiting.

18.10   The goals of pharmacotherapy for migraine headaches are to stop migraines in progress and to prevent them from occurring. Triptans, ergot alkaloids, and a number of drugs from other classes are used for migraines.

NCLEX-RN® REVIEW QUESTIONS

1 The nurse teaches the client relaxation techniques and guided imagery as an adjunct to medication for treatment of pain. The nurse explains that the major benefit of these techniques is that they:

1. Are less costly.
2. Allow lower doses of drugs with fewer side effects.
3. Can be used at home.
4. Do not require self-injection.

2 The nurse recognizes that opioid analgesics exert their action by interacting with a variety of opioid receptors. Drugs such as morphine act by:

1. Activating kappa and blocking mu receptors.
2. Inhibiting mu and kappa receptors.
3. Activating mu and kappa receptors.
4. Blocking sigma and delta receptors.

3 A client admitted with hepatitis B is prescribed Vicodin 2 tablets for pain. The appropriate nursing action is to:

1. Administer the drug as ordered.
2. Administer one tablet only.
3. Question the physician about the order.
4. Hold the drug until the physician arrives.

4 The nurse administers morphine sulfate 4 mg IV to a client for treatment of severe pain. Which of the following assessments require immediate nursing interventions? (Select all that apply.)

1. The client's blood pressure is 110/70 mm Hg.
2. The client is drowsy.
3. The client's pain is unrelieved in 15 minutes.
4. The client's respiratory rate is 10 breaths per minute.
5. The client becomes unresponsive.

5 Nursing intervention for a client receiving opioid analgesics over an extended period should include:

1. Referring the client to a drug treatment center.
2. Encouraging increased fluids and fiber in the diet.
3. Monitoring for GI bleeding.
4. Teaching the client to self-assess blood pressure.

CRITICAL THINKING QUESTIONS

1. A client is on a patient-controlled analgesia (PCA) pump to manage postoperative pain related to recent orthopedic surgery. The PCA is set to deliver a basal rate of morphine of 6 mg/h. The nurse discovers the client to be unresponsive with a respiratory rate of 8 breaths per minute and oxygen saturation of 84%. What is the nurse's initial response? What are the nurse's subsequent actions?

2. A 64-year-old client has had a long-standing history of migraine headaches as well as coronary artery disease, type 2 diabetes, and hypertension. On review of the medical history, the nurse notes that this client has recently started on sumatriptan (Imitrex), prescribed by the client's new neurologist. What intervention and teaching should be done for this client?

3. A 58-year-old client with a history of a recent MI is on beta-blocker and anticoagulant therapy. The client also has a history of arthritis, and during a recent flare-up began taking aspirin because it helped control pain in the past. What teaching or recommendation would the nurse have for this client?

See Appendix D for answers and rationales for all activities.

EXPLORE
MediaLink

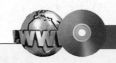

www.prenhall.com/adams

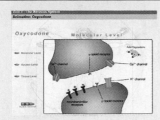

NCLEX-RN® review, case studies, and other interactive resources for this chapter can be found on the companion website at www.prenhall.com/adams. Click on "Chapter 18" to select the activities for this chapter. For animations, more NCLEX-RN® review questions, and an audio glossary, access the accompanying Prentice Hall Nursing MediaLink DVD-ROM in this textbook.

PRENTICE HALL NURSING MEDIALINK DVD-ROM

- **Animations**
  Mechanism in Action: Morphine (*Astramorph*)
  Mechanism in Action: Naproxen (*Naprosyn, Naprolen*)
  Mechanism in Action: Oxycodone (*OxyContin*)
- **Audio Glossary**
- **NCLEX-RN® Review**

COMPANION WEBSITE

- **NCLEX-RN® Review**
- **Dosage Calculations**
- **Case Study:** Pain management
- **Care Plan:** Client who is receiving morphine to control pain following surgery

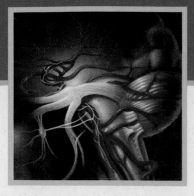

CHAPTER 19

Drugs for Local and General Anesthesia

DRUGS AT A GLANCE

LOCAL ANESTHETICS
Amides
  ➲ *lidocaine (Xylocaine)*
Esters
GENERAL ANESTHETICS
Inhalation Agents
Gases
  ➲ *nitrous oxide*
Volatile Liquids
  ➲ *halothane (Fluothane)*
Intravenous Agents
Barbiturate and Barbiturate-like Agents
  ➲ *thiopental (Pentothal)*
Opioids
Benzodiazepines
ADJUNCTS TO ANESTHESIA
Barbiturate and Barbiturate-like Agents
Opioids
Neuromuscular-blocking Agents
  ➲ *succinylcholine (Anectine)*

OBJECTIVES

After reading this chapter, the student should be able to:

1. Compare and contrast the five major clinical techniques for administering local anesthetics.
2. Describe differences between the two major chemical classes of local anesthetics.
3. Explain why epinephrine and sodium hydroxide are sometimes included in local anesthetic cartridges.
4. Identify the actions of general anesthetics on the CNS.
5. Compare and contrast the two primary ways that general anesthesia may be induced.
6. Identify the four stages of general anesthesia.
7. For each of the drug classes listed in Drugs at a Glance, know representative drug examples, and explain their mechanisms of action, primary actions, and important adverse effects.
8. Categorize drugs used for anesthesia based on their classification and drug action.
9. Use the Nursing Process to care for clients who are receiving anesthesia.

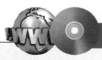

MediaLink

www.prenhall.com/adams

NCLEX-RN® review, case studies, and other interactive resources for this chapter can be found on the companion website at www.prenhall.com/adams. Click on "Chapter 19" to select the activities for this chapter. For animations, more NCLEX-RN® review questions, and an audio glossary, access the accompanying Prentice Hall Nursing MediaLink DVD-ROM in this textbook.

KEY TERMS

amide *page 246*

balanced anesthesia *page 249*

ester *page 246*

general anesthesia *page 245*

local anesthesia *page 245*

neuroleptanalgesia *page 255*

neuromuscular blocker *page 257*

surgical anesthesia *page 250*

Anesthesia is a medical procedure performed by administering drugs that cause a loss of sensation. **Local anesthesia** occurs when sensation is lost to a limited part of the body without loss of consciousness. **General anesthesia** requires different classes of drugs that cause loss of sensation to the entire body, usually resulting in a loss of consciousness. This chapter examines drugs used for both local and general anesthesia.

LOCAL ANESTHESIA

Local anesthesia is loss of sensation to a relatively small part of the body without loss of consciousness to the client. This procedure may be necessary when a relatively brief dental or medical procedure is performed.

19.1 Regional Loss of Sensation Using Local Anesthetics

Although local anesthesia often results in a loss of sensation to a small, limited area, it sometimes affects relatively large portions of the body, such as an entire limb. Thus, some local anesthetic treatments are more accurately called *surface* anesthesia or *regional* anesthesia, depending on how the drugs are administered and their resulting effects.

The five major routes for applying local anesthetics are shown in ● Figure 19.1. The method employed is dependent on the location and extent of the desired anesthesia. For example, some local anesthetics are applied topically before a needle stick or minor skin surgery. Others are used to block sensations to large areas such as a limb or the lower abdomen. The different methods of local and regional anesthesia are summarized in Table 19.1.

LOCAL ANESTHETICS

Local anesthetics are drugs that produce a rapid loss of sensation to a limited part of the body. They produce their therapeutic effect by blocking the entry of sodium ions into neurons.

19.2 Mechanism of Action of Local Anesthetics

The mechanism of action of local anesthetics is well known. Recall that the concentration of sodium ions is normally higher on the outside of neurons than on the inside. A rapid influx of sodium ions into cells is necessary for neurons to fire.

Local anesthetics act by blocking sodium channels, as illustrated in Pharmacotherapy Illustrated 19.1 (see page 247). Because the blocking of sodium channels is a nonselective process, both sensory and motor impulses are affected. Thus, both sensation and muscle activity will temporarily diminish in the area treated with the local anesthetic. Because of their mechanism of action, local anesthetics are sometimes called *sodium channel blockers*.

During a medical or surgical procedure, it is essential that the action of the anesthetic last long enough to complete the procedure. Small amounts of epinephrine

---

PHARMFACTS

Anesthesia and Anesthetics

- More than 20 million people receive general anesthetics each year in the United States.
- About half of all general anesthetics are administered by a nurse anesthetist.
- The first medical applications of anesthetics were in 1842, using ether, and, in 1846, using nitrous oxide.
- Herbal products may interact with anesthetics; St. John's wort may intensify or prolong the effects of some opioids and anesthetics.

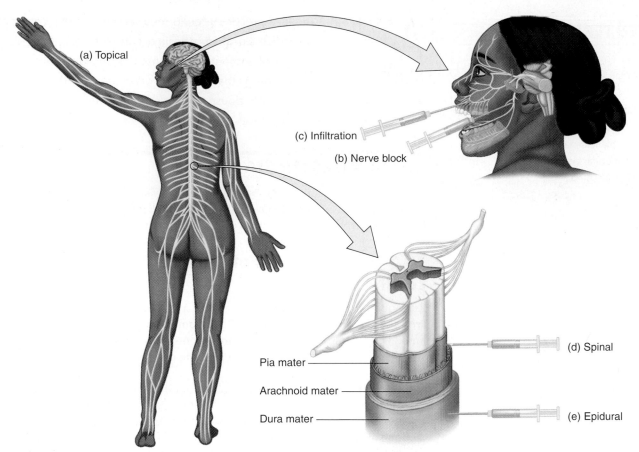

● **Figure 19.1** Techniques for applying local anesthesia: (a) topical; (b) nerve block; (c) infiltration; (d) spinal; and (e) epidural

are sometimes added to the anesthetic solution to constrict blood vessels in the immediate area where the local anesthetic is applied. This keeps the anesthetic in the area longer, thus extending the duration of action of the drug. The addition of epinephrine to lidocaine (Xylocaine), for example, increases the duration of its local anesthetic effect from 20 minutes to as long as 60 minutes. This is important for dental or surgical procedures that take longer than 20 minutes; otherwise, a second injection of the anesthetic would be necessary.

Sodium hydroxide is sometimes added to anesthetic solutions to increase the effectiveness of the anesthetic in regions that have extensive local infection or abscesses. Bacteria tend to acidify an infected site, and local anesthetics are less effective in an acidic environment. Adding alkaline substances such as sodium hydroxide or sodium bicarbonate neutralizes the region and creates a more favorable environment for the anesthetic.

19.3 Classification of Local Anesthetics

Local anesthetics are classified by their chemical structures; the two major classes are **esters** and **amides** (Table 19.2) (see page 248). The terms *ester* and *amide* refer to types of chemical linkages found within the anesthetic molecules, as illustrated in ● Figure 19.2 (see page 248). Although esters and amides have

TABLE 19.1	Methods of Local Anesthetic Administration	
Route	**Formulation/Method**	**Description**
epidural anesthesia	injection into epidural space of spinal cord	most commonly used in obstetrics during labor and delivery
infiltration (field block) anesthesia	direct injection into tissue immediate to the surgical site	drug diffuses into tissue to block a specific group of nerves in a small area close to the surgical site
nerve block anesthesia	direct injection into tissue that may be distant from the operation site	drug affects nerve bundles serving the surgical area; used to block sensation in a limb or large area of the face
spinal anesthesia	injection into the cerebral spinal fluid (CSF)	drug affects large, regional area such as the lower abdomen and legs
topical (surface) anesthesia	creams, sprays, suppositories, drops, and lozenges	applied to mucous membranes including the eyes, lips, gums, nasal membranes, and throat; very safe unless absorbed

19.1 Mechanism of Action of Local Anesthetics

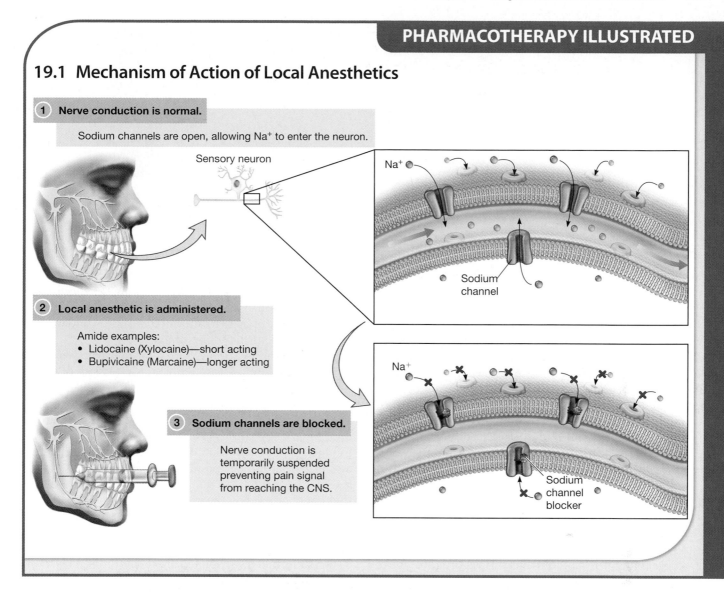

1 **Nerve conduction is normal.**

Sodium channels are open, allowing Na⁺ to enter the neuron.

Sensory neuron

Na⁺

Sodium channel

2 **Local anesthetic is administered.**

Amide examples:
- Lidocaine (Xylocaine)—short acting
- Bupivicaine (Marcaine)—longer acting

Na⁺

3 **Sodium channels are blocked.**

Nerve conduction is temporarily suspended preventing pain signal from reaching the CNS.

Sodium channel blocker

---

equal efficacy, important differences exist. A small number of miscellaneous agents are neither esters nor amides.

Cocaine was the first local anesthetic widely used for medical procedures. Cocaine is a natural ester, found in the leaves of the plant *Erythroxylon coca*, native to the Andes Mountains of Peru. As late as the 1880s, cocaine was routinely used for eye surgery, nerve blocks, and spinal anesthesia. Although still available for local anesthesia, cocaine is a Schedule II drug and rarely used therapeutically in the United States. The abuse potential of cocaine is discussed in Chapter 12 ∞.

Another ester, procaine (Novocain), was the drug of choice for dental procedures from the mid-1900s until the 1960s, until the development of the amide anesthetics led to a significant decline in the use of the drug. One ester, benzocaine (Solarcaine, others) is used as a topical, OTC agent for treating a large number of painful conditions, including sunburn, insect bites, hemorrhoids, sore throat, and minor wounds.

Amides have largely replaced the esters because they produce fewer side effects and generally have a longer duration of action. Lidocaine (Xylocaine) is the most widely used amide for short surgical procedures requiring local anesthesia.

Adverse effects of local anesthetics are uncommon. Allergy is rare. When it does occur, it is often due to sulfites, which are added as preservatives to prolong the shelf life of

NATURAL THERAPIES

Cloves and Anise as Natural Dental Remedies

One natural remedy for tooth pain is oil of cloves. Extracted from the plant *Eugenia*, eugenol is the chemical extract found in cloves thought to produce its numbing effect. It works especially well for cavities. The herb is applied by soaking a piece of cotton and packing it around the gums close to the painful area. Dentists sometimes recommend it for temporary relief of a toothache. Clove oil has an antiseptic effect that has been reported to kill bacteria, fungi, and helminths. Another natural remedy is oil of anise, scientific name *Pimpinella*, for jaw pain caused by nerve pressure or gritting of teeth. Anise oil is an antispasmodic agent, which means it relaxes intense muscular pressure around the jaw angle, cheeks, and throat area. Its extra benefits are that it is also a natural expectorant, cough suppressant, and breath freshener. The pharmacological effects of anise are thought to be due to the chemical anethole, which is similar in structure to natural catecholamines.

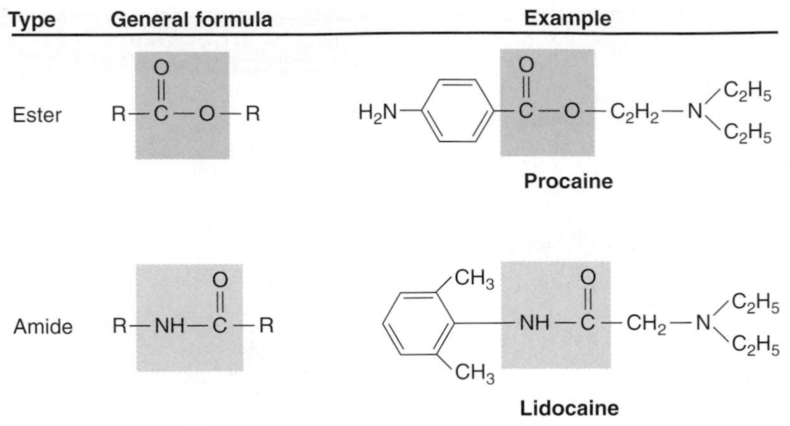

Type	General formula	Example

● **Figure 19.2** Chemical structures of ester and amide local anesthetics

the anesthetic, or to methylparaben, which may be added to retard bacterial growth in anesthetic solutions. Early signs of adverse effects of local anesthetics include symptoms of CNS stimulation such as restlessness or anxiety. Later effects, such as drowsiness and unresponsiveness, are due to CNS depression. Cardiovascular effects, including hypotension and dysrhythmias, are possible. Clients with a history of cardiovascular disease are often given forms of local anesthetics that contain no epinephrine to reduce the potential effects of this sympathomimetic on the heart and blood pressure. CNS and cardiovascular side effects are not expected unless the local anesthetic is absorbed rapidly or is accidentally injected directly into a blood vessel.

NURSING CONSIDERATIONS

The role of the nurse in local anesthetic administration involves careful monitoring of a client's condition and providing education as it relates to the prescribed drug treatment. Although the physician usually administers these medications when an area needs to be anesthetized for a medical procedure,

the nurse often assists. The nurse's role may include preparing the area to be anesthetized, and monitoring the effectiveness of the medication by assessing pain and comfort levels. Check for the presence of broken skin, infection, burns, and wounds at the site of anesthetic administration.

Contraindications for these drugs include hypersensitivity to local anesthetics; sepsis and blood dyscrasias; untreated sinus bradycardia; and severe degrees of atrioventricular, sinoatrial, and intraventricular heart block in the absence of a pacemaker. Local anesthetics should be used with caution over large body areas, in clients with extensive surface trauma, and in severe skin disorders, because the medication may be absorbed and result in systemic effects. Unless specifically formulated for optic use, local anesthetics should not be used on the eyes.

Adverse reactions are rare; nonetheless, monitor clients for cardiac palpitations and difficulty breathing or swallowing. Assess vital signs during the procedure and report any changes immediately. Monitor the client for local reactions such as irritation, rash, and for signs of CNS excitation, such as for example, restlessness or anxiety.

TABLE 19.2	**Selected Local Anesthetics**	
Chemical Classification	**Drug**	**General Adverse Effects**
esters	benzocaine (Americaine, Solarcaine, others) chloroprocaine (Nesacaine) procaine (Novocain) tetracaine (Pontocaine)	*CNS depression* Respiratory arrest, circulatory failure, anaphylactoid reaction
amides	articaine (Septodont) bupivacaine (Marcaine) dibucaine (Nupercaine, Nupercainal) etidocaine (Duranest) levobupivacaine (Chirocaine) ⊕ lidocaine (Xylocaine) mepivacaine (Carbocaine) prilocaine (Citanest) ropivacaine (Naropin)	Difficulty breathing or swallowing, respiratory depression and arrest, convulsions, anaphylactoid reaction
miscellaneous agents	dyclonine (Dyclone) pramoxine (Tronothane)	*Burning, stinging, sensation at application site* Respiratory or cardiac arrest

Italics indicate common adverse effects; underlining indicates serious adverse effects.

Pr PROTOTYPE DRUG | Lidocaine *(Xylocaine)* | Local Anesthetic Amide

ACTIONS AND USES

Lidocaine, the most frequently used injectable local anesthetic, acts by blocking neuronal pain impulses. It is injected as a nerve block, for spinal and epidural anesthesia. It acts by blocking sodium channels located within the membranes of neurons.

Lidocaine may be given IV, IM, or subcutaneously to treat dysrhythmias, as discussed in Chapter 23 ∞. A topical form is also available.

ADMINISTRATION ALERTS

- Solutions of lidocaine containing preservatives or epinephrine are intended for local anesthesia only, and must never be given parenterally for dysrhythmias.
- Do not apply topical lidocaine to large skin areas or to broken or abraded areas, because significant absorption may occur. Do not allow it to come in contact with the eyes.
- For spinal or epidural block, use only preparations specifically labeled for IV use.
- Pregnancy category B.

PHARMACOKINETICS

Onset: 45–90 sec IV; 5–15 min IM; 2–5 min topical

Peak: < 30 min

Half-life: 1.5–2 h

Duration: 10–20 min IV; 60–90 min IM; 30–60 min topical; more than 100 min injected for anesthesia

ADVERSE EFFECTS

When lidocaine is used for anesthesia, side effects are uncommon. An early symptom of toxicity is CNS excitement, leading to irritability and confusion. Serious adverse effects include convulsions, respiratory depression, and cardiac arrest. Until the effect of the anesthetic diminishes, clients may injure themselves by biting or chewing areas of the mouth that have no sensation following a dental procedure.

Contraindications: Lidocaine should be avoided in cases of sensitivity to amide-type local anesthetics. Application or injection of lidocaine anesthetic is also contraindicated in the presence of severe trauma or sepsis, blood dyscrasias, dysrhythmias, sinus bradycardia, and severe degrees of heart block.

INTERACTIONS

Drug–Drug: Barbiturates may decrease the activity of lidocaine. Increased effects of lidocaine occur if taken concurrently with cimetidine, quinidine, and beta-blockers. If lidocaine is used on a regular basis, its effectiveness may diminish when used with other medications.

Lab Tests: Unknown.

Herbal/Food: Unknown.

Treatment of Overdose: Emergency medical attention is needed because of the many associated substantive symptoms such as breathing difficulty, swelling of the lips, chest pain, irregular heart beat, nausea, vomiting, tremors, and seizure activity.

 See the Companion Website for a Nursing Process Focus specific to this drug.

Lidocaine viscous is used to anesthetize the throat for some procedures, such as endoscopy. After such procedures, monitor the client for return of the gag reflex before offering water to drink or anything to eat.

Carefully monitor clients receiving an epidural or spinal anesthesia for the presence of a spinal headache. These frequently occur when the spinal dura mater has been punctured multiple times, and spinal fluid leaks. The current treatment for spinal headaches that are not resolved with over-the-counter (OTC) analgesics is an autologous blood patch. This is the most rapid, reliable, and beneficial method of treatment. Assist clients with ambulation until the effects of the epidural or spinal anesthesia have been resolved.

Client Teaching. Client education as it relates to local anesthesia drugs should include the goals of therapy; the reasons for obtaining baseline data such as vital signs and the existence of underlying disorders, and possible drug side effects. Include the following points when teaching clients about local anesthesia drugs:

- Use benzocaine (Solarcaine, others) cautiously on inflamed skin or mucous membranes, because it may increase irritation.
- Report headache that occurs after epidural or spinal anesthesia.
- Immediately report cardiac palpitations and difficulty breathing or swallowing during use of anesthetics.

- Do not eat or drink anything until the healthcare provider indicates you can do so.

GENERAL ANESTHESIA

General anesthesia is a loss of sensation throughout the entire body, accompanied by a loss of consciousness. General anesthetics are applied when it is necessary for clients to remain still and without pain for a longer time than could be achieved with local anesthetics.

19.4 Characteristics of General Anesthesia

The goal of general anesthesia is to provide a rapid and complete loss of sensation. Signs of general anesthesia include total analgesia and loss of consciousness, memory, and body movement. Although these signs are similar to those of sleeping, general anesthesia and sleep are not exactly the same. General anesthetics depress most nervous activity in the brain, whereas sleeping depresses only very specific areas. In fact, some brain activity actually increases during sleep, as described in Chapter 14 ∞.

General anesthesia is rarely achieved with a single drug. Instead, multiple medications are used to rapidly induce unconsciousness, cause muscle relaxation, and maintain deep anesthesia. This approach, called **balanced anesthesia,**

NURSING PROCESS FOCUS Clients Receiving Local Anesthesia

Assessment	Potential Nursing Diagnoses
Prior to administration: ■ Assess for allergies to amide-type local anesthetics. ■ Check for the presence of broken skin, infection, burns, and wounds where medication is to be applied. ■ Assess for character, duration, location, and intensity of pain where medication is to be applied.	■ Aspiration, Risk for ■ Injury, Risk for ■ Knowledge, Deficient, related to drug use

Planning: Client Goals And Expected Outcomes

The client will:
■ Experience no pain during surgical procedure.
■ Experience no side effects or adverse reactions to anesthesia.

Implementation

Interventions and (Rationales)	Client Education/Discharge Planning
■ Monitor for cardiovascular side effects. (These may occur if anesthetic is absorbed.)	■ Instruct client to report any unusual heart palpitations. If medication is being used on a regular basis, instruct client to see a healthcare provider regularly.
■ Monitor skin or mucous membranes for infection or inflammation. (Condition could be worsened by the drug.)	■ Instruct client to report irritation or increase in discomfort in areas where medication is used.
■ Monitor for length of effectiveness. (Local anesthetics are effective for 1 to 3 hours.)	■ Instruct client to report any discomfort during procedure.
■ Obtain information and monitor use of other medications. (There is always the potential for severe drug interactions).	■ Instruct client to report use of any medication to the healthcare provider.
■ Provide for client safety. (There is a potential for injury related to lack of sensation in the area being treated.)	■ Instruct client that having no feeling in the anesthetized area requires taking extra caution to avoid injury, including heat-related injury.
■ Monitor for gag reflex. (Xylocaine viscous may interfere with swallowing reflex.)	Instruct client to: ■ Not eat within 1 hour of administration. ■ Not chew gum while any portion of mouth or throat is anesthetized, to prevent biting injuries.

Evaluation of Outcome Criteria

Evaluate the effectiveness of drug therapy by confirming that client goals and expected outcomes have been met (see "Planning").
■ The client feels no pain during surgical procedure.
■ The client experiences no side effects or adverse reactions to the anesthesia.

∞ See Table 19.2 for a list of drugs to which these nursing actions apply.

allows a lower dose of inhalation anesthetic, thus making the procedure safer for the client.

General anesthesia is a progressive process that occurs in distinct phases. The most efficacious medications can quickly induce all four stages, whereas others are able to induce only stage 1. Stage 3 is where most major surgery occurs; thus it is called **surgical anesthesia.** When seeking surgical anesthesia, it is desirable to progress through stage 2 as rapidly as possible, as this stage produces distressing symptoms. These stages are listed in Table 19.3.

GENERAL ANESTHETICS

General anesthetics are drugs that rapidly produce unconsciousness and total analgesia. These drugs are usually administered by the IV or inhalation routes. To supplement the effects of a general anesthetic, adjunct drugs are given before, during, and after surgery.

19.5 Pharmacotherapy With Inhaled General Anesthetics

There are two primary methods of inducing general anesthesia. Intravenous agents are usually administered first because they act within a few seconds. After the client loses consciousness, inhaled agents are used to maintain the anesthesia. During short surgical procedures or those requiring lower stages of anesthesia, the IV agents may be used alone.

Inhaled general anesthetics, listed in Table 19.4, may be gases or volatile liquids. These agents produce their effects by preventing the flow of sodium into neurons in the CNS, thus delaying nerve impulses and producing a dramatic reduction in neural activity. The exact mechanism is not exactly known, although it is likely that gamma-aminobutyric acid (GABA) receptors in the brain are activated. It is not

TABLE 19.3	Stages of General Anesthesia
Stage	**Characteristics**
1	Loss of pain: The client loses general sensation but may be awake. This stage proceeds until the client loses consciousness.
2	Excitement and hyperactivity: The client may be delirious and try to resist treatment. Heart rate and breathing may become irregular and blood pressure can increase. IV agents are administered here to calm the client.
3	Surgical anesthesia: Skeletal muscles become relaxed and delirium stabilizes. Cardiovascular and breathing activities stabilize. Eye movements slow and the client becomes still. Surgery begins here and remains until the procedure ends.
4	Paralysis of the medulla region in the brain (responsible for controlling respiratory and cardiovascular activity): If breathing or the heart stops, death could result. This stage is usually avoided during general anesthesia.

the same mechanism as is known for local anesthetics. There is some inconclusive evidence suggesting that the mechanism may be related to that of some antiseizure drugs. There is not a specific receptor that binds to general anesthetics, and they do not seem to affect neurotransmitter release.

GASEOUS GENERAL ANESTHETICS

The only gas used routinely for anesthesia is nitrous oxide, commonly called *laughing gas.* Nitrous oxide is used for dental procedures and for brief obstetrical and surgical procedures. It may also be used in conjunction with other general anesthetics, making it possible to decrease their dosages with greater effectiveness.

Nitrous oxide should be used cautiously in myasthenia gravis, as it may cause respiratory depression and prolonged hypnotic effects. Clients with cardiovascular disease, especially those with increased intracranial pressure, should be monitored carefully, because the hypnotic effects of the drug may be prolonged or potentiated.

Pr PROTOTYPE DRUG | Nitrous Oxide | General Anesthetic, Gas

ACTIONS AND USES

The main action of nitrous oxide is analgesia caused by suppression of pain mechanisms in the CNS. This agent has a low potency and does not produce complete loss of consciousness or profound relaxation of skeletal muscle. Because nitrous oxide does not induce surgical anesthesia (stage 3), it is commonly combined with other surgical anesthetic agents. Nitrous oxide is ideal for dental procedures because the client remains conscious and can follow instructions while experiencing full analgesia.

ADMINISTRATION ALERT

- Establish an IV if one is not already in place in case emergency medications are needed.

PHARMACOKINETICS

Onset: 2–5 min

Peak: < 10 min

Half-life: Variable

Duration: Clients recover from anesthesia rapidly after nitrous oxide is discontinued.

ADVERSE EFFECTS

When used in low to moderate doses, nitrous oxide produces few adverse effects. At higher doses, clients exhibit some adverse signs of stage 2 anesthesia such as anxiety, excitement, and combativeness. Lowering the inhaled dose will quickly reverse these adverse effects. As nitrous oxide is exhaled, the client may temporarily have some difficulty breathing at the end of a procedure. Nausea and vomiting following the procedure are more common with nitrous oxide than with other inhalation anesthetics.

Some general anesthetics infrequently produce liver damage. Nitrous oxide has the potential to be abused by users (sometimes medical personnel) who enjoy the relaxed, sedated state that the drug produces.

Contraindications: This drug is contraindicated in clients with impaired level of consciousness, head injury, inability to comply with instructions, decompression sickness (nitrogen narcosis, air embolism, air transport), undiagnosed abdominal pain or marked distention, bowel obstruction, hypotension, shock, chronic obstructive pulmonary disease, cyanosis, or chest trauma with pneumothorax.

INTERACTIONS

Drug–Drug: Sympathomimetics and phosphodiesterase inhibitors may exacerbate dysrhythmias.

Lab Tests: Unknown.

Herbal/Food: Some have claimed that milk thistle taken before and after anesthesia may lower the potential risk of liver damage. Herbal products such as ginger may also provide benefit.

Treatment of Overdose: Metoclopramide may help reduce the symptoms of nausea and vomiting associated with inhalation of nitrous oxide.

 See the Companion Website for a Nursing Process Focus specific to this drug.

TABLE 19.4   Inhaled General Anesthetics

Type	Drug	General Adverse Effects
gas	 nitrous oxide	*Dizziness, drowsiness nausea, euphoria, vomiting*
		Malignant hyperthermia, apnea, cyanosis
volatile liquid	desflurane (Suprane) enflurane (Ethrane) halothane (Fluothane) isoflurane (Forane) methoxyflurane (Penthrane) sevoflurane (Ultane)	*Drowsiness, nausea, vomiting* Myocardial depression, marked hypotension, pulmonary vasoconstriction, hepatotoxicity

Italics indicate common adverse effects, <u>underlining</u> indicates serious adverse effects.

VOLATILE LIQUID GENERAL ANESTHETICS

The volatile anesthetics are liquid at room temperature but are converted into a vapor and inhaled to produce their anesthetic effects. Commonly administered volatile agents are halothane (Fluothane), enflurane (Ethrane), and isoflurane (Forane). The most potent of these is halothane (Fluothane). Some general anesthetics enhance the sensitivity of the heart to drugs such as epinephrine, norepinephrine, dopamine, and serotonin. Most volatile liquids depress cardiovascular and respiratory function. Because it has less effect on the heart and does not damage the liver, isoflurane (Forane) has become the most widely used inhalation anesthetic. The volatile liquids are excreted almost entirely by the lungs, through exhalation.

Pr PROTOTYPE DRUG | Halothane *(Fluothane)* | Volatile Anesthetic

ACTIONS AND USES

Halothane produces a potent level of surgical anesthesia that is rapid in onset. Although potent, halothane does not produce as much muscle relaxation or analgesia as other volatile anesthetics. Therefore, halothane is primarily used with other anesthetic agents including muscle relaxants and analgesics. Nitrous oxide is sometimes combined with halothane.

PHARMACOKINETICS

Onset: 2–5 min

Peak: < 10 min; the minimum alveolar concentration (MAC) is 0.75%. MAC is reduced in elderly clients.

Half-life: Variable

Duration: Halothane's duration of action is variable owing to its lipid solubility. Clients recover from anesthesia rather rapidly after halothane is discontinued (variable among different age groups; elderly clients take longer to recover).

ADVERSE EFFECTS

Halothane moderately sensitizes the heart muscle to epinephrine; therefore, dysrhythmias are a concern. This agent lowers blood pressure and the respiration rate. It also overcomes reflex mechanisms that normally keep the contents of the stomach from entering the lungs. Because of potential hepatotoxicity, use of halothane has declined.

Malignant hyperthermia is a rare but potentially fatal adverse effect triggered by all inhalation anesthetics. It causes muscle rigidity and severe temperature elevation (up to 43 °C). This risk is greatest when halothane is used with succinylcholine.

Halothane dilates the cerebral vasculature and may, in certain conditions, increase intracranial pressure.

Contraindications: Halothane is contraindicated in clients with a history of significant or malignant hyperthermia after previous halothane exposure. It should be used with caution in clients with hepatic function impairment, dysrhythmias, head injury, myasthenia gravis, or pheochromocytoma.

INTERACTIONS

Drug–Drug: Excessive hypotension may occur when halothane is combined with antihypertensive drugs. Halothane potentiates action of nondepolarizing neuromuscular blocking agents.

Levodopa taken concurrently increases the level of dopamine in the CNS, and should be discontinued 6 to 8 hours before halothane administration.

Skeletal muscle weakness, respiratory depression, or apnea may occur if halothane is administered concurrently with polymyxins, lincomycin, or aminoglycosides.

Lab Tests: Unknown.

Herbal/Food: Unknown.

Treatment of Overdose: No specific therapy is available; clients are treated symptomatically.

See the Companion Website for a Nursing Process Focus specific to this drug.

NURSING PROCESS FOCUS   Clients Receiving General Anesthesia

Assessment	Potential Nursing Diagnoses
Prior to administration: ■ Obtain a complete health history including allergies, drug history, and possible drug interactions. ■ Assess for presence or history of severe respiratory, cardiac, renal, or liver disorders. ■ Obtain baseline vital signs. ■ Obtain blood work including a complete blood count and chemistry panel. ■ Assess client's knowledge of procedure and level of anxiety.	■ Anxiety, related to surgical procedure ■ Gas Exchange, Impaired ■ Knowledge, Deficient, related to drug use ■ Nausea, related to drug side effect ■ Sensory Perception, Disturbed ■ Breathing Pattern, Ineffective ■ Cardiac Output, Decreased

Planning: Client Goals and Expected Outcomes

The client will:
- Experience adequate anesthesia during surgical procedure.
- Experience no side effects or adverse reactions to anesthesia.
- Demonstrate an understanding of perioperative procedures.

Implementation

Interventions and (Rationales)	Client Education/Discharge Planning
■ Preoperatively, assess knowledge level of preoperative and postoperative procedures. Ensure that client has accurate information and questions are answered. (Teaching reduces client anxiety.)	Instruct client about: ■ Preoperative and postoperative instructions. ■ What the client will see, hear, and feel prior to surgery. ■ The recovery room process. ■ What the client and family will see and hear postoperatively. ■ The operative facilities, if possible.
■ Preoperatively, assess emotional state. (Clients who are fearful or extremely anxious may be more difficult to induce and maintain under anesthesia.)	■ Instruct client about using stress-reduction techniques such as deep breathing, imagery, and distraction.
■ Monitor preoperative status. (Noncompliance with preoperative instructions may result in serious problems for the client.)	Instruct client to: ■ Not ingest food or beverages prior to surgery to prevent risk of aspiration, nausea, and vomiting. ■ Stop taking medications 24 hours prior to surgery as ordered by the healthcare provider. ■ Refrain from drinking alcohol 24 hours prior to surgery.
■ Postoperatively, monitor for respiratory difficulty and adequate O_2–CO_2 exchange. (Anesthetics cause respiratory depression.)	■ Inform client to report shortness of breath, difficulty breathing, or dizziness.
■ Monitor recovery from anesthesia. Evaluate level of consciousness, nausea, vomiting, and pain. (Failure to control pain, nausea, and vomiting can result in a longer recovery period.)	■ Instruct client about possible side effects and to report any discomfort immediately.
■ Monitor vital signs. (Respiratory status may be impaired leading to prolonged apnea, respiratory depression, and cyanosis. Blood pressure may decrease to levels that cause shock.)	■ Advise client to report heart palpitations, dizziness, difficulty breathing, or faintness.

Evaluation of Outcome Criteria

Evaluate the effectiveness of drug therapy by confirming that client goals and expected outcomes have been met (see "Planning").
- The client experiences adequate anesthesia during surgical procedure.
- The client experiences no side effects or adverse reactions to anesthesia.
- The client states an understanding of perioperative procedures.

∞ *See Tables 19.4 and 19.5 for lists of drugs to which these nursing actions apply.*

HOME & COMMUNITY CONSIDERATIONS

Postanesthesia Follow-up Care

Clients are kept in the inpatient or outpatient hospital or clinic setting until the effects of an anesthesia are resolved. Clients may return to the home environment following certain outpatient surgeries, dental, and diagnostic procedures using conscious sedation before the effects of the sedation have worn off. Clients are required to have someone with them for 24 hours to monitor and assist their needs. Usually, the nurse or another healthcare provider follows up with the client via phone.

NURSING CONSIDERATIONS

The role of the nurse in general anesthesia therapy involves careful monitoring of the client's condition and providing education as it relates to the prescribed drug treatment. General anesthesia is primarily used for lengthy surgical procedures and involves significant risks. Inform the client that anesthesia will be administered by highly trained personnel, either an anesthesiologist or a nurse anesthetist, and that you will assist to help ensure client safety. Preoperatively, assess vital signs, lab tests, health history, level of knowledge concerning the procedure, and the presence of anxiety. Assess the client for the use of alcohol or other CNS depressants within the previous 24 hours, because these products potentiate anesthetic effects. Obtain information concerning the use of other medications.

Nitrous oxide has a rapid onset and recovery, with minimal side effects, such as nausea and vomiting. Determine the client's knowledge level and offer reassurance to alleviate the client's anxiety.

In the immediate postoperative period, monitor the client for side effects of the general anesthesia such as nausea and vomiting, CNS depression, respiratory difficulty, vital sign changes, and complications related to the procedure such as bleeding or impending shock.

Use of halothane (Fluothane) is contraindicated in clients who have had this drug within the previous 14 to 21 days because it can cause halothane hepatitis if used frequently. Do not give halothane to pregnant women (category D) or to clients with diminished hepatic functioning, because it can be hepatotoxic. Caution should be used in clients with cardiac conditions, especially bradycardia and dysrhythmias, because the medication decreases blood pressure and sensitizes the myocardium to catecholamines, which can lead to serious dysrhythmias.

Lifespan Considerations.   Children are usually more sensitive to anesthesia than adults because their body systems are not fully developed. Therefore, medication dosages used must be carefully calculated. Some drugs used for anesthesia, such as neuromuscular blockers, are not recommended for use by children younger than age 2.

Nurses must understand that children who are undergoing surgery have fears and concerns about surgery and anesthesia. A child's age and developmental level play a critical role in his or her thoughts about receiving anesthesia. Children younger than age 1 are usually not concerned about what will be happening, but they will display separation anxiety when separated from family members. Fear of needles, of the unknown, and of injury to their body integrity begins during the toddler stage and continues throughout childhood. Children often perceive the anxieties of their parents, so it is imperative that caregivers remain calm. Holding the child through induction of anesthesia might help alleviate fears. Local anesthetic creams can be rubbed on the skin to remove the pain of needles.

Elderly clients are also more affected by anesthesia than are younger adults. Because of the changes in drug metabolism that occur with advancing age, these clients are particularly sensitive to the effects of barbiturates and general anesthetics. This increases the chances of side effects; therefore, elderly clients should be monitored closely. Elderly clients are also especially sensitive to the effects of local anesthetics. Sedative-hypnotic drugs used preoperatively may cause increased confusion or excitement in elderly clients; therefore, the risk for injury increases. Monitoring elderly clients to prevent falls is extremely important.

The use of anesthesia during pregnancy must be carefully evaluated for the potential effect on the fetus. It is imperative that any drug given to expectant mothers is also given to fetuses. The use of any type of anesthesia during the pregnancy or during the labor and birth has an anesthetic effect on the fetus. Anesthesia may slow or even stop labor, reducing the ability of the woman to push during the birth, or resulting in a neonate that is sedated at birth. Timing of an anesthesia given during the labor and birth is critical to prevent a "narcan" newborn.

Client Teaching.   Client education as it relates to general anesthesia drugs should include the goals of therapy, the reasons for obtaining baseline data such as vital signs and the existence of underlying disorders, and possible drug side effects. Include the following points when teaching clients about general anesthesia drugs:

- Stop taking medications and herbal and dietary supplements 24 hours prior to surgery or as directed by the healthcare provider.
- Discontinue alcohol use 24 hours prior to surgery.
- Do not eat or drink after having anesthesia until the healthcare provider indicates that you can do so.
- Postoperatively, practice deep breathing as instructed by the healthcare provider.

IV ANESTHETICS

IV anesthetics are used either alone, for short procedures, or in combination with inhalation anesthetics.

19.6 Pharmacotherapy With IV Anesthetics

Intravenous anesthetics, listed in Table 19.5, are important supplements to general anesthesia. Although occasionally used alone, they are often administered with inhaled general anesthetics. Concurrent administration of IV and inhaled anesthetics allows the dose of the inhaled agent to be

Pr PROTOTYPE DRUG | Thiopental *(Pentothal)* | IV Anesthetic

ACTIONS AND USES

Thiopental is the oldest IV anesthetic. It is used for brief medical procedures and to rapidly induce unconsciousness prior to administering inhaled anesthetics. It is classified as an ultrashort-acting barbiturate, having an onset time of less than 30 seconds and a duration of only 10 to 30 minutes. Unlike some anesthetic agents, it has very low analgesic properties.

ADMINISTRATION ALERT

- Pregnancy category C.

PHARMACOKINETICS

Onset: 30–60 sec

Peak: 10–30 min

Half-life: 12 min

Duration: 20–30 min

ADVERSE EFFECTS

Like other barbiturates, thiopental can produce severe respiratory depression when used in high doses. It is used with caution in clients with cardiovascular disease because of its ability to depress the myocardium and cause dysrhythmias. Clients may experience emergence delirium postoperatively. This causes hallucinations, confusion, and excitability.

Contraindications: Thiopental should not be administered to clients with hypersensitivity to barbiturates or with veins unsuitable for IV administration. Variegate porphyria or acute intermittent porphyria are contraindications. In these cases, thiopental or other barbiturates can cause nerve demyelination and CNS lesions, which may lead to pain, weakness, and life-threatening paralysis.

INTERACTIONS

Drug–Drug: Thiopental interacts with many other drugs. For example, use with CNS depressants potentiates respiratory and CNS depression. Phenothiazines increase the risk of hypotension.

Lab Tests: Unknown.

Herbal/Food: Kava and valerian may potentiate sedation.

Treatment of Overdose: Because the half-life of thiopental is very brief, overdose is easily managed in the surgical suite by discontinuing the drug and assisting ventilation until respirations return to normal.

 See the Companion Website for a Nursing Process Focus specific to this drug.

reduced, thus lowering the potential for serious side effects. Furthermore, when IV and inhaled anesthetics are combined, they provide greater analgesia and muscle relaxation than could be provided by the inhaled anesthetic alone. When IV anesthetics are administered alone, they are generally reserved for medical procedures that take less than 15 minutes.

Drugs employed as IV anesthetics include barbiturates, opioids, and benzodiazepines. Opioids offer the advantage of superior analgesia. Combining the opioid fentanyl (Sublimaze) with the antipsychotic agent droperidol (Inapsine) produces a state known as **neuroleptanalgesia.** In this state,

clients are conscious, though insensitive to pain and unconnected with surroundings. The premixed combination of these two agents is marketed as Innovar. A similar conscious, dissociated state is produced with ketamine (Ketalar).

NURSING CONSIDERATIONS

The role of the nurse in drug therapy with IV anesthetics involves careful monitoring of a client's condition and providing education as it relates to the prescribed drug treatment. IV sedation is used to decrease anxiety and fear secondary to

TABLE 19.5 Intravenous Anesthetics

Chemical Classification	Drug	General Adverse Effects
barbiturates and barbiturate-like agents	etomidate (Amidate) methohexital sodium (Brevital) propofol (Diprivan)	<u>Circulatory or respiratory depression with apnea, laryngospasm, anaphylaxis</u>
benzodiazepines	diazepam (Valium) lorazepam (Ativan) midazolam hydrochloride (Versed)	<u>Cardiovascular collapse, laryngospasm</u>
opioids	alfentanil hydrochloride (Alfenta) fentanyl citrate (Sublimaze, others) remifentanil hydrochloride (Ultiva) sufentanil citrate (Sufenta)	*Nausea, GI disturbances* <u>Marked CNS depression</u>
miscellaneous	ketamine (Ketalar)	*Dissociation, increased blood pressure and pulse rate, delirium, hallucinations, confusion, excitement*

Italics indicate common adverse effects; <u>underlining</u> indicates serious adverse effects.

confinement by the mask used for inhalation anesthesia. Assist the healthcare provider in completing a thorough assessment, including medical history prior to selecting an anesthetic or combination of anesthetics. Administer medications other than anesthesia during preoperative, perioperative, or postoperative periods, including antianxiety agents, sedatives, analgesics, opioids, and anticholinergics that may be ordered. IV anesthetics are contraindicated in clients with drug sensitivity, because allergic reactions can result, ranging from hives to respiratory arrest. Assess the suitability of an IV access site.

Carefully monitor clients with cardiovascular disease, because IV anesthetics can cause depression of the myocardium leading to dysrhythmias. Also carefully monitor clients with respiratory disorders, because respiratory depression may result in high levels of anesthetic in the blood. Thiopental (Pentothal) should be used with caution in clients with seizure disorders, increased intracranial pressure, neurological disorders, and myxedema.

Using general anesthetics causes CNS depression. During the postoperative period, monitor the client for vital sign changes, hallucinations, confusion, and excitability. Other side effects or reactions that should be assessed include respiratory difficulties, shivering and trembling, nausea or vomiting, headache, and somnolence. Preoperative teaching is vital to the client's understanding of the anesthetic and the entire surgical experience and helps allay fears and anxiety of the client and caregivers.

Client Teaching. Client education as it relates to general anesthetics should include the goals of therapy, the reasons for obtaining baseline data such as vital signs and the existence of underlying cardiovascular disorders, and possible drug side effects. Include the following points when teaching clients about general anesthetics:

- Medications may be administered preoperatively to assist with the sedation process.
- Vital signs and assessments will occur on a routine basis until they are stable.
- Do not eat or drink until the healthcare provider indicates that you can do so.
- Immediately report any difficulty breathing, and nausea or discomfort following the procedure.

19.7 Nonanesthetic Drugs as Adjuncts to Surgery

A number of drugs are used either to complement the effects of general anesthetics or to treat anticipated side effects of the anesthesia. These agents, listed in Table 19.6,

TABLE 19.6 Selected Adjuncts to Anesthesia

Chemical Classification	Drug	General Adverse Effects
barbiturates and barbiturate-like agents	amobarbital (Amytal) butabarbital sodium (Butisol) pentobarbital (Nembutal) secobarbital (Seconal)	*Drowsiness, lethargy, hangover* Respiratory depression, laryngospasm
opioids	alfentanil hydrochloride (Alfenta) fentanyl citrate (Duragesic, Actiq, others) fentanyl/droperidol (Innovar) remifentanil hydrochloride (Ultiva) sufentanil citrate (Sufenta)	*Sedation* Circulatory depression, cardiac arrest, respiratory depression or arrest
anticholinergic	bethanechol chloride (Duvoid, Urabeth, Urecholine)	*Salivation, abdominal craniping, sweating* Transient complete heart block
dopamine blocker	droperidol (Inapsine)	*Postoperative drowsiness, extrapyramidal symptoms, hypotension, tachycardia* Laryngospasm, bronchospasm
phenothiazine	promethazine (Phenazine, Phenergan, others)	*Blurred vision, dry mouth* Respiratory depression, agranulocytosis
neuromuscular blocker	ⓟ succinylcholine chloride (Anectine)	*Muscle fasciculations, bradycardia* Respiratory depression, malignant hyperthermia
neuromuscular blocker	tubocurarine	*Hypotension* Malignant hyperthermia, respiratory depression, apnea, circulatory collapse

Italics indicate common adverse effects; underlining indicates serious adverse effects.

are called *adjuncts* to anesthesia. They may be given prior to, during, or after surgery.

The preoperative drugs given to relieve anxiety and to provide mild sedation include barbiturates or benzodiazepines. Opioids such as morphine may be given to counteract pain that the client will experience after surgery. Anticholinergics such as atropine may be administered to dry secretions and to suppress the bradycardia caused by some anesthetics.

During surgery, the primary adjuncts are the **neuromuscular blockers**. So that surgical procedures can be carried out safely, it is necessary to administer drugs that cause skeletal muscles to totally relax. Administration of these drugs also allows the amount of anesthetic to be reduced. Neuromuscular blocking agents are classified as *depolarizing* blockers or *nondepolarizing* blockers. The only depolarizing blocker is succinylcholine (Anectine), which works by binding to acetylcholine receptors at neuromuscular junctions to cause total skeletal muscle relaxation. Succinylcholine is used in surgery for ease of tracheal intubation. Mivacurium (Mivacron) is the shortest acting of the nondepolarizing blockers, whereas tubocurarine is a longer acting neuromuscular blocking agent. The nondepolarizing blockers cause muscle paralysis by competing with acetylcholine for cholinergic receptors at neuromuscular junctions. Once attached to the receptor, the nonpolarizing blockers prevent muscle contraction.

Pr PROTOTYPE DRUG | Succinylcholine *(Anectine)* | Neuromuscular Blocker

ACTIONS AND USES

Like the natural neurotransmitter acetylcholine, succinylcholine acts on cholinergic receptor sites at neuromuscular junctions. At first, depolarization occurs, and skeletal muscles contract. After repeated contractions, however, the membrane is unable to repolarize as long as the drug stays attached to the receptor. Effects are first noted as muscle weakness and muscle spasms. Eventually, paralysis occurs. Succinylcholine is rapidly broken down by the enzyme pseudocholinesterase; when the IV infusion is stopped, the duration of action is only a few minutes. Use of succinylcholine reduces the amount of general anesthetic needed for procedures.

ADMINISTRATION ALERT

- Pregnancy category C.

PHARMACOKINETICS

Onset: 0.5–1 min IV; 2–3 min IM

Peak: Unknown

Half-life: Unknown

Duration: 2–3 min IV; 10–30 min IM

ADVERSE EFFECTS

Succinylcholine can cause complete paralysis of the diaphragm and intercostal muscles; thus, mechanical ventilation is necessary during surgery. Bradycardia and respiratory depression are expected adverse effects. If doses are high, the ganglia are affected, causing tachycardia, hypotension, and urinary retention.

Clients with certain genetic defects may experience rapid onset of extremely high fever with muscle rigidity—a serious condition known as malignant hyperthermia.

Succinylcholine should be employed with caution in clients with fractures or muscle spasms, because the initial muscle fasciculations may cause additional trauma. Neuromuscular blockade may be prolonged in clients with hypokalemia, hypocalcemia, or low plasma pseudocholinesterase levels.

Contraindications: Succinylcholine should be used with extreme caution in clients with severe burns or trauma neuromuscular diseases, or glaucoma. Succinylcholine is contraindicated in clients with a family history of malignant hyperthermia or conditions of pulmonary, renal, cardiovascular, metabolic, or hepatic dysfunction.

INTERACTIONS

Drug–Drug: Additive skeletal muscle blockade will occur if succinylcholine is given concurrently with clindamycin, aminoglycosides, furosemide, lithium, quinidine, or lidocaine. The effect of succinylcholine may be increased if given concurrently with phenothiazines, oxytocin, promazine, tacrine, or thiazide diuretics. The effect of succinylcholine is decreased if given with diazepam.

If this drug is given concurrently with halothane or nitrous oxide, an increased risk of bradycardia, dysrhythmias, sinus arrest, apnea, and malignant hyperthermia exists. If succinylcholine is given concurrently with cardiac glycosides, there is increased risk of cardiac dysrhythmias. If narcotics are given concurrently with succinylcholine, there is increased risk of bradycardia and sinus arrest.

Lab Tests: Unknown.

Herbal/Food: Unknown.

Treatment of Overdose: Treatment may involve drug therapy for the following symptoms: weakness, lack of coordination, watery eyes and mouth, tremors, and seizures. Problems with breathing require emergency medical measures.

 See the Companion Website for a Nursing Process Focus specific to this drug.

Postoperative drugs include analgesics for pain and antiemetics such as promethazine (Phenergan, others) for the nausea and vomiting that sometimes occur during recovery from the anesthetic. Occasionally a parasympathomimetic such as bethanechol (Urecholine) is administered to stimulate the smooth muscle of the bowel and the urinary tract to begin peristalsis following surgery. Bethanechol is featured as a prototype drug in Chapter 13 ∞.

NURSING CONSIDERATIONS

The role of the nurse in neuromuscular blocker therapy involves careful monitoring of a client's condition and providing education as it relates to the prescribed drug treatment. Neuromuscular blocking agents are used so that the client experiences complete skeletal muscle relaxation during the surgical procedure. Continuous use is not recommended because of potential side effects. Clients should be aware that these drugs are used only in a controlled acute care setting, usually during surgery, by a skilled professional.

In preparation for use of succinylcholine, assess for the presence/history of hepatic or renal dysfunction, neuromuscular disease, fractures, myasthenia gravis, malignant hyperthermia, glaucoma, or penetrating eye injuries. Use of this drug is contraindicated with these conditions. Use in children under 2 years is contraindicated because it can cause dysrhythmias and malignant hyperthermia.

Mivacurium (Mivacron) is used for intubation and is contraindicated for persons with renal or hepatic disease, fluid and electrolyte imbalances, neuromuscular disorders, respiratory disease, or obesity. It should be used cautiously in elderly clients and children. It should not be used during pregnancy or lactation. An anesthesiologist may administer the drug during cesarean section.

Prior to using any neuromuscular blocker, assess physical status including vital signs, reflexes, muscle tone and response, pupil size and reactivity, ECG, lung sounds, bowel sounds, affect, and level of consciousness. Monitor for hypotension, tachycardia, prolonged apnea, bronchospasm, respiratory depression, paralysis, and hypersensitivity

Client Teaching. Client education as it relates to neuromuscular blockers should include the goals of therapy, the reasons for obtaining baseline data such as vital signs and the existence of underlying hepatic or renal disorders, and possible drug side effects. Include the following points when teaching clients about neuromuscular blockers:

- During the procedure, you will not be able to move or speak because of paralysis.

- You may be awake and aware during the procedure; therefore, an antianxiety medication may also be administered to help you relax.

- A healthcare provider will be with you until the effects of the medication have subsided.

- Your healthcare provider will assess your need for pain medications during this time.

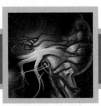

CHAPTER REVIEW

KEY CONCEPTS

The numbered key concepts provide a succinct summary of the important points from the corresponding numbered section within the chapter. If any of these points are not clear, refer to the numbered section within the chapter for review.

19.1 Regional loss of sensation is achieved by administering local anesthetics topically or through the infiltration, nerve block, spinal, or epidural routes.

19.2 Local anesthetics act by blocking sodium channels in neurons. Epinephrine is sometimes added to prolong the duration of anesthetic action.

19.3 Local anesthetics are classified as amides or esters. The amides, such as lidocaine (Xylocaine), have generally replaced the esters owing to their greater safety.

19.4 General anesthesia produces a complete loss of sensation accompanied by loss of consciousness. This state is usually achieved through the use of multiple medications.

19.5 Inhaled general anesthetics are used to maintain surgical anesthesia. Some, such as nitrous oxide, have low efficacy, whereas others, such as halothane (Fluothane), can induce deep anesthesia.

19.6 IV anesthetics are used either alone, for short procedures, or in combination with inhalation anesthetics.

19.7 Numerous nonanesthetic medications, including opioids, antianxiety agents, barbiturates, and neuromuscular blockers, are administered as adjuncts to surgery.

NCLEX-RN® REVIEW QUESTIONS

1 The client received lidocaine viscous before a gastroscopy was performed. Priority nursing assessment includes:

1. Return of gag reflex.
2. Ability to urinate.
3. Abdominal pain.
4. Ability to stand.

2 The nurse observes a coworker preparing to administer a solution of lidocaine and epinephrine to a client with multiple premature ventricular contractions. The appropriate action by the nurse is to:

1. Document administration of the drug.
2. Notify the nursing supervisor of the error.
3. Do nothing; the drug choice is correct.
4. Prevent the administration and give a plain lidocaine solution.

3 The nurse establishes a nursing diagnosis of Knowledge Deficient, Perioperative Procedures. What is the first action the nurse should take when implementing the plan?

1. Give the client a tour of the hospital.
2. Discuss the plan with the client and significant others.
3. Assess the level of knowledge of perioperative procedures.
4. Give pamphlets to read related to perioperative procedure.

4 The nurse recognizes the main action of nitrous oxide is to:

1. Provide total relaxation of skeletal muscles.
2. Induce loss of consciousness.
3. Cause analgesia by suppressing the pain mechanism in the CNS.
4. Induce stage 3 anesthesia.

5 The nurse should assess the client for which of the following side effects if succinylcholine (Anectine) is used as an adjunct to anesthesia? (Select all that apply.)

1. Bradycardia
2. Severe headache
3. Hypertension
4. Respiratory depression
5. Urinary frequency

CRITICAL THINKING QUESTIONS

1. An elderly client requires local anesthesia for a 3-cm laceration to the distal fourth metacarpal of the left hand. The healthcare provider requests lidocaine (Xylocaine) 1% with epinephrine. What is the nurse's response?

2. A client who has a history of heart failure is on digoxin (Lanoxin) and has a history of mild renal failure. The healthcare provider asks the nurse to prepare succinylcholine (Anectine) IV as an anesthetic for this client who

is having an outclient procedure. What is the nurse's response?

3. The nurse is reviewing the chart of a client who has recently had abdominal surgery. The client is 67 years old, has been on digoxin (Lanoxin), ibuprofen, St. John's wort, and Maalox daily. Which of the information would indicate that this client may require closer monitoring (and why)? Which is a priority?

See Appendix D for answers and rationales for all activities.

EXPLORE MediaLink

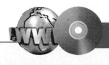

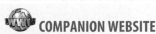
www.prenhall.com/adams

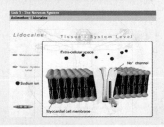

NCLEX-RN® review, case studies, and other interactive resources for this chapter can be found on the companion website at www.prenhall.com/adams. Click on "Chapter 19" to select the activities for this chapter. For animations, more NCLEX-RN® review questions, and an audio glossary, access the accompanying Prentice Hall Nursing MediaLink DVD-ROM in this textbook.

PRENTICE HALL NURSING MEDIALINK DVD-ROM

- **Animation**
  Mechanism in Action: Lidocaine (*Xylocaine*)
- **Audio Glossary**
- **NCLEX-RN® Review**

COMPANION WEBSITE

- **NCLEX-RN® Review**
- **Dosage Calculations**
- **Case Study:** Client receiving anesthetics
- **Care Plan:** Client who received halothane during surgery

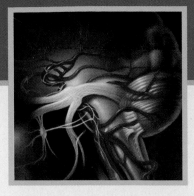

CHAPTER 20

Drugs for Degenerative Diseases of the Nervous System

DRUGS AT A GLANCE

DRUGS FOR PARKINSON'S DISEASE
Dopaminergic Agents
   👁 *levodopa (Larodopa)*
Cholinergic Blockers (Anticholinergics)
   👁 *benztropine (Cogentin)*
DRUGS FOR ALZHEIMER'S DISEASE
Acetylcholinesterase Inhibitors
   👁 *donepezil (Aricept)*
Combination NMDA Drug Therapy

OBJECTIVES

After reading this chapter, the student should be able to:

1. Identify the most common degenerative diseases of the central nervous system (CNS).
2. Describe symptoms of Parkinson's disease.
3. Explain the neurochemical basis for Parkinson's disease, focusing on the roles of dopamine and acetylcholine in the brain.
4. Describe the nurse's role in the pharmacological management of Parkinson's disease and Alzheimer's disease.
5. For each of the drug classes listed in Drugs at a Glance, know representative drug examples, and explain their mechanisms of action, primary action, and important adverse effects.
6. Describe symptoms of Alzheimer's disease and explain theories about why these symptoms develop.
7. Explain the goals of pharmacotherapy for Alzheimer's disease and the efficacy of existing medications.
8. Categorize drugs used in the treatment of Alzheimer's disease and Parkinson's disease based on their classification and mechanism of action.
9. Use the Nursing Process to care for clients receiving drug therapy for degenerative diseases of the CNS.

MediaLink 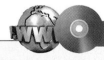 **www.prenhall.com/adams**

KEY TERMS

acetylcholinesterase (AchE) *page 269*

Alzheimer's disease (AD) *page 268*

amyloid plaques *page 269*

bradykinesia *page 262*

corpus striatum *page 262*

dementia *page 268*

hippocampus *page 269*

neurofibrillary tangle *page 269*

parkinsonism *page 261*

substantia nigra *page 262*

Degenerative diseases of the CNS are often difficult to deal with pharmacologically. Medications are unable to stop or reverse the progressive nature of these diseases; they can offer only symptomatic relief. Parkinson's disease and Alzheimer's disease, the two most common debilitating and progressive conditions, are the focus of this chapter.

20.1 Degenerative Diseases of the Central Nervous System

Degenerative diseases of the CNS include a diverse set of disorders differing in their causes and outcomes. Some, such as Huntington's disease, are quite rare, affect younger clients, and are caused by chromosomal defects. Others, such as Alzheimer's disease, affect millions of people, mostly elderly clients and have a devastating economic and social impact. Table 20.1 lists the major degenerative disorders of the CNS.

The etiology of most neurological degenerative diseases is unknown. Most progress from very subtle signs and symptoms early in the course of the disease, to profound neurological and cognitive deficits. In their early stages, these disorders may be quite difficult to diagnose. With the exception of Parkinson's disease, pharmacotherapy provides only minimal benefit. Currently, medication is unable to cure any of the degenerative diseases of the CNS.

PARKINSON'S DISEASE

Parkinson's disease is a degenerative disorder of the CNS caused by death of neurons that produce the brain neurotransmitter dopamine. It is the second most common degenerative disease of the nervous system, affecting more than 1.5 million Americans. Pharmacotherapy is often successful at reducing some of the distressing symptoms of this disease.

20.2 Characteristics of Parkinson's Disease

Parkinson's disease affects primarily clients older than 50 years of age; however, even teenagers can develop the disorder. Men are affected slightly more than women. The disease is progressive, with the expression of full symptoms often taking many years. The symptoms of Parkinson's disease, or **parkinsonism,** are summarized as follows:

- *Tremors* The hands and head develop a palsylike motion or shakiness when at rest; pin rolling is a common behavior in progressive states, in which clients rub the thumb and forefinger together in a circular motion.
- *Muscle rigidity* Stiffness may resemble symptoms of arthritis; clients often have difficulty bending over or moving limbs. Some clients develop a rigid

---

TABLE 20.1 Degenerative Diseases of the Central Nervous System

Disease	Description
Alzheimer's disease	progressive loss of brain function characterized by memory loss, confusion, and dementia
amyotrophic lateral sclerosis	progressive weakness and wasting of muscles caused by destruction of motor neurons
Huntington's chorea	autosomal-dominant genetic disorder resulting in progressive dementia and involuntary, spasmodic movements of limb and facial muscles
multiple sclerosis	demyelination of neurons in the central nervous system (CNS), resulting in progressive weakness, visual disturbances, mood alterations, and cognitive deficits
Parkinson's disease	progressive loss of dopamine in the CNS causing tremor, muscle rigidity, and abnormal movement and posture

PharmFacts

Degenerative Diseases of the Central Nervous System

- More than 1.5 million Americans have Parkinson's disease.
- Most clients with Parkinson's disease are older than age 50.
- More than 50% of Parkinson's clients who have difficulty with voluntary movement are younger than 60.
- More men than women develop Parkinson's disease.
- More than 4 million Americans have Alzheimer's disease.
- Alzheimer's disease mainly affects clients older than age 65.
- Of all clients with dementia, 60% to 70% have Alzheimer's disease.
- More than 49,000 Americans die annually of Alzheimer's disease.

poker face. These symptoms may be less noticeable at first, but progress to become obvious in later years.

- *Bradykinesia* The most noticeable of all symptoms, **bradykinesia** is marked by difficulty chewing, swallowing, or speaking. Clients with Parkinson's disease have difficulties initiating movement and controlling fine muscle movements. Walking often becomes difficult. Clients shuffle their feet without taking normal strides.

- *Postural instability* Clients may be humped over slightly and easily lose their balance. Stumbling results in frequent falls with associated injuries.

Although Parkinson's disease is a progressive neurological disorder primarily affecting muscle movement, other health problems often develop in these clients, including anxiety, depression, sleep disturbances, dementia, and disturbances of the autonomic nervous system such as difficulty urinating and performing sexually. Several theories have been proposed to explain the development of parkinsonism. Because some clients with Parkinson's symptoms have a family history of this disorder, a genetic link is highly probable. Numerous environmental toxins also have been suggested as a cause, but results have been inconclusive. Potentially harmful agents include carbon monoxide, cyanide, manganese, chlorine, and pesticides. Viral infections, head trauma, and stroke have also been proposed as causes of parkinsonism.

Symptoms of parkinsonism develop because of degeneration and destruction of dopamine-producing neurons found within an area of the brain known as the **substantia nigra.** Under normal circumstances, neurons in the substantia nigra supply dopamine to the **corpus striatum,** a region of the brain that controls unconscious muscle movement.

Balance, posture, muscle tone, and involuntary muscle movement depend on the proper balance of the neurotransmitters dopamine (inhibitory) and acetylcholine (stimulatory) in the corpus striatum. If dopamine is absent, acetylcholine has a more dramatic stimulatory effect in this area. For this reason, drug therapy for parkinsonism focuses not only on restoring dopamine function but also on blocking the effect of acetylcholine within the corpus striatum. Thus, when the brain experiences a loss of dopamine within the substantia nigra or an overactive cholinergic influence in the corpus striatum, parkinsonism results.

Extrapyramidal side effects (EPS) develop for the same neurochemical reasons as Parkinson's disease. Recall from Chapter 17 ∞ that antipsychotic drugs act through a blockade of dopamine receptors. Treatment with certain antipsychotic drugs may induce parkinsonism-like symptoms, or EPS, by interfering with the same neural pathway and functions affected by the lack of dopamine.

EPS may occur suddenly and become a medical emergency. With acute EPS, clients' muscles may spasm or become locked up. Fever and confusion are other signs and symptoms of this reaction. If acute EPS occurs in a healthcare facility, short-term medical treatment can be provided by administering parenteral diphenhydramine (Benadryl). If EPS is recognized outside the healthcare setting, the client should immediately be taken to the emergency room, because untreated acute episodes of EPS can be fatal.

PARKINSONISM DRUGS

Antiparkinsonism agents are given to restore the balance of dopamine and acetylcholine in specific regions of the brain. These drugs include dopaminergic agents and anticholinergics (cholinergic blockers). Dopaminergic agents are listed in Table 20.2.

DOPAMINERGICS

These drugs either restore dopamine function or stimulate dopamine receptors located within the brain. Recent efforts have focused on the use of dopamine agonists for the initial treatment of Parkinson's disease.

20.3 Treating Parkinsonism With Dopaminergic Drugs

The goal of pharmacotherapy for Parkinson's disease is to increase the ability of the client to perform normal daily activities of living (ADLs) such as eating, walking, dressing, and bathing. Although pharmacotherapy does not cure this disorder, symptoms may be dramatically reduced in some clients.

TABLE 20.2 Dopaminergic Drugs Used for Parkinsonism

Drug	Route and Adult Dose (max dose where indicated)	Adverse Effects
amantadine (Symmetrel)	PO; 100 mg 1–2 times/day	*Dizziness, light-headedness, difficulty concentrating, confusion, anxiety, headache, sleep dysfunction, fatigue, nausea, vomiting, constipation, orthostatic hypotension, choreiform and involuntary movements, dystonia, dyskinesia*
bromocriptine (Parlodel)	PO; 1.25–2.5 mg/day up to 100 mg/day in divided doses	
carbidopa-levodopa (Sinemet)	PO; 1 tablet containing 10 mg carbidopa/100 mg levodopa or 25 mg carbidopa/100 mg levodopa tid (max: 6 tabs/day)	
entacapone (Comtan)	PO; 200 mg given with levodopa/carbidopa up to 8 times/day	
levodopa (L-Dopa, Larodopa)	PO; 500 mg–1 g/day; may be increased by 100–750 mg every 3–7 days	<u>Acute MI, shock, neuroleptic malignant syndrome, agranulocytosis, depression with suicidal tendencies, EPS, fulminant liver failure, severe hepatocellular injury</u>
pergolide (Permax)	PO; Start with 0.05 mg/day for 2 days; increase by 0.1 or 0.15 mg/day q3 days for 12 days; then increase by 0.25 mg every third day (max: 5 mg/day)	
pramipexole dihydrochloride (Mirapex)	PO; Start with 0.125 mg tid for 1 wk; double this dose for the next week; continue to increase by 0.25 mg/dose tid every week to a target dose of 1.5 mg tid	
ropinirole hydrochloride (Requip)	PO; Start with 0.25 mg tid; may increase by 0.25 mg/dose tid every week to a target dose of 1 mg tid	
selegiline hydrochloride (L-Deprenyl, Eldepryl)	PO; 5 mg/dose bid; doses greater than 10 mg/day are potentially toxic	
tolcapone (Tasmar)	PO; 100 mg tid (max: 600 mg/day)	

Italics indicate common adverse effects; <u>underlining</u> indicates serious adverse effects.

Drug therapy attempts to restore the functional balance of dopamine and acetylcholine in the corpus striatum of the brain. Dopaminergic drugs are used to increase dopamine levels in this region. The drug of choice for parkinsonism is levodopa (Larodopa), a dopaminergic drug that has been used more extensively than any other medication for this disorder. As shown in Pharmacotherapy Illustrated 20.1 (see page 264), levodopa is a precursor of dopamine synthesis. Supplying it directly leads to increased biosynthesis of dopamine within the nerve terminals. Whereas levodopa can cross the blood–brain barrier, dopamine cannot; thus, dopamine itself is not used for therapy. The effectiveness of levodopa can be "boosted" by combining it with carbidopa. This combination, marketed as Sinemet, makes more levodopa available to enter the CNS.

Several additional approaches to enhancing dopamine are used in treating parkinsonism. Tolcapone (Tasmar), entacapone (Comtan), and selegiline (Carbex, Eldepryl) inhibit enzymes that normally destroy levodopa and dopamine. Bromocriptine (Parlodel), pergolide (Permax), pramipexole (Mirapex), and ropinirole (Requip) directly activate the dopamine receptor and are called *dopamine agonists*. Amantadine (Symmetrel), an antiviral agent, causes the release of dopamine from its nerve terminals. All these drugs are considered adjuncts to the pharmacotherapy of parkinsonism because they are not as effective as levodopa.

Recent guidelines have focused on dopamine agonists as the initial line of treatment for Parkinson's disease. For example, some studies have purported ropinirole (Requip) to be more than twice as effective in controlling dyskinesia. Clients taking ropinirole alone may also experience less progressive dyskinesia symptoms. However, in terms of activities of daily living (ADLs), some have reported that L-dopa may still better control motor symptoms. Others have suggested that L-dopa taken alone may produce no greater long-term therapeutic advantage than dopamine agonists. Pramipexole (Mirapex) and ropinirole (Requip) have proven to be safe and effective for the initial sole therapy and when combined with L-dopa. The side effects of pramipexole and ropinirole are intense and may include nausea and constipation, headache, orthostatic hypotension, nasal congestion, sudden sleep attacks, and hallucinations.

Other drugs reducing the requirements for L-dopa include the catechol-O-methyl transferase (COMT) inhibitors. Like L-dopa, these agents increase concentrations of existing dopamine in the brain and improve motor fluctuations

NATURAL THERAPIES

Ginkgo Biloba and Garlic for Treatment of Dementia

Ginkgo biloba has been used for many years to improve memory. In Europe, an extract of this herb is already approved for the treatment of dementia. In U.S. studies, 120 mg of ginkgo taken daily has been shown to improve mental functioning and stabilize Alzheimer's disease. In other studies, positive clinical results were seen after 4 weeks and 6 months of treatment (Sierpina, Wollschlaeger et al., 2003). Clients need to speak with their healthcare provider before taking this herb. Although most clients can take ginkgo without problems, those on anticoagulants may have an increased risk for bleeding. Ginkgo biloba extract is often standardized to contain 24% flavonoids and 6% terpenoids. A typical dose is 80 to 240 mg per day.

Garlic also shows promise as a natural treatment for dementia. In a study that used aged garlic extract, researchers felt there was "compelling evidence" to support the use of garlic not only to prevent cognitive decline but also to improve learning and memory retention (Borek, 2006). Garlic can potentiate the effects of anticoagulants, so clients taking these medications should limit their intake of garlic. Garlic is often standardized to percent allicin, an active ingredient. A typical dose is 2 to 5 g of fresh garlic or 400 to 1200 mg of garlic powder daily.

PHARMACOTHERAPY ILLUSTRATED

20.1 Antiparkinson Drugs Focus on Restoring Dopamine Function and Blocking Cholinergic Activity in the Nigrostriatal Pathway

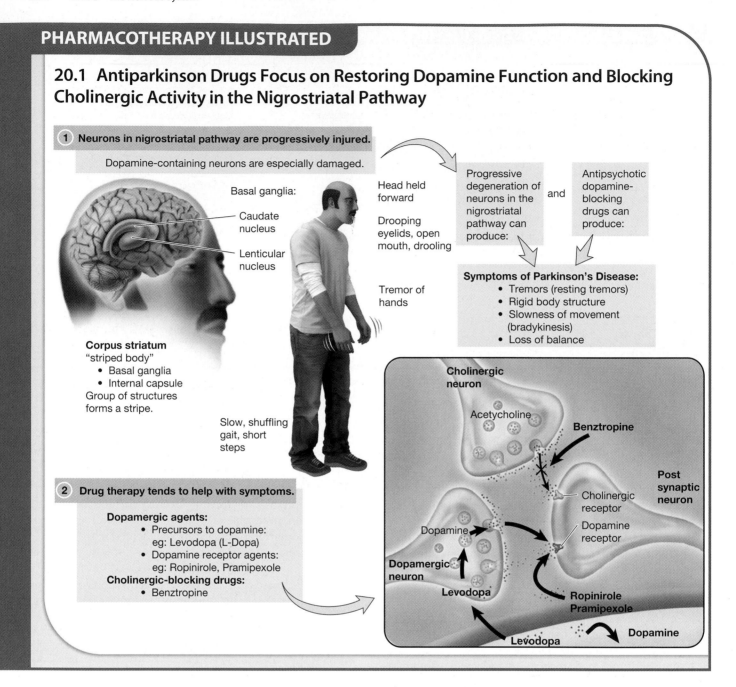

1 Neurons in nigrostriatal pathway are progressively injured.

Dopamine-containing neurons are especially damaged.

Basal ganglia:
— Caudate nucleus
— Lenticular nucleus

Corpus striatum
"striped body"
• Basal ganglia
• Internal capsule
Group of structures
forms a stripe.

Head held forward

Drooping eyelids, open mouth, drooling

Tremor of hands

Slow, shuffling gait, short steps

Progressive degeneration of neurons in the nigrostriatal pathway can produce: **and** Antipsychotic dopamine-blocking drugs can produce:

Symptoms of Parkinson's Disease:
• Tremors (resting tremors)
• Rigid body structure
• Slowness of movement (bradykinesis)
• Loss of balance

2 Drug therapy tends to help with symptoms.

Dopamergic agents:
• Precursors to dopamine:
  eg: Levodopa (L-Dopa)
• Dopamine receptor agents:
  eg: Ropinirole, Pramipexole
Cholinergic-blocking drugs:
• Benztropine

Cholinergic neuron
Acetycholine
Benztropine
Cholinergic receptor
Dopamine receptor
Post synaptic neuron
Dopamine
Dopamergic neuron
Levodopa
Ropinirole Pramipexole
Levodopa
Dopamine

---

relating to the wearing-off effect. An example of this drug class is entacapone (Comtan). Side effects of COMT inhibitors include mental confusion and hallucination, nausea and vomiting, cramps, headache, diarrhea, and possible liver damage.

NURSING CONSIDERATIONS

The role of the nurse in dopaminergic therapy for parkinsonism involves careful monitoring of a client's condition and providing education as it relates to the prescribed drug treatment. Prior to initiating drug therapy, take the client's health history. Those with narrow-angle glaucoma, undiagnosed skin lesions, or history of hypersensitivity should not take dopaminergic agents.

Dopaminergics should be used cautiously in clients with severe cardiac, renal, liver, or endocrine diseases; mood disorders; or history of seizures or ulcers; or in those who are pregnant or lactating. Obtain baseline and periodic blood tests including a complete blood count (CBC) and liver and renal function studies. Assess baseline vital signs, especially blood pressure, mental status, and symptoms of Parkinson's disease. Fully evaluate all other medications taken by the client for compatibility with dopaminergic agonists.

During initial treatment, closely monitor blood pressure, pulse, and respirations, because these drugs may cause hypotension and tachycardia. Clients expected to take the drug long term should additionally be tested for diabetes and acromegaly. Carefully monitor clients for excessive

Pr PROTOTYPE DRUG | Levodopa *(Larodopa)* | Dopaminergic Agent

ACTIONS AND USES

Levodopa restores the neurotransmitter dopamine in extrapyramidal areas of the brain, thus relieving some Parkinson's symptoms. To increase its effect, levodopa is often combined with other medications, such as carbidopa, which prevent its enzymatic breakdown. Up to 6 months may be needed to achieve maximum therapeutic effects.

ADMINISTRATION ALERTS

- The client may be unable to self-administer medication and may need assistance.
- Administer exactly as ordered.
- Abrupt withdrawal of drug can result in parkinsonism crisis or neuroleptic malignant syndrome (NMS).
- Pregnancy category C.

PHARMACOKINETICS

Onset: < 30 min

Peak: 1–3 h

Half-life: 1 h

Duration: Variable

ADVERSE EFFECTS

Side effects of levodopa include uncontrolled and purposeless movements such as extending the fingers and shrugging the shoulders, involuntary movements, loss of appetite, nausea, and vomiting. Muscle twitching and spasmodic winking are early signs of toxicity. Orthostatic hypotension is common in some clients. The drug should be discontinued gradually, because abrupt withdrawal can produce acute parkinsonism.

Contraindications: Levodopa is contraindicated in the treatment of narrow-angle glaucoma, particularly in clients with suspicious pigmented lesions or a history of melanoma. This medication should be avoided in cases of acute psychoses and severe psychoneurosis within 2 weeks of therapy with MAOI.

INTERACTIONS

Drug–Drug: Levodopa interacts with many drugs. For example, tricyclic antidepressants decrease effects of levodopa, increase postural hypotension, and may increase sympathetic activity, with hypertension and sinus tachycardia. Levodopa cannot be used if a MAOI was taken within 14 to 28 days, because concurrent use may precipitate hypertensive crisis. Haloperidol taken concurrently may antagonize therapeutic effects of levodopa. Methyldopa may increase toxicity. Antihypertensives may cause increased hypotensive effects. Anticonvulsants may decrease therapeutic effects of levodopa. Antacids containing magnesium, calcium, or sodium bicarbonate may increase levodopa absorption, which could lead to toxicity. Pyridoxine reverses antiparkinsonism effects of levodopa.

Lab Tests: Abnormalities in lab tests may include elevations of liver function tests such as alkaline phosphatase, aspartate aminotransferase (AST), alanine aminotransferase (ALT), lactic dehydrogenase, and bilirubin. Abnormalities in blood urea nitrogen and positive Coombs' test have also been reported.

Herbals/Food: Kava may worsen symptoms of Parkinson's.

Treatment of Overdose: General supportive measures should be taken along with immediate gastric lavage. Intravenous fluids should be administered judiciously and an adequate airway maintained.

MediaLink

Mechanism in Action: Levodopa

---

daytime sleepiness, eye twitching, involuntary movements, hand tremors, fatigue, anxiety, mood changes, confusion, agitation, nausea, vomiting, anorexia, dry mouth, and constipation. Muscle twitching and mood changes may indicate toxicity and should be reported at once. Assist the client with drug administration and activities of daily living (ADLs), including ambulation, at the initiation of therapy. It is normal for the client's urine and perspiration to darken in color.

Client Teaching.   Client education as it relates to dopaminergic drugs should include the goals of therapy, the reasons for obtaining baseline data such as vital signs and the existence of underlying disorders such as glaucoma or renal disease, and possible drug side effects. Include the following points when teaching clients about dopaminergic drugs:

- Increase fiber and fluid intake to prevent constipation.
- Avoid foods high in pyridoxine (vitamin B_6) such as beef, liver, ham, pork, egg yolks, sweet potatoes, and

oatmeal, because they will decrease the effects of these medications.

- Avoid all over-the-counter (OTC) drugs and fortified cereals because of the possible presence of pyridoxine.
- Immediately report muscle spasm, spasmodic winking, and an increase in bradykinesia.
- It may be several months before the full therapeutic effect of pharmacotherapy is achieved.
- Do not abruptly stop taking the drug, because parkinsonian crisis may occur.
- Change positions slowly to prevent dizziness or fainting.

ANTICHOLINERGICS

These drugs inhibit the action of acetylcholine in the brain. They are used early in the course of therapy for Parkinsonism disease.

NURSING PROCESS FOCUS Clients Receiving Levodopa (Larodopa)

Assessment	Potential Nursing Diagnoses
Prior to administration: ▪ Obtain a complete health history including allergies, drug history, and possible drug interactions. ▪ Obtain baseline evaluation of severity of Parkinson's disease to determine medication effectiveness. ▪ Obtain baseline vital signs, especially blood pressure and pulse.	▪ Fall, Risk for ▪ Knowledge, Deficient, related to drug therapy ▪ Mobility, Physical, Impaired ▪ Self-Care Deficit: Feeding, Toileting ▪ Constipation

Planning: Client Goals and Expected Outcomes

The client will:
▪ Report increased ease of movement and decreased symptoms of Parkinson's disease.
▪ Demonstrate an understanding of the drug's action by accurately describing drug side effects and precautions.
▪ Immediately report side effects and adverse reactions.
▪ Adhere to the medication regimen.

Implementation

Interventions and (Rationales)	Client Education/Discharge Planning
▪ Monitor vital signs closely when the dose is being adjusted. (Hypotension could occur as a result of dose adjustment. Dysrhythmias can occur in clients predisposed to cardiac problems.)	▪ Instruct client and caregiver to report signs of hypotension, dizziness, light-headedness, feelings that heart is racing or skipping beats, or dyspnea; and have ECG and vital signs taken periodically.
▪ Provide for client safety. (Orthostatic hypotension may occur.)	▪ Instruct client to change position slowly and to resume normal activities slowly.
▪ Monitor for behavior changes. (Drug increases risk of depression or suicidal thoughts and may cause other mood disturbances such as aggressiveness and confusion.)	▪ Instruct client and caregiver to watch for and report immediately any signs of changes in behavior or mood and seek counseling or a support group to help deal with these feelings; assist client in finding such resources if needed.
▪ Monitor for symptoms of overdose. (Muscle twitching and blepharospasm are early symptoms.)	▪ Instruct client and caregiver to be aware of newly occurring muscle twitching, including muscles of eyelids, and to report them immediately.
▪ Monitor for improved functional status followed by a loss of therapeutic effects (on–off phenomenon), due to changes in dopamine levels that may last only minutes or days. (This usually occurs in clients on long-term levodopa therapy.)	▪ Instruct client and caregiver to immediately report rapid, unpredictable changes in motor symptoms, which can be corrected with changes in levodopa dosage schedule.
▪ Evaluate diet. (Absorption of levodopa decreases with high-protein meals or high consumption of pyridoxine-containing foods.)	▪ Instruct client to take on empty stomach; eat food 15 minutes after if necessary to decrease GI upset; avoid taking levodopa with high-protein meals; avoid high consumption of foods containing vitamin B_6 (pyridoxine) such as bananas, wheat germ, green vegetables, liver, and legumes; and avoid vitamin B_6 in multivitamins, fortified cereals, and antinauseants.
▪ Monitor glucose levels in clients with diabetes mellitus. (Loss of glycemic control may occur in the diabetic client.)	▪ Instruct diabetic client to consistently self-monitor blood glucose levels, have periodic lab studies, and report symptoms of hypoglycemia or hyperglycemia.
▪ Monitor for decreased kidney or liver function. (Decrease in these functions may slow metabolism and excretion of drug, possibly leading to overdose or toxicity.)	▪ Instruct client to keep all appointments for liver and kidney function tests during therapy.
▪ Monitor for side effects in elderly clients. (Elderly clients may experience more rapid and severe side effects, especially those affecting the cardiovascular system.)	▪ Instruct elderly client to report any symptoms involving cardiovascular system, including changes in heart rate, dizziness, faintness, edema, or palpitations.
▪ Monitor for other drug-related changes. (Drug may cause urine and perspiration to darken in color, but it is not a sign of overdose or toxicity.)	▪ Inform client that urine may darken and sweat may be dark colored, but not to be alarmed.

NURSING PROCESS FOCUS Clients Receiving Levodopa (Larodopa) *(Continued)*

Evaluation of Outcome Criteria

Evaluate effectiveness of drug therapy by confirming that client goals and expected outcomes have been met (see "Planning").

- The client reports increased ease of movement and decreased symptoms of Parkinson's disease.
- The client demonstrates an understanding of the drug's action by accurately describing drug side effects and precautions.
- The client accurately states signs and symptoms to be reported to the healthcare provider.
- The client adheres to the medication regimen.

20.4 Treating Parkinsonism With Anticholinergics

A second approach to changing the balance between dopamine and acetylcholine in the brain is to give cholinergic blockers, or anticholinergics. By blocking the effect of acetylcholine, anticholinergics inhibit the overactivity of this neurotransmitter in the corpus striatum of the brain. These agents are listed in Table 20.3.

Anticholinergics such as atropine were the first agents used to treat parkinsonism. The large number of peripheral side effects has limited the uses of this drug class. The anticholinergics now used for parkinsonism are centrally acting and produce fewer side effects. Although anticholinergics act on the CNS, autonomic effects such as dry mouth, blurred vision, tachycardia, urine retention, and constipation are still troublesome. The centrally acting anticholinergics are not as effective as levodopa at relieving severe symptoms of parkinsonism. They are used early in the course of the disease when symptoms are less severe, in clients who cannot tolerate levodopa, and in combination therapy with other antiparkinsonism drugs.

NURSING CONSIDERATIONS

The following content provides nursing considerations that apply to anticholinergics when given to treat parkinsonism. For the complete nursing process applied to anticholinergic therapy, see "Nursing Process Focus: Clients Receiving Anticholinergic Therapy, page 148" in Chapter 13 ∞.

The role of the nurse in anticholinergic therapy for parkinsonism involves careful monitoring of a client's condition and providing education as it relates to the prescribed drug treatment. Carefully evaluate and monitor clients taking this class of drugs (as with those taking dopaminergic drugs). Before a client begins treatment, obtain a thorough health history. Clients younger than age 3 and those with known hypersensitivity, narrow-angle glaucoma, myasthenia gravis, or obstruction of the urinary or gastrointestinal tract should not take cholinergic blockers. These drugs should be used carefully in elderly clients because of slowed metabolism, and used cautiously with clients who have dysrhythmias, benign prostatic hypertrophy (BPH), or in pregnant or lactating women. Before treatment begins, obtain a history of medications taken and a complete physical to include CBC, liver and renal function studies, vital signs, mental status, and progression of Parkinson's disease to establish baseline data. These tests should be repeated throughout the treatment to help determine effectiveness of the drug.

Client Teaching. Client education as it relates to anticholinergics should include the goals of therapy, the reasons for obtaining baseline data such as vital signs and the existence of underlying disorders such as prostatic disease, and possible drug side effects. Include the following points when teaching clients about anticholinergics:

- Increase fiber and fluid intake to prevent constipation.
- To help relieve dry mouth, take frequent drinks of cool liquids, suck on sugar-free hard candy or ice chips, and chew sugar-free gum.
- Take with food or milk to prevent GI upset.
- Be evaluated by an eye specialist periodically, because anticholinergics may promote glaucoma development.
- Avoid driving, because drowsiness may occur.

MediaLink Alzheimer's Information

TABLE 20.3 Anticholinergic Drugs and Drugs With Anticholinergic Activity Used for Parkinsonism		
Drug	**Route and Adult Dose (max dose where indicated)**	**Adverse Effects**
℞ benztropine mesylate (Cogentin)	PO; 0.5–1 mg/day; gradually increase as needed (max: 6 mg/day)	*Sedation, nausea, constipation, dry mouth, blurred vision, drowsiness, dizziness, tachycardia, hypotension, nervousness*
biperiden hydrochloride (Akineton)	PO; 2 mg 1–4 times/day	
diphenhydramine hydrochloride (Benadryl) (see page 583 for the Prototype Drug box ∞)	PO; 25–50 mg tid–qid (max: 300 mg/day)	
		<u>Paralytic ileus, cardiovascular collapse</u>
procyclidine hydrochloride (Kemadrin)	PO; 2.5 mg tid after meals; may be increased to 5 mg tid if tolerated, with an additional 5 mg at bedtime (max: 45–60 mg/day)	
trihexyphenidyl hydrochloride (Artane)	PO; 1 mg on Day 1; 2 mg on Day 2; then increase by 2 mg every 3–5 days up to 6–10 mg/day (max: 15 mg/day)	

Italics indicate common adverse effects; <u>underlining</u> indicates serious adverse effects.

- Do not abruptly stop taking the drug, because withdrawal symptoms such as tremors, insomnia, and restlessness may occur.
- Avoid alcohol use.
- Immediately report disorientation, depression, hallucinations, confusion, memory impairment, nervousness, psychoses, vision changes, nausea/vomiting, urine retention, or dysuria.
- Wear dark glasses and avoid bright sunlight as necessary.

ALZHEIMER'S DISEASE

Alzheimer's disease is a devastating, progressive, degenerative disease that generally begins after age 60. By age 85, as many as 50% of the population may be affected. Pharmacotherapy has limited success in improving the cognitive function of clients with Alzheimer's disease.

20.5 Characteristics of Alzheimer's Disease

Alzheimer's disease (AD) is responsible for 70% of all dementia. **Dementia** is a degenerative disorder characterized by progressive memory loss, confusion, and inability

to think or communicate effectively. Consciousness and perception are usually unaffected. Known causes of dementia include multiple cerebral infarcts, severe infections, and toxins. Although the cause of most dementia is unknown, it is usually associated with cerebral atrophy or other structural changes within the brain. The client generally lives 5 to 10 years following diagnosis; AD is the fourth leading cause of death.

Despite extensive, ongoing research, the etiology of Alzheimer's disease remains unknown. The early-onset

---

Pr **PROTOTYPE DRUG** | Benztropine *(Cogentin)* | Cholinergic Blocker

ACTIONS AND USES

Benztropine acts by blocking excess cholinergic stimulation of neurons in the corpus striatum. It is used for relief of parkinsonism symptoms and for the treatment of EPS brought on by antipsychotic pharmacotherapy. This medication suppresses tremors but does not affect tardive dyskinesia.

ADMINISTRATION ALERTS

- The client may be unable to self-administer medication and may need assistance.
- Benztropine may be taken in divided doses, two to four times a day, or the entire day's dose may be taken at bedtime.
- If muscle weakness occurs, the dose should be reduced.
- Pregnancy category C.

PHARMACOKINETICS

Onset: 15 min IM/IV; 1 h PO

Peak: 1–2 h

Half-life: 2–3 h

Duration: 6–10 h

ADVERSE EFFECTS

As expected from its autonomic action, benztropine can cause typical anticholinergic side effects such as dry mouth, constipation, and tachycardia. Adverse general effects include sedation, drowsiness, dizziness, restlessness, irritability, nervousness, and insomnia.

Contraindications: Contraindications include narrow-angle glaucoma, myasthenia gravis, and obstructive diseases of the genitourinary and GI tracts.

INTERACTIONS

Drug–Drug: Benztropine interacts with many drugs. For example, benztropine should not be taken with alcohol, tricyclic antidepressants, MAOIs, phenothiazines, procainamide, or quinidine because of combined sedative effects. OTC cold medicines and alcohol should be avoided. Other drugs that enhance dopamine release or activation of the dopamine receptor may produce additive effects. Haloperidol decreases effectiveness.

Antihistamines, phenothiazines, tricyclics, and disopyramide quinidine may increase anticholinergic effects, and antidiarrheals may decrease absorption.

Lab Tests: Unknown.

Herbal/Food: Unknown.

Treatment of Overdose: Physostigmine salicylate, 1 to 2 mg subcutaneously or IV, will reverse symptoms of anticholinergic intoxication. A second injection may be given after 2 hours, if required. Otherwise, treatment is symptomatic and supportive.

 See the Companion Website for a Nursing Process Focus specific to this drug.

TABLE 20.4	Acetylcholinesterase Inhibitors Used for Alzheimer's Disease	
Drug	**Route and Adult Dose (max dose where indicated)**	**Adverse Effects**
⊕ donepezil hydrochloride (Aricept)	PO; 5–10 mg at bedtime	*Headache, dizziness, insomnia, nausea, diarrhea, vomiting, muscle cramps, anorexia, abdominal pain*
galantamine (Reminyl)	PO; Initiate with 4 mg bid for at least 4 wk; if tolerated, may increase by 4 mg bid q4wk to target dose of 12 mg bid (max: 8–16 mg bid)	<u>Hepatotoxicity</u>
rivastigmine tartrate (Exelon)	PO; Start with 1.5 mg bid with food; may increase by 1.5 mg bid q2wk if tolerated; target dose 3–6 mg bid (max: 12 mg bid)	
tacrine (Cognex)	PO; 10 mg qid; increase in 40 mg/day increments not sooner than every 6 wk (max: 160 mg/day)	

Italics indicate common adverse effects; <u>underlining</u> indicates serious adverse effects.

familial form of this disorder, accounting for about 10% of cases, is associated with gene defects on chromosome 1, 14, or 21. Chronic inflammation and excess free radicals may cause neuron damage. Environmental, immunological, and nutritional factors, as well as viruses, are considered possible sources of brain damage.

Although the cause may be unknown, structural damage in the brain of Alzheimer's clients has been well documented. **Amyloid plaques** and **neurofibrillary tangles,** found within the brain at autopsy, are present in nearly all clients with AD. It is suspected that these structural changes are caused by chronic inflammatory or oxidative cellular damage to the surrounding neurons. There is a loss in both the number and function of neurons.

Alzheimer's clients experience a dramatic loss of ability to perform tasks that require acetylcholine as the neurotransmitter. Because acetylcholine is a major neurotransmitter within the **hippocampus,** an area of the brain responsible for learning and memory, and other parts of the cerebral cortex, neuronal function within these brain areas is especially affected. Thus, an inability to remember and to recall information is among the early symptoms of AD. Symptoms of this disease are as follows:

- Impaired memory and judgment
- Confusion or disorientation
- Inability to recognize family or friends
- Aggressive behavior
- Depression
- Psychoses, including paranoia and delusions
- Anxiety

DRUGS FOR ALZHEIMER'S DISEASE

Drugs are used to slow memory loss and other progressive symptoms of dementia. Some drugs are given to treat associated symptoms such as depression, anxiety, or psychoses. The acetylcholinesterase inhibitors are the most widely used class of drugs for treating AD. These agents are listed in Table 20.4. Memantine (Namenda), the first of a new class of drugs called glutamergic inhibitors, was approved in October 2003.

ACETYLCHOLINESTERASE INHIBITORS (PARASYMPATHOMIMETICS)

The FDA has approved only a few drugs for AD. The most effective of these medications act by intensifying the effect of acetylcholine at the cholinergic receptor, as shown in Pharmacotherapy Illustrated 20.2.

20.6 Treating Alzheimer's Disease With Acetylcholinesterase Inhibitors

Acetylcholine is naturally degraded in the synapse by the enzyme **acetylcholinesterase (AchE).** When AchE is inhibited, acetylcholine levels become elevated and produce a more profound effect on the receptor. As described in Chapter 13 ∞, the AchE inhibitors are indirect-acting parasympathomimetics.

The goal of pharmacotherapy in the treatment of AD is to improve function in three domains: ADLs, behavior, and cognition. Although the AchE inhibitors improve all three domains, their efficacy is modest, at best. These agents do not cure AD—they only slow its progression. Therapy is begun as soon as the diagnosis of AD is established. These agents are ineffective in treating the severe stages of this disorder, probably because so many neurons have died; increasing the level of acetylcholine is effective only if there are functioning neurons present. Often, as the disease progresses, the AchE inhibitors are discontinued; their therapeutic benefit does not outweigh their expense or the risks of side effects.

All acetylcholinesterase inhibitors used to treat AD have equal efficacy. Side effects are those expected of drugs that enhance the parasympathetic nervous system (Chapter 13 ∞). The GI system is most affected, with nausea, vomiting, and diarrhea being reported. Of the agents available for AD, tacrine (Cognex) is associated with hepatotoxicity. Rivastigmine (Exelon) is associated with weight loss, a potentially serious side effect in some elderly clients. When therapy is discontinued doses of the AchE inhibitors should be lowered gradually.

In 2003, memantine (Namenda) was approved by the Food and Drug Administration (FDA) for treatment of moderate to severe AD. Its mechanism of action differs from that of the cholinesterase inhibitors. Unlike cholinesterase inhibitors that

PHARMACOTHERAPY ILLUSTRATED

20.2 Alzheimer's Drugs Work by Intensifying the Effect of Acetylcholine at the Receptor

1 **Alzheimers disease**

Characterized by abnormal structures in the brain:
- Neurons die.
- The brain shrinks.
- Memory is lost.

Amyloid plaques

Neurofibrillary tangles

Unhealthy neuronal structure

Healthy neuronal structure

2 **Drug therapy focuses on restoring or enhancing acetylcholine's role in the brain.**

- Cholinesterase inhibitors
  eg: donepezil

3 **Factors responsible for brain cell death include excessive transmission of glutamate.**

Drug therapy:
- N-methyl-D-aspartate (NMDA) receptor agents
  eg: memantine

Combination drug therapy:
- Donepezil and memantine

Cholinergic neuron

Normally:

1 Ach is released.

2 Ach binds with its receptor.

3 The action of Ach is terminated by AchE.

4 If AchE is *inhibited*, Ach is *not* broken down as quickly and produces a more dramatic effect.

AchE = acetylcholinesterase

Pyruvate

AcetylCoA + Choline

Acetylcholine (Ach)

1

Choline + Acetate

Ach **2**

4

3 AchE

Normal role of acetylcholine in a vast array of brain functions, including the ability to speak, move, see, think, and remember

Cholinergic receptor

Neuron with cholinergic receptor

---

address the cholinergic defect in the brains of AD clients, memantine reduces the abnormally high levels of glutamate. Glutamate exerts its neural effects through interaction with the *N*-methyl-D-aspartate (NMDA) receptor. When bound to the receptor, glutamate causes calcium to enter neurons, producing an excitatory effect. Too much glutamate in the brain may be responsible for brain cell death. Mematine may have a protective function in reducing neuronal calcium overload.

Because memantine and cholinesterase inhibitors act by different mechanisms, they may be taken in combination. Donepezil and memantine are approved for the treatment of progressive AD and are marketed under the brand name Aricept. When taken together, these drugs do not interfere with each other's absorption, distribution, metabolism, or elimination. There is evidence that memantaine may be effective in the treatment of vascular dementia.

Although acetylcholinesterase inhibitors have been the mainstay in the treatment of AD dementia, several other agents are being investigated for their possible benefit in delaying the progression of AD. Because at least some of the neuronal changes in AD are caused by oxidative cellular

Pr PROTOTYPE DRUG | Donepezil *(Aricept)* | Acetylcholinesterase Inhibitor

ACTIONS AND USES

Donepezil is an AchE inhibitor that improves memory in cases of mild to moderate Alzheimer's dementia by enhancing the effects of acetylcholine in neurons in the cerebral cortex that have not yet been damaged. Clients should receive pharmacotherapy for at least 6 months prior to assessing maximum benefits of drug therapy. Improvement in memory may be observed as early as 1 to 4 weeks following medication. The therapeutic effects of donepezil are often short-lived, and the degree of improvement is modest, at best. An advantage of donepezil over other drugs in its class is that its long half-life permits it to be given once daily.

ADMINISTRATION ALERTS

- Give medication prior to bedtime.
- Medication is most effective when given on a regular schedule.
- Pregnancy category C.

PHARMACOKINETICS

Onset: < 20 min

Peak: 3–4 h

Half-life: Unknown

Duration: Variable

ADVERSE EFFECTS

Common side effects of donepezil are vomiting, diarrhea, and darkened urine. CNS side effects include insomnia, syncope, depression, headache, and irritability. Musculoskeletal side effects include muscle cramps, arthritis, and bone fractures. Generalized side effects include headache, fatigue, chest pain, increased libido, hot flashes, urinary incontinence, dehydration, and blurred vision.

Unlike with tacrine, hepatotoxicity has not been observed. Clients with bradycardia, hypotension, asthma, hyperthyroidism, or active peptic ulcer disease should be monitored carefully.

Contraindications: Donepezil is contraindicated in clients with GI bleeding and jaundice.

INTERACTIONS

Drug–Drug: Anticholinergics will be less effective. Donepezil interacts with several other drugs. For example, bethanechol causes a synergistic effect. Phenobarbital, phenytoin, dexamethasone, and rifampin may speed elimination of donepezil. Quinidine or ketoconazole may inhibit metabolism of donepezil. Because donepezil acts by increasing cholinergic activity, two parasympathomimetics should not be administered concurrently.

Lab Tests: Unknown.

Herbal/Food: Unknown.

Treatment of Overdose: Anticholinergics such as atropine may be used as an antidote for donezepil overdosage. Intravenous atropine sulfate titrated to effect is recommended: an initial dose of 1 to 2 mg IV with subsequent doses based on clinical response.

 See the Companion Website for a Nursing Process Focus specific to this drug.

damage, antioxidants such as vitamin E are being examined for their effects in AD clients. Other agents currently being examined are anti-inflammatory agents, such as the COX-2 inhibitors, estrogen, and ginkgo biloba.

Agitation occurs in the majority of clients with AD. This may be accompanied by delusions, paranoia, hallucinations, or other psychotic symptoms. Atypical antipsychotic agents such as risperidone (Risperdal) and olanzapine (Zyprexa) may be used to control these episodes. Conventional antipsychotics such as haloperidol (Haldol) are occasionally prescribed, though extrapyramidal side effects often limit their use. The pharmacotherapy of psychosis is presented in Chapter 17 ∞.

Anxiety and depression, although not as common as agitation, may occur in AD clients. Anxiolytics such as buspirone (BuSpar) or some of the benzodiazepines are used to control unease and excessive apprehension (Chapter 14 ∞). Mood stabilizers such as sertraline (Zoloft), citalopram (Celexa), or fluoxetine (Prozac) are given when major depression interferes with daily activities (Chapter 16 ∞).

NURSING CONSIDERATIONS

The following content provides nursing considerations that apply to acetylcholinesterase inhibitors when given to treat Alzheimer's disease. For the complete Nursing Process applied to acetylcholinesterase inhibitor therapy, see "Nursing Process Focus: Clients Receiving Parasympathomimetic Therapy," page 145 in Chapter 13 ∞.

The role of the nurse in AchE inhibitor (parasympathomimetic) therapy for AD involves careful monitoring of the client's condition and providing education as it relates to the prescribed drug treatment. Prior to the initiation of drug therapy, take the client's health history. Young children and those with hypersensitivity should not take AchE inhibitors. Clients with narrow-angle glaucoma or undiagnosed skin lesions should not take rivastigmine (Exelon). All AchE inhibitors should be used cautiously in clients with severe cardiac, renal, liver, or respiratory diseases (such as asthma or COPD); a history of seizures; GI bleeding, or peptic ulcers; and in those who are pregnant or lactating. Obtain baseline and periodic lab tests, including a CBC and liver and renal function tests. Assess baseline vital signs and carefully monitor them throughout treatment, because these medications may cause hypotension. Assess mental status and other signs of AD at baseline to help determine effectiveness of medication. Fully evaluate all other medications taken by the client to determine possible interactions with AchE inhibitors.

Monitor clients for side effects or reactions such as changes in mental status, mood changes, dizziness, confusion, insomnia, nausea, vomiting, and anorexia. Additionally, monitor those taking tacrine (Cognex) for urinary frequency, hepatotoxicity, and GI bleeding.

Nurses may care for clients with AD in acute-care or long-term care facilities, or may provide support and education for caregivers in the home. Families and clients who are able to understand must be made aware that currently available medications may slow the progression of the disease but not effect a cure.

Client Teaching. Client education as it relates to AchE inhibitors should include the goals of therapy, the reasons for obtaining baseline data such as vital signs and the existence of underlying disorders such as glaucoma or ulcers, and possible drug side effects. Include the following points when teaching clients about acetylcholinesterase inhibitors:

- Take the drug with food or milk to decrease GI disturbances.

- Take the drug strictly as prescribed, or serious side effects may result.

- Report any changes in mental status or mood.

- Report dizziness, confusion, insomnia, constipation, nausea, urinary frequency, GI bleeding, vomiting, seizures, or anorexia.

- Keep scheduled appointments with the healthcare provider.

- To help relieve dry mouth, take frequent drinks of cool liquids, suck on sugar-free hard candy, or chew sugar-free gum.

- Increase fiber and fluid intake to prevent constipation.

- Recognize and report severe nausea and vomiting, sweating, salivation, hypotension, bradycardia, convulsions, and increased muscle weakness (especially respiratory muscles).

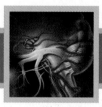

CHAPTER REVIEW

KEY CONCEPTS

The numbered key concepts provide a succinct summary of the important points from the corresponding numbered section within the chapter. If any of these points are not clear, refer to the numbered section within the chapter for review.

20.1 Degenerative diseases of the nervous system such as Parkinson's disease and Alzheimer's disease cause a progressive loss of neuron function.

20.2 Parkinson's disease is characterized by symptoms of tremors, muscle rigidity, and postural instability and ambulation caused by the destruction of dopamine-producing neurons found within the corpus striatum. The underlying biochemical problem is lack of dopamine activity and a related overactivity of acetylcholine.

20.3 The most commonly used medications for parkinsonism attempt to restore levels of dopamine in the corpus striatum

of the brain. Levodopa (Larodopa) is the drug of choice for Parkinson's disease.

20.4 Centrally acting anticholinergic drugs are sometimes used to relieve symptoms of parkinsonism, although they are less effective than levodopa (Larodopa).

20.5 Alzheimer's disease is a progressive degenerative disease of older adults. Primary symptoms include disorientation, confusion, and memory loss.

20.6 Acetylcholinesterase inhibitors are used to slow the progression of Alzheimer's disease symptoms. These agents have minimal efficacy, and do not cure the dementia.

NCLEX-RN® REVIEW QUESTIONS

1 The family member caring for a client with Parkinson's disease at home notifies the nurse that the client is demonstrating extrapyramidal symptoms. The nurse should instruct the caregiver to:

1. Give dyphenhydramine (Benadryl) 25 mg PO.
2. Transport the client to the emergency department.
3. Increase the dosage of antiparkinsonism drugs.
4. Make an appointment with the healthcare provider for evaluation.

2 The client asks what can be expected from drug therapy for treatment of parkinsonism. The best response by the nurse would be that:

1. A cure can be expected within 6 months.
2. Symptoms can be reduced and the ability to perform ADLs can be improved.
3. Disease progression will be stopped.
4. EPS will be prevented.

3 Levodopa (Laradopa) is prescribed for a client with Parkinson's disease. At discharge the nurse should include the following teaching points:

1. Monitor blood pressure every 2 hours for the first 2 weeks.
2. Expect the urine color to be orange.
3. Report the development of diarrhea.
4. Keep scheduled lab appointments for liver and renal function tests.

4 The nurse discussed the disease process of Alzheimer's with the client and caregiver. What does the nurse explain is the cause of AD?

1. The cause is unknown. Amyloid plaques and neurofibrillary tangles have been found in the brain at autopsy.
2. The cause is unknown. Chronic small intracranial bleeds have been found on CT scans.
3. Loss of circulation to the brain has been found on CT scans.
4. Loss of dopamine receptors is thought to occur as a part of the aging process.

5 An overdose of drugs to treat AD may occur if they are taken improperly or if decreased liver or renal function occurs. The nurse assesses the client for signs of overdose, which include (select all that apply):

1. Bradycardia and muscle weakness.
2. Tachycardia and hypertension.
3. Nausea and vomiting.
4. Emotional withdrawal and tachypnea.
5. Hypotension and increased muscle strength.

CRITICAL THINKING QUESTIONS

1. A 58-year-old Parkinson's client is placed on levodopa (Larodopa). In obtaining her health history, the nurse notes that the client takes Mylanta on a regular basis for mild indigestion, and multivitamins daily (vitamins A, B_6, D, and E). She also has a history of diabetes mellitus type 2. What should the nurse include in teaching for this client?

2. A client is on levodopa and benztropine (Cogentin). During a regular office follow-up, the client tells the nurse that she is going to Arizona in July to visit her grandchildren. What teaching is important for this client?

3. A 67-year-old Alzheimer's client is on donepezil (Aricept) and has a history of congestive heart failure, diabetes mellitus type 2, and hypertension. The client's wife asks the nurse if this new medicine is appropriate for her husband to take. How should the nurse respond? What teaching should be done?

See Appendix D for answers and rationales for all activities.

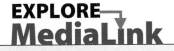 **EXPLORE MediaLink**

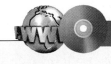 www.prenhall.com/adams

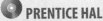

NCLEX-RN® review, case studies, and other interactive resources for this chapter can be found on the companion website at www.prenhall.com/adams. Click on "Chapter 20" to select the activities for this chapter. For animations, more NCLEX-RN® review questions, and an audio glossary, access the accompanying Prentice Hall Nursing MediaLink DVD-ROM in this textbook.

PRENTICE HALL NURSING MEDIALINK DVD-ROM

- **Animation**
  Mechanism in Action: Levodopa (*Larodopa*)
- **Audio Glossary**
- **NCLEX-RN® Review**

 ### COMPANION WEBSITE

- **NCLEX-RN® Review**
- **Dosage Calculations**
- **Case Study:** Client taking dopaminergic drug for parkinsonism
- **Care Plan:** Client with Parkinson's disease who is receiving levodopa-carbidopa

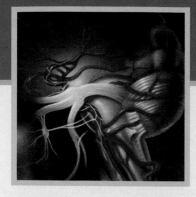

CHAPTER 21

Drugs for Neuromuscular Disorders

DRUGS AT A GLANCE

CENTRALLY ACTING MUSCLE RELAXANTS
- *cyclobenzaprine (Cycoflex, Flexeril)*

DIRECT-ACTING ANTISPASMOTICS
- *dantrolene sodium (Dantrium)*

OBJECTIVES

After reading this chapter, the student should be able to:

1. Identify the different body systems contributing to muscle movement.
2. Discuss nonpharmacological therapies used to treat muscle spasms and spasticity.
3. Explain the goals of pharmacotherapy with skeletal muscle relaxants.
4. Describe the nurse's role in the pharmacological management of muscle spasms.
5. Compare and contrast the roles of the following drug categories in treating muscle spasms and spasticity: centrally acting skeletal muscle relaxants and direct-acting antispasmodics.
6. For each of the drug classes listed in Drugs at a Glance, know representative drugs, and explain their mechanisms of action, primary actions, and important adverse effects.
7. Use the Nursing Process to care for clients who are receiving drug therapy for muscle spasms.

MediaLink

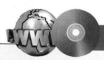

www.prenhall.com/adams

NCLEX-RN® review, case studies, and other interactive resources for this chapter can be found on the companion website at www.prenhall.com/adams. Click on "Chapter 21" to select the activities for this chapter. For animations, more NCLEX-RN® review questions, and an audio glossary, access the accompanying Prentice Hall Nursing MediaLink DVD-ROM in this textbook.

KEY TERMS

clonic spasm *page 275*
dystonia *page 277*
muscle spasms *page 275*
spasticity *page 276*
tonic spasm *page 275*

Disorders associated with movement are some of the most difficult conditions to treat because their underlying mechanisms span other important systems in the body: the nervous, muscular, endocrine, and skeletal systems. Proper body movement depends not only on intact neural pathways but also on proper functioning of muscles, bones, and joints (Chapter 47 ∞), which in turn depends on the levels of minerals such as sodium, potassium, and calcium in the bloodstream (Chapters 31 and 47 ∞). This chapter focuses on the pharmacotherapy of muscular disorders associated with muscle spasms and spasticity. Many of the drugs used to treat muscle spasms are distinct from those used for spasticity.

MUSCLE SPASMS

Muscle spasms are involuntary contractions of a muscle or group of muscles. The muscles become tightened and develop a fixed pattern of resistance, resulting in a diminished level of functioning.

21.1 Causes of Muscle Spasms

Muscle spasms are a common condition usually associated with excessive use of and local injury to the skeletal muscle. Other causes of muscle spasms include overmedication with antipsychotic drugs (Chapter 17 ∞), epilepsy, hypocalcemia, pain, and debilitating neurological disorders. Clients with muscle spasms may experience inflammation, edema, and pain at the affected muscle, loss of coordination, and reduced mobility. When a muscle goes into spasm, it locks in a contracted state. A single, prolonged contraction is a **tonic spasm,** whereas multiple, rapidly repeated contractions are **clonic spasms.** Treatment of muscle spasms involves both nonpharmacological and pharmacological therapies.

21.2 Pharmacological and Nonpharmacological Treatment of Muscle Spasms

Treating a client with complaints of muscle spasms requires a careful history and physical exam to determine the etiology. After a determination has been made, nonpharmacological therapies are normally used in conjunction with medications. Nonpharmacological measures may include immobilization of the affected muscle, application of heat or cold, hydrotherapy, ultrasound, supervised exercises, massage, and manipulation.

Pharmacotherapy for muscle spasm may include combinations of analgesics, anti-inflammatory agents, and centrally acting skeletal muscle relaxants. Most skeletal muscle relaxants relieve symptoms of muscular stiffness and rigidity

---

PHARMFACTS

Muscle Spasms

- More than 12 million people worldwide have muscle spasms.
- Muscle spasms severe enough for drug therapy are often found in patients who have other debilitating disorders such as stroke, injury, neurodegenerative diseases, or cerebral palsy.
- Cerebral palsy is usually associated with events that occur before or during birth, but may be acquired during the first few months or years of life as the result of head trauma or infection.
- Dystonia affects about 250,000 people in the United States; it is the third most common movement disorder, following essential tremor and Parkinson's disease.
- Researchers have recognized multiple forms of inheritable dystonia and identified at least 10 genes or chromosomal locations responsible for the various manifestations.

resulting from muscular injury. They help improve mobility in cases in which clients have restricted movements. The therapeutic goals are to minimize pain and discomfort, increase range of motion, and improve the client's ability to function independently.

CENTRALLY ACTING SKELETAL MUSCLE RELAXANTS

Many muscle relaxants generate their effects by inhibiting motor neurons within the brain and/or spinal cord. Thus, the origin of drug action is within the central nervous system.

21.3 Treating Muscle Spasms at the Level of the Central Nervous System

Skeletal muscle relaxants act at various levels of the central nervous system (CNS). Although their exact mechanisms are not fully understood, it is believed that they generate their effects within the brain and/or spinal cord by inhibiting upper motor neuron activity, causing CNS depressant effects, or altering simple spinal reflexes.

Antispasmodic drugs are used to treat local spasms resulting from muscular injury and may be prescribed alone or in combination with other medications to reduce pain and increase range of motion. Commonly used centrally acting medications include baclofen (Lioresal), cyclobenzaprine (Cycoflex, Flexeril), tizanidine (Zanaflex), and benzodiazepines such as diazepam (Valium), clonazepam (Klonopin), and lorazepam (Ativan), as summarized in Table 21.1. All the centrally acting agents have the potential to cause sedation.

Baclofen (Lioresal), structurally similar to the inhibitory neurotransmitter gamma-aminobutyric acid (GABA), produces its effect by a mechanism that is not fully known. It inhibits neuronal activity within the brain and possibly the spinal cord, although there is some question as to whether the spinal effects of baclofen are associated with (gamma aminobutyric acid GABA). Baclofen may be used to reduce muscle spasms in patients with multiple sclerosis, cerebral palsy, or spinal cord injury. Common side effects of baclofen are drowsiness, dizziness, weakness, and fatigue. Baclofen is often a drug of first choice owing to its wide safety margin.

Tizanidine (Zanaflex) is a centrally acting alpha$_2$-adrenergic agonist that inhibits motor neurons mainly at the spinal cord level. Patients receiving high doses report drowsiness; thus, it also affects some neural activity within the brain. Though uncommon, one adverse effect of tizanidine is hallucinations. The most frequent side effects are dry mouth, fatigue, dizziness, and sleepiness. Tizanidine is as efficacious as baclofen and is considered by some to be a drug of first choice.

As discussed in Chapter 14 ∞, benzodiazepines inhibit both sensory and motor neuron activity by enhancing the effects of GABA. Common adverse side effects include drowsiness and ataxia (loss of coordination). Benzodiazepines are usually prescribed for muscle relaxation when baclofen and tizanidine fail to produce adequate relief.

SPASTICITY

Spasticity is a condition in which certain muscle groups remain in a continuous state of contraction, usually resulting from damage to the CNS. The contracted muscles become

TABLE 21.1	**Centrally Acting Skeletal Muscle Relaxants**	
Drug	**Route and Adult Dose (max dose where indicated)**	**Adverse Effects**
baclofen (Lioresal)	PO; 5 mg tid (max: 80 mg/day)	*Drowsiness, dizziness, dry mouth, sedation, ataxia, light-headedness, urinary hesitancy or retention, hypotension, bradycardia*
Ⓟ cyclobenzaprine hydrochloride (Cycoflex, Flexeril)	PO; 10–20 mg bid–qid (max: 60 mg/day)	
carisoprodol (Soma)	PO; 350 mg tid	<u>Edema of tongue, anaphylactic reaction, respiratory depression, coma, laryngospasm, cardiovascular collapse</u>
chlorphenesin (Maolate)	PO; 800 mg tid until effective; reduce to 400 mg qid or less	
chlorzoxazone (Paraflex, Parafon Forte)	PO; 250–500 mg tid–qid (max: 3 g/day)	
clonazepam (Klonopin)	PO; 1.5 mg tid, may be increased in increments of 0.5–1.0 mg q3 days	
diazepam (Valium) (see page 177 for the Prototype Drug Box ∞)	PO; 4–10 mg bid–qid IM/IV; 2–10 mg, repeat if needed in 3–4 h IV pump; administer emulsion at 5 mg/min	
lorazepam (Ativan) (see page 163 for the Prototype Drug Box ∞)	PO; 1–2 mg bid–tid (max: 10 mg/day)	
metaxalone (Skelaxin)	PO; 800 mg tid–qid (max: 10 mg/day)	
methocarbamol (Robaxin)	PO; 1.5 g qid for 2–3 days; then reduce to 1 g qid	
orphenadrine citrate (Banflex, Flexon, Myolin, Norflex)	PO; 100 mg bid	
tizanidine (Zanaflex)	PO; 4–8 mg tid–qid (max: 36 mg/day)	

Italics indicate common adverse effects; <u>underlining</u> indicates serious adverse effects.

Pr PROTOTYPE DRUG | Cyclobenzaprine *(Cycoflex, Flexeril)* | Centrally Acting Muscle Relaxant

ACTIONS AND USES

Cyclobenzaprine relieves muscle spasms of local origin without interfering with general muscle function. This drug acts by depressing motor activity primarily in the brainstem; limited effects also occur in the spinal cord. Cyclobenzaprine increases circulating levels of norepinephrine, blocking presynaptic uptake. Its mechanism of action is similar to that of tricyclic antidepressants (Chapter 16 ∞). The drug causes muscle relaxation in cases of acute muscle spasticity, but it is not effective in cases of cerebral palsy or diseases of the brain and spinal cord. This medication is meant to provide therapy for only 2 to 3 weeks.

ADMINISTRATION ALERTS

- The drug is not recommended for pediatric use.
- Maximum effects may take 1 to 2 weeks.
- Pregnancy category B.

PHARMACOKINETICS

Onset: 1 h

Peak: 3–8 h

Half-life: 1–3 days

Duration: 12–14 h

ADVERSE EFFECTS

Adverse reactions to cyclobenzaprine include drowsiness, blurred vision, dizziness, dry mouth, rash, and tachycardia. One reaction, although rare, is swelling of the tongue.

Contraindications: Cyclobenzaprine should be used with caution in clients with MI, dysrhythmias, or severe cardiovascular disease.

INTERACTIONS

Drug–Drug: Alcohol, phenothiazines, and other CNS depressants may cause additive sedation. Cyclobenzaprine should not be used within 2 weeks of a monoamine oxidase inhibitor (MAOI) therapy because hyperpyretic crisis and convulsions may occur.

Lab Tests: Unknown.

Herbal/Food: Unknown.

Treatment of Overdose: The intravenous administration of 1 to 3 mg of physostigmine salicylate is reported to reverse symptoms of poisoning by drugs with anticholinergic activity. Physostigmine may be helpful in the treatment of cyclobenzaprine overdose.

 See the Companion Website for a Nursing Process Focus specific to this drug.

MediaLink   Mechanism in Action: Cyclobenzaprine

---

stiff with increased muscle tone. Other signs and symptoms may include mild to severe pain, exaggerated deep tendon reflexes, muscle spasms, scissoring (involuntary crossing of the legs), and fixed joints.

21.4 Causes and Treatment of Spasticity

Spasticity usually results from damage to the motor area of the cerebral cortex that controls muscle movement. Etiologies most commonly associated with this condition include neurological disorders such as cerebral palsy, severe head injury, spinal cord injury or lesions, and stroke. **Dystonia,** a chronic neurological disorder, is characterized by involuntary muscle contraction that forces body parts into abnormal, occasionally painful movements or postures. It affects the muscle tone of the arms, legs, trunk, neck, eyelids, face, or vocal cords. Spasticity can be distressing and greatly affect an individual's quality of life, whether the condition is short or long term. In addition to causing pain, impaired physical mobility influences the ability to perform activities of daily living (ADLs) and diminishes the client's sense of independence.

Effective treatment for spasticity includes both physical therapy and medications. Medications alone are not adequate in reducing the complications of spasticity. Regular and consistent physical therapy exercises have been shown to decrease the severity of symptoms. Types of treatment includes muscle stretching to help prevent contractures,

muscle-group strengthening exercises, and repetitive-motion exercises for improvement of accuracy. In extreme cases, surgery to release tendons or to sever the nerve–muscle pathway has occasionally been used. Drugs effective in the treatment of spasticity include several classifications of antispasmodics that act at the level of the CNS, neuromuscular junction, or muscle tissue.

NATURAL THERAPIES

Cayenne for Muscular Tension

Cayenne (*Capsicum annum*), also known as chili pepper, paprika, or red pepper, has been used as a remedy for muscle tension. Applied in a cream base, it is commonly used to relieve muscle spasms in the shoulder and areas of the arm. Capsaicin, the active ingredient in cayenne, diminishes the chemical messengers that travel through the sensory nerves, thereby decreasing the sensation of pain (Nelson, Ragan, et al. 2004). Its effect accumulates over time, so creams containing capsaicin need to be applied regularly to be effective. Although no known medical condition exists that would prevent the use of cayenne, it should never be applied over broken skin. External use of full-strength cayenne should be limited to no more than 2 days because it may cause skin inflammation, blisters, and ulcers. It also needs to be kept away from eyes and mucous membranes to avoid burns. Hands must be washed thoroughly after use. Capsaicin cream (0.025% to 0.075%) may be applied directly to the affected area up to four times a day.

Cayenne is also taken by clients for digestive problems, but evidence of effectiveness for this indication is lacking. It is available in capsules, 30 to 120 mg, taken three times daily, or as a tea by adding 1/4 to 1/2 tsp of powder to a cup of boiling water.

PHARMACOTHERAPY ILLUSTRATED

21.1 Mechanism of Action of Direct-acting Antispasmodics

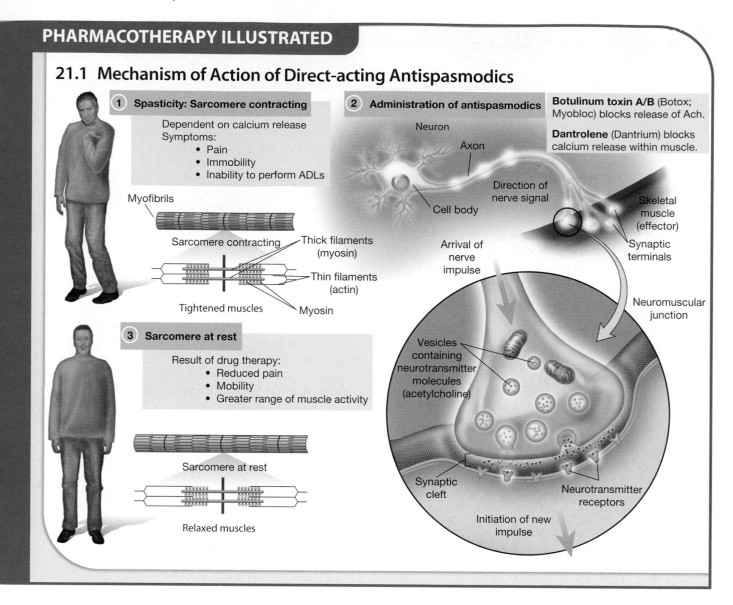

1 Spasticity: Sarcomere contracting

Dependent on calcium release
Symptoms:
- Pain
- Immobility
- Inability to perform ADLs

Myofibrils

Sarcomere contracting

Thick filaments (myosin)

Thin filaments (actin)

Tightened muscles

Myosin

3 Sarcomere at rest

Result of drug therapy:
- Reduced pain
- Mobility
- Greater range of muscle activity

Sarcomere at rest

Relaxed muscles

2 Administration of antispasmodics

Botulinum toxin A/B (Botox; Myobloc) blocks release of Ach.

Dantrolene (Dantrium) blocks calcium release within muscle.

Neuron

Axon

Direction of nerve signal

Cell body

Arrival of nerve impulse

Skeletal muscle (effector)

Synaptic terminals

Neuromuscular junction

Vesicles containing neurotransmitter molecules (acetylcholine)

Synaptic cleft

Neurotransmitter receptors

Initiation of new impulse

DIRECT-ACTING ANTISPASMODICS

A few centrally acting drugs effective in the treatment of general muscles spasms have already been covered: baclofen (Lioresal) and diazepam (Valium). These and other skeletal muscle relaxants are effective in treating spasticity as well. As shown in Pharmacotherapy Illustrated 21.1, dantrolene (Dantrium) is a direct-acting drug. The direct-acting drugs produce an antispasmodic effect at the level of the neuromuscular junction and skeletal muscle.

21.5 Treating Muscle Spasms Directly at the Muscle Tissue

Dantrolene relieves spasticity by interfering with the release of calcium ions in skeletal muscle. Other direct-acting drugs include botulinum toxin type A (Botox, Dysport) and botulinum toxin type B (Myobloc), used to offer significant relief of symptoms to people with dystonia; and quinine sulfate (Quinamm, Quiphile), which is used to treat leg cramps. Direct-acting drugs are summarized in Table 21.2.

Botulinum toxin is an unusual drug because, in higher quantities, it acts as a poison. *Clostridium botulinum* is the bacterium responsible for food poisoning or botulism. At lower doses, however, this drug is safe and effective as a muscle relaxant for patients with dystonia. It produces its effect by blocking the release of acetylcholine from cholinergic nerve terminals (Chapter 13 ∞).

Because of the extreme weakness associated with botulinum, therapies may be needed to improve muscle strength. To circumvent major problems with mobility or posture, botulinum toxin is often applied to small muscle groups. Sometimes this drug is administered with centrally acting oral medications to increase functional use of a range of muscle groups.

Drawbacks to botulinum therapy are its delayed and limited effects. The treatment is mostly effective within 6 weeks and lasts for only 3 to 6 months. Another drawback

TABLE 21.2   Direct-acting Antispasmodic Drugs

Drug	Route and Adult Dose (max dose where indicated)	Adverse Effects
NEUROMUSCULAR JUNCTION		
botulinum toxin type A (Botox, Dysport)	25 units injected directly into target muscle (max: 30-day dose should not exceed 200 units)	*Headache, dysphagia, ptosis, local muscle weakness, pain, muscle tenderness*
botulinum toxin type B (Myobloc)	2,500–5,000 units/dose injected directly into target muscle; doses should be divided among muscle groups	<u>Anaphylaxis, dysphagia, death</u>
quinine sulfate (Quinamm, Quiphile)	PO; 260–300 mg in the evening	
SKELETAL MUSCLE		
dantrolene sodium (Dantrium)	PO; 25 mg/day; increase to 25 mg bid–qid; may increase every 4–7 days up to 100 mg bid–tid	*Muscle weakness, dizziness, diarrhea* <u>Hepatic necrosis</u>

Italics indicate common adverse effects; <u>underlining</u> indicates serious adverse effects.

is pain; botulinum is injected directly into the muscle. Pain associated with injections is usually blocked by a local anesthetic.

NURSING CONSIDERATIONS

The role of the nurse in antispasmodic therapy involves careful monitoring of a client's condition and providing education as it relates to the prescribed drug treatment. Assess compliance with drug use, side effects, and expected outcomes. Centrally acting drugs such as cyclobenzaprine and chlorzoxazone should be avoided in clients with liver disease. Prior to beginning therapy assess for myasthenia gravis and narrow angle glaucoma because cyclobenzaprine and orphenadrine are contraindicated for these disorders. Perform a baseline assessment of the extent of muscle pain, stiffness, spasticity and rigidity because relief of these symptoms is used to gauge the success of pharmacotherapy.

Although dantrolene is a direct-acting muscle relaxant, its effects and precautions are similar to those of centrally acting drugs and is contraindicated in clients with liver disease, compromised pulmonary function, or cardiac dysfunction. Assess for jaundice and monitor hepatic laboratory values regularly during dantrolene therapy because the drug is hepatotoxic. The nurse should also be

---

Pr PROTOTYPE DRUG | Dantrolene Sodium *(Dantrium)* | Direct-acting Antisposmodic

ACTIONS AND USES

Dantrolene is often used for spasticity, especially for spasms of the head and neck. It directly relaxes muscle spasms by interfering with the release of calcium ions from storage areas inside skeletal muscle cells. It does not affect cardiac or smooth muscle. Dantrolene is especially useful for muscle spasms when they occur after spinal cord injury or stroke and in cases of cerebral palsy or multiple sclerosis, and occasionally for the treatment of muscle pain after heavy exercise. It is also used for the treatment of malignant hyperthermia.

ADMINISTRATION ALERTS

- Use oral suspension within several days because it does not contain a preservative.
- IV solution has a high pH and therefore is extremely irritating to tissue.
- Pregnancy category C.

PHARMACOKINETICS

Onset: 1–2 h

Peak: 5 h

Half-life: 4–8 h IV; 8–9 h PO

Duration: Variable

ADVERSE EFFECTS

Adverse effects include muscle weakness, drowsiness, dry mouth, dizziness, nausea, diarrhea, tachycardia, erratic blood pressure, photosensitivity, and urinary retention.

Contraindications: Clients with impaired cardiac or pulmonary function or hepatic disease should not take this drug.

INTERACTIONS

Drug–Drug: Dantrolene interacts with many other drugs. For example, it should not be taken with OTC cough preparations and antihistamines, alcohol, or other CNS depressants. Verapamil and other calcium channel blockers taken with dantrolene increase the risk of ventricular fibrillation and cardiovascular collapse.

Lab Tests: Unknown.

Herbal/Food: Unknown.

Treatment of Overdose: For acute overdosage, general supportive measures should be used.

 See the Companion Website for a Nursing Process Focus specific to this drug.

NURSING PROCESS FOCUS Clients Receiving Drugs for Muscle Spasms or Spasticity

Assessment	Potential Nursing Diagnoses
Prior to administration: ■ Obtain a complete health history including allergies, drug history, and possible drug interactions. ■ Obtain a complete physical examination. ■ Establish baseline level of consciousness and vital signs.	■ Pain (acute/chronic), related to muscle spasms ■ Physical Mobility, Impaired, related to acute/chronic pain ■ Injury, Risk for, related to drug side effects ■ Knowledge, Deficient, related to drug therapy

Planning: Client Goals and Expected Outcomes

The client will:
■ Report a decrease in pain, increase in range of motion, and reduction of muscle spasms.
■ Exhibit no adverse effects from the therapeutic regimen.
■ Demonstrate an understanding of the drug's action by accurately describing drug side effects and precautions.

Implementation

Interventions and (Rationales)	Client Education/Discharge Planning
■ Monitor LOC and vital signs. (Some skeletal muscle relaxants alter the client's LOC. Others within this class may alter blood pressure and heart rate.)	Instruct client to: ■ Avoid driving and other activities requiring mental alertness until effects of the medication are known. ■ Report any significant change in sensorium, such as slurred speech, confusion, hallucinations, or extreme lethargy. ■ Report palpitations, chest pain, dyspnea, unusual fatigue, weakness, and visual disturbances. ■ Avoid using other CNS depressants such as alcohol that will intensify sedation.
■ Monitor pain and determine location, duration, and precipitating factors. (Drugs should diminish client's pain.)	Instruct client to: ■ Report the development of new sites of muscle pain. ■ Use relaxation techniques, deep breathing, and meditation methods to facilitate relaxation and reduce pain.
■ Monitor for withdrawal reactions. (Abrupt withdrawal of baclofen may cause visual hallucinations, paranoid ideation, and seizures.)	■ Advise client not to abruptly discontinue treatment.
■ Monitor muscle tone, range of motion, and degree of muscle spasm. (This will determine effectiveness of drug therapy.)	■ Instruct client to perform gentle range-of-motion exercises, only to the point of mild physical discomfort, throughout the day.
■ Provide additional pain relief measures such as positional support, gentle massage, and moist heat or ice packs. (Drugs alone may not be sufficient in providing pain relief.)	■ Instruct client in complementary pain interventions such as positioning, gentle massage, and the application of heat or cold to the painful area.
■ Monitor for side effects such as drowsiness, dry mouth, dizziness, nausea, vomiting, faintness, headache, nervousness, diplopia, and urinary retention. (Cyclobenzaprine may cause these side effects.)	Instruct client to: ■ Report side effects. ■ Take medication with food to decrease GI upset. ■ Report signs of urine retention such as a feeling of urinary bladder fullness, distended abdomen, and discomfort.
■ Monitor for side effects such as muscle weakness, dry mouth, dizziness, nausea, diarrhea, tachycardia, erratic blood pressure, photosensitivity, and urine retention. (These adverse effects occur with certain drugs in this class.)	Instruct client: ■ That frequent mouth rinses, sips of water, and sugar-free candy or gum may help relieve dry mouth. ■ That medication may cause a decrease in muscle strength, and dosage may need to be reduced. ■ To use sunscreen and protective clothing when outdoors.

Evaluation of Outcome Criteria

Evaluate the effectiveness of drug therapy by confirming that patient goals and expected outcomes have been met (see "Planning").
■ The client reports a decrease in pain, increase in range of motion, and reduction of muscle spasm.
■ The client is free of adverse effects from the therapeutic regimen.
■ The client demonstrates an understanding of the drug's action by accurately describing drug side effects and precautions.

∞ *See Tables 21.1 and 21.2 for lists of drugs to which these nursing actions apply.*

SPECIAL CONSIDERATIONS

The New Fountain of Youth?

Seen as the new fountain of youth, botulinum toxin type A (Botox Cosmetic) injections were approved by the FDA for the temporary improvement in the appearance of moderate to severe frown lines (vertical lines between the brows) in adult patients aged 65 years or younger. It works to relax frown muscles by blocking nerve impulses that trigger wrinkle-causing muscle contractions, creating a smooth appearance between the brows. Administered in a few tiny injections of purified protein, this minimally invasive treatment is simple and quick, and delivers dramatic results with minimal discomfort. Results can be seen as early as 24 to 48 hours after injection, and the effect lasts up to 4 months. Injections should not be repeated more than once every 3 months. Side effects include headache, nausea, flulike symptoms, temporary eyelid drooping, mild pain, erythema at the injection site, and muscle weakness. According to the American Society for Aesthetic Plastic Surgery (ASAPS), Botox injections are the fastest growing cosmetic procedure in the industry. Plastic surgery events known as Botox parties—as well as seminars, evenings, and socials—are seen to be a key element of Botox marketing in much of the United States.

aware that a client with spasticity may not be able to self-medicate, and caregiver assistance may be required.

Lifespan Considerations. The disease processes and injuries that contribute to muscle spasms and spasticity may occur at any time throughout the client's lifespan. Although a stroke is usually associated with elderly clients, and cerebral palsy with events that occur in utero or during the birth process, either of these conditions may occur at other times in the lifespan. Because these conditions affect all age groups, the caregiver must be aware of the contraindications and adverse effects for all age groups. Nurses must also consider that some of the drugs used to treat these conditions are not recommended for pediatric clients or for women of childbearing age because of the effects on the fetus.

Client Teaching. Client education as it relates to centrally acting and direct-acting antispasmodics should include the goals of therapy, the reasons for obtaining baseline data such as vita signs and the existence of underlying cardiac or pulmonary disorders, and possible drug side effects. Include the following points when teaching clients about centrally acting and direct-acting antispasmodics:

- Avoid driving and other hazardous activities until effects of the medication are known.
- Immediately report changes in sensorium, palpitations, chest pain, dyspnea, unusual fatigue, visual disturbances, or signs of urine retention.
- Do not take any other prescribed drugs, OTC medications, herbal therapies, or vitamin supplements without notifying your healthcare provider.
- Discontinue alcohol use.
- Perform gentle range-of-motion exercises, only to the point of mild physical discomfort, throughout the day.
- Do not discontinue the drug suddenly because seizures may occur.

HOME & COMMUNITY CONSIDERATIONS

Muscle Relaxant Therapy in the Home Setting

Muscle spasms and spasticity are conditions that may affect clients throughout their lifespan. In today's society many of the clients who in the past resided in nursing homes and institutions are now being cared for at home by family members and home heath agencies. Also, the neurological diseases that affect young adults are being treated in the home/community setting. Thus, all age groups are able to be with their family members and live as normal a life as possible. The main factor to remember is that education and support for caregivers is extremely important to ensuring that clients are compliant with their therapy and that caregivers are competent to administer the therapy.

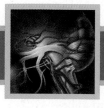

CHAPTER REVIEW

KEY CONCEPTS

The numbered key concepts provide a succinct summary of the important points from the corresponding numbered section within the chapter. If any of these points are not clear, refer to the numbered section within the chapter for review.

21.1 Muscle spasms, involuntary contractions of a muscle or group of muscles, most commonly occur because of localized trauma to the skeletal muscle.

21.2 Muscle spasms can be treated through nonpharmacological and pharmacological therapies.

21.3 Many muscle relaxants treat muscle spasms at the level of the CNS, generating their effect within the brain and/or spinal cord, usually by inhibiting upper motor neuron activity, causing sedation, or altering simple reflexes.

21.4 Spasticity, a condition in which selected muscles are continuously contracted, results from damage to the CNS. Effective treatment for spasticity includes both physical therapy and medications.

21.5 Some antispasmodic drugs used for spasticity act directly on muscle tissue, relieving spasticity by interfering with the release of calcium ions.

NCLEX-RN® REVIEW QUESTIONS

1 Cyclobenzaprine (Cycoflex, Flexeril) is prescribed for a client with muscle spasms of the lower back. Appropriate nursing intervention would include (select all that apply):

1. Assessing the heart rate for tachycardia.
2. Providing for client safety.
3. Encouraging frequent ambulation.
4. Providing oral suction for excessive oral secretions.
5. Assessing for rash.

2 The client is scheduled to receive botulinum toxin type B (Myoblocare) for treatment of muscle spasticity. Client education needed to prepare the client for the injections includes that:

1. Relief of muscle spasms should occur within several days.
2. Drowsiness may occur.
3. A rapid return of energy is to be expected.
4. Local anesthesia will be given to decrease the pain of the injections.

3 Prior to administration of cyclobenzaprine (Cycoflex, Flexeril), the nurse notes that the client's liver enzymes are elevated. The appropriate action would be to:

1. Hold the medication and report the elevation to the physician.
2. Give the medication as ordered.
3. Place the lab report on the medical record and await instructions from the physician.
4. Give the medication as ordered. Collect a blood sample for liver enzymes in 6 hours.

4 A client who was prescribed dantrolene sodium (Dantrium) reports taking verapamil (Calan) as part of the drug regimen. Appropriate nursing intervention includes:

1. Monitoring neurological status.
2. Holding the drug until the physician arrives.
3. Monitoring closely for cardiac dysrhythmias.
4. Monitoring renal function.

5 Which of the following statements made by the client prescribed dantrolene sodium (Dantrium) indicates an understanding of the side effects of the drug?

1. "I will be able to drive myself home from the hospital."
2. "I will not be concerned if I cannot empty my bladder; it's probably my prostate."
3. "I will be able to do my regular work as soon as I get home."
4. "I will report frequent changes in my blood pressure to my doctor."

CRITICAL THINKING QUESTIONS

1. A 46-year-old male quadriplegic client has been experiencing severe spasticity in the lower extremities, making it difficult for him to maintain position in his electric wheelchair. Prior to the episodes of spasticity, the client was able to maintain a sitting posture. The risks and benefits of therapy with dantrolene (Dantrium) have been explained to him, and he has decided that the benefits outweigh the risks. What assessments should the nurse make to determine whether the treatment is beneficial?

2. A 52-year-old breast cancer survivor is taking tamoxifen (Nolvadex) and has experienced leg and foot cramps "almost nightly." She states that these cramps have markedly decreased the quality of her sleep and that she is ready to "just stop taking" the tamoxifen to end the leg cramps. The nurse is aware that tamoxifen is considered important in the chemoprevention of breast cancer. What variety of treatment modalities can be offered this client to promote her comfort and decrease the chance that she will stop therapy?

3. A 32-year-old cotton farmer injured his lower back while unloading a truck at a farm cooperative. His healthcare provider started him on cyclobenzaprine (Flexeril) 10 mg tid for 7 days and referred him to outpatient physical therapy. After 4 days, the client reports back to the office nurse that he is constipated and having trouble emptying his bladder. Discuss the cause of these side effects.

See Appendix D for answers and rationales for all activities.

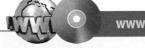

EXPLORE MediaLink

www.prenhall.com/adams

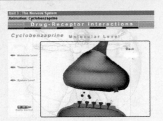

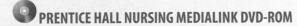

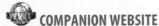

NCLEX-RN® review, case studies, and other interactive resources for this chapter can be found on the companion website at www.prenhall.com/adams. Click on "Chapter 21" to select the activities for this chapter. For animations, more NCLEX-RN® review questions, and an audio glossary, access the accompanying Prentice Hall Nursing MediaLink DVD-ROM in this textbook.

PRENTICE HALL NURSING MEDIALINK DVD-ROM

- **Animation**
  Mechanism in Action: Cyclobenzaprine (*Cycoflex, Flexeril*)
- **Audio Glossary**
- **NCLEX-RN® Review**

COMPANION WEBSITE

- **NCLEX-RN® Review**
- **Dosage Calculations**
- **Case Study:** Treating muscle spasms
- **Care Plan:** Female client who is paraplegic secondary to a skiing accident

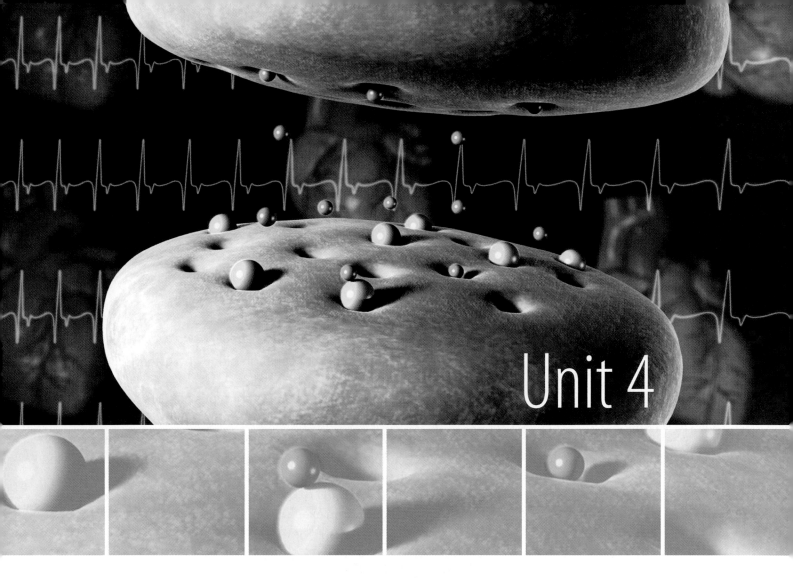

Unit 4

The Cardiovascular and Urinary Systems

CHAPTER 22 Drugs for Lipid Disorders

CHAPTER 23 Drugs for Hypertension

CHAPTER 24 Drugs for Heart Failure

CHAPTER 25 Drugs for Angina Pectoris and Myocardial Infarction

CHAPTER 26 Drugs for Dysrhythmias

CHAPTER 27 Drugs for Coagulation Disorders

CHAPTER 28 Drugs for Hematopoietic Disorders

CHAPTER 29 Drugs for Shock

CHAPTER 30 Diuretic Therapy and Drugs for Renal Failure

CHAPTER 31 Drugs for Fluid Balance, Electrolyte, and Acid–Base Disorders

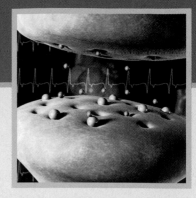

CHAPTER 22

Drugs for Lipid Disorders

DRUGS AT A GLANCE

HMG-COA REDUCTASE INHIBITORS
 ☞ *atorvastatin (Lipitor)*
BILE ACID RESINS
 ☞ *cholestyramine (Questran)*
NICOTINIC ACID
FIBRIC ACID AGENTS
 ☞ *gemfibrozil (Lopid)*
CHOLESTEROL ABSORPTION INHIBITORS

OBJECTIVES

After reading this chapter, the student should be able to:

1. Summarize the link between high blood cholesterol, LDL levels, and cardiovascular disease.
2. Compare and contrast the different types of lipids.
3. Illustrate how lipids are transported through the blood.
4. Compare and contrast the different types of lipoproteins.
5. Give examples of how cholesterol and LDL levels can be controlled through nonpharmacological means.
6. For each of the drug classes listed in Drugs at a Glance, know representative drug examples, and explain their mechanisms of action, primary actions, and important adverse effects.
7. Categorize antilipidemic drugs based on their classifications and mechanisms of action.
8. Explain the nurse's role in the pharmacological management of lipid disorders.
9. Use the Nursing Process to care for clients receiving drug therapy for lipid disorders.

MediaLink

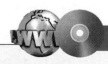

www.prenhall.com/adams

NCLEX-RN® review, case studies, and other interactive resources for this chapter can be found on the companion website at www.prenhall.com/adams. Click on "Chapter 22" to select the activities for this chapter. For animations, more NCLEX-RN® review questions, and an audio glossary, access the accompanying Prentice Hall Nursing MediaLink DVD-ROM in this textbook.

KEY TERMS

apoprotein *page 289*

atherosclerosis *page 287*

bile acid resin *page 293*

dyslipidemia *page 289*

high-density lipoprotein (HDL) *page 289*

HMG-CoA reductase *page 291*

hypercholesterolemia *page 289*

hyperlipidemia *page 289*

lecithin *page 287*

lipoprotein *page 289*

low-density lipoprotein (LDL) *page 289*

phospholipid *page 287*

reverse cholesterol transport *page 289*

rhabdomyolysis *page 291*

steroid *page 287*

sterol nucleus *page 287*

triglyceride *page 287*

very low-density lipoprotein (VLDL) *page 289*

Research during the 1960s and 1970s brought about a nutritional revolution as new knowledge about lipids and their relationship to obesity and cardiovascular disease allowed people to make more intelligent lifestyle choices. Since then, advances in the diagnosis of lipid disorders have helped identify those clients at greatest risk for cardiovascular disease and those most likely to benefit from pharmacologic intervention. Research in pharmacology has led to safe, effective drugs for lowering lipid levels, thus decreasing the risk of cardiovascular-related diseases. As a result of this knowledge and through advancements in pharmacology, the incidence of death due to most cardiovascular diseases has been declining, although cardiovascular disease remains the leading cause of death in the United States.

22.1 Types of Lipids

The three types of lipids important to humans are illustrated in ● Figure 22.1. The most common are the **triglycerides,** or neutral fats, which form a large family of different lipids all having three fatty acids attached to a chemical backbone of glycerol. Triglycerides are the major storage form of fat in the body and the only type of lipid that serves as an important energy source. They account for 90% of total lipids in the body.

A second class, the **phospholipids,** is formed when a phosphorus group replaces one of the fatty acids in a triglyceride. This class of lipids is essential to building plasma membranes. The best-known phospholipids are **lecithins,** which are found in high concentration in egg yolks and soybeans. Once promoted as a natural treatment for high cholesterol levels, controlled studies have not shown lecithin to be of any benefit for this disorder. Likewise, lecithin has been proposed as a remedy for nervous system diseases such as Alzheimer's disease and bipolar disorder, but there is no definite evidence to support these claims.

The third class of lipids is the **steroids,** a diverse group of substances having a common chemical structure called the **sterol nucleus,** or ring. Cholesterol is the most widely known of the steroids, and its role in promoting **atherosclerosis** has been clearly demonstrated. Cholesterol is a natural and vital component of plasma membranes. Unlike the triglycerides that provide fuel for the body during times of energy need, cholesterol serves as the building block for a number of essential biochemicals, including vitamin D, bile acids, cortisol, estrogen, and testosterone. Although cholesterol is clearly essential for life, the body needs only minute amounts of it. Moreover, the liver is able to synthesize adequate amounts of cholesterol from other chemicals; it is not necessary to provide additional cholesterol in the diet. Dietary cholesterol is obtained solely from animal products; humans do not metabolize the sterols produced by plants. The American Heart Association recommends intake of less than 300 mg of dietary cholesterol per day.

MediaLink

How Can I Lower My Cholesterol by Changing My Diet?

PHARMFACTS

High Blood Cholesterol

- The incidence of high blood cholesterol increases until age 65, at which time it levels off.
- More than 100 million Americans are estimated to have total blood cholesterol levels of 200 mg/dl or above. This is 40% to 50% of the adult population.
- Moderate alcohol intake does not reduce LDL-cholesterol, but it does increase HDL-cholesterol.
- Prior to menopause, high blood cholesterol occurs more frequently in men. After age 50, higher percentages of women have elevated cholesterol than men.
- To lower blood cholesterol, both dietary cholesterol and saturated fats must be reduced.
- Familial hypercholesterolemia affects 1 in 500 people and is a genetic disease that predisposes people to high cholesterol levels.

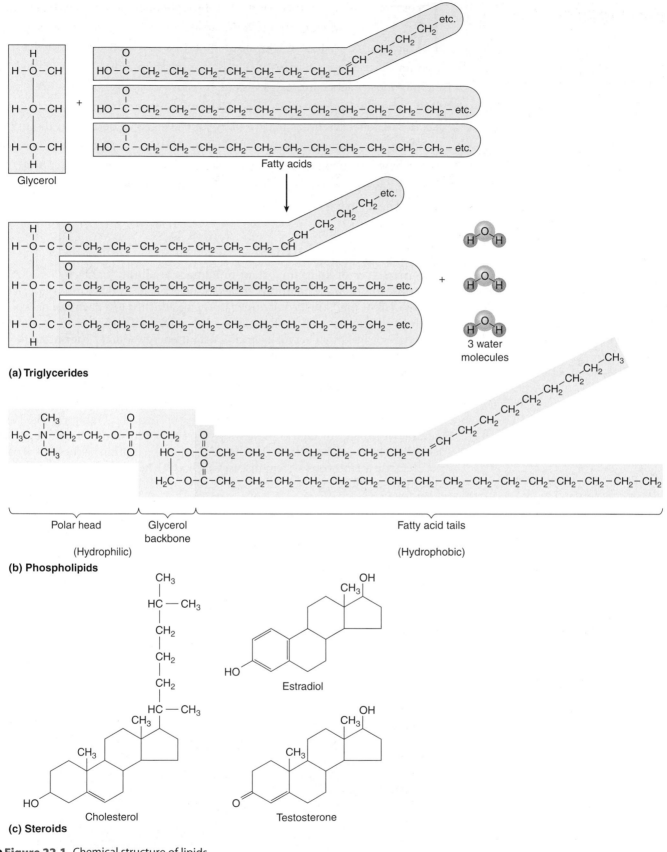

(a) Triglycerides

(b) Phospholipids

Polar head

Glycerol
backbone

(Hydrophilic)

Fatty acid tails

(Hydrophobic)

Fatty acids

3 water
molecules

Glycerol

(c) Steroids

Cholesterol

Estradiol

Testosterone

● **Figure 22.1** Chemical structure of lipids

22.2 Lipoproteins

Because lipid molecules are not soluble in plasma, they must be specially packaged for transport through the blood. To accomplish this transport, the body forms complexes called **lipoproteins,** which consist of various amounts of cholesterol, triglycerides, and phospholipids, along with a protein carrier. The protein component is called an **apoprotein** (*apo-* means "separated from or derived from").

The three most common lipoproteins are classified according to their composition, size, and weight or density, which is due primarily to the amount of apoprotein present in the complex. Each type varies in lipid and apoprotein makeup and serves a different function in transporting lipids from sites of synthesis and absorption to sites of utilization. For example, **high-density lipoprotein (HDL)** contains the most apoprotein, up to 50% by weight. The highest amount of cholesterol is carried by **low-density lipoprotein (LDL).** ● Figure 22.2 illustrates the three basic lipoproteins and their compositions.

To understand the pharmacotherapy of lipid disorders, it is important to learn the functions of the major lipoproteins and their roles in transporting cholesterol. LDL transports cholesterol from the liver to the tissues and organs, where it is used to build plasma membranes or to synthesize other steroids. Once in the tissues, cholesterol can also be stored for later use. Storage of cholesterol in the lining of blood vessels, however, is not desirable because it contributes to plaque buildup and atherosclerosis. LDL is often called "bad" cholesterol, because this lipoprotein contributes significantly to plaque deposits and coronary artery disease. **Very low–density lipoprotein (VLDL)** is the primary carrier of triglycerides in the blood. Through a series of steps, VLDL is reduced in size to become LDL. Lowering LDL levels in the blood has been shown to decrease the incidence of coronary artery disease.

HDL is manufactured in the liver and small intestine and assists in the transport of cholesterol away from the body tissues and back to the liver in a process called **reverse cholesterol transport.** The cholesterol component of the HDL is then broken down to unite with bile that is subsequently excreted in the feces. Excretion via bile is the only route the body uses to remove cholesterol. Because HDL transports cholesterol for destruction and removes it from the body, it is considered "good" cholesterol.

Hyperlipidemia, the general term meaning "high levels of lipids in the blood," is a major risk factor for cardiovascular disease. Elevated blood cholesterol, or **hypercholesterolemia,** is the type of hyperlipidemia that is most familiar to the general public. **Dyslipidemia** is the term that refers to abnormal (excess or deficient) levels of lipoproteins. Most clients with these disorders are asymptomatic and do not seek medical intervention until cardiovascular disease produces symptoms such as chest pain or signs of hypertension. Statistics suggest that more than half the adult

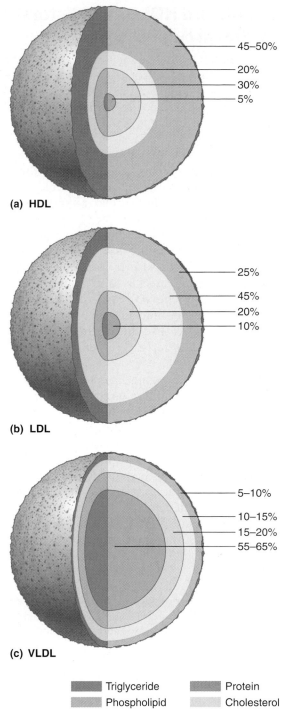

(a) HDL — 45–50%, 20%, 30%, 5%

(b) LDL — 25%, 45%, 20%, 10%

(c) VLDL — 5–10%, 10–15%, 15–20%, 55–65%

■ Triglyceride   ■ Protein
■ Phospholipid   ■ Cholesterol

● **Figure 22.2** Composition of lipoproteins: (a) HDL; (b) LDL; (c) VLDL

population in the United States have total cholesterol levels above 200 mg/dl and that two thirds of these clients are unaware of their hyperlipidemia.

The etiology of hyperlipidemia may be inherited or acquired. Certainly, diets high in saturated fats and lack of exercise contribute greatly to hyperlipidemia and resulting cardiovascular diseases. However, genetics determines ones ability to metabolize lipids and contributes to high lipid levels in substantial numbers of clients.

22.3 LDL and HDL as Predictors of Cardiovascular Disease

Although high serum cholesterol is associated with cardiovascular disease, it is not adequate to simply measure total cholesterol in the blood. Because some cholesterol is being transported for destruction, a more accurate profile is obtained by measuring LDL and HDL. The goal in maintaining normal cholesterol levels is to maximize the HDL and minimize the LDL. This goal is sometimes stated as a ratio of LDL to HDL. If the ratio is greater than 5.0 (5 times more LDL than HDL), the male client is considered at risk for cardiovascular disease. The normal ratio in women is slightly lower, at 4.5.

Scientists have further divided LDL into subclasses of lipoproteins. For example, one variety found in LDL, called lipoprotein (a), has been strongly associated with plaque formation and heart disease. It is likely that further research will discover other varieties, with the expectation that drugs will be designed to be more selective toward the "bad" lipoproteins. Table 22.1 gives the optimal, borderline, and high laboratory values for each of the major lipids and lipoproteins.

Establishing treatment guidelines for dyslipidemia has been difficult, as the condition has no symptoms, and the progression to cardiovascular disease may take decades. Based on years of research, the National Cholesterol Education Program (NCEP), an expert panel of the National Heart, Lung, and Blood Institute, recently revised the recommended treatment guidelines for dyslipidemia. The new guidelines are based on accumulated evidence that reducing "borderline" high cholesterol levels can result in fewer heart attacks and fewer deaths. Optimal levels of LDL cholesterol have been lowered from 130 mg/dl to 100 mg/dl. HDL cholesterol should now be at least 40 mg/dl, compared with

SPECIAL CONSIDERATIONS

Pediatric Dyslipidemias

Most people consider dyslipidemia a condition that occurs with advancing age. Dyslipidemias, however, are also a concern for some pediatric clients. Children at risk include those with a family history of premature coronary artery disease or dyslipidemia, and those who have hypertension, diabetes, or are obese. Lipid levels fluctuate in children and tend to be higher in girls. Nutritional intervention, regular physical activity, and risk factor management are warranted when the LDL level reaches 110 to 129 mg/dl. More aggressive dietary therapy and pharmacotherapy may be warranted in pediatric clients with LDL levels above 130 mg/dl. The long-term effects of lipid-lowering drugs in children have not been clearly established; therefore, drug therapy is not recommended below 10 years of age. Cholestyramine (Questran) and colestipol (Colestid) are the only approved drugs for hypercholesterolemia in children, although side effects sometimes result in poor compliance. Research into the use of niacin and low-dose statin pharmacotherapy in children is continuing.

the previous 35 mg/dl. In addition, the NCEP guidelines recommend that high cholesterol levels be treated more aggressively in people with diabetes, and that hormone replacement therapy not be considered as an alternative to cholesterol-lowering medications. The new guidelines will likely lead to more widespread use of medications to treat dyslipidemia.

22.4 Controlling Lipid Levels Through Lifestyle Changes

Lifestyle changes should always be included in any treatment plan for reducing blood lipid levels. Many clients with borderline laboratory values can control their dyslipidemia entirely through nonpharmacological means. It is important to note that all the lifestyle factors for reducing blood

TABLE 22.1	Standard Laboratory Lipid Profiles	
Type of Lipid	**Laboratory Value (mg/dl)**	**Standard**
total cholesterol	<200	desirable
	200–239	borderline high
	>239	high
LDL cholesterol	<100	optimal
	100–129	near or above optimal
	130–159	borderline high
	160–189	high
	>190	very high
HDL cholesterol	<40	low
	>60	high
triglycerides	<150	normal
	150–199	borderline high
	200–499	high
	>500	very high

lipid levels also apply to cardiovascular disease in general. Because many clients taking lipid-lowering drugs also have underlying cardiovascular disease, these lifestyle changes are particularly important. To emphasize the importance of lifestyle changes, clients should be taught that *all* drugs used for hyperlipidemia have side effects and, to the extent possible, that maintaining normal lipid values *without* pharmacotherapy should be a therapeutic goal. Following are the most important lipid-reduction lifestyle interventions:

- Monitor blood lipid levels regularly, as recommended by the healthcare provider.
- Maintain weight at an optimum level.
- Implement a medically supervised exercise plan.
- Reduce dietary saturated fats and cholesterol.
- Increase soluble fiber in the diet, as found in oat bran, apples, beans, grapefruit, and broccoli.
- Reduce or eliminate tobacco use.

Nutritionists recommend that the intake of dietary fat be less than 30% of the total caloric intake. Cholesterol intake should be reduced as much as possible but not exceed 300 mg/day. It is interesting to note that restriction of dietary cholesterol alone will not result in a significant reduction in blood cholesterol levels. This is because the liver reacts to a low-cholesterol diet by making more cholesterol and by inhibiting its excretion when saturated fats are present. Thus, the client must reduce saturated fat in the diet, as well as cholesterol, to control the amount made by the liver and to ultimately lower blood cholesterol levels.

The use of plant sterols and stanols is now recommended by the NCEP to reduce blood cholesterol levels. These plant lipids have a similar structure to cholesterol and therefore compete with that substance for absorption in the digestive tract. When the body absorbs the plant sterols, cholesterol is excreted from the body. When less cholesterol is delivered to the liver, LDL uptake increases, thereby decreasing serum LDL (the "bad" cholesterol) level. Plant sterols and stanols may be obtained from a variety of sources including wheat, corn, rye, oats, and rice, as well as nuts and olive oil. Commercially, stanols and sterols are available in products fortified with Reducol, found in margarines, salad dressings, certain cereals, and some fruit juices. According to the AHA, the recommended daily intake of plant sterols or stanols is 2 to 3 g.

HMG-CoA REDUCTASE INHIBITORS/STATINS

The statin class of antihyperlipidemics interferes with a critical enzyme in the synthesis of cholesterol. These agents, listed in Table 22.2, are first-line drugs in the treatment of lipid disorders.

22.5 Pharmacotherapy With Statins

In the late 1970s, compounds isolated from various species of fungi were found to inhibit cholesterol production in human cells in the laboratory. This class of drugs, known as the *statins*, has since revolutionized the treatment of lipid disorders. Statins can produce a dramatic 20% to 40% reduction in LDL-cholesterol levels. In addition to dropping the LDL-cholesterol level in the blood, statins can also lower triglyceride and VLDL levels, and raise the level of "good" HDL cholesterol.

Cholesterol is manufactured in the liver by a series of more than 25 metabolic steps, beginning with acetyl CoA, a two-carbon unit that is produced in the breakdown of fatty acids. Of the many enzymes involved in this complex pathway, **HMG-CoA reductase** (3-hydroxy-3-methylglutaryl coenzyme A reductase) serves as the primary regulatory site for cholesterol biosynthesis. Under normal conditions, this enzyme is controlled through negative feedback: High levels of LDL cholesterol in the blood will shut down production of HMG-CoA reductase, thus turning off the cholesterol pathway. ● Figure 22.3 illustrates selected steps in cholesterol biosynthesis and the importance of HMG-CoA reductase.

The statins act by inhibiting HMG-CoA reductase, which results in less cholesterol biosynthesis. As the liver makes less cholesterol, it responds by making more LDL receptors on the surface of liver cells. The greater number of LDL receptors in liver cells results in increased removal of LDL from the blood. Blood levels of both LDL and cholesterol are reduced. The drop in lipid levels is not permanent, however, so clients need to remain on these drugs during the remainder of their lives or until their hyperlipidemia can be controlled through dietary or lifestyle changes. Statins have been shown to slow the progression of coronary artery disease and to reduce mortality from cardiovascular disease. The mechanisms of action of the statins and other drugs for dyslipdidemia are illustrated in Pharmacotherapy Illustrated 22.1 (see page 294).

All the statins are given orally and are tolerated well by most clients. Minor side effects include headache, fatigue, muscle or joint pain, and heartburn. Severe myopathy and rhabdomyolysis are rare but serious adverse effects of the statins. **Rhabdomyolysis** is a breakdown of muscle fibers usually due to muscle trauma or ischemia. The mechanism by which statins cause this disorder is unknown. During rhabdomyolysis, contents of muscle cells spill into the systemic circulation causing potentially fatal acute renal failure. Macrolide antibiotics such as erythromycin, azole antifungals, fibric acid agents, and certain immunosuppressants should be avoided during statin therapy, since these interfere with statin metabolism and increase the risk of severe myopathy.

Many statins should be administered in the evening because cholesterol biosynthesis in the body is higher at night.

TABLE 22.2   Drugs for Dyslipidemias

Drug	Route and Adult Dose (max dose where indicated)	Adverse Effects
HMG-COA REDUCTASE INHIBITORS		
℗ atorvastatin (Lipitor)	PO; 10–80 mg/day	*Headache, dyspepsia, abdominal cramping, myalgia, rash or pruritus*
fluvastatin (Lescol)	PO; 20 mg/day (max: 80 mg/day)	
lovastatin (Mevacor)	PO; 20–40 mg/day in 1 or 2 doses	Rhabdomyolysis, severe myositis
pravastatin (Pravachol)	PO; 10–40 mg/day	
rosuvastatin (Crestor)	PO; 5–40 mg/day	
simvastatin (Zocor)	PO; 5–40 mg/day	
BILE ACID–BINDING AGENTS		
℗ cholestyramine (Questran)	PO; 4–8 g bid–qid ac and at bedtime	*Constipation, nausea, vomiting, abdominal pain, bloating, dyspepsia*
colesevelam (Welchol)	PO; 1,350 mg/day	
colestipol (Colestid)	PO; 5–15 g bid–qid ac and at bedtime	GI tract obstruction, vitamin deficiencies due to poor absorption
FIBRIC ACID AGENTS		
clofibrate (Atromid-S)	PO; 2 g/day in 2 to 4 divided doses	*Abdominal pain, rash, myalgia, fatigue, flulike syndrome, dyspepsia, nausea, vomiting, asthenia*
fenofibrate (Tricor)	PO; 54 mg/day (max: 160 mg/day)	
℗ gemfibrozil (Lopid)	PO; 600 mg bid (max: 1,500 mg/day)	Cholelithiasis, pancreatitis
OTHER AGENTS		
ezetimibe (Zetia)	Hyperlipidemia: PO; 10 mg/day	*Arthralgia, fatigue, abdominal pain, diarrhea*
		No serious side effects
niacin (Niac, Nicobid, others)	Hyperlipidemia: PO; 1.5–3.0 g/day in divided doses (max: 6 g/day) Niacin deficiency: PO; 10–20 mg/day	*Flushing, nausea, pruritus, headache, bloating, diarrhea*
		Dysrhythmias

Italics indicate common adverse effects; underlining indicates serious adverse effects.

Atorvastatin and rosuvastatin have longer half-lives and are effective regardless of the time of day they are taken.

Much research is ongoing to determine other therapeutic effects of drugs in the statin class. For example, statins block the vasoconstrictive effect of the A-beta protein, a significant protein involved in Alzheimer's disease. Cholesterol and A-beta protein have similar effects on blood vessels, causing them to constrict. Preliminary research suggests that the statins may protect against dementia by inhibiting the protein and thus slowing dementia caused by blood vessel constriction. Research also suggests that the statins may have the ability to lower the incidence of colorectal cancer.

NURSING CONSIDERATIONS

The role of the nurse in statin therapy for hyperlipidemia involves careful monitoring of a patient's condition and providing education as it relates to the prescribed drug treatment. First assess the client's laboratory tests for triglyceride, total cholesterol, LDL, and HDL levels. Although statin drugs are effective in reducing blood lipid levels, there can be serious adverse effects in some clients. Assess for pregnancy; statins should not be used in clients who may become pregnant, or are pregnant or breast-feeding.

Because liver dysfunction may occur with the use of statin drugs, monitor liver function tests before and during the first few months of therapy. Statin drugs should not be used in clients with active liver disease or unexplained elevations in liver function tests. Take a careful social history to assess alcohol use, because statins require cautious use in clients who drink large quantities of alcohol. Alcohol use should be restricted or discontinued while clients are taking this medication. Assess for complaints of muscle pain, tenderness, and weakness, which could indicate myopathy. Monitor creatine phosphokinase (CPK) levels if myopathy is suspected, and discontinue the drug if the levels are elevated. Statin therapy may also be discontinued if muscle weakness persists even without CPK elevation.

Assess the client for complaints of nausea, vomiting, heartburn, dyspepsia, abdominal cramping, and diarrhea, which are common but less serious side effects. Administer statins with the evening meal to help alleviate GI upset.

Lifespan Considerations.   Explain to women of childbearing age the importance of using effective birth control when taking statins. Instruct them to stop taking the medication if they suspect pregnancy.

Client Teaching.   Client education as it relates to statins should include the goals of therapy, the reasons for obtaining

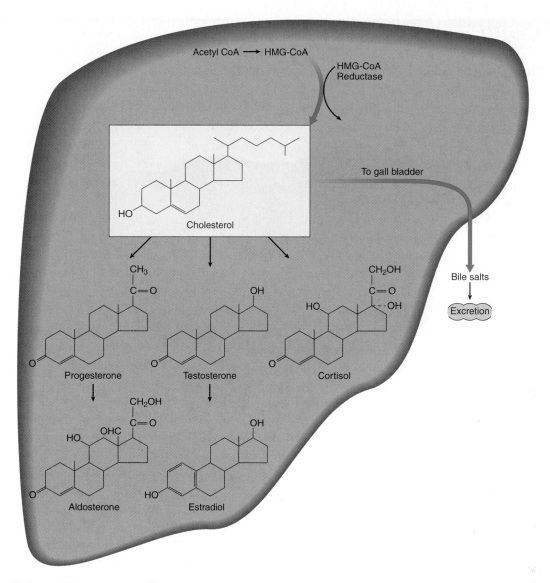

● **Figure 22.3** Cholesterol biosynthesis and excretion

baseline data such as vital signs and the existence of under-lying cardiac and hepatic disorders, and possible drug side effects. Include the following points when teaching clients about HMG-CoA reductase inhibitors:

- Keep all scheduled laboratory visits for liver function tests.
- Do not take other prescription drugs and OTC medications, herbal remedies, or vitamins and minerals without notifying your healthcare provider, because some antibiotics and immunosuppressants can increase the risk of severe myopathy.
- Avoid alcohol use.
- Practice reliable contraception and notify your health-care provider if pregnancy is planned or suspected.
- Immediately report unexplained muscle pain, tenderness, or weakness, especially if accompanied by malaise or fever.
- Immediately report unexplained numbness, tingling, weakness, or pain in feet or hands.
- Take the drug with the evening meal to prevent GI disturbances.

BILE ACID RESINS

Bile acid resins bind bile acids, thus increasing the excretion of cholesterol in the stool. They are sometimes used in combination with the statins. These agents are shown in Table 22.2.

22.6 Bile Acid Resins for Reducing Cholesterol and LDL Levels

Prior to the discovery of the statins, the primary means of lowering blood cholesterol was through use of bile acid–binding drugs. These drugs, called **bile acid resins** or sequestrants, bind bile acids, which contain a high concentration of cholesterol. Because of their large size, resins are not absorbed from the small intestine, and the bound bile acids and cholesterol are eliminated in the feces. The liver responds to the loss of cholesterol by making more LDL receptors, which removes even more cholesterol from the blood in a mechanism similar to that of the statin drugs.

PHARMACOTHERAPY ILLUSTRATED

22.1 Mechanism of Action of Lipid-lowering Drugs

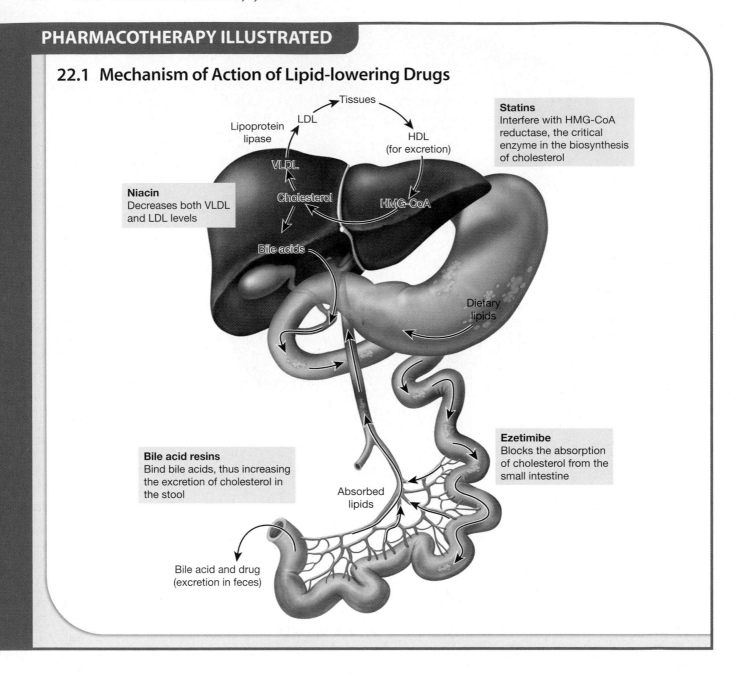

Statins
Interfere with HMG-CoA reductase, the critical enzyme in the biosynthesis of cholesterol

Niacin
Decreases both VLDL and LDL levels

Ezetimibe
Blocks the absorption of cholesterol from the small intestine

Bile acid resins
Bind bile acids, thus increasing the excretion of cholesterol in the stool

Tissues
LDL
Lipoprotein lipase
HDL (for excretion)
VLDL
Cholesterol
HMG-CoA
Bile acids
Dietary lipids
Absorbed lipids
Bile acid and drug (excretion in feces)

The bile acid resins are capable of producing a 20% drop in LDL cholesterol. They are no longer considered first-line drugs for dyslipidemia, although they are sometimes combined with statins for clients who are unable to achieve sufficient response from the statins alone.

The bile acid sequestrants tend to cause more frequent side effects than statins. Because they are not absorbed into the systemic circulation, side effects are limited to the GI tract, such as bloating and constipation. In addition to binding bile acids, these agents can also bind other drugs, such as digoxin and warfarin, thus increasing the potential for drug–drug interactions.

A new bile acid–binding agent, colesevelam (Welchol), was recently approved. This agent has more bile acid–binding capacity than the older resins and is formulated in smaller tablets that are easier to swallow. In addition, fewer tablets per day are required.

NURSING CONSIDERATIONS

The role of the nurse in bile acid sequestrant therapy for hyperlipidemia involves careful monitoring of the client's condition and providing education as it relates to the prescribed drug regimen. Because bile acid resins act in the GI tract and are not absorbed, they have no systemic side effects. They can, however, cause significant GI effects such as constipation, abdominal pain, bloating, nausea, vomiting, diarrhea, and steatorrhea. Take a careful history for past GI disorders such as peptic ulcer disease, hemorrhoids, inflammatory bowel disease, or chronic constipation. Bile acid sequestrants may worsen or aggravate these conditions. Also assess for a history of dysphagia or esophageal stricture, because this medication can cause obstruction. Be sure to assess bowel sounds during therapy. These drugs are generally not used during pregnancy or lactation (pregnancy category C).

Pr PROTOTYPE DRUG | Atorvastatin *(Lipitor)* | HMG-CoA Reductase Inhibitor/Statin

ACTIONS AND USES

The primary indication for atorvastatin is hypercholesterolemia. The statins act by inhibiting HMG-CoA reductase. As the liver makes less cholesterol, it responds by making more LDL receptors on the surface of liver cells. The greater number of LDL receptors in liver cells results in increased removal of LDL from the blood. Blood levels of both LDL and cholesterol are reduced, although at least 2 weeks of therapy is required before these effects are realized.

ADMINISTRATION ALERTS

- Administer with food to decrease GI discomfort.
- May be taken at any time of the day.
- Pregnancy category X.

PHARMACOKINETICS

Onset: 2 wk

Peak: Plasma concentration, 1–2 h; cholesterol reduction, 2–4 wk

Half-life: 14 h (20–30 h for active metabolites)

Duration: Unknown

ADVERSE EFFECTS

Side effects of atorvastatin are rarely severe enough to cause discontinuation of therapy and include GI complaints such as intestinal cramping, diarrhea, and constipation. A small percentage of clients experience liver damage; thus, hepatic function is monitored during the first few months of therapy.

Contraindications: Contraindications include serious liver disease, unexplained persistent elevations of serum transaminases, and prior hypersensitivity to the drug.

INTERACTIONS

Drug–Drug: Atorvastatin interacts with many other drugs. For example, it may increase digoxin levels by 20%, as well as increase levels of norethindrone and ethinyl estradiol (oral contraceptives). Erythromycin may increase atorvastatin levels 40%. Risk of rhabdomyolysis increases with concurrent administration of atorvastatin with macrolide antibiotics, cyclosporine, azole antifungals, and niacin.

Lab Tests: May increase serum transaminase and creatine kinase levels.

Herbal/Food: Grapefruit juice inhibits the metabolism of statins, allowing them to reach toxic levels. Since HMG-CoA reductase inhibitors also decrease the synthesis of coenzyme Q10 (CoQ10), clients may benefit from CoQ10 supplements. Manifestations of CoQ10 deficiency include high blood pressure, congestive heart failure, low energy.

Treatment of Overdose: There is no specific treatment for overdose.

 See the Companion Website for a Nursing Process Focus specific to this drug.

MediaLink

Mechanism in Action: Atorvastatin

Administer other medications, including vitamins and minerals, more than 1 hour before or 4 hours after the client takes a bile acid sequestrant to prevent decreased absorption of the medicines. Mix cholestyramine (Questran) powder with 60 to 180 ml of water, noncarbonated beverages, highly liquid soups, or pulpy fruits (applesauce, crushed pineapple) to prevent esophageal irritation. Place the contents of the packet of resin on the surface of fluid. Allow it to stand without stirring for 2 minutes, occasionally twirling the glass, and then stir slowly (to prevent foaming) to form a suspension. Have the client drink the medication immediately after stirring. Do not allow the client to inhale the powder, because it may irritate mucous membranes.

Lifespan Considerations. Colestipol and cholestyramine are the only antilipidemic drugs that are approved for use in children.

Client Teaching. Client education as it relates to bile acid resins should include the goals of therapy, the reasons for obtaining baseline data such as vital signs and the existence of underlying GI disorders, and possible drug side effects. Include the following points when teaching clients about bile acid resins:

- Take medication before meals.
- Take other medication 1 hour before or 4 hours after taking bile acid resins to avoid interference with absorption of other drugs.
- Follow a high-bulk diet and drink lots of fluids to decrease constipation and bloating.
- Take vitamin supplements to replace folic acid, fat-soluble vitamins, and vitamin K, because bile acid resins decrease the absorption of vitamins and minerals and can lead to hypokalemia.
- Do not take other prescription drugs and OTC medications, herbal remedies, or vitamins or minerals without notifying the healthcare provider.
- Immediately report yellowing of skin or whites of eyes, severe constipation, flatulence, nausea, heartburn, straining with passing of stools, tarry stools, or abnormal bleeding.

NATURAL THERAPIES

Coenzyme Q10 and Statins

Coenzyme Q10 (CoQ10) is a vitamin-like substance found in most animal cells. It is an essential component in the cell's mitochondria for producing energy or ATP. Because the heart requires high levels of ATP, a sufficient level of CoQ10 is essential to that organ. Supplementation with CoQ10 is especially important to some clients taking the HMG-CoA reductase inhibitors (statins), as these drugs significantly lower blood levels of CoQ10. Coenzyme Q10 and cholesterol share the same metabolic pathways. Inhibition of the enzyme HMG-CoA reductase concurrently decreases CoQ10 levels. Many of the adverse effects of statins may be due to the decrease in CoQ10 levels, including muscle weakness and rhabdomyolysis.

Foods richest in this substance are pork, sardines, beef heart, salmon, broccoli, spinach, and nuts. Elderly people appear to have an increased need for CoQ10. Although CoQ10 can be synthesized by the body, many amino acids and other substances are required for this synthesis; thus clients having nutritional deficiencies may need supplementation.

NURSING PROCESS FOCUS Clients Receiving HMG-CoA Reductase Inhibitor Therapy

Assessment	Potential Nursing Diagnoses
Prior to administration: ■ Obtain a complete health history including allergies, drug history, and possible drug interactions. ■ Obtain baseline liver function tests, lipid studies, and a pregnancy test in women of childbearing age.	■ Knowledge, Deficient, related to need for altered lifestyle ■ Noncompliance, related to dietary and drug regimen ■ Pain, Chronic, related to drug-induced myopathy ■ Health Maintenance, Impaired, related to insufficient knowledge of actions and effects of prescribed drug therapy

Planning: Client Goals and Expected Outcomes

The client will:
■ Demonstrate improved knowledge about appropriate lifestyle changes.
■ Demonstrate improved compliance to dietary and drug regimen.
■ Immediately report skeletal muscle pain, unexplained muscle soreness, or weakness.
■ Demonstrate an understanding of the drug's action by accurately describing drug side effects and precautions.
■ Have cholesterol levels and LDL to HDL ratios and liver enzymes within normal ranges.

Implementation

Interventions (and Rationales)	Client Education/Discharge Planning
■ Monitor blood cholesterol and triglyceride levels at intervals during therapy. (These levels determine effectiveness of therapy).	■ Advise client of the importance of keeping appointments for laboratory testing.
■ Monitor client compliance with dietary regimen. (Maintenance of controlled saturated-fat diet is essential to effectiveness of medications.)	■ Provide client with information needed to maintain low–saturated fat, low-cholesterol diet.
■ Monitor client for alcohol abuse. (Excessive alcohol intake may result in liver damage and interfere with drug effectiveness.)	■ Instruct client to avoid or limit alcohol use.
■ Monitor creatinine phosphokinase (CPK) level. (Elevated CPK may indicate impending myopathy.)	■ Instruct client to immediately report symptoms of leg or muscle pain.
■ Obtain client's smoking history. (Smoking increases risk of cardiovascular disease and may decrease HDL levels.)	■ Encourage client to cease smoking, if appropriate.

Evaluation of Outcome Criteria

Evaluate the effectiveness of drug therapy by confirming that client goals and expected outcomes have been met (see "Planning").
■ The client demonstrates increased knowledge about lifestyle changes
■ The client demonstrates compliance with appropriate lifestyle changes.
■ The client immediately reports skeletal muscle pain, unexplained muscle soreness, or weakness.
■ The client demonstrates an understanding of the drug's action by accurately describing drug side effects and precautions.
■ The client's cholesterol levels and LDL to HDL ratios and liver enzymes are within normal range.

∞ *See Table 22.2 for a list of drugs to which these nursing actions apply.*

NICOTINIC ACID (NIACIN)

Nicotinic acid is a vitamin that is occasionally used to lower lipid levels. It has a number of side effects that limit its use. The dose for nicotinic acid is given in Table 22.2.

22.7 Pharmacotherapy With Nicotinic Acid

Nicotinic acid, or niacin, is a B complex vitamin. Its ability to lower lipid levels, however, is unrelated to its role as a vitamin because much higher doses are needed to produce its antilipidemic effects. For lowering cholesterol, the usual dose of niacin is 2 to 3 g/day. When taken as a vitamin, the dose is only 25 mg/day. The primary effect of nicotinic acid is to decrease VLDL levels, and because LDL is synthesized from VLDL, the client experiences a reduction in LDL levels. It also has the desirable effects of reducing triglycerides and increasing HDL levels. As with other lipid-lowering drugs, maximum therapeutic effects may take a month or longer to achieve.

Although effective at reducing LDL levels by as much as 20%, nicotinic acid produces more side effects than the statins. Flushing and hot flashes occur in almost every client. In addition, a variety of uncomfortable intestinal effects such as nausea, excess gas, and diarrhea are commonly reported. More serious side effects such as hepatotoxicity and gout are possible. Niacin is not usually prescribed for clients with diabetes mellitus, because the drug can raise fasting glucose levels. Because of these adverse effects, nicotinic acid is most often used in lower

Pr **PROTOTYPE DRUG** | Cholestyramine *(Questran)* | Bile Acid Resin

ACTIONS AND USES

Cholestyramine is a powder that is mixed with fluid before being taken once or twice daily. It is not absorbed or metabolized once it enters the intestine; thus, it does not produce any systemic effects. It may take 30 days or longer to produce its maximum effect. Questran binds with bile acids (containing cholesterol) in an insoluble complex that is eliminated in the feces. Cholesterol levels decline owing to fecal loss.

ADMINISTRATION ALERTS

- Mix thoroughly with liquid and have the client drink it immediately to avoid potential irritation or obstruction in the GI tract.
- Give other drugs more than 2 hours before or 4 hours after client takes cholestyramine.
- Pregnancy category C.

PHARMACOKINETICS

Onset: 24–48 h

Peak: 1–3 wk

Half-life: Unknown

Duration: 2–4 wk

ADVERSE EFFECTS

Although cholestyramine rarely produces serious side effects, clients may experience constipation, bloating, gas, and nausea that sometimes limit its use.

Contraindications: This drug is contraindicated in clients with total biliary obstruction and in those with prior hypersensitivity to the drug.

INTERACTIONS

Drug–Drug: Because cholestyramine can bind to other drugs, such as digoxin, penicillins, thyroid hormone, and thiazide diuretics, and interfere with their absorption, it should not be taken at the same time as these other medications. Cholestyramine may increase the effects of anticoagulants by decreasing the levels of vitamin K in the body.

Lab Tests: Serum aspartate aminotransferase (AST), phosphorus, chloride, and alkaline phosphatase (ALP) levels may increase. Serum calcium, sodium, and potassium levels may decrease.

Herbal/Food: Taking cholestyramine with food interferes with the absorption of the following essential nutrients: Beta-carotene, calcium, folic acid, iron, magnesium, vitamin B_{12}, vitamin D, vitamin E, vitamin K, and zinc; manifestations of nutrient depletion include weakened immune system, cardiovascular problems, and osteoporosis.

Treatment of Overdose: There is no specific treatment for overdose.

 See the Companion Website for a Nursing Process Focus specific to this drug.

---

doses in combination with a statin or bile acid–binding agent, because the beneficial effects of these drugs are additive. Taking one aspirin tablet 30 minutes prior to niacin administration can reduce uncomfortable flushing in many clients.

Because niacin is available without a prescription, clients should be instructed not to attempt self-medication with this drug. One form of niacin available OTC as a vitamin supplement called nicotinamide has no lipid-lowering effects. Clients should be informed that if nicotinic acid is to be used to lower cholesterol, it should be done under medical supervision.

NURSING CONSIDERATIONS

The role of the nurse in niacin therapy for hyperlipidemia involves careful monitoring of a client's condition and providing education as it relates to the prescribed drug regimen. Assess liver function prior to and during therapy to monitor risk of liver toxicity, particularly when clients are taking sustained-release formulas. Clients with elevated liver enzymes, a history of liver disease, or peptic ulcers should not take niacin to lower lipids, because this medication can worsen these conditions. In clients predisposed to gout, nicotinic acid may increase uric acid levels and precipitate acute gout.

Administer one aspirin 30 minutes prior to the nicotinic acid dose to help decrease a flushing response with pruritus, which can occur 1 to 2 hours after taking the drug. Aspirin helps decrease prostaglandin release that may cause a flushing effect, which decreases with time. Monitor blood sugar levels of diabetic clients more frequently until the effect of nicotinic acid is known, because the drug can affect glycemic control. Give the medication with food to help decrease GI side effects.

Client Teaching. Client education as it relates to nicotinic acid should include the goals of therapy; the reasons for obtaining baseline data such as vital signs and the existence of underlying cardiac, hepatic, and renal disorders; and possible drug side effects. Include the following points when teaching clients about nicotinic acid:

- Do not take megadoses of niacin because of the risk of serious toxic effects.
- Take niacin with cold water, because hot beverages increase flushing.
- Take with or after meals to prevent GI upset.
- Do not take other prescription drugs and OTC medications, herbal remedies, or vitamins or minerals without notifying the healthcare provider.
- Immediately report flank, joint, or stomach pain; skin color changes (advise client to stay out of the sun if skin changes occur); and yellowing of the whites of eyes.

FIBRIC ACID AGENTS

Once widely used to lower lipid levels, the fibric acid agents have been largely replaced by the statins. They are sometimes used in combination with the statins. The fibric acid agents are shown in Table 22.2.

22.8 Pharmacotherapy With Fibric Acid Agents

The first fibric acid agent, clofibrate (Atromid-S), was widely prescribed until a 1978 study determined that it did not reduce mortality from cardiovascular disease. In fact, clofibrate was found to *increase* overall mortality compared with a control group. Although clofibrate is now rarely prescribed, two other fibric acid agents, fenofibrate (Tricor) and gemfibrozil (Lopid), are sometimes indicated for clients with excessive triglyceride and VLDL levels. They are drugs of choice for treating severe hypertriglyceridemia. Combining a fibric acid agent with a statin results in greater decreases in triglyceride levels than using either drug used alone. The mechanism of action of the fibric acid agents is largely unknown.

NURSING CONSIDERATIONS

The role of the nurse in fibric acid therapy for hypertriglyceridemia involves careful monitoring of the client's condition and providing education as it relates to the prescribed drug regimen. Prior to administering fibric acid, assess the client for complaints of abdominal pain, nausea, and vomiting. These are the most common adverse effects of the drug therapy, so knowing baseline complaints will enable you to determine if later complaints are a result of drug therapy or an underlying problem. Obtain an accurate drug history. Using fibric acid agents with statin drugs increases the risk of myositis. Using these agents with warfarin (Coumadin) may potentiate the effects of the anticoagulant, so lower warfarin doses will be needed. Monitor prothrombin time and international normalized ratio (PT/INR) more frequently until these values stabilize. Assess for pregnancy, because fibric acid is generally not used in lactation or pregnancy (category B). Assess for history of gallbladder or biliary disease. Clofibrate has a tendency to concentrate bile and cause gallbladder disease. This increase in gallbladder disease has not been seen with other fibric acid agents, but drugs in this class are generally not used in clients with preexisting gallbladder or biliary disease.

Administer the medication with meals to decrease GI distress. Monitor client for signs of increased clotting time, such as bruising and bleeding from gums, nose, and vagina. Monitor for side effects such as symptoms of cholelithiasis or cholecystitis.

Client Teaching.   Client education as it relates to fibric acid therapy should include the goals of therapy, the reasons for obtaining baseline data such as vital signs and the existence of underlying cardiac and renal disorders, and possible drug side effects. Include the following points when teaching clients about fibric acid agents:

- Keep all scheduled medical follow-up visits and laboratory visits for testing.
- Immediately report unusual bruising or bleeding, right upper quadrant pain, changes in stool color, or muscle cramping.

CHOLESTEROL ABSORPTION INHIBITORS

In the early 2000s, a new class of drugs was discovered that inhibits the absorption of cholesterol. There is only one drug in this class, ezetimibe (Vytorin), which is listed in Table 22.2.

Pr PROTOTYPE DRUG | Gemfibrozil (Lopid) | Fibric Acid Agent

ACTIONS AND USES

Effects of gemfibrozil include up to a 50% reduction in VLDL with an increase in HDL. The mechanism of achieving this action is unknown. It is less effective than the statins at lowering LDL; thus, it is not a drug of first choice for reducing LDL levels. Gemfibrozil is taken orally at 600 to 1,200 mg/day.

ADMINISTRATIVE ALERT

- Administer with meals to decrease GI distress.
- Pregnancy category B.

PHARMACOKINETICS

Onset: 1–2 h

Peak: 1–2 h

Half-life: 1.5 h

Duration: 2–4 mo

ADVERSE EFFECTS

Gemfibrozil produces few serious adverse effects, but it may increase the likelihood of gallstones and occasionally affect liver function. The most common side effects are GI related: diarrhea, nausea, and cramping.

Contraindications: Gemfibrozil is contraindicated in clients with hepatic impairment, severe renal dysfunction, or preexisting gallbladder disease, or those with prior hypersensitivity to the drug.

INTERACTIONS

Drug–Drug: Concurrent use of gemfibrozil with oral anticoagulants may potentiate anticoagulant effects. Use with lovastatin increases the risk of myopathy and rhabdomyolysis.

Lab Tests: May increase liver enzyme values, and CPK and serum glucose levels. May decrease hemoglobin (Hgb), hematocrit (Hct), and WBC counts.

Herbal/Food: Fatty foods may decrease the efficacy of gemfibrozil.

Treatment of Overdose: There is no specific treatment for overdose.

 See the Companion Website for a Nursing Process Focus specific to this drug.

22.9 Pharmacotherapy With Cholesterol Absorption Inhibitors

Cholesterol is absorbed from the intestinal lumen by cells in the jejunum of the small intestine. Ezetimibe blocks this absorption by as much as 50%, causing less cholesterol to enter the blood. Unfortunately the body responds by synthesizing more cholesterol; thus, a statin may be administered concurrently.

When given as monotherapy, ezetimibe produces a modest reduction in LDL of about 20%. Adding a statin to the therapeutic regimen reduces LDL by an *additional* 15% to 20%. Vytorin is a combination tablet containing fixed-dose combinations of ezetimibe and simvastatin. Because bile acid sequestrants inhibit the absorption of ezetimibe, these drugs should not be taken together.

AVOIDING MEDICATION ERRORS

The nurse administers the following oral medications ordered for a 64-year-old man: tetracycline 500 mg bid, digoxin 0.25 mg/day, and cholestyramine (Questran) 4 g bid ac and at bed time. At 8 A.M., before breakfast, the nurse administers tetracycline 500 mg, Lanoxin 0.25 mg, and cholestyramine 4 mg. What should the nurse have done differently?
See Appendix D for the suggested answer.

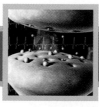

CHAPTER REVIEW

KEY CONCEPTS

The numbered key concepts provide a succinct summary of the important points from the corresponding numbered section within the chapter. If any of these points are not clear, refer to the numbered section within the chapter for review.

22.1 Lipids can be classified into three types, based on their chemical structures: triglycerides, phospholipids, and sterols. Triglycerides and cholesterol are blood lipids that can lead to atherosclerotic plaque.

22.2 Lipids are carried through the blood as lipoproteins; VLDL and LDL are associated with an increased incidence of cardiovascular disease, whereas HDL exerts a protective effect.

22.3 Blood lipid profiles are important diagnostic tools in guiding the therapy of dyslipidemias.

22.4 Before starting pharmacotherapy for hyperlipidemia, clients should seek to control the condition through lifestyle changes such as restriction of dietary saturated fats and cholesterol, increased exercise, and smoking cessation.

22.5 Statins, which inhibit HMG-CoA reductase, a critical enzyme in the biosynthesis of cholesterol, are drugs of first choice in reducing blood lipid levels.

22.6 The bile acid resins bind bile and cholesterol and accelerate their excretion. These agents can reduce cholesterol and LDL levels but are not drugs of choice owing to their side effects.

22.7 Nicotinic acid, or niacin, can reduce LDL levels, but side effects limit its usefulness.

22.8 Fibric acid agents lower triglyceride levels but have little effect on LDL. They are not drugs of choice because of their potential side effects.

22.9 The newest class of antilipidemic drugs includes ezetimibe, which acts by inhibiting the absorption of cholesterol across the small intestine.

NCLEX-RN® REVIEW QUESTIONS

1 The nurse assesses the client on HMG-CoA reductase inhibitors for:

1. Constipation.
2. Muscle weakness and pain.
3. Hemorrhoids.
4. Hypokalemia.

2 When evaluating the effectiveness of nicotinic acid, the nurse would monitor for:

1. Increased VLDL levels and increased LDL levels.
2. Increased VLDL levels and decreased LDL levels.
3. Decreased VLDL levels and decreased LDL levels.
4. Maintenance of VLDL and LDL levels.

3 The nurse is providing care to a client on nicotinic acid and realizes which of the following are side effects of the medication? (Select all that apply.)

1. Nausea
2. Diarrhea
3. Constipation
4. Excess flatulence
5. Flushing and hot flashes

4 The nurse teaches the client with a diagnosis of hyperlipidemia about lipids in the body. The nurse informs the client that the major storage form of fat in the body is:

1. Phospholipids.
2. Steroids.
3. Triglycerides.
4. Lecithins.

5 The nurse evaluates the effectiveness of drug therapy for hyperlipidemia. Effective therapy is evidenced by:

1. HDL, 35 mg/dl; LDL, 130 mg/dl.
2. HDL, 38 mg/dl; LDL, 135 mg/dl.
3. HDL, 40 mg/dl; LDL, 100 mg/dl.
4. HDL, 25 mg/dl; LDL, 175 mg/dl.

CRITICAL THINKING QUESTIONS

1. Identify the plan of care for a client with hyperlipidemia who has been prescribed atorvastatin (Lipitor).

2. A client is put on cholestyramine (Questran) for elevated lipids. What teaching is important for this client?

3. A male diabetic client presents to the emergency department with complaints of being flushed and having "hot flashes."

The client admits to self-medicating with niacin for elevated lipids. What is the nurse's response?

See Appendix D for answers and rationales for all activities.

EXPLORE
MediaLink

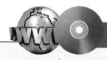 www.prenhall.com/adams

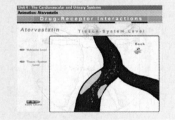

NCLEX-RN® review, case studies, and other interactive resources for this chapter can be found on the companion website at www.prenhall.com/adams. Click on "Chapter 22" to select the activities for this chapter. For animations, more NCLEX-RN® review questions, and an audio glossary, access the accompanying Prentice Hall Nursing MediaLink DVD-ROM in this textbook.

PRENTICE HALL NURSING MEDIALINK DVD-ROM

- **Animation**
  Mechanism in Action: Atorvastatin (*Lipitor*)
- **Audio Glossary**
- **NCLEX-RN® Review**

COMPANION WEBSITE

- **NCLEX-RN® Review**
- **Dosage Calculations**
- **Case Study:** Controlling lipid levels
- **Care Plan:** Client with elevated LDH levels

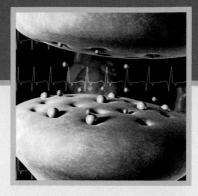

CHAPTER 23

Drugs for Hypertension

DRUGS AT A GLANCE

DIURETICS
- *hydrochlorothiazide (HydroDIURIL)*

CALCIUM CHANNEL BLOCKERS
- *nifedipine (Procardia)*

DRUGS AFFECTING THE RENIN–ANGIOTENSIN SYSTEM

Angiotensin-converting Enzyme (ACE) Inhibitors
- *enalapril (Vasotec)*

Angiotensin-receptor Blockers

ADRENERGIC ANTAGONISTS

Alpha-adrenergic Blockers
- *doxazosin (Cardura)*

BETA-ADRENERGIC BLOCKERS

CENTRALLY ACTING AGENTS

DIRECT VASODILATORS
- *hydralazine (Apresoline)*

OBJECTIVES

After reading this chapter, the student should be able to:

1. Explain how hypertension is classified.
2. Summarize the long-term consequences of untreated hypertension.
3. Explain the effects of cardiac output, peripheral resistance, and blood volume on blood pressure.
4. Discuss how the vasomotor center, baroreceptors, chemoreceptors, emotions, and hormones influence blood pressure.
5. Discuss the role of therapeutic lifestyle changes in the management of hypertension.
6. Differentiate between drug classes used for the primary treatment of hypertension and those secondary agents reserved for persistent hypertension.
7. Describe the nurse's role in the pharmacological management of clients receiving drugs for hypertension.
8. For each of the drug classes listed in Drugs at a Glance, know representative drug examples, and explain their mechanisms of drug action, primary actions, and important adverse effects.
9. Use the Nursing Process to care for clients receiving antihypertensive drugs.

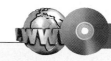

MediaLink

www.prenhall.com/adams

NCLEX-RN® review, case studies, and other interactive resources for this chapter can be found on the companion website at www.prenhall.com/adams. Click on "Chapter 23" to select the activities for this chapter. For animations, more NCLEX-RN® review questions, and an audio glossary, access the accompanying Prentice Hall Nursing MediaLink DVD-ROM in this textbook.

KEY TERMS

aldosterone *page 317*

angiotensin II *page 317*

angiotensin-converting enzyme (ACE)
  page 317

antidiuretic hormone (ADH) *page 304*

baroreceptors *page 304*

benign prostatic hyperplasia (BPH) *page 322*

calcium channel blocker (CCB) *page 311*

cardiac output *page 303*

chemoreceptors *page 304*

diuretic *page 304*

electrolytes *page 308*

hypertension (HTN) *page 302*

orthostatic hypotension *page 309*

peripheral resistance *page 304*

reflex tachycardia *page 314*

renin–angiotensin system *page 305*

stroke volume *page 303*

vasomotor center *page 304*

Cardiovascular disease (CVD), which includes all conditions affecting the heart and blood vessels, is the most frequent cause of death in the United States. Hypertension, or high blood pressure, is the most common of the cardiovascular diseases. According to the American Heart Association, high blood pressure is associated with more than 150,000 deaths in the United States each year. Although mild hypertension (HTN) can often be controlled with lifestyle modifications, moderate to severe HTN requires pharmacotherapy.

Because nurses encounter numerous clients with this condition, having an understanding of the underlying principles of antihypertensive therapy is essential. By improving public awareness of hypertension and teaching the importance of early intervention, the nurse can contribute significantly to reducing cardiovascular mortality.

23.1 Definition and Classification of Hypertension

Hypertension (HTN) is defined as the consistent elevation of systemic arterial blood pressure. The diagnosis of chronic HTN is rarely made on a single blood pressure measurement. A client with a sustained systolic blood pressure of greater than 140 mm Hg or diastolic pressure of greater than 90 to 99 mm Hg after multiple measurements are made over several clinic visits is said to have HTN.

Many attempts have been made to further define HTN, to develop guidelines for treatment. In 2003 the National High Blood Pressure Education Program Coordinating Committee of the National Heart, Lung, and Blood Institute of the National Institutes of Health determined the need for new guidelines that addressed the relationship between blood pressure and the risk of cardiovascular disease. This committee issued The Seventh Report of the Joint National Committee on Prevention, Detection, Evaluation, and Treatment of High Blood Pressure (JNC-7), which has become the standard for treating HTN. The recommendations from Committee Report JNC-7 are summarized in Table 23.1.

In addition to classifying HTN into three categories—prehypertension, Stage 1, and Stage 2—the JNC-7 report issued remarkable data regarding the disease.

• The risk of cardiovascular disease beginning at 115/75 mm Hg doubles with each additional increment of 20/10 mm Hg.

• Individuals with a systolic blood pressure of 120 to 139 mm Hg or a diastolic blood pressure of 80 to 89 mm Hg should be considered as prehypertensive.

PHARMFACTS

Statistics of Hypertension

- Prehypertension (120–139/80–89 mm Hg) affects approximately 22% of the adult population, or nearly 45 million people.
- High blood pressure affects more than 50 million U.S. adults, or approximately 1 in 4 Americans.
- People with diabetes are 2 to 3 times more likely to have hypertension than nondiabetics.
- Hypertension is responsible for more than 35 million office visits each year.
- African Americans have the highest rate (33%) of hypertension.
- Among people with HTN, more than 32% do not realize they have the condition.
- Hypertension is the most common complication of pregnancy.
- Approximately 40,000 Americans die of HTN per year; it is a contributing factor in 223,000 additional deaths each year.

TABLE 23.1   Classification and Management of Hypertension in Adults

BP Classification	SBP* mm Hg	DBP* mm Hg	Lifestyle Modification	Initial Drug Therapy Without Compelling Indication	With Compelling Indication
Normal	<120	and <80	Encourage		
Prehypertension	120–139	or 80–89	Yes	No antihypertensive drug indicated.	Drug(s) for compelling indications‡
Stage 1 hypertension	140–159	or 90–99	Yes	Thiazide-type diuretics for most. May consider ACEI, ARB, BB, CCB, or combination.	Drug(s) for the compelling indications:‡ Other antihypertensive drugs (diuretics, ACEI, ARB, BB, CCB) as needed).
Stage 2 hypertension	≥160	or ≥100	Yes	Two-drug combination for most† (usually thiazide-type diuretic and ACEI or ARB or BB or CCB).	

DBP, diastolic blood pressure; SBP, systolic blood pressure.
Drug abbreviations: ACEI, angiotensin-converting enzyme inhibitor; ARB, angiotensin-receptor blocker; BB, beta blocker; CCB, calcium channel blocker.
*Treatment determined by highest BP category.
†Initial combined therapy should be used cautiously in those at risk for orthostatic hypotension.
‡Treat patients with chronic kidney disease or diabetes to BP goal of <130/80 mm Hg.
Compelling indications include HF, post-MI, high risk for coronary artery disease, diabetes, chronic kidney disease, and recurrent stroke prevention.
Source: JNC-7 Express. (2003) The Seventh Report of the Joint National Committee on Prevention, Detection, Evaluation and Treatment of High Blood Pressure by National High Blood Pressure Education Program, National Heart, Lung & Blood Institute. Retrieved November 1, 2006, from www.nhlbi.nih.gov.

These clients should be strongly encouraged by the nurse to adopt health-promoting lifestyle modifications to prevent CVD.

• Clients with prehypertension are at increased risk for progression to HTN; those in the 130 to 139/80 to 89 mm Hg blood pressure range are at twice the risk for developing HTN as those with lower values.

Blood pressure changes throughout the lifespan, gradually and continuously rising from childhood through adulthood. What is considered normal blood pressure at one age may be considered abnormal in someone older or younger. Table 23.2 shows the normal variation in blood pressure in clients that occurs throughout the life span. Hypertension has the greatest impact on elderly clients, affecting approximately 30% of those older than 50 years, 64% of men older than age 65, and 75% of women older than age 75.

23.2 Factors Responsible for Blood Pressure

Although many factors can influence blood pressure, the three factors responsible for creating the pressure are cardiac output, blood volume, and peripheral resistance. These are shown in ● Figure 23.1. An understanding of these factors is essential for relating the pathophysiology of HTN to its pharmacotherapy.

The volume of blood pumped per minute is the **cardiac output.** The higher the cardiac output, the higher the blood pressure. Cardiac output is determined by heart rate and **stroke volume,** the amount of blood pumped by a ventricle in one contraction. This is important to pharmacology, because

TABLE 23.2   Variation in Blood Pressure Thoughout the Lifespan

Age (years)	Men (mm Hg)	Women (mm Hg)
1	96/66	95/65
5	92/62	92/62
10	103/69	103/70
20–24	123/76	116/72
30–34	126/79	120/75
40–44	129/81	127/80
50–54	135/83	137/84
60–64	142/85	144/85
70–74	145/82	159/85
80+	145/82	157/83

MediaLink   The American Society of Hypertension

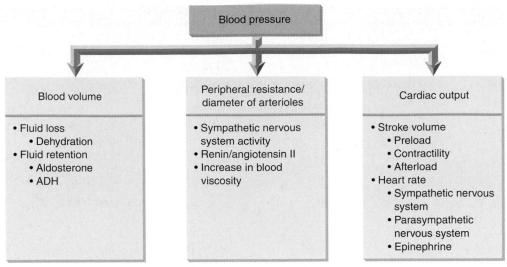

● Figure 23.1 Primary factors affecting blood pressure

drugs that change the cardiac output, stroke volume, or heart rate have the potential to influence a client's blood pressure.

As blood flows at high speeds through the vascular system, it exerts force against the walls of the vessels. Although the inner layer of the blood vessel lining, the endothelium, is extremely smooth, friction reduces the velocity of the blood. This friction in the arteries is called **peripheral resistance.** Arteries have smooth muscle in their walls that when constricted, will cause the inside diameter or lumen to become smaller, thus creating more resistance and higher pressure. A large number of drugs affect vascular smooth muscle, causing vessels to constrict, thus raising blood pressure. Other drugs cause the smooth muscle to relax, thereby opening the lumen and lowering blood pressure. The role of the autonomic nervous system in controlling peripheral resistance is explained in Chapter 13 ∞.

The third factor responsible for blood pressure is the total amount of blood in the vascular system, or blood volume. Although an average person maintains a relatively constant blood volume of approximately 5 L, this value can change owing to many regulatory factors, certain disease states, and pharmacotherapy. More blood in the vascular system will exert additional pressure on the walls of the arteries and raise blood pressure. Drugs are frequently used to adjust blood volume. For example, infusion of intravenous fluids increases blood volume and raises blood pressure. This factor is used to advantage when treating hypotension due to shock (Chapter 29 ∞). In contrast, substances known as **diuretics** can cause fluid loss through urination, thus decreasing blood volume and lowering blood pressure.

23.3 Physiological Regulation of Blood Pressure

It is critical that the body maintain a normal range of blood pressure and that it has the ability to safely and rapidly change pressure as it proceeds through daily activities such

as sleep and exercise. Hypotension can cause dizziness and lack of adequate urine formation, whereas extreme hypertension can cause blood vessels to rupture, or restrict blood flow to critical organs. ● Figure 23.2 illustrates how the body maintains homeostasis during periods of blood pressure change.

The central and autonomic nervous systems are intimately involved in regulating blood pressure. On a minute-to-minute basis, a cluster of neurons in the medulla oblongata called the **vasomotor center** regulates blood pressure. Nerves travel from the vasomotor center to the arteries, where the smooth muscle is directed to either constrict (raise blood pressure) or relax (lower blood pressure). Sympathetic outflow from the vasomotor center stimulates alpha$_1$-adrenergic receptors on arterioles, causing vasoconstriction (Chapter 13 ∞).

Receptors in the aorta and the internal carotid artery act as sensors to provide the vasomotor center with vital information on conditions in the vascular system. **Baroreceptors** have the ability to sense pressure within blood vessels, whereas **chemoreceptors** recognize levels of oxygen and carbon dioxide, and the pH in the blood. The vasomotor center reacts to information from baroreceptors and chemoreceptors by raising or lowering blood pressure accordingly. With aging or certain disease states such as diabetes, the baroreceptor response may be diminished.

Emotions can also have a profound effect on blood pressure. Anger and stress can cause blood pressure to rise, whereas mental depression and lethargy may cause it to fall. Strong emotions, if present for a prolonged time period, may become important contributors to chronic hypertension.

A number of hormones and other agents affect blood pressure on a daily basis. When given as medications, some of these agents may have a profound effect on blood pressure. For example, injection of epinephrine or norepinephrine will immediately raise blood pressure. **Antidiuretic**

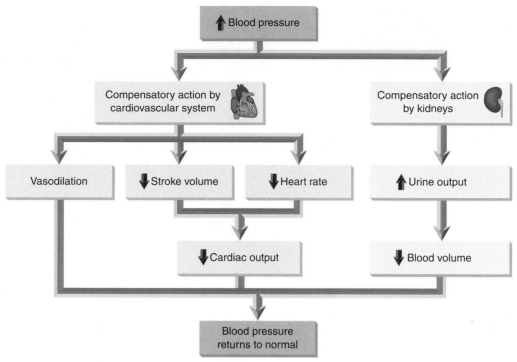

● **Figure 23.2** Blood pressure homeostasis

hormone (ADH) is a potent vasoconstrictor that can also increase blood pressure by raising blood volume. The **renin–angiotensin system** is particularly important in the pharmacotherapy of hypertension and is discussed in Section 23.9. A summary of the various nervous and hormonal factors influencing blood pressure is shown in ● Figure 23.3.

23.4 Etiology and Pathogenesis of Hypertension

Hypertension is a complex disease that is caused by a combination of genetic and environmental factors. For the large majority of hypertensive clients, no specific cause can be identified. Hypertension having no identifiable cause is called *primary, idiopathic,* or *essential,* and accounts for 90% of all cases.

In some cases, a specific cause *can* be identified. This type is called *secondary hypertension,* and accounts for 10% of all HTN. Certain diseases, such as Cushing's syndrome, hyperthyroidism, chronic renal impairment, pheochromocytoma, or arteriosclerosis are associated with elevated blood pressure. Certain drugs are also associated with HTN, including corticosteroids, oral contraceptives, estrogen, erythropoietin, and sibutramine. The therapeutic goal for secondary HTN is to treat the condition causing the blood pressure elevation. In many cases, correcting the comorbid condition will cure HTN and return blood pressure to normal.

Because chronic HTN may produce no identifiable symptoms, many people are not aware of their condition. Failure to control this condition, however, can result in serious consequences. Four target organs are most often affected by prolonged or improperly controlled HTN: the heart, brain, kidneys, and retina.

One of the most serious consequences of chronic HTN is that the heart must work harder to pump blood to the organs and tissues. The excessive cardiac workload can cause the heart to fail and the lungs to fill with fluid, a condition known as *heart failure* (HF). Drug therapy of HF is covered in Chapter 24 ∞.

High blood pressure over a prolonged period adversely affects the vascular system. Damage to the blood vessels supplying blood and oxygen to the brain can result in transient ischemic attacks and cerebral vascular accidents or strokes. Chronic HTN damages arteries in the kidneys, leading to a progressive loss of renal function. Vessels in the retina can rupture or become occluded, resulting in visual impairment and even blindness.

The importance of treating this disorder in its prehypertensive stage cannot be overstated. If the disease is allowed to progress unchecked, the long-term damage to target organs caused by HTN may be irreversible. This is especially critical in clients with diabetes and those with chronic kidney disease, as these clients are particularly susceptible to the long-term consequences of HTN.

23.5 Nonpharmacological Management of Hypertension

When a client is first diagnosed with HTN, a comprehensive medical history is necessary to determine whether the disease can be controlled without the use of drugs. Therapeutic lifestyle changes should be recommended for all clients

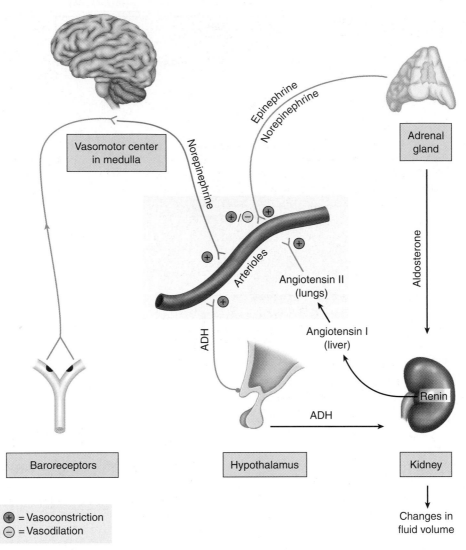

Vasomotor center in medulla

Norepinephrine

Epinephrine
Norepinephrine

Adrenal gland

Aldosterone

$\oplus$/$\ominus$

$\oplus$

Arterioles

$\oplus$

Angiotensin II (lungs)

ADH

Angiotensin I (liver)

Renin

Baroreceptors

Hypothalamus

ADH

Kidney

Changes in fluid volume

$\oplus$ = Vasoconstriction
$\ominus$ = Vasodilation

● **Figure 23.3** Hormonal and nervous factors influencing blood pressure

MediaLink Dietary Modifications for the Hypertensive Patient

with prehypertension or hypertension. Of greatest importance is maintaining optimum weight, since obesity is closely associated with dyslipidemia and hypertension. Even in obese clients, a 10- to 20-lb weight loss often produces a measurable decrease in blood pressure. Combining a safe weight loss program with proper nutrition can delay the progression from prehypertension to hypertension.

In many cases, implementing positive lifestyle changes may eliminate the need for pharmacotherapy altogether. Even if pharmacotherapy is required, it is important that the clients continue their lifestyle modifications so that dosages can be minimized, thus lowering the potential for drug side effects. The nurse is key to educating clients how to control HTN. Because all blood pressure medications have potential side effects, it is important that clients attempt to control their disease though nonpharmacological means to the greatest extent possible. Important nonpharmacological methods for controlling hypertension are as follows:

- Limit intake of alcohol.
- Restrict salt consumption.
- Reduce intake of saturated fat and cholesterol and increase consumption of fresh fruits and vegetables.
- Increase aerobic physical activity.
- Discontinue use of tobacco products.
- Explore measures for dealing with stress.
- Maintain optimum weight.

23.6 Factors Affecting the Selection of Antihypertensive Drugs

The goal of antihypertensive therapy is to reduce the morbidity and mortality associated with chronic HTN. Research has confirmed that maintaining blood pressure within normal ranges reduces the risk of hypertension-related diseases such as stroke and heart failure. Several strategies that are used to achieve this goal are summarized in Pharmacotherapy Illustrated 23.1.

The pharmacological management of hypertension is individualized to the client's risk factors, comorbid medical

PHARMACOTHERAPY ILLUSTRATED

23.1 Mechanism of Action of Antihypertensive Drugs

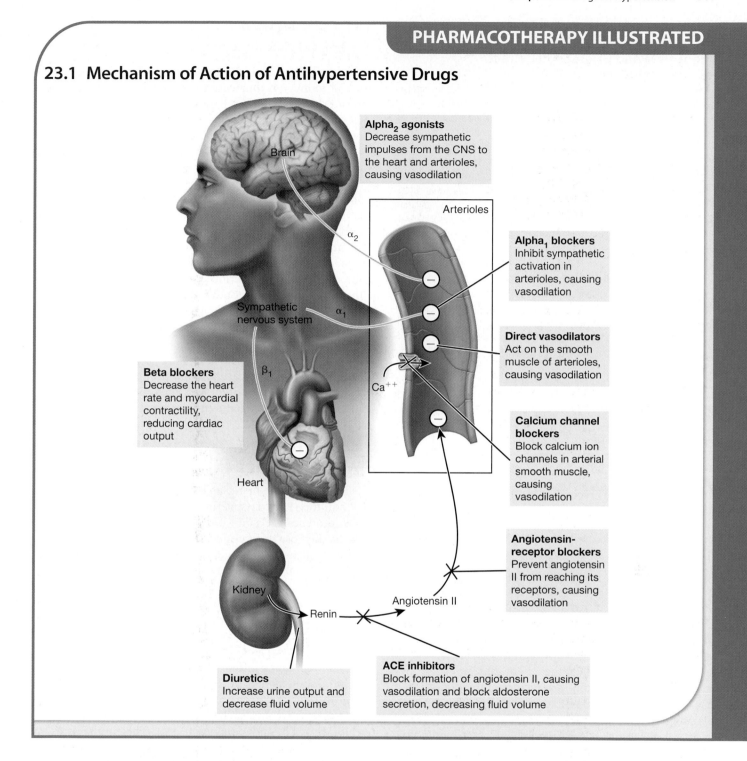

Alpha₂ agonists
Decrease sympathetic impulses from the CNS to the heart and arterioles, causing vasodilation

Brain

Arterioles

α_2

Alpha₁ blockers
Inhibit sympathetic activation in arterioles, causing vasodilation

Sympathetic nervous system

α_1

Direct vasodilators
Act on the smooth muscle of arterioles, causing vasodilation

Beta blockers
Decrease the heart rate and myocardial contractility, reducing cardiac output

β_1

Ca^{++}

Calcium channel blockers
Block calcium ion channels in arterial smooth muscle, causing vasodilation

Heart

Angiotensin-receptor blockers
Prevent angiotensin II from reaching its receptors, causing vasodilation

Kidney

Angiotensin II

Renin

Diuretics
Increase urine output and decrease fluid volume

ACE inhibitors
Block formation of angiotensin II, causing vasodilation and block aldosterone secretion, decreasing fluid volume

conditions, and degree of blood pressure elevation. Client responses to antihypertensive medications vary widely because of the many complex genetic and environmental factors affecting blood pressure. A large number of antihypertensive drugs are available, and choice of therapy is often based on the experience of the clinician. Although antihypertensive treatment varies, there are several principles that guide pharmacotherapy.

In most cases, low doses of the initial drug are prescribed and the client is reevaluated, after an appropriate time interval. If necessary, dosage is adjusted to maintain optimum blood pressure. The following drug classes are considered primary antihypertensive agents:

- Diuretics
- Angiotensin-converting enzyme (ACE) inhibitors
- Angiotensin II receptor blockers
- Beta-adrenergic antagonists
- Calcium channel blockers

Chocolate and Grape Seed Extract for Hypertension

New research suggests that two antioxidant-rich products, dark chocolate and grape seed extract, may be effective at lowering blood pressure.

Researchers believe that dark chocolate improves blood pressure through the regulation of nitric oxide production (E.L. Ding, Hutfless, X. Ding, & Girotra, 2006; Buijsse, Feskens, Kok, & Krombaut, 2006; Vlachopoulos et al., 2005; Grassi, Lippi, Necozione, Derileri, & Ferri 2005). The beneficial antioxidants are also found in cocoa. However, it is important to note that only *dark* chocolate infers these benefits. Also important is the fact that chocolate contains large quantities of sugar, so patients with insulin regulation problems should severely limit their consumption of or avoid chocolate altogether. There are several brands of high-quality, minimally processed dark chocolate available that contain small amounts of sugar; these would be the best choices.

Research has shown that grape seed extract helps improve blood pressure by strengthening capillaries, arteries, and veins (Chang et al., 2006). In a recent clinical trial at the University of California–Davis, patients who received between 150 and 300 mg of grape seed extract experienced an average drop of 12 mm Hg in systolic pressure, and 8 mm Hg in diastolic pressure. Grape seed extract has received the GRAS (generally recognized as safe) certification from the FDA and has no known side effects. The best products are those that use the whole grape seed extract, rather than the isolated compounds.

Patients should be advised not to rely on any supplement or food to treat hypertension without frequent measurements of blood pressure to be certain therapy is effective.

The JNC-7 Report recommends thiazide diuretics as the initial drugs for mild to moderate HTN. Clients with a compelling condition, however, may benefit from a second drug, either in combination with the diuretic or in place of the diuretic. The JNC-7 Report lists the following as compelling conditions: heart failure, post–myocardial infarction, high risk for coronary artery disease, diabetes, chronic kidney disease, and recurrent stroke prevention.

Prescribing two antihypertensives concurrently results in additive or synergistic blood pressure reduction, and is common practice when managing resistant HTN. This is often necessary when the client has not responded to the initial medication, has a compelling condition, or has a very high, sustained blood pressure. The advantage of using two drugs is that lower doses of each may be used, resulting in fewer side effects and better client compliance. Drug manufacturers sometimes combine two drugs into a single pill or capsule to improve client compliance. The majority of these combinations include a thiazide diuretic, usually hydrochlorothiazide (HCTZ). Selected combination antihypertensives are listed in Table 23.3.

Certain antihypertensive classes cause more side effects and are generally prescribed only when first-line agents do not produce a satisfactory response. The alternative antihypertensive drug classes include the following:

- Alpha$_1$-adrenergic antagonists
- Alpha$_2$-adrenergic agonists
- Direct-acting vasodilators
- Peripheral adrenergic antagonists

Convincing clients to change established lifestyle habits, spend money on medication, and take drugs on a regular basis when they feel well is a difficult task for the nurse. Clients with limited incomes or those who do not have health insurance are especially at risk for noncompliance. The prescriber should consider generic forms of these drugs to reduce cost and increase compliance.

Further reducing compliance is the occurrence of undesirable side effects. Some of the antihypertensive drugs cause embarrassing side effects such as impotence, which may go unreported. Others cause fatigue and generally make the client feel sicker than they were before therapy was initiated. The nurse should teach the client the importance of treating the disease to avoid serious long-term consequences. Furthermore, the nurse should teach clients to report drug side effects promptly so that dosage can be adjusted, or the drug changed, and treatment may continue without interruption.

DIURETICS

Diuretics act by increasing urine production and output. They are widely used in the treatment of hypertension and heart failure. These agents are listed in Table 23.4.

23.7 Treating Hypertension With Diuretics

Diuretics were the first class of drugs used to treat hypertension in the 1950s. Despite many advances in pharmacotherapy, diuretics are still considered first-line drugs for this disease because they produce few adverse effects and are very effective at controlling mild to moderate hypertension. In addition, clinical research has clearly demonstrated that thiazide diuretics reduce HTN-related morbidity and mortality. Although sometimes used alone, they are frequently prescribed with drugs from other antihypertensive classes to enhance their effectiveness. Diuretics are also used to treat heart failure (Chapter 24 ∞) and kidney disorders (Chapter 30 ∞).

Although many different diuretics are available for HTN, all produce a similar outcome: the reduction of blood volume through the urinary excretion of water and electrolytes. **Electrolytes** are ions such as sodium (Na^+), calcium (Ca^{2+}), chloride (Cl^-), and potassium (K^+). The mechanisms by which diuretics reduce blood volume, specifically where and how the kidney is affected, differ among the various classes of diuretics and are discussed in Chapter 30 ∞. When a drug changes urine composition or output, electrolyte depletion and dehydration are possible; the specific electrolyte lost is dependent on the mechanism of action of the particular drug. Potassium loss (hypokalemia) is of particular concern for loop and thiazide diuretics.

Thiazide and *thiazide-like* diuretics have been the mainstay for the pharmacotherapy of hypertension for decades. The thiazide diuretics are inexpensive, and most are available in generic formulations. They are safe drugs, with urinary potassium loss being the primary adverse effect.

TABLE 23.3   Combination Drugs Commonly Used to Treat Hypertension

Trade Name	Thiazide Diuretic	Adrenergic Agent	Potassium-sparing Diuretic	ACE Inhibitor or Angiotensin II Blocker	Other
Alazide	hydrochlorothiazide		spironolactone		
Aldactazide	hydrochlorothiazide		spironolactone		
Aldoril	hydrochlorothiazide				methyldopa
Apresazide	hydrochlorothiazide				hydralazine
Capozide	hydrochlorothiazide			captopril	
Combipres	chlorthalidone				clonidine
Diupres	chlorothiazide				reserpine
Dyazide	hydrochlorothiazide		triamterene		
Hydropres	hydrochlorothiazide				reserpine
Hyzaar	hydrochlorothiazide			losartan	
Inderide	hydrochlorothiazide	propranolol			
Lopressor	hydrochlorothiazide	metoprolol			
Lotensin	hydrochlorothiazide			benazepril	
Minizide	polythiazide	prazosin			
Moduretic	hydrochlorothiazide		amiloride		
Tarka				trandolapril	verapamil
Timolide	hydrochlorothiazide	timolol			
Uniretic	hydrochlorothiazide			moexipril	
Vaseretic	hydrochlorothiazide			enalapril	
Zestoretic	hydrochlorothiazide			lisinopril	
Ziac	hydrochlorothiazide	bisoprolol			

The prototype drug in this class, hydrochlorothiazide, is highlighted in this chapter.

Although the *potassium-sparing diuretics* produce only a modest diuresis, their primary advantage is that they do not cause potassium depletion. Thus, they are beneficial when clients are at risk of developing hypokalemia owing to their medical condition or to the use of thiazide or loop diuretics. The primary concern when using potassium-sparing diuretics is the possibility of retaining *too much* potassium. Taking potassium supplements with potassium-sparing diuretics may result in dangerously high potassium levels in the blood (hyperkalemia) and lead to cardiac conduction abnormalities. Concurrent use with an ACE inhibitor or angiotensin II receptor blocker significantly increases the potential for the development of hyperkalemia. Spironolactone is featured as a prototype drug for this class in Chapter 30 ∞.

The *loop diuretics* cause more diuresis, and thus a greater reduction in blood pressure, than the thiazides or potassium-sparing diuretics. Although this makes them very effective at reducing blood pressure, they are not ideal agents for HTN maintenance therapy. The risk of side effects such as hypokalemia and dehydration is greater because of their ability to remove large amounts of fluid from the body in a short time period. Because of their higher toxicity, loop diuretics are often reserved for more serious cases of hypertension. Furosemide is the only loop diuretic in widespread use, and it is presented as a prototype for heart failure in Chapter 24 ∞.

NURSING CONSIDERATIONS

The role of the nurse in diuretic therapy for HTN involves careful monitoring of a client's condition and providing education as it relates to the prescribed drug treatment. Assess kidney function and urine output before initiating therapy because most diuretics are contraindicated in clients who are unable to produce urine (anuria). Diuretics decrease circulating blood volume, causing the potential development of dehydration and hypovolemia. Therefore, monitor clients for **orthostatic hypotension,** dizziness and light-headedness when changing positions.

Because diuretics change fluid and electrolyte balance in the body, carefully monitor laboratory values for electrolytes and weigh the client daily. Report an increase or decrease of more than 2 lb in a 24-hour period. Monitor intake and output and assess fluid loss that may occur owing to high fever or exercise. Assess ankles and lower legs for pitting edema, which signifies fluid retention and may indicate pulmonary edema. Auscultate breath and heart sounds when taking vital signs. Report "crackles" and murmurs immediately because these may indicate impending heart failure. Monitor sodium and potassium levels carefully during diuretic therapy. If

TABLE 23.4   Diuretics for Hypertension

Drug	Route and Adult Dose (max dose where indicated)	Adverse Effects
POTASSIUM-SPARING AGENTS		
amiloride (Midamor)	PO; 5–20 mg in a single dose or 2 divided doses (max: 20 mg/day)	*Minor hyperkalemia, headache, fatigue, gynecomastia*
spironolactone (Aldactone) (see page 432 for the Prototype Drug box ∞)	PO; 25–100 mg/day (max: 200 mg/day)	Dysrhythmias (from hyperkalemia), dehydration, hyponatremia, agranulocytosis and other blood dyscrasias
triamterene (Dyrenium)	PO; 100 mg bid (max: 300 mg/day)	
THIAZIDE AND THIAZIDE-LIKE AGENTS		
benzthiazide (Aquatab, others)	PO; 25–200 mg/day	*Minor hypokalemia, fatigue*
chlorothiazide (Diuril) (see page 430 for the Prototype Drug box ∞)	PO; 250–500 mg/day (max: 2 g/day)	Serious hypokalemia, electrolyte depletion, dehydration, hypotension, hyponatremia, hyperglycemia, coma, blood dyscrasias
chlorthalidone (Hygroton)	PO; 50–100 mg/day (max: 100 mg/day)	
hydrochlorothiazide (HydroDIURIL, HCTZ)	PO; 12.5–100 mg/day (max: 5 mg/day)	
indapamide (Lozol)	PO; 2.5–5.0 mg/day	
metolazone (Diulo, others)	PO; 5–20 mg/day	
polythiazide (Renese)	PO; 1–4 mg/day	
trichlormethiazide (Diurese, others)	PO; 1–4 mg/day	
LOOP/HIGH-CEILING AGENTS		
bumetanide (Bumex)	PO; 0.5–2.0 mg/day (max: 10 mg/day)	*Minor hypokalemia, postural hypotension, tinnitus, nausea, diarrhea, dizziness, fatigue*
furosemide (Lasix) (see page 336 for the Prototype Drug box ∞)	PO; 20–80 mg/day (max: 600 mg/day)	Serious hypokalemia, blood dyscrasias, dehydration, ototoxicity, electrolyte imbalances, circulatory collapse
torsemide (Demadex)	PO; 4–20 mg/day	

Italics indicate common adverse effects; underlining indicates serious adverse effects.

hypokalemia develops, hold non-potassium-sparing diuretics and notify the physician prior to administration. Because diuretics can reduce the renal excretion of lithium, monitor lithium levels frequently. Assess kidney function and urine output, since most diuretics are contraindicated in clients who are unable to produce urine (anuria).

Because diuretics cause frequent urination, assess the client's ability to safely ambulate to the bathroom, and obtain a urinal or bedside commode, if needed. Answer call lights promptly to assist clients with urgency due to diuretic therapy. Administer diuretics early in the day so sleep is not interrupted by frequent urination.

Photosensitivity is also a side effect of many diuretics because when the drug is absorbed into the bloodstream, it also enters the skin. This may occur 10 to 14 days after therapy is initiated.

For clients receiving *potassium-sparing diuretics*, restrict the use of salt substitutes and potassium-rich foods. Assess for pregnancy, as these drugs are contraindicated for pregnant or lactating women. Take a thorough history to determine previous gout or kidney stones, since diuretics can increase the likelihood of both. Routinely monitor uric acid levels. Monitor blood tests for agranulocytosis and anemia. Assess for fever, rash, and sore throat, especially in clients with low white cell counts. For spironolactone (Aldactone) assess for gynecomastia (breast enlargement) and testicular atrophy in males, or accelerated hair growth (hirsutism) in females.

For clients on *thiazide and thiazide-like diuretics*, monitor laboratory values (K^+, Cl^-, Na^+, Ca^{2+}, Mg^{2+}, CBC, BUN, creatinine, cholesterol, and serum lipids) closely. Because these drugs may cause excess potassium excretion, ensure that clients have adequate potassium in their diet; potassium supplements may be necessary. Monitor blood glucose levels in diabetic clients, because these diuretics can cause hyperglycemia and decrease the effectiveness of oral antidiabetic drugs. Monitor uric acid levels and assess clients for signs and symptoms of gout. Clients with hyperlipidemia may experience an increase in blood lipid values.

Assess for pregnancy or recent birth because thiazide and thiazide-like diuretics cross the placenta and are secreted into breast milk. Determine whether the client has systemic lupus erythematosus (SLE), since thiazide and thiazide-like diuretics may cause exacerbations. Assess digoxin levels frequently, because loss of potassium and magnesium caused by thiazide diuretics increases the risk of digoxin toxicity.

For clients taking *loop diuretics*, monitor for severe potassium loss, hypovolemia, and hypotension. Monitor blood pressure frequently, especially with IV administration. Because loop diuretics are ototoxic, assess for hearing loss, which occurs more frequently in clients with renal insufficiency or when high doses are administered. Hearing loss usually reverses when the drug is discontinued. Monitor glucose and uric acid levels for increases.

Pr PROTOTYPE DRUG | Hydrochlorothiazide *(HydroDIURIL)* | Thiazide Diuretic

ACTIONS AND USES

Hydrochlorothiazide (HCTZ) is the most widely prescribed diuretic for hypertension. Like many diuretics, it produces few adverse effects and is effective at producing a 10 to 20 mm Hg reduction in blood pressure. Clients with severe HTN or a compelling condition may require the addition of a second drug from a different class to control the disease. Hydrochlorothiazide is the most common agent found in fixed-dose combination drugs for HTN.

Hydrochlorothiazide acts on the kidney tubule to decrease the reabsorption of Na$^+$. Normally, more than 99% of the sodium entering the kidney is reabsorbed by the body. When HCTZ blocks this reabsorption, more Na$^+$ is sent into the urine. When sodium moves across the tubule, water flows with it; thus, blood volume decreases and blood pressure falls. The volume of urine produced is directly proportional to the amount of sodium reabsorption blocked by the diuretic.

ADMINISTRATION ALERT

- Administer the drug early in the day to prevent nocturia.
- Pregnancy category B.

PHARMACOKINETICS

Onset: 2 h

Peak: 4 h

Half-life: 5.6–14.8 h

Duration: 45–120 min

ADVERSE EFFECTS

The most common side effects of HCTZ are potential electrolyte imbalances; K$^+$ is lost along with the Na$^+$. Because hypokalemia may cause conduction abnormalities in the heart, clients are usually instructed to increase their potassium intake as a precaution.

Contraindications: Contraindications include anuria and prior hypersensitivity to thiazides or sulfonamides.

INTERACTIONS

Drug–Drug: When given concurrently, other antihypertensives have additive or synergistic effects with HCTZ on blood pressure. Thiazides may reduce the effectiveness of anticoagulants, sulfonylureas, and antidiabetic drugs including insulin. Cholestyramine and colestipol decrease the absorption of HCTZ and reduce its effectiveness. HCTZ increases the risk of renal toxicity from NSAIDs. Corticosteroids and amphotericin B increase potassium loss when given with HCTZ. Hypokalemia caused by HCTZ may increase digoxin toxicity. Hydrochlorothiazide decreases the excretion of lithium and can lead to lithium toxicity.

Lab Tests: HCTZ may increase serum glucose, cholesterol, bilirubin, triglyceride, and calcium levels. The drug may decrease serum magnesium, potassium, and sodium levels.

Herbal/Food: Ginkgo biloba may produce a paradoxical increase in blood pressure.

Treatment of Overdose: Overdose is manifested as electrolyte depletion, which is treated with infusions of fluids containing electrolytes. Infusion of fluids will also prevent dehydration and hypotension.

 See the Companion Website for a Nursing Process focus specific to this drug.

Lifespan Considerations. Elderly clients taking thiazide and thiazide-like diuretics are at increased risk of electrolyte imbalances owing to physiological changes in the kidneys related to aging.

Client Teaching. Client education as it relates to diuretics should include the goals of therapy, the reasons for obtaining baseline data such as vital signs and the existence of underlying hepatic and renal disorders, and possible drug side effects. Include the following points when teaching clients about diuretics:

- Keep all scheduled laboratory visits for electrolyte levels and organ function tests.
- Do not use salt substitutes (which contain potassium) or sports drinks when taking potassium-sparing diuretics.
- If taking lithium, keep all scheduled visits for lithium-level tests.
- If taking loop or thiazide diuretics, include high potassium foods in the diet, such as bananas, orange juice, and apricots.
- Report signs or symptoms of gout.
- If taking a drug that causes photosensitivity, wear protective clothing when outdoors in sunlight.
- If diabetic, monitor glucose levels carefully and report changes immediately.

- Check blood pressure daily and notify your healthcare provider if your blood pressure is 90/60 mm Hg or less.
- Report nausea, vomiting, bleeding, abdominal pain, or jaundice because these could indicate liver toxicity.
- Weigh yourself at the same time each day, and report a weight gain or loss of more than 2 lb in 24 hours.

CALCIUM CHANNEL BLOCKERS

Calcium channel blockers exert beneficial effects on the heart and blood vessels by blocking calcium ion channels. They are used in the treatment of HTN and other cardiovascular diseases. These agents are listed in Table 23.5.

23.8 Treating Hypertension With Calcium Channel Blockers

Calcium channel blockers (CCBs) comprise a group of drugs used to treat angina pectoris, dysrhythmias, and HTN. When CCBs were first approved for the treatment of angina in the early 1980s, it was quickly noted that a "side effect" was the lowering of blood pressure in hypertensive clients. CCBs are usually not used as monotherapy for chronic HTN. They are, however, useful in treating certain populations such as the elderly and African Americans, who

NURSING PROCESS FOCUS Clients Receiving Diuretic Therapy

Assessment	Potential Nursing Diagnoses
Prior to administration: ■ Obtain a complete health history including allergies, drug history, and possible drug interactions. ■ Obtain baseline vital signs. ■ Auscultate chest sounds for rales or rhonchi indicative of pulmonary edema. ■ Assess lower limbs for edema; note character/level (e.g., "++ pitting"). ■ Obtain blood and urine specimens for laboratory analysis.	■ Fluid Volume, Excess ■ Fluid Volume, Deficient, Risk for ■ Urinary Elimination, Impaired, related to diuretic use ■ Fatigue ■ Health Maintenance, Ineffective

Planning: Client Goals and Expected Outcomes

The client will:
■ Exhibit a reduction in systolic and diastolic blood pressure.
■ Demonstrate an understanding of the drug's action by accurately describing drug side effects and precautions.
■ Maintain normal serum electrolyte levels during drug therapy.

Implementation

Interventions and (Rationales)	Client Education/Discharge Planning
■ Monitor laboratory values. (Diuretic therapy affects the results of certain laboratory tests.)	Instruct client to: ■ Inform laboratory personnel of diuretic therapy when providing blood or urine samples. ■ Carry a wallet card or wear medical identification jewelry to indicate diuretic therapy.
■ Monitor vital signs, especially blood pressure. Take blood pressure sitting, lying, and standing to detect orthostatic hypotension. (Diuretics reduce circulating blood volume, resulting in lowered blood pressure.)	Instruct client to: ■ Monitor blood pressure prior to taking the diuretic. ■ Stop medication if blood pressure is 90/60 mm Hg or below, and immediately notify healthcare provider.
■ Ensure client safety. Observe for changes in level of consciousness. Monitor ambulation until effects of drug are known. (Postural hypotension may occur.)	Instruct client to: ■ Call for assistance prior to getting out of bed or attempting to walk alone. ■ Always rise slowly and avoid sudden position changes. ■ Avoid driving or other activities requiring mental alertness or physical coordination until effects of the drug are known. ■ Report dizziness or light-headedness.
■ Measure intake and output, and record daily weights. (Diuresis is indicated by output greater than intake, and weight loss.)	Instruct client to: ■ Immediately report any severe shortness of breath, frothy sputum, profound fatigue, or edema in extremities. ■ Weigh at the same time (before breakfast) every day and report weight loss or gain of more than 2 lb in 24 hours. ■ Consume enough *plain* water to remain adequately, but not overly, hydrated. ■ Avoid excessive heat that contributes to excessive sweating and fluid loss. ■ Note that increased urine output and decreased weight indicate that the drug is working.
■ Monitor nutritional status. (Electrolyte imbalances may occur.)	For clients taking potassium-*wasting* diuretics, instruct to: ■ Eat foods high in potassium such as bananas, apricots, kidney beans, sweet potatoes, and peanut butter. For clients taking potassium-*sparing* diuretics, instruct to: ■ Avoid foods high in potassium. ■ Consult with nurse before using vitamin/mineral supplements or electrolyte-fortified sports drinks.
■ Observe for signs of hyperglycemia. Use with caution in clients with diabetes. (Diuretics can cause hyperglycemia, especially in diabetics.)	■ Instruct client to report signs and symptoms of diabetes mellitus or elevated blood sugar to healthcare provider.

NURSING PROCESS FOCUS   Clients Receiving Diuretic Therapy (*Continued*)

Implementation

Interventions and (Rationales)	Client Education/Discharge Planning
▪ Monitor liver and kidney function. *(Most diuretics are metabolized by the liver and excreted by the kidneys.)*	Instruct client to: ▪ Immediately report symptoms of metabolic imbalances: nausea and vomiting, profound weakness, lethargy, muscle cramps, depression/disorientation, hallucinations, heart palpitations, numbness or tingling in limbs, extreme thirst, or changes in urine output. ▪ Keep all scheduled laboratory visits for tests.
▪ Observe for hypersensitivity reaction. (Some clients may be sensitive to diuretics.)	▪ Instruct client to immediately seek medical attention for difficulty breathing, throat tightness, hives or rash, muscle cramps, or tremors.
▪ Observe for signs of infection. (Certain diuretics may decrease white blood cell counts and the body's ability to fight infection.)	▪ Instruct client to report any flulike symptoms: shortness of breath, fever, sore throat, malaise, joint pain, or profound fatigue.
▪ Monitor hearing and vision. (Loop diuretics are ototoxic. Thiazide diuretics increase serum digitalis levels, which may produce visual changes.)	Instruct client to: ▪ Report changes in hearing such as ringing or buzzing in the ears or becoming "hard of hearing." ▪ Report dimness of sight or seeing halos or "yellow vision."
▪ Monitor for alcohol and caffeine use. (Alcohol increases the hypotensive action of some thiazide diuretics. Caffeine is a mild diuretic that could increase diuresis.)	▪ Instruct client to restrict consumption of alcohol and caffeine to prevent potentiation of drug.
▪ Monitor reactivity to light exposure. (Drug causes photosensitivity.)	Instruct client to: ▪ Limit exposure to the sun. ▪ Wear dark glasses and light-colored, loose-fitting clothes when outdoors.

Evaluation of Outcome Criteria

Evaluate the effectiveness of drug therapy by confirming that client goals and expected outcomes have been met (see "Planning").
- The client's blood pressure is within normal limits.
- The client demonstrates an understanding of the drug's action by accurately describing drug side effects and precautions.
- The client's serum electrolyte levels are stable.

∞ *See Table 23.4 for a list of drugs to which these nursing actions apply.*

---

are sometimes less responsive to drugs in other antihypertensive classes.

Contraction of muscle is regulated by the amount of calcium ion inside the cell. When calcium enters the cell through channels in the plasma membrane, muscular contraction occurs. CCBs block these channels and inhibit Ca^{2+} from entering the cell, limiting muscular contraction. At low doses, CCBs relax arterial smooth muscle, lowering peripheral

TABLE 23.5   Calcium Channel Blockers for Hypertension

Drug	Route and Adult Dose (max dose where indicated)	Adverse Effects
SELECTIVE: FOR BLOOD VESSELS		
amlodipine (Norvasc)	PO; 5–10 mg/day (max: 10 mg/day)	*Flushed skin, headache, dizziness, peripheral edema, light-headedness, nausea, diarrhea*
felodipine (Plendil)	PO; 5–10 mg/day (max: 20 mg/day)	
nicardipine (Cardene)	PO; 20–40 mg/day (max: 120 mg/day)	<u>Hepatotoxicity, MI, CHF, confusion, mood changes</u>
⊙ nifedipine (Procardia, Adalat)	PO; 10–20 mg tid (max: 180 mg/day)	
NONSELECTIVE: FOR BOTH BLOOD VESSELS AND HEART		
diltiazem (Cardizem, Dilacor, Tiamate, Triassic) (see page 354 for the Prototype Drug box ∞)	PO; 60–120 mg sustained release bid	
isradipine (DynaCirc)	PO; 1.25–10 mg bid (max: 20 mg/day)	
nisoldipine (Nisocor)	PO; 10–20 mg bid (max: 40 mg/day)	
verapamil (Calan, Isoptin, Verelan) (see page 373 for the Prototype Drug box ∞)	PO; 80–160 mg tid (max: 360 mg/day)	

Italics indicate common adverse effects; <u>underlining</u> indicates serious adverse effects.

resistance and decreasing blood pressure. Some CCBs such as nifedipine (Procardia) are *selective* for calcium channels in arterioles, whereas others such as verapamil (Calan) affect channels in *both* arterioles and the myocardium. CCBs vary in their potency and by the frequency and types of side effects produced. Verapamil (Calan) is featured as a prototype anti-dysrhythmic in Chapter 26 ∞, and diltiazem (Cardizem) as an antianginal in Chapter 25 ∞.

NURSING CONSIDERATIONS

The role of the nurse in calcium channel blocker therapy for HTN involves careful monitoring of a client's condition and providing education as it relates to the prescribed drug treatment. Because CCBs affect the coronary arteries and myocardial contractility, obtain baseline ECG, heart rate, and blood pressure prior to therapy. During therapy, monitor vital signs regularly for effects on heart rate and blood pressure. Obtain a thorough health history to detect heart dysrhythmias because CCBs are contraindicated in clients with certain types of heart conditions such as sick sinus syndrome or third-degree AV blocks without the presence of a pacemaker. Assess the client closely for changes in vital signs and symptoms that could indicate CHF or **reflex tachycardia,** a condition that occurs when the heart rate increases owing to the rapid fall in blood pressure created by the drug. Tachycardia and hypotension are most pronounced with IV administration of CCBs. Assess for the possibility of pregnancy, because CCBs are pregnancy category C.

Avoid giving the client grapefruit juice, which increases absorption of these drugs from the GI tract, causing greater-than-expected effects from the dose. If grapefruit juice is taken with a sustained-release CCB, it could result in rapid toxic overdose, which is a medical emergency. Assess the client for complaints of dizziness, headache, or flushing, which are minor side effects. Some CCBs reduce myocardial contractility and can worsen heart failure. Evaluate any complaints of chest pain, which could indicate cardiac compromise or CHF.

Client Teaching. Client education as it relates to calcium channel blockers should include the goals of therapy, the reasons for obtaining baseline data such as vital signs and underlying disorders, and possible drug side effects. Include the following points when teaching clients about calcium channel blockers:

- Check blood pressure daily. Notify your healthcare provider if your blood pressure is 90/60 mm Hg or less.
- Immediately report chest pain, palpitations, or a "racing heart."
- Report dizziness or light-headedness.
- Rise slowly from a sitting or lying position to prevent dizziness.
- Weigh yourself at the same time each day and report a weight gain or loss of more than 2 lb in 24 hours.

Pr PROTOTYPE DRUG | Nifedipine *(Procardia)* | Calcium Channel Blocker

ACTIONS AND USES

Nifedipine is a CCB generally prescribed for HTN and variant or vasospastic angina. It is occasionally used to treat Raynaud's phenomenon and hypertrophic cardiomyopathy. Nifedipine acts by selectively blocking calcium channels in myocardial and vascular smooth muscle, including those in the coronary arteries. This results in less oxygen utilization by the heart, an increase in cardiac output, and a fall in blood pressure. It is available as capsules and as extended-release tablets (XL).

ADMINISTRATION ALERTS

- Do not administer immediate-release formulations of nifedipine if an impending MI is suspected, or within 2 weeks following a confirmed MI.
- Administer nifedipine capsules or tablets whole. If capsules or extended-release tablets are chewed, divided, or crushed, the entire dose will be delivered at once.
- Pregnancy category C.

PHARMACOKINETICS

Onset: 10–30 min PO

Peak: 30 min

Half-life: 2–5 h

Duration: 4–8 h (24 h extended release)

ADVERSE EFFECTS

Side effects of nifedipine are generally minor and related to vasodilation such as headache, dizziness, and flushing. Fast-acting forms of nifedipine can cause reflex tachycardia. To avoid rebound hypotension, the drug should be discontinued gradually. In rare cases, nifedipine may cause a paradoxical increase in anginal pain, possibly related to hypotension or heart failure.

Contraindications: The only contraindication is prior hypersensitivity to nifedipine.

INTERACTIONS

Drug–Drug: When given concurrently, other antihypertensives have additive effects with nifedipine on blood pressure. Concurrent use of nifedipine with a beta-blocker increases the risk of congestive heart failure. Nifedipine may increase serum levels of digoxin, leading to bradycardia and digoxin toxicity. Alcohol potentiates the vasodilating action of nifedipine, and could lead to syncope caused by a severe drop in blood pressure.

Lab Tests: May increase values for the following lab tests: alkaline phosphatase, LDH, ALT, CPK, and AST.

Herbal/Food: Grapefruit juice may enhance the absorption of nifedipine. Melatonin may increase blood pressure and heart rate.

Treatment of Overdose: The most likely sign of overdosage is hypotension, which is treated with vasopressors. Calcium infusions may be indicated.

 See the Companion Website for a Nursing Process Focus specific for this drug.

NURSING PROCESS FOCUS   Clients Receiving Calcium Channel Blocker Therapy

Assessment	Potential Nursing Diagnoses
Prior to administration: ■ Obtain a complete health history including recent cardiac events and any incidence of angioedema, allergies, drug history, and possible drug interactions. ■ Obtain baseline ECG and vital signs. ■ Assess neurological status and level of consciousness. ■ Ausculatate chest sounds for rales or rhonchi indicative of pulmonary edema. ■ Assess lower limbs for edema; note character/level.	■ Health Maintenance, Ineffective ■ Knowledge, Deficient, related to drug therapy ■ Cardiac Output, Decreased ■ Tissue Perfusion, Altered

Planning: Client Goals and Expected Outcomes

The client will:
■ Exhibit a reduction in systolic and diastolic blood pressure.
■ Exhibit a stable pulse without reflex tachycardia.
■ Demonstrate an understanding of the drug's action by accurately describing drug side effects and precautions.

Implementation

Interventions and (Rationales)	Client Education/Discharge Planning
■ Monitor vital signs and ECG during initial therapy. (CCBs dilate the arteries, reducing blood pressure.)	Instruct client to: ■ Monitor blood pressure and ensure the proper use of home equipment. ■ Stop medication if blood pressure is 90/60 mm Hg or below, and immediately notify the healthcare provider. ■ Immediately report palpitations or rapid heartbeat.
■ Observe for changes in level of consciousness, dizziness, fatigue, postural hypotension. (Vasodilation occurs.)	■ Instruct client to report dizziness or light-headedness.
■ Observe for paradoxical increase in chest pain or angina symptoms. (Severe hypotension may cause this.)	■ Instruct client to report chest pain or other angina-like symptoms.
■ Obtain blood pressure readings in sitting, standing, and supine positions. (It is important to monitor fluctuations in blood pressure.)	■ Instruct client to always rise slowly and avoid sudden position changes.
■ Monitor for signs of heart failure. (CCBs can decrease myocardial contractility, increasing the risk of heart failure.)	■ Instruct client to immediately report any severe shortness of breath, frothy sputum, profound fatigue, or swelling of extremities. These may be signs of heart failure or fluid accumulation in the lungs.
■ Measure intake and output, and record daily weights. (Edema is a side effect of some CCBs.)	■ Instruct client to weigh daily at the same time each day. Report weight gain of greater than 2 lb in 24 hours.
■ Observe for hypersensitivity reaction.	■ Instruct client to immediately seek medical attention for difficulty breathing, throat tightness, hives or rash, muscle cramps, or tremors.
■ Monitor liver and kidney function. (CCBs are metabolized in the liver and excreted by the kidneys.)	Instruct client to: ■ Immediately report signs of liver toxicity: nausea, vomiting, anorexia, bleeding, severe upper or abdominal pain, heartburn, jaundice, or a change in the color or character of stools ■ Immediately report signs of renal toxicity: fever, flank pain, changes in urine output, color, or character (cloudy, with sediment, etc.) ■ Keep scheduled appointments for laboratory testing.
■ Observe for constipation. (CCBs may cause constipation.)	Instruct client to: ■ Maintain adequate fluid and fiber intake to facilitate stool passage ■ Use a bulk laxative or stool softener, as recommended by the healthcare provider.
■ Monitor for safe ambulation until response to drug is known. (Postural hypotension may occur.)	■ Instruct client to avoid driving or other activities requiring mental alertness or physical coordination until effects of drug are known.

(Continued)

NURSING PROCESS FOCUS Clients Receiving Calcium Channel Blocker Therapy (*Continued*)

Evaluation of Outcome Criteria

Evaluate the effectiveness of drug therapy by confirming that client goals and expected outcomes have been met (see "planning").

- The client's blood pressure is within normal limits.
- The client's pulse is stable without reflex tachycardia.
- The client demonstrates an understanding of the drug's action by describing drug side effects and precautions.

∞ *See Table 23.5 for a list of drugs to which these nursing actions apply.*

- Immediately report severe shortness of breath, profound fatigue, frothy sputum, or swelling of extremities.
- Immediately seek medical help for throat tightness, difficulty breathing, hives, rash, or muscle tremors.
- Report nausea, vomiting, bleeding, abdominal pain, or jaundice because these could indicate liver toxicity.
- Report fever, flank pain, or changes in color, amount, or character of urine, because these could indicate kidney toxicity.
- Do not take a CCB with grapefruit juice.

DRUGS AFFECTING THE RENIN–ANGIOTENSIN SYSTEM

Drugs that affect the renin–angiotensin pathway decrease blood pressure and increase urine volume. They are widely used in the pharmacotherapy of HTN, heart failure, and myocardial infarction. These agents are listed in Table 23.6.

23.9 Treating Hypertension With ACE Inhibitors and Angiotensin Receptor Blockers

The renin–angiotensin system is a key homeostatic mechanism controlling blood pressure and fluid balance. This mechanism is illustrated in ● Figure 23.4. Renin is an enzyme secreted by specialized cells in the kidney when blood pressure falls, or when there is a decrease in Na^+ flowing through the kidney tubules. Once in the blood, renin converts the inactive liver protein angiotensinogen to angiotensin I. When it passes through the lungs, angiotensin

TABLE 23.6 ACE Inhibitors and Angiotensin II Receptor Blockers for Hypertension		
Drug	**Route and Adult Dose (max dose where indicated)**	**Adverse effects**
ACE INHIBITORS		
benazepril (Lotensin)	PO; 10–40 mg in a single dose or divided doses (max: 40 mg/day)	*Headache, dizziness, orthostatic hypotension, rash*
captopril (Capoten)	PO; 6.25–25 mg tid (max: 450 mg/day)	
enalapril (Vasotec)	PO; 5–40 mg in a single dose or 2 divided doses (max: 40 mg/day)	<u>Angioedema, acute renal failure, first-dose phenomenon</u>
fosinopril (Monopril)	PO; 5–40 mg/day (max: 80 mg/day)	
lisinopril (Prinivil, Zestoretic, Zestril) (see page 334 for the Prototype Drug box ∞)	PO; 10 mg/day (max: 80 mg/day)	
moexipril (Univasc)	PO; 7.5–30 mg/day (max: 30 mg/day)	
perindopril (Aceon)	PO; 4 mg/day (max: 8 mg/day)	
quinapril (Accupril)	PO; 10–20 mg/day (max: 80 mg/day)	
ramipril (Altace)	PO; 2.5–5 mg/day (max: 20 mg/day)	
trandolapril (Mavik)	PO; 1–4 mg/day (max: 8 mg/day)	
ANGIOTENSIN II RECEPTOR BLOCKERS		
candesartan (Atacand)	PO; start at 16 mg/day (range: 8–32 mg divided once or twice daily)	
eprosartan (Teveten)	PO; 600 mg/day or 400 mg qid–bid (max: 800 mg/day)	
irbesartan (Avapro)	PO; 150–300 mg/day (max: 300 mg/day)	
losartan (Cozaar)	PO; 25–50 mg in a single dose or 2 divided doses (max: 100 mg/day)	
olmesartan medoxomil (Benicar)	PO; 20–40 mg/day	
telmisartan (Micardis)	PO; 40 mg/day (max: 80 mg/day)	
valsartan (Diovan)	PO; 80 mg/day (max: 320 mg/day)	

Italics indicate common adverse effects; <u>underlining</u> indicates serious adverse effects.

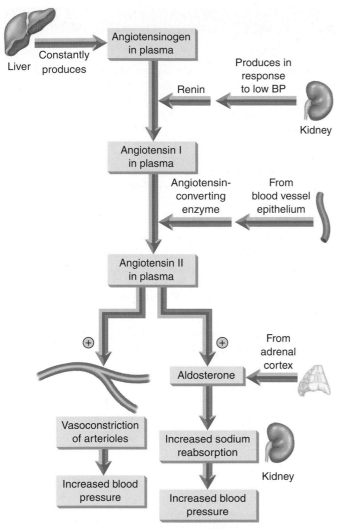

● **Figure 23.4** The renin–angiotensin pathway

Side effects of ACE inhibitors are usually minor and include persistent cough and postural hypotension, particularly following the first few doses of the drug. Hyperkalemia may occur and can be a major concern for diabetics, those with renal impairment, and clients taking potassium-sparing diuretics. Though rare, the most serious adverse effect of ACE inhibitors is the development of angioedema. When it does occur, angioedema most often develops within hours or days after beginning ACE inhibitor therapy.

A second method of altering the renin–angiotensin system is to block the action of angiotensin II *after* it is formed. The angiotensin II receptor blockers (ARBs) block receptors for angiotensin II in arteriolar smooth muscle and in the adrenal gland, thus causing blood pressure to fall. Their effects of arteriolar dilation and increased sodium excretion by the kidneys are similar to those of the ACE inhibitors. Angiotensin II receptor blockers have relatively few side effects, most of which are related to hypotension. Unlike the ACE inhibitors, they do not cause cough, and angioedema is even more rare in the ARBs. Drugs in this class are often combined with drugs from other classes in the management of HTN.

Two new methods of altering the renin–angiotensin system show promise for the pharmacotherapy of HTN. Eplerenone (Inspra) is the first aldosterone receptor blocker approved for HTN. This drug prevents aldosterone from reaching its receptors in the kidneys, resulting in less sodium reabsorption and a fall in blood pressure. In addition, several vasopeptidase inhibitors are completing final clinical trials. These new agents cause both vasodilation and diuresis. In clinical trials, vasopeptidase inhibitors appear to be as effective as or more effective than conventional antihypertensives. Omapatrilat (Vanlev) is the best studied of these agents and the most likely to receive approval.

NURSING CONSIDERATIONS

The role of the nurse in ACE-inhibitor therapy for HTN involves careful monitoring of a client's condition and providing education as it relates to the prescribed drug treatment. Assess baseline vital signs. ACE inhibitors are given to lower blood pressure and treat heart failure. The first dose of an ACE inhibitor, especially by the IV route, can cause severe hypotension. When possible, administer the first dose at bedtime to avoid first-dose phenomenon. Monitor blood pressure carefully with IV administration and be prepared to treat loss of consciousness if it occurs.

A life-threatening side effect of ACE inhibitors is angioedema, leading to laryngeal swelling that can cause asphyxia. Assess for severe paroxysms of dry coughing and stridor, both symptoms of possible angioedema. Monitor the client closely, especially during IV administration. Keep the emergency cart and oxygen on standby during initiation of IV ACE-inhibitor therapy.

Another serious side effect of these drugs is neutropenia or agranulocytosis. Monitor lab values closely for a decrease in white blood cells and assess for signs of possible infection. Also monitor a client's potassium level because

I is converted to **angiotensin II,** one of the most potent natural vasoconstrictors known. The enzyme responsible for the final step in this system is **angiotensin-converting enzyme (ACE).** The intense vasoconstriction of arterioles caused by angiotensin II raises blood pressure by increasing peripheral resistance.

Angiotensin II also stimulates the secretion of **aldosterone,** a hormone from the adrenal cortex. The primary action of aldosterone is to increase sodium reabsorption in the kidney. The enhanced sodium reabsorption causes the body to retain water, increasing blood volume and raising blood pressure. Thus, angiotensin II increases blood pressure through two distinct mechanisms: direct vasoconstriction and an increase in water retention.

First detected in the venom of pit vipers in the 1960s, inhibitors of ACE have been approved for HTN since the 1980s. Since then, drugs in this class have become key agents in the treatment of HTN. ACE inhibitors block the effects of angiotensin II, decreasing blood pressure through two mechanisms: lowering peripheral resistance and decreasing blood volume. Some ACE inhibitors have become primary drugs for the treatment of heart failure and myocardial infarction, as discussed in Chapters 4 and 27 ∞, respectively.

Pr PROTOTYPE DRUG | Enalapril *(Vasotec)* | ACE Inhibitor

ACTIONS AND USES

Enalapril is one of the most frequently prescribed ACE inhibitors for HTN. Unlike captopril (Capoten), the first ACE inhibitor to be marketed, enalapril has a prolonged half-life, which permits administration once or twice daily. It is available as oral tablets and as an IV injection. Enalapril acts by reducing angiotensin II and aldosterone levels to produce a significant reduction in blood pressure with few side effects. Enalapril may be used by itself or in combination with other antihypertensives to minimize side effects.

ADMINISTRATION ALERTS

- May produce a first-dose phenomenon resulting in profound hypotension, which may result in syncope.
- Pregnancy category D.

PHARMACOKINETICS

Onset: 1 h PO; 15 min IV

Peak: 4–8 h PO; 4 h IV

Half-life: 2 h

Duration: 12–24 h PO; 4 h IV

ADVERSE EFFECTS

Unlike diuretics, ACE inhibitors such as enalapril have little effect on electrolyte balance; and unlike beta-adrenergic blockers, they cause few cardiac side effects. Enalapril may cause orthostatic hypotension when the client moves quickly from a supine to an upright position. A rapid fall in blood pressure may occur following the first dose. Other side effects include headache and dizziness. ACE inhibitors can cause life-theatening angioedema, neutropenia, or agranulocytosis.

Contraindications: Enalapril is contraindicated in clients with prior hypersensitivity and should not be administered during pregnancy or lactation.

INTERACTIONS

Drug–Drug: When given concurrently, other antihypertensives have additive effects with enalapril on blood pressure. Thiazide diuretics increase potassium loss. Potassium supplements or potassium-sparing diuretics increase the risk of hyperkalemia. Enalapril may induce lithium toxicity by reducing renal clearance of lithium. NSAIDs may reduce the hypotensive action of ACE inhibitors.

Lab Tests: May increase values of the following: BUN, alkaline phosphatase, serum potassium, serum creatinine, ALT, and AST; may cause positive ANA titer

Herbal/Food: Unknown.

Treatment of Overdose: The most likely sign of overdosage is hypotension, which is treated with an IV infusion of normal saline solution.

 See the Companion Website for a Nursing Process Focus specific to this drug.

NURSING PROCESS FOCUS Clients Receiving ACE-inhibitor Therapy

Assessment	Potential Nursing Diagnoses
Prior to administration: - Obtain a complete health history including recent cardiac events and any incidence of angioedema, allergies, drug history, and possible drug interactions. - Obtain baseline ECG and vital signs. - Assess neurological status and level of consciousness. - Obtain blood and urine specimens for laboratory analysis.	- Injury, Risk for, related to orthostatic hypotension - Knowledge, Deficient, related to drug therapy - Nutrition imbalanced: more than body requirements, related to hyperkalemia

Planning: Client Goals and Expected Outcomes

The client will:
- Exhibit a reduction in systolic and diastolic blood pressure.
- Maintain normal serum electrolyte levels during drug therapy.
- Demonstrate an understanding of the drug's action by accurately describing drug side effects and precautions.

Implementation

Interventions and (Rationales)	Client Education/Discharge Planning
- Monitor for profound hypotension. (ACE inhibitors can cause first- dose phenomenon with initial doses.)	Instruct client: - About the first-dose phenomenon and reassure that this effect diminishes with continued therapy. - To immediately report feelings of faintness because rapid reduction in blood pressure can cause changes in consciousness. - To rest in the supine position beginning 1 hour after administration and for 3 to 4 hours after the first dose.

NURSING PROCESS FOCUS Clients Receiving ACE-inhibitor Therapy *(Continued)*

Implementation

Interventions and (Rationales)	Client Education/Discharge Planning
■ Observe for hypersensitivity reaction, particularly angioedema. (Angioedema may occur at any time during ACE inhibitor therapy, but is generally expected shortly after initiation of therapy.)	Instruct client: ■ To immediately seek medical attention for difficulty breathing, throat tightness, muscle cramps, hives or rash, or tremors. These symptoms can occur on the first dose or much later as a delayed reaction. ■ That angioedema can be life theatening and to call emergency medical services if severe dyspnea or hoarseness is accompanied by swelling of the face or mouth.
■ Monitor for neutropenia and signs of infection. (ACE inhibitors can lower white blood cell count and decrease the ability to fight infection.)	■ Instruct client to immediately report any flulike symptoms such as fever, sore throat, malaise, and joint pain.
■ Monitor for changes in level of consciousness, dizziness, drowsiness, or light-headedness. (ACE inhibitors can cause decreased circulation to the brain owing to vasodilation.)	Instruct client to: ■ Report dizziness or fainting that persists beyond the first dose, as well as unusual sensations such as numbness and tingling, or other changes in the face or limbs. Sudden collapse is possible. ■ Contact the healthcare provider before the next scheduled dose of the drug, if fainting occurs.
■ Monitor for persistent dry cough or changes in cough pattern. (ACE inhibitors affect the proinflammatory action of bradykinin. A change in cough may indicate another disease process.)	Instruct client to: ■ Expect persistent dry cough. ■ Sleep with head elevated if cough becomes troublesome when in supine position. ■ Use nonmedicated sugar-free lozenges or hard candies to relieve cough. ■ Immediately report any change in the character or frequency of cough. Any cough accompanied by shortness of breath, fever, or chest pain should be reported *immediately* because it may indicate MI.
■ Monitor for hyperkalemia. (Reduced aldosterone levels, especially in clients with CHF, impaired kidney function, and diabetes, may cause hyperkalemia.)	Instruct client to: ■ Immediately report signs of hyperkalemia: nausea, irregular heartbeat, profound fatigue/muscle weakness, and slow or faint pulse. ■ Avoid consuming electrolyte-fortified snacks, or sports drinks that may contain potassium. ■ Avoid using salt substitute (KCl) to flavor foods. ■ Consult the healthcare provider before taking any nutritional supplements containing potassium.
■ Monitor for liver and kidney function. (ACE inhibitors are metabolized by the liver and excreted by the kidneys.)	Instruct client to: ■ Report signs of liver toxicity: nausea, vomiting, anorexia, diarrhea, rash, jaundice, abdominal pain, tenderness or distention, or change in the color or character of stools. ■ Immediately stop drug and contact healthcare provider if jaundice occurs. ■ Keep all scheduled laboratory visits for testing.
■ Monitor for safe ambulation until response to drug is known. (The drugs may cause postural hypotension.)	Instruct client to: ■ Avoid driving or other activities requiring mental alertness or physical coordination until effects of drug are known. ■ Always rise slowly and avoid sudden position changes.

Evaluation of Outcome Criteria

Evaluate the effectiveness of drug therapy by confirming that client goals and expected outcomes have been met (see "Planning").

■ The client's blood pressure is within normal limits.

■ The client's serum electrolyte levels remain normal during drug therapy.

■ The client demonstrates an understanding of the drug's action by accurately describing drug side effects and precautions.

∞ *See Table 23.6 under "ACE Inhibitors" for a list of drugs to which these nursing actions apply.*

hyperkalemia may occur, especially in clients with CHF, impaired kidney function, and diabetes.

Assess for common, though less serious, side effects such as hypotension, dizziness, headache, and a "tickling," nonproductive cough. The cough is generally due to the action of ACE inhibitors on the vasodilator bradykinin. Assess frequency and type of cough. Assess for the possibility of pregnancy, since ACE inhibitors are contraindicated in pregnancy (category D).

Client Teaching. Client education as it relates to ACE inhibitors should include the goals of therapy, the reasons for obtaining baseline data such as vital signs and underlying disorders such as renal and hepatic disease, and possible drug side effects. Include the following points when teaching clients about ACE inhibitors:

- Call for emergency medical help if difficult breathing, hives, rash, muscle cramps or tremors, swelling of the tongue or face, or hoarseness occurs. These are signs of angioedema and are life threatening.

- Report flulike symptoms of sore throat, fever, joint pain, and malaise, which may indicate infection.

- Immediately report any chest pain, fever, or shortness of breath, because these symptoms can indicate a heart attack.

- Expect a persistent, dry cough. Report a cough that becomes productive. Sleep with the head of the bed elevated if the cough worsens.

- Suck on hard candies to help relieve cough.

- Report any nausea, muscle weakness, and heart palpitations because these may indicate high potassium levels.

- Avoid foods and drinks high in potassium, including sports drinks and salt substitutes.

- Take the first few doses of the medication at bedtime, to avoid the "first-dose" phenomenon.

- Report nausea, vomiting, bleeding, abdominal pain or jaundice because these could indicate liver toxicity.

- Report fever, flank pain, or changes in color, amount or character of urine, because these may indicate kidney toxicity.

ADRENERGIC ANTAGONISTS

The adrenergic receptor has been a site of pharmacological action in the treatment of HTN since the first such drugs were developed for this disorder in the 1950s. Blockade of adrenergic receptors results in a number of therapeutic effects on the heart and vessels, and these autonomic drugs are used for a wide variety of cardiovascular disorders. Table 23.7 lists the adrenergic antagonists used for hypertension.

23.10 Treating Hypertension With Adrenergic Antagonists

As discussed in Chapter 13 ∞, the autonomic nervous system controls involuntary functions of the body such as heart rate, pupil size, and smooth muscle contraction, including that in the bronchi and arterial walls. Stimulation of the sympathetic division causes fight-or-flight responses such as faster heart rate, an increase in blood pressure, and bronchodilation. Peripheral blood vessels are innervated only by sympathetic nerves.

Antihypertensive drugs have been developed that affect the sympathetic division through a number of distinct mechanisms, although all have in common the effect of lowering blood pressure. These mechanisms include the following:

- Blockade of $beta_1$-adrenergic receptors in the heart
- Blockade of $alpha_1$-adrenergic receptors in the arterioles
- Nonselective blockade of both $alpha_1$- and beta-adrenergic receptors
- Stimulation of $alpha_2$-receptors in the brainstem (centrally acting)
- Blockade of peripheral adrenergic neurons

The earliest drugs for HTN were nonselective agents that blocked nerve transmission at the ganglia or at both alpha- and beta-adrenergic receptors. Although these nonselective agents revolutionized the treatment of HTN, they produced significant side effects. These drugs are rarely used today, because the selective agents are more efficacious and better tolerated by clients.

Of the five subclasses of adrenergic antagonists, only the *beta-adrenergic blockers* are considered first-line drugs for the pharmacotherapy of HTN. By decreasing the heart rate and contractility, they reduce cardiac output and lower systemic blood pressure. Some of their antihypertensive effect is also caused by blockade of $beta_1$-receptors in the juxtaglomerular apparatus, which inhibits the secretion of renin and the formation of angiotensin II.

Beta-blockers have several other important therapeutic applications. By decreasing the cardiac workload, beta-blockers can ease the symptoms of angina pectoris (Chapter 25 ∞). By slowing conduction through the myocardium, beta-blockers are able to treat certain types of dysrhythmias (Chapter 26 ∞). Other therapeutic uses include the treatment of heart failure, myocardial infarction (Chapter 25), and migraines (Chapter 18 ∞). Prototypes of beta-adrenergic antagonists can be found for carvedilol (Coreg) in Chapter 24, propranolol (Inderal) in Chapter 25, metoprolol (Lopressor) and atenolol (Tenormin) in Chapter 27, and timolol (Timoptic) in Chapter 49 ∞.

TABLE 23.7   Adrenergic Antagonists for Hypertension

Drug	Route and Adult Dose (max dose where indicated)	Adverse Effects
BETA-ADRENERGIC ANTAGONISTS		
atenolol (Tenormin): beta$_1$ (see page 353 for the Prototype Drug box ∞)	PO; 25–50 mg/day (max: 100 mg/day)	*Fatigue, insomnia, drowsiness, impotence or decreased libido, bradycardia and confusion*
bisoprolol (Zebeta): beta$_1$	PO; 2.5–5 mg/day (max: 20 mg/day)	
metoprolol (Toprol, Lopressor): beta$_1$	PO; 50–100 mg/day–bid (max: 450 mg/day)	Agranulocytosis, laryngospasm, Stevens–Johnson syndrome, anaphylaxis; if the drug is abruptly withdrawn, palpitations, rebound hypertension, dysrhythmias, MI
propranolol (Inderal): beta$_1$ and beta$_2$ (see page 369 for the Prototype Drug box ∞)	PO; 10–30 mg tid or daily (max: 320 mg/day) IV; 0.5–3.0 mg of q4h PRN	
timolol (Betimol, others): beta$_1$ and beta$_2$ (see page 776 for the Prototype Drug box ∞)	PO; 15–45 mg tid (max: 60 mg/day)	
ALPHA$_1$-ADRENERGIC ANTAGONISTS		
doxazosin (Cardura)	PO; 1 mg at bedtime; may increase to 16 mg/day in a single dose or 2 divided doses (max: 16 mg/day)	*Orthostatic hypotension, dizziness, headache, fatigue*
prazosin (Minipress) (see page 141 for the Prototype Drug box ∞)	PO; 1 mg at bedtime; may increase to 1 mg bid–tid (max: 20 mg/day)	First-dose phenomenon, tachycardia, dyspnea
terazosin (Hytrin)	PO; 1 mg at bedtime; may increase 1–5 mg/day (max: 20 mg/day)	
ALPHA$_2$-ADRENERGIC AGONISTS		
clonidine (Catapres)	PO; 0.1 mg bid–tid (max: 0.8 mg/day)	*Peripheral edema, sedation, depression, headache, dry mouth, decreased libido*
guanabenz (Wytensin)	PO; 4 mg bid; may increase by 4–8 mg/day q1–2 wk (max: 32 mg bid)	
methyldopa (Aldomet)	PO; 250 mg bid or tid (max: 3 g/day)	Hepatotoxicity, hemolytic anemia, granulocytopenia
ALPHA$_1$- AND BETA-BLOCKERS (CENTRALLY ACTING)		
carteolol (Cartrol, Ocupress)	PO; 2.5 mg/day; may increase to 5–10 mg if needed (max: 10 mg/day)	*Headache, drowsiness, anxiety, depression, lethargy, impotence*
labetalol (Trandate, Normodyne)	PO; 100 mg bid; may increase to 200–400 mg bid (max: 1200–2400 mg/day)	Bradycardia, may worsen heart failure and mask symptoms of hypoglycemia
ADRENERGIC NEURON BLOCKERS (PERIPHERALLY ACTING)		
guanadrel (Hylorel)	PO; 5 mg bid; may increase to 20–75 mg/day in 2–4 divided doses	*Fatigue, dizziness, edema, nasal congestion, drowsiness, bradycardia*
guanethidine (Ismelin)	PO; 10 mg daily; may increase by 10 mg q5–7 days up to 300 mg/day (start with 25–50 mg/day in hospitalized patients, increase by 25–50 mg q1–3 days)	Respiratory depression, bronchospasm, mental depression
reserpine (Serpasil)	PO; 1.5 mg daily initially; may reduce to 0.1–0.25 mg/day	

Italics indicate common adverse effects; underlining indicates serious adverse effects.

The *alpha$_1$-adrenergic antagonists* lower blood pressure directly by blocking sympathetic receptors in arterioles, causing the vessels to dilate. The alpha-blockers are not first-line drugs for HTN because long-term clinical trials have shown them to be less effective at reducing the incidence of serious cardiovascular events than diuretics. When used to treat HTN, the alpha-blockers should be used concurrently with other classes of antihypertensives, such as the diuretics. Prototypes for alpha-blockers include prazosin (Minipress), discussed in Chapter 13, and tamsulosin (Flomax), discussed in Chapter 46 ∞.

The side effects of adrenergic blockers are generally predictable extensions of the fight-or-flight response. At low doses, the beta-blockers are well tolerated, and serious adverse effects are uncommon. As the dosage is increased, beta-blockers will slow the heart rate and cause bronchoconstriction, they should be used with caution in clients with asthma or heart failure. Many clients report fatigue and activity intolerance at higher doses, because the reduction in heart rate causes the heart to become less responsive to exertion. The alpha$_1$-adrenergic blockers tend to cause orthostatic hypotension when a person moves quickly from a supine to an upright position. Dizziness, nausea, bradycardia, and dry mouth are also common. Less common, though sometimes a major cause of noncompliance, is the effect of adrenergic blockers on male sexual function. These agents can cause decreased libido and erectile dysfunction (impotence). Because abrupt cessation of beta-blocker therapy can result in rebound HTN, angina, and MI, drug doses should be tapered over several weeks.

The *alpha₂-adrenergic agonists* decrease the outflow of sympathetic nerve impulses from the central nervous system to the heart and arterioles. In effect, this produces the same responses as inhibition of the alpha₁-receptor: slowing of the heart rate and conduction velocity, and dilation of the arterioles. The alpha₂-agonists cause sedation, dizziness, and other CNS effects. With the exception of methyldopa (Aldomet), which is sometimes a preferred agent for treating HTN occurring during pregnancy, these drugs are rarely prescribed.

The final class of adrenergic agents for HTN, *adrenergic neuron blockers*, inhibits the synthesis or release of norepinephrine (NE) in sympathetic neurons. The adrenergic neuron blocking agents such as reserpine have mostly historical interest, as they are rarely prescribed in clinical practice owing to the development of safer medications.

NURSING CONSIDERATIONS

The role of the nurse in adrenergic antagonist therapy for HTN involves careful monitoring of a patient's condition and providing education as it is related to the prescribed drug treatment. Obtain baseline vital signs and monitor blood pressure during therapy. Assess client's blood pressure changes as dosage is increased. Assess apical pulse rate and blood pressure before administering these medications. Hold the medicine if the pulse is below 60 beats per minute or the blood pressure is 90/60 mm Hg or below, and notify the healthcare provider. Assess the client's ability to tolerate activity by gradually increasing ambulation frequency and distance. Monitor cardiac response by assessing heart rate, rhythm, heart sounds, and ECG. Observe for bradycardia and heart block. Assess for orthostatic hypotension and other side effects such as dizziness, nausea, and dry mouth.

Observe clients with diabetes for signs and symptoms of hypoglycemia. Monitor finger-stick blood glucose levels at regular intervals, since symptoms of hypoglycemia may not be apparent in clients taking beta-adrenergic blockers.

Alpha₁-adrenergic Blockers

Alpha₁-adrenergic blockers are prescribed for hypertension and **benign prostatic hypertrophy (BPH)** because they relax smooth muscle in the prostate and bladder neck, thus reducing urethral resistance. The first-dose phenomenon, including syncope, can occur. Assess blood pressure prior to and routinely during therapy because the client may experience hypotension with the first few doses of these medications, and orthostatic hypotension may persist throughout treatment. Assess for common side effects such as weakness, dizziness, headache, and GI complaints such as nausea and vomiting. Elderly clients are especially prone to the hypotensive and hypothermic effects related to vasodilation caused by these drugs. Drugs in this group range from pregnancy category B (prazosin) to C (terazosin). See "Nursing Process Focus: Client Receiving Adrenergic Blocker Therapy," page 142 in Chapter 13 ∞.

Pr **PROTOTYPE DRUG** | Doxazosin *(Cardura)* | Alpha₁-adrenergic Blocker

ACTIONS AND USES

Doxazosin is a selective alpha₁-adrenergic blocker available only as tablets. Because it is selective for blocking alpha₁-receptors in vascular smooth muscle, it has few adverse effects on other autonomic organs and is preferred over nonselective beta-blockers. Doxazosin dilates arteries and veins and is capable of causing a rapid, profound fall in blood pressure. Clients who have difficulty urinating owing to an enlarged prostate (BPH) sometimes receive this drug to relieve symptoms of dysuria.

ADMINISTRATION ALERTS

- May produce a first-dose phenomenon resulting in profound hypotension, and possible syncope.
- The first-dose phenomenon can reoccur when medication is resumed after a period of withdrawal and with dosage increases.
- Pregnancy category B.

PHARMACOKINETICS

Onset: 2 h

Peak: 2–6 h

Half-life: 9–12 h

Duration: 24 h

ADVERSE EFFECTS

On starting doxazosin therapy, some clients experience serious orthostatic hypotension, although tolerance often develops to this side effect after a few doses. Dizziness and headache are also common side effects, although they are rarely severe enough to cause discontinuation of therapy.

Contraindications: Doxazosin is contraindicated in clients with prior hypersensitivity to alpha blockers.

INTERACTIONS

Drug–Drug: When given concurrently, other antihypertensives have additive effects with doxazosin on blood pressure. Oral cimetidine may cause a mild increase (10%) in the half-life of doxazosin.

Lab Tests: Unknown.

Herbal/Food: Unknown.

Treatment of Overdose: The most likely sign of overdosage is hypotension, which is treated with a vasopressor and/or IV infusion of fluids.

 See the Companion Website for a Nursing Process Focus specific to this drug.

NURSING PROCESS FOCUS   Clients Receiving Beta-adrenergic Antagonist Therapy

Assessment	Potential Nursing Diagnoses
Prior to administration: • Obtain a complete health history including allergies, drug history, and possible drug interactions. • Assess vital signs, urinary output, and cardiac output (initially and throughout therapy). • Assess for presence of respiratory disease, including asthma and COPD.	• Knowledge, Deficient, related to drug therapy • Cardiac Output, Decreased • Injury, Risk for, related to orthostatic hypotension • Sexual Dysfunction • Noncompliance, related to therapeutic regimen

Planning: Client Goals and Expected Outcomes

The client will:
• Exhibit a reduction in systolic and diastolic blood pressure.
• Exhibit stable cardiac output and pulse rate.
• Demonstrate an understanding of the drug's action by accurately describing drug side effects and precautions.

Implementation

Interventions and (Rationales)	Client Education/Discharge Planning
• Monitor vital signs and pulse, observe for signs of bradycardia, heart failure, or pulmonary edema. (Beta-blockers decrease heart rate and cardiac output.)	• Instruct client to monitor pulse and blood pressure daily.
• Monitor for orthostatic hypotension. (Beta-blockers cause orthostatic hypotension.)	Instruct client to: • Stop medication and notify healthcare provider if pulse falls below 60 beats per minute or blood pressure is 90/60 mm Hg or below. • Rise slowly from a sitting or lying position to avoid dizziness.
• Observe for drowsiness, fatigue, and weakness. (These are side effects of beta-blockers.)	Instruct client to: • Report side effects such as difficulty in breathing, dizziness, confusion, fatigue, weakness, and impotence. • Avoid driving or other activities requiring mental alertness or physical coordination until effects of the drug are known.
• In diabetic clients, monitor for hypoglycemia. (Some beta-blockers may lower blood glucose levels.)	Instruct the diabetic client to: • Check finger-stick blood glucose levels at regular intervals and report signs of hypoglycemia and/or consistent fasting blood glucose levels below 70 mg/dl.
• Monitor for effects on the heart, especially with exertion. (Beta-blockers can decrease cardiac output.)	Instruct client to: • Begin exercise or other exertion slowly and to determine tolerance to increased activity. • Report chest pain, shortness of breath, fainting, or palpitations with exertion. • Keep all scheduled laboratory visits and appointments for cardiac evaluations such as ECGs.

Evaluation of Outcome Criteria

Evaluate the effectiveness of drug therapy by confirming that client goals and expected outcomes have been met (see "Planning"):
• The client's blood pressure is within normal limits.
• The client's cardiac output and pulse rate remain stable.
• The client demonstrates an understanding of the drug's action by describing drug side effects and precautions.

∞ *See Table 23.7 under "Beta-Blockers" for a list of drugs to which these nursing actions apply.*

Alpha₂-adrenergic Agonists

Alpha$_2$-agonists are centrally acting and have multiple side effects, thus these drugs are usually reserved to treat hypertension uncontrolled by other drugs. Assess for the presence of common adverse effects such as orthostatic hypotension, sedation, decreased libido, impotence, sodium/water retention, and dry mouth. Alpha$_2$-agonists are pregnancy category C; these drugs are distributed into breast milk.

Beta-adrenergic Blockers

Some beta-adrenergic blockers decrease heart rate and affect myocardial conduction and contractility. Assess for signs of respiratory distress, including shortness of breath and wheezing, in clients on nonspecific beta-blocking drugs. These side effects tend to occur at high doses.

Because beta-blockers affect myocardial contractility, monitor heart rate, rhythm, and sounds, as well as ECG.

TABLE 23.8	Direct-acting Vasodilators for Hypertension	
Drug	**Route and Adult Dose (max dose where indicated)**	**Adverse Effects**
diazoxide (Hyperstat IV)	IV; 1–3 mg/kg push (max: 150 mg)	*Orthostatic hypotension, fluid retention, headache, palpitations*
hydralazine (Apresoline)	PO; 10–50 mg qid (max: 300 mg/day)	
minoxidil (Loniten)	PO; 5–40 mg/day in a single dose or divided doses (max: 100 mg/day)	<u>Lupus-like reaction (hydralazine), severe hypotension, MI, dysrhythmias, shock</u>
nitroprusside (Nitropress)	IV; 1.5–10 mcg/kg/min	

Italics indicate common adverse effects; <u>underlining</u> indicates serious adverse effects.

MediaLink Herbal Therapies for Hypertension

Assess for bradycardia, heart block, and fatigue and activity intolerance. Beta-blockers cause the heart rate to become less responsive to exertion.

Client Teaching. Client education as it relates to these drugs should include the goals of therapy, the reasons for obtaining baseline data such as vital signs and the existence of underlying disorders, and possible drug side effects. Include the following points when teaching patients about adrenergic antagonists:

- Rise slowly from a sitting or lying position to prevent dizziness.
- Monitor pulse and blood pressure daily, and notify healthcare provider if pulse is below 60 beats per minute and blood pressure is 90/60 mm Hg or below.
- Report dizziness, shortness of breath, fatigue, confusion, or weakness.
- If diabetic, check finger-stick blood glucose at regular intervals, and report fasting blood glucose consistently below 70 mg/dl. The usual signs of hypoglycemia may not be experienced when taking these medications.

DIRECT VASODILATORS

Drugs that directly affect vascular smooth muscle are highly effective at lowering blood pressure but produce too many side effects to be drugs of first choice. These agents are listed in Table 23.8.

23.11 Treating Hypertension With Direct Vasodilators

Many of the antihypertensive classes discussed thus far lower blood pressure through indirect means by affecting enzymes (ACE inhibitors), autonomic nerves (alpha- and beta-blockers), or fluid volume (diuretics). It would seem that a more efficient way to reduce blood pressure would be to cause a direct relaxation of vascular smooth muscle; unfortunately, the direct vasodilator drugs have the potential to produce serious adverse effects.

Direct vasodilators produce reflex tachycardia, a compensatory response to the sudden decrease in blood pressure caused by the drug. Reflex tachycardia forces the heart to work harder, and blood pressure increases, counteracting the effect of the antihypertensive drug. Clients with coro-

nary artery disease could experience an acute angina attack. Fortunately, reflex tachycardia can be prevented by the concurrent administration of a beta-adrenergic blocker, such as propranolol.

A second potentially serious side effect of direct vasodilator therapy is sodium and water retention. As the kidney retains more sodium and water, blood volume increases, thus raising blood pressure and canceling the antihypertensive action of the vasodilator. A diuretic may be administered concurrently with a direct vasodilator to prevent fluid retention.

One direct-acting vasodilator, nitroprusside (Nitropress), is a drug of choice for hypertensive emergency, a condition in which diastolic pressure is greater than 120 mm Hg, and there is evidence of target-organ damage, usually to the heart, kidney, or brain. This potentially life-threatening condition must be controlled quickly. Nitroprusside, with a half-life of only 2 minutes, has the ability to lower blood pressure almost instantaneously on IV administration. Care must be taken not to decrease blood pressure too quickly because overtreatment can result in hypotension and severe restriction of blood flow to the cerebral, coronary, or renal vascular capillaries. It is essential to continuously monitor clients receiving this drug. Other drugs for hypertensive emergencies include diazoxide (a direct vasodilator), nicardipine (a calcium channel blocker), and enalaprilat (an ACE inhibitor).

NURSING CONSIDERATIONS

Direct vasodilators are utilized primarily in emergency situations when it is necessary to reduce blood pressure quickly. In the critical care or emergency department setting, monitor vital signs, ECG, and pulse oximetry continuously while the drug is being infused. Assess for increased heart rate due to reflex tachycardia. Auscultate blood pressure every 5 to 15 minutes during the drug infusion if the client is not on continuous monitoring.

Obtain a thorough history to detect hypersensitivity, coronary artery disease, rheumatic mitral valve disease, cerebrovascular disease, renal insufficiency, or systemic lupus erythematosus, all of which could contraindicate the use of direct vasodilators. A rare but upsetting side effect is *priapism,* a sustained, painful penile erection unrelieved by orgasm. If not treated promptly, permanent impotence may result. Put clients at ease and display a matter-of-fact demeanor to relieve embarrassment in this situation.

During repeated treatment with IV diazoxide (Hyperstat), assess clients for signs of fluid retention, such as edema of the extremities, face, and eyes. Monitor lab values for elevation in sodium levels. Administer concurrent diuretics as ordered to minimize this side effect.

During therapy with minoxidil (Loniten), monitor blood pressure and pulse in both arms in three positions (lying, sitting, and standing) to assess for orthostatic hypotension. Inform clients that body hair normally changes in length, thickness, and pigmentation during use and will reverse when the drug is discontinued.

Administer nitroprusside IV *only* with 5% dextrose in water (D5W) and never with any other drugs or diluents. Reconstituted nitroprusside solution is brown and considered stable for up to 24 hours, but the drug is exceptionally light sensitive. Wrap the IV bag and tubing in an opaque substance such as aluminum foil; also label the wrap on the bag itself. Check the solution periodically and discard it if the color of the solution changes.

Lifespan Considerations. Intravenous diazoxide (Hyperstat) may be used during hypertensive emergencies in labor and delivery. When this medication is used, assess the newborn closely for hyperbilirubinemia; thrombocytopenia and altered carbohydrate metabolism may also be side effects.

Client Teaching. Client education as it relates to these drugs should include the goals of therapy, the reasons for obtaining baseline data such as vital signs and underlying disorders, and possible drug side effects. Include the following points when teaching clients about direct vasodilators:

- Immediately report priapism (painful, sustained penile erection) because it is a medical emergency that could cause permanent impotence.
- Minoxidil therapy may cause reversible changes in the color and texture of body hair as a side effect.
- Report dizziness, palpitations, or faintness during IV administration.
- Report headache or signs of stroke, such as facial drooping, slurred speech, or numbness in extremities.
- Monitor blood pressure daily and report readings 90/60 mm Hg or below or above 140/90 mm Hg.
- Do not drive until effects of the drug are known.
- Rise slowly from a sitting or lying position to prevent dizziness.

Pr PROTOTYPE DRUG | Hydralazine *(Apresoline)* | Direct Vasodilator

ACTIONS AND USES

Hydralazine was one of the first oral antihypertensive drugs marketed in the United States. It acts through a direct vasodilation of arterial smooth muscle; it has no effect on veins. Although hydralazine produces an effective reduction in blood pressure, drugs in other antihypertensive classes have largely replaced it owing to safety concerns. The drug is available as tablets and in parenteral formulations for the treatment of hypertensive emergency.

ADMINISTRATION ALERTS

- Abrupt withdrawal of drug may cause rebound hypertension and anxiety.
- Pregnancy category C.

PHARMACOKINETICS

Onset: 20–30 min PO; 10–30 min IM, 5–20 min IV

Peak: Unknown

Half-life: 3–7 h

Duration: 2–6 h

ADVERSE EFFECTS

Hydralazine may produce serious side effects, including severe reflex tachycardia. Clients taking hydralazine often receive a beta-adrenergic blocker to counteract this effect on the heart. Rarely, the drug may produce a lupus-like syndrome that may persist for 6 months or longer. Sodium and fluid retention is a potentially serious adverse effect. Because of these side effects, the use of hydralazine is limited mostly to clients whose HTN cannot be controlled with other, safer medications.

Contraindications: Because of its effects on the heart, hydralazine is contraindicated in clients with angina, rheumatic heart disease, MI, or tachycardia. Clients with lupus should not receive hydralazine, as the drug can worsen symptoms.

INTERACTIONS

Drug–Drug: When given concurrently, other antihypertensives have additive or synergistic effects with hydralazine on blood pressure. Use with MAO inhibitors may potentiate hypotensive action.

Lab Tests: May produce false positive Coombs tests.

Herbal/Food: Unknown.

Treatment of Overdose: The most likely sign of overdosage is hypotension, which is treated with a vasopressor and/or an IV infusion of fluids.

 See the Companion Website for a Nursing Process Focus specific to this drug.

NURSING PROCESS FOCUS Clients Receiving Direct Vasodilator Therapy

Assessment	Potential Nursing Diagnoses
Prior to administration: - Obtain a complete health history including allergies, drug history, possible drug interactions, and especially impaired cardiac/cerebral circulation. - Obtain an ECG and vital signs. - Auscultate heart and chest sounds. - Assess neurological status and level of consciousness. - Obtain blood and urine specimens for laboratory analysis.	- Tissue Perfusion, Ineffective - Fluid Volume, Excess - Injury, Risk for, related to orthostatic hypotension - Skin Integrity, Risk for Impaired, related to infiltration of IV medication - Knowledge, deficient, related to drug therapy

Planning: Client Goals and Expected Outcomes

The client will:
- Exhibit a reduction in systolic and diastolic blood pressure.
- Demonstrate an understanding of the drug's action by accurately describing drug side effects and precautions.

Implementation

Interventions and (Rationales)	Client Education/Discharge Planning
- Observe for signs and symptoms of lupus. (These are side effects of the drug.)	- Instruct client to report classic "butterfly rash" over the nose and cheeks, muscle aches, and fatigue when taking hydralazine.
- Monitor vital signs every 5 to 15 minutes and titrate infusion based on prescribed parameters and be prepared to treat reflex tachycardia if it occurs. (These drugs cause rapid hypotension and reflex tachycardia.)	Instruct client: - About the purpose of treatment and reassure the client during emergency care. - To report feelings of rapid heart rate, dizziness, or faintness.
- Observe for IV infiltration. (Direct vasodilators can cause tissue destruction if infiltration occurs.)	- Instruct client to report any burning or stinging pain, swelling, warmth, redness, or tenderness at IV insertion site.
- Monitor cardiac/cerebral circulation. (Hypotension produced by vasodilators may further compromise individuals who already suffer from ischemia.)	Instruct client to: - Report angina-like symptoms: chest, arm, back and/or neck pain, palpitations. - Report faintness, dizziness, drowsiness, any sensation of cold, numbness, tingling, pale or dusky look to the hands and feet. - Report headache or signs of stroke: facial drooping, visual changes, limb weakness, or paralysis. - Monitor vital signs (especially blood pressure) daily after discharge.
- Monitor for hypotension and dizziness. (Direct vasodilators may cause decreased circulation to the brain.)	Instruct client to: - Avoid driving or other activities requiring mental alertness or physical coordination until effects of the drug are known. - Rise from a sitting or lying position slowly to avoid dizziness.
- Evaluate for needed lifestyle modifications. (Lifestyle modifications are effective in reducing HTN.)	- Instruct client to comply with additional interventions for HTN such as weight reduction, modification of sodium intake, smoking cessation, exercise, and stress management.
- Discontinue medication gradually. (Abrupt withdrawal of drug may cause rebound hypertension and anxiety.)	- Instruct client to not stop taking drug suddenly.

Evaluation of Outcome Criteria

Evaluate the effectiveness of drug therapy by confirming that client goals and expected outcomes have been met (see "Planning").
- The client's blood pressure is within normal limits.
- The client demonstrates an understanding of the drug's actions by accurately describing drug side effects and precautions.

∞ *See Table 23.8 for a list of drugs to which these nursing applications apply.*

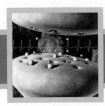

CHAPTER REVIEW

KEY CONCEPTS

The numbered key concepts provide a succinct summary of the important points from the corresponding numbered section within the chapter. If any of these points are not clear, refer to the numbered section within the chapter for review.

23.1 High blood pressure is classified as essential (primary) or secondary. Uncontrolled hypertension can lead to chronic and debilitating disorders such as stroke, heart attack, and heart failure.

23.2 The three primary factors controlling blood pressure are cardiac output, peripheral resistance, and blood volume.

23.3 Many factors help regulate blood pressure, including the vasomotor center, baroreceptors and chemoreceptors in the aorta and internal carotid arteries, and the renin–angiotensin system.

23.4 Hypertension has recently been redefined as a sustained blood pressure of 140/90 mm Hg after multiple measurements made over several clinic visits. A person with sustained blood pressure of 120–139/80–89 mm Hg is said to be prehypertensive, and is at increased risk of developing hypertension.

23.5 Because antihypertensive medications may have uncomfortable side effects, lifestyle changes such as proper diet and exercise should be implemented prior to and during pharmacotherapy to allow lower drug doses.

23.6 Pharmacotherapy of HTN often begins with low doses of a single medication. If this medication proves ineffec-

tive, a second agent from a different class may be added to the regimen.

23.7 Diuretics are often the first-line medications for HTN because they have few side effects and can control minor to moderate hypertension.

23.8 Calcium channel blockers block calcium ions from entering cells and cause smooth muscle in arterioles to relax, thus reducing blood pressure. CCBs have emerged as major drugs in the treatment of hypertension.

23.9 Blocking the renin–angiotensin system prevents the intense vasoconstriction caused by angiotensin II. These drugs also decrease blood volume, which enhances their antihypertensive effect.

23.10 Antihypertensive autonomic agents are available that block $alpha_1$-adrenergic receptors, block $beta_1$- and/or $beta_2$-adrenergic receptors, or stimulate $alpha_2$-adrenergic receptors in the brainstem (centrally acting).

23.11 A few medications lower blood pressure by acting directly to relax arteriolar smooth muscle, but these are not widely used owing to their numerous side effects.

NCLEX-RN® REVIEW QUESTIONS

1 The client, prescribed furosemide (Lasix) as an adjunct to treatment of hypertension, returns for follow-up. Which of the following is the most objective data for determining the effectiveness of the drug therapy?

1. Absence of edema in lower extremities.
2. Weight loss of 6 lb.
3. Blood pressure log notes blood pressure 120/70 mm Hg to 134/88 mm Hg since discharge.
4. Frequency of voiding of at least 6 times per day.

2 The nurse prepares to administer hydrochlorothiazide (HydroDIURIL) 25 mg to a client with hypertension. The potassium lab result is 2.5 mEq. The nurse's best action is to:

1. Hold the medication and notify the healthcare provider.
2. Administer the drug with orange juice.
3. Administer the drug as ordered.
4. Give the client a banana and recheck the potassium level.

3 The client is on two antihypertensive drugs. The nurse recognizes that the advantage of combination therapy is:

1. The blood pressure will decrease faster.
2. There will be fewer side effects and greater client compliance.
3. There is less daily medication dosing.
4. Combination therapy will treat the client's other medical conditions.

4 The class of antihypertensives that affects the renin-angiotensin pathway to increase urine is the:

1. Calcium channel blockers
2. Adrenergic blockers
3. ACE inhibitors
4. Direct acting vasodilators

5 The nurse is preparing to administer the first dose of enalapril (Vasotec). Identify potential adverse effects of this medication. (Select all that apply.)

1. Reflux hypertension
2. Hyperkalemia
3. Persistent cough
4. Angioedema
5. Hypotension

CRITICAL THINKING QUESTIONS

1. A 74-year-old client has a history of hypertension, mild renal failure, and angina. The client is on a low-sodium, low-protein diet. The most recent BP is 106/84. Should the nurse give the client benazepril (Lotensin) as scheduled? Provide rationale for the decision.

2. A client with diabetes is on atenolol (Tenormin) for hypertension. Identify a teaching plan for this client.

3. A client is having a hypertensive crisis (230/130), and the BP needs to be lowered. The client has an IV drip of nitroprusside (Nitropress) initiated. How much would the nurse want to lower this client's BP? Identify three nursing interventions that are crucial when administering this medication.

See Appendix D for answers and rationales for all activities.

EXPLORE
MediaLink

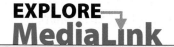
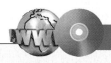

www.prenhall.com/adams

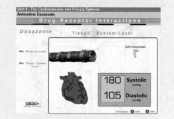

NCLEX-RN® review, case studies, and other interactive resources for this chapter can be found on the companion website at www.prenhall.com/adams. Click on "Chapter 23" to select the activities for this chapter. For animations, more NCLEX-RN® review questions, and an audio glossary, access the accompanying Prentice Hall Nursing MediaLink DVD-ROM in this textbook.

 PRENTICE HALL NURSING MEDIA LINK DVD-ROM

- **Animations**
  Mechanism in Action: Nifedipine (*Procardia*)
  Mechanism in Action: Doxazosin (*Cardura*)
- **Audio Glossary**
- **NCLEX-RN® Review**

 COMPANION WEBSITE

- **NCLEX-RN® Review**
- **Dosage Calculations**
- **Case Study:** Client with hypertension
- **Care Plan:** Client who takes enalapril for hypertension

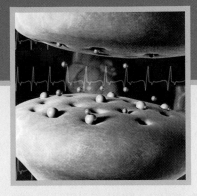

CHAPTER 24

Drugs for Heart Failure

DRUGS AT A GLANCE

ANGIOTENSIN-CONVERTING ENZYME (ACE) INHIBITORS AND ANGIOTENSIN-RECEPTOR BLOCKERS
   💿 *lisinopril (Prinivil, Zestril)*

DIURETICS
   💿 *furosemide (Lasix)*

BETA-ADRENERGIC BLOCKERS (ANTAGONISTS)
   💿 *metoprolol (Lopressor)*

VASODILATORS
   💿 *isosorbide dinitrate (Isordil, Sorbitrate, Dilatrate)*

CARDIAC GLYCOSIDES
   💿 *digoxin (Lanoxin, Lanoxicaps)*

PHOSPHODIESTERASE INHIBITORS
   💿 *milrinone (Primacor)*

OBJECTIVES

After reading this chapter, the student should be able to:

1. Identify the major diseases associated with heart failure.
2. Relate how the classic symptoms associated with heart failure may be caused by weakened heart muscle.
3. Explain how preload and afterload affect cardiac function.
4. Describe the nurse's role in the pharmacological management of heart failure.
5. For each of the drug classes listed in Drugs at a Glance, know representative drug examples, and explain their mechanisms of action, primary actions, and important adverse effects.
6. Categorize heart failure drugs based on their classification and mechanisms of action.
7. Use the Nursing Process to care for clients who are receiving drug therapy for heart failure.

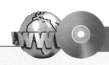

MediaLink　　　www.prenhall.com/adams

NCLEX-RN® review, case studies, and other interactive resources for this chapter can be found on the companion website at www.prenhall.com/adams. Click on "Chapter 24" to select the activities for this chapter. For animations, more NCLEX-RN® review questions, and an audio glossary, access the accompanying Prentice Hall Nursing MediaLink DVD-ROM in this textbook.

KEY TERMS

afterload *page 331*

cardiac output *page 331*

cardiac remodeling *page 331*

contractility *page 331*

Frank–Starling law *page 331*

heart failure (HF) *page 330*

inotropic effect *page 336*

peripheral edema *page 331*

phosphodiesterase *page 341*

preload *page 331*

Heart failure is one of the most common and fatal of the cardiovascular diseases, and its incidence is expected to increase as the population ages. Despite the dramatic decline in mortality for most cardiovascular disease (CVD) that has occurred over the past two decades, the death rate for heart failure has only recently begun to decrease. Although improved treatment of myocardial infarction (MI) and hypertension (HTN) has led to declines in mortality due to heart failure, approximately one in five clients still dies within 1 year of diagnosis of heart failure, and 50% die within 5 years. Historically, this condition was called *congestive heart failure;* however, because not all incidences of this disease are associated with congestion, the more appropriate name is heart failure.

24.1 The Etiology of Heart Failure

Heart failure (HF) is the inability of the ventricles to pump enough blood to meet the body's metabolic demands. Heart failure can be caused by any disorder that affects the heart's ability to receive or eject blood. Whereas weakening of cardiac muscle is a natural consequence of aging, the process can be caused or accelerated by the following:

- Mitral stenosis
- MI
- Chronic HTN
- Coronary artery disease (CAD)
- Diabetes mellitus

Because there is no cure for heart failure, the treatment goals are to prevent, treat, or remove the underlying *causes* when possible. Controlling lipid levels and keeping blood pressure within normal limits reduces the incidences of CAD and MI. Maintaining blood glucose within normal values reduces the cardiovascular consequences of uncontrolled diabetes. Thus, for many clients, HF is a preventable condition; controlling associated diseases will greatly reduce the risk of eventual HF. No longer is therapy of HF focused on endstages of the disorder. Pharmacotherapy is now targeted at *prevention* and *slowing the progression* of HF. This change in emphasis has led to significant improvements in survival and the quality of life for clients with HF.

PHARMFACTS

Heart Failure

- Heart failure (HF) increases with age. It affects:
  2% of those 40 to 50 years old
  5% of those 60 to 69 years old
  10% of those older than age 70
- More than 42,000 people die of HF each year.
- The incidence of sudden death is as much as nine times higher in clients with HF than in the general population.
- Heart failure is the most common hospital discharge diagnosis in clients aged 65 or older.
- African Americans have one and a half to two times the incidence of HF as whites.
- Heart failure occurs slightly more frequently in men than in women.
- Heart failure is twice as frequent in hypertensive clients and five times as frequent in persons who have experienced a heart attack.

24.2 Cardiovascular Changes in Heart Failure

Although a number of diseases can lead to heart failure, the result is the same: The heart is unable to pump the volume of blood required to meet the metabolic needs of the body. To understand how medications act on the weakened myocardium, it is essential to understand the underlying cardiac physiology.

The right side of the heart receives blood from the venous system and pumps it to the lungs, where the blood receives oxygen and releases carbon dioxide. The blood returns to the left side of the heart, which pumps it to the rest of the body via the aorta. The amount of blood received by the right side should exactly equal that sent out by the left side. If the heart is unable to completely empty the left ventricle, HF may occur. The amount of blood pumped by each ventricle per minute is the **cardiac output.** The relationship between cardiac output and blood pressure is explained in Chapter 23 ∞.

Although many variables affect cardiac output, the two most important factors are **preload** and **afterload.** Just before the chambers of the heart contract (systole), they are filled to their maximum capacity with blood. The degree to which the myocardial fibers are stretched just prior to contraction is called preload. The more these fibers are stretched, the more forcefully they will contract, a principle called the **Frank–Starling law.** This is somewhat similar to a rubber band; the more it is stretched, the more forcefully it will snap back. The strength of contraction of the heart is called **contractility.** Up to a physiological limit, *drugs that increase preload and contractility will increase the cardiac output.*

Drugs that *increase* contractility are called *positive inotropic agents.* Examples of positive inotropic agents include epinephrine, norepinephrine, thyroid hormone, and dopamine. Drugs that *decrease* contractility are called *negative inotropic agents.* Examples include quinidine and beta-adrenergic antagonists such as propranolol.

The second important factor affecting cardiac output is *afterload,* the degree of pressure in the aorta that must be overcome for blood to be ejected from the left ventricle. The most common cause of increased afterload is an increase in peripheral resistance due to HTN. The greater afterload caused by chronic HTN creates an increased workload on the heart, which explains why clients with chronic HTN are more likely to experience HF. *Lowering blood pressure creates less afterload, resulting in less workload for the heart.*

In HF, the myocardium becomes weakened, and the heart cannot eject all the blood it receives. This impairment may occur on the left side, the right side, or on both sides of the heart. If it occurs on the left side, excess blood accumulates in the left ventricle. The wall of the left ventricle thickens and enlarges (hypertrophy) in an attempt to compensate for the increased workload. Over time, changes in the size, shape, and structure of the myocardial cells (myocytes) occur, a process known as **cardiac remodeling.** Because the left ventricle has limits to its ability to compensate for the increased preload, blood "backs up" into the lungs, resulting in the classic symptoms of cough and shortness of breath. Left heart failure is sometimes called *congestive heart failure (CHF).* The pathophysiology of HF is shown in ● Figure 24.1.

Although left heart failure is more common, the right side of the heart can also weaken, either simultaneously with the left side or independently of the left side. In right heart failure, the blood backs up into veins, resulting in **peripheral edema** and engorgement of organs such as the liver.

Through proper pharmacotherapy and lifestyle modifications, many clients with HF can be maintained in an asymptomatic state for years. When the heart reaches a stage at which it can no longer handle the workload, *cardiac decompensation* occurs and classic symptoms of HF appear, such as dyspnea on exertion, fatigue, pulmonary congestion,

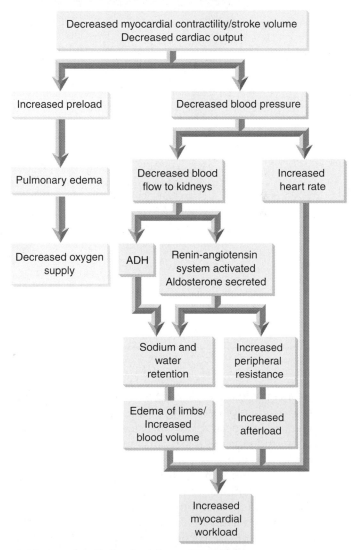

● **Figure 24.1** Pathophysiology of heart failure

PHARMACOTHERAPY ILLUSTRATED

24.1 Mechanisms of Action of Drugs Used for Heart Failure

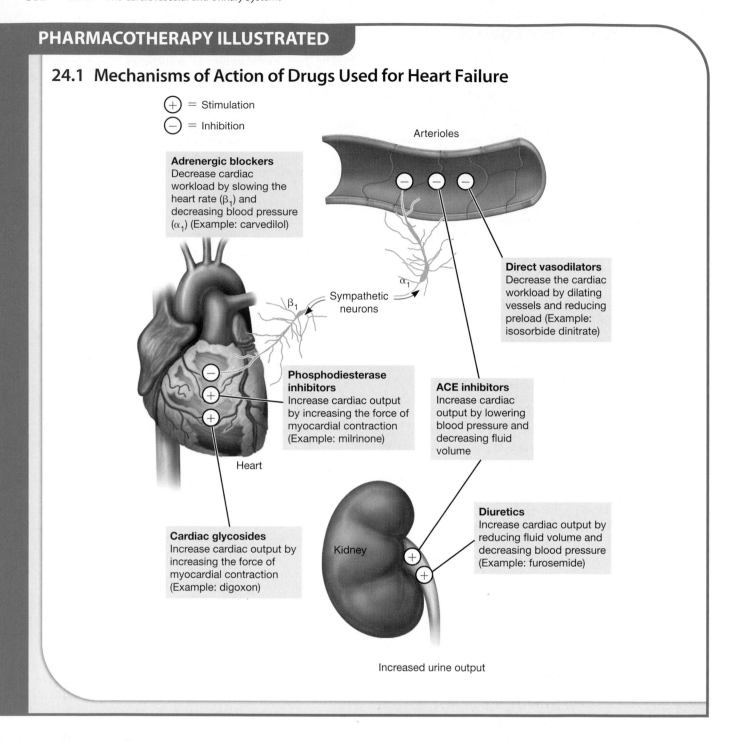

$\oplus$ = Stimulation

$\ominus$ = Inhibition

Adrenergic blockers
Decrease cardiac workload by slowing the heart rate (β_1) and decreasing blood pressure (α_1) (Example: carvedilol)

Arterioles

Sympathetic neurons

β_1

α_1

Direct vasodilators
Decrease the cardiac workload by dilating vessels and reducing preload (Example: isosorbide dinitrate)

Phosphodiesterase inhibitors
Increase cardiac output by increasing the force of myocardial contraction (Example: milrinone)

ACE inhibitors
Increase cardiac output by lowering blood pressure and decreasing fluid volume

Heart

Cardiac glycosides
Increase cardiac output by increasing the force of myocardial contraction (Example: digoxon)

Kidney

Diuretics
Increase cardiac output by reducing fluid volume and decreasing blood pressure (Example: furosemide)

Increased urine output

and peripheral edema. Lung congestion causes cough and orthopnea (difficulty breathing when recumbent). When pulmonary edema occurs, the client feels as if he or she is suffocating, and extreme anxiety may result. The condition often worsens at night.

The most common reason why clients experience decompensation is noncompliance with sodium and water restrictions. The second most common reason is noncompliance with drug therapy. The nurse must stress to clients the importance of sodium restriction and drug compliance to maintain a properly functioning heart. Cardiac events such as MI or myocardial ischemia can also precipitate acute HF.

PHARMACOTHERAPY OF HEART FAILURE

Drugs can relieve the symptoms of heart failure by a number of different mechanisms, including slowing the heart rate, increasing contractility, and reducing its workload. These mechanisms are shown in Pharmacotherapy Illustrated 24.1.

ACE INHIBITORS

Drugs affecting the renin–angiotensin system lower blood pressure and reduce the afterload on the heart. They are often drugs of choice in the treatment of heart failure. The ACE inhibitors used for HF are listed in Table 24.1.

TABLE 24.1 Drugs for Heart Failure

Drug	Route and Adult Dose (max dose where indicated)	Adverse Effects
ACE INHIBITORS		
captopril (Capoten)	PO; 6.25–12.5 mg tid (max: 450 mg/day)	*Headache, dizziness, orthostatic hypotension, cough*
enalapril (Vasotec) (see page 318 for the Prototype Drug box ∞)	PO; 2.5 mg qid–bid (max: 40 mg/day)	
fosinopril (Monopril)	PO; 5–40 mg/day (max: 40 mg/day)	<u>Severe hypotension (first-dose phenomenon), syncope, angioedema, blood dyscrasias</u>
lisinopril (Prinivil, Zestoretic, Zestril)	PO; 10 mg/day (max: 80 mg/day)	
quinapril (Accupril)	PO; 10–20 mg/day (max: 40 mg/day)	
ramipril (Altace)	PO; 2.5–5.0 mg bid (max: 10 mg/day)	
LOOP OR HIGH-CEILING DIURETICS		
bumetanide (Bumex)	PO; 0.5–2 mg/day (max: 10 mg/day)	*Electrolyte imbalances, orthostatic hypotension*
furosemide (Lasix)	PO; 20–80 mg in a single dose or divided doses (max: 600 mg/day)	<u>Severe hypotension, dehydration, hypokalemia, hyponatremia, ototoxicity</u>
torsemide (Demadex)	PO; 10–20 mg/day (max: 200 mg/day)	
THIAZIDE AND THIAZIDE-LIKE DIURETICS		
hydrochlorothiazide (HydroDIURIL, HCTZ) (see page 311 for the Prototype Drug box ∞)	PO; 25–200 mg in a single dose or 3 divided doses (max: 200 mg/day)	*Electrolyte imbalances, orthostatic hypotension* <u>Severe hypotension, dehydration, hypokalemia, hyponatremia</u>
POTASSIUM-SPARING DIURETIC (ALDOSTERONE ANTAGONIST)		
spironolactone (Aldactone) (see page 432 for the Prototype Drug box ∞)	PO; 5–200 mg in divided doses (max: 200 mg/day)	*Hyperkalemia, gynecomastia in men, fatigue* <u>Dysrhythmias due to hyperkalemia</u>
BETA-ADRENERGIC BLOCKERS		
carvedilol (Coreg)	PO; 3.125 mg bid for 2 wk (max: 25 mg bid if <85 kg or 50 mg bid if >85 kg)	*Fatigue, insomnia, drowsiness, impotence or decreased libido, bradycardia, confusion*
metoprolol extended release (Toprol-XL)	PO; 25 mg/day for 2 wk; 12.5 mg/day for severe cases (max: 200 mg/day)	<u>Agranulocytosis, laryngospasm, Stevens–Johnson syndrome, anaphylaxis; if the drug is abruptly withdrawn, palpitations, rebound hypertension, life-threatening dysrhythmias, or myocardial ischemia may occur</u>
VASODILATORS		
hydralazine (Apresoline) (see page 325 for the Prototype Drug box ∞)	PO; 10–50 mg qid (max: 300 mg/day)	*Headache, flushing of face, orthostatic hypotension, dizziness, reflex tachycardia*
isosorbide dinitrate (Isordil, Sorbitrate, Dilatate)	PO; 2.5–30 mg qid, administer with meals and at nighttime (max: 160 mg/day)	<u>Fainting, severe headache, severe hypotension with overdose, lupuslike reaction (hydralazine)</u>
CARDIAC GLYCOSIDE		
digoxin (Lanoxin, Lanoxicaps)	PO; 0.125–0.5 mg/day	*Nausea, vomiting, headache, and visual disturbances such as seeing halos, a yellow-green tinge, or blurring* <u>Dysrhythmias, AV block</u>
PHOSPHODIESTERASE INHIBITORS		
inamrinone (Inocor)	IV; 0.75 mg/kg bolus given slowly over 2–3 min; then 5–10 mcg/kg/min (max: 10 mg/kg/day)	*Headache, hypotension* <u>Dysrhythmias</u>
milrinone (Primacor)	IV; 50 mcg over 10 min; then 0.375–0.75 mcg/kg/min	

Italics indicate common adverse effects; <u>underlining</u> indicates serious adverse effects.

24.3 Treatment of Heart Failure With ACE Inhibitors and Angiotensin-receptor Blockers

ACE inhibitors were approved for the treatment of hypertension in the 1980s. Since then, research studies have clearly demonstrated that they can slow the progression of heart failure and reduce mortality from this disease. Because of their relative safety, they have replaced digoxin as drugs of choice for the treatment of chronic HF. Indeed, unless specifically contraindicated, all clients with HF and many clients at high risk for HF should receive an ACE inhibitor.

The two primary actions of the ACE inhibitors are to *lower peripheral resistance* and *inhibit aldosterone secretion,* which reduces blood volume. The resultant reduction of arterial blood pressure diminishes the afterload, thus increasing cardiac output. An additional effect of the ACE inhibitors is dilation of veins. This action, which is probably not directly related to their inhibition of angiotensin, decreases pulmonary congestion and reduces peripheral edema. The combined reductions in preload, afterload, and blood volume substantially decrease the workload on the heart and allow it to work more efficiently for the HF client. Clients taking ACE inhibitors experience fewer HF-related symptoms, hospitalizations, and treatment failures. Several ACE inhibitors have been shown to reduce mortality following acute MI when therapy is started soon after the onset of symptoms (Chapter 25 ∞).

Another mechanism for blocking the effects of angiotensin is the use of angiotensin-receptor blockers (ARBs). The actions of the ARBs are similar to those of the ACE inhibitors, as would be expected, since both classes inhibit angiotensin. In clients with HF, ARBs show equivalent efficacy to the ACE inhibitors. Valsartan (Diovan) and candesartan (Atacand) were approved to treat HF in 2005. Because research has not yet demonstrated a clear advantage of ARBs over other medications, their use in the treatment of HF is usually reserved for clients unable to tolerate the side effects of ACE inhibitors.

NURSING CONSIDERATIONS

The role of the nurse in ACE inhibitor therapy for HF involves careful monitoring of a client's condition and providing education as it relates to the prescribed drug treatment. Prior to therapy, complete a thorough health

---

Pr   PROTOTYPE DRUG | Lisinopril *(Prinivil, Zestril)* | ACE Inhibitor

ACTIONS AND USES

Because of its value in the treatment of both HF and hypertension, lisinopril has become one of the most commonly prescribed drugs. Lisinopril acts by inhibiting angiotensin-converting enzyme and decreasing aldosterone secretion. Blood pressure is decreased and cardiac output is increased. As with other ACE inhibitors, 2 to 3 weeks of therapy may be required to reach maximum efficacy, and several months of therapy may be needed for cardiac function to return to normal.

ADMINISTRATION ALERTS

- Measure blood pressure just prior to administering lisinopril to be certain that effects are lasting for 24 hours and to determine whether the client's blood pressure is within acceptable range.
- Safety and efficacy have been established in the use of this medication in the treatment of pediatric clients.
- Geriatric clients may have higher blood levels related to renal failure.
- Pregnancy category C (first trimester) or D (second and third trimesters). Use during the second and third trimesters of pregnancy may result in injury or death to the fetus. Discontinue use as soon as pregnancy is suspected.

PHARMACOKINETICS

Onset: 1 h

Peak: 6–8 h

Half-life: 12 h

Duration: 24 h

ADVERSE EFFECTS

Lisinopril is tolerated well by most clients. The most common side effects are dizziness, headache, and cough. Hyperkalemia may occur during therapy; thus, electrolyte levels are usually monitored periodically. Other side effects include taste disturbances, chest pain, nausea, vomiting, diarrhea, and hypotension. Though rare, angioedema is a serious adverse effect.

Contraindications: Lisinopril is contraindicated in clients who have previously experienced angioedema due to ACE inhibitor therapy. It should not be used during pregnancy because it is a category D drug during the second and third trimesters.

INTERACTIONS

Drug–Drug: Indomethacin and other NSAIDs may interact with lisinopril, causing decreased antihypertensive activity. Because of the additive hypotensive action of lisinopril and diuretics, combined therapy with these or other antihypertensive drugs should be carefully monitored. When lisinopril is taken concurrently with potassium-sparing diuretics, hyperkalemia may result. Lisinopril may increase lithium levels and cause lithium toxicity.

Lab Tests: May cause positive ANA titer and increase values of the following: BUN, serum bilirubin, serum alkaline phosphatase, AST and ALT.

Herbal/Food: Avoid excessive intake of high potassium foods because of the possibility of hyperkalemia.

Treatment of Overdose: Overdose causes hypotension, which is treated with the administration of normal saline or a vasopressor.

 See the Companion Website for a Nursing Process Focus specific to this drug.

MediaLink   **Mechanism in Action: Lisinopril**

history. These drugs are contraindicated in pregnancy, lactation, and history of angioedema. Obtain a complete blood count (CBC) before starting therapy, and repeat it every month for the first 3 to 6 months of treatment. Thereafter, obtain a CBC at periodic intervals for 1 year. Hold medication if the neutrophil count drops below 1,000/mm^3, because these drugs may cause neutropenia.

Diuretics should be discontinued before the nurse initially administers ACE inhibitors to prevent severe hypotension. Because ACE inhibitors can cause severe hypotension with initial doses, monitor the client closely for several hours afterward. If severe hypotension does occur, place the client in a supine position and notify the healthcare provider. A lower dose is indicated for elderly clients and those with renal insufficiency. Use with caution in clients with impaired kidney function, hyperkalemia, and those with autoimmune diseases, especially systemic lupus erythematosus (SLE).

Client Teaching.   Client education as it relates to ACE inhibitors used to treat HF should include the goals of therapy, the reasons for obtaining baseline data such as vital signs and the existence of underlying cardiac and renal disorders, and possible drug side effects. Include the following points when teaching clients about ACE inhibitors:

- Do not take any other prescription or OTC drugs, herbal remedies, or dietary supplements without notifying your healthcare provider.

- Be aware that it may take weeks or months for maximum therapeutic response to be reached.

- Follow prescribed dietary modifications, including sodium and potassium restrictions, to prevent side effects of hyperkalemia and hyponatremia.

- Do not take salt or potassium supplements unless ordered by the healthcare provider.

- Avoid driving until the effects of the drug are known.

Please refer to "Nursing Process Focus: Clients Receiving ACE Inhibitor Therapy," page 319 in Chapter 23 ∞, for additional information.

DIURETICS

Diuretics increase urine flow, thereby reducing blood volume and cardiac workload. They are widely used in the treatment of cardiovascular disease. Selected diuretics are listed in Table 24.1.

24.4 Treatment of Heart Failure With Diuretics

Diuretics are common drugs for the treatment of clients with HF because they produce few adverse effects and are effective at reducing blood volume, peripheral edema, and pulmonary congestion. As diuretics reduce fluid volume and lower blood pressure, the workload on the heart is reduced, and cardiac output increases. Diuretics are rarely used alone but rather are prescribed in combination with

ACE inhibitors or other HF drugs. Because clinical research has not demonstrated their effectiveness in slowing the progression of HF or in decreasing mortality associated with the disease, diuretics are indicated only when there is evidence of fluid retention. In clients presenting with fluid retention, especially with symptoms of severe pulmonary congestion or peripheral edema, diuretics are essential medications.

Of the diuretic classes, the loop diuretics such as furosemide (see Prototype Drug box, page 336) are most commonly prescribed for HF because of their effectiveness in removing fluid from the body. Loop diuretics are also able to function in clients with renal impairment, an advantage for many clients with decompensated HF. Another major advantage in acute HF is that loop diuretics act quickly, especially IV formulations, which work within minutes.

Thiazide diuretics are also used in the pharmacotherapy of HF. Because they are less effective than the loop diuretics, thiazides are generally reserved for clients with mild to moderate HF. They are sometimes combined with loop diuretics to achieve a more effective diuresis in clients with acute HF.

Most potassium-sparing diuretics have limited roles in the treatment of HF because of their low efficacy. Spironolactone, however, is an exception. In addition to being a potassium-sparing diuretic, spironolactone is classified as an *aldosterone antagonist*. Clinical research has demonstrated that spironolactone blocks deleterious effects of aldosterone on the heart. Spironolactone has been shown to decrease mortality due to sudden death, as well as progression to advanced HF.

NURSING CONSIDERATIONS

The role of the nurse in diuretic therapy for heart failure involves careful monitoring of a client's condition and providing education as it relates to the prescribed drug treatment. Prior to initiation of diuretic therapy, question the client about history of kidney disease. Diuretics are contraindicated in clients with renal dysfunction, fluid and electrolyte depletion, hepatic coma, pregnancy, and lactation. Use diuretics cautiously in clients with hepatic cirrhosis and nephritic syndrome and in infants and older adults.

Monitor potassium levels closely, because potassium-wasting diuretics cause hypokalemia with diuresis. Closely observe elderly clients for weakness, hypotension, and confusion. Monitor for electrolyte imbalance, elevated blood urea nitrogen (BUN), hyperglycemia, and anemia, which can all be side effects of diuretics. Monitor vital signs as well as intake and output carefully to establish the effectiveness of the medication. Rapid and excessive diuresis can result in dehydration, hypovolemia, and circulatory collapse.

Client Teaching.   Client education as it relates to diuretics should include the goals of therapy, the reasons for obtaining baseline data such as vital signs and the existence

Pr PROTOTYPE DRUG | Furosemide *(Lasix)* | Loop Diuretic

ACTIONS AND USES

Furosemide is often used in the treatment of acute HF because it has the ability to remove large amounts of excess fluid from the client in a short period. When given IV, diuresis begins within 5 minutes, giving clients quick relief from their distressing symptoms. Furosemide acts by preventing the reabsorption of sodium and chloride in the loop of Henle region of the nephron. Compared with other diuretics, furosemide is particularly beneficial when cardiac output and renal flow are severely diminished.

ADMINISTRATION ALERTS

- Check client's serum potassium levels before administering drug. If potassium levels are falling or are below normal, notify physician before administering.
- Due to the prolonged half-life in premature infants and neonates, the drug must be used with caution.
- Geriatric clients may be more sensitive to the usual adult dose.
- Pregnancy category C.

PHARMACOKINETICS

Onset: 30–60 min PO; 5 min IV

Peak: 60–70 min PO; 20–60 min IV

Half-life: 30–60 min

Duration: 6–8 h PO; 2 h IV

ADVERSE EFFECTS

Side effects of furosemide, like those of most diuretics, involve potential electrolyte imbalances, the most important of which is hypokalemia. Because furosemide is so efficacious, fluid loss must be carefully monitored to avoid possible dehydration and hypotension.

Contraindications: Contraindications include hypersensitivity to furosemide or sulfonamides, anuria, hepatic coma, or severe fluid or electrolyte depletion.

INTERACTIONS

Drug–Drug: Because hypokalemia may cause dysrhythmias in clients taking cardiac glycosides, combination therapy with digoxin must be carefully monitored. Concurrent use with corticosteroids, amphotericin B, or other potassium-depleting drugs can result in hypokalemia. When given with lithium, elimination of lithium is decreased, causing higher risk of toxicity. Furosemide may diminish the hypoglycemic effects of sulfonylureas and insulin.

Lab Tests: Furosemide may increase values for the following: blood glucose, BUN, serum amylase, cholesterol, triglycerides and serum electrolytes.

Herbal/Food: Unknown.

Treatment of Overdose: Overdose will result in hypotension and severe fluid and electrolyte loss. Fluid and electrolyte infusions and treatment with a vasopressor may be necessary.

See the Companion Website for a Nursing Process Focus specific to this drug.

---

of underlying renal disorders, and possible drug side effects. Include the following points when teaching clients about diuretics:

- Keep sodium intake to no more than 4,000 mg daily.
- Report weight loss of more than 2 lb/week.
- Report fatigue and muscle cramping.
- Change positions slowly to avoid dizziness.

See "Nursing Process Focus: Clients Receiving Diuretic Therapy," page 312 in Chapter 23 ∞, for additional information.

BETA-ADRENERGIC BLOCKERS (ANTAGONISTS)

Only two beta-blockers are approved for the treatment of HF—carvedilol (Coreg) and metoprolol extended release (Toprol-XL). The doses of these agents are listed in Table 24.1. They reduce the cardiac workload by decreasing afterload.

24.5 Treatment of Heart Failure With Beta-adrenergic Blockers

Cardiac glycosides and other drugs that produce a *positive* **inotropic effect** increase the strength of myocardial contraction and are often used to reverse symptoms of HF.

It may seem surprising, then, to find beta-adrenergic blockers—drugs that exhibit a *negative* inotropic effect—prescribed for this disease. Although this class of drugs does indeed have the potential to worsen HF, they have become standard therapy for many clients with this chronic disorder.

Clients with HF have excessive activation of the sympathetic nervous system, which damages the heart and leads to progression of the disease. Beta-adrenergic antagonists block the cardiac actions of the sympathetic nervous system, thus slowing the heart rate and reducing blood pressure. Workload on the heart is decreased; after several months of therapy, heart size, shape, and function return to normal in some clients. Extensive clinical research has demonstrated that the proper use of beta-blockers can dramatically reduce the number of HF-associated hospitalizations and deaths.

To benefit clients with HF, however, beta-blockers must be administered in a very specific manner. Initial doses must be 1/10 to 1/20 of the target dose. Doses are doubled every 2 weeks until the optimum dose is reached. If therapy is begun with too high a dose, or the dose is increased too rapidly, beta-blockers can worsen HF. Beta-blockers are rarely used as monotherapy for this disease, but instead are usually combined with other agents, especially ACE inhibitors.

Pr **PROTOTYPE DRUG** | Metoprolol *(Lopressor)* | Beta-adrenergic Blocker

ACTIONS AND USES

Metoprolol is a selective beta$_1$-adrenergic blocker available in tablet, sustained-release tablet, and IV forms. At high doses, it may also affect beta$_2$-receptors in bronchial smooth muscle. The drug acts by reducing sympathetic stimulation of the heart, thus decreasing cardiac workload. Metoprolol has been found to slow the progression of HF and to significantly reduce the long-term consequences of the disease. It is usually combined with other HF drugs such as ACE inhibitors. Metoprolol is also approved for angina, hypertension, and MI.

ADMINISTRATION ALERTS

- During IV administration, monitor ECG, blood pressure, and pulse frequently.
- Assess pulse and blood pressure before oral administration. Hold if pulse is below 60 beats per minute or if client is hypotensive.
- Advise client not to crush or chew sustained-release tablets.
- Safety and efficacy have not established in the use of this drug for pediatric clients.
- Pregnancy category C.

PHARMACOKINETICS

Onset: 10–15 min; sustained release, unknown

Peak: 1.5–4 h; 6–12 h sustained release

Half-life: 3–4 h

Duration: 6 h (24 h sustained release)

ADVERSE EFFECTS

Because it is selective for blocking beta$_1$-receptors in the heart, metoprolol has few adverse effects on other autonomic targets and thus is preferred over nonselective beta-blockers such as propranolol for clients with respiratory disorders. Side effects are generally minor and relate to its autonomic activity, such as slowing of the heart rate and hypotension. Because of its multiple effects on the heart, clients with heart failure should be carefully monitored.

Contraindications: This agent is contraindicated in asthma, cardiogenic shock, sinus bradycardia, heart block greater than first degree, and overt cardiac failure.

INTERACTIONS

Drug–Drug: Concurrent use with digoxin may result in bradycardia. Oral contraceptives may cause increased metoprolol effects. Alcohol or antihypertensives may result in additive hypotension. Metoprolol may enhance the hypoglycemic effects of insulin and oral hypoglycemic agents.

Lab Tests: Metoprolol may increase values for the following: uric acid, lipids, potassium, bilirubin, alkaline phosphatase, creatinine, and antinuclear antibody.

Herbal/Food: Unknown.

Treatment of Overdose: Atropine or isoproterenol can be used to reverse bradycardia. Hypotension may be reversed by a vasopressor such as parenteral dopamine or dobutamine.

 See the Companion Website for a Nursing Process Focus specific to this drug.

The basic pharmacology of the beta-blockers is presented in Chapter 13 ∞. Other uses of the beta-adrenergic blockers are discussed elsewhere in this text: for hypertension in Chapter 23 ∞, for dysrhythmias in Chapter 26, and for angina/myocardial infarction in Chapter 25 ∞.

NURSING CONSIDERATIONS

The role of the nurse in beta-adrenergic blocker therapy involves careful monitoring of a client's condition and providing education as it relates to the prescribed drug treatment. Beta-adrenergic blockers are contraindicated in clients with decompensated heart failure, chronic obstructive pulmonary disease (COPD), bradycardia, or heart block. Beta-blockers are also contraindicated in pregnant or lactating clients. Use with caution in clients with diabetes, peripheral vascular disease, and hepatic impairment. Caution is needed with elderly clients, who may need a reduced dose.

Monitor for worsening signs and symptoms of HF and for signs of hepatic toxicity. Liver function tests should be performed periodically. Notify the physician if signs or symptoms of liver impairment become apparent.

Client Teaching.   Client education as it relates to beta-adrenergic blockers should include the goals of therapy, the

reasons for obtaining baseline data such as vital signs and the existence of underlying liver disorders, and possible drug side effects. Include the following points when teaching clients regarding beta-adrenergic blockers:

- Monitor blood pressure and pulse. Notify the healthcare provider if pulse rate is less than 50 beats/minute.
- Immediately report signs and symptoms of worsening HF, such as shortness of breath, edema of feet and ankles, and chest pain.
- Do not suddenly stop taking the drug without consulting the healthcare provider.
- If diabetic, monitor serum glucose carefully, because these drugs may cause changes in blood glucose levels.
- Immediately report significant side effects such as fainting, difficulty breathing, weight gain, and slow, irregular heart rate.

See "Nursing Process Focus: Clients Receiving Beta-adrenergic Antagonist Therapy" on page 323 in Chapter 23 ∞ for additional information.

VASODILATORS

Through their hypotensive effects, vasodilators play a minor role in the pharmacotherapy of HF. They are also used for hypertension and angina pectoris. Doses for the vasodilators are listed in Table 24.1.

24.6 Treatment of Heart Failure With Direct Vasodilators

The two drugs in this class, hydralazine (Apresoline) and isosorbide dinitrate (Isordil), act directly to relax blood vessels and lower blood pressure. Hydralazine acts on arterioles. It is an effective antihypertensive drug, although it is not a drug of first choice for this indication. Isosorbide dinitrate (Isordil) is an organic nitrate that acts on veins. The drug is not very effective as monotherapy, and tolerance develops to its actions with continued use.

Because the two drugs act synergistically, isosorbide dinitrate is often combined with hydralazine in the treatment of HF. The high incidence of side effects, including reflex tachycardia and orthostatic hypotension, however, limits their use to clients who cannot tolerate ACE inhibitors. Hydralazine is featured as a prototype drug in Chapter 23 ∞.

NURSING CONSIDERATIONS

The role of the nurse in the care of clients receiving drug therapy with hydralazine for the treatment of hypertension is discussed in Chapter 23 (see "Nursing Considerations,"

page 325, and "Nursing Process Focus: Clients Receiving Direct Vasodilator Therapy," page 326 ∞).

CARDIAC GLYCOSIDES

Cardiac glycosides were once used as arrow poisons by African tribes and as medicines by the ancient Egyptians and Romans. Their value in treating heart disorders has been known for over 2,000 years. The chemical classification draws its name from three sugars, or glycosides, which are attached to a steroid nucleus. Information on the cardiac glycosides is provided in Table 24.1.

24.7 Treatment of Heart Failure With Cardiac Glycosides

Extracted from the beautiful flowering plants *Digitalis purpurea* (purple foxglove) and *Digitalis lanata* (white foxglove), drugs from this class are sometimes called *digitalis glycosides*. Until the discovery of ACE inhibitors, cardiac glycosides were the mainstay of HF treatment. The cardiac glycosides cause the heart to beat more forcefully and more slowly, improving cardiac output. The two primary cardiac glycosides—digoxin and digitoxin—are quite similar in efficacy; the primary difference is that the latter has a more prolonged half-life. Digitoxin is no longer available in the United States.

Although the cardiac glycosides clearly produce symptomatic improvement in clients, they do not reduce mortality

---

Pr PROTOTYPE DRUG | Isosorbide Dinitrate *(Isordil, others)* | Organic Nitrate Vasodilator

ACTIONS AND USES

Isosorbide dinitrate acts directly and selectively on veins to cause venodilation. This reduces venous return (preload), thus decreasing cardiac workload. The resultant improvement in cardiac output reduces pulmonary congestion and peripheral edema and improves exercise tolerance. Isosorbide dinitrate also dilates the coronary arteries to bring more oxygen to the myocardium. Isosorbide dinitrate belongs to a class of drugs called organic nitrates that are widely used in the treatment of angina.

ADMINISTRATION ALERTS

- Do not confuse this drug with isosorbide (Ismotic), an oral osmotic diuretic.
- If administered sublingually, advise client not to eat, drink, talk, or smoke while tablet is dissolving.
- Safety and efficacy has not been established with this drug in pediatric clients.
- Pregnancy category C.

PHARMACOKINETICS

Onset: 2–5 min sublingual; 30 min sustained release

Peak: Unknown

Half-life: Unknown

Duration: 1–2 h sublingual; 6–8 h sustained release

ADVERSE EFFECTS

Common side effects of isosorbide dinitrate include headache, mostly at the initiation of therapy, and reflex tachycardia. Orthostatic hypotension can cause dizziness and falling, particularly in older adults.

Contraindications: The drug should not be administered to clients with high intracranial pressure, severe anemia or who have shown hypersensitivity to nitrates.

INTERACTIONS

Drug–Drug: Concurrent use with alcohol, phenothiazines, or antihypertensives can cause serious hypotension. Sildenafil (Viagra) should not be taken concurrently with nitrates because serious hypotension may result.

Lab Tests: May increase urine vanillylmandelic acid and catecholamine levels.

Herbal/Food: Unknown.

Treatment of Overdose: Overdose will cause hypotension, which is treated with the administration of normal saline. Vasopressors should not be used because they may worsen symptoms.

 See the Companion Website for a Nursing Process Focus specific to this drug.

Pr PROTOTYPE DRUG | Digoxin (Lanoxin) | Cardiac Glycoside

ACTIONS AND USES

The primary benefit of digoxin is its ability to increase the contractility or strength of myocardial contraction—a positive inotropic action. Digoxin accomplishes this by inhibiting Na^+-K^+ ATPase, the critical enzyme responsible for pumping sodium ion out of the myocardial cell in exchange for potassium ion. As sodium accumulates, calcium ions are released from their storage areas in the cell. The release of calcium ion produces a more forceful contraction of the myocardial fibers.

By increasing myocardial contractility, digoxin directly increases cardiac output, thus alleviating symptoms of HF and improving exercise tolerance. The improved cardiac output results in increased urine production and a desirable reduction in blood volume, relieving distressing symptoms of pulmonary congestion and peripheral edema.

In addition to its positive inotropic effect, digoxin affects impulse conduction in the heart. Digoxin has the ability to suppress the sinoatrial (SA) node and slow electrical conduction through the atrioventricular (AV) node. Because of these actions, digoxin is sometimes used to treat dysrhythmias, as discussed in Chapter 26 ∞.

ADMINISTRATION ALERTS

- Take apical pulse for 1 full minute, noting rate, rhythm, and quality before administering. If pulse is below the parameter established by the physician (usually 60 beats per minute), withhold the dose and notify the healthcare provider.
- Check for recent serum digoxin level results before administering. If level is higher than the parameter established by the physician (usually 1.8 ng/ml), withhold the dose and notify the healthcare provider.
- Use with caution in the geriatric and pediatric populations because of immature or impaired renal and hepatic systems.
- Pregnancy category A.

PHARMACOKINETICS

Onset: Onset 30–90 min PO; 5–30 min IV

Peak: 4–6 h PO; 1.5 h IV

Half-life: 3–4 days

Duration: 6–8 days

ADVERSE EFFECTS

The most dangerous adverse effect of digoxin is its ability to create dysrhythmias, particularly in clients who have hypokalemia or impaired renal function. Because diuretics can cause hypokalemia and are often used to treat HF, concurrent use of digoxin and diuretics must be carefully monitored. Other adverse effects of digoxin therapy include nausea, vomiting, anorexia, and visual disturbances such as seeing halos, a yellow-green tinge, or blurring. Periodic serum drug levels should be obtained to determine whether the digoxin concentration is within the therapeutic range.

Contraindications: Clients with AV block or ventricular dysrhythmias unrelated to HF should not receive digoxin, as the drug may worsen these conditions. Digoxin should be administered with caution to elderly clients because these clients experience a higher incidence of adverse effects. Clients with renal impairment should receive lower doses of digoxin, because the drug is excreted by this route. The drug should be used with caution in clients with MI, cor pulmonale, or hypothyroidism.

INTERACTIONS

Drug–Drug: Digoxin interacts with many drugs. Concurrent use of digoxin with diuretics can cause hypokalemia and increase the risk of dysrhythmias. Use with ACE inhibitors, spironolactone, or potassium supplements can lead to hyperkalemia and reduce the therapeutic action of digoxin. Administration of digoxin with other positive inotropic agents can cause additive effects on heart contractility. Concurrent use with beta-blockers may result in additive bradycardia. Antacids and cholesterol-lowering drugs can decrease the absorption of digoxin. If calcium is administered IV together with digoxin, it can increase the risk of dysrhythmias. Quinidine, verapamil, amiodarone, and alprazolam will decrease the distribution and excretion of digoxin, thus increasing the risk of digoxin toxicity.

Lab Tests: Unknown.

Herbal/Food: Ginseng may increase the risk of digoxin toxicity. Mahuang and ephedra may induce dysrhythmias.

Treatment of Overdose: Digoxin overdose can be fatal. Specific therapy involves IV infusion of digoxin immune fab (Digibind), which contains antibodies specific for digoxin.

 See the Companion Website for a Nursing Process Focus specific to this drug.

---

from HF. Because of the development of safer and more effective drugs such as ACE inhibitors, cardiac glycosides are now primarily used for more advanced stages of HF, in combination with other agents.

The margin of safety between a therapeutic dose and a toxic dose of digitalis is quite narrow, and severe adverse effects may result from unmonitored treatment. Digitalization refers to a procedure in which the dose of cardiac glycoside is gradually increased until tissues become saturated with the drug, and the symptoms of HF diminish. If the client is critically ill, digitalization can be accomplished rapidly with IV doses in a controlled clinical environment, in which side adverse effects are carefully monitored. Clients who are treated outside the hospital may experience digitalization with digoxin over a period of 7 days, using oral dosing. In either case, the goal is to

determine the proper dose of drug that may be administered without undue adverse effects. Frequent serum digoxin levels should be obtained during therapy, and the dosage adjusted based on the laboratory results and the client's clinical response.

NURSING CONSIDERATIONS

The role of the nurse in cardiac glycoside therapy involves careful monitoring of a client's condition and providing education as it relates to the prescribed drug treatment. Prior to beginning therapy with cardiac glycosides, evaluate the client for ventricular dysrhythmias not caused by HF and for any history of hypersensitivity to cardiac glycosides. Assess the client's renal function, because the drug is excreted by the kidneys. Administer these drugs with

NURSING PROCESS FOCUS Clients Receiving Cardiac Glycoside Therapy

Assessment	Potential Nursing Diagnoses
Prior to administration: - Obtain a complete health history including allergies, drug history, and possible drug interactions. - Assess vital signs, urine output, and cardiac output, initially and throughout therapy. - Determine the reason the medication is being administered.	- Tissue Perfusion, Ineffective, related to impaired cardiac status - Cardiac Output, Decreased - Fluid Volume, Excess - Knowledge, Deficient, related to drug therapy

Planning: Client Goals and Expected Outcomes

The client will:
- Report decreased symptoms of cardiac decompensation related to fluid overload.
- Exhibit evidence of improved organ perfusion, including kidney, heart, and brain.
- Demonstrate an understanding of the drug's action by accurately describing drug side effects and precautions.
- Immediately report side effects such as nausea, vomiting, diarrhea, heart rate below 60 beats per minute, and vision changes.

Implementation

Interventions and (Rationales)	Client Education/Discharge Planning
- Monitor ECG for rate and rhythm changes during initial digitalization therapy. (Digoxin has a strong positive inotropic effect.)	Instruct client to: - Count pulse for 1 full minute and record pulse with every dose. - Contact the healthcare provider if pulse rate is less than 60 or greater than 100 beats per minute.
- Observe for side effects such as nausea, vomiting, diarrhea, anorexia, shortness of breath, vision changes, and leg muscle cramps. (These are signs of toxicity.)	- Instruct client to report side effects immediately to prevent toxicity.
- Weigh client daily. (Weight gain could indicate worsening of heart failure.)	- Instruct client to report weight gain of 2 lb or more per day.
- Administer precise ordered dose at same time each day. (Overdose may cause serious toxicity.)	Instruct client to: - Take as directed; do not double doses. - Not discontinue drug without the advice of the healthcare provider.
- Monitor serum drug level and report level greater than 1.8 ng/ml. (Serum drug levels help determine therapeutic concentration and toxicity.)	- Instruct client to keep scheduled laboratory visits for testing.
- Monitor levels of potassium, magnesium, calcium, BUN, and creatinine. (Hypokalemia predisposes the client to digoxin toxicity.)	- Instruct client to consume foods high in potassium such as bananas, apricots, kidney beans, sweet potatoes, and peanut butter.
- Monitor for signs and symptoms of digoxin toxicity. (Early assessment may help prevent severe toxicity.)	- Instruct client to immediately report visual changes, mental depression, palpitations, weakness, loss of appetite, vomiting, and diarrhea.

Evaluation of Outcome Criteria

Evaluate the effectiveness of drug therapy by confirming that client goals and expected outcomes have been met (see "Planning").
- The client verbalizes decreased symptoms of cardiac decompensation related to fluid overload.
- The client exhibits evidence of improved organ perfusion, including kidney, heart, and brain.
- The client demonstrates an understandings of the drug's action by accurately describing drug side effects and precautions.
- The client reports nausea, vomiting, heart rate less than 60 beats per minute, and vision changes.

∞ *See Table 24.1, under "Cardiac Glycosides," for a list of drugs to which these nursing actions apply.*

caution in elderly clients; those with acute MI, incomplete heart block, and renal insufficiency; or in pregnant or lactating mothers.

Monitor the client for side effects such as fatigue, drowsiness, dizziness, visual disturbances, anorexia, nausea, and vomiting. Advise clients to carry or wear identification describing their medical diagnosis and drug regimen. Monitor potassium levels, because hypokalemia predisposes the client to serious digoxin toxicity. Do not give clients antacids or antidiarrheal medications within 2 hours of cardiac glycoside administration, because they decrease the absorption of digoxin. Cardiac glycosides interact with many other drugs, so be vigilant in observing for drug–drug interactions. Caution must be used when administering nephrotoxic drugs with digoxin, due to the potential for a rapid buildup of digoxin in the blood.

It is common for dysrhythmias to occur when high doses of digoxin are administered. Prepare to administer digoxin immune Fab (Digibind) in the case of a life-threatening dysrhythmia. This drug binds and subsequently removes digoxin from the body and prevents toxic effects of overdose.

Client Teaching.   Client education as it relates to cardiac glycosides should include the goals of therapy, the reasons for obtaining baseline data such as vital signs and the existence of underlying renal disorders, and possible drug side effects. Include the following points when teaching clients about cardiac glycosides:

- Keep all scheduled laboratory visits to determine whether the drug is within therapeutic range.
- Immediately report signs of toxicity such as nausea, vomiting, anorexia, and visual disturbances, (e.g., seeing halos, a yellow-green tinge, or blurring).
- Report a pulse rate that is less than 60 beats/minute or greater than 100 beats/minute.
- Weigh self daily and report a weight gain of 2 lb or more per day.
- Consume foods high in potassium such as bananas, apricots, kidney beans, sweet potatoes, and peanut butter.
- Do not take any other prescription or OTC drugs, herbal remedies, or dietary supplements without notifying your healthcare provider.

PHOSPHODIESTERASE INHIBITORS

Phosphodiesterase inhibitors have a brief half-life and are used for the short-term control of acute heart failure. The doses of these agents are listed in Table 24.1.

24.8 Treatment of Heart Failure With Phosphodiesterase Inhibitors and Other Inotropic Agents

Advanced HF can be a medical emergency, and prompt, effective treatment is necessary to avoid organ failure or death. In addition to high doses of diuretics, use of positive inotropic drugs is often necessary. The two primary classes of inotropic agents used for decompensated HF are phosphodiesterase inhibitors and beta-adrenergic agonists.

In the 1980s, two drugs became available that block the enzyme **phosphodiesterase** in cardiac and smooth muscle. Blocking phosphodiesterase has the effect of increasing the amount of calcium available for myocardial contraction. The inhibition results in two main actions

---

Pr PROTOTYPE DRUG | Milrinone *(Primacor)* | Phosphodiesterase Inhibitor

ACTIONS AND USES

Of the two phosphodiesterase inhibitors available, milrinone is generally preferred because it has a shorter half-life and fewer side effects. It is given only intravenously and is primarily used for the short-term therapy of advanced HF. The drug has a rapid onset of action. Immediate effects of milrinone include an increased force of myocardial contraction and an increase in cardiac output.

ADMINISTRATION ALERTS

- When this medication is administered IV, a microdrip set and an infusion pump should be used.
- Safety and efficacy have not established in the geriatric and pediatric populations.
- Pregnancy category C.

PHARMACOKINETICS

Onset: 2–10 min

Peak: 10 min

Half-life: 3–6 h

Duration: Variable

ADVERSE EFFECTS

The most serious side effect of milrinone is ventricular dysrhythmia, which may occur in 1 of every 10 clients taking the drug. The client's ECG is usually monitored continuously during the infusion of the drug. Blood pressure is also continuously monitored during the infusion to avoid hypotension.

Contraindications: The only contraindication to milrinone is previous hypersensitivity to the drug. Milrinone should be used with caution in clients with preexisting dysrhythmias.

INTERACTIONS

Drug–Drug: Milrinone interacts with disopyramide, causing excessive hypotension. Caution should be used when administering milrinone with digoxin, dobutamine, or other inotropic drugs, since their positive inotropic effects on the heart may be additive.

Lab Tests: Unknown.

Herbal/Food: Unknown.

Treatment of Overdose: Overdose causes hypotension, which is treated with the administration of normal saline or a vasopressor.

 *See the Companion Website for a Nursing Process Focus specific to this drug.*

that benefit clients with HF: a positive inotropic action and vasodilation. Cardiac output is increased because of the increase in contractility and the decrease in left ventricular afterload. Because of their toxicity, phosphodiesterase inhibitors are normally reserved for clients who have not responded to ACE inhibitors or cardiac glycosides, and they are generally used for only 2 to 3 days. Prior to 2000, inamrinone was called amrinone. The name was changed to prevent medication errors: the name amrinone looked and sounded too similar to amiodarone, an antidysrhythmic drug.

Beta-adrenergic agonists used for HF include isoproterenol (Isuprel), epinephrine, norepinephrine, dopamine, and dobutamine. Dobutamine is often the drug of choice in this class because it has the ability to increase myocardial contractility rapidly and effectively, with minimal changes to heart rate or blood pressure. This is important because increases in heart rate or blood pressure increase the oxygen demands on the heart and possibly worsen HF. Therapy with dobutamine is usually limited to 72 hours. The two most common side effects of beta-agonists are tachycardia and dysrhythmias. The basic pharmacology of the beta-adrenergic agonists was presented in Chapter 13. Epinephrine is featured as a prototype drug for anaphylaxis on page 420 in Chapter 29, and dopamine is featured as a prototype drug for shock on page 417 in Chapter 29 ∞.

NURSING CONSIDERATIONS

The role of the nurse in drug therapy with phosphodiesterase inhibitors involves careful monitoring of a client's condition and providing education as it relates to the prescribed drug treatment. Prior to administration of phosphodiesterase inhibitors, assess potassium levels. If hypokalemia is present, it should be corrected before administering these drugs. Evaluate the client for a history of renal impairment and dysrhythmias. Obtain baseline vital signs, especially blood pressure, because these drugs can cause hypotension. During IV administration, continuously monitor the client for ventricular dysrhythmias such as ectopic beats, supraventricular dysrhythmias, premature ventricular contractions (PVCs), ventricular tachycardia, and ventricular fibrillation. If these drugs are ordered for elderly, pregnant, or pediatric clients, consult the healthcare

HOME & COMMUNITY CONSIDERATIONS

Increasing Compliance in Heart Failure Treatment

Heart failure is a chronic disease, and most of the care is through the home and community bases. Clients and/or their caregivers must be monitored for compliance with the drug therapy regimen. Since these drugs are capable of creating as many lifestyle changes as the disease itself, noncompliance is seen frequently. The drugs are also expensive, which can create problems in both the geriatric and pediatric populations, especially in low-income families. These clients must be counseled and helped with gaining access to community assistance to prevent this problem.

NATURAL THERAPIES

Hawthorn for Heart Failure

Hawthorn (sometimes spelled *hawthorne*) is a bush found throughout the United States, Canada, Europe, and Asia. It is one of the most commonly used herbs, and is used frequently to treat HF. The research supports its use in HF. In a meta-analysis of randomized clinical trials, it was concluded that there is a significant benefit from hawthorn extract as an adjunctive treatment for chronic heart failure (Pittler, Schmidt, & Ernst 2003). Its cardiovascular effects are believed to be due to its antioxidant flavonoid components, which increase the integrity of the blood vessel walls, improve coronary blood flow, and increase oxygen utilization (Chang, Dao, & Shas 2005).

Reported adverse effects include nausea, vomiting, and dizziness. Because hawthorn is effective at reducing blood pressure, this vital sign must be monitored, and clients should be aware of this side effect, especially if they are concurrently taking an antihypertensive medication.

Many HF clients use digoxin to treat their condition, so concurrent use with hawthorn is a concern. An interaction study, however, showed that at dosages of 0.25 mg of digoxin per day and 450 mg of hawthorn twice daily, hawthorn did not significantly alter the pharmacokinetic parameters for digoxin (Tankanow, et al., 2003).

provider, because safety has not been established in these populations or conditions.

Client Teaching. Client education as it relates to phosphodiesterase inhibitors should include the goals of therapy, the reasons for obtaining baseline data such as vital signs and the existence of underlying cardiac and renal disorders, and possible drug side effects. Include the following points when teaching clients about phosphodiesterase inhibitors:

- Immediately report irregular, fast heartbeat; pain or swelling at the infusion site; and fever of 101 °F or higher.
- Immediately report any increase in chest pain that might indicate angina.

24.9 Newer Agents for Heart Failure

In 2001, the first new medication for HF in more than 10 years was approved. Nesiritide (Natrecor) is a small-peptide hormone, produced through recombinant DNA technology, that is structurally identical to endogenous human beta-type natriuretic peptide (hBNP).

In healthy individuals, the atria secrete atrial natriuretic peptide (ANP) in response to increasing blood pressure. As a natural component of homeostasis, ANP is a hormone that acts on the kidneys to increase the excretion of sodium and water and return blood pressure to normal levels. When heart failure occurs, the ventricles begin to secrete hBNP in response to the increased stretch on the ventricular walls. hBNP has the same action as ANP: diuresis and renal excretion of sodium. In therapeutic doses, hBNP also causes vasodilation, with also contributes to reduced preload. By reducing preload and afterload, hBNP compensates for diminished cardiac function.

Nesiritide (Natrecor) has limited uses because of its ability to cause severe hypotension. The drug is given by IV infusion, and clients require continuous monitoring. It is approved for clients with acutely decompensated heart failure.

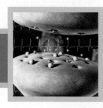

CHAPTER REVIEW

KEY CONCEPTS

The numbered key concepts provide a succinct summary of the important points from the corresponding numbered section within the chapter. If any of these points are not clear, refer to the numbered section within the chapter for review.

24.1 Heart failure is closely associated with chronic hypertension, coronary artery disease, and diabetes.

24.2 The body attempts to compensate for HF by increasing cardiac output. Preload and afterload are two primary factors determining cardiac output.

24.3 ACE inhibitors improve HF by reducing peripheral edema and increasing cardiac output. They are drugs of choice for the treatment of HF.

24.4 Diuretics relieve symptoms of HF by reducing fluid overload and decreasing blood pressure.

24.5 Beta-adrenergic blockers slow the heart rate and decrease blood pressure. They can dramatically reduce hospitalizations and increase the survival of clients with HF.

24.6 Vasodilators can relieve symptoms of HF by reducing preload and decreasing the cardiac workload.

24.7 Cardiac glycosides increase the force of myocardial contraction and were once drugs of choice for HF. Because of their low safety margin, and the development of more effective drugs, their use has declined.

24.8 Phosphodiesterase inhibitors and other inotropic agents increase the force of contraction and improve cardiac output. They are used for the short-term therapy of acute HF.

24.9 Human beta-natriuretic peptide (hBNP) is a natural hormone secreted by the ventricles of clients with HF. Through recombinant DNA technology, this hormone is now available as nesiritide (Natrecor) for the treatment of acute HF.

NCLEX-RN® REVIEW QUESTIONS

1 The client is prescribed digoxin (Lanoxin) for treatment of HF. Which of the following statements by the client indicates the need for further teaching?

1. "I may notice my heart rate decrease."
2. "I may feel tired during early treatment."
3. "This drug will help my heart muscle pump less."
4. "My heart rate will speed up."

2 The nurse reviews lab studies of a client receiving digoxin (Lanoxin). Intervention by the nurse is required if the results include a:

1. Serum digoxin level of 1.2 ng/dl.
2. Serum potassium level of 3.0 mEq/L.
3. Hemoglobin of 14.4 g/dl.
4. Serum sodium level of 140 mEq/L.

3 Nursing interventions during initial therapy with ACE inhibitors must include:

1. Monitoring ECG.
2. Monitoring intake and output.
3. Monitoring blood pressure.
4. Monitoring serum levels.

4 The teaching plan for a client receiving thiazide diuretics should include:

1. Taking apical pulse.
2. Including citrus fruits, melons, and vegetables in diet.
3. Decreasing potassium-rich food in the diet.
4. Checking blood pressure three times a day.

5 Lisinopril (Prinivil) is part of the treatment regimen for a client with HF. The nurse monitors the client for the side effects of this drug which may include (select all that apply):

1. Hyperkalemia.
2. Hypokalemia.
3. Cough.
4. Dizziness.
5. Headache.

CRITICAL THINKING QUESTIONS

1. A client is newly diagnosed with mild heart failure. The client has been started on digoxin (Lanoxin). What objective evidence would indicate that this drug has been effective?

2. A 69-year-old client has a sudden onset of acute pulmonary edema. The client has no past cardiac history, is allergic to sulfa antibiotics, and routinely takes no medications. The healthcare provider orders furosemide (Lasix) to relieve the pulmonary congestion. What interventions are essential in the care of this client?

3. A client who is diabetic and hypertensive is started on ACE inhibitors for mild heart failure. What teaching is important for this client?

See Appendix D for answers and rationales for all activities.

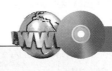

EXPLORE MediaLink

www.prenhall.com/adams

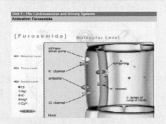

NCLEX-RN® review, case studies, and other interactive resources for this chapter can be found on the companion website at www.prenhall.com/adams. Click on "Chapter 24" to select the activities for this chapter. For animations, more NCLEX-RN® review questions, and an audio glossary, access the accompanying Prentice Hall Nursing MediaLink DVD-ROM in this textbook.

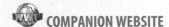

PRENTICE HALL NURSING MEDIALINK DVD-ROM

- **Animations**
  Mechanism in Action: Digoxin (*Lanoxin*)
  Mechanism in Action: Lisinopril (*Prinivil*)
  Mechanism in Action: Furosemide (*Lasix*)
- **Audio Glossary**
- **NCLEX-RN® Review**

COMPANION WEBSITE

- **NCLEX-RN® Review**
- **Dosage Calculations**
- **Case Study:** Client taking cardiac glycosides
- **Care Plan:** Client with congestive heart failure who is taking digoxin

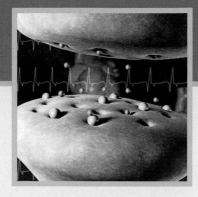

Drugs for Angina Pectoris and Myocardial Infarction

DRUGS AT A GLANCE

ORGANIC NITRATES
  ↪ *nitroglycerin (Nitrostat)*
BETA-ADRENERGIC BLOCKERS (ANTAGONISTS)
  ↪ *atenolol (Tenormin)*
CALCIUM CHANNEL BLOCKERS
  ↪ *diltiazem (Cardizem)*
THROMBOLYTICS
  ↪ *reteplase (Retavase)*
ADJUNCT DRUGS FOR MYOCARDIAL INFARCTION

OBJECTIVES

After reading this chapter, the student should be able to:

1. Explain the relationship between atherosclerosis and coronary artery disease.
2. Describe the blood supply to the myocardium.
3. Explain the pathophysiology of angina pectoris and myocardial infarction.
4. Describe the nurse's role in the pharmacological management of clients with angina and myocardial infarction.
5. Explain mechanisms by which drugs can be used to decrease cardiac oxygen demand and relieve angina pain.
6. For each of the drug classes listed in Drugs at a Glance, know representative drug examples, and explain their mechanism of action, primary actions, and important adverse effects.
7. Categorize drugs used in the treatment of angina and myocardial infarction based on their classification and mechanism of action.
8. Use the Nursing Process to care for clients who are receiving drug therapy for angina and myocardial infarction.

MediaLink

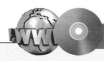

www.prenhall.com/adams

NCLEX-RN® review, case studies, and other interactive resources for this chapter can be found on the companion website at www.prenhall.com/adams. Click on "Chapter 25" to select the activities for this chapter. For animations, more NCLEX-RN® review questions, and an audio glossary, access the accompanying Prentice Hall Nursing MediaLink DVD-ROM in this textbook.

KEY TERMS

anastomoses *page 346*
angina pectoris *page 346*
atherosclerosis *page 346*
coronary artery bypass graft (CABG)
   surgery *page 348*
coronary artery disease (CAD) *page 346*
glycoprotein IIb/IIIa *page 358*
myocardial infarction (MI) *page 355*
myocardial ischemia *page 346*
percutaneous transluminal coronary
   angioplasty (PTCA) *page 348*
plaque *page 346*
silent angina *page 347*
stable angina *page 347*
unstable angina *page 347*
vasospastic (Prinzmetal's) angina *page 347*

The tissues and organs of the body are dependent on a continuous arterial supply of oxygen and other vital nutrients to support life and health. With its high metabolic requirements, the heart in particular demands a steady source of oxygen. Should the arterial blood supply become compromised, cardiovascular function may become impaired, resulting in angina pectoris, myocardial infarction (MI), and possibly death. This chapter focuses on the pharmacological interventions related to angina pectoris and MI.

25.1 Etiology of Coronary Artery Disease and Myocardial Ischemia

Coronary artery disease (CAD) is one of the leading causes of mortality in the United States. The primary defining characteristic of CAD is narrowing or occlusion of a coronary artery. The narrowing deprives cells of needed oxygen and nutrients, a condition known as **myocardial ischemia.** If the ischemia develops over a long period of time, the heart may compensate for its inadequate blood supply, and the client may experience no symptoms. Indeed, coronary arteries may be occluded as much as 50% or more and cause no symptoms. As CAD progresses, however, the myocardium does not receive enough oxygen to meet the metabolic demands of the heart, and symptoms of angina begin to appear. Persistent myocardial ischemia may lead to heart attack.

The most common etiology of CAD in adults is **atherosclerosis,** the presence of **plaque**—a fatty, fibrous material within the walls of the coronary arteries. Plaque develops progressively over time, producing varying degrees of intravascular narrowing, and a situation that results in partial or total blockage of the vessel. In addition, the plaque impairs normal vessel elasticity, and the coronary vessel is unable to dilate properly when the myocardium needs additional blood or oxygen, such as during periods of exercise. Plaque accumulation occurs gradually, over periods of 40 to 50 years in some individuals, but actually begins to accrue early in life. The development of atherosclerosis is illustrated in ●Figure 25.1.

25.2 Blood Supply to the Myocardium

The heart, from the moment it begins to function in utero until death, works to distribute oxygen and nutrients via its nonstop pumping action. It is the hardest working organ in the body, functioning continually during both activity and rest. Because the heart is a muscle, it needs a steady supply of nourishment to sustain itself and maintain the systemic circulation in a balanced state of equilibrium. Any disturbance in blood flow to the vital organs or the myocardium itself—even for brief episodes—can result in life-threatening consequences.

The myocardium receives its blood via the right and left coronary arteries, which arise within the aortic sinuses at the base of the aorta. These arteries further diverge into smaller branches that encircle the heart, bringing the myocardium a continuous supply of oxygen and nutrients.

Numerous smaller vessels, known as **anastomoses,** serve as natural communication networks among the coronary arteries. In the event that one of the coronary vessels becomes restricted or blocked, blood flow to the myocardium may remain relatively uncompromised because these channels can bypass the block.

ANGINA PECTORIS

25.3 Pathogenesis of Angina Pectoris

Angina pectoris is acute chest pain caused by insufficient oxygen to a portion of the myocardium. More than 6 million Americans have angina pectoris, with over 350,000 new cases occurring each year. It is more prevalent in those over 55 years of age.

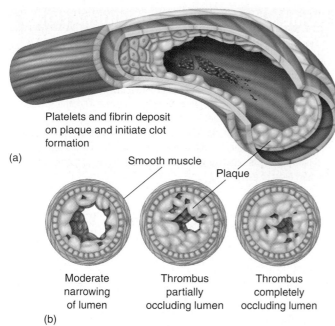

(a)

Platelets and fibrin deposit
on plaque and initiate clot
formation

Smooth muscle

Plaque

Moderate	Thrombus	Thrombus
narrowing	partially	completely
of lumen	occluding lumen	occluding lumen

(b)

● **Figure 25.1** Atherosclerosis in the coronary arteries
Source: Mulvihill, Marylou; Zelman, Mark; Holdaway, Paul;
Tompary, Elaine; Raymond, Jill, Human Diseases: A Systematic
Approach, 6th Edition, © 2006, p.115. Reprinted by permission
of Pearson Education, Inc., Upper Saddle River, NJ.

The classic presentation of angina pectoris is steady, intense pain in the anterior chest, sometimes accompanied by a crushing or constricting sensation. Typically, the discomfort radiates to the left shoulder and proceeds down the left arm. It may also extend posterior to the thoracic spine or move upward to the jaw. In some clients, the pain is experienced in the midepigastrium or abdominal area. Accompanying the discomfort is severe emotional distress—a feeling of panic with fear of impending death. There is usually pallor, dyspnea with cyanosis, diaphoresis, tachycardia, and elevated blood pressure.

Angina pain is usually precipitated by physical exertion or emotional excitement—events associated with *increased myocardial oxygen demand*. Narrowed coronary arteries containing atherosclerotic deposits prevent the proper flow of oxygen and nutrients to the stressed myocardium. Angina pectoris episodes are usually of short duration. With physical rest and/or stress reduction, the increased demands on the heart diminish, and the discomfort subsides within 5 to 10 minutes.

There are several types of angina. When angina occurrences are fairly predictable as to frequency, intensity, and duration, the condition is described as classic or **stable angina.** The pain associated with stable angina is usually relieved by rest.

A second type of angina, known as **vasospastic** or **Prinzmetal's angina** occurs when the decreased myocardial blood flow is caused by *spasms* of the coronary arteries. The vessels undergoing spasms may or may not contain atherosclerotic plaque. Vasospastic angina pain occurs most often during periods of rest, although it may occur unpredictably, and be unrelated to rest or activity.

Silent angina is a form of the disease that occurs in the absence of angina pain. One or more coronary arteries are occluded, but the client remains asymptomatic. Although the mechanisms underlying silent angina are not completely understood, the condition is associated with a high risk for acute MI and sudden death.

When episodes of angina arise more frequently, become more intense, and occur during periods of rest, the condition is called **unstable angina.** Unstable angina is a type of acute coronary syndrome in which a portion of plaque within a coronary artery ruptures. A thrombus quickly builds on the displaced plaque, and the artery becomes in serious danger of occlusion. This condition is a medical emergency requiring aggressive medical intervention because it is associated with an increased risk for MI.

Angina pain often parallels the signs and symptomatology of a heart attack. It is extremely important that the nurse be able to accurately identify the characteristics that differentiate the two conditions, because the pharmacological interventions related to angina differ considerably from those of MI. Angina, although painful and distressing, rarely leads to a fatal outcome, and the chest pain is usually immediately relieved by nitroglycerin. Myocardial infarction, however, carries a high mortality rate if appropriate treatment is delayed. Pharmacological intervention must be initiated immediately and systematically maintained in the event of MI.

The nurse should understand that a number of conditions—many unrelated to cardiac pathology—may cause chest pain. These include gallstones, peptic ulcer disease, esophageal reflux, biliary disease, pneumonia, musculoskeletal injuries, and certain cancers. When a person presents with chest pain, the foremost objective for the healthcare provider is to quickly determine the cause of the pain so that proper, effective interventions can be delivered. This determination incorporates a detailed individual and family health history and a complete physical examination with laboratory workup and other diagnostic tests. All healthcare providers work collaboratively to quickly determine the cause of chest pain.

PHARMFACTS

Angina Pectoris

- The incidence of angina peaks in the 75 to 84 age group. Other incidences include:
  4% of those 65 to 74 years old
  6% of those 75 to 84 years old
  4% of those over age 85
- 20% of the deaths due to cardiovascular disease are attributed to smoking.

Myocardial Infarction

- More than 1.1 million Americans experience a new or recurrent MI each year.
- About one third of the clients experiencing MIs will die from them.
- About 60% of the clients who died suddenly of MI had no previous symptoms of the disease.
- More than 20% of men and 40% of women will die from MI within 1 year after being diagnosed.

25.4 Nonpharmacological Management of Angina

A combination of variables influence the development and progression of angina, including dietary patterns and lifestyle choices. The nurse is instrumental in teaching clients how to prevent coronary artery disease as well as how to lower the rate of recurrence of angina episodes. Such support includes the formulation of a comprehensive plan of care that incorporates psychosocial support and an individualized teaching plan. The client needs to understand the causes of angina, identify the conditions and situations that trigger it, and develop motivation to modify behaviors associated with the disease.

Listing therapeutic lifestyle behaviors that modify the development and progression of cardiovascular disease (CVD) may seem repetitive, as the student has encountered these same factors in chapters on hypertension, hyperlipidemia, and heart disease. However, the importance of prevention and management of CVD through nonpharmacological means cannot be overemphasized. Practicing healthy lifestyle habits can *prevent* CAD in many individuals and *slow the progression* of the disease in those who have plaque buildup. The following factors have been shown to reduce the incidence of CAD.

- Limit alcohol consumption to small or moderate amounts.
- Eliminate foods high in cholesterol or saturated fats.
- Keep blood cholesterol and other lipid indicators within the normal ranges.
- Keep blood pressure within normal range.
- Exercise regularly and maintain optimum weight.
- Keep blood glucose levels within normal range.
- Do not use tobacco.

When the coronary arteries are significantly obstructed, the two most common interventions are **percutaneous transluminal coronary angioplasty (PTCA)**, with stent insertion, and **coronary artery bypass graft (CABG) surgery.** PTCA is a procedure whereby the area of narrowing is dilated using either a balloon catheter or a laser. The basic procedure is to place a catheter, with a small inflatable balloon on the end, within the narrowed section of the artery. Inflation of the balloon catheter pushes the plaque against the arterial wall, reestablishing normal blood flow. Because the artery may return to its original narrowed state

SPECIAL CONSIDERATIONS

The Influence of Gender and Ethnicity on Angina

Angina occurs more frequently in females than males, but the prevalence of MI is higher among men than women. Among ethnic groups, the incidence of angina is highest amongst African Americans, followed by Hispanic Americans and Caucasians, and lowest in Asian populations. African American females have twice the risk of angina compared with African American males.

HOME & COMMUNITY CONSIDERATIONS

CPR and Other Education for Heart Disease

Coronary heart disease is the number one killer in the United States. For this reason it is imperative that individuals learn CPR and encourage others to become certified. In addition, nurses should educate those in their communities on methods to lower their risks for coronary heart disease. Education pertaining to positive lifestyle changes, controlling hypertension, and smoking cessation are all important issues to decrease an individual's risk. Lifestyle changes such as decreasing dietary fat intake, increasing intake of fruit and vegetables, and participating in regular exercise are essential to limiting one's risk for coronary heart disease.

after the procedure, a stent is sometimes used in conjunction with a balloon angioplasty. Angioplasty with stenting typically relieves 90% of the original blockage in the artery. The client usually receives aspirin therapy 2 hours prior to the procedure and heparin for 24 hours after the completion of angioplasty to minimize the risk of thrombus formation.

Coronary bypass surgery is reserved for severe cases of coronary blockage that cannot be dealt with by less invasive treatment modalities. A portion of a vein from the leg or chest is used to create a "bypass artery." One end of the graft is sewn to the aorta and the other end to the coronary artery beyond the narrowed area. Blood from the aorta then flows through the new grafted vessel to the heart muscle, "bypassing" the blockage in the coronary artery. The result is increased blood flow to the heart muscle, which reduces angina and the risk of MI.

25.5 Goals for the Pharmacotherapy of Angina

There are several desired therapeutic outcomes for a client receiving pharmacotherapy for angina. A primary goal is to reduce the intensity and frequency of angina episodes. Additionally, successful pharmacotherapy should improve exercise tolerance and allow the client to participate more actively in activities of daily living. Long-term goals include extending the client's lifespan by preventing serious consequences of ischemic heart disease such as dysrhythmias, heart failure, and MI. To be most effective, pharmacotherapy must be accompanied by therapeutic lifestyle changes that promote a healthy heart.

Although various drug classes are used to treat the disease, antianginal medications may be placed into two basic categories: those that *terminate* an acute angina episode in progress, and those that decrease the *frequency* of angina episodes. The primary means by which antianginal drugs accomplish these goals is to reduce the myocardial demand for oxygen. This may be accomplished by the following mechanisms.

- Slowing the heart rate
- Dilating veins so the heart receives less blood (reduced preload)

- Causing the heart to contract with less force (reduced contractility)
- Lowering blood pressure, thus offering the heart less resistance when ejecting blood from its chambers (reduced afterload)

The pharmacotherapy of angina uses three classes of drugs: organic nitrates, beta-adrenergic antagonists, and calcium channel blockers. Rapid-acting organic nitrates are drugs of choice for terminating an acute angina episode. Beta-adrenergic blockers are drugs of choice for prophylactic treatment, although calcium channel blockers are used when beta-blockers are not tolerated well by a client. Long-acting nitrates, given by the oral or transdermal routes, are effective alternatives. Persistent angina requires drugs from two or more classes, such as a beta-adrenergic blocker combined with a long-acting nitrate or calcium channel blocker. Pharmacotherapy Illustrated 25.1 illustrates the mechanisms of action of drugs used to prevent and treat coronary artery disease.

ORGANIC NITRATES

25.6 Treating Angina With Organic Nitrates

After their medicinal properties were discovered in 1857, the organic nitrates became the mainstay for the treatment of angina. Their mechanism of action is the result of the formation of nitric acid, a potent vasodilator, in vascular smooth muscle.

The primary therapeutic action of the organic nitrates is their ability to relax both arterial and venous smooth muscle. Dilation of veins reduces the amount of blood returning to the heart (preload), so the chambers contain a smaller volume. With less blood for the ventricles to pump, cardiac output is reduced and the workload on the heart is decreased, thereby lowering myocardial oxygen demand. The therapeutic outcome is that chest pain is alleviated and episodes of angina become less frequent. The organic nitrates are shown in Table 25.1.

PHARMACOTHERAPY ILLUSTRATED

25.1 Mechanisms of Action of Drugs Used to Treat Angina

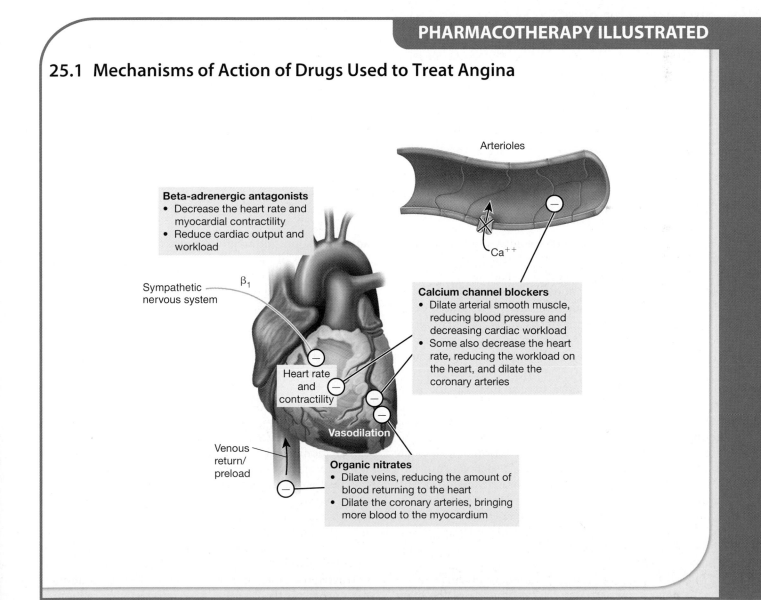

TABLE 25.1 Selected Drugs for Angina and Myocardial Infarction

Drug	Route and Adult Dose (max dose where indicated)	Adverse Effects
ORGANIC NITRATES		
amyl nitrite	Inhalation; 1 ampule (0.18–0.3 ml) PRN	*Headache, postural hypotension, flushing of face, dizziness, rash (transdermal patch), tolerance*
isosorbide dinitrate (Iso-Bid, Isordil, Sorbitrate, Dilatate) (see page 338 for the Prototype Drug box ∞)	PO; 2.5–30 mg qid	
isosorbide mononitrate (Imdur, ISMO, Monoket)	PO; 20 mg qid	Anaphylaxis, circulatory collapse due to hypotension, syncope due to orthostatic hypotension
ⓟ nitroglycerin (Nitrostat, Nitro-Dur, Nitro-Bid, others)	SL; 1 tablet (0.3–0.6 mg) or 1 spray (0.4–0.8 mg) q3–5min (max: 3 doses in 15 min)	
BETA-ADRENERGIC BLOCKERS		
ⓟ atenolol (Tenormin)	PO; 25–50 mg/day (max: 100 mg/day)	*Fatigue, insomnia, drowsiness, impotence or decreased libido, bradycardia, and confusion*
metoprolol (Lopressor, Toprol XL)	PO; 100 mg bid (max: 400 mg/day)	
propranolol (Inderal, Inderal LA) (see page 369 for the Prototype Drug box ∞)	PO; 10–20 mg bid–tid (max: 320 mg/day)	Agranulocytosis, laryngospasm, Stevens–Johnson syndrome, anaphylaxis; if the drug is abruptly withdrawn, palpitations, rebound hypertension, life-threatening dysrhythmias, or MI may occur
timolol maleate (Betimol, Blocadren) (see page 776 for the Prototype Drug box ∞)	PO; 15–45 mg tid (max: 60 mg/day)	
CALCIUM CHANNEL BLOCKERS		
amlodipine (Norvasc)	PO; 5–10 mg/day (max: 10 mg/day)	*Flushed skin, headache, dizziness, peripheral edema, light-headedness, nausea, diarrhea*
bepridil (Vascor)	PO; 200 mg/day (max: 360 mg/day)	
ⓟ diltiazem (Cardizem, Dilacor XR, Tiamate, Tiazac)	PO; 30 mg qid (max: 360 mg/day)	Hepatotoxicity, MI, CHF, confusion, mood changes
nicardipine (Cardene)	PO; 20–40 mg tid or 30–60 mg SR bid (max: 120 mg/day)	
nifedipine (Adalat, Procardia) (see page 314 for the Prototype Drug box ∞)	PO; 10–20 mg tid (max: 180 mg/day)	
verapamil (Calan, Covera-HS, Isoptin, Verelan) (see page 373 for the Prototype Drug box ∞)	PO; 80 mg tid–qid (max: 480 mg/day)	

Italics indicate common adverse effects; underlining indicates serious adverse effects.

Organic nitrates also have the ability to dilate coronary arteries, which was once thought to be their primary mechanism of action. It seems logical that dilating a partially occluded coronary artery would allow more oxygen to reach the ischemic tissue. Although this effect does indeed occur, it is no longer considered the primary mechanism of nitrate action in *stable* angina. This action, however, is crucial in treating *vasospastic* angina, in which the chest pain is caused by coronary artery spasm. The organic nitrates can relax these spasms, allowing more oxygen to reach the myocardium, thereby terminating the pain.

Organic nitrates are of two types, short acting and long acting. The short-acting nitrates, such as nitroglycerin, are taken sublingually to quickly terminate an acute angina episode. Long-acting nitrates, such as isosorbide dinitrate (Isordil), are taken orally or delivered through a transdermal patch to decrease the frequency and severity of angina episodes. Long-acting organic nitrates are also occasionally used to treat symptoms of heart failure, and their role in the treatment of this disease is discussed in Chapter 22 ∞.

Tolerance is a common and serious problem with the long-acting organic nitrates. The magnitude of the tolerance depends on the dosage and the frequency of drug administration. Although tolerance develops rapidly, after only 24 hours of therapy in some clients, it also disappears rapidly when the drug is withheld. Clients are often instructed to remove the transdermal patch for 6 to 12 hours each day or withhold the nighttime dose of the oral medications to delay the development of tolerance. Because the oxygen demands of the heart during sleep are diminished, the client with stable angina experiences few angina episodes during this drug-free interval.

NURSING CONSIDERATIONS

The role of the nurse in nitrate therapy for angina involves careful monitoring of a client's condition and providing education as it relates to the prescribed drug treatment. Obtain the client's baseline blood pressure reading prior to administering nitrates. Nitrates are contraindicated for clients with a diagnosis of cardiac tamponade and pericarditis because these conditions affect cardiac output, and vasodilation can cause severe hypotension. Nitrates are also contraindicated in clients with a diagnosis of head injury, shock, and increased intracranial pressure because the vasodilation is detrimental to these clients. Use nitrates with caution in clients with severe liver or kidney disease or early MI.

Alcohol intake is contraindicated with nitrates because alcohol may cause severe hypotension and cardiovascular collapse. The combination of sustained-release nitrates such as isosorbide dinitrate (Isordil, others) or isosorbide mononitrate (Imdur, others) with the ingestion of alcohol may cause severe cardiovascular complications.

If hypotension occurs, withhold the client's nitrates or remove topical forms of nitrate until blood pressure has returned to normal. Monitor blood pressure frequently during nitrate therapy to assess for hypotension. IV nitrates have the greatest risk for causing severe hypotension. Titrate infusions of nitrates to effect desired pain relief or to reach a specific blood pressure level. Hold other forms of nitrates and remove topical nitrates during the IV infusion.

Client Teaching.   Client education as it relates to nitrates should include the goals of therapy, the reasons for obtaining baseline data such as vital signs and the existence of underlying renal and cardiac disorders, and possible drug side effects. Include the following points when teaching clients about nitrates:

- Avoid or limit alcohol use; flushing, weakness, and fainting may occur as a result of hypotension.
- When using transdermal patches, rotate the sites and wash skin thoroughly after patch removal.
- When taking a sublingual nitrate, allow the tablet to dissolve under the tongue without chewing or swallowing the medication.

- Sit or lie down when taking a sublingual nitrate to prevent dizziness.
- If chest discomfort is not relieved after three doses of nitroglycerin, call the emergency medical system (EMS or 911 if available).
- Immediately report blurred vision, dry mouth, or severe headache, which may indicate overdose.
- Keep medication in its original container, away from heat, light, and moisture.
- Replace sublingual nitrate prescriptions every 6 months.

BETA-ADRENERGIC BLOCKERS (ANTAGONISTS)

Beta-adrenergic antagonists or blockers reduce the cardiac workload by slowing heart rate and reducing contractility.

25.7 Treating Angina With Beta-adrenergic Blockers

These drugs are as effective as the organic nitrates in decreasing the frequency and severity of angina episodes caused by exertion. Unlike with the organic nitrates, tolerance does not develop to the antianginal effects of the beta-blockers. They are ideal for clients who have both hypertension *and* coronary artery disease owing to their antihypertensive action. They are considered drugs of choice for the prophylaxis of chronic angina. The beta-blockers

---

Pr PROTOTYPE DRUG | Nitroglycerin *(Nitrostat, Nitro-Bid, Nitro-Dur, others)* | Organic Nitrate

ACTIONS AND USES

Nitroglycerin, the oldest and most widely used organic nitrate, can be delivered by a number of different routes: sublingual, oral, translingual, IV, transmucosal, transdermal, topical, and extended-release forms. It may be taken while an acute angina episode is in progress or just prior to physical activity. When given sublingually, it reaches peak plasma levels in 2–4 minutes, thus terminating angina pain rapidly. Chest pain that does not respond to two or three doses of sublingual nitroglycerin may indicate MI.

ADMINISTRATION ALERTS

- For IV administration, use a glass IV bottle and special IV tubing, because plastic absorbs nitrates significantly, thus reducing client dose.
- Cover IV bottle to reduce degradation of nitrates due to light exposure.
- Use gloves when applying nitroglycerin paste or ointment to prevent self-administration.
- Pregnancy category C.

PHARMACOKINETICS

Onset: 1–3 min sublingual; 2–5 min buccal; 40–60 min transdermal patch

Peak: 4–8 min sublingual; 4–10 min buccal; 1–2 h transdermal patch

Half-life: 1–4 min

Duration: 30–60 min sublingual; 2 h buccal; 18–24 h transdermal patch

ADVERSE EFFECTS

The side effects of nitroglycerin are usually cardiovascular in nature and rarely life threatening. Because nitroglycerin can dilate cerebral vessels, headache is a common side effect and may be severe. Occasionally the venous dilation caused by nitroglycerin produces reflex tachycardia. Some healthcare providers prescribe a beta-adrenergic blocker to diminish this undesirable increase in heart rate. The side effects of nitroglycerin often diminish after a few doses.

Contraindications: Nitroglycerin should not be given to clients with preexisting hypotension or with high intracranial pressure or head trauma. Drugs in this class are contraindicated in pericardial tamponade and constrictive pericarditis because the heart cannot increase cardiac output to maintain blood pressure when vasodilation occurs. Sustained-release forms of the medicines should not be given to clients with glaucoma.

INTERACTIONS

Drug–Drug: Concurrent use with sildenafil (Viagra) may cause life-threatening hypotension and cardiovascular collapse. Use with alcohol and antihypertensive drugs may cause additive hypotension.

Lab Tests: May increase values of urinary catecholamines and VMA concentrations.

Herbal/Food: Unknown.

Treatment of Overdose: Hypotension may be reversed with administration of IV normal saline. If methemoglobinemia is suspected, methylene blue may be administered.

NURSING PROCESS FOCUS Clients Receiving Nitroglycerin

Assessment	Potential Nursing Diagnoses
Prior to administration: ■ Obtain a complete health history including allergies, drug and alcohol history, and possible drug interactions. ■ Obtain vital signs, ECG, and frequency and severity of angina. ■ Obtain history of cardiac disorders and serum labs, including cardiac enzymes, CBC, BUN, creatinine, and liver enzymes. ■ Assess if client has taken sildenafil (Viagra) in past 24 hours, because it may cause MI.	■ Tissue Perfusion, Ineffective, related to hypotension due to drug. ■ Injury, Risk for, dizziness or syncope related to hypotension ■ Pain, Acute (headache) related to adverse effects of drug ■ Knowledge, Deficient, related to drug therapy

Planning: Client Goals and Expected Outcomes

The client will:
■ Experience relief or prevention of chest pain.
■ Immediately report chest pain unrelieved by nitroglycerin.
■ Demonstrate an understanding of the drug's actions by accurately describing drug side effects and precautions.

Implementation

Interventions and (Rationales)	Client Education/Discharge Planning
■ Assess client's level of pain, including location, quality and intensity. (Assessment aids in determining drug dose.)	Instruct client: ■ If after three doses, chest pain has not subsided, to call for emergency services. ■ To sit or lie down prior to taking nitroglycerin and maintain position for a few minutes. ■ Not to ingest any alcohol while taking nitroglycerin.
■ Monitor ECG, blood pressure, and pulse. (Assessment aids in determining drug dose.)	■ Inform client to monitor blood pressure and pulse daily.
■ Assess for headache. (Nitrates commonly cause headache.)	■ Inform client that headache is a common side effect that usually resolves over time.
■ Assess for use of sildenafil. (The combination may lead to severe hypotension.)	■ Instruct client to not take sildenafil (Viagra) within 24 hours after taking nitrates, and wait 24 hours after taking Viagra to resume nitrate therapy.

Evaluation of Outcome Criteria

Evaluate the effectiveness of drug therapy by confirming that client goals and expected outcomes have been met (see "Planning").
■ The client is free of chest pain.
■ The client verbalizes the importance of notifying the healthcare provider of unrelieved chest pain.
■ The client demonstrates an understanding of the drug's action by accurately describing drug side effects and precautions.

used for angina are shown in Table 25.1. Beta-blockers are widely used in medicine, and additional details may be found in Chapters 13, 23, 24, and 26 ∞.

NURSING CONSIDERATIONS

The role of the nurse in beta-adrenergic antagonist therapy for angina involves careful monitoring of a client's condition and providing education as it relates to the prescribed drug treatment. Prior to administration of beta-blockers, assess apical heart rate, especially if the client is taking digoxin (Lanoxin), because both drugs slow AV conduction. Beta-blockers lower blood pressure; thus, take vital signs prior to administration and monitor them during treatment to prevent hypotension. Assess and continually monitor respiratory status during administration of beta-blockers. Side effects usually occur with high doses of beta-blockers.

Because beta-adrenergic antagonists slow heart rate and conduction, they are contraindicated in bradycardia, second- and third-degree heart block, overt heart failure, and cardiogenic shock. Use beta-blockers cautiously in clients with the following conditions: heart failure (taking digoxin and diuretics), asthma, COPD, and impaired renal function. Warn diabetic clients that initial symptoms indicative of hypoglycemia, such as palpitations, diaphoresis, and nervousness, may not be evident while taking beta-blockers. Monitor serum glucose levels in diabetic clients, because insulin doses may need to be adjusted.

Do not discontinue beta-blockers abruptly, because with long-term use the heart becomes accustomed to the catecholamines blocked by these medications. When beta-blockers are discontinued abruptly, the adrenergic receptors are stimulated, causing excitation. This may exacerbate angina and cause tachycardia or MI in clients with cardiovascular disease. Assess for fatigue during exercise because the blockade effect prevents the heart rate from increasing during physical activity. Determine cardiac status by assessing heart rate and ECG readings before administering beta-blockers.

Client Teaching. Client education as it relates to beta-blocker therapy for angina should include the goals of therapy, the reasons for obtaining baseline data such as vital signs and the existence of underlying disorders, and possible drug side effects. Include the following points when teaching clients about beta-blockers:

- Rise slowly from a sitting or lying position to prevent dizziness.
- Report dizziness and light-headedness.
- Do not discontinue the medication abruptly; this may cause angina or MI.
- Do not take other prescription drugs, OTC medications, herbal remedies, or vitamins or minerals without notifying the healthcare provider.
- Check pulse rate daily. Stop medication if pulse rate is 60 beats per minute or lower, and contact the healthcare provider immediately.
- Report symptoms of depression or fatigue
- Check blood pressure daily and notify your healthcare provider if it is 90/60 mm Hg or less.

- Keep additional clothing nearby because beta-blockers may increase sensitivity to cold.

CALCIUM CHANNEL BLOCKERS

25.8 Treating Angina With Calcium Channel Blockers

Blockade of calcium channels has a number of effects on the heart, most of which are similar to those of beta-blockers. Like beta-blockers, calcium channel blockers (CCBs) are used for a number of cardiovascular conditions, including hypertension (Chapter 23) and dysrhythmias (Chapter 26 ∞). The calcium channel blockers used for angina are shown in Table 25.1.

CCBs have several cardiovascular actions that benefit the client with angina. Most important, CCBs relax arteriolar smooth muscle, thus lowering blood pressure. This reduction in afterload decreases myocardial oxygen demand. Some of the CCBs also slow conduction velocity through the heart, decreasing heart rate and contributing to the reduced cardiac workload. An additional effect of the CCBs is their ability to dilate the coronary arteries, bringing more oxygen to the myocardium. This is especially important in clients with vasospastic angina. Because they are able to relieve the acute vasospasms of variant angina, CCBs are considered drugs of choice for this condition. For stable angina, they may

---

Pr PROTOTYPE DRUG | Atenolol *(Tenormin)* | Beta-adrenergic Blocker

ACTIONS AND USES

Atenolol is one of the most frequently prescribed drugs in the United States owing to its relative safety and effectiveness in treating a number of chronic disorders, including heart failure, hypertension, angina, and MI. The drug selectively blocks beta$_1$-adrenergic receptors in the heart. Its effectiveness in angina is attributed to its ability to slow heart rate and reduce contractility, both of which lower myocardial oxygen demand. As with other beta-blockers, therapy generally begins with low doses, which are gradually increased until the therapeutic effect is achieved. Because of its 7- to 9-hour half-life, it may be taken once daily.

ADMINISTRATION ALERTS

- During IV administration, monitor ECG continuously; blood pressure and pulse should be assessed before, during, and after dose is administered.
- Assess pulse and blood pressure before oral administration. Hold if pulse is below 60 beats per minute or if client is hypotensive.
- Atenolol may precipitate bronchospasm in susceptible clients with initial doses.
- Pregnancy category D.

PHARMACOKINETICS

Onset: 1 h

Peak: 2–4 h

Half-life: 1–4 min

Duration: 24 h

ADVERSE EFFECTS

Being a cardioselective beta$_1$-adrenergic blocker, atenolol has few adverse effects on the lung. The most common side effects of atenolol include fatigue, weakness, bradycardia, and hypotension.

Contraindications: Because atenolol slows heart rate, it should not be used in clients with severe bradycardia, AV heart block, cardiogenic shock, or decompensated heart failure. Owing to its vasodilation effects, it is contraindicated in clients with severe hypotension.

INTERACTIONS

Drug–Drug: Concurrent use with calcium channel blockers may result in excessive cardiac suppression. Use with digoxin may slow AV conduction, leading to heart block. Concurrent use of atenolol with other antihypertensives may result in additive hypotension. Anticholinergics may cause decreased absorption from the GI tract.

Lab Tests: Atenolol may increase values of the following blood tests: uric acid, lipids, potassium, creatinine, and antinuclear antibody.

Herbal/Food: Unknown.

Treatment of Overdose: Atenolol can be removed from the systemic circulation by hemodialysis. Atropine or isoproterenol may be used to reverse bradycardia.

 See the Companion Website for a Nursing Process Focus specific to this drug.

be used as monotherapy in clients unable to tolerate beta-blockers. In clients with persistent symptoms, CCBs may be combined with organic nitrates or beta-blockers.

NURSING CONSIDERATIONS

The role of the nurse in CCB therapy for angina involves careful monitoring of a client's condition and providing education as it relates to the prescribed drug treatment. Assess vital signs before administering CCBs because of their effects on blood pressure and heart rate. Do not give CCBs to clients who are hypotensive and/or have a heart rate of 60 beats per minute or less. Take blood pressure readings from both arms and while the client is lying, sitting, and then standing to assess for orthostatic hypotension. Because CCBs affect myocardial conduction, do not administer to clients with sick sinus syndrome or third-degree AV block without a pacemaker. Obtain an ECG prior to administration to assess for any conduction disturbances.

Some CCBs reduce myocardial contractility and can worsen heart failure. Assess for signs of deteriorating heart failure such as increased peripheral edema, shortness of breath, and pulmonary congestion. Obtain daily weights for heart-failure clients to assess for fluid retention (a sudden increase in weight of 2 lb or more). CCBs can cause constipation, so assess bowel function and take measures to reduce the incidence of constipation. Give extended-release capsules whole, because splitting or crushing may cause a rapid absorption of the drug, resulting in severe hypotension.

Client Teaching.   Client education as it relates to CCBs should include the goals of therapy, the reasons for obtaining baseline data such as vital signs and the existence of underlying renal or hepatic disorders, and possible drug side effects. Include the following points when teaching clients about CCBs:

- Keep all scheduled laboratory visits for testing and physician visits for monitoring.
- Monitor blood pressure and pulse daily. Stop drug if blood pressure falls below 90/60 mmHg or if heart rate is 60 beats per minute or less, and immediately notify the healthcare provider.
- Record frequency and severity of each angina attack and bring the record to each physician visit.
- Rise slowly from a sitting or lying position to prevent dizziness.
- Immediately notify your healthcare provider if you experience any symptoms of heart failure such as sudden weight gain, swelling in the legs, decreased heart rate, and shortness of breath.
- Do not abruptly stop taking the medication, because angina or MI may result.
- Take extended-release tablets on an empty stomach, and do not split or crush medication.
- Take measures to avoid constipation.
- Report weakness or unusual fatigue to your healthcare provider.

Pr **PROTOTYPE DRUG** | Diltiazem *(Cardizem)* | Calcium Channel Blocker

ACTIONS AND USES

Like other calcium channel blockers, diltiazem inhibits the transport of calcium into myocardial cells. It has the ability to relax both coronary and peripheral blood vessels, bringing more oxygen to the myocardium and reducing cardiac workload. It is useful in the treatment of atrial dysrhythmias and hypertension, as well as stable and vasospastic angina. When given as sustained-release capsules, it is administered once daily.

ADMINISTRATION ALERTS

- During IV administration, the client must be continuously monitored, and cardioversion equipment must be available.
- Extended-release tablets and capsules should not be crushed or split.
- Pregnancy category C.

PHARMACOKINETICS

Onset: 30–60 min (2–3 h sustained release)

Peak: 2–3 h (6–11 h sustained release)

Half-life: 3.5–9 h

Duration: 6–8 h (12 h sustained release)

ADVERSE EFFECTS

Side effects of diltiazem are generally not serious and are related to vasodilation: headache, dizziness, and edema of the ankles and feet. Abrupt withdrawal may precipitate an acute anginal episode.

Contraindications: Diltiazem is contraindicated in clients with AV heart block, sick sinus syndrome, severe hypotension, or bleeding aneurysm, or those undergoing intracranial surgery. Use with caution in clients with renal or hepatic impairment.

INTERACTIONS

Drug–Drug: Concurrent use of diltiazem with other cardiovascular drugs, particularly digoxin or beta-adrenergic blockers, may cause partial or complete heart block, heart failure, or dysrhythmias. Diltiazem may increase digoxin or quinidine levels when taken concurrently. Additive hypotension may occur if used with beta-blockers or antihypertensives.

Lab Tests: Unknown.

Herbal/Food: Herbal supplements such as dong quai and ginger may interfere with blood clotting.

Treatment of Overdose: Atropine or isoproterenol may be used to reverse bradycardia. Hypotension may be reversed by a vasopressor such as parenteral dopamine or dobutamine.

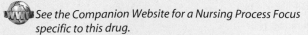 *See the Companion Website for a Nursing Process Focus specific to this drug.*

See also "Nursing Process Focus: Clients Receiving Calcium Channel Blocker Therapy," page 315 in Chapter 23 ∞, for the complete Nursing Process applied to clients receiving calcium channel blockers.

MYOCARDIAL INFARCTION

25.9 Diagnosis of Myocardial Infarction

Heart attacks or **myocardial infarctions (MIs)** are responsible for a substantial number of deaths each year. Some clients die before reaching a medical facility for treatment, and many others die within 48 hours following the initial MI. Clearly, MI is a serious and frightening disease and one responsible for a large percentage of sudden deaths.

The primary cause of myocardial infarction is advanced coronary artery disease. Plaque buildup can severely narrow one or more branches of the coronary arteries. Pieces of unstable plaque can break off and lodge in a small vessel serving a portion of the myocardium. Exposed plaque activates the clotting cascade, resulting in platelet aggregation and adherence (Chapter 27 ∞). A new clot quickly builds on the existing plaque, making obstruction of the vessel imminent.

Deprived of its oxygen supply, this area of myocardium becomes ischemic, and myocytes begin to die in about 20 minutes unless the blood supply is quickly restored. The death of myocardial tissue, which may be irreversible, releases certain "marker" enzymes, which can be measured in the blood to confirm the client has experienced an MI.

Extreme chest pain is usually the first symptom of MI, and the one that drives most clients to seek medical attention. An electrocardiogram can give important clues as to the extent and location of the MI. The infarcted region of the myocardium is nonconducting, producing abnormalities of Q waves, T, waves and S-T segments (Chapter 26 ∞). Laboratory test results are used to aid in diagnosis and monitor progress after an MI. Table 25.2 describes some of these important laboratory values.

Early diagnosis of MI, and prompt pharmacotherapy, can significantly reduce mortality and the long-term disability associated with MI. The pharmacological goals for treating a client with an acute MI are as follows:

- Restore blood supply (reperfusion) to the damaged myocardium as quickly as possible through the use of thrombolytics.
- Reduce myocardial oxygen demand with organic nitrates, beta-blockers, or CCBs to prevent additional infarctions.
- Control or prevent associated dysrhythmias with beta-blockers or other antidysrhythmics.
- Reduce post-MI mortality with aspirin and ACE inhibitors.
- Manage severe MI pain and associated anxiety with narcotic analgesics.

THROMBOLYTICS

25.10 Treating Myocardial Infarction With Thrombolytics

In treating MI, thrombolytic therapy is administered to dissolve clots obstructing the coronary arteries, thus restoring circulation to the myocardium. Quick restoration of cardiac circulation reduces mortality caused by acute MI. After the clot is successfully dissolved, anticoagulant therapy is initiated to prevent the formation of additional clots. Dosages

TABLE 25.2 Changes in Blood Test Values With Acute MI

Blood Test	Initial Elevation after MI	Peak Elevation after MI	Duration of Elevation	Normal Range
cholesterol			4 wk, during stress response	200 mg/dl
CK = creatine kinase/CPK = creatinine phosphokinase	3–8 h	12–24 h	2–4 days	males: 12–80 units/L females: 10–70 units/L
	4–8 h	8–24 h	2–3 days	0%–3% of CK
ESR	first week		several weeks	
glucose			duration of stress response	fasting: 80–120 mg/dl
LDH, LDH1 = lactase dehydrogenase	8–72 h	3–6 days	8–14 days	45–90 units/L
myoglobin	1–3 h	4–6 h	1–2 days	0–85 ng/ml
troponin I	2–4 h	24–36 h	7–10 days	3.1 mcg/L
troponin T	2–4 h	24–36 h	10–14 days	0.01–0.1ng/L
WBC	few hours	3–7 days	$4.8–10.8 \times 10^3$ mcg/L	

ESR, erythrocyte sedimentation rate; WBC, white blood cell (count).

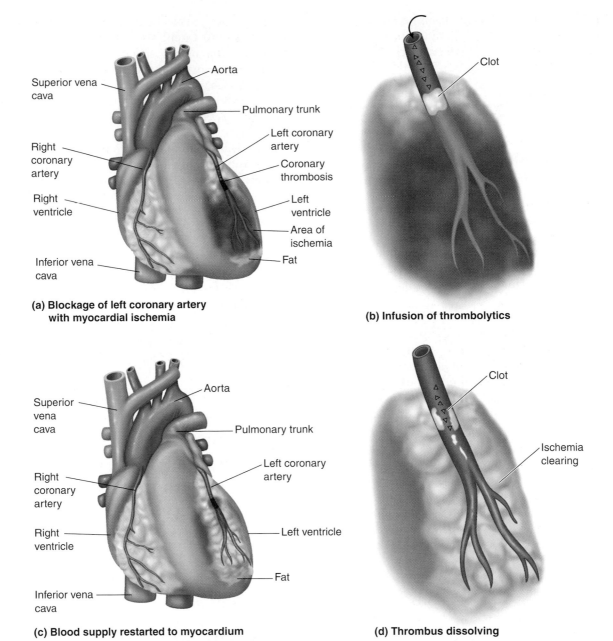

(a) Blockage of left coronary artery with myocardial ischemia

Superior vena cava
Aorta
Pulmonary trunk
Left coronary artery
Coronary thrombosis
Right coronary artery
Right ventricle
Left ventricle
Area of ischemia
Inferior vena cava
Fat

(b) Infusion of thrombolytics

Clot

(c) Blood supply restarted to myocardium

Superior vena cava
Aorta
Pulmonary trunk
Left coronary artery
Right coronary artery
Right ventricle
Left ventricle
Inferior vena cava
Fat

(d) Thrombus dissolving

Clot
Ischemia clearing

● **Figure 25.2** Blockage and reperfusion following myocardial infarction: (a) blockage of left coronary artery with myocardial ischemia; (b) infusion of thrombolytics; (c) blood supply returning to myocardium; (d) thrombus dissolving and ischemia clearing.
Source: Figures (a) and (c): Mulvihill, Marylou; Zelman, Mark; Holdaway, Paul; Tompary, Elaine; Raymond, Jill, Human Diseases: A Systematic Approach, 6th Edition, © 2006, p.105. Reprinted by permission of Pearson Education, Inc., Upper Saddle River, NJ.

and descriptions of the various thrombolytics are given in Chapter 27 on page 388 ∞. ● Figure 25.2 illustrates the pathogenesis and treatment of MI.

Thrombolytics are most effective when administered from 20 minutes to 12 hours after the onset of MI symptoms. If administered after 24 hours, the drugs are mostly ineffective. In addition, research has suggested that clients older than age 75 do not experience reduced mortality from these drugs. Because thrombolytic therapy is expensive and has the potential to produce serious side effects, it is important to identify circumstances that contribute to successful therapy. The development of clinical practice guidelines to identify those clients who

benefit most from thrombolytic therapy is an ongoing process.

Thrombolytics have a narrow margin of safety between dissolving clots and producing serious adverse effects. Although therapy is usually targeted to a single thrombus in a specific artery, once infused in the blood, the drugs travel to all vessels and may cause adverse effects anywhere in the body. The primary risk of thrombolytics is excessive bleeding due to interference with the normal clotting process. Vital signs must be monitored continuously; signs of bleeding call for discontinuation of therapy. Because these drugs are rapidly destroyed in the blood, stopping the infusion normally results in the rapid termination of adverse effects.

The role of the nurse in thrombolytic therapy for MI involves careful monitoring of a client's condition and providing education as it relates to the prescribed drug regimen. Assess for conditions that would contraindicate thrombolytic therapy, including recent trauma, biopsies, surgery, lumbar puncture, GI bleeding, postpartum (within 10 days), cerebral hemorrhage, bleeding disorders, and thrombocytopenia, because thrombolytics place the client at increased risk for bleeding. Do not administer to clients with septic thrombophlebitis, because the favorable clot would be dissolved by thrombolytics, resulting in client injury. Use with caution in any condition in which bleeding could be a significant hazard, such as severe renal or liver disease.

Start IV lines and arterial lines and insert a Foley catheter prior to beginning therapy to decrease the chance of bleeding from those sites. Monitor vital signs, intake and output, and changes in laboratory values (hematocrit, hemoglobin, platelets, and coagulation studies) that may indicate bleeding. Because cerebral hemorrhage is a concern, assess for changes in mental and neurological status. Monitor cardiac function and assess for dysrhythmia, because cardiac tissue perfusion is reestablished after MI. Obtain tests such as complete blood cell count, international normalized ratio, prothrombin time, and partial thromboplastin time to assess for internal bleeding. The client has an increased risk of bleeding 2 to 4 days posttherapy.

Client Education. Client education as it relates to thrombolytic therapy should include the goals of therapy, the reasons for obtaining baseline data such as vital signs and the existence of underlying cardiac and renal disorders, and possible drug side effects. Include the following points when teaching clients about thrombolytics:

- Avoid touching IV sites to prevent bleeding.
- Keep physical activity to a minimum during infusion.
- Report bleeding from old IV sites, gums, rectum, vagina, nose, and urine. Continue to assess for 4 days postinfusion.

See Nursing Process Focus: "Clients Receiving Anticoagulant Therapy," page 384 in Chapter 27 ∞.

25.11 Drugs for Symptoms and Complications of Acute Myocardial Infarction

The most immediate needs of the client with MI are to ensure that the heart continues functioning and that permanent damage from the infarction is minimized. In addition to thrombolytic therapy to restore perfusion to the myocardium, drugs from several other classes are administered soon after the onset of symptoms, to prevent reinfarction and ultimately to reduce mortality from the episode.

Pr PROTOTYPE DRUG | Reteplase *(Retavase)* | Thrombolytic

ACTIONS AND USES

Prepared through recombinant DNA technology, reteplase acts by cleaving plasminogen to form plasmin. Plasmin then degrades the fibrin matrix of thrombi. Reteplase is one of the newer thrombolytics. Like other drugs in this class, reteplase should be given as soon as possible after the onset of MI symptoms. Administered by IV bolus, it usually acts within 20 minutes. A second bolus may be injected 30 minutes after the first, if needed to clear the thrombus. After the clot has been dissolved, heparin therapy is started to prevent additional clots from forming.

ADMINISTRATION ALERTS

- Must be reconstituted just prior to use with diluent provided by manufacturer; swirl to mix—do not shake.
- Do not give any other drug simultaneously through the same IV line.
- Reteplase and heparin are incompatible and must never be combined in the same solution.
- Pregnancy category C.

PHARMACOKINETICS

Onset: Immediate

Peak: Unknown

Half-life: 13–16 min

Duration: Unknown

ADVERSE EFFECTS

The most serious side effects of reteplase relate to internal bleeding. Bleeding may be prolonged at injection sites and catheter insertion sites. Dysrhythmias may occur during myocardial reperfusion.

Contraindications: Reteplase is contraindicated in clients with active bleeding or history of CVA, or who have had recent surgical procedures.

INTERACTIONS

Drug–Drug: Concurrent therapy with aspirin, anticoagulants, and platelet aggregation inhibitors will produce an additive anticoagulant effect and increase the risk of bleeding.

Lab Tests: Reteplase degrades plasminogen in blood samples, thus decreasing serum plasminogen and fibrinogen levels.

Herbal/Food: Ginkgo biloba may increase the risk of bleeding.

Treatment of Overdose: There is no specific treatment for overdose.

 See the Companion Website for a Nursing Process Focus specific to this drug.

ANTIPLATELET AND ANTICOAGULANT DRUGS

Unless contraindicated, 160 to 325 mg of aspirin is given as soon as an MI is suspected. Aspirin use in the weeks following an acute MI dramatically reduces mortality, probably owing to its antiplatelet action. The low doses used in maintenance therapy (75–150 mg/day) rarely cause GI bleeding.

The adenosine diphosphate (ADP)–receptor blockers clopidogrel (Plavix) and ticlopidine (Ticlid) are effective antiplatelet agents that are approved for the prevention of thrombotic stroke and MI. Because these drugs are considerably more expensive than aspirin, they are usually considered for clients allergic to aspirin or who are at risk for GI bleeding from aspirin.

Glycoprotein IIb/IIIa inhibitors are antiplatelet agents with a mechanism of action distinct from that of aspirin. These agents are sometimes indicated for unstable angina or MI, or for clients undergoing PTCA. The most common drug in this class, abciximab (ReoPro), is infused at the time of PTCA, and continued for 12 hours after the procedure is completed.

On diagnosis of MI in the emergency room, clients are immediately placed on the anticoagulant heparin to prevent additional thrombi from forming. Heparin therapy is generally continued for 48 hours, or until PTCA is completed, at which time clients are switched to warfarin (Coumadin). An alternative is to administer a low molecular weight heparin, such as enoxaparin (Lovenox). The student should refer to Chapter 27 ∞ for a comparison of the different coagulation modifiers and the dosages for these medications.

NITRATES

The value of organic nitrates in treating angina was discussed in Section 25.6. Nitrates have additional uses in the client with a suspected MI. At the initial onset of chest pain, sublingual nitroglycerin is administered to assist in the diagnosis, and three doses may be taken 5 minutes apart. Pain that persists 5–10 minutes after the initial dose may indicate an MI, and the client should seek immediate medical assistance.

Clients with persistent pain, heart failure, or severe hypertension may receive IV nitroglycerin for 24 hours following the onset of pain. The arterial and venous dilation produced by the drug reduces myocardial oxygen demand. Organic nitrates also relieve coronary artery vasospasm, which may be present during the acute stage of MI. On the client's discharge from the hospital, organic nitrates are discontinued, unless they are needed for relief of stable angina pain.

BETA-ADRENERGIC BLOCKERS

Beta-blockers reduce myocardial oxygen demand, which is critical for clients experiencing a recent MI. In addition, they slow impulse conduction through the heart, thereby suppressing dysrhythmias, which are serious and sometimes fatal complications following an MI. Research has clearly demonstrated that beta-blockers can reduce MI-associated mortality if they are administered within 8 hours of MI onset. These drugs may initially be administered IV, and then switched to oral dosing for chronic therapy. Unless contraindicated, beta-blocker therapy continues for the remainder of the client's life. For clients unable to tolerate beta-blockers, calcium channel blockers are an alternative.

ANGIOTENSIN-CONVERTING ENZYME (ACE) INHIBITORS

Clinical research has demonstrated increased survival for clients administered the ACE inhibitors captopril (Capoten) or lisinopril (Prinivil, Zestoretic) following an acute MI. These drugs are most effective when therapy is started within 24 hours after the onset of symptoms. Oral doses are normally begun after thrombolytic therapy is completed and the client's condition has stabilized. IV therapy may be used during the early stages of MI pharmacotherapy.

Pain Management

The pain associated with an MI can be debilitating. Pain control is essential to ensure client comfort and to reduce stress. Narcotic analgesics such as morphine sulfate or meperidine (Demerol) are given to ease extreme pain and to sedate the anxious client. Pharmacology of the narcotic analgesics was presented in Chapter 18 ∞.

NATURAL THERAPIES

Ginseng and Myocardial Ischemia

Ginseng is one of the oldest known herbal remedies, with at least six species being reported to have medicinal properties. *Panax ginseng* is distributed throughout China, Korea, and Siberia, whereas *Panax quinquefolius* is native to Canada and the United States. The plant's popularity has led to its extinction from certain regions, and much of the available ginseng is now grown commercially.

Standardization of ginseng focuses on a group of chemicals called *ginsenosides*, although there are many other chemicals in the root, which is the harvested portion of the plant. The German *Commission E Monographs* recommend a dose of 20 to 30 mg ginsenosides. This value is sometimes reported as a percent, with 5% being the recommended standard of ginsenosides.

There are differences in chemical composition among the various species of ginseng; American ginseng is not considered equivalent to Siberian ginseng. Ginseng is reported to be a calcium channel antagonist. By increasing the conversion of L-arginine to nitric oxide, ginseng improves blood flow to the heart in times of low oxygen supply, such as with myocardial ischemia. The nurse should caution clients who take ginseng, because herb–drug interactions are possible with warfarin and loop diuretics.

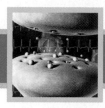

CHAPTER REVIEW

KEY CONCEPTS

The numbered key concepts provide a succinct summary of the important points from the corresponding numbered section within the chapter. If any of these points are not clear, refer to the numbered section within the chapter for review.

25.1 Coronary artery disease includes both angina and myocardial infarction. It is caused by narrowing of the arterial lumen due to atherosclerotic plaque.

25.2 The myocardium requires a continuous supply of oxygen from the coronary arteries to function properly.

25.3 Angina pectoris is the narrowing of a coronary artery, resulting in a lack of sufficient oxygen to the heart muscle. Chest pain on emotional or physical exertion is the most characteristic symptom, although some forms of angina do not cause pain.

25.4 Angina management may include nonpharmacological therapies such as diet and lifestyle modifications, angioplasty, or surgery.

25.5 Goals for the pharmacotherapy of angina are to terminate acute attacks and prevent future episodes. They are usually achieved by reducing cardiac workload.

25.6 The organic nitrates relieve angina by dilating veins and coronary arteries. They are drugs of choice for terminating acute episodes of stable angina.

25.7 Beta-adrenergic blockers relieve anginal pain by decreasing the oxygen demands on the heart. They are drugs of choice for prophylaxis of stable angina.

25.8 Calcium channel blockers relieve angina by dilating the coronary vessels and reducing the workload on the heart. They are drugs of first choice for treating vasospastic angina.

25.9 The early diagnosis of myocardial infarction increases chances of survival. Early pharmacotherapy antidysrhythmics targeted reducing the workload on the heart and inhibiting fatal dysrhythmias.

25.10 If given within hours after the onset of MI, thrombolytic agents can dissolve clots and restore perfusion to affected regions of the myocardium.

25.11 A number of additional drugs are used to treat the symptoms and complications of acute MI. These include antiplatelet and anticoagulant agents, beta-blockers, glycoprotein IIB/IIIA inhibitors, analgesics, and ACE inhibitors.

NCLEX-RN® REVIEW QUESTIONS

1 The client is being discharged with nitroglycerin (Nitrostat). Client education would include the instructions:

1. "Swallow 3 tablets immediately for pain and call 911."
2. "Put 1 tablet under your tongue for chest pain. If pain does not subside, you may repeat in 5 minutes, taking no more than 3 tablets."
3. "Call your physician when you have chest pain. He will tell you how many tablets to take."
4. "Place 3 tablets under your tongue and call 911."

2 The teaching plan for a client with angina includes the action of antianginal agents. The nurse teaches that these drugs:

1. Increase heart rate.
2. Increase preload.
3. Increase contractility.
4. Decrease afterload.

3 The nurse recognizes that the mechanism of action of beta-adrenergic blockers in the treatment of angina is:

1. Slowed heart rate and decreased contractility.
2. Increased contractility and heart rate.
3. Relaxation of arterial and venous smooth muscle.
4. Decreased peripheral resistance.

4 The client should remove the transdermal nitroglycerin patch at night to:

1. Prevent overdose.
2. Prevent adverse reactions.
3. Assure the dosage is appropriate.
4. Delay development of tolerance.

5 Put the following nursing interventions in order for a client who is experiencing chest pain.

1. Administer nitroglycerin sublingual.
2. Assess heart rate and blood pressure.
3. Assess for hypotension.
4. Assess location, quality, and intensity of pain.
5. Document interventions and outcomes.

CRITICAL THINKING QUESTIONS

1. A client on the medical unit is complaining of chest pain (4 on a scale of 10), has a history of angina, and is requesting his PRN nitroglycerin spray. The client's blood pressure is 96/60 mm Hg at present. Identify what the nurse should do.

2. A client is recovering from an acute MI and has been put on atenolol (Tenormin). What teaching should the client receive prior to discharge from the hospital?

3. A client with chest pain has been given the calcium channel blocker diltiazem (Cardizem) IV for a heart rate of 118 beats per minute. Blood pressure at this time is 100/60 mm Hg. What precautions should the nurse take?

See Appendix D for answers and rationales for all activities.

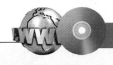

EXPLORE
MediaLink

www.prenhall.com/adams

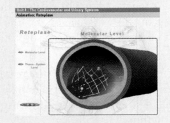

NCLEX-RN® review, case studies, and other interactive resources for this chapter can be found on the companion website at www.prenhall.com/adams. Click on "Chapter 25" to select the activities for this chapter. For animations, more NCLEX-RN® review questions, and an audio glossary, access the accompanying Prentice Hall Nursing MediaLink DVD-ROM in this textbook.

PRENTICE HALL NURSING MEDIALINK DVD-ROM

- **Animation**
  Mechanism in Action: Reteplase (*Retavase*)
- **Audio Glossary**
- **NCLEX-RN® Review**

COMPANION WEBSITE

- **NCLEX-RN® Review**
- **Dosage Calculations**
- **Case Study:** Client receiving nitrates for angina
- **Care Plan:** Client with stable angina, type 2 diabetes, erectile dysfunction, and treatment with nitroglycerine

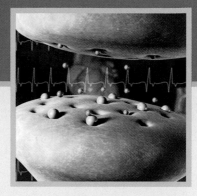

CHAPTER 26

Drugs for Dysrhythmias

DRUGS AT A GLANCE

SODIUM CHANNEL BLOCKERS
- 🔊 *procainamide (Procan, Procanbid, Pronestyl)*

BETA-ADRENERGIC BLOCKERS
- 🔊 *propranolol (Inderal)*

POTASSIUM CHANNEL BLOCKERS
- 🔊 *amiodarone (Cordarone)*

CALCIUM CHANNEL BLOCKERS
- 🔊 *verapamil (Calan)*

OBJECTIVES

After reading this chapter, the student should be able to:

1. Explain how rhythm abnormalities can affect cardiac function.
2. Illustrate the flow of electrical impulses through the normal heart.
3. Classify dysrhythmias based on their location and type of rhythm abnormality.
4. Explain how an action potential is controlled by the flow of sodium, potassium, and calcium ions across the myocardial membrane.
5. Identify the importance of nonpharmacological therapies in the treatment of dysrhythmias.
6. Identify the primary mechanisms of antidysrhythmic drugs.
7. Describe the nurse's role in the pharmacological management of clients with dysrhythmias.
8. Know representative drug examples for each of the drug classes listed in Drugs at a Glance, and explain their mechanisms of action, primary actions, and important adverse effects.
9. Categorize antidysrhythmic drugs based on their classification and mechanism of action.
10. Use the Nursing Process to care for clients receiving drug therapy for dysrhythmias.

MediaLink 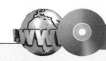 www.prenhall.com/adams

NCLEX-RN® review, case studies, and other interactive resources for this chapter can be found on the companion website at www.prenhall.com/adams. Click on "Chapter 26" to select the activities for this chapter. For animations, more NCLEX-RN® review questions, and an audio glossary, access the accompanying Prentice Hall Nursing MediaLink DVD-ROM in this textbook.

KEY TERMS

action potential *page 363*

atrioventricular bundle *page 364*

atrioventricular (AV) node *page 363*

automaticity *page 363*

bundle branches *page 364*

calcium ion channel *page 364*

cardioversion/defibrillation *page 364*

depolarization *page 364*

dysrhythmias *page 362*

ectopic foci/pacemakers *page 364*

electrocardiogram (ECG) *page 364*

fibrillation *page 362*

implantable cardioverter defibrillators (ICD)
  page 364

polarized *page 364*

potassium ion channel *page 364*

Purkinje fibers *page 364*

refractory period *page 365*

sinoatrial (SA) node *page 363*

sinus rhythm *page 363*

sodium ion channel *page 364*

Dysrhythmias are abnormalities of electrical conduction that may result in disturbances in heart rate or cardiac rhythm. Sometimes called *arrhythmias,* they encompass a number of different disorders that range from harmless to life threatening. Diagnosis is often difficult because clients often must be connected to an electrocardiograph (ECG) and be experiencing symptoms in order to determine the exact type of rhythm disorder. Proper diagnosis and optimum pharmacotherapy can significantly affect the frequency of dysrhythmias and their consequences.

26.1 Frequency of Dysrhythmias in the Population

Whereas some dysrhythmias produce no symptoms and have negligible effects on cardiac function, others are life threatening and require immediate treatment. Typical symptoms include dizziness, weakness, decreased exercise tolerance, shortness of breath, and fainting. Clients may report palpitations or a sensation that their heart has skipped a beat. Persistent dysrhythmias are associated with increased risk of stroke and heart failure. Severe dysrhythmias may result in sudden death. Because asymptomatic clients may not seek medical attention, it is difficult to estimate the frequency of the disease, although it is likely that dysrhythmias are quite common in the population.

26.2 Classification of Dysrhythmias

Dysrhythmias are classified by a number of different methods. The simplest method is to name dysrhythmias according to the *type* of rhythm abnormality produced and its *location*. Dysrhythmias that originate in the atria are sometimes referred to as *supraventricular*. Atrial **fibrillation,** a complete disorganization of rhythm, is the most common type of dysrhythmia. Those that originate in the ventricles are generally more serious, as they are more likely to interfere with the normal function of the heart. A summary of common dysrhythmias and a brief description of each abnormality are given in Table 26.1. Although a correct diagnosis of the type of dysrhythmia is sometimes difficult, it is essential for effective treatment.

Dysrhythmias can occur in both healthy and diseased hearts. Although the actual cause of most dysrhythmias is elusive, they are closely associated with certain conditions, primarily heart disease and myocardial infarction. The following are diseases and conditions associated with dysrhythmias.

- Hypertension
- Cardiac valve disease such as mitral stenosis

PHARMFACTS

Dysrhythmias

- Dysrhythmias are responsible for more than 44,000 deaths each year.
- Atrial dysrhythmias occur more commonly in men than in women.
- The incidence of atrial dysrhythmias increases with age. They affect:
  $<0.5\%$ of those aged 25 to 35
  1.5% of those up to age 60
  9% of those over age 75
- About 15% of strokes occur in clients with atrial dysrhythmias.
- A large majority of sudden cardiac deaths are thought to be caused by ventricular dysrhythmias.
- Atrial fibrillation affects 1.5 to 2.2 million people in the United States.

TABLE 26.1   Types of Dysrhythmias

Name of Dysrhythmia	Description
atrial or ventricular flutter and/or fibrillation	very rapid, uncoordinated beats; atrial may require treatment but is not usually fatal; ventricular flutter or fibrillation requires immediate treatment
atrial or ventricular tachycardia	rapid heart beat greater than 150 beats per minute; ventricular tachycardia is more serious than atrial tachycardia
heart block	area of nonconduction in the myocardium; may be partial or complete; classified as first, second, or third degree
premature atrial or premature ventricular contractions (PVCs)	an extra beat often originating from a source other than the SA node; not normally serious unless it occurs in high frequency
sinus bradycardia	slow heart beat, less than 50 beats per minute; may require a pacemaker

- Coronary artery disease
- Medications such as digoxin
- Low potassium levels in the blood
- Myocardial infarction
- Stroke
- Diabetes mellitus
- Congestive heart failure

26.3 Conduction Pathways in the Myocardium

Although there are many types of dysrhythmias, all have in common a defect in the *generation* or *conduction* of electrical impulses across the myocardium. These electrical impulses, or **action potentials,** carry the signal for the cardiac muscle cells to contract and are precisely coordinated for the chambers to beat in a synchronized manner. For the heart to function properly, the atria must contract simultaneously, sending their blood into the ventricles. Following atrial contraction, the right and left ventricles then must contract simultaneously.

Lack of synchronization of the atria and ventricles or of the right and left sides of the heart may have profound consequences. The total time for the electrical impulse to travel across the heart is about 0.22 second. The normal conduction pathway in the heart is illustrated in ● Figure 26.1.

Normal control of synchronization begins in a small area of tissue in the wall of the right atrium known as the **sinoatrial (SA) node.** The SA node or *pacemaker* of the heart has a property called **automaticity,** the ability of certain cells to spontaneously generate an action potential. The SA node generates a new action potential approximately 75 times per minute under resting conditions. This is referred to as the normal **sinus rhythm.** The SA node is greatly influenced by the activity of the sympathetic and parasympathetic divisions of the autonomic nervous system.

On leaving the SA node, the action potential travels quickly across both atria to the **atrioventricular (AV) node.** The AV node also has the property of automaticity, although less so than the SA node. Should the SA node malfunction, the AV node has the ability to spontaneously generate action potentials and continue the heart's contraction at a rate of 40 to 60 beats per minute. Impulse conduction

MediaLink

Childhood Dysrhythmias

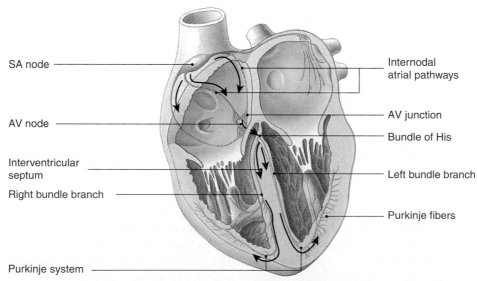

SA node

Internodal atrial pathways

AV junction

AV node

Bundle of His

Interventricular septum

Left bundle branch

Right bundle branch

Purkinje fibers

Purkinje system

● **Figure 26.1** Normal conduction pathway in the heart   *Source: Pearson Education/PH College.*

through the AV node, compared with other areas in the heart, is slow. This allows the atrial contraction enough time to completely empty blood into the ventricles, thereby optimizing cardiac output.

As the action potential leaves the AV node it travels rapidly to the **atrioventricular bundle,** or *bundle of His.* The impulse is then conducted down the right and left **bundle branches** to the **Purkinje fibers,** which carry the action potential to all regions of the ventricles almost simultaneously. Should the SA and AV nodes become nonfunctional, cells in the AV bundle and Purkinje fibers can continue to generate myocardial contractions at a rate of about 30 beats per minute.

Although action potentials normally begin at the SA node and spread across the myocardium in a coordinated manner, other regions of the heart may begin to initiate beats. These areas, known as **ectopic foci** or **ectopic pacemakers,** may send impulses across the myocardium that compete with those from the normal conduction pathway. Although healthy hearts often experience an extra beat without incident, ectopic foci in diseased hearts have the potential to cause the types of dysrhythmias noted in Table 26.1.

It is important to understand that the underlying purpose of this conduction system is to keep the heart beating in a regular, synchronized manner so that cardiac output can be maintained. Some dysrhythmias occur sporadically, elicit no symptoms, and do not affect cardiac output. These types of abnormalities may go unnoticed by the client, and rarely require treatment. Others, however, profoundly affect cardiac output, result in client symptoms, and have the potential to produce serious if not mortal consequences. It is these types of dysrhythmias that require pharmacotherapy.

26.4 The Electrocardiograph

The wave of electrical activity across the myocardium can be measured using the electrocardiograph. The graphic recording from this device, or **electrocardiogram (ECG),** is useful in diagnosing many types of heart conditions, including dysrhythmias.

Three distinct waves are produced by a normal ECG: the P wave, the QRS complex, and the T wave. Changes to the wave patterns or in their timing can reveal certain pathologies. For example, an exaggerated R wave suggests enlargement of the ventricles, and a flat T wave indicates ischemia to the myocardium. Elevated S–T segments are used to guide the pharmacotherapy of MI. A normal ECG and its relationship to impulse conduction in the heart is shown in ● Figure 26.2.

26.5 Nonpharmacological Therapy of Dysrhythmias

The therapeutic goals of antidysrhythmic pharmacotherapy are to *terminate* existing dysrhythmias or to *prevent* abnormal rhythms to reduce the risks of sudden death, stroke, or other complications resulting from the disease. Because they can cause serious side effects, antidysrhythmic drugs are normally reserved for clients experiencing overt symptoms or for those whose condition cannot be controlled by other means. Treating asymptomatic dysrhythmias with medications provides little or no benefit to the client. Healthcare providers use several nonpharmacological strategies to eliminate dysrhythmias.

The more serious types of dysrhythmias are corrected through electrical shock of the heart, a treatment called elective **cardioversion,** or **defibrillation.** The electrical shock momentarily stops all electrical impulses in the heart, both normal and abnormal. The temporary cessation of electrical activity often allows the SA node to automatically return conduction to a normal sinus rhythm.

Other types of nonpharmacological treatment include identification and destruction of the myocardial cells responsible for the abnormal conduction through a surgical procedure called *catheter ablation.* Cardiac pacemakers are sometimes implanted to correct the types of dysrhythmias that cause the heart to beat too slowly. **Implantable cardioverter defibrillators (ICD)** are placed in clients to restore normal rhythm by either pacing the heart or giving it an electric shock when dysrhythmias occur. In addition, the ICD is capable of storing information regarding the heart rhythm for the healthcare provider to evaluate.

26.6 Sodium, Potassium, and the Myocardial Action Potential

Because most antidysrhythmic drugs act by interfering with myocardial action potentials, a firm grasp of this phenomenon is necessary for understanding drug mechanisms. Action potentials occur in both nervous and cardiac muscle cells owing to differences in the concentration of certain ions found inside and outside the cell. Under resting conditions, Na^+ and Ca^{++} are found in higher concentrations *outside* myocardial cells, and K^+ is found in higher concentration *inside* these cells. These imbalances are, in part, responsible for the slight negative charge (80 to 90 mV) inside a myocardial cell membrane relative to the outside of the membrane. A cell having this negative membrane potential is called **polarized.**

An action potential begins when **sodium ion channels** located in the plasma membrane open and Na^+ rushes *into* the cell producing a rapid **depolarization,** or loss of membrane potential. During this period, Ca^{++} also enters the cell through **calcium ion channels,** although the influx is slower than that of sodium. The entry of Ca^{++} into the cells is a signal for the release of additional intracellular calcium that is held in storage inside the sarcoplasmic reticulum. It is this large increase in intracellular Ca^{++} that is responsible for the contraction of cardiac muscle.

During depolarization, the inside of the plasma membrane temporarily reverses its charge, becoming positive. The cell returns to its polarized state by the removal of Na^+ from the cell via the sodium pump and movement of K^+ back into the cell through **potassium ion channels.** In cells located in the SA and AV nodes, it is the influx of Ca^{++}, rather than Na^+, that generates the rapid depolarization of the membrane.

Although it may seem complicated to learn the different ions involved in an action potential, understanding the process is

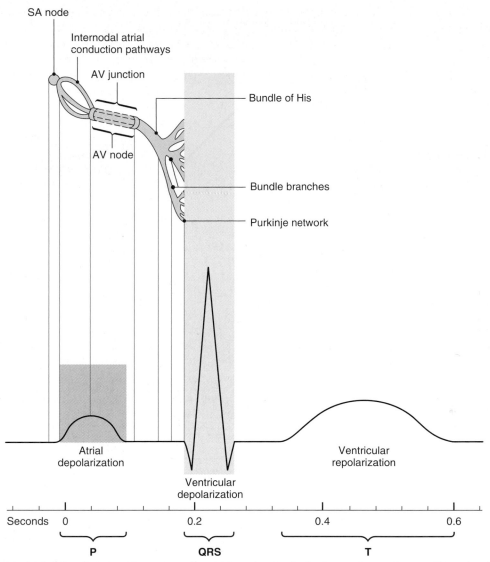

SA node

Internodal atrial
conduction pathways

AV junction

Bundle of His

AV node

Bundle branches

Purkinje network

Atrial
depolarization

Ventricular
depolarization

Ventricular
repolarization

Seconds   0   0.2   0.4   0.6

P   QRS   T

● **Figure 26.2** Relationship of the electrocardiogram to electrical conduction in the heart   *Source: Pearson Education/PH College.*

very important to cardiac pharmacology. Blocking potassium, sodium, or calcium ion channels is a pharmacological strategy used to terminate or prevent dysrhythmias. ● Figure 26.3 illustrates the flow of ions during the action potential.

The pumping action of the heart requires alternating periods of contraction and relaxation of cardiac muscle. There is a brief period of time following depolarization, and most of repolarization, during which the cell cannot initiate another action potential. This time, known as the **refractory period,** ensures that the myocardial cell finishes contracting before a second action potential begins. Some antidysrhythmic agents produce their effects by prolonging the refractory period.

26.7 Mechanisms and Classification of Antidysrhythmic Drugs

Antidysrhythmic drugs act by altering specific electrophysiologic properties of the heart. They do this through two basic mechanisms: blocking flow through ion channels (conduction) or altering autonomic activity (automaticity).

Antidysrhythmic drugs are grouped according to the stage in which they affect the action potential. These drugs fall into four primary classes, referred to as classes I, II, III, and IV, and a fifth group that includes miscellaneous drugs not acting by one of the first four mechanisms. The five categories of antidysrhythmics and their mechanisms are listed in Table 26.2.

The use of antidysrhythmic drugs has significantly declined in recent years. Research studies have found that the use of antidysrhythmic medications for prophylaxis can actually *increase* client mortality. This is because there is a narrow margin between a therapeutic effect and a toxic effect with drugs that affect cardiac rhythm. They have the ability not only to *correct* dysrhythmias but also to worsen or even *create* new dysrhythmias. These prodysrhythmic effects have resulted in less use of drugs in class I and increased use of drugs in class II and class III (specifically, amiodarone).

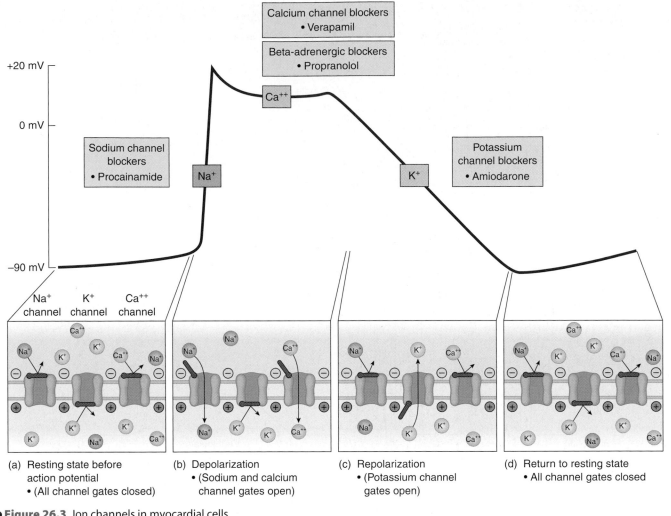

● **Figure 26.3** Ion channels in myocardial cells

Another reason for the decline in antidysrhythmic drug use is the success of nonpharmacological techniques. Research has demonstrated that catheter ablation and implantable defibrillators are more successful in managing certain types of dysrhythmias than is the prophylactic use of medications.

SODIUM CHANNEL BLOCKERS (CLASS I)

The first medical use of quinidine, a sodium channel blocker, was recorded in the 18th century. This is the largest class of antidysrhythmics. The sodium channel blockers are listed in Table 26.3.

Class	Actions	Indications
TABLE 26.2 **Classification of Antidysrhythmics**		
I: Sodium channel blockers		
IA example: procainamide	delays repolarization; slows conduction velocity; increases duration of the action potential	atrial fibrillation, premature atrial contractions, PVCs, ventricular tachycardia
IB example: lidocaine	accelerates repolarization; slows conduction velocity; decreases duration of action potential	severe ventricular dysrhythmias
IC example: flecainide	no significant effect on repolarization; slows conduction velocity	severe ventricular dysrhythmias
II: Beta-adrenergic antagonists example: propranolol	slows conduction velocity; decreases automaticity; prolongs refractory period	atrial flutter and fibrillation, tachydysrhythmia, ventricular dysrhythmias
III: Potassium channel blockers example: amiodarone	slows repolarization; increases duration of action potential; prolongs refractory period	severe atrial and ventricular dysrhythmias
IV: Calcium channel blockers example: verapamil	slows conduction velocity; decreases contractility; prolongs refractory period	paroxysmal supraventricular tachycardia, supraventricular tachydysrhythmia

TABLE 26.3 Antidysrhythmic Drugs

Drug	Route and Adult Dose (max dose where indicated)	Adverse Effects
CLASS IA: SODIUM CHANNEL BLOCKERS		
disopyramide phosphate (Norpace, NAPAmide)	PO; 100–200 mg qid (max: 800 mg/day); therapeutic serum drug level is 2–5 mcg/ml	*Nausea, vomiting, diarrhea, dry mouth, urinary retention*
ⓟ procainamide HCl (Pronestyl, Procan, others)	PO; 1 g loading dose followed by 250–500 mg q3h	
quinidine gluconate (Duraquin, Quinaglute)	PO; 200–600 mg tid–qid (max: 3–4 g/day)	May produce new dysrhythmias or worsen existing ones; hypotension, blood dyscrasias (quinidine) and lupus (procainamide)
quinidine polygalacturonate (Cardioquin)	PO; 275–825 mg q3–4h for 4 or more doses until dysrhythmia terminates; then 137.5–275 mg bid–tid	
quinidine sulfate (Quinidex, others)	PO; 200–600 mg tid–qid (max: 3–4 g/day); therapeutic serum drug level is 2–5 mcg/ml	
CLASS IB: SODIUM CHANNEL BLOCKERS		
lidocaine (Xylocaine) (see page 249 for the Prototype Drug box ∞)	IV; 1–4 mg/min infusion; no more than 200–300 mg should be infused in a 1–h period	*Nausea, vomiting, drowsiness, dizziness, lethargy*
mexiletine (Mexitil)	PO; 200–300 mg tid (max: 1,200 mg/day)	May produce new dysrhythmias or worsen existing ones; hypotension, bradycardia, CNS toxicity (lidocaine), malignant hyperthermia (lidocaine), status epilepticus if abruptly withdrawn (phenytoin)
phenytoin (Dilantin) (see page 179 for the Prototype Drug box ∞)	IV; 50–100 mg every 10–15 min until dysrhythmia is terminated (max: 1 g/day)	
tocainide (Tonocard)	PO; 400–600 mg tid (max 2.4 g/day)	
CLASS IC: SODIUM CHANNEL BLOCKERS		
flecainide (Tambocor)	PO; 100 mg bid; increase by 500 mg bid every 4 days (max: 400 mg/day)	*Nausea, vomiting, dizziness, headache*
propafenone (Rythmol)	PO; 150–300 mg tid (max: 900 mg/day)	May produce new dysrhythmias or worsen existing ones; hypotension, bradycardia
CLASS II: BETA-ADRENERGIC BLOCKERS		
acebutolol (Sectral)	PO; 200–600 mg bid (max: 1,200 mg/day)	*Fatigue, insomnia, drowsiness, impotence or decreased libido, bradycardia, and confusion*
esmolol (Brevibloc)	IV; 50 mcg /kg/min maintenance dose (max: 200 mcg /kg/min)	
ⓟ propranolol (Inderal)	PO; 10–30 mg tid–qid (max: 320 mg/day); 0.5–3.1 mg IV q4h or PRN	Agranulocytosis, laryngospasm, Stevens–Johnson syndrome, anaphylaxis; if the drug is abruptly withdrawn, palpitations, rebound hypertension, life-threatening dysrhythmias, or myocardial ischemia may occur
CLASS III: POTASSIUM CHANNEL BLOCKERS		
ⓟ amiodarone (Cordarone, Pacerone)	PO; 400–600 mg/day in 1–2 divided doses (max: 1,600 mg/day as loading dose)	*Blurred vision (amiodarone), photosensitivity, nausea, vomiting, anorexia*
bretylium (Bertylol)	IV; rapid injection or 1–2 mg /min as continuous infusion	May produce new dysrhythmias or worsen existing ones; hypotension, bradycardia, pneumonia-like syndrome (amiodarone), angioedema (dofetilide), CNS toxicity (ibutilide)
dofetilide (Tikosyn)	PO; 125–500 mcg bid based on creatinine clearance	
ibutilide (Corvert)	IV; 1 mg infused over 10 min	
sotalol (Betapace)*	PO; 80 mg bid (max: 320 mg/day)	
CLASS IV: CALCIUM CHANNEL BLOCKERS		
diltiazem (Cardizem, others) (see page 354 for the Prototype Drug box ∞)	IV; 5–10 mg/h continuous infusion (max: 15 mg/h) for a maximum of 24 h	*Flushed skin, headache, dizziness, peripheral edema, light-headedness, nausea, diarrhea*
ⓟ verapamil (Calan, others) (see page 373 for the Prototype Drug box ∞)	PO; 240–480 mg/day in divided doses; 5–10 mg IV direct: may repeat in 15–30 min if needed	Hepatotoxicity, MI, CHF, confusion, mood changes
adenosine (Adenocard, Adenoscan)	IV; 6–12 mg given as a bolus injection	*Facial flushing, dyspnea* May produce new dysrhythmias or worsen existing ones

(Continued)

TABLE 26.3 **Antidysrhythmic Drugs** *(Continued)*		
Drug	**Route and Adult Dose (max dose where indicated)**	**Adverse Effects**
MISCELLANEOUS ANTIDYSRHYTHMICS		
digoxin (Lanoxin) (see page 339 for the Prototype Drug box ∞)	PO; 0.125–0.5 mg qid; therapeutic serum drug level is 0.8–2 ng/ml	*Nausea, vomiting, headache, and visual disturbances* <u>May produce new dysrhythmias or worsen existing ones</u>

Italics indicate common adverse effects; <u>underlining</u> indicates serious adverse effects.
*Sotalol is a beta-blocker, but because its cardiac effects are similar to those of amiodarone, it is considered in class III.

26.8 Treating Dysrhythmias With Sodium Channel Blockers

Sodium channel blockers, the class I drugs, are divided into three subgroups, IA, IB, and IC, based on subtle differences in their mechanism of action. Because the action potential is dependent on the opening of sodium ion channels, a blockade of these channels will prevent depolarization. The spread of the action potential across the myocardium will slow, and areas of ectopic pacemaker activity will be suppressed.

The sodium channel blockers are similar in structure and action to local anesthetics. In fact, lidocaine is a class I antidysrhythmic that is a prototype local anesthetic in Chapter 19 ∞. This anesthetic-like action slows impulse conduction across the heart. Some, such as quinidine and procainamide, are effective against many types of dys-

rhythmias. The remaining class I drugs are more specific, and indicated only for life-threatening ventricular dysrhythmias. Although a prototype for many decades, quinidine (Quinidex, others) is rarely used today owing to the availability of safer antidysrhythmics.

The side effects of the sodium blockers vary with each individual drug. All these agents can cause new dysrhythmias or worsen existing ones. The reduced heart rate caused by the drug can result in hypotension, dizziness, and syncope. Some class I drugs have significant anticholinergic side effects such as dry mouth, constipation, and urinary retention. Lidocaine can cause CNS toxicity such as drowsiness, confusion, and convulsions. Special precautions should be taken with older adults, as anticholinergic side effects may worsen urinary hesitancy in clients with prostate enlargement.

Pr PROTOTYPE DRUG | Procainamide *(Procan, Procanbid, Pronestyl)* | Sodium Channel Blocker/ Class IA Antidysrhythmic

ACTIONS AND USES

Procainamide is chemically related to the local anesthetic procaine. Like other drugs in this class, procainamide blocks sodium ion channels in myocardial cells, thus reducing automaticity and slowing conduction of the action potential across the myocardium. This slight delay in conduction velocity prolongs the refractory period and can suppress dysrhythmias. Procainamide is referred to as a broad-spectrum drug because it has the ability to correct many different types of atrial and ventricular dysrhythmias. Procainamide is available in capsule, extended-release tablet, IV, and IM formulations. The therapeutic serum drug level is 4–8 mcg/ml.

ADMINISTRATION ALERTS

- Use the supine position during IV administration because severe hypotension may occur.
- Do not break or crush extended-release tablets
- Pregnancy category C.

PHARMACOKINETICS (PO)

Onset: 30 min

Peak: 1–1.5 h

Half-life: 3 h

Duration: 3 h (8 h sustained release)

ADVERSE EFFECTS

Nausea, vomiting, abdominal pain, and headache are common during procainamide therapy. High doses may produce CNS effects such as confusion or psychosis. Like all antidysrhythmic drugs, procainamide has the ability to produce new dysrhythmias or worsen existing ones. A lupus-like syndrome may occur in 30% to 50% of clients taking the drug over a year.

Contraindications: Procainamide is contraindicated in clients with complete AV block, severe CHF, blood dyscrasias, and myasthenia gravis.

INTERACTIONS

Drug–Drug: Additive cardiac depressant effects may occur if procainamide is administered with other antidysrhythmics. Additive anticholinergic side effects will occur if procainamide is used concurrently with anticholinergic agents.

Lab Tests: May increase values for the following: AST, ALT, serum alkaline phosphatase, LDH, and serum bilirubin. False-positive Coombs and ANA titers may occur.

Herbal/Food: Unknown.

Treatment of Overdose: Treatment is targeted to reversing hypotension with vasopressors, and preventing dysrhythmias.

 See the *Companion Website for a Nursing Process Focus* specific to this drug.

Pr PROTOTYPE DRUG | Propranolol (Inderal) | Beta-adrenergic Antagonist/Class II Antidysrhythmic

ACTIONS AND USES

Until 1978, propranolol was the only beta-blocker approved to treat dysrhythmias. Propranolol is a nonselective beta-adrenergic blocker, affecting beta$_1$-receptors in the heart, and beta$_2$-receptors in pulmonary and vascular smooth muscle. Propranolol reduces heart rate, slows myocardial conduction velocity, and lowers blood pressure. Propranolol is most effective against tachycardia caused by excessive sympathetic stimulation. It is approved to treat a wide variety of diseases, including hypertension, angina, and migraine headaches, and for prevention of myocardial infarction. The drug is available in tablet, extended-release capsules, and IV formulations. The therapeutic serum drug level is 50–100 ng/ml.

ADMINISTRATION ALERTS

- Abrupt discontinuation may cause MI, severe hypertension, and ventricular dysrhythmias because of a potential rebound effect.
- If pulse is less than 60 beats per minute, notify the physician.
- Pregnancy category C.

PHARMACOKINETICS (PO)

Onset: 0.5–1 h

Peak: 1–2 h (6 h extended release)

Half-life: 3–5 h

Duration: 6–12 h (24 h extended release)

ADVERSE EFFECTS

Common side effects of propranolol include fatigue, hypotension, and bradycardia. Because of the ability of propranolol to slow the heart rate, clients with other cardiac disorders such as heart failure must be carefully monitored. Side effects such as diminished libido and impotence may result in noncompliance in male clients. Propranolol should be used cautiously in diabetics owing to its hypoglycemic effects. This drug should be used with caution in clients with reduced renal output, because the drug may accumulate to toxic levels in the blood and cause dysrhythmias.

Contraindications: Because of its depressive effects on the heart, propranolol is contraindicated in cardiogenic shock, sinus bradycardia, greater than first-degree heart block, and heart failure. Owing to its constriction of smooth muscle in the airways, the drug is contraindicated in clients with COPD or asthma.

INTERACTIONS

Drug–Drug: Concurrent administration with other beta-blockers may produce additive effects on the heart, and bradycardia or hypotension may result. Because both propranolol and calcium channel blockers suppress myocardial contractility, concurrent use may lead to additive bradycardia. Phenothiazines can add to the hypotensive effects of propranolol. Propranolol should not be given within 2 weeks of an MAO inhibitor, as severe bradycardia and hypotension could result. Use of ethanol or antacids containing aluminum hydroxide gel will slow the absorption of propranolol and reduce its therapeutic effects. Administration of beta-adrenergic agonists such as albuterol (Proventil) will antagonize the actions of propranolol.

Lab Tests: May give a false increase for urinary catecholamines.

Herbal/Food: Unknown.

Treatment of Overdose: Treatment is targeted to reversing hypotension with vasopressors, and bradycardia with atropine or isoproterenol.

 See the Companion Website for a Nursing Process Focus specific to this drug.

MediaLink   Mechanism in Action: Propranolol

NURSING CONSIDERATIONS

The role of the nurse in sodium blocker therapy for dysrhythmias involves careful monitoring of a client's condition and providing education as it relates to the prescribed drug treatment. Obtain a complete health history and physical examination, including baseline ECG, vital signs, hepatic and renal function tests, and electrolyte values, before initiating therapy because class I antidysrhythmics have profound effects on the heart. Assess for heart failure, hypotension, myasthenia gravis, and renal or hepatic impairment, because these are contraindications for class I antidysrhythmic therapy. Obtain a thorough drug history, because these agents interact with a large number of other drugs, including digoxin (Lanoxin), cimetidine, anticonvulsants, nifedipine, and warfarin.

During pharmacotherapy, monitor the client for changes in the ECG such as an increase in P–R and Q–T intervals and widening of the QRS complex. Monitor blood pressure frequently, because some agents can cause hypotension. Other drugs in this class can cause arterial embolism. This adverse effect is related to the formation of small blood clots in the atrium while the client is being treated for atrial fibrillation. Monitor the client for changes in level of consciousness and respiratory status, and immediately report abnormal findings to the physician.

Monitor drug plasma levels during therapy, and check the client for diarrhea, which occurs in approximately one third of clients on quinidine. This adverse effect is due to quinidine's chemical relation to quinine in structure and action. Diarrhea may be intense, so implement appropriate interventions related to the diarrhea to maintain fluid and electrolyte balance.

Client Teaching.   Client education as it relates to sodium channel blockers should include the goals of therapy, the reasons for obtaining baseline data such as vital signs and underlying cardiac and renal disorders, and possible drug side effects. Include the following points when teaching clients about calcium channel blockers:

- Do not skip doses of the medications, even if feeling well. Do not take two doses at a time if the first dose is missed.
- Avoid the use of alcohol, caffeine, and tobacco.
- Keep all scheduled visits for laboratory tests.
- Immediately report the following symptoms: shortness of breath, signs of bleeding, excessive bruising, fever, nausea, persistent headache, changes to vision or hearing, diarrhea, or dizziness.

NURSING PROCESS FOCUS Clients Receiving Antidysrhythmic Therapies

Assessment	Potential Nursing Diagnoses
Prior to administration: ▪ Obtain a complete health history including allergies, drug history, and possible drug interactions. ▪ Assess to determine if cardiac alteration is producing a symptomatic effect on cardiac output. Assessment should include vital signs, level of consciousness, urinary output, skin temperature, and peripheral pulses. ▪ Obtain baseline ECG to compare throughout therapy.	▪ Ineffective Tissue Perfusion, related to cardiac conduction abnormality ▪ Knowledge Deficit, related to drug therapy ▪ Risk for Injury, related to adverse effects of drug ▪ Decreased Cardiac Output, R/T cardiac conduction abnormality

Planning: Client Goals and Expected Outcomes

The client will:
▪ Exhibit improved cardiac output as evidenced by stabilization of heart rate, heart rhythm, sensorium, urine output, and vital signs.
▪ Demonstrate an understanding of the drug's action by accurately describing drug side effects and precautions.
▪ Be free of preventable adverse effects.

Implementation

Interventions and (Rationales)	Client Education/Discharge Planning
▪ Monitor cardiac rate and rhythm continuously if administering drug IV. (IV route is used when rapid therapeutic effects are needed. Constant monitoring is needed to detect serious dysrhythmias.)	▪ Instruct client about need for continuous ECG monitoring when administering the medication intravenously.
▪ Monitor IV site. (Administer all parenteral medication via infusion pump.)	▪ Instruct client to report any burning or stinging pain, swelling, warmth, redness, or tenderness at the IV insertion site.
▪ Investigate possible causes of the dysrhythmia such as electrolyte imbalances, hypoxia, pain, anxiety, caffeine ingestion, and tobacco use.	Instruct client to: ▪ Maintain a diet low in sodium and fat with sufficient potassium. ▪ Report illness such as flu, vomiting, diarrhea, and dehydration to healthcare provider to avoid adverse effects. ▪ Restrict use of caffeine and tobacco products.
▪ Observe for side effects specific to the antidysrhythmic used. (Side effects may indicate overdosage.)	Instruct client to: ▪ Report adverse effects specific to prescribed antidysrhythmic. ▪ Report palpitations, chest pain, dyspnea, unusual fatigue, weakness, and visual disturbances.
▪ Monitor for proper use of medication. (Improper use may result in dysrhythmias, hypotension, or bradycardia.)	Instruct client to: ▪ Never discontinue the drug abruptly. ▪ Take the drug exactly as prescribed, even if feeling well. ▪ Take pulse prior to taking the drug. (Instruct client regarding the normal range and rhythm of pulse; instruct to consult the healthcare provider regarding "reportable" pulse.)

Evaluation of Outcome Criteria

Evaluate the effectiveness of drug therapy by confirming that client goals and expected outcomes have been met (see "Planning").
▪ The client's heart rate, heart rhythm, sensorium, urine output, and vital signs are stable, evidencing improved cardiac output.
▪ The client demonstrates an understanding of the drug's action by accurately describing drug side effects and precautions.
▪ The client is free of preventable adverse effects.

∞ *See Table 26.3 for a list of drugs (classes I–IV) to which these nursing actions apply.*

BETA-ADRENERGIC ANTAGONISTS/BLOCKERS (CLASS II)

Beta-adrenergic antagonists are widely used for cardiovascular disorders. Their ability to slow the heart rate and conduction velocity can suppress several types of dysrhythmias. The beta-blockers are listed in Table 26.3.

26.9 Treating Dysrhythmias With Beta-adrenergic Antagonists

Beta-adrenergic blockers are used to treat a large number of cardiovascular diseases, including hypertension, MI, heart failure, and dysrhythmias. As expected from their effects on the autonomic nervous system, beta-blockers slow the heart rate and decrease conduction velocity through the AV node. Myocardial automaticity is reduced, and many types of dysrhythmias are stabilized. The main value of beta-blockers as antidysrhythmic agents is to treat atrial dysrhythmias associated with heart failure. In post-MI clients, beta-blockers decrease the likelihood of sudden death owing to their antidysrhythmic effects. The basic pharmacology of beta-adrenergic antagonists is explained in Chapter 13 ∞.

Only a few beta-blockers are approved for dysrhythmias, because of potential side effects. Blockade of beta-receptors in the heart may result in bradycardia. Hypotension may cause dizziness and possible syncope. Those beta-blockers that affect $beta_2$-adrenergic receptors will also affect the lung, possibly causing bronchospasm. This is of particular concern in clients with asthma, or in elderly clients with chronic obstructive pulmonary disease (COPD). Abrupt discontinuation of beta-blockers can lead to dysrhythmias and hypertension.

NURSING CONSIDERATIONS

The role of the nurse in beta-blocker therapy for dysrhythmias involves careful monitoring of a client's condition and providing education as it relates to the prescribed drug treatment. All drugs in this class are contraindicated in clients with heart block, severe bradycardia, AV block, and asthma. Because beta-blockers decrease contractions of the myocardium and lessen the speed of conduction through the AV node, they predispose clients with preexisting heart conditions to a significant decrease in heart rate that may not be well tolerated. Assess vital signs, because the most common adverse reaction to these drugs is hypotension. Monitor for hypoglycemia. There is an increased incidence of hypoglycemia in clients with type 1 diabetes mellitus, because beta-blockers may inhibit glycogenolysis.

Lifespan Considerations. Monitor elderly clients for cognitive dysfunction and depression, as well as hallucinations and psychosis, which are more likely with higher doses. These reactions appear to be related to the lipid solubility of this medication and its ability to cross the blood–brain barrier.

Client Teaching. Client education as it relates to beta-blockers should include the goals of therapy, the reasons for obtaining baseline data such as vital signs and the existence of underlying cardiac and renal disorders, and possible drug

side effects. Include the following points when teaching clients about beta-blockers:

- Take pulse rate prior to taking the drug and report a pulse rate less than 60 beats per minute to the healthcare provider.
- Rise slowly from a sitting or lying position to prevent dizziness.
- Immediately report the following symptoms: shortness of breath, feeling of skipping a heartbeat, painful or difficult urination, frequent night-time urination, weight gain of 2 lf or more, dizziness, insomnia, drowsiness, or confusion.

POTASSIUM CHANNEL BLOCKERS (CLASS III)

Although a small class of drugs, the potassium channel blockers have important applications in the treatment of dysrhythmias. These drugs prolong the duration of the action potential and reduce automaticity. The potassium channel blockers are listed in Table 26.2.

26.10 Treating Dysrhythmias With Potassium Channel Blockers

The drugs in class III exert their actions by blocking potassium ion channels in myocardial cells. After the action potential has passed and the myocardial cell is in a depolarized state, repolarization depends on replacement of potassium inside the cell. By blocking potassium channels, the class III medications delay repolarization of the myocardial cells and lengthen the refractory period, which tends to stabilize dysrhythmias. Most drugs in this class have multiple actions and also affect adrenergic receptors or sodium channels. For example, in addition to blocking potassium channels, sotalol (Betapace) is considered a beta-adrenergic blocker.

The potassium channel blockers are reserved for serious dysrhythmias. Amiodarone (Cordarone, Pacerone) is one of the more frequently used drugs in this class, and is featured as a class III antidysrhythmic prototype in this chapter. It has been used to treat many different types of atrial and ventricular dysrhythmias. Dofetilide (Tikosyn) and ibutilide (Corvert) are given to terminate atrial flutter or fibrillation. Sotalol (Betapace) is approved for specific types of atrial and ventricular dysrhythmias, when safer drugs have failed to terminate the dysrhythmia. Bretylium is rarely used, but has an important indication in treating severe ventricular dysrhythmias when other therapies have failed.

Drugs in this class have limited uses because of potentially serious side effects. Like other antidysrhythmics, potassium channel blockers slow the heart rate, resulting in serious bradycardia and possible hypotension. These side effects occur in a significant number of clients. These agents can worsen dysrhythmias, especially following the first few doses. Older adults with preexisting heart failure must be carefully monitored because they are particularly at risk for adverse cardiac side effects of potassium channel blockers.

Amiodarone can produce pulmonary toxicity in a significant number of clients. Sotalol and ibutilide can produce torsades de pointes, a type of ventricular tachycardia that can become rapidly fatal if not recognized and treated. Treatment of torsades de pointes includes IV magnesium sulfate or potassium chloride.

NURSING CONSIDERATIONS

The role of the nurse in potassium channel blocker therapy for dysrhythmias involves careful monitoring of a client's condition and providing education as it relates to the prescribed drug treatment. All drugs in this class should be used cautiously in clients with heart block. Obtain the client's baseline ECG and vital signs. For amiodarone, obtain baseline chest x-ray and pulmonary function tests, as this drug has pulmonary toxicity.

During therapy, assess the client's vital signs and ECG continuously during IV therapy. Withhold the medication if pulse rate is 60 beats per minute or lower, or if systolic blood pressure falls below 90 mm Hg. Assess for signs of pulmonary toxicity with amiodarone, including cough and dyspnea. Assess the client for weight gain, decreased urine output, dyspnea and lung crackles, as these may indicate worsening congestive heart failure. Monitor serum drug levels, as appropriate. Additional information can be found in "Nursing Process Focus: Clients Receiving Antidysrhythmic Therapies," on page 370.

Lifespan Considerations. These drugs are not recommended for use during pregnancy (category C or D) or lactation.

Client Teaching. Client education as it relates to potassium channel blockers should include the goals of therapy, the reasons for obtaining baseline data such as vital signs and the existence of underlying cardiac and renal disorders, and possible drug side effects. Include the following points when teaching clients about potasssium channel blockers:

- Have regular eye exams because of the risk for possible vision changes.
- Avoid prolonged sun exposure and use sunscreen.
- Take medication with food or a small snack.
- Immediately report shortness of breath, feeling that the heart has skipped a beat, cough, vision changes, yellow eyes and skin color (jaundice), right upper abdominal pain, and dizziness.

Pr **PROTOTYPE DRUG** | Amiodarone *(Cordarone)* | Potassium Channel Blocker/ Class III Antidysrhythmic

ACTIONS AND USES

Amiodarone is structurally similar to thyroid hormone. It is approved for the treatment of resistant ventricular tachycardia that may prove life threatening, and it has become a drug of choice for the treatment of atrial dysrhythmias in clients with heart failure. In addition to blocking potassium ion channels, some of this drug's actions on the heart relate to its blockade of sodium ion channels. Its onset of action may take several weeks when given orally. Its effects, however, can last 4 to 8 weeks after the drug is discontinued, since it has an extended half-life that may exceed 100 days. It is available as tablets or as an IV infusion. The therapeutic serum level of amiodarone is 0.5–2.5 mcg/ml.

ADMINISTRATION ALERTS

- Hypokalemia and hypomagnesemia should be corrected prior to initiating therapy.
- Pregnancy category D.

PHARMACOKINETICS (PO)

Onset: 2–3 d to 1–3 wk

Peak: 3–7 h

Half-life: 15–100 d

Duration: 10–150 d

ADVERSE EFFECTS

The most serious adverse effect from amiodarone occurs in the lung, with the drug causing a pneumonia-like syndrome. Amiodarone may also cause blurred vision, rashes, photosensitivity, nausea, vomiting, anorexia, fatigue, dizziness, and hypotension. This medication is concentrated by certain tissues; thus, adverse effects may be slow to resolve.

Contraindications: Amiodarone is contraindicated in clients with severe bradycardia, cardiogenic shock, sick sinus syndrome, severe sinus node dysfunction, or third-degree AV block.

INTERACTIONS

Drug–Drug: Amiodarone can increase serum digoxin levels by as much as 70%. Amiodarone greatly enhances the actions of anticoagulants:, thus, the dose of warfarin must be cut by as much as half. Use with beta-adrenergic blockers or calcium channel blockers may potentiate sinus bradycardia, sinus arrest, or AV block. Amiodarone may increase phenytoin levels two- to threefold.

Lab Tests: May increase values for the following tests: nuclear antibody, ALT, AST and serum alkaline phosphatase, T_4.

Herbal/Food: Use with echinacea may cause an increased risk of hepatotoxicity. Aloe may cause an increased effect of amiodarone.

Treatment of Overdose: Treatment is targeted to reversing hypotension with vasopressors, and bradycardia with atropine or isoproterenol.

 See the Companion Website for a Nursing Process Focus specific to this drug.

CALCIUM CHANNEL BLOCKERS (CLASS IV)

Like beta-blockers, the calcium channel blockers are widely prescribed for various cardiovascular disorders. By slowing conduction velocity, they are able to stabilize certain dysrhythmias. The antidysrhythmic calcium channel blockers are listed in Table 26.3.

26.11 Treating Dysrhythmias With Calcium Channel Blockers

Although about 10 calcium channel blockers (CCBs) are available to treat cardiovascular diseases, only a limited number have been approved for dysrhythmias. A few CCBs such as diltiazem (Cardizem) and verapamil (Calan) block calcium ion channels in both the heart and arterioles; the remainder are specific to calcium channels in vascular smooth muscle. Diltiazem is a prototype drug for the treatment of angina, as discussed in Chapter 25 ∞. The basic pharmacology of this drug class is presented in Chapter 23 ∞.

Blockade of calcium ion channels has a number of effects on the heart, most of which are similar to those of beta-adrenergic blockers. Effects include reduced automaticity in the SA node and slowed impulse conduction through the AV node. This slows the heart rate and prolongs the refractory period. Calcium channel blockers are effective only against supraventricular dysrhythmias.

Calcium channel blockers are safe medications that are well tolerated by most clients. As with other antidysrhythmics, bradycardia and hypotension are common adverse effects. Because the cardiac effects of CCBs are almost identical with those of beta-adrenergic blockers, clients concurrently taking drugs from both classes are especially at risk for bradycardia and possible heart failure. Because older clients often have multiple cardiovascular disorders, such as hypertension, heart failure, and dysrhythmias, it is not unusual to find elderly clients taking drugs from multiple classes.

NURSING CONSIDERATIONS

The role of the nurse in calcium channel blocker therapy for dysrhythmias involves careful monitoring of a client's condition and providing education as it relates to the prescribed drug treatment. Never initiate calcium channel blocker therapy in clients with sick sinus syndrome, heart block, severe hypotension, cardiogenic shock, or severe congestive heart failure. Obtain the client's baseline ECG and vital signs. Obtain a thorough drug history, because CCBS may interact with other drugs, especially beta-adrenergic blockers, to cause additive effects on blood pressure and heart rate. Vital signs should be monitored regularly during CCB therapy to avoid hypotension and bradycardia. Assess the client for weight gain, decreased urine output, dyspnea and lung crackles, as these drugs may worsen congestive heart failure.

Pr PROTOTYPE DRUG | Verapamil *(Calan)* | Calcium Channel Blocker/Class IV Antidysrhythmic

ACTIONS AND USES

Verapamil was the first CCB approved by the FDA. It acts by inhibiting the flow of calcium ions both into myocardial cells and in vascular smooth muscle. In the heart, this action slows conduction velocity and stabilizes dysrhythmias. In the vessels, calcium channel blockade lowers blood pressure, reducing cardiac workload. Verapamil also dilates the coronary arteries, an action that is important when the drug is used to treat angina (Chapter 25 ∞). The drug is available in oral, oral extended-release, and IV formulations. The therapeutic serum level is 0.08–0.3 mcg/ml.

ADMINISTRATION ALERTS

- Do not dissolve or allow clients to chew capsule contents.
- For IV administration, inspect drug preparation to make sure solution is clear and colorless.
- Pregnancy category C.

PHARMACOKINETICS (PO)

Onset: 1–2 h

Peak: 30–90 min (4–8 h extended release)

Half-life: 2–8 h

Duration: 3–7 h PO (24 h extended release)

ADVERSE EFFECTS

Side effects are generally minor and include headache, constipation, and hypotension. Because verapamil can cause bradycardia, clients with heart failure should be carefully monitored.

Contraindications: Verapamil is contraindicated in clients with AV heart block, sick sinus syndrome, severe hypotension, or bleeding aneurysm, or those undergoing intracranial surgery. Use with caution in clients with renal or hepatic impairment.

INTERACTIONS

Drug–Drug: Verapamil has the ability to elevate blood levels of digoxin. Since digoxin and verapamil both slow conduction through the AV node, their concurrent use must be carefully monitored to avoid bradycardia. Use with antihypertensive drugs, including beta blockers, may cause additive hypotension.

Lab Tests: Unknown.

Herbal/Food: Grapefruit juice may increase verapamil levels. Hawthorn may have additive hypotensive effects.

Treatment of Overdose: Treatment is targeted to reversing hypotension with vasopressors. Calcium salts may be administered to increase the amount of calcium available to the myocardium and arterioles.

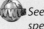 *See the Companion Website for a Nursing Process Focus specific to this drug.*

NATURAL THERAPIES

Magnesium for Dysrhythmias

Magnesium may be effective in the treatment of certain cardiac dysrhythmias in those who are magnesium deficient (Ueshima, 2005; Piotrowski & Kalus, 2004). Additional research has shown that magnesium supplementation reduces the risk of arrhythmia after cardiac surgery (Beattie & Elliot, 2005). Magnesium deficiency is associated with a number of dysrhythmias, including atrial fibrillation, premature atrial and ventricular beats, ventricular tachycardia, and ventricular fibrillation (Tong & Rude, 2005). The mechanism of magnesium's antidysrhythmic action is not fully understood but may be related to its role in maintaining intracellular potassium. It may also be related to its role as a natural calcium channel blocker. Magnesium may be administered intravenously or in liquid or capsule form. Foods that are rich in magnesium include unpolished grains, nuts, and green vegetables.

Lifespan Considerations. Because CCBs cause vasodilation of peripheral arterioles and decrease total peripheral vascular resistance, some clients, especially the elderly, may not be able to tolerate rapid changes in blood pressure caused by the CCBs. These drugs are not recommended for use during pregnancy (category C) or lactation.

Client Teaching. Client education as it relates to CCBs used to treat dysrhythmias should include the goals of therapy, the reasons for obtaining baseline data such as vital signs and underlying disorders, and possible drug side effects. Include the following points when teaching clients about CCBs:

- Report any sensations that the heart has skipped a beat.
- Take blood pressure frequently and report changes (either low blood pressure or elevated blood pressure).
- Take pulse frequently and notify the healthcare provider if pulse rate falls below 60 beats per minute.
- Report shortness of breath or swelling in the ankles or feet.

HOME & COMMUNITY CONSIDERATIONS

Clients Taking Antidysrhythmics

Clients taking antidysrhythmics who live alone should have a medical alert system in place to contact a healthcare provider in the case of dysrhythmias.

AVOIDING MEDICATION ERRORS

During a morning assessment, the nurse observes that a surgical client has developed an irregular heart rate of 120 beats per minute. The nurse notifies the resident physician, who orders a stat electrocardiogram. A ventricular arrhythmia is detected and the physician tells the nurse to administer lidocaine 150 mg as a single bolus to be followed by a continuous infusion of 1 g of lidocaine in 500 ml of 5% dextrose in water. The nurse isn't sure what the usual loading dose is. What should the nurse do?
See Appendix D for the suggested answer.

- Rise slowly from a sitting or lying position to prevent dizziness.
- Eat foods high in fiber.
- Do not take verapamil with grapefruit juice.

26.12 Miscellaneous Drugs for Dysrhythmias

Several other drugs are occasionally used to treat specific dysrhythmias, but do not act by the mechanisms previously described. These miscellaneous agents are listed in Table 26.3. Although digoxin (Lanoxin) is primarily used to treat heart failure, it is also prescribed for certain types of atrial dysrhythmias owing to its ability to decrease automaticity of the SA node and slow conduction through the AV node. Because excessive levels of digoxin can produce serious dysrhythmias, and interactions with other medications are common, clients must be carefully monitored during therapy. Additional information on the mechanism of action and the adverse effects of digoxin may be found in Chapter 24 ∞, where this drug is featured as a prototype cardiac glycoside for heart failure.

Adenosine (Adenocard) is a naturally occurring nucleoside. When given as a 1- to 2-second bolus IV injection, adenosine terminates serious atrial tachycardia by slowing conduction through the AV node and decreasing automaticity of the SA node. Its only indication is a specific dysrhythmia known as paroxysmal supraventricular tachycardia (PSVT), for which it is a drug of choice. Although dyspnea is common, side effects are generally self-limiting because of its 10-second half-life.

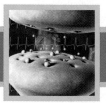

CHAPTER REVIEW

KEY CONCEPTS

The numbered key concepts provide a succinct summary of the important points from the corresponding numbered section within the chapter. If any of these points are not clear, refer to the numbered section within the chapter for review.

26.1 The frequency of dysrhythmias in the population is difficult to predict because many clients experience no symptoms. Persistent or severe dysrhythmias may be lethal.

26.2 Dysrhythmias are classified by the location (atrial or ventricular) or type (flutter, fibrillation, or block) of rhythm abnormality produced. Atrial fibrillation is the most common type of dysrhythmia.

26.3 The electrical conduction pathway from the SA node, to the AV node, to the bundle branches and Purkinje fibers keeps the heart beating in a synchronized manner. Some myocardial cells in these regions have the property of automaticity.

26.4 The electrocardiograph may be used to record electrophysiologic events in the heart and to diagnose dysrhythmias.

26.5 Nonpharmacological therapy of dysrhythmias, including cardioversion, ablation, and implantable cardioverter defibrillators, are often the treatments of choice.

26.6 Changes in sodium and potassium levels generate the action potential in myocardial cells. Depolarization occurs when sodium (and calcium) rushes in; repolarization occurs when sodium ions are removed and potassium ions are restored inside the cell.

26.7 Antidysrhythmic drugs are classified by their mechanism of action, namely, classes I through IV. The use of antidysrhythmic drugs has been declining.

26.8 Sodium channel blockers, the largest group of antidysrhythmics, act by slowing the rate of impulse conduction across the heart.

26.9 Beta-adrenergic blockers act by reducing automaticity as well as by slowing conduction velocity across the myocardium.

26.10 Potassium channel blockers act by prolonging the refractory period of the heart.

26.11 Calcium channel blockers act by reducing automaticity and by slowing myocardial conduction velocity. Their actions and effects are similar to those of the beta-blockers.

26.12 Digoxin and adenosine are used for specific dysrhythmias but do not act by blocking ion channels.

NCLEX-RN® REVIEW QUESTIONS

1 A client with a diagnosis of cardiac dysrhythmias and a history of type I diabetes mellitus is placed on propranolol (Inderal) therapy. The client asks the nurse if the drug will affect insulin needs. The best response by the nurse would be that:

1. The drug will have no effect on insulin needs.
2. The drug may cause hypoglycemia.
3. The drug may cause hyperglycemia.
4. The client should ask the physician this question.

2 The nurse adjusts the plan of care for a client of Asian descent who is receiving propranolol to include increased monitoring of:

1. Heart rate.
2. Blood pressure.
3. Glucose.
4. Potassium.

3 Sodium channel blockers:

1. Reduce automaticity.
2. Slow the impulse conduction.
3. Prolong the refractory period.
4. Increase impulse conduction.

4 Common side effects of antidysrhythmic medications include (select all that apply):

1. Hypotension.
2. Hypertension.
3. Dizziness.
4. Weakness.
5. Panic attacks.

5 The nurse in the telemetry unit explains the mechanism of myocardial contraction as:

1. Increased calcium outside myocardial cells.
2. Increased potassium outside myocardial cells.
3. Increased calcium inside myocardial cells.
4. Increased potassium inside myocardial cells.

CRITICAL THINKING QUESTIONS

1. A client with a history of COPD and tachycardia has recently been placed on propranolol (Inderal) to control the tachydysrhythmia. What is a priority for the nurse in monitoring this client?

2. A client is started on amiodarone (Cordarone) for cardiac dysrhythmias. This client is also on digoxin (Lanoxin), warfarin (Coumadin), and insulin. What is a priority teaching for this client?

3. A client is on verapamil (Calan) and digoxin (Lanoxin). What is a priority that this client needs to be monitored for?

See Appendix D for answers and rationales for all activities.

EXPLORE
MediaLink

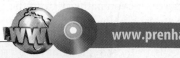

www.prenhall.com/adams

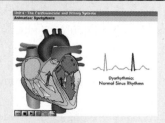

NCLEX-RN® review, case studies, and other interactive resources for this chapter can be found on the companion website at www.prenhall.com/adams. Click on "Chapter 26" to select the activities for this chapter. For animations, more NCLEX-RN® review questions, and an audio glossary, access the accompanying Prentice Hall Nursing MediaLink DVD-ROM in this textbook.

PRENTICE HALL NURSING MEDIALINK DVD-ROM

- **Animations**
  Mechanism in Action: Propranolol (*Inderal*)
  Mechanism in Action: Amiodarone (*Cordarone*)
- **Audio Glossary**
- **NCLEX-RN® Review**

COMPANION WEBSITE

- **NCLEX-RN® Review**
- **Dosage Calculations**
- **Case Study:** Client taking a sodium channel blocker
- **Care Plan:** Client with atrial fibrillation who is being treated with propranolol

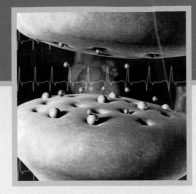

CHAPTER 27

Drugs for Coagulation Disorders

DRUGS AT A GLANCE

ANTICOAGULANTS
Parenteral Anticoagulants
  heparin (Heplock)
Oral Anticoagulants
  warfarin (Coumadin)
ANTIPLATELET AGENTS
ADP Receptor Blockers
  clopidogrel (Plavix)
Glycoprotein IIb/IIIa Receptor Antagonists
Agents for Intermittent Claudication
THROMBOLYTICS
  alteplase (Activase)
HEMOSTATICS
  aminocaproic acid (Amicar)

OBJECTIVES

After reading this chapter, the student should be able to:

1. Construct a diagram illustrating the important steps of hemostasis and fibrinolysis.
2. Describe thromboembolic disorders that are indications for coagulation modifiers.
3. Identify the primary mechanisms by which coagulation modifiers act.
4. Explain how laboratory testing of coagulation parameters is used to monitor anticoagulant pharmacotherapy.
5. Describe the nurse's role in the pharmacological management of coagulation disorders.
6. For each of the classes listed in Drugs at a Glance, know representative drug examples, and explain the mechanism of drug action, primary actions, and important adverse effects.
7. Categorize coagulation-modifying drugs based on their classification and mechanism of action.
8. Use the Nursing Process to care for clients receiving drug therapy for coagulation disorders.

MediaLink

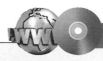

www.prenhall.com/adams

NCLEX-RN® review, case studies, and other interactive resources for this chapter can be found on the companion website at www.prenhall.com/adams. Click on "Chapter 27" to select the activities for this chapter. For animations, more NCLEX-RN® review questions, and an audio glossary, access the accompanying Prentice Hall Nursing MediaLink DVD-ROM in this textbook.

KEY TERMS

activated partial thromboplastin time (aPTT) *page 380*

anticoagulant *page 381*

antithrombin III *page 381*

clotting factors *page 378*

coagulation *page 378*

coagulation cascade *page 378*

embolus *page 380*

fibrin *page 379*

fibrinogen *page 379*

fibrinolysis *page 379*

glycoprotein IIb/IIIa *page 386*

hemophilia *page 380*

hemostasis *page 378*

hemostatics *page 381*

intermittent claudication *page 386*

low-molecular-weight heparin (LMWH) *page 381*

plasmin *page 379*

plasminogen *page 379*

prothrombin *page 379*

prothrombin activator *page 378*

prothrombin time (PT) *page 380*

thrombin *page 379*

thrombocytopenia *page 380*

thromboembolic disorders *page 380*

thrombolytics *page 381*

thrombus *page 380*

tissue plasminogen activator (TPA) *page 379*

von Willebrand's disease (vWD) *page 380*

Hemostasis, or the stopping of blood flow, is an essential mechanism that protects the body from both external and internal injury. Without efficient hemostasis, bleeding from wounds or internal injuries would lead to shock and perhaps death. Too much clotting, however, can be just as dangerous. The physiological processes of hemostasis must maintain a delicate balance between fluidity and coagulation.

A number of diseases and conditions can affect hemostasis, including myocardial infarction (MI), cerebrovascular accident (CVA), venous thrombus, valvular heart disease, and indwelling catheters. Because these disorders are so prevalent, nurses frequently administer and monitor coagulation-modifying drugs.

27.1 The Process of Hemostasis

Hemostasis is a complex process involving a number of **clotting factors** that are activated in a series of sequential steps, sometimes referred to as a *cascade*. Drugs may be used to modify several of these steps.

When a blood vessel is injured, a series of events initiate the clotting process. The vessel spasms, causing constriction, which limits the flow of blood to the injured area. Platelets become sticky, adhering to each other and to the damaged vessel. Aggregation is facilitated by adenosine diphosphate (ADP), the enzyme thrombin, and thromboxane A_2. Adhesion is made possible by platelet receptor sites (glycoprotein IIb/IIIa) and von Willebrand's factor. As the bound platelets break down, they release substances that attract more platelets to the area. The flow of blood is reduced, thus allowing the process of **coagulation,** the formation of an insoluble clot, to occur. The basic steps of hemostasis are shown in ● Figure 27.1.

When collagen is exposed at the site of injury, the damaged cells initiate a series of complex reactions called the **coagulation cascade.** Coagulation occurs when fibrin threads create a meshwork that traps blood constituents so that they develop a clot. During the cascade, various plasma proteins circulating in an inactive state are converted to their active forms. Two separate pathways, along with numerous biochemical processes, lead to coagulation. The *intrinsic* pathway is activated in response to injury. The *extrinsic* pathway is activated when blood leaks out of a vessel and enters tissue spaces. The two pathways have common steps, and the outcome is the same—the formation of the fibrin clot. The steps in each coagulation cascade are shown in ● Figure 27.2.

Near the end of the common pathway, a chemical called **prothrombin activator** or prothrombinase is formed. Prothrombin activator converts the clotting factor

PHARMFACTS

Clotting Disorders

- Liver disease is a common cause of coagulation disorders, because this organ supplies many of the clotting factors.
- Von Willebrand's disease (vWD) is the most common hereditary bleeding disorder, caused by a deficiency of the protein von Willebrand factor (vWF), which plays a role in platelet aggregation and acts as a carrier for factor VIII.
- More than 2 million clients each year develop a deep vein thrombosis (DVT).
- More than 60,000 clients each year die of pulmonary emboli.
- Hemophilia A, or classic hemophilia, is a hereditary condition in which a person lacks clotting factor VIII; it accounts for 80% of all hemophilia cases.
- Hemophilia B, or "Christmas disease," is a hereditary absence of clotting factor IX.
- More than 15,000 people in the United States have hemophilia A or B.

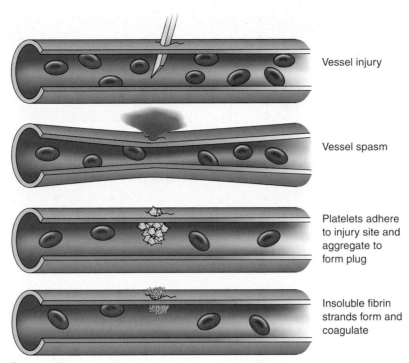

● **Figure 27.1** Basic steps in hemostasis

prothrombin to an enzyme called **thrombin.** Thrombin then converts **fibrinogen,** a plasma protein, to long strands of **fibrin.** The fibrin strands provide a framework for the clot. Thus, two of the factors essential to clotting, thrombin and fibrin, are formed only *after* injury to the vessels. The fibrin strands form an insoluble web over the injured area to stop blood loss. Normal blood clotting occurs in approximately 6 minutes.

It is important to note that several clotting factors, including fibrinogen, are proteins made by the liver, which constantly circulate through the blood in an *inactive* form. Vitamin K, which is made by bacteria residing in the large intestine, is required for the liver to make four of the clotting factors. Because of the crucial importance of the liver in creating these clotting factors, clients with serious hepatic impairment often have abnormal coagulation.

27.2 Removal of Blood Clots

Hemostasis is achieved once a blood clot is formed, protecting the body from excessive hemorrhage. The clot, however, may restrict blood flow to the affected area; circulation must eventually be restored so that the tissue can resume normal activities. The process of clot removal is called **fibrinolysis.** It is initiated within 24 to 48 hours of clot formation and continues until the clot is dissolved.

Fibrinolysis also involves several cascading steps. When the fibrin clot is formed, nearby blood vessel cells secrete the enzyme **tissue plasminogen activator (TPA).** TPA converts the inactive protein **plasminogen,** which is present in the fibrin clot, to its active enzymatic form, **plasmin.** Plasmin then digests the fibrin strands to remove the clot. The body normally regulates fibrinolysis such that *unwanted* fibrin clots are removed, whereas fibrin present in wounds is left to maintain hemostasis. The steps of fibrinolysis are shown in ● Figure 27.3.

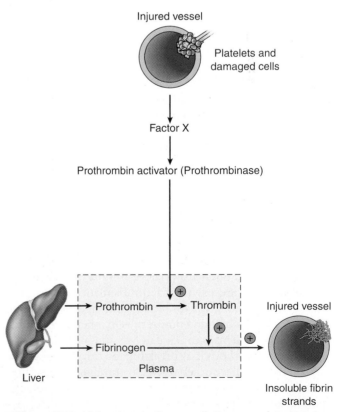

● **Figure 27.2** Major steps in the coagulation cascade: common pathway

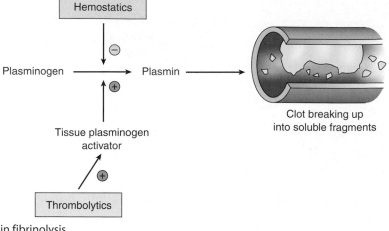

● **Figure 27.3** Primary steps in fibrinolysis

NATURAL THERAPIES

Garlic for Cardiovascular Health

Garlic (*Allium sativum*) is one of the best-studied herbs. Several different substances, known as *alliaceous oils*, have been isolated from garlic and shown to have pharmacological activity. Dosage forms include eating prepared garlic oil or the fresh bulbs from the plant. Aged garlic extracts have shown the most therapeutic effect in trials (Allison, Lowe, & Rahman 2006).

Garlic has been shown to decrease the aggregation or "stickiness" of platelets, thus producing an anticoagulant effect (Rahman & Lowe, 2006). Platelet aggregation on roughened walls of arteries damaged by atherosclerosis commonly initiates the formation of blood clots that lead to heart attacks and strokes. Clients taking anticoagulant medications should limit their intake of garlic to avoid bleeding complications. Garlic also has hypoglycemic effects, so oral antidiabetic dosages may need to be adjusted.

27.3 Diseases of Hemostasis

To diagnose a bleeding disorder, a thorough health history and physical examination is necessary. Laboratory tests measuring coagulation must be obtained. These usually include whole blood clotting time, **prothrombin time (PT)**, thrombin time, **activated partial thromboplastin time (aPTT),** liver function tests, and, in some instances, a bleeding time. Platelet count is also important when assessing bleeding disorders. Additional tests may be indicated, based on the results of these laboratory analyses.

Thromboembolic disorders occur when the body forms undesirable clots. Once a stationary clot, called a **thrombus,** forms in a vessel, it often grows larger as more fibrin is added. Arterial thrombi are particularly problematic because they deprive an area of adequate blood flow, causing tissue ischemia. Cessation of blood flow results in infarction, and tissue death results. This is the case in MIs and many CVAs.

Pieces of a thrombus may break off and travel through the bloodstream to affect other vessels. A traveling clot is called an **embolus.** Thrombi in the venous system usually form in the veins of the legs in susceptible clients owing to sluggish blood flow, a condition called *deep vein thrombosis (DVT).* Thrombi can form in the atria during atrial fibrillation. An embolus from the right atrium will cause pulmonary emboli, whereas an embolus from the left atrium will cause a CVA or an arterial infarction elsewhere in the body. Arterial thrombi and emboli can also occur following surgical procedures, and arterial punctures such as angiography. Clients with indwelling catheters and mechanical heart valves are susceptible to thrombi formation and frequently receive prophylactic anticoagulant therapy. Thromboembolic disorders are the most common indications for pharmacotherapy with anticoagulants.

Bleeding disorders are characterized by abnormal clot formation. The most common nonhereditary bleeding disorder is a deficiency of platelets known as **thrombocytopenia,** which results from any condition that suppresses bone marrow function. Certain drugs such as immunosuppressants and most of the drugs used for cancer chemotherapy can cause this condition.

Hemophilias are bleeding disorders caused by genetic deficiencies in certain clotting factors. They are typified by prolonged coagulation times, which result in persistent bleeding that can be acute. The classic form, hemophilia A, is caused by a lack of clotting factor VIII and accounts for approximately 80% of all cases. Hemophilia B is caused by a deficiency of factor IX; about 20% of those afflicted with hemophilia have this type. Hemophilia is treated by administering the absent clotting factor and, in acute situations, by transfusing fresh frozen plasma. **von Willebrand's disease (vWD)** is the most

HOME & COMMUNITY CONSIDERATIONS

Clients Taking Anticoagulant Therapy

The drugs given for coagulation disorders require intensive client education. The client is at a high risk for severe bleeding complications. Take into consideration the educational level and ability of the client to understand the importance of the discharge instructions. To ensure that all levels of learning capabilities are covered, include written, verbal, audio/visual, and demonstration methods of client teaching. If the client is unable to understand the instructions because of age, cognitive impairment, or sensory impairment, ensure that a responsible person has received and understands the discharge instructions.

TABLE 27.1   Mechanisms of Action of Coagulation Modifiers

Type of Modification	Mechanism	Drug Classification
prevention of clot formation	inhibition of specific clotting factors	anticoagulants
prevention of clot formation	inhibition of platelet actions	antiplatelet agents
removal of an existing clot	dissolution of clot by the drug	thrombolytics
promotion of clot formation	inhibition of fibrin destruction	hemostatics

common inherited bleeding disease. This disorder results in a decrease in quantity or quality of von Willebrand factor (vWF), which has a role in platelet aggregation. This type of bleeding disorder is treated with factor VIII concentrate as well as desmopressin (DDAVP), which promotes the release of stored vWF. For the most severely affected clients, plasma products containing vWF may be required.

27.4 Mechanisms of Coagulation Modification

Drugs can modify hemostasis by four basic mechanisms, as summarized in Table 27.1. The most commonly prescribed coagulation modifiers are the **anticoagulants,** which are used to prevent the formation of clots. These drugs can either inhibit specific clotting factors in the coagulation cascade or diminish the clotting action of platelets. Regardless of the mechanism, all anticoagulant drugs will increase the normal clotting time.

Once an abnormal clot has formed in a blood vessel, it may be critical to remove it quickly to restore normal tissue function. This is particularly important for vessels serving the heart, lungs, and brain. A specific class of drugs, the **thrombolytics,** are used to dissolve such life-threatening clots.

Occasionally, it is necessary to *promote* the formation of clots with drugs called **hemostatics.** These drugs inhibit the normal removal of fibrin, thus keeping the clot in place for a longer period. Hemostatics are used to speed clot formation, thereby limiting bleeding from a surgical site.

To prevent serious adverse effects, pharmacotherapy with coagulation modifiers is individualized to each client. Drug–drug interactions are common with anticoagulants, and can either increase or diminish the anticoagulant effect. Serious kidney or liver disease can cause toxicity. Clients require regular physical assessment and laboratory monitoring.

ANTICOAGULANTS

Anticoagulants are drugs used to prolong bleeding time and thereby prevent blood clots from forming. They are widely used in the treatment of thromboembolic disease.

27.5 Pharmacotherapy With Parenteral and Oral Anticoagulants

By inhibiting certain clotting factors, anticoagulants lengthen clotting time and prevent thrombi from forming or growing larger. Thromboembolic disease can be life

threatening; thus, therapy is often begun by administering anticoagulants intravenously or subcutaneously to achieve a rapid onset of action. As the disease stabilizes, the client is switched to oral anticoagulants, with careful monitoring of appropriate coagulation laboratory studies. The most common parenteral anticoagulant is heparin.

Anticoagulants act by a number of different mechanisms, as illustrated in Figure 27.4. These drugs are often referred to as *blood thinners,* which is a misnomer, because they do not change the viscosity of the blood. Instead, anticoagulants impart a negative charge to the surface of the platelets, which inhibits the clumping action or aggregation of these cells. The most commonly prescribed anticoagulants are heparin and warfarin (Coumadin). Heparin acts by enhancing the inhibitory actions of **antithrombin III.** Warfarin acts by inhibiting the hepatic synthesis of coagulation factors II, VII, IX, and X. Table 27.2 lists the primary anticoagulants.

In recent years, the heparin molecule has been shortened and modified to create a new class of drugs called **low-molecular-weight heparins (LMWHs).** The mechanism of action of these agents is similar to that of heparin, except

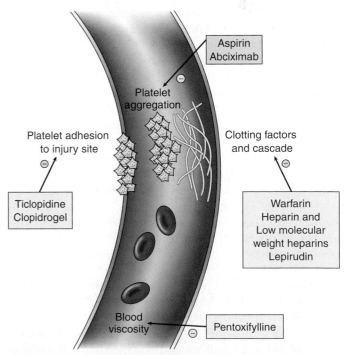

● **Figure 27.4** Mechanisms of action of anticoagulants

TABLE 27.2 Anticoagulants

Drug	Route and Adult Dose (max dose where indicated)	Adverse Effects
anisindione (Miradon)	PO; 300 mg Day 1,200 mg Day 2, then 100 mg/day thereafter; adjust dose to maintain desired PT level (dose range: 25–250 mg)	*Nausea, vomiting, transient thrombocytopenia (heparin), anemia (fondaparinux)*
fondaparinux (Arixta)	Subcutaneous; 2.5 mg/day starting at least 6 h postop for 5–9 days	
● heparin (Heplock)	IV infusion; 5,000–40,000 units/day Subcutaneous; 15,000–20,000 units bid	Hemorrhage, anaphylaxis (heparin)
● warfarin (Coumadin)	PO; 2–15 mg/day	
LOW-MOLECULAR-WEIGHT HEPARINS (LMWHS)		
ardeparin (Normiflo)	Subcutaneous; 50 units/kg bid for 14 days	*Nausea, vomiting, allergic reactions (rash, urticaria), pain at injection site*
dalteparin (Fragmin)	Subcutaneous; 2,500–5,000 units/day for 5–10 days	
danaparoid (Orgaran)	Subcutaneous; 750 units bid for 7–10 days	Hemorrhage, anaphylaxis, thrombocytopenia
enoxaparin (Lovenox)	Subcutaneous; 30 mg bid for 7–10 days	
tinzaparin (Innohep)	Subcutaneous; 175 units/kg daily for at least 6 days	
DIRECT THROMBIN INHIBITORS		
argatroban (Acova, Novastan)	IV; 2 mcg/kg/min (max: 10 mcg/kg/min)	*Fever, nausea, allergic skin reactions, hepatic impairment, minor bleeding, back pain (bivalirudin)*
bivalirudin (Angiomax)	IV; 1 mg/kg initial bolus followed by 2.5 mg/kg/h for 4 h (max: continue at 0.2 mg/kg/h up to 20 h)	
desirudin (Iprivask)	Subcutaneous; 15 mg bid	Serious internal hemorrhage
lepirudin (Refludan)	IV; 0.4 mg/kg initial bolus (max: 44 mg), followed by 0.15 mg/kg/h (max: 16.5 mg/h) for 2–10 days	

Italics indicate common adverse effects; <u>underlining</u> indicates serious adverse effects.

their inhibition is more specific to active factor X (see Figure 27.2). LMWHs possess the same degree of anticoagulant activity as heparin but have several advantages. Their duration of action is two to four times longer than that of heparin. The LMWHs also produce a more stable response than heparin; thus fewer follow-up lab tests are needed, and family members or the client can be trained to give the necessary SC injections at home. These anticoagulants are also less likely to cause thrombocytopenia. LMWHs have become the drugs of choice for a number of clotting disorders, including the prevention of DVT following surgery.

Other parenteral anticoagulants include the direct thrombin inhibitors argatroban (Acova, Novastan), bivalirudin (Angiomax), and lepirudin (Refludan). These agents bind to the active site of thrombin, preventing the formation of fibrin clots. They act on both clot-bound and circulating thrombin. These agents are infused until a therapeutic aPTT value is obtained, usually one and a half to three times the control value. The thrombin inhibitors have limited therapeutic uses. Bivalirudin is administered in combination with aspirin to prevent thrombi in clients undergoing angioplasty. Argatroban and lepirudin are indicated for prevention or treatment of thrombocytopenia induced by heparin therapy. Desirudin (Iprivask) is a newer antithrombin agent that is given subcutaneously 15 minutes prior to hip replacement surgery for prophylaxis of DVT.

The most common, and potentially serious, adverse effect of all the anticoagulant agents is bleeding. Clients who have recently experienced a traumatic injury or surgery are especially at risk. Specific antagonists may be administered to reverse the anticoagulant effects: protamine sulfate is used for heparin, and vitamin K is administered for warfarin (see the drug prototype features in this chapter).

NURSING CONSIDERATIONS

The role of the nurse in anticoagulant therapy for thrombotic and thromboembolic disorders involves careful monitoring of the client's condition and providing education as it relates to the prescribed drug treatment. Anticoagulants are frequently given to reduce the risk for DVT after any surgery, illness, or injury that restricts mobility. When the body's ability to form blood clots is altered by medications, it is imperative that the nurse be aware of the potential serious effects that could occur in the other body systems.

The most serious side effect of anticoagulants is bleeding. Assess the client for signs of bleeding, including bruising, nosebleeds, excessive menstrual flow, "coffee-grounds" emesis, tarry stools, tea-colored urine, bright red bleeding from the rectum, dizziness, fatigue, or pale pasty-looking skin. The risk of bleeding is dose dependent: the higher the dose, the higher the risk.

Hypotension accompanied by declining complete blood count (CBC) values [red blood cells (RBCs), platelets, hemoglobin, and hematocrit] may signal internal bleeding. Lumbar pain and unilateral abdominal wall bulges or swelling could indicate retroperitoneal hemorrhage. Guaiac tests can be performed on stool to identify occult blood. Use of heparin during breast-feeding can trigger bleeding from the nipples and should be avoided. Use of warfarin during pregnancy is contraindicated because it can cause hemorrhage or other abnormalities in the fetus.

Monitoring laboratory values during anticoagulant therapy is essential to ensure client safety. For heparin, aPTT is measured, with normal values ranging from 25 to 40 seconds. For therapeutic anticoagulation, the aPTT should be one to two times the client's baseline. During continuous intravenous heparin therapy, the aPTT is measured daily and 6 to 8 hours after any changes in dosage.

Prothrombin time is a laboratory test used to monitor effectiveness of warfarin. The normal PT range is 12 to 15 seconds. During therapeutic anticoagulation, PT should increase to one to two times the client's baseline. Because laboratory testing methods for PT vary, prothrombin time is also reported as an international normalized ratio (INR) value; INR values of 2.0 to 3.5 are considered therapeutic. PT is measured daily until the therapeutic dose is determined, and then the frequency of testing is decreased to weekly or monthly as therapy progresses.

When a client is transitioning from IV heparin to oral warfarin, the two drugs must be administered simultaneously for 2 to 3 days. Heparin has a brief half-life (90 minutes), whereas warfarin has a half-life of 1 to 3 days. The aPTT returns to normal within 2 to 3 hours following discontinuation of heparin; thus, concomitant pharmacotherapy is necessary to ensure continuous therapeutic anticoagulation. During this transition, there is increased risk of bleeding, due to the potentiated action of the combined drugs.

Give LMWHs subcutaneously, with dosage calculations based on the client's weight rather than laboratory values. Follow manufacturers' recommendations for sites of injection. There is an increased risk of bleeding if the drugs are injected into muscle. For example, enoxaparin (Lovenox) is given in the subcutaneous tissue of the anterolateral or posterolateral abdominal wall (the "love handles"). To administer the drug safely, grasp a skin fold between the thumb and forefinger, insert a 3/8-inch needle fully at a 90° angle, and hold the skin fold throughout the injection. For exceptionally lean clients, use a longer needle and carefully insert it at a 45° angle to avoid inadvertent IM injection of the medication. To prevent tissue injury and bruising, never aspirate or massage an injection site.

Lifespan Considerations. Instruct elderly clients, menstruating women, and those with peptic ulcer disease, alcoholism, or kidney or liver disease that they have an increased risk for bleeding. Clients with diabetes, high blood pressure, or hypercholesterolemia are at increased risk for developing microscopic clots, despite anticoagulant therapy.

Pr PROTOTYPE DRUG | Heparin *(Heplock)* | Anticoagulant *(Parenteral)*

ACTIONS AND USES

Heparin is a natural substance found in the liver and in the lining of blood vessels. Its normal function is to prolong coagulation time, thereby preventing excessive clotting within blood vessels. As a result, it prevents the enlargement of existing clots and the formation of new ones. The binding of heparin to antithrombin III inactivates several clotting factors and inhibits thrombin activity. The onset of action for IV heparin is immediate, whereas subcutaneous heparin may take up to 1 hour to achieve a therapeutic effect. This drug is also called *unfractionated* heparin, to distinguish it from the LMWHs.

ADMINISTRATION ALERTS

- Heparin is poorly absorbed by the GI mucosa because of rapid metabolism by the hepatic enzyme heparinase. Therefore, it must be given either sc or through iv bolus injection or continuous infusion.
- When administering heparin subcutaneously, never draw back the syringe plunger once the needle has entered the skin; never massage the site after injection. Doing either can contribute to bleeding or tissue damage.
- IM administration is contraindicated owing to bleeding risk.
- Pregnancy category C.

PHARMACOKINETICS (SUBCUTANEOUS)

Onset: 20–60 min

Peak: 2 h

Half-life: 90 min

Duration: 8–12 h

ADVERSE EFFECTS

Abnormal bleeding may occur during heparin therapy. Should aPTT become prolonged or toxicity be observed, stopping the infusion will result in diminished anticoagulant activity within hours.

Contraindications: Heparin should not be administered to clients with active internal bleeding, bleeding disorders, severe hypertension, recent trauma, intracranial hemorrhage, or bacterial endocarditis.

INTERACTIONS

Drug–Drug: Oral anticoagulants, including warfarin, potentiate the action of heparin. Drugs that inhibit platelet aggregation, such as aspirin, indomethacin, and ibuprofen, may induce bleeding. Nicotine, digoxin, tetracyclines, or antihistamines may inhibit anticoagulation.

Lab Tests: The following values may be increased: free fatty acids, AST, and ALT. Serum cholesterol and triglycerides may be decreased.

Herbal/Food: Herbal supplements such as arnica or ginkgo may increase the risk of bleeding.

Treatment of Overdose: If serious hemorrhage occurs, a specific antagonist, protamine sulfate, may be administered IV (1 mg for every 100 units of heparin) to neutralize the anticoagulant activity of heparin. Protamine sulfate has an onset of action of 5 minutes and is also an antagonist to the LMWHs.

 See the Companion Website for a Nursing Process Focus specific to this drug.

Pr PROTOTYPE DRUG | Warfarin (Coumadin) | Anticoagulant (Oral)

ACTIONS AND USES

Unlike with heparin, the anticoagulant activity of warfarin can take several days to reach its maximum effect. This explains why heparin and warfarin therapy are overlapped. Warfarin inhibits the action of vitamin K. Without adequate vitamin K, the synthesis of clotting factors II, VII, IX, and X is diminished. Because these clotting factors are normally circulating in the blood, it takes several days for their plasma levels to fall, and for the anticoagulant effect of warfarin to appear. Another reason for the slow onset is that 99% of the warfarin is bound to plasma proteins and is thus unavailable to produce its effect. The therapeutic range of serum warfarin levels varies from 1 to 10 mcg/ml, to achieve an INR value of 2.0–3.0.

ADMINISTRATION ALERTS

- If life-threatening bleeding occurs during therapy, the anticoagulant effects of warfarin can be reduced by IM or subcutaneous administration of its antagonist, vitamin K_1.
- Pregnancy category X.

PHARMACOKINETICS (PO)

Onset: 2–7 days

Peak: 0.5–3 days

Half-life: 0.5–3 days

Duration: 3–5 days

ADVERSE EFFECTS

The most serious adverse effect of warfarin is abnormal bleeding. On discontinuation of therapy, the anticoagulant activity of warfarin may persist for up to 10 days.

Contraindications: Clients with recent trauma, active internal bleeding, bleeding disorders, intracranial hemorrhage, severe hypertension, bacterial endocarditis, or severe hepatic or renal impairment should not take warfarin.

INTERACTIONS

Drug–Drug: Extensive protein binding is responsible for numerous drug–drug interactions, including an increased effect of warfarin with alcohol, NSAIDs, diuretics, SSRIs and other antidepressants, steroids, antibiotics and vaccines, and vitamins (e.g., vitamin K). During warfarin therapy the client should not take any other prescription or OTC drugs unless approved by the healthcare provider.

Lab Tests: Unknown.

Herbal/Food: Herbal supplements such as arnica, feverfew, garlic, and ginger may increase the risk of bleeding.

Treatment of Overdose: The specific treatment for overdose is oral or parenteral administration of vitamin K_1. When administered IV, vitamin K_1 can reverse the anticoagulant effects of warfarin within 6 hours.

 See the Companion Website for a Nursing Process Focus specific to this drug.

Heparin and the LWMHs are the only anticoagulant therapies that should be given during pregnancy. These molecules are too large to cross the placenta.

Client Teaching. Client education as it relates to anticoagulants should include the goals of therapy; the reasons for obtaining baseline data such as vital signs, laboratory values, and the existence of underlying renal or hepatic disorders; and possible drug side effects. Include the following points when teaching clients about anticoagulants:

- Immediately report burning, stinging, warmth, excessive bruising, or evidence of swelling or pain at heparin injection or IV insertion sites.
- Take warfarin at the same time each day.
- Avoid suddenly increasing your intake of vitamin K–rich foods (cabbage, cauliflower, broccoli, asparagus, lettuce, turnip greens or kale, onions, spinach, fish, or liver) when taking warfarin.
- Avoid strenuous or hazardous activities that could result in bleeding injuries.
- Immediately report any bleeding, nosebleeds, excessive menstrual flow, bleeding of the gums, or bruising with minor injury to the skin.
- Limit intake of garlic to prevent bleeding complications.

ANTIPLATELET AGENTS

Antiplatelet drugs cause an anticoagulant effect by interfering with various aspects of platelet function—primarily platelet aggregation. Unlike the anticoagulants, which are used primarily to prevent thrombosis in veins, antiplatelet agents are used to prevent clot formation in arteries. The antiplatelet agents are listed in Table 27.3.

27.6 Inhibition of Platelet Function

Platelets are a key component of hemostasis: too few platelets or diminished platelet function can profoundly increase bleeding time. The following four types of drugs are classified as antiplatelet agents:

- Aspirin
- ADP receptor blockers
- Glycoprotein IIb/IIIa receptor antagonists
- Agents for intermittent claudication

Aspirin deserves special mention as an antiplatelet agent. Because it is available over the counter, clients may not consider aspirin a potent medication; however, its anticoagulant activity is well documented. Aspirin acts by binding irreversibly to the enzyme cyclooxygenase in platelets. This binding inhibits the formation of thromboxane A_2, a powerful inducer of platelet aggregation. The anticoagulant effect of a single dose of aspirin may persist for as long as a week. Concurrent use of aspirin with other coagulation modifiers should be avoided, unless medically approved. Aspirin is featured as a drug prototype for pain relief in Chapter 18 ∞, and is also indicated for prevention of strokes and MI in Chapter 25 ∞, and reduction of inflammation in Chapter 33 ∞.

NURSING PROCESS FOCUS Clients Receiving Anticoagulant Therapy

Assessment	Potential Nursing Diagnoses
Prior to administration: ▪ Obtain a complete health history including recent surgeries or trauma, allergies, drug history, and possible drug interactions. ▪ Obtain vital signs and assess in context of client's baseline values.	▪ Injury, Risk for (bleeding), related to adverse effects of anticoagulant therapy ▪ Activity Intolerance (Contact Sports) ▪ Tissue Perfusion, Ineffective, related to hemorrhage ▪ Tissue Integrity, Impaired ▪ Infection, Risk for ▪ Knowledge, Deficient, related to drug therapy

Planning: Client Goals and Expected Outcomes

The client will:
▪ Experience a decrease in blood coagulation as evidenced by laboratory values.
▪ Demonstrate an understanding of the drug's action by accurately describing drug side effects and precautions.

Implementation

Interventions and (Rationales)	Client Education/Discharge Planning
▪ Monitor for adverse clotting reaction(s). (Heparin can cause thrombus formation with thrombocytopenia, or "white clot syndrome." Warfarin may cause cholesterol microemboli that result in gangrene, localized vasculitis, or "purple toes syndrome.")	Instruct client to: ▪ Immediately report sudden dyspnea, chest pain, temperature or color change in the hands, arms, legs, or feet.
▪ Observe for skin necrosis, changes in blue or purple mottling of the feet that blanches with pressure or fades when the legs are elevated. (Clients on anticoagulant therapy remain at risk for developing emboli resulting in CVA or PE.)	Instruct client to: ▪ Check pulses in the ankle daily. ▪ Protect feet from injury by wearing loose-fitting socks; avoid going barefoot.
▪ Use with caution in clients with GI, renal and/or liver disease, alcoholism, diabetes, hypertension, hyperlipidemia, and in the elderly and premenopausal women. (Clients with CAD, diabetes, hypertension, and hyperlipidemia are at increased risk for developing cholesterol microemboli.)	▪ Instruct elderly clients, menstruating women, and those with peptic ulcer disease, alcoholism, or kidney or liver disease that they have an increased risk of bleeding.
▪ Monitor for signs of bleeding: flulike symptoms, excessive bruising, pallor, epistaxis, hemoptysis, hematemesis, menorrhagia, hematuria, melena, frank rectal bleeding, or excessive bleeding from wounds or in the mouth. (Bleeding is a sign of anticoagulant overdose.)	Instruct client to: ▪ Immediately report flulike symptoms (dizziness, chills, weakness, pale skin); blood coming from a cough, the nose, mouth, or rectum; menstrual "flooding"; "coffee grounds" vomit; tarry stools; excessive bruising; bleeding from wounds that cannot be stopped within 10 minutes; all physical injuries. ▪ Avoid all contact sports and amusement park rides that cause intense or violent bumping or jostling. ▪ Use a soft toothbrush and an electric shaver.
▪ Monitor vital signs. (Increase in heart rate accompanied by low blood pressure or subnormal temperature may signal bleeding.)	▪ Instruct client to immediately report palpitations, fatigue, or feeling faint, which may signal low blood pressure related to bleeding.
▪ Monitor laboratory values: aPTT and PTT for therapeutic values. (Heparin may cause significant elevations of aspartate aminotransferase (AST) and alanine transaminase (ALT), because the drug is metabolized by the liver.)	Instruct client to: ▪ Always inform laboratory personnel of heparin therapy when providing samples. ▪ Carry a wallet card or wear medical ID jewelry indicating heparin therapy.
▪ Monitor CBC, especially in premenopausal women. (Changes in CBC may indicate excessive bleeding.)	▪ Instruct client to keep a "pad count" during menstrual periods to estimate blood losses.

Evaluation of Outcome Criteria

Evaluate the effectiveness of drug therapy by confirming that client goals and expected outcomes have been met (see "Planning").
▪ The client's laboratory values exhibit a decrease in blood coagulation.
▪ The client demonstrates an understanding of the drug's action by accurately describing drug side effects and precautions.

∞ *See Table 27.2 for a list of drugs to which these nursing actions apply.*

TABLE 27.3 Antiplatelet Agents

Drug	Route and Adult Dose (max dose where indicated)	Adverse Effects
aspirin (ASA, acetylsalicylic acid) (see page 235 for the Prototype Drug box ∞)	PO; 80 mg/day to 650 mg bid	*Nausea, vomiting, diarrhea, abdominal pain*
dipyridamole (Persantine)	PO; 75–100 mg/day	Increased clotting time, GI bleeding (aspirin), CNS effects (dipyridamole), anaphylaxis (aspirin)
ADP RECEPTOR BLOCKERS		
clopidogrel (Plavix)	PO; 75 mg/day	*Dyspepsia, abdominal pain, rash, and diarrhea*
ticlopidine (Ticlid)	PO; 250 mg bid	Increased clotting time, GI bleeding, blood dyscrasias
GLYCOPROTEIN IIB/IIIA RECEPTOR ANTAGONISTS		
abciximab (ReoPro)	IV; 0.25 mg/kg initial bolus over 5 min; then 10 mcg/kg/min for 12 h	*Dyspepsia, dizziness, pain at injection site*
eptifibatide (Integrilin)	IV; 180 mcg/kg initial bolus over 1–2 min; then 2 mcg/kg/min for 24–72 h	Hemorrhage, thrombocytopenia
tirofiban (Aggrastat)	IV; 0.4 mcg/kg/min for 30 min; then 0.1 mcg/kg/min for 12–24 h	
AGENTS FOR INTERMITTENT CLAUDICATION		
cilostazol (Pletal)	PO; 100 mg bid	*Dyspepsia, nausea, vomiting, dizziness*
pentoxifylline (Trental)	PO; 400 mg tid	Tachycardia and palpitations (cilostazol), CNS effects (pentoxifylline)

Italics indicate common adverse effects; underlining indicates serious adverse effects.

The ADP receptor blockers are a small group of drugs that irreversibly alter the plasma membrane of platelets. This alteration changes the binding of ADP to its receptor on platelets so they are unable to receive the chemical signals required for them to aggregate. Both ticlopidine (Ticlid) and clopidogrel (Plavix) are given orally to prevent thrombi formation in clients who have experienced a recent thromboembolic event such as a stroke or MI. Ticlopidine (Ticlid) can cause life-threatening neutropenia and agranulocytosis. Clopidogrel (Plavix) is much safer, having side effects comparable to those of aspirin.

Glycoprotein IIb/IIIa receptor antagonists are relatively new additions to the treatment of thromboembolic disease. **Glycoprotein IIb/IIIa** is an enzyme necessary for platelet aggregation. These drugs are used to prevent thrombi in clients experiencing a recent MI, stroke, or percutaneous transluminal coronary angioplasty (PTCA). Although these drugs are the most effective antiplatelet agents, they are very expensive. Another major disadvantage is that they can be given only by the IV route.

Intermittent claudication (IC) is a condition caused by lack of sufficient blood flow to skeletal muscles in the lower limbs. Ischemia of skeletal muscles causes severe pain on walking, particularly in the calf muscles. Although some of the therapies for myocardial ischemia are beneficial in treating IC, two drugs are approved *only* for this disorder. Pentoxifylline (Trental) acts on RBCs to reduce their viscosity and increase their flexibility, thus allowing them to enter vessels that are partially occluded and reduce hypoxia and pain in the muscle. Pentoxifylline also has antiplatelet action and is sometimes classified as a hemorheological drug. Cilostazol (Pletal) inhibits platelet aggregation and promotes vasodilation, which brings additional blood to ischemic muscles. Both drugs are given orally and show only modest improvement in IC symptoms. Exercise and therapeutic lifestyle changes are necessary for maximum benefit.

NURSING CONSIDERATIONS

The role of the nurse in antiplatelet therapy for thrombotic and thromboembolic disorders involves careful monitoring of a client's condition and providing education as it relates to the prescribed drug treatment. Drugs affecting platelet aggregation increase the risk of bleeding when the client sustains trauma or undergoes medical procedures or surgery. These drugs are sometimes given concurrently with anticoagulants, which further increases bleeding risk. Injection or venipuncture sites will require prolonged direct pressure to control bleeding. Observe the client for ecchymoses, and monitor bleeding time following venipunctures. Bleeding lasting more than 10 minutes may require special medical or nursing interventions, such as suturing or "sandbagging" a large venipuncture site.

AVOIDING MEDICATION ERRORS

A breast-feeding mother develops thrombophlebitis. Warfarin (Coumadin) 2 mg once a day is ordered. What should the nurse question about this order? *See Appendix D for the suggested answer.*

Aspirin (ASA) may cause gastritis or GI bleeding owing to inhibition of prostaglandins in the GI tract (prostaglandins increase bicarbonate and mucous layer production). Aspirin and ticlopidine (Ticlid) may cause nausea and GI upset. Nursing interventions for ASA therapy can be found in "Nursing Process Focus: Clients Receiving NSAID Therapy," page 236 in Chapter 18 ∞.

Lifespan Considerations. Use antiplatelet agents cautiously in premenopausal women and elderly clients, because excessive bleeding may occur.

Client Teaching. Client education as it relates to antiplatelet agents should include the goals of therapy; the reasons for obtaining baseline data such as vital signs, laboratory tests, and the existence of underlying hepatic or renal disorders; and possible drug side effects. Include the following points when teaching clients about antiplatelet agents:

- Avoid strenuous or hazardous activities that could result in bleeding injuries.
- Do not take OTC products containing aspirin unless otherwise directed by a healthcare provider.
- If taking antiplatelet agents concurrently with anticoagulants, be aware that the risk of bleeding is greater.
- Immediately report any bleeding, nosebleeds, excessive menstrual flow, bleeding of the gums, or bruising with minor injury to the skin.

THROMBOLYTICS

Thrombolytics promote fibrinolysis, or clot destruction, by converting plasminogen to plasmin. The enzyme plasmin digests fibrin and breaks down fibrinogen, prothrombin, and other plasma proteins and clotting factors. Unlike the anticoagulants, which can only *prevent* clots, thrombolytics actually *dissolve* the insoluble fibrin within intravascular emboli and thrombi.

27.7 Pharmacotherapy With Thrombolytics

It is often mistakenly believed that the purpose of anticoagulants such as heparin or warfarin (Coumadin) is to dissolve preexisting clots, but this is not the case. A totally different class of drugs is needed for this purpose. The thrombolytics, listed in Table 27.4, are administered for disorders in which an intravascular clot has already formed, such as in acute MI, pulmonary embolism, acute ischemic CVA, and DVT.

The goal of thrombolytic therapy is to quickly restore blood flow to the tissue served by the blocked vessel. Delays in reestablishing circulation may result in ischemia and permanent tissue damage. The therapeutic effect of thrombolytics is greater when they are administered as soon as possible after clot formation occurs, preferably within 4 hours.

Thrombolytics are nonspecific—that is, they will dissolve whatever clots they encounter. Because clotting is a natural and desirable process to prevent excessive bleeding, thrombolytics have a narrow margin of safety between dissolving "normal" and "abnormal" clots. Vital signs must be monitored continuously, and signs of bleeding call for discontinuation of therapy. Because these drugs are rapidly destroyed in the bloodstream, discontinuation of the infusion normally results in the immediate termination of thrombolytic activity. After the clot is successfully dissolved with the thrombolytic, anticoagulant therapy is generally initiated to prevent the re-formation of clots.

Pr PROTOTYPE DRUG | Clopidogrel Bisulfate *(Plavix)* | Antiplatelet Agent

ACTIONS AND USES

Clopidogrel prolongs bleeding time by inhibiting platelet aggregation. Although its only approved use is to reduce the risk of stroke due to thrombi, it may also be given to prevent thrombi formation in clients with coronary artery stents, and to prevent postoperative deep vein thromboses. Because the drug is expensive, it is usually prescribed for clients unable to tolerate aspirin, which has similar anticoagulant activity. It is given orally.

ADMINISTRATION ALERTS

- Tablets should not be crushed or split
- Discontinue drug at least 7 days prior to surgery
- Pregnancy Category B.

PHARMACOKINETICS (PO)

Onset: 1–2 h

Peak: 2 h

Half-life: 8 h

Duration: Unknown

ADVERSE EFFECTS

Clopidogrel has no serious adverse effects. Common side effects are flu-like syndrome, headache, dizziness, and rash or pruritus.

Contraindications: Clopidogrel is contraindicated in clients with active bleeding.

INTERACTIONS

Drug–Drug: Use with anticoagulants or NSAIDs, including aspirin, may increase the risk of bleeding.

Lab Tests: Bleeding time is prolonged.

Herbal/Food: Use with feverfew, ginkgo, ginger or garlic may increase the risk of bleeding.

Treatment of Overdose: In cases of poisoning, platelet transfusions may be necessary to prevent hemorrhage.

 See the Companion Website for a Nursing Process Focus specific to this drug.

TABLE 27.4   Thrombolytics

Drug	Route and Adult Dose (max dose where indicated)	Adverse Effects
alteplase (Activase, TPA)	IV; begin with 60 mg; then infuse 20 mg/h over next 2 h	*Superficial bleeding at injection sites, allergic reactions*
anistreplase (Eminase)	IV; 30 units over 2–5 min	
reteplase (Retavase) (see page 357 for the Prototype Drug box) ∞	IV; 10 units over 2 min; repeat dose in 30 min	<u>Serious internal bleeding, intracranial hemorrhage</u>
streptokinase (Kabikinase)	IV; 250,000–1.5 million units over a short time	
tenecteplase (TNKase)	IV; 30–50 mg infused over 5 sec	

Italics indicate common adverse effects; <u>underlining</u> indicates serious adverse effects.

Since the discovery of streptokinase, the first thrombolytic, there have been a number of ensuing generations of thrombolytics. The newer drugs such as tenecteplase (TNKase) have a more rapid onset and longer duration and are reported to have fewer side effects than older drugs in this class. TPA, marketed as alteplase (Activase), has replaced urokinase as the drug of choice in clearing thrombosed central intravenous lines. Because urokinase was obtained from pooled human donors and had a small risk for being contaminated with viruses, it was removed from the market.

NURSING CONSIDERATIONS

The role of the nurse in thrombolytic therapy involves careful monitoring of a client's condition and providing education as it relates to the prescribed drug treatment.

Thrombolytics are generally administered in the critical care setting or emergency department. First, identify underlying conditions that exclude the client from receiving thrombolytics, such as recent trauma, surgery or biopsies, arterial emboli, recent cerebral embolism, hemorrhage, thrombocytopenia, septic thrombophlebitis, or childbirth (within 10 days). Obtain baseline coagulation tests (aPTT, bleeding time, PT, and/or INR) prior to therapy. Obtain baseline hematocrit, hemoglobin, and platelet counts to compare with later values and assess for bleeding. Cerebral hemorrhage is a major concern; thus, assess for changes in level of consciousness and check neurological status. When giving thrombolytics following an MI, observe for dysrhythmias that may occur, because these drugs reestablish cardiac tissue perfusion. Do not give these drugs by IM injections because of the risk of bleeding.

Pr **PROTOTYPE DRUG** | Alteplase *(Activase)* | Thrombolytic

ACTIONS AND USES

Produced through recombinant DNA technology, alteplase is identical with the enzyme human tissue plasminogen activator (TPA). As with other thrombolytics, the primary action of alteplase is to convert plasminogen to plasmin, which then dissolves fibrin clots. To achieve maximum effect, therapy should begin immediately after the onset of symptoms. Alteplase does not exhibit the allergic reactions seen with streptokinase. An off-label use is for restoration of patency of IV catheters.

ADMINISTRATION ALERTS

- Drug must be given within 6 hours of onset of symptoms of MI and within 3 hours of thrombotic CVA for maximum effectiveness.
- Avoid parenteral injections during alteplase infusion to decrease risk of bleeding.
- Pregnancy category C.

PHARMACOKINETICS

Onset: Immediate

Peak: 5–10 min after infusion is discontinued

Half-life: 30 min

Duration: 3 h

ADVERSE EFFECTS

The most common side effect of alteplase is bleeding, which may occur superficially or internally. Intracranial bleeding is a rare, though possible, adverse effect. Signs of bleeding such as spontaneous ecchymoses, hematomas, or epistaxis should immediately be reported to the healthcare provider.

Contraindications: Active internal bleeding, history of CVA within the past 2 months, recent trauma or surgery, severe uncontrolled hypertension, intracranial neoplasm, or arteriovenous malformation.

INTERACTIONS

Drug–Drug: Concurrent use with anticoagulants, antiplatelet agents or NSAIDs, including aspirin, may increase the risk of bleeding.

Lab Tests: Alteplase will increase PT and aPTT.

Herbal/Food: Herbal supplements such as ginkgo may increase the risk of bleeding.

Treatment of Overdose: There is no specific treatment for overdose.

 See the Companion Website for a Nursing Process Focus specific to this drug.

NURSING PROCESS FOCUS Clients Receiving Thrombolytic Therapy

Assessment	Potential Nursing Diagnoses
Prior to administration: ■ Obtain a complete health history including recent surgeries or trauma, allergies, drug history, and possible drug interactions. ■ Obtain vital signs and assess in context of client's baseline values. ■ Assess lab values: aPTT, PT, hemoglobin (Hgb), hematocrit (Hct), platelet count.	■ Injury, Risk for (bleeding), related to adverse effects of thrombolytic therapy ■ Tissue Perfusion, Ineffective, related to increase in size of thrombus due to ineffective thrombolytic therapy ■ Knowledge, Deficient, related to drug therapy

Planning: Client Goals and Expected Outcomes

The client will:
■ Experience preexisting blood clot(s) dissolution as evidenced by laboratory values.
■ Demonstrate an understanding of the drug's action by accurately describing drug side effects and precautions.

Implementation

Interventions and (Rationales)	Client Education/Discharge Planning
■ If necessary, start IV lines, arterial line, or Foley catheter prior to beginning therapy. (This decreases the risk of bleeding from those sites).	■ Instruct client about procedures and their necessity prior to beginning thrombolytic therapy.
■ Monitor vital signs every 15 minutes during first hour of infusion, and then every 30 minutes during remainder of infusion. (Changes in vital signs may indicate bleeding.)	■ Instruct client that frequent vital signs must be taken.
■ Move client as little as possible during the infusion. (This is done to prevent internal injury.)	■ Instruct client that activity will be limited during infusion, and that pressure dressing may be needed to prevent any active bleeding.
■ If given for thrombotic CVA, monitor neurological status frequently. (A change in neurological status could indicate increased intercranial pressure.)	■ Advise client about assessments and why they are necessary.
■ Monitor cardiac response while medication is infusing. (Dysrhythmias may occur with reperfusion of myocardium.)	■ Advise client that cardiac rhythm will be monitored during therapy.
■ Monitor blood tests (Hct, Hgb, platelet counts) for indications of blood loss due to internal bleeding. (The client has an increased risk of bleeding for 2 to 4 days postinfusion.)	■ Instruct client about increased risk for bleeding, activity restriction, and frequent monitoring during this time.

Evaluation of Outcome Criteria

Evaluate the effectiveness of drug therapy by confirming that client goals and expected outcomes have been met (see "Planning").
■ The client's laboratory values reflect that preexisting blood clots have dissolved.
■ The client demonstrates an understanding of the drug's actions by accurately describing drug side effects and precautions.

∞ *See Table 27.4 for a list of drugs to which these nursing actions apply.*

Be aware that these drugs are given in acute situations when time for client teaching may be limited and the client may be unable to focus on information related to the stress of the situation.

Client Teaching.   Client education as it relates to thrombolytic therapy should include the goals of therapy; the reasons for obtaining baseline data such as vital signs, laboratory values, and the existence of underlying disorders (recent trauma, recent cerebral embolism, hemorrhage, thrombocytopenia, or recent childbirth); and possible drug side effects. Include the following points when teaching clients about thrombolytics:

• There is an increased risk for bleeding with thrombolytic agents. Immediately report nosebleeds, excessive

menstrual flow, bleeding of the gums, or bruising with minor injury to the skin.

• Avoid strenuous or hazardous activities that could result in bleeding injuries.

• Expect vital signs to be taken and assessments to be made frequently to identify potential complications.

HEMOSTATICS

Hemostatics, also called *antifibrinolytics,* have an action opposite that of anticoagulants: they shorten bleeding time. The class name *hemostatics* comes from the durgs' ability to slow blood flow. They are used to prevent excessive bleeding following surgery.

> **Pr PROTOTYPE DRUG | Aminocaproic Acid (Amicar) | Hemostatic**
>
> ### ACTIONS AND USES
>
> Aminocaproic acid acts by inactivating plasminogen, the precursor of the enzyme plasmin that digests the fibrin clot. Aminocaproic acid is prescribed in situations in which there is excessive bleeding because clots are being dissolved prematurely. During acute hemorrhages, the drug can be given IV to reduce bleeding in 1 to 2 hours. It is also available in tablet form. It is most commonly prescribed following surgery to reduce postoperative bleeding. The therapeutic serum level is 100–400 mcg/ml.
>
> ### ADMINISTRATION ALERTS
>
> - May cause hypotension and bradycardia when given IV. Assess vital signs frequently and place client on cardiac monitor to assess for dysrhythmias.
> - Pregnancy category C.
>
> > **PHARMACOKINETICS (PO)**
> >
> > **Onset:** Unknown
> >
> > **Peak:** 2 h
> >
> > **Half-life:** Unknown
> >
> > **Duration:** Unknown
>
> ### ADVERSE EFFECTS
>
> Because aminocaproic acid tends to stabilize clots, it should be used cautiously in clients with a history of thromboembolic disease. Side effects are generally mild.
>
> **Contraindications:** Aminocaproic acid is contraindicated in clients with disseminated intravascular clotting or severe renal impairment.
>
> ### INTERACTIONS
>
> **Drug–Drug:** Hypercoagulation may occur with concurrent use of estrogens and oral contraceptives.
>
> **Lab Tests:** Unknown.
>
> **Herbal/Food:** Unknown.
>
> **Treatment of Overdose:** There is no treatment for overdose.
>
> *See the Companion Website for a Nursing Process Focus specific to this drug.*

27.8 Pharmacotherapy With Hemostatics

The final class of coagulation modifiers, the hemostatics, is a small group of drugs used to prevent and treat excessive bleeding from surgical sites. All the hemostatics have very specific indications for use, and none are commonly prescribed. Although their mechanisms differ, all drugs in this class prevent fibrin from dissolving, thus enhancing the stability of the clot. The hemostatics are listed in Table 27.5.

NURSING CONSIDERATIONS

The role of the nurse in hemostatic drug therapy for bleeding disorders involves careful monitoring of a client's condition and providing education as it relates to the prescribed drug treatment. Assess the client for clotting. Changes in peripheral pulses, paresthesias, positive Homans' sign, and prominence of superficial veins indicate clotting in peripheral arterial or venous vasculature. Chest pain and shortness of breath may indicate pulmonary thrombus or embolus. Use is contraindicated in clients with disseminated intravascular clotting and severe renal impairment.

Administer hemostatic agents intravenously. Frequently monitor injection sites for thrombophlebitis and extravasation. These drugs may affect the muscles, causing wasting and weakness. Identify and report the presence of myopathy and myoglobinuria, which manifests as reddish brown urine.

Client Teaching. Client education as it relates to hemostatic agents should include the goals of therapy; the reasons for obtaining baseline data such as vital signs, diagnostic procedures, laboratory tests, and the existence of underlying disorders; and possible drug side effects. Include the following points when teaching clients about hemostatic agents:

- Immediately report renewed bleeding episodes.
- Avoid the use of aspirin or OTC medications containing aspirin.

TABLE 27.5 Hemostatics		
Drug	**Route and Adult Dose (max dose where indicated)**	**Adverse Effects**
Pr aminocaproic acid (Amicar)	IV; 4–5 g for 1 h, then 1–1.25 g/h until bleeding is controlled	*Allergic skin reactions, headache*
aprotinin (Trasylol)	IV; 1 ml (10,000 Kallikrein inactivator units [KIU]) as a test dose; then 500,000 KIV/h unit client leaves OR	<u>Anaphylaxis, thrombosis. bronchospasm, nephrotoxicity</u>
tranexamic acid (Cyklokapron)	PO; 25 mg/kg qid	

Italics indicate common adverse effects; <u>underlining</u> indicates serious adverse effects.

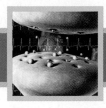

CHAPTER REVIEW

KEY CONCEPTS

The numbered key concepts provide a succinct summary of the important points from the corresponding numbered section within the chapter. If any of these points are not clear, refer to the numbered section within the chapter for review.

27.1 Hemostasis is a complex process involving multiple steps and a large number of enzymes and clotting factors. The final product is a fibrin clot that stops blood loss.

27.2 Fibrinolysis, or removal of a blood clot, is an enzymatic process initiated by the release of TPA. Plasmin digests the fibrin strands, thus restoring circulation to the injured area.

27.3 Diseases of hemostasis include thromboembolic disorders caused by thrombi and emboli, thrombocytopenia, and bleeding disorders such as hemophilia and von Willebrand's disease.

27.4 The normal coagulation process can be modified by a number of different mechanisms, including inhibiting specific clotting factors, dissolving fibrin, and inhibiting platelet function.

27.5 Anticoagulants are used to prevent thrombi from forming or enlarging. The primary drugs in this category are heparin (parenteral) and warfarin (oral), although low-molecular-weight heparins and thrombin inhibitors are also available.

27.6 Several drugs prolong bleeding time by interfering with the aggregation of platelets. Antiplatelet drugs include aspirin, ADP blockers, glycoprotein IIb/IIIa receptor antagonists, and miscellaneous agents for treating intermittent claudication.

27.7 Thrombolytics are used to dissolve existing intravascular clots in clients with MI or CVA.

27.8 Hemostatics or antifibrinolytics are used to promote the formation of clots in clients with excessive bleeding from surgical sites.

NCLEX-RN® REVIEW QUESTIONS

1 The nurse's understanding of the clotting mechanism is important in administering anticoagulant drugs. The nurse understands that which of the following clotting factors are formed after injury to the vessels?

1. Fibrin, vitamin K
2. Thromboplastin, fibrinogen
3. Prothrombin, thrombin
4. Thrombin, fibrin

2 The client receiving heparin therapy asks how the "blood thinner" works. The best response by the nurse would be:

1. "Heparin makes the blood less viscous."
2. "Heparin does not thin the blood but prevents platelets from clumping."
3. "Heparin decreases the number of platelets so that blood clots more slowly."
4. "Heparin dissolves the clot."

3 Nursing interventions for a client receiving enoxaparin (Lovenox) may include (select all that apply):

1. Teaching the client or family to give subcutaneous injections at home.
2. Teaching the client or family not to take any OTC drugs without first consulting with the healthcare provider.
3. Teaching the client to observe for unexplained bleeding such as pink, red, or dark brown urine or bloody gums.
4. Teaching the client to monitor for the development of DVT.
5. Teaching the importance of drinking grapefruit juice daily.

4 The nurse receives the client's lab values throughout warfarin drug therapy. The expected therapeutic level is:

1. aPTT of 25 to 40 seconds.
2. aPTT one to two times the client's baseline level.
3. PT one to two times the client's baseline.
4. INR of 0.5 to 1.5.

5 A patient is receiving a thrombolytic agent, alteplase (Activase), following an acute myocardial infarction. Which condition is most likely attributed to thrombolytic therapy with this agent?

1. Skin rash with urticaria
2. Wheezing with labored respiratons
3. Bruising and epistaxis
4. Temperature elevation of 100.8 °F

CRITICAL THINKING QUESTIONS

1. The nurse is working on a medical unit in which a client suddenly develops left-sided weakness and garbled speech. The nurse calls the healthcare provider, who diagnoses the client with a CVA and orders heparin 5,000 units IV and a heparin drip to run at 1,000 units per hour. What should the nurse do?

2. A client has had an acute MI and has received alteplase (Activase) to lyse the clot. What nursing actions should have been taken prior to administering the medication to the client?

3. A client is receiving enoxaparin subcutaneously after being diagnosed with thrombophlebitis. What precautions should be taken when giving this medication?

See Appendix D for answers and rationales for all activities.

EXPLORE MediaLink

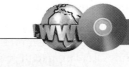

www.prenhall.com/adams

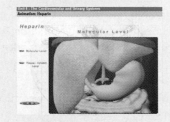

NCLEX-RN® review, case studies, and other interactive resources for this chapter can be found on the companion website at www.prenhall.com/adams. Click on "Chapter 27" to select the activities for this chapter. For animations, more NCLEX-RN® review questions, and an audio glossary, access the accompanying Prentice Hall Nursing MediaLink DVD-ROM in this textbook.

PRENTICE HALL NURSING MEDIA LINK DVD-ROM

- **Animations**
  Mechanism in Action: Warfarin (*Coumadin*)
  Mechanism in Action: Heparin (*Heplock*)
- **Audio Glossary**
- **NCLEX-RN® Review**

COMPANION WEBSITE

- **NCLEX-RN® Review**
- **Dosage Calculations**
- **Case Study:** Client taking anticoagulants
- **Care Plan:** Client taking warfarin after deep vein thrombosis

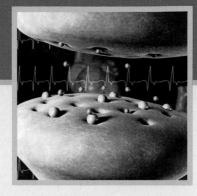

CHAPTER 28

Drugs for Hematopoietic Disorders

DRUGS AT A GLANCE

HEMATOPOIETIC GROWTH FACTORS

Erythropoietin
- *epoetin alfa (Epogen, Procrit)*

Colony-stimulating Factors
- *filgrastim (Neupogen)*

Platelet Enhancers

ANTIANEMIC AGENTS
- *cyanocobalamin (Crystamine, others): vitamin B₁₂*

Folic Acid

Iron Salts
- *ferrous sulfate (Feosol, others)*

OBJECTIVES

After reading this chapter, the student should be able to:

1. Describe the process of hematopoiesis.
2. Explain how hematopoiesis is regulated.
3. Explain why hematopoietic agents are often administered to clients following chemotherapy or organ transplant.
4. Identify the method by which colony-stimulating factors are named.
5. Classify types of anemia based on their causes.
6. Identify the role of intrinsic factor in the absorption of vitamin B_{12}.
7. Compare and contrast anemias caused by vitamin B_{12} and folate deficiency.
8. Describe the metabolism, storage, and transfer of iron in the body.
9. Describe the nurse's role in the pharmacological management of hematopoietic disorders.
10. For each of the drug classes listed in Drugs at a Glance, know representative drugs, and explain their mechanism of drug action, primary actions, and important adverse effects.
11. Categorize drugs used in the treatment of hematopoietic disorders based on their classification and mechanism of action.
12. Use the Nursing Process to care for clients who are receiving drug therapy for hematopoietic disorders.

MediaLink

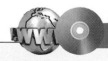

www.prenhall.com/adams

NCLEX-RN® review, case studies, and other interactive resources for this chapter can be found on the companion website at www.prenhall.com/adams. Click on "Chapter 28" to select the activities for this chapter. For animations, more NCLEX-RN® review questions, and an audio glossary, access the accompanying Prentice Hall Nursing MediaLink DVD-ROM in this textbook.

KEY TERMS

anemia *page 401*

colony-stimulating factor (CSF) *page 398*

erythropoietin *page 395*

ferritin *page 403*

folic acid/folate *page 402*

hematopoiesis *page 394*

hemosiderin *page 403*

intrinsic factor *page 401*

pernicious (megaloblastic) anemia *page 402*

stem cell *page 394*

thrombopoietin *page 399*

transferrin *page 403*

The blood serves all other cells in the body and is the only fluid tissue. Because of its diverse functions, diseases affecting blood constituents have widespread effects on the body. Correspondingly, drugs for treating blood disorders will affect cells in many different tissues. Pharmacology of the hematopoietic system is a small, though emerging, branch of medicine.

28.1 Hematopoiesis

Blood is a highly dynamic tissue; more than 200 billion new blood cells are formed every day. The process of blood cell formation is called **hematopoiesis,** or hemopoiesis. Hematopoiesis occurs primarily in red bone marrow and requires B vitamins, vitamin C, copper, iron, and other nutrients.

Hematopoiesis is responsive to the demands of the body. For example, the production of white blood cells can increase to 10 times the normal number in response to infection. The number of red blood cells can increase as much as 5 times normal in response to anemia or hypoxia. Homeostatic control of hematopoiesis is influenced by a number of hormones and growth factors, which allow for points of pharmacological intervention. The process of hematopoiesis is illustrated in ● Figure 28.1.

The process of hematopoiesis begins with a **stem cell,** which is capable of maturing into any type of blood cell. The specific path taken by the stem cell, whether it becomes an erythrocyte, leukocyte, or platelet, depends on the internal needs of

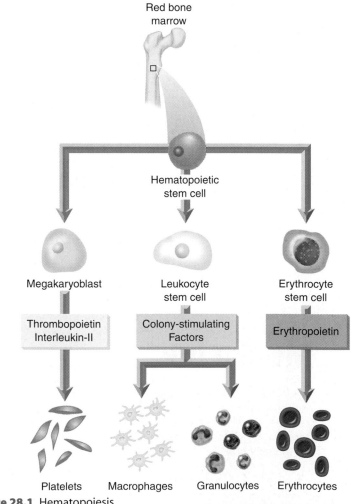

●**Figure 28.1** Hematopoiesis

the body. Regulation of hematopoiesis occurs through messages from hormones such as erythropoietin, chemicals secreted by leukocytes known as colony-stimulating factors, and other circulating substances. Through recombinant DNA technology, some of these growth agents are now available in sufficient quantity to be used as medications.

HEMATOPOIETIC GROWTH FACTORS

Natural hormones that promote some aspect of blood formation are called *hematopoietic growth factors*. Several growth factors, shown in Table 28.1, are used pharmacologically to stimulate erythrocyte, leukocyte, or platelet production.

HUMAN ERYTHROPOIETIN AND RELATED DRUGS

28.2 Pharmacotherapy With Erythropoietin

The process of red blood cell formation, or *erythropoiesis*, is regulated primarily by the hormone **erythropoietin.** Secreted by the kidney, erythropoietin travels to the bone marrow, where it interacts with receptors on hematopoietic stem cells with the message to increase erythrocyte production. Erythropoietin also stimulates the production of hemoglobin, which is required for a functional erythrocyte. The primary signal for the increased secretion of erythropoietin is a reduction in oxygen reaching the kidneys. Serum levels of erythropoietin may increase as much as 1,000-fold in response to severe hypoxia. Hemorrhage, chronic obstructive pulmonary disease, anemia, or high altitudes may cause this hypoxia. Erythropoietin is marketed as epoetin alfa (Epogen, Procrit).

Darbepoetin alfa (Aranesp) is a newer agent that is closely related to epoetin alfa. It has the same pharmacological action, efficacy, and safety profile; however, it has an extended duration of action that allows it to be administered once weekly. Darbepoietin alfa is approved for the treatment of anemia associated with chemotherapy or chronic renal failure.

NURSING CONSIDERATIONS

The role of the nurse in erythropoietin therapy involves careful monitoring of a client's condition and providing education as it relates to the prescribed drug treatment.

TABLE 28.1 Hematopoietic Growth Factors

Drug	Route and Adult Dose (max dose where indicated)	Adverse Effects
epoetin alfa (Epogen): erythropoietin	Subcutaneous/IV; 3–500 units/kg/dose 3 times/wk, usually starting with 50–100 units/kg/dose until target Hct range of 30%–33% (max: 36%) is reached. Hct should not increase by more than 4 points in any 2-week period.	*Headache, fever, nausea, diarrhea and edema* Hypertension, seizures
darbepoetin alfa (Aranesp)	Subcutaneous/IV; 0.45 mcg/kg once per wk	
COLONY-STIMULATING FACTORS		
filgrastim (Neupogen): granulocyte-CSF	IV; 5 mcg/kg/day by 30-min infusion, may increase by 5 mcg/kg/day (max: 30 mcg/kg/day); 5 mcg/kg/day subcutaneous as single dose, may increase by 5 mcg/kg/day (max: 20 mcg/kg/day)	*Flulike syndrome, fever, dyspnea* Bone pain, arthralgia, thrombocytopenia, pericardial effusion (sargramostim)
pegfilgrastim (Neulasta)	Subcutaneous; 6 mg once per chemotherapy cycle at least 24 h after chemotherapy	
sargramostim (Leukine): granulocyte-macrophage-CSF	IV; 250 mcg/m²/day infused over 2 h for 21 days, begin 2–4 h after bone marrow transfusion and not less than 24 h after last dose of chemotherapy or 12 h after last radiation therapy	
PLATELET ENHANCER		
oprelvekin (Neumega)	Subcutaneous; 50 mcg/kg once daily starting 6–24 h after completing chemotherapy	*Edema, fever, headache, dizziness, dyspnea, rash, nausea, vomiting* Tachycardia, dysrhythmias

Italics indicate common adverse effects; underlining indicates serious adverse effects.

Pr PROTOTYPE DRUG | Epoetin Alfa *(Epogen, Procrit)* | Hematopoietic Growth Factor

ACTIONS AND USES

Epoetin alfa is made through recombinant DNA technology and is functionally identical to human erythropoietin. Because of its ability to stimulate erythropoiesis, epoetin alfa is effective in treating disorders caused by a deficiency in red blood cell formation. Clients with chronic renal failure often cannot secrete enough endogenous erythropoietin, and benefit from epoetin administration. Epoetin is sometimes given to clients undergoing cancer chemotherapy to counteract the anemia caused by antineoplastic agents. It is occasionally prescribed for clients prior to blood transfusions or surgery, and to treat anemia in HIV-infected clients. Epoetin alfa is usually administered 3 times per week until a therapeutic response is achieved.

ADMINISTRATION ALERTS

- The subcutaneous route is generally preferred over IV, since lower doses are needed and absorption is slower.
- Do not shake vial, because this may deactivate the drug. Visibly inspect solution for particulate matter.
- Pregnancy category C.

PHARMACOKINETICS (SUBCUTANEOUS)

Onset: 7–14 days

Peak: Unknown

Half-life: 413 h

Duration: Unknown

ADVERSE EFFECTS

The most serious adverse effect of epoetin alfa is hypertension, which may occur in as many as 30% of clients receiving the drug. An antihypertensive drug may be indicated. The risk of thromboembolic events is increased. Common side effects include headache, fever, nausea, diarrhea, and edema.

Clients who are on dialysis may require increased doses of heparin. Transient ischemic attacks (TIAs), heart attacks, and strokes have occurred in chronic renal failure clients on dialysis who are being treated with epoetin alfa.

The effectiveness of epoetin alfa will be greatly reduced in clients with iron deficiency or other vitamin-depleted states. Most clients receive iron supplements during therapy to compensate for the increased red blood cell production.

Contraindications: Contraindications include uncontrolled hypertension, and known hypersensitivity to mammalian cell products.

INTERACTIONS

Drug–Drug: There are no clinically significant drug interactions with epoetin alfa.

Lab Tests: Unknown.

Herbal/Food: Unknown.

Treatment of Overdose: Overdose may lead to polycythemia (too many erythrocytes), which can be corrected by phlebotomy.

Hematopoietic growth factors are used to stimulate erythrocyte, leukocyte, or platelet production. Epoetin alfa (Epogen, Procrit) may be prescribed to treat complications of disease processes such as cancer, AIDS, and chronic renal failure.

Although epoetin alfa does not cure the primary disease condition, it helps reduce the anemia that dramatically affects the client's ability to perform daily activities. Assess for food or drug allergies, because epoetin alfa is contraindicated in individuals who are hypersensitive to many protein-based products. Also assess for a history of uncontrolled hypertension, because the drug can raise blood pressure to dangerous levels. Obtain baseline laboratory tests, especially a CBC, and vital signs. Hematocrit and hemoglobin levels provide indicators for evaluating the drug's effectiveness.

Because this drug increases the risk of thromboembolic disease, monitor the client for early signs of stroke or heart attack. Clients on dialysis are at higher risk for TIA, stroke, and MI and may need increased doses of heparin while receiving epoetin alfa. Monitor for side effects such as nausea and vomiting, constipation, medication site reaction, and headache.

Lifespan Considerations. Premature infants are sensitive to benzyl alcohol, which may be present in multidose formulations of epoetin alfa. Premature infants must be given the preservative-free formulation to prevent "fetal gasping" syndrome. Epoetin alfa should be used with caution in pregnant and lactating clients (pregnancy category C).

Client Teaching. Client education as it relates to erythropoietin should include the goals of therapy, the reasons for obtaining baseline data such as vital signs and the existence of underlying cardiac and hepatic disorders and allergies, and possible drug side effects. Include the following points when teaching clients about hematopoietic growth factors:

- Monitor blood pressure daily during drug therapy.
- Keep all scheduled laboratory appointments for hematologic studies.

HOME & COMMUNITY CONSIDERATIONS

Treating Clients With Hematopoietic Disorders

Clients treated for hematopoietic disorders are frequently managed outside the hospital setting. Care may be provided by the client and in many instances family members and other caregivers. However, factors that have led to the need for this therapy may limit the client's ability to assume this responsibilty, especially during initial therapy. Children are commonly affected by these disorders; therefore, care must be provided by parents. The nurse should assure that adequate teaching is provided to the client and caregivers for safe administration of medications as well as detection and reporting of side effects and adverse reactions. The nurse visiting the client in a home-care setting should obtain a complete medical history, including an evaluation of the client and/or caregiver's understanding of the treatment requirements. Assessment of the client's response to treatment is essential at each home visit or return to the medical office. Appropriate nursing interventions should be implemented to ensure client needs are met. Effective communication among the nurse, client, caregivers, physician, and other healthcare providers is vital to providing optimal care of clients receiving hematopoietic therapy.

NURSING PROCESS FOCUS   Clients Receiving Epoetin Alfa

Assessment	Potential Nursing Diagnoses
Prior to administration: ▪ Obtain complete health history including allergies, drug history, and possible drug reactions. ▪ Assess reason for drug administration such as presence/history of anemia secondary to chronic renal failure, malignancy, chemotherapy, autologous blood donation, and HIV-infected clients treated with zidovudine. ▪ Assess vital signs, especially blood pressure. ▪ Assess complete blood count, specifically hematocrit and hemoglobin levels, to establish baseline values.	▪ Tissue Perfusion, Ineffective, related to ineffective response to drug ▪ Injury, (weakness, dizziness, syncope), Risk for, related to anemia ▪ Injury, Risk for, related to seizure activity secondary to drug ▪ Activity Intolerance, related to RBC deficiency ▪ Knowledge, Deficient, related to drug therapy

Planning: Client Goals and Expected Outcomes

The client will:

▪ Exhibit an increase in hematocrit level and improvement in anemia-related symptoms.

▪ Immediately report severe headache, chest pain, confusion, numbness, or loss of movement in an extremity.

▪ Demonstrate an understanding of the drug's action by accurately describing drug side effects and precautions.

Implementation

Interventions and (Rationales)	Client Education/Discharge Planning
▪ Monitor vital signs, especially blood pressure. (The rate of hypertension is directly related to the rate of rise of the hematocrit. Clients who have existing hypertension are at higher risk for stroke and seizures. Hypertension is also much more likely in clients with chronic renal failure.)	▪ Instruct client to periodically monitor blood pressure using proper monitoring equipment. Consistent increases in blood pressure should be reported immediately.
▪ Monitor for side effects, especially symptoms of neurological or cardiovascular events. (Headache, seizures, and hypertension have been related to drug usage.)	▪ Instruct client to report side effects such as nausea, vomiting, constipation, redness/pain at injection site, confusion, numbness, chest pain, and difficulty breathing.
▪ Monitor client's ability to self-administer medication. (Inability to self-administer medication requires the nurse to arrange for someone else to administer the medication.)	▪ Instruct client in the technique for subcutaneous injection if client is to self-administer the medication, and on the proper disposal of needles and syringes.
▪ Monitor laboratory values such as hematocrit and hemoglobin to evaluate effectiveness of treatment. (Increases in hematocrit and hemoglobin values indicate increased RBC production.)	▪ Instruct client to keep all laboratory appointments for testing and to adjust activities according to the latest hematocrit value.
▪ Monitor client for signs of seizure activity. (Seizures result in a rapid rise in the hematocrit—especially during first 90 days of treatment.)	▪ Instruct client to avoid driving or performing hazardous activities until the effects of the drug are known.
▪ Monitor client for signs of thrombus such as swelling, warmth, and pain in an extremity. (As hematocrit rises, there is an increased chance of thrombus formation, particularly for clients with chronic renal failure.)	Instruct client to: ▪ Report any increase in size, pain, and/or warmth in an extremity. ▪ Monitor for signs and symptoms of blood clots. ▪ Avoid rubbing or massaging calves and to report leg discomfort.
▪ Monitor dietary intake. Ensure adequate intake of all essential nutrients. (Response to this medication is minimal if blood levels of iron, folic acid, and vitamin B_{12} are deficient.)	Instruct client to: ▪ Maintain adequate dietary intake of essential vitamins and nutrients. ▪ Continue to follow necessary dietary restrictions if receiving renal dialysis.

Evaluation of Outcome Criteria

Evaluate the effectiveness of drug therapy by confirming that client goals and expected outcomes have been met (see "Planning").

▪ The client exhibits an increase in hematocrit level and improvement in anemia-related symptoms.

▪ The client reports severe headache, chest pain, confusion, numbness, or loss of movement in an extremity.

▪ The client demonstrates an understanding of the drug's action by accurately describing drug side effects and precautions.

- Use proper subcutaneous injection techniques if self-administering the medication.

- Immediately report if you experience nausea, vomiting, constipation, redness or pain at injection site, confusion, numbness, chest pain, or difficulty breathing.

- Maintain adequate dietary intake of essential vitamins and nutrients.

COLONY-STIMULATING FACTORS

Colony-stimulating factors are natural substances that stimulate the production of blood cells. Several have application to pharmacotherapy.

28.3 Pharmacotherapy With Colony-stimulating Factors

Control of white blood cell (WBC) production, or *leukopoiesis,* is more complicated than erythropoiesis because of the many different types of leukocytes in the blood. The two basic categories of WBC growth factors are interleukins and **colony-stimulating factors (CSFs).** Because the primary action of the interleukins is to modulate the immune system rather than enhance leukopoiesis, they are presented in Chapter 32 ∞. One interleukin stimulates the production of platelets and is discussed in Section 28.4.

The colony-stimulating factors are active at very low concentrations. It is believed that each stem cell stimulated by these growth factors is capable of producing as many as 1,000 mature leukocytes. The growth factors not only increase the production of leukocytes but also activate existing white blood cells. Examples of enhanced functions include increased migration of leukocytes to antigens, increased antibody toxicity, and increased phagocytosis.

CSFs are named according to the types of blood cells that they stimulate. For example, granulocyte colony-stimulating factor (G-CSF) increases the production of neutrophils, the most common type of granulocyte. Granulocyte/macrophage colony-stimulating factor (GM-CSF) stimulates both neutrophil and macrophage production. The process of identifying the many endogenous CSFs, determining their normal functions, and discovering their potential value as therapeutic agents is an emerging area of pharmacology.

Made through recombinant DNA technology, several CSFs are now available as medications. The goal of CSF therapy is to produce a rapid increase in the number of neutrophils in clients who have suppressed immune systems (neutropenia). CSF therapy shortens the length of time clients are susceptible to life-threatening infections. Indications include clients undergoing chemotherapy or receiving transplants, or who have certain malignancies.

Filgrastim (Neupogen) is similar to natural G-CSF and is primarily used for chronic neutropenia or neutropenia secondary to chemotherapy. Pegfilgrastim (Neulasta) is a form of filgrastim with a molecule of polyethylene glycol (PEG) attached. The PEG decreases the renal excretion of the molecule, allowing it to remain in the body with a sustained

duration of action. Sargramostim (Leukine) is similar to natural GM-CSF and is used to treat neutropenia in clients treated for acute myelogenous leukemia, and clients who are having autologous bone marrow transplantation. Doses for these agents are given in Table 28.1.

NURSING CONSIDERATIONS

The role of the nurse in colony-stimulating factor (CSF) therapy involves careful monitoring of a client's condition and providing education as it relates to the prescribed drug treatment. Obtain a health history, especially checking for myeloid cancers such as leukemia, because filgrastim (Neupogen) may stimulate proliferation of these malignant cells. Prior to administration of filgrastim, assess for hypersensitivity to certain foreign proteins, specifically those in *Escherichia coli.* Because of filgrastim's structural components, the drug is contraindicated in clients with this type of hypersensitivity. Do not administer this drug simultaneously with chemotherapy. Obtain a baseline CBC with differential and platelet count to evaluate drug effectiveness. Use of filgrastim may cause dysrhythmias and tachycardia; therefore, perform a thorough initial and ongoing cardiac assessment.

Assess for hypertension and skeletal pain, which are adverse effects of filgrastim therapy. Monitor ECG readings for abnormal ST-segment depression, which is also a side effect of the drug. See "Nursing Process Focus: Clients Receiving Filgrastim" for further details on this drug.

Prior to administering sargramostim (Leukine), review results of the CBC. This drug is contraindicated when excessive leukemic myeloid blasts are present in blood or bone marrow. Obtain a health history, specifically for any known hypersensitivity to GM-CSF or yeast products. Use sargramostim cautiously in clients with cardiac disease such as dysrhythmias or HF, because this agent may cause supraventricular dysrhythmias. This is usually a temporary side effect that disappears when the drug is discontinued. Use the drug with caution in clients with kidney and liver impairment.

It is often difficult to assess the adverse effects of CSF medications because the symptoms may be attributed to the chemotherapy or to the disease itself. A serious side effect of sargramostim is respiratory distress that occurs during the IV infusion the first time the drug is administered. This appears to be related to the trapping of granulocytes in the pulmonary circulation. The client develops difficulty breathing, tachycardia, low blood pressure, and light-headedness. If these symptoms occur, notify the physician and follow protocol related to continuing the infusion.

Client Teaching. Client education as it relates to CSF therapy should include the goals of therapy, the reasons for obtaining baseline data such as vital signs and the existence of underlying cardiac and malignant disorders or allergies, and possible drug side effects. Include the following points when teaching clients about CSF therapy:

- Wash hands frequently.

- Avoid people with infections such as colds and flu.

Pr **PROTOTYPE DRUG** | Filgrastim *(Neupogen)* | Colony-stimulating Factor

ACTIONS AND USES

Filgrastim is human G-CSF produced through recombinant DNA technology. Its two primary actions are to increase neutrophil production in the bone marrow and to enhance the phagocytic and cytotoxic functions of existing neutrophils. This is particularly important for clients with neutropenia, a reduction in circulating neutrophils that often results in severe bacterial and fungal infections. Administration of filgrastim will shorten the length of neutropenia in cancer clients whose bone marrow has been suppressed by antineoplastic agents or in clients following organ transplants. It may also be used in clients with AIDS-related immunosuppression. It is administered subcutaneously or by slow IV infusion.

ADMINISTRATION ALERTS

- Do not administer within 24 hours before or after chemotherapy with cytotoxic agents because this will greatly decrease the effectiveness of filgrastim.
- Pregnancy category C.

PHARMACOKINETICS (SUBCUTANEOUS)

Onset: 4 h

Peak: 2–8 h

Half-life: 1.4–7.2 h

Duration: 1 wk

ADVERSE EFFECTS

Bone pain is a common side effect of high-dose filgrastim therapy. A small percentage of clients may develop an allergic reaction. Frequent laboratory tests are conducted to ensure that excessive numbers of neutrophils, or leukocytosis, does not occur.

Contraindications: The only contraindication is hypersensitivity to *E. coli* proteins.

INTERACTIONS

Drug–Drug: Because antineoplastic drugs and colony-stimulating factors produce opposite effects, filgrastim is not administered until at least 24 hours after a chemotherapy session.

Lab Tests: Values for the following may be increased: leukocyte alkaline phosphatase, serum alkaline phosphatase, uric acid, and LDH.

Herbal/Food: Unknown.

Treatment of Overdose: There is no treatment for overdose.

- Immediately report chest pain or palpitations, respiratory difficulty, nausea, vomiting, fever, chills, and malaise.
- Keep all scheduled physician and laboratory testing appointments.
- Immediately report if bone pain does not respond to prescribed medications.
- Use proper injection techniques if self-administering this medication.

PLATELET ENHANCERS

Patients with anemia can often benefit from drugs that enhance platelet production or function. A few drugs have been developed for this function.

28.4 Pharmacotherapy With Platelet Enhancers

The production of platelets, or *thrombocytopoiesis*, begins when megakaryocytes in the bone marrow start shedding membrane-bound packets. These packets enter the bloodstream and become platelets. A single megakaryocyte can produce thousands of platelets.

Megakaryocyte activity is controlled by the hormone **thrombopoietin,** which is produced by the liver. Thrombopoietin is not available as a medication, although it is currently undergoing clinical trials.

Oprelvekin (Neumega) is a drug, produced through recombinant DNA technology that stimulates the production of megakaryocytes and thrombopoietin. Although it differs slightly from endogenous interleukin-2, the two are considered functionally equivalent. Oprelvekin is used to stimulate the production of platelets in clients who are at risk for thrombocytopenia caused by cancer chemotherapy. The onset of action is 5 to 9 days, and therapy generally continues until the platelet count returns to greater than 100,000/mcl. Platelet counts will remain elevated for about 7 days after the last dose. Oprelvekin is given only only by the SC route. Its primary side effect is fluid retention, which can be a concern for clients with existing cardiac or renal disease.

NURSING CONSIDERATIONS

The role of the nurse in platelet enhancer therapy involves careful monitoring of a client's condition and providing education as it relates to the prescribed drug treatment. Obtain a complete health history including hypersensitivity and history of cardiac disease. Do not give oprelvekin to clients with hypersensitivity to this drug. Use with caution in clients with cardiac disease, especially HF, dysrhythmias, and left ventricular dysfunction, since fluid retention is a common side effect.

Do not give oprelvekin within 24 hours of chemotherapy, because the cytotoxic effects of the antineoplastic agents decrease the effectiveness of the drug. Adverse effects are related to fluid retention and may be severe, and include pleural effusion and papilledema. Advise clients to report

NURSING PROCESS FOCUS Clients Receiving Filgrastim (Neupogen)

Assessment	Potential Nursing Diagnoses
Prior to administration: ▪ Obtain a complete health history including allergies, drug history, and possible drug reactions. ▪ Assess reason for drug administration such as presence/history of severe bacterial or fungal infections, chemotherapy-induced neutropenia, or AIDS-related immunosuppression. ▪ Assess vital signs. ▪ Assess complete blood count, specifically WBCs with differential, to establish baseline values.	▪ Infection, Risk for, related to impaired immune defense (low WBC) ▪ Injury, Risk for, related to side effects of drug therapy ▪ Knowledge, Deficient, related to drug therapy

Planning: Client Goals and Expected Outcomes

The client will:
▪ Exhibit an increase in leukocyte levels and experience a decrease in the incidence of infection.
▪ Demonstrate an understanding of the drug's action by accurately describing drug side effects and precautions.
▪ Immediately report nausea, vomiting, fever, chills, malaise, and skeletal pain, and allergic-type responses such as rash, urticaria, wheezing, and dyspnea.

Implementation

Interventions and (Rationales)	Client Education/Discharge Planning
▪ Monitor vital signs. (Myocardial infarction and dysrhythmias have occurred in a small number of clients, because the drug has been known to cause abnormal ST-segment depression.)	▪ Instruct client to report any chest pain or palpitations.
▪ Monitor for signs and symptoms of infection and limit the client's exposure to pathogenic microorganisms. (Clients are more susceptible to infection until WBC response is achieved.)	Instruct client to: ▪ Wash hands frequently. ▪ Avoid crowds and people with colds, flu, and infections. ▪ Cook all foods completely and thoroughly. ▪ Clean surfaces touched by raw foods. ▪ Wash fresh fruits and vegetables thoroughly. ▪ Limit exposure to children and animals.
▪ Monitor complete blood count with differential until WBC count is at an acceptable level. (Filgrastim increases neutrophil proliferation and differentiation within the bone marrow.)	▪ Instruct client to take necessary precautions to avoid infection based on WBC status.
▪ Monitor hepatic status during pharmacotherapy. (Filgrastim may cause an elevation in liver enzymes.)	▪ Instruct client to keep all laboratory appointments.
▪ Assess for bone pain. (Drug works by stimulating bone marrow cells.)	▪ Instruct client to report any pain not relieved by OTC analgesics.
▪ Monitor for significant side effects and allergic-type reactions. (Client may be hypersensitive to *E. coli*.)	Instruct client to immediately report: ▪ Side effects such as nausea, vomiting, fever, chills, and malaise. ▪ Symptoms of allergic reaction such as rash, urticaria, wheezing, and dyspnea.
▪ Monitor client's ability to self-administer medication. (Improper injection techniques can lead to infection.)	Instruct client about: ▪ Self-injection techniques. ▪ Proper disposal of needles and syringes.

Evaluation of Outcome Criteria

Evaluate the effectiveness of drug therapy by confirming that client goals and expected outcomes have been met (see "Planning").
▪ The client exhibits an increase in leukocyte levels and experience a decrease in the incidence of infection.
▪ The client demonstrates an understanding of the drug's action by accurately describing drug side effects and precautions.
▪ The client reports nausea, vomiting, fever, chills, malaise, and skeletal pain, and allergic-type responses such as rash, urticaria, wheezing, and dyspnea.

edema and to avoid activities that could cause bleeding until the platelet count has returned to normal.

Withhold oprelvekin for 12 hours before or after radiation therapy, because the breakdown of cells after radiation will decrease the effectiveness of the medication. Monitor clients with a history of edema, because this drug aggravates fluid retention, and oprelvekin may cause pleural effusion or congestive heart failure.

Client Teaching.   Client education as it relates to platelet enhancer therapy should include the goals of therapy, the reasons for obtaining baseline data such as vital signs and the existence of underlying cardiac and hepatic disorders, and possible drug side effects. Include the following points when teaching clients about platelet enhancer therapy:

- Immediately report edema and difficulty breathing.
- Report changes in urinary output, especially a decrease.
- Report increased bruising or the presence of blood in the urine.
- Avoid activities that may produce injury.
- Monitor blood pressure and heart rate daily.
- Weigh daily and report any weight gain of 2 lb within 24 hours.
- Keep all scheduled physician and laboratory testing appointments.

ANEMIAS

Anemia is a condition in which red blood cells have a diminished capacity to carry oxygen. Although there are many different causes of anemia, they fall into one of the following categories:

- Blood loss due to hemorrhage
- Increased erythrocyte destruction
- Impaired erythrocyte production

Anemia is considered a sign, rather than a distinct disease. For therapy to be successful, the underlying pathology must be identified and treated.

28.5 Classification of Anemias

Classification of anemia is generally based on a description of the erythrocyte's size and color. Sizes are described as normal (normocytic), small (microcytic), or large (macro-cytic). Color is based on the amount of hemoglobin present and is described as normal red (normochromic) or light red (hypochromic). This classification is shown in Table 28.2.

Each type of anemia has specific characteristics, but all have common signs and symptoms. If the anemia occurs gradually, the client may remain asymptomatic, except during periods of physical exercise. As the condition progresses, the client often exhibits pallor, a paleness of the skin and mucous membranes due to hemoglobin deficiency. Decreased exercise tolerance, fatigue, and lethargy occur because insufficient oxygen reaches muscles. Dizziness and fainting are common as the brain does not receive enough oxygen to function properly. The respiratory and cardiovascular systems compensate for the oxygen depletion by increasing respiration rate and heart rate. Chronic or severe disease can result in heart failure.

ANTIANEMIC AGENTS

Depending on the type of anemia, several vitamins and minerals may be given to enhance the oxygen-carrying capacity of blood. The most common antianemic agents are cyanocobalamin (Crystamine, others), folic acid (Folvite, others) and ferrous sulfate (Feosol, others). These agents are listed in Table 28.3.

VITAMIN B$_{12}$ AND FOLIC ACID

Vitamin B$_{12}$ and folic acid are dietary nutrients essential for rapidly dividing cells. Because erythropoiesis occur at a continuously high rate throughout the lifespan, deficiencies in these nutrients often manifest as anemias.

28.6 Pharmacotherapy With Vitamin B$_{12}$ and Folic Acid

Vitamin B$_{12}$ is an essential component of two coenzymes that are required for normal cell growth and DNA replication. Vitamin B$_{12}$ is not synthesized by either plants or animals; only bacteria can make this substance. Because only minuscule amounts of vitamin B$_{12}$ are required (3 mcg/day), deficiency of this vitamin is usually not due to insufficient dietary intake. Instead, the most common cause of vitamin B$_{12}$ deficiency is absence of **intrinsic factor,** a protein secreted by stomach cells. Intrinsic factor is required for vitamin B$_{12}$ to be absorbed from the intestine. ● Figure 28.2 illustrates the metabolism of vitamin B$_{12}$. Inflammatory diseases of the stomach or surgical removal of the stomach

TABLE 28.2	Classification of Anemia	
Morphology	**Description**	**Examples**
macrocytic-normochromic	large, abnormally shaped erythrocytes with normal hemoglobin concentration	pernicious anemia, folate-deficiency anemia
microcytic-hypochromic	small, abnormally shaped erythrocytes with decreased hemoglobin concentration	iron-deficiency anemia, thalassemia
normocytic-normochromic	destruction or depletion of normal erythroblasts or mature erythrocytes	aplastic anemia, hemorrhagic anemia, sickle-cell anemia, hemolytic anemia

MediaLink

Anemia

TABLE 28.3 Antianemic Agents

Drug	Route and Adult Dose (max dose where indicated)	Adverse Effects
cyanocobalamin (Crystamine, others)	IM/deep subcutaneous; 30 mcg/day for 5–10 days; then 100–200 mcg/mo	*Diarrhea, hypokalemia, rash* <u>Anaphylaxis</u>
folic acid (Folvite)	PO/IM/subcutaneous/IV; <1 mg/day	No side effects
IRON SALTS		
ferrous fumarate (Feostat, others)	PO; 200 mg tid or qid	*Nausea, heartburn, constipation, dark stools*
ferrous gluconate (Fergon, others)	PO; 325–600 mg qid; may be gradually increased to 650 mg qid as needed and tolerated	<u>Cardiovascular collapse, aggravation of peptic ulcers or ulcerative colitis, hepatic necrosis, anaphylaxis (iron dextran)</u>
ferrous sulfate (Feosol, others)	PO; 750–1500 mg/day in 1–3 divided doses	
iron dextran (Dexferrum, others)	IM/IV; dose is individualized and determined from a table supplied by the drug manufacturer that correlates body weight to hemoglobin values (max: 100 mg within 24 h)	

Italics indicate common adverse effects; <u>underlining</u> indicates serious adverse effects.

may result in deficiency of intrinsic factor. Inflammatory diseases of the small intestine that affect food and nutrient absorption may also cause vitamin B_{12} deficiency. Because vitamin B_{12} is found primarily in foods of animal origin, strict vegetarians may require a vitamin supplement to avoid deficiency.

The most profound consequence of vitamin B_{12} deficiency is a condition called **pernicious** or **megaloblastic anemia,** which affects both the hematologic and nervous systems. The hematopoietic stem cells produce abnormally large erythrocytes that do not fully mature. Red blood cells are most affected, though lack of maturation of all blood cell types may occur in severe disease. The symptoms of pernicious anemia are often nonspecific and develop slowly, sometimes over decades. Nervous system symptoms may include memory loss, confusion, unsteadiness, tingling or numbness in the limbs, delusions, mood disturbances, and even hallucinations in severe deficiencies. Permanent nervous system damage may result if the disease remains untreated. Pharmacotherapy includes the administration of cyanocobalamin, a form of vitamin B_{12} (see the prototype drug feature in this chapter).

Folic acid, or folate, is a B-complex vitamin essential for normal DNA and RNA synthesis. As with B_{12} deficiency, insufficient folic acid can manifest itself as anemia. In fact, the metabolism of vitamin B_{12} and folic acid are intricately linked; a B_{12} deficiency will create a lack of activated folic acid.

Unlike vitamin B_{12}, folic acid does not require intrinsic factor for intestinal absorption, and the most common cause of folate deficiency is insufficient dietary intake. This deficiency is often observed in chronic alcoholism, since alcohol interferes with folate metabolism in the liver. Fad diets and absorption diseases of the small intestine can also result in folate anemia. Hematopoietic signs of folate deficiency are the same as those for B_{12} deficiency; however, no neurological signs are present. Folate deficiency during pregnancy has been linked to neural birth defects such as spina bifida. Treatment is often accomplished by increasing the dietary

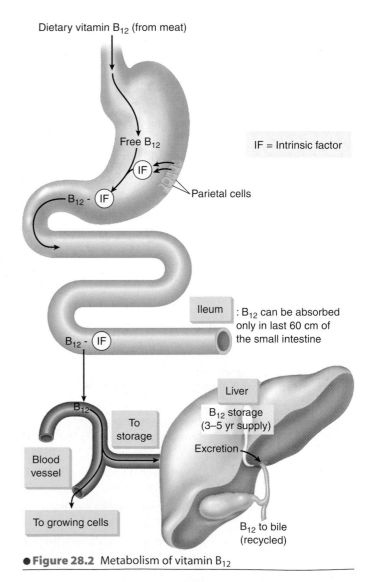

Dietary vitamin B_{12} (from meat)

IF = Intrinsic factor

Free B_{12}

IF

B_{12} - IF

Parietal cells

Ileum : B_{12} can be absorbed only in last 60 cm of the small intestine

B_{12} - IF

Liver

B_{12} storage (3–5 yr supply)

B_{12}

To storage

Excretion

Blood vessel

To growing cells

B_{12} to bile (recycled)

●**Figure 28.2** Metabolism of vitamin B_{12}

intake of folic acid through fresh green vegetables, dried beans, and wheat products. In cases when adequate dietary intake cannot be achieved, therapy with folate sodium (Folvite) or folic acid is warranted. Folic acid is discussed further in Chapter 38 ∞, where it is found as a drug prototype for water-soluble vitamins.

NURSING CONSIDERATIONS

The role of the nurse in antianemia therapy involves careful monitoring of a client's condition and providing education as it relates to the prescribed drug treatment. Antianemic agents are given to enhance the oxygen-carrying capacity of blood. Clients with anemia commonly experience fatigue, intolerance to activity, dizziness, and fainting. Clients with advanced anemia may experience chest pain, difficulty breathing, and pallor. Obtain a complete health history including ability to perform activities of daily living, fatigue, chest pain, palpitations, dyspnea, cold intolerance, and skin color changes. Although most vitamin B_{12} deficiencies are caused by a lack of intrinsic factor, investigate the possibility of inadequate dietary intake of the vitamin. Prior to administration assess for other causes of anemia including GI dysfunction, GI surgery, tapeworm infestation, and gluten enteropathy.

Prior to and at regular intervals during treatment, monitor the CBC to evaluate the effectiveness of vitamin B_{12} therapy. This drug is not an effective treatment for iron-deficiency anemias. Cyanocobalamin is contraindicated in clients with severe pulmonary disease and is used cautiously in clients with heart disease.

Monitor potassium levels during pharmacotherapy, because hypokalemia is a possible side effect of this drug. Assess clients for additional side effects such as itching, rash, or flushing. Clients taking this drug may develop pulmonary edema and heart failure, so monitor cardiovascular status.

Client Teaching.   Client education as it relates to antianemia therapy should include the goals of therapy, the reasons for obtaining baseline data such as vital signs and underlying cardiac and hepatic disorders or allergies, and possible drug side effects. Include the following points when teaching clients about vitamin B_{12} and folic acid therapy:

- Keep all scheduled laboratory visits to evaluate the effectiveness of therapy and possible medication side effects.
- Immediately report any shortness of breath or edema.
- Allow for rest breaks to conserve energy.
- Eat a well-balanced nutritious diet.

IRON

Iron is a mineral essential to the function of several biological molecules. Of all the iron in the body, 60% to 80% is associated with hemoglobin inside erythrocytes. Iron is also essential for a number of mitochondrial enzymes involved in metabolism and energy production in the cell. Because free iron is toxic, the body binds the mineral to the protein complexes **ferritin, hemosiderin,** and **transferrin.** Ferritin and hemosiderin maintain iron stores *inside* cells, whereas transferrin *transports* iron to sites in the body where it is needed.

Pr PROTOTYPE DRUG | Cyanocobalamin *(Crystamine, others)* | Antianemic Agent/Vitamin Supplement

ACTIONS AND USES

Cyanocobalamin is a purified form of vitamin B_{12} that is administered in deficiency states. Treatment of vitamin B_{12} deficiency is most often by weekly, biweekly, or monthly IM or SC injections. In 2005, a nasal spray formulation (Nascobol) was approved which provides for the convenience of once-weekly dosing and which is beneficial in clients who are unable to take oral cyanocobalamin because of malabsorptive conditions. Although oral B_{12} supplements are available, they are effective only in clients having sufficient intrinsic factor and normal absorption in the small intestine. Parenteral administration rapidly reverses most signs and symptoms of B_{12} deficiency, usually within a few days or weeks. If the disease has been prolonged, symptoms may take longer to resolve, and some neurological damage may be permanent. In most cases, treatment must often be maintained for the remainder of the client's life.

ADMINISTRATION ALERTS

- If PO preparations are mixed with fruit juices, administer quickly because ascorbic acid affects the stability of vitamin B_{12}.
- Pregnancy category A (C when used parenterally).

PHARMACOKINETICS

Because vitaimin B_{12} is a natural substance, it is difficult to obtain pharmacokinetic values.

ADVERSE EFFECTS

Side effects from cyanocobalamin are uncommon. Hypokalemia is possible; thus, serum potassium levels are monitored periodically. A small percentage of clients receiving B_{12} exhibit rashes, itching, or other signs of allergy. Anaphylaxis is possible, though rare.

Contraindications: Contraindications include sensitivity to cobalt and folic acid–deficiency anemia.

INTERACTIONS

Drug–Drug: Drug interactions with cyanocobalamin include a decrease in absorption when given concurrently with alcohol, aminosalicylic acid, neomycin, and colchicine. Chloramphenicol may interfere with therapeutic response to cyanocobalamin.

Lab Tests: Unknown.

Herbal/Food: Unknown.

Treatment of Overdose: No overdosage has been reported.

 See the Companion Website for a Nursing Process Focus specific to this drug.

28.7 Pharmacotherapy With Iron

The most common cause of nutritional anemia is iron deficiency. A primary cause of iron-deficiency anemia is acute or chronic blood loss, such as may occur from peptic ulcer disease, and dietary deficiency. Certain individuals have an increased demand for iron, including those who are pregnant, experiencing heavy menstruation, or undergoing intensive athletic training. These conditions may require more than the recommended daily allowance (RDA) of iron (Chapter 42 ∞). The most significant effect of iron deficiency is a reduction in erythropoiesis, resulting in symptoms of anemia.

After erythrocytes die, nearly all the iron in their hemoglobin is incorporated into transferrin and recycled for later use. Because of this efficient recycling, only about 1 mg of iron is excreted from the body per day, making daily dietary iron requirements in most individuals quite small. Iron balance is maintained by increased absorption of the mineral from the proximal small intestine. In the United States and Canada, iron deficiency most commonly occurs in women of childbearing age owing to blood losses during menses and pregnancy. Because iron is found in greater quantities in meat products, vegetarians are at higher risk of iron-deficiency anemia.

Ferrous sulfate (Feosol, others), ferrous gluconate (Fergon, others), and ferrous fumarate (Feostat, others) are commonly used oral iron supplements. Slow-release products, called carbonyl iron (Feosol-caps, Ferronyl), are more expensive but are less dangerous following accidental exposure in children because there is a longer period for intervention before toxic effects materialize. Iron dextran (Dexferrum, others) is a parenteral supplement that may be used when the client is unable to take oral preparations. Because iron oxidizes vitamin C, many iron supplements contain this vitamin. Vitamin C also is believed to enhance iron absorption. Depending on the degree of iron depletion and the amount of iron supplement that can be tolerated by the client without significant side effects, 3 to 6 months of therapy may be required.

NURSING CONSIDERATIONS

The role of the nurse in iron pharmacotherapy involves careful monitoring of a client's condition and providing education as it relates to the prescribed drug regimen. Iron therapy is given to alleviate symptoms of anemia caused by blood loss or dietary deficiency. Before initiating therapy with these drugs, the nurse should obtain vital signs and a CBC, including hemoglobin and hematocrit levels, to establish baseline values. The nurse should obtain a health history, assessing for peptic ulcer, regional enteritis, ulcerative colitis, and cirrhosis of the liver, because presence of these disorders may be the source of the client's symptoms. Oral iron preparations may be contraindicated because of the effect on the gastric mucosa. The nurse should also obtain a complete dietary assessment.

Iron dextran can be given as an IM injection or as an IV infusion and is often used for clients who cannot tolerate

---

Pr PROTOTYPE DRUG | Ferrous Sulfate *(Feosol, others)* | Antianemic Agent/Iron Supplement

ACTIONS AND USES

Ferrous sulfate is an iron supplement containing about 30% elemental iron. It is available in a wide variety of dosage forms to prevent or rapidly reverse symptoms of iron-deficiency anemia. Other forms of iron include ferrous fumarate, which contains 33% elemental iron, and ferrous gluconate, which contains 12% elemental iron. The doses of these various preparations are based on their iron content.

Laboratory evaluation of hemoglobin or hematocrit values is conducted regularly, as excess iron is toxic. Although a positive therapeutic response may be achieved in 48 hours, therapy may continue for several months.

ADMINISTRATION ALERTS

- When administering IV, be careful to prevent infiltration, as iron is highly irritating to tissues.
- Use the Z-track method (deep muscle) when giving IM.
- Do not crush tablet or empty contents of capsule when administering.
- Do not give tablets or capsules within 1 hour of bedtime.
- Pregnancy category A.

PHARMACOKINETICS

Because iron is a natural substance, it is difficult to obtain pharmacokinetic values.

ADVERSE EFFECTS

The most common side effect of ferrous sulfate is GI upset. Taking the drug with food will diminish GI upset but can decrease the absorption of iron by as much as 70%. In addition, antacids should not be taken with ferrous sulfate because they also reduce absorption of the mineral. Ideally, iron preparations should be administered 1 hour before or 2 hours after a meal. Iron preparations may darken stools, but this is a harmless side effect. Constipation is common; therefore, an increase in dietary fiber may be indicated. Excessive doses of iron are very toxic, and the nurse should advise clients to take the medication exactly as directed.

Contraindications: These drugs should not be used in hemolytic anemia without documentation of iron deficiency, or hemochromatosis, peptic ulcer, regional enteritis, and ulcerative colitis.

INTERACTIONS

Drug–Drug: Absorption is reduced when oral iron salts are given concurrently with antacids, proton-pump inhibitors, or calcium supplements. Iron decreases the absorption of tetracyclines, fluoroquinolones, and etidronate. It is advisable to take iron supplements at least 1 hour before or after other medications.

Lab Tests: May decrease serum calcium level and increase serum bilirubin.

Herbal/Food: Food, especially dairy products, will inhibit absorption.

Treatment of Overdose: The antidote for acute iron intoxication is deferoxamine (Desferal). This parenteral agent binds iron, which is subsequently removed by the kidneys, turning the urine a reddish brown color.

NURSING PROCESS FOCUS Clients Receiving Ferrous Sulfate (*Feosol, others*)

Assessment	Potential Nursing Diagnoses
Prior to administration: ■ Obtain a complete health history including allergies, drug history, possible drug reactions, history of peptic ulcer disease, or recent blood loss. ■ Assess reason for drug administration such as presence/history of anemia, or prophylaxis during infancy, childhood, and pregnancy. ■ Assess complete blood count, specifically hematocrit and hemoglobin levels, to establish baseline values. ■ Assess vital signs.	■ Nutrition, Risk for Imbalanced, related to inadequate iron intake ■ Gas Exchange, Risk for Impaired, related to low RBC count resulting in decreased oxygenation ■ Injury (weakness, dizziness, syncope), Risk for, related to anemia ■ Knowledge Deficient, related to drug therapy

Planning: Client Goals and Expected Outcomes

The client will:
■ Exhibit an increase in hematocrit level and improvement in anemia-related symptoms.
■ Demonstrate an understanding of the drug's action by accurately describing drug side effects and precautions.
■ Immediately report significant side effects such as GI distress.

Implementation

Interventions and (Rationales)	Client Education/Discharge Planning
■ Monitor vital signs, especially pulse. (Increased pulse is an indicator of decreased oxygen content in the blood.)	■ Instruct client to monitor pulse rate and report irregularities and changes in rhythm.
■ Monitor complete blood count to evaluate effectiveness of treatment. (Increases in hematocrit and hemoglobin values indicate increased RBC production.)	Instruct client: ■ On the need for initial and continuing laboratory blood monitoring. ■ To keep all laboratory appointments.
■ Monitor changes in stool. (The drug may cause constipation, change stool color, and cause false positives when stool is tested for occult blood.)	Instruct client: ■ That stool color may change to dark green or black, and this is not a cause for alarm. ■ On measures to relieve constipation, such as including high-fiber vegetables and grains in diet, and increasing fluid intake and exercise.
■ Plan activities and allow for periods of rest to help client conserve energy. (Diminished iron levels result in decreased formation of hemoglobin, leading to weakness and fatigue.)	Instruct client to: ■ Rest when feeling tired, and avoid overexertion. ■ Plan activities to avoid fatigue.
■ Administer medication on an empty stomach (if tolerated) at least 1 hour before bedtime.(Lack of food in the stomach maximizes absorption; taking closer to bedtime may increase the chance of GI distress.)	Instruct client: ■ Not to crush or chew sustained-release preparations. ■ That medication may cause GI upset. ■ To take medication with food if GI upset becomes a problem. ■ To take at least 1 hour before bedtime.
■ Administer liquid iron preparations through a straw or place on the back of the tongue. (This drug stains the teeth.)	Instruct client to: ■ Dilute liquid medication before using and to use a straw to take medication. ■ Rinse the mouth after swallowing to decrease the chance of staining the teeth.
■ Monitor dietary intake. (This ensure adequate intake of foods high in iron.)	■ Instruct client to increase intake of iron-rich foods such as liver, egg yolks, brewer's yeast, wheat germ, and muscle meats.
■ Monitor for potential for child access to medication. (Iron poisoning can be fatal to young children.)	■ Advise parents to store iron-containing vitamins out of reach of children and in childproof containers.

Evaluation of Outcome Criteria

Evaluate the effectiveness of drug therapy by confirming that client goals and expected outcomes have been met (see "Planning").
■ The client exhibits an increase in hematocrit level and improvement in anemia-related symptoms.
■ The client demonstrates an understanding of the drug's action by accurately describing drug side effects and precautions.
■ The client immediately reports significant side effects such as GI distress.

oral iron preparations. Prior to administration of an infusion, the client must receive a test dose to determine possible allergic reaction, which may cause respiratory arrest and circulatory collapse. Vital signs must be monitored during the test dose infusion.

Assess for GI complaints because nausea, vomiting, constipation, and diarrhea are common reactions with administration of oral iron preparations. Taking oral iron with food reduces GI distress but also greatly reduces absorption. Assess for other common adverse reactions of iron dextran such as headache, muscle pain, and joint pain, which are more severe when the drug is given IV. Iron dextran appears to increase bone density in the joints, which is the probable cause of the muscle and joint pain.

Lifespan Considerations.   Iron deficiency and iron-deficiency anemia have been identified as significant problems among children 1 to 2 years of age. Inadequate iron intake and storage is the main reason for this condition. Extremely low levels of iron can cause permanent mental and psychomotor impairment; therefore, prevention is of utmost importance. Primary prevention of iron deficiency can be accomplished by daily supplementation of 10 mg of elemental iron with iron-fortified vitamins, iron drops, or an iron-fortified nutritional drink. Accidental overdosing with products containing iron is one of the leading causes of fatal poisoning in children. It is extremely important that iron be kept out of the reach of children. If overdosing occurs, caregivers should call the healthcare provider or poison control center. Pregnant women have an increased demand for iron. Adequate dietary intake and supplementation should be advised. Women experiencing increased or excessive menstrual flow are at risk for iron-deficiency anemia. Correction of the cause, increased dietary intake, and iron supplements may be required.

Client Teaching.   Client education as it relates to iron therapy should include the goals of therapy, the reasons for obtaining baseline data such as vital signs and the existence of underlying cardiac and hepatic disorders, allergy history, and possible drug side effects. Include the following points when teaching clients about iron therapy:

- Take oral preparations with food if GI distress occurs.
- Use a straw or place liquid preparations on back of tongue to prevent staining teeth.
- Keep all iron preparations out of reach of children.
- Maintain adequate dietary intake of iron-rich foods.
- Expect stools to turn dark green or black during therapy.
- Immediately report any evidence of GI bleeding.

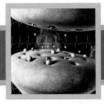

CHAPTER REVIEW

KEY CONCEPTS

The numbered key concepts provide a succinct summary of the important points from the corresponding numbered section within the chapter. If any of these points are not clear, refer to the numbered section within the chapter for review.

28.1 Hematopoiesis is the process of blood cell production that begins with primitive stem cells that reside in bone marrow. Homeostatic control of hematopoiesis is maintained through hormones and growth factors.

28.2 Erythropoietin is a hormone that stimulates the production of red blood cells when the body experiences hemorrhage or hypoxia. Epoetin alfa is a synthetic form of erythropoietin used to treat specific anemias.

28.3 Colony-stimulating factors (CSFs) are growth factors that stimulate the production of leukocytes. They are used to reduce the duration of neutropenia in clients undergoing chemotherapy or organ transplantation.

28.4 Platelet enhancers stimulate the activity of megakaryocytes and thrombopoietin, and increase the production of platelets. Oprelvekin, the only drug in this class, is prescribed for clients with thrombocytopenia.

28.5 Anemias are disorders in which the oxygen-carrying capacity of the blood is reduced owing to hemorrhage, excessive erythrocyte destruction, or insufficient erythrocyte synthesis.

28.6 Deficiencies in either vitamin B_{12} or folic acid can lead to pernicious anemia. Treatment with cyanocobalamin can reverse symptoms of pernicious anemia in many clients, although some degree of nervous system damage may be permanent.

28.7 Iron deficiency is the most common cause of nutritional anemia and can be successfully treated with iron supplements.

NCLEX-RN® REVIEW QUESTIONS

1 An elderly client diagnosed with iron-deficiency anemia will be taking ferrous sulfate (Ferralyn) 1 g PO daily in 3 divided doses. The drug is available as 325-mg tablets. How many tablets will the nurse administer per dose? Write your answer below.

_____

2 Erythropoietin regulates the process of red blood cell (RBC) formation. The nurse understands this mechanism is activated by a reduction of oxygen reaching the:

1. Brain.
2. Heart.
3. Kidneys.
4. Lungs.

3 The client with a diagnosis of cancer is receiving epoetin alfa (Epogen, Procrit) as part of the treatment regimen. The nurse evaluates the effectiveness of this drug by:

1. Assessing the client's energy level.
2. Monitoring the hematocrit and hemoglobin level.
3. Monitoring the client's blood pressure.
4. Assessing the client's level of consciousness.

4 The nursing plan of care for a client receiving epoetin alfa (Epogen, Procrit) should include careful monitoring for symptoms of:

1. Angina, or a change in level of consciousness.
2. Severe hypotension.
3. Impaired liver function.
4. Severe diarrhea.

5 The nurse explains to the client that the development of pernicious anemia is caused by:

1. Bone marrow depression.
2. Lack of intrinsic factor, vitamin B_{12} deficiency.
3. Iron deficiency.
4. Blood loss.

CRITICAL THINKING QUESTIONS

1. A client newly diagnosed with renal failure asks the nurse why he must receive injections of epoetin alfa (Epogen, Procrit). Develop teaching points to describe the indications for this drug.

2. A client is receiving filgrastim (Neupogen). What nursing interventions are appropriate to safely administer this drug and provide client safety throughout therapy?

3. A client is receiving ferrous sulfate (Feosol, others). What teaching should the nurse provide to this client?

See Appendix D for answers and rationales for all activities.

EXPLORE
MediaLink

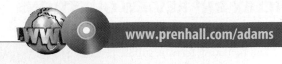

www.prenhall.com/adams

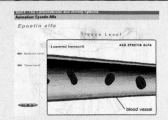

NCLEX-RN® review, case studies, and other interactive resources for this chapter can be found on the companion website at www.prenhall.com/adams. Click on "Chapter 28" to select the activities for this chapter. For animations, more NCLEX-RN® review questions, and an audio glossary, access the accompanying Prentice Hall Nursing MediaLink DVD-ROM in this textbook.

PRENTICE HALL NURSING MEDIALINK DVD-ROM

- **Animation**
  Mechanism in Action: Epoetin alfa (*Epogen, Procrit*)
- **Audio Glossary**
- **NCLEX-RN® Review**

COMPANION WEBSITE

- **NCLEX-RN® Review**
- **Dosage Calculations**
- **Case Study:** Erythropoietin and erythrocyte production
- **Care Plan:** Client with chronic renal failure secondary to diabetes mellitus treated with epoetin alfa

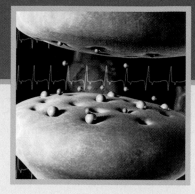

CHAPTER 29

Drugs for Shock

DRUGS AT A GLANCE

FLUID REPLACEMENT AGENTS
Blood and Blood Products
Crystalloid Solutions
Colloid Solutions
- 🔊 *normal serum albumin (Albuminar, Albutein)*

VASOCONSTRICTORS/
VASOPRESSORS
- 🔊 *norepinephrine (Levarterenol, Levophed)*

INOTROPIC AGENTS
- 🔊 *dopamine (Dopastat, Inotropin)*

DRUGS FOR ANAPHYLAXIS
- 🔊 *epinephrine (Adrenalin)*

OBJECTIVES

After reading this chapter, the student should be able to:

1. Compare and contrast the different types of shock.
2. Relate the general symptoms of shock to their physiological causes.
3. Explain the initial treatment priorities for a client who is in shock.
4. Compare and contrast the use of colloids and crystalloids in fluid replacement therapy.
5. List the drugs used in the pharmacotherapy of anaphylaxis and discuss their indications.
6. For each of the classes shown in Drugs at a Glance, know representative drug examples, and explain their mechanism of action, primary actions, and important adverse effects.
7. Categorize drugs used in the treatment of shock based on their classification and mechanism of action.
8. Use the steps of the Nursing Process to care for clients who are receiving drug therapy for shock.

MediaLink

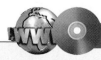 www.prenhall.com/adams

NCLEX-RN® review, case studies, and other interactive resources for this chapter can be found on the companion website at www.prenhall.com/adams. Click on "Chapter 29" to select the activities for this chapter. For animations, more NCLEX-RN® review questions, and an audio glossary, access the accompanying Prentice Hall Nursing MediaLink DVD-ROM in this textbook.

KEY TERMS

anaphylactic shock *page 410*

cardiogenic shock *page 410*

colloids *page 411*

crystalloids *page 411*

hypovolemic shock *page 410*

inotropic agent *page 417*

neurogenic shock *page 410*

oncotic pressure *page 411*

septic shock *page 410*

shock *page 410*

Shock is a condition in which vital tissues and organs are not receiving enough blood to function properly. Without adequate oxygen and other nutrients, cells cannot carry out normal metabolic processes. Shock is considered a medical emergency; failure to reverse the causes and symptoms of shock may lead to irreversible organ damage and death. This chapter examines how drugs are used to aid in the treatment of different types of shock, including anaphylatic.

29.1 Characteristics of Shock

Shock is a collection of signs and symptoms, many of which are nonspecific. Although symptoms vary somewhat among the different kinds of shock, some similarities exist. The client appears pale and may claim to feel sick or weak without reporting specific complaints. Behavioral changes are often some of the earliest symptoms and may include restlessness, anxiety, confusion, depression, and apathy. Lack of sufficient blood flow to the brain may cause unconsciousness. Thirst is a common complaint. The skin may feel cold or clammy. Without immediate treatment, multiple body systems will be affected and respiratory or renal failure may result. ● Figure 29.1 shows common symptoms of a client in shock.

The central problem in most types of shock is the inability of the cardiovascular system to send sufficient blood to the vital organs, with the heart and brain being affected early in the progression of the disease. Assessing the client's cardiovascular status will often give important clues for a diagnosis of shock. Blood pressure is usually low and cardiac output diminished. Heart rate may be rapid with a weak, thready pulse. Breathing is usually rapid and shallow. ● Figure 29.2 (page 412) illustrates the physiological changes that occur during circulatory shock.

29.2 Causes of Shock

Shock is often classified by naming the underlying pathological process or organ system causing the disease. Table 29.1 lists the different types of shock and their primary causes.

Diagnosis of shock is rarely based on nonspecific symptoms. A careful medical history, however, may give the nurse valuable clues as to what type of shock may be present. For example, obvious trauma or bleeding would suggest **hypovolemic shock,** related to volume depletion. If trauma to the brain or spinal cord is evident, **neurogenic shock,** a type of distributive shock caused by a sudden loss of nerve impulse communication, may be suspected. A history of heart disease would suggest **cardiogenic shock,** which is caused by inadequate cardiac output due to pump failure. A recent infection may indicate **septic shock,** a type of distributive shock caused by the presence of bacteria and toxins in the blood. A history of allergy with a sudden onset of symptoms following food or drug intake may suggest **anaphylactic shock,** the most severe

PHARMFACTS

Shock

- Cardiogenic shock, because it responds poorly to treatment, is the most lethal form of shock and has an 80% to 100% mortality rate.
- Hypovolemic shock carries a 10% to 31% mortality rate.
- With anaphylactic or distributive shock, death can ensue within minutes if treatment is not available to treat the condition: Neurogenic shock is a form of distributive shock.
- It is estimated that 500 to 1000 cases of fatal anaphylactic shock occur each year in the United States.
- Septic shock, usually caused by gram-negative bacteria, has a mortality rate of 40% to 70% but can be as high as 90%, depending on the causative organism.

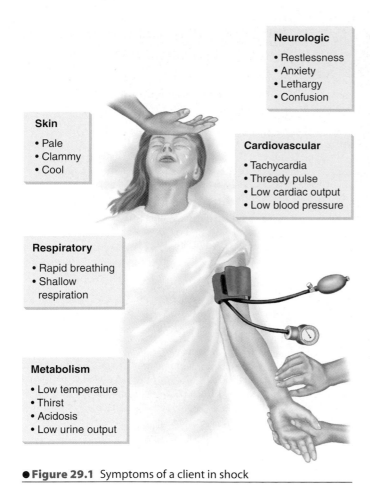

Neurologic

- Restlessness
- Anxiety
- Lethargy
- Confusion

Skin

- Pale
- Clammy
- Cool

Cardiovascular

- Tachycardia
- Thready pulse
- Low cardiac output
- Low blood pressure

Respiratory

- Rapid breathing
- Shallow respiration

Metabolism

- Low temperature
- Thirst
- Acidosis
- Low urine output

● **Figure 29.1** Symptoms of a client in shock

type I allergic response. The pharmacotherapy of anaphylaxis is included in Section 29.7 (page 413).

29.3 Treatment Priorities for Shock

Shock is treated as a medical emergency, and the first goal is to maintain basic life support. Rapid identification of the underlying cause, followed by aggressive treatment, is essential, because the client's condition may deteriorate rapidly without specific, emergency measures. The initial nursing interventions of maintaining the ABCs of life support—airway, breathing, and circulation—to sustain normal blood pressure are critical. The client is immediately connected to a cardiac monitor, and a pulse oximeter is applied. Blood pressure readings are taken on the arm opposite the pulse oximeter, as peripheral vasoconstriction with the inflation of the BP cuff will alter oximetry readings. Unless contraindicated, oxygen is administered at 15 L/min via a nonrebreather mask. Neurological status and level of consciousness are monitored. Additional nursing interventions consist of keeping the client quiet and warm and offering psychological support and reassurance.

The remaining therapies for shock depend on the specific cause of the condition. The two primary pharmacotherapeutic goals are to restore normal fluid volume and composition and to maintain adequate blood pressure. For anaphylaxis, an additional therapeutic goal is to prevent or stop the hypersensitive inflammatory response.

FLUID REPLACEMENT AGENTS

Certain agents are used to replace blood or other fluids lost during hypovolemic shock. Fluid replacement therapy includes blood, blood products, colloids, and crystalloids, as listed in Table 29.2 (page 413).

29.4 Treating Shock With IV Infusion Therapy

Hypovolemic shock can be triggered by a number of conditions, including hemorrhage, extensive burns, severe dehydration, persistent vomiting or diarrhea, and intensive diuretic therapy. If the client has lost significant blood or other body fluids, immediate maintenance of blood volume through the IV infusion of fluid and electrolytes or blood products is essential.

Blood or blood products may be administered to restore fluid volume, depending on the clinical situation. Whole blood is indicated for the treatment of acute, massive blood loss (depletion of more than 30% of the total volume) when there is a need to replace plasma volume *and* supply red blood cells to increase the oxygen-carrying capacity.

The administration of whole blood has been largely replaced with the use of blood components. A single unit of whole blood can be separated into its specific constituents (red and white blood cells, platelets, plasma proteins, fresh frozen plasma, and globulins), which can be used to treat more than one client. The supply of blood products depends on human donors and requires careful cross matching to ensure compatibility between the donor and the recipient. Whole blood, despite being carefully screened, has the potential to transmit serious infections such as hepatitis or HIV.

Because it is safer to administer only the needed components, rather than whole blood, other products are often used to expand volume and to sustain blood pressure. These are of two basic types: colloids and crystalloids. Colloid and crystalloid infusions are often used when up to one third of an adult's blood volume has been lost.

Colloids are proteins or other large molecules that stay suspended in the blood for a long period because they are too large to easily cross membranes. While circulating they draw water molecules from the cells and tissues into the blood vessels through their ability to increase plasma **oncotic pressure.** Blood-product colloids include normal human serum albumin, plasma protein fraction, and serum globulins. The non-blood-product colloids are dextran (40, 70, and high molecular weight) and hetastarch (Hespan). These agents are administered to provide life-sustaining support following massive hemorrhage and to treat shock, as well as to treat burns, acute liver failure, and neonatal hemolytic disease.

Crystalloids are IV solutions that contain electrolytes in concentrations resembling those of plasma. Unlike colloids, crystalloid solutions can readily leave the blood and enter cells. They are used to replace fluids that have been lost and to promote urine output. Common crystalloids used in shock include normal saline, lactated Ringer's, Plasmalyte,

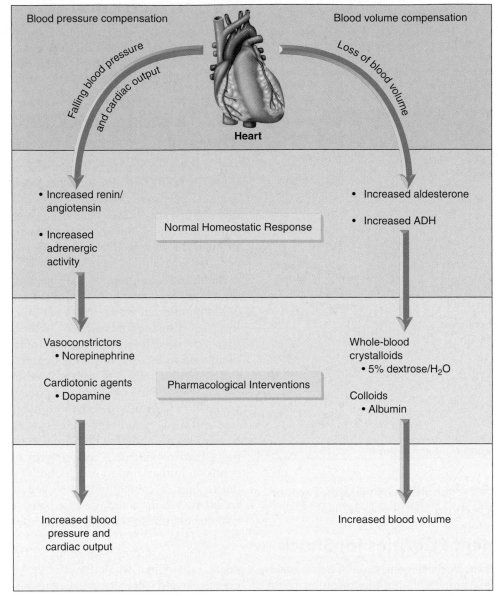

Blood pressure compensation

Blood volume compensation

Falling blood pressure and cardiac output

Loss of blood volume

Heart

- Increased renin/ angiotensin
- Increased adrenergic activity

Normal Homeostatic Response

- Increased aldesterone
- Increased ADH

Vasoconstrictors
- Norepinephrine

Cardiotonic agents
- Dopamine

Pharmacological Interventions

Whole-blood crystalloids
- 5% dextrose/H_2O

Colloids
- Albumin

Increased blood pressure and cardiac output

Increased blood volume

● **Figure 29.2** Physiological changes during circulatory shock: pharmacological intervention

TABLE 29.1	Common Types of Shock	
Type of Shock	**Definition**	**Underlying Pathology**
anaphylactic	acute allergic reaction	severe reaction to allergen such as penicillin, nuts, shellfish, or animal proteins
cardiogenic	failure of the heart to pump sufficient blood to tissues	left heart failure, myocardial ischemia, MI, dysrhythmias, pulmonary embolism, myocardial or pericardial infection
hypovolemic	loss of blood volume	hemorrhage, burns, profuse sweating, excessive urination, vomiting, or diarrhea
neurogenic	vasodilation due to overstimulation of the parasympathetic or understimulation of the sympathetic nervous systems	trauma to spinal cord or medulla, severe emotional stress or pain, drugs that depress the central nervous system
septic	multiple organ dysfunction as a result of pathogenic organisms in the blood resulting in vasodilation and changes in permeability of capillaries; often a precursor to acute respiratory distress syndrome and disseminated intravascular coagulation	widespread inflammatory response to bacterial, fungal, or parasitic infection

TABLE 29.2   Fluid Replacement Agents

Agent	Examples
blood products	• whole blood • plasma protein fraction • fresh frozen plasma • packed red blood cells
colloids	• plasma protein fraction (Plasmanate, Plasma-Plex, Plasmatein, PPF, Protenate) • dextran 40 (Gentran 40, Hyskon, Rheomacrodex) or dextran 70 (Macrodex) • hetastarch (Hespan) • normal serum albumin, human (Albuminar, Albutein, Buminate, Plasbumin)
crystalloids	• normal saline (0.9% sodium chloride) • lactated Ringer's • Plasmalyte • hypertonic saline (3% sodium chloride) • 5% dextrose in water (D5W)*

* Not used for shock

and hypertonic saline. Additional information on the role of crystalloids and colloids in correcting fluid balance disorders is included in Chapter 31 ∞.

NURSING CONSIDERATIONS

The role of the nurse in crystalloid and colloid therapy involves careful monitoring of a client's condition and providing education as it relates to the prescribed drug treatment. Crystalloid and colloid therapies are used to re-place fluids and raise blood pressure, so first assess the blood pressure and cardiovascular status. Because hypertonic and isotonic colloids can pull fluid into the vascular space, circulatory overload is a serious complication. Monitoring for blood pressure changes is essential; pressure may increase with a healthy heart, or decrease if the heart fails, resulting in fluid overload. Monitor breath sounds; crackles will be heard with pulmonary congestion. Monitor for changes in oxygenation that may become evident before breath sounds change. Also monitor intake, output, and body

---

Pr   PROTOTYPE DRUG | Normal Serum Albumin *(Albuminar, Albutein, Buminate, Plasbumin)* | Fluid Replacement Agent/Colloid

ACTIONS AND USES

Normal serum albumin is a protein extracted from whole blood, plasma, or placental human plasma that contains 96% albumin and 4% globulins and other proteins. Albumin naturally comprises about 60% of all blood proteins. Its normal functions are to maintain plasma oncotic pressure and to shuttle certain substances through the blood, including a substantial number of drug molecules. After extraction from blood or plasma, albumin is sterilized to remove possible contamination by the hepatitis viruses or HIV.

Administered IV, albumin increases the oncotic pressure of the blood and causes fluid to move from the tissues to the general circulation. It is used to restore plasma volume in hypovolemic shock, or to restore blood proteins in clients with hypoproteinemia. It has an immediate onset of action and is available in concentrations of 5% and 25%.

ADMINISTRATION ALERTS

- Infuse higher concentrations more slowly because the risk of a large, rapid fluid shift is greater.
- Use a large-gauge (16- to 20-gauge) IV cannula for administration of the drug.
- Pregnancy category C.

PHARMACOKINETICS

Because albumin is a natural substance, it is difficult to obtain pharmacokinetic values for supplements.

ADVERSE EFFECTS

Because albumin is a natural blood product, allergic reactions are possible. However, coagulation factors, antibodies, and most other blood proteins have been removed; therefore, the incidence of allergic reactions from albumin is not high. Signs of allergy include fever, chills, rash, dyspnea, and possibly hypotension. Protein overload may occur if excessive albumin is infused.

Contraindications: Contraindications include severe anemia or cardiac failure in the presence of normal or increased intravascular volume, and allergy to albumin.

INTERACTIONS

Drug–Drug: Unknown.

Lab Tests: May increase serum alkaline phosphatase.

Herbal/Food: Unknown.

Treatment of Overdose: There is no treatment for overdose.

 See the Companion Website for a Nursing Process Focus specific to this drug.

weight to assess fluid retention or loss. These products are used with caution in lactation and pregnancy (category C).

Anaphylactic reactions may occur with the use of plasma protein fraction (Plasmanate), dextran 75 (Gentran 75), dextran 70 (Macrodex), and hetastarch (Hespan). Signs and symptoms of an allergic response may include periorbital edema, urticaria, wheezing, and difficulty breathing. The use of dextran, a high-molecular-weight polysaccharide, is further limited because it can interfere with coagulation and platelet adhesion. Hetastarch, a synthetic starch resembling human glycogen, can increase the prothrombin time (PT), partial thromboplastic time (PTT), and bleeding time when given in large doses, thus limiting its use in conditions in which normal clotting is essential. Clients with renal failure exhibiting anuria or oliguria are at great risk for fluid overload because of the fluid shift that will occur and their inability to rid the body of excess fluid through urination.

Client Teaching.   Client education as it relates to crystalloid and colloids therapy should include the goals of therapy, the reasons for obtaining baseline data such as vital signs, and the existence of underlying disorders such as cardiac and renal disorders, and possible drug side effects. Include the following points when teaching clients about crystalloid and colloid therapy.

- Immediately report difficulty breathing, wheezing, or itching.
- Report changes in sensorium such as light-headedness, drowsiness, or dizziness.
- Report signs of edema such as swelling of the feet or ankles.

VASOCONSTRICTORS/VASOPRESSORS

In some types of shock, the most serious medical challenge facing the client is hypotension, which may become so profound as to cause collapse of the circulatory system. Vasoconstrictors are drugs for maintaining blood pressure when vasodilation has caused hypotension but fluids have not been lost (i.e., anaphylactic shock) and when fluid replacement agents have proved ineffective. These agents are listed in Table 29.3.

29.5 Treating Shock With Vasoconstrictors/Vasopressors

In the early stages of shock, the body compensates for the initial fall in blood pressure by activating the sympathetic nervous system. This sympathetic activity produces vasoconstriction, which raises blood pressure and increases the rate and force of myocardial contractions. The purpose of these compensatory measures is to maintain blood flow to vital organs such as the heart and brain, and to decrease flow to other organs, including the kidneys and liver.

The body's ability to compensate is limited, however, and profound hypotension may develop as shock progresses. In severe cases, fluid replacement agents alone are not effective at raising blood pressure, and other medications are indicated. Historically, sympathomimetic vasoconstrictors, also known as *vasopressors*, have been used to stabilize blood pressure in shock clients. When given intravenously, these drugs have rapid onsets with short durations, and will immediately raise blood pressure. Because of side effects and potential organ damage due to the rapid and intense vasoconstriction, vasopressors are used only after fluid and electrolyte restoration has failed to raise blood pressure. These drugs are considered critical care agents: The infusions are continuously monitored and adjusted to ensure the desired therapeutic effect has been achieved without significant adverse effects. Therapy is discontinued as soon as the client's condition stabilizes. Discontinuation of vasopressor therapy is always gradual, owing to the possibility of rebound hypotension and undesirable cardiac effects.

Sympathomimetics used for shock include norepinephrine (Levarterenol, Levophed), isoproterenol (Isuprel), phenylephrine (Neo-Synephrine), and mephentermine (Wyamine). These agents activate *alpha*-adrenergic receptors. Sympathomimetics that are more selective for *beta₁*-adrenergic receptors have beneficial cardiac effects (Section 29.6). The use of the nonselective sympathomimetic epinephrine is associated with the treatment of anaphylaxis (Section 29.7). The basic pharmacology of the sympathomimetics is presented in Chapter 13 ∞.

TABLE 29.3 Vasoconstrictors for Shock		
Drug	**Route and Adult Dose (max dose where indicated)**	**Adverse Effects**
NONSELECTIVE ALPHA- AND BETA-ADRENERGIC AGENTS		
mephentermine (Wyamine) ⊕ norepinephrine (Levarterenol, Levophed)	IV; 20–60 mg as an infusion (1.2 mg/ml of D5W) IV; 8–12 mcg/min until pressure stabilizes, then 2–4 mcg/min for maintenance	*Restlessness, anxiety, palpitations, nausea, vomiting, headache* Tachycardia or bradycardia (overdose), hypertension
SELECTIVE ALPHA-ADRENERGIC AGENTS		
phenylephrine (Neo-Synephrine, others) (see page 138 for the Prototype Drug box ∞)	IV; 0.1–0.18 mg/min until pressure stabilizes, then 0.04–0.06 mg/min for maintenance	*Palpitations, tingling or coldness of extremities, nervousness* Severe peripheral vasoconstriction, tachycardia or bradycardia (overdose), hypertension, dysrhythmias, necrosis at injection site

Italics indicate common adverse effects; underlining indicates serious adverse effects.

Pr PROTOTYPE DRUG | Norepinephrine *(Levarterenol, Levophed)* | Vasoconstrictor/Sympathomimetic

ACTIONS AND USES

Norepinephrine is a sympathomimetic that acts directly on alpha-adrenergic receptors in vascular smooth muscle to immediately raise blood pressure. To a lesser degree, it also stimulates beta$_1$-receptors in the heart, thus producing a positive inotropic response that may increase cardiac output. Its primary indications are acute shock and cardiac arrest. Norepinephrine is the vasopressor of choice for septic shock because reseach has demonstrated that it significantly decreases mortality. It is given by the IV route and has a duration of only 1 to 2 minutes after the infusion is terminated.

ADMINISTRATION ALERTS

- Start an infusion only after ensuring the patency of the IV. Monitor the flow rate continuously.
- Keep phentolamine available in case of extravasation.
- Do not abruptly discontinue infusion.
- Pregnancy category D.

PHARMACOKINETICS

Onset: 1–2 min

Peak: 1–2 min

Half-life: Unknown

Duration: Unknown

ADVERSE EFFECTS

Norepinephrine is a powerful vasoconstrictor; thus, continuous monitoring of the client's blood pressure is required to detect hypertension. When first administered, reflex bradycardia is sometimes experienced. It also has the ability to produce various types of dysrhythmias, although less so than other vasopressors. Blurred vision and photophobia are signs of overdose.

Contraindications: Norepinephrine should not be administered to clients who are experiencing hypotension due to blood volume deficits because vasoconstriction already exists in such clients. Norepinephrine may cause additional, severe peripheral and visceral vasoconstriction with decreased urine output. Norepinephrine is not usually given to clients with mesenteric or peripheral vascular thrombosis, because there is an increased risk of increasing ischemia and worsening the infarction.

INTERACTIONS

Drug–Drug: Alpha- and beta-blockers may antagonize the drug's vasopressor effects. Conversely, ergot alkaloids and tricyclic antidepressants may potentiate vasopressor effects. Digoxin, halothane, and cyclopropane may increase the risk of dysrhythmias.

Lab Tests: Unknown.

Herbal/Food: Unknown.

Treatment of Overdose: Discontinuing the infusion usually results in rapid reversal of adverse effects such as hypertension.

 See the Companion Website for a Nursing Process Focus specific to this drug.

NURSING CONSIDERATIONS

The role of the nurse in vasoconstrictor therapy for hypotension related to shock involves careful monitoring of a client's condition and providing education as it relates to the prescribed drug treatment. Because the client is experiencing shock, initially assess blood pressure and heart rate. Also assess the client's history for cardiovascular disease, in particular (vasoconstrictors are contraindicated in severe cardiovascular disease), obtain an ECG reading, and monitor urine output. Place the client on telemetry for the duration of intravenous therapy. Because vasoconstrictors may increase intraocular pressure, assess for a history of narrow-angle glaucoma.

In addition to knowing the adverse effects described in the Prototype Drug box for norepinephrine, also be aware that other drugs in this class could cause additional side effects. Phenylephrine (Neo-Synephrine) will cause necrosis of tissue if extravasation occurs. Ensure IV patency prior to beginning the infusion, and monitor the IV site during infusion. Monitor blood pressure and titrate the IV rate if blood pressure is elevated. Monitor urine output, because extreme vasoconstriction may lead to decreased renal perfusion. Assess for severe headache because this is often an early sign of overdose with vasopressors.

Closely monitor the client for chest pain and ECG changes. Dosages are usually reduced if the heart rate exceeds 110 beats per minute. During drug administration, monitor mental status changes, skin temperature of extremities, and color of ear lobes, nail beds, and lips.

Client Teaching. Client education as it relates to vasoconstrictor therapy should include the goals of therapy, the reasons for obtaining baseline data such as vital signs and the existence of underlying cardiac disorders, and possible drug side effects. Include the following points when teaching clients about vasoconstrictors:

- Immediately report any pain or burning at the IV site.
- Immediately report blanching or blueness of fingers.
- Immediately report chest pain or palpitations.

See "Nursing Process Focus: Clients Receiving Sympathomimetic Therapy," page 139 in Chapter 13 ∞, for the complete Nursing Process applied to caring for clients receiving sympathomimetics (beta-adrenergic agonists).

INOTROPIC AGENTS

Inotropic agents, also called *cardiotonic drugs,* increase the force of contraction of the heart. In the treatment of shock, they are used to increase the cardiac output. The inotropic agents are listed in Table 29.4.

NURSING PROCESS FOCUS   Clients Receiving IV Fluid Replacement Therapy for Shock

Assessment	Potential Nursing Diagnoses
Prior to administration: ■ Obtain a complete health history, including allergies, drug history, and possible drug interactions. ■ Assess breath sounds and vital signs. ■ Assess renal function (BUN and creatinine). ■ Assess level of consciousness. ■ Assess knowledge level about medications.	■ Injury, Risk for, related to allergic reaction to drug ■ Fluid Volume, Excess, related to increased intravascular volume ■ Tissue Perfusion, Ineffective, related to adverse effects of drug ■ Knowledge, Deficient, related to drug therapy

Planning: Client Goals and Expected Outcomes

The client will:
■ Immediately report difficulty breathing, itching, or flushing.
■ Maintain urine output of at least 50 ml/h.
■ Maintain systolic blood pressure greater than 90 mm Hg.
■ Remain alert and oriented.
■ Demonstrate an understanding of the drug's action by accurately describing drug side effects and precautions.

Implementation

Interventions and (Rationales)	Client Education/Discharge Planning
■ Monitor respiratory status. (Effects of drugs and rapid infusion may result in fluid overload.)	Instruct client to: ■ Report any signs of respiratory distress. ■ Report changes in sensorium such as light-headedness, drowsiness, or dizziness.
■ Monitor intake and output for changes in renal function. (Renal function is decreased with shock.)	■ Instruct client concerning rationale for Foley catheter insertion.
■ Monitor electrolytes. (Crystalloid drugs may cause hypernatremia and resulting fluid retention.)	■ Instruct client to report any evidence of edema.
■ Observe client for signs of allergic reactions. (Administration of blood and blood products could cause allergic reactions.)	Instruct client: ■ To report itching, rash, chills, and difficulty breathing. ■ That frequent blood draws are necessary to monitor possible complications of drug administration.
■ Observe urine for changes in color. (Adverse reaction to blood [hemolysis] could cause hematuria.)	■ Instruct client to notify the healthcare provider if changes in urine color occur.

Evaluation of Outcome Criteria

Evaluate the effectiveness of drug therapy by confirming that client goals and expected outcomes have been met (see "Planning").
■ The client is free of itching, flushing, and shortness of breath.
■ The client maintains urine output of at least 50 ml/h.
■ The client's systolic blood pressure is greater than 90 mm Hg.
■ The client is alert and oriented.
■ The client demonstrates an understanding of the drug's action by accurately describing drug side effects and precautions.

∞ *See Table 29.2 for a list of the drugs to which these nursing actions apply.*

TABLE 29.4 **Inotropic Drugs for Shock**		
Drug	**Route and Adult Dose (max dose where indicated)**	**Adverse Effects**
digoxin (Lanoxin, Lanoxicaps) (see page 339 for the Prototype Drug box ∞)	IV; digitalizing dose 2.5–5 mcg q6h for 24 h; maintenance dose 0.125–0.5 mg/day	*Nausea, vomiting, headache, and visual disturbances such as halos, a yellow/green tinge, or blurring* Dysrhythmias, AV block
dobutamine (Dobutrex) 🔵 dopamine (Dopastat, Intropin)	IV; infused at a rate of 2.5–40 mcg/kg/min for a max of 72 h IV; 1.5 mcg/kg/min initial dose; may be increased to 30 mcg/kg/min	*Headache, palpitations, nausea, vomiting, changes in blood pressure (hypotension or hypertension)* Dysrhythmias, gangrene, severe hypertension

Italics indicate common adverse effects; <u>underlining</u> indicates serious adverse effects.

29.6 Treating Shock With Inotropic Agents

As shock progresses, the heart may begin to fail; cardiac output decreases, lowering the amount of blood reaching vital tissues and deepening the degree of shock. **Inotropic agents** have the potential to reverse the cardiac symptoms of shock by increasing the strength of myocardial contraction. For example, digoxin (Lanoxin) increases myocardial contractility and cardiac output, thus quickly bringing critical tissues their essential oxygen. Chapter 22 ∞ should be reviewed, because digoxin and other medications prescribed for heart failure are sometimes used for the treatment of shock.

Dobutamine (Dobutrex) is a selective beta$_1$-adrenergic agent that has value in the short-term treatment of certain types of shock, owing to its ability to cause the heart to beat more forcefully. Dobutamine is especially beneficial when the primary cause of shock is related to heart failure, rather than hypovolemia. The resulting increase in cardiac output assists in maintaining blood flow to vital organs. Dobutamine has a half-life of only 2 minutes and is given only as an IV infusion.

Dopamine (Dopastat, Inotropin) activates both beta- and alpha-adrenergic receptors. Dopamine is utilized at different dosage levels and will have different effects based on the receptors most affected. It is primarily used in shock conditions to increase blood pressure by causing peripheral

---

Pr PROTOTYPE DRUG | Dopamine *(Dopastat, Inotropin)* | Inotropic Agent

ACTIONS AND USES

Dopamine is the immediate metabolic precursor to norepinephrine. Although dopamine is classified as a sympathomimetic, its mechanism of action is dependent on the dose. At low doses, the drug selectively stimulates dopaminergic receptors, especially in the kidneys, leading to vasodilation and an increased blood flow through the kidneys. This makes dopamine of particular value in treating hypovolemic and cardiogenic shock. At higher doses, dopamine stimulates beta$_1$-adrenergic receptors, causing the heart to beat more forcefully and increasing cardiac output. Another beneficial effect of dopamine when given in higher doses is its ability to stimulate alpha-adrenergic receptors, thus causing vasoconstriction and raising blood pressure.

ADMINISTRATION ALERTS

- Give this drug as a continuous infusion only.
- Ensure patency of the IV prior to beginning infusion.
- Keep phentolamine readily available as the antidote for extravasation.
- Pregnancy category C.

PHARMACOKINETICS

Onset: 1–2 min

Peak: Unknown

Half-life: 2 min

Duration: Less than 10 min

ADVERSE EFFECTS

Because of dopamine's profound effects on the cardiovascular system, clients receiving the drug must be continuously monitored for signs of dysrhythmias and hypertension. Side effects are normally self-limiting because of the short half-life of the drug. Dopamine is a vesicant drug that can cause severe, irreversible damage if the drug infiltrates.

Contraindications: Dopamine is contraindicated in patients with pheochromocytoma or ventricular fibrillation.

INTERACTIONS

Drug–Drug: Concurrent administration with MAO inhibitors or ergot alkaloids increase alpha-adrenergic effects. Phenytoin may decrease dopamine action. Beta-blockers may inhibit the inotropic effects of dopamine. Alpha-blockers inhibit peripheral vasoconstriction. Digoxin and many anesthetics increase the risk of dysrhythmias.

Lab Tests: Unknown.

Herbal/Food: Unknown.

Treatment of Overdose: Discontinuing the infusion usually results in rapid reversal of adverse effects such as hypertension. The short-acting alpha-adrenergic blocker phentolamine may be administered to stabilize the client's condition.

 See the Companion Website for a Nursing Process Focus specific to this drug.

vasoconstriction (alpha₁ activation) and increasing the force of myocardial contraction (beta₁ activation). Dopamine has the potential to cause dysrhythmias and is given only as an IV infusion.

NURSING CONSIDERATIONS

The role of the nurse in inotropic therapy for shock involves careful monitoring of a client's condition and providing education as it relates to the prescribed drug treatment. Prior to administration, assess for history of cardiovascular disease and obtain an ECG. Also assess blood pressure, pulse, urine output, and body weight.

Because inotropic agents worsen dysrhythmias, they are contraindicated in clients with ventricular tachycardia. Increased myocardial contractility may precipitate heart failure; therefore, inotropic agents are also contraindicated in hypertrophic idiopathic subaortic stenosis.

Safe use during pregnancy and lactation has not been established (category C). Use inotropic agents cautiously in clients who are hypertensive because these drugs increase blood pressure. With atrial fibrillation, a rapid ventricular response may increase heart rate excessively. Hypovolemia should be corrected with whole blood or plasma volume expanders prior to the start of dopamine infusion.

Inotropic medications may be used separately or concurrently with other antishock agents. Inotropic medication is administered only as a continuous infusion, and the dosage is calculated in micrograms per kilograms per minute. Always infuse these medications via an IV pump. IV pump technology is such that some pumps will automate calculations, and most have the ability to deliver dosages to a tenth of a milliliter. Despite the automated calculations, ensure that the medication is infusing at the correct milliliters per minute. To calculate the IV rate, multiply the ordered dose times the client's weight in kilograms times 60 (to get micrograms per hour); then divide this amount by the concentration of the infusion (micrograms/milliliter). The result is the milliliters/hour to be administered. Weigh the client each morning and recalculate the dose each day, based on the current weight.

Monitor the client's cardiac rhythm prior to and during the infusion of inotropic drugs. Assess blood pressure frequently. If a pressure-monitoring catheter is in place, assess pulmonary wedge pressure and cardiac output to keep these parameters within normal ranges. Use a large vein for IV infusion; a central line is preferable. Extravasation of dopamine (Dopastat, Inotropin) can cause severe localized vasoconstriction, resulting in sloughing of tissue and tissue necrosis if not reversed with phentolamine (Regitine) injections at the site of the infiltration. If extravasation occurs, discontinue the IV, restart it in another site, and administer the antidote. If infiltration occurs, dobutamine (Dobutrex) can be irritating to the vein and surrounding tissues, although it causes less severe vasoconstriction than dopamine.

Monitor renal function closely, including urine output, BUN, and creatinine levels. With improved cardiac output, renal function should improve and urine output increase. Low doses of dopamine increase renal perfusion and should enhance urine output. Foley catheters may be employed to ensure accurate measurement of urine output.

Client Teaching. Client education as it relates to inotropic drug therapy for shock should include the goals of therapy, the reasons for obtaining baseline data such as vital signs and the existence of underlying cardiac and renal disorders, and possible drug side effects. Explain frequent monitoring and any catheter placement.

Include the following points when teaching clients about inotropic agents:

- Expect that continuous cardiac monitoring will occur during administration of the medication.
- Immediately report chest pain, difficulty breathing, palpitations, or headache.
- Immediately report burning or pain at the IV site.
- Immediately report numbness or tingling in the extremities.

See "Nursing Process Focus: Clients Receiving Sympathomimetic Therapy," page 139 in Chapter 13 ∞, for the complete Nursing Process applied to caring for clients receiving beta-adrenergic agonists.

ANAPHYLAXIS

Anaphylaxis is a potentially fatal condition in which body defenses produce a hyperresponse to a foreign chemical known as an *antigen* or *allergen*. On first exposure, the allergen produces no symptoms; however, the body responds by becoming highly sensitized for a subsequent exposure. During anaphylaxis, the body responds quickly, often just minutes after exposure to the allergen, by releasing massive amounts of histamine and other mediators of the inflammatory response. The client may experience itching, hives, and a tightness in the throat or chest. Swelling occurs around the larynx, causing a nonproductive cough and the voice to become hoarse. As anaphylaxis progresses, the client experiences a rapid fall in blood pressure and difficulty breathing due to bronchoconstriction. The hypotension causes reflex tachycardia. Without medical intervention, anaphylaxis leads to a profound state of shock, which is often fatal. ● Figure 29.3 illustrates the symptoms of anaphylaxis.

29.7 Pharmacotherapy of Anaphylaxis

The pharmacotherapy of anaphylaxis is symptomatic and involves supporting the cardiovascular system and preventing further hyperresponse by body defenses. Various medications are used to treat the symptoms of anaphylaxis, depending on the severity of the symptoms.

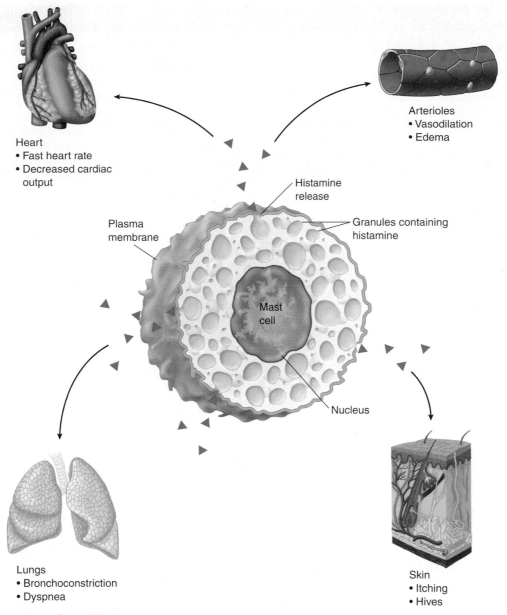

Heart
• Fast heart rate
• Decreased cardiac output

Arterioles
• Vasodilation
• Edema

Histamine release

Granules containing histamine

Plasma membrane

Mast cell

Nucleus

Lungs
• Bronchoconstriction
• Dyspnea

Skin
• Itching
• Hives

● **Figure 29.3** Symptoms of anaphylaxis

Epinephrine, 1:1000, given subcutaneously or IM, is an initial drug of choice because it can rapidly reverse hypotension. If necessary, the dose may be repeated up to three times at 10- to 15-minute intervals. Antihistamines such as diphenhydramine (Benadryl) may be administered IM or IV to prevent further release of histamine. A bronchodilator such as albuterol (Ventolin, Proventil) is often administered by inhalation to relieve the acute shortness of breath caused by histamine release. High-flow oxygen is usually administered. Systemic glucocorticoids such as hydrocortisone are given to dampen the *delayed* inflammatory response that may occur several hours after the initial event.

Nearly all drugs have the capability to *cause* anaphylaxis. Although this is a rare adverse drug effect, the nurse must be prepared to quickly deal with anaphylaxis by understanding the indications and doses of the various drugs on the emergency cart. The most common drugs causing anaphylaxis include the following:

• Antibiotics, especially penicillins, cephalosporins, and sulfonamides

• NSAIDs, such as aspirin, ibuprofen, and naproxen

• ACE inhibitors

• Opioid analgesics

• Iodine-based contrast media used for radiographic exams

Although obtaining a client history of drug allergy is helpful in predicting some adverse drug reactions, anaphylaxis may occur without a previously reported incident. However, previous severe hypersensitivity to a drug is always a contraindication to the future use of that or closely related drugs in the same class. Unless the drug is the only one available to treat the client's condition, the drug should not be administered.

Pr PROTOTYPE DRUG | Epinephrine *(Adrenalin)* | Sympathomimetic/Anaphylaxis Drug

ACTIONS AND USES

Subcutaneous or IV epinephrine is a drug of choice for anaphylaxis because it can reverse many of the distressing symptoms within minutes. Epinephrine is a nonselective adrenergic agonist, stimulating both alpha- and beta-adrenergic receptors. Almost immediately after injection, blood pressure rises owing to stimulation of alpha$_1$-receptors. Activation of beta$_2$-receptors in the bronchi opens the airways and relieves the client's shortness of breath. Cardiac output increases owing to stimulation of beta$_1$-receptors in the heart. In addition to the SC and IM routes, inhalation and ophthalmic preparations are available.

ADMINISTRATION ALERTS

- Parenteral epinephrine is an irritant that may cause tissue damage if extravasation occurs.
- Pregnancy category C.

PHARMACOKINETICS

Onset: 3–5 min (subcutaneously); 5–10 min IM

Peak: 20 min

Half-life: Unknown

Duration: 1–4 h

ADVERSE EFFECTS

When administered parenterally, epinephrine may cause serious adverse effects. Hypertension and dysrhythmias may occur rapidly; therefore, the client should be monitored carefully following injection.

Contraindications. In life-threatening conditions such as anaphylaxis, there are no absolute contraindications for the use of epinephrine. The drug must be used with caution, however, in clients with dysrhythmias, cerebrovascular insufficiency, hyperthyroidism, narrow-angle glaucoma, hypertension, or coronary ischemia, because epinephrine may worsen these conditions.

INTERACTIONS

Drug–Drug: Epinephrine may result in hypotension if used with phenothiazines or oxytocin. There may be additive cardiovascular effects with other sympathomimetics. MAO inhibitors, tricyclic antidepressants, and alpha- and beta-adrenergic agents inhibit the actions of epinephrine. Epinephrine will decrease the effects of beta-blockers. Some general anesthetics may sensitize the heart to the effects of epinephrine.

Lab Tests: May decrease serum potassium level.

Herbal/Food: Unknown.

Treatment of Overdose: Overdose may be serious, an alpha- and beta-adrenergic blockers are indicated. If blood pressure remains high, a vasodilator may be administered.

 See the Companion Website for a Nursing Process Focus specific to this drug.

If a drug must be given for which the client has a known allergy, the client may be *pretreated* with antihistamines or glucocorticoids to suppress the inflammatory response. If time permits, clients may be desensitized. Desensitization for penicillin and cephalosporin allergy, which takes about 6 hours, has been shown to be effective in preventing severe allergic reactions to these antibiotics. A typical desensitization regimen would involve administering an initial dose of 0.01 mg of the antibiotic and observing the client for allergy. The dose may then be doubled every 15 to 20 minutes until the full dose has been achieved. Desensitization has also been achieved for clients with aspirin-induced asthma who require aspirin therapy for another condition.

NURSING CONSIDERATIONS

The role of the nurse in vasoconstrictor therapy for anaphylaxis involves careful monitoring of a client's condition and providing education as it relates to the prescribed drug treatment. Vasoconstrictors such as epinephrine (Adrenalin) are given as an emergency response to severe allergic reactions. Although epinephrine is contraindicated for known hypersensitivity to this drug, in life-threatening situations there are no absolute contraindications to its use. Prior to administration, assess the blood pressure and symptoms of allergic response (bronchospasm, hives, and dyspnea).

Administer epinephrine with caution to clients with cardiac disease or a history of cerebral atherosclerosis because it can cause intracranial bleeding, dysrhythmias, or pulmonary edema—resulting from a steep rise in blood pressure—and peripheral vascular constriction combined with cardiac stimulation. Administer epinephrine with caution to clients with hyperthyroidism; epinephrine exacerbates tachycardia.

This drug is frequently administered in the emergency department setting because resuscitative equipment must be readily accessible. Parenteral epinephrine is irritating to tissues; thus, closely monitor IV sites for signs of extravasation. Continuously monitor vital signs, including ECG, during epinephrine infusions. Auscultate breath sounds before and after epinephrine injection to monitor improvement in bronchoconstriction (wheezing). Monitor clients with a history of closed-angle glaucoma for visual changes as a result of changes in intraocular pressure.

Client Teaching.   Client education as it relates to anaphylaxis therapy should include the goals of therapy, the reasons for obtaining baseline data such as vital signs, ECG, and the existence of underlying cardiac and respiratory disorders, and possible drug side effects. Include the following points when teaching clients about clients regarding epinephrine:

- Seek emergency medical attention immediately if a single auto-injection of epinephrine fails to bring relief.

- Immediately report burning, irritation, tenderness, swelling, or hardness at IV or IM injection sites.
- Immediately report changes in level of consciousness, particularly feeling faint.
- Immediately report palpitations, chest pain, nausea, vomiting, sweating, weakness, dizziness, confusion, blurred vision, headache, anxiety, or sense of impending doom.

See "Nursing Process Focus: Clients Receiving Sympathomimetic Therapy," page 139 in Chapter 13 ∞, for more information.

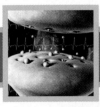

HOME & COMMUNITY CONSIDERATIONS

Recurrent Anaphylaxis

Clients with a history of recurrent anaphylaxis may be prescribed epinephrine to be self-administered intramuscularly via an automatic injectable device (EpiPen). Instruct these clients regarding safe "pen" storage and disposal and the proper injection technique. Encourage clients to use the medication-free "trainer" auto-inject pen to practice the technique. Advise clients to expect some medication to remain in the pen following injection and to report all episodes requiring pen usage to their healthcare provider. Advise clients to wear a MedicAlert bracelet stating "allergy" and to carry a medication allergy list in wallet or purse.

CHAPTER REVIEW

KEY CONCEPTS

The numbered key concepts provide a succinct summary of the important points from the corresponding numbered section within the chapter. If any of these points are not clear, refer to the numbered section within the chapter for review.

29.1 Shock is a clinical syndrome characterized by the inability of the cardiovascular system to pump enough blood to meet the metabolic needs of the tissues. Key body systems affected by shock are the nervous, renal, and cardiovascular systems.

29.2 Shock is often classified by the underlying pathological process or by the organ system that is primarily affected, including cardiogenical, hypovolemic, neurogenic, septic, and anaphylactic shock.

29.3 The initial treatment of shock involves administration of basic life support, replacement of lost fluid, and maintenance of blood pressure.

29.4 During hypovolemic shock, crystalloids replace lost fluids and electrolytes; colloids expand plasma volume and maintain blood pressure. Whole blood may be indicated in cases of massive hemorrhage.

29.5 Vasoconstrictors are critical care drugs sometimes needed during severe shock to maintain blood pressure. These drugs are sympathomimetics that strongly activate alpha-adrenergic receptors in arterioles.

29.6 Inotropic drugs are useful in reversing the decreased cardiac output resulting from shock by increasing the strength of myocardial contraction.

29.7 Anaphylaxis is a serious hypersensitivity response to an allergen that is treated with a large number of different drugs, including sympathomimetics, antihistamines, and glucocorticoids. Common drugs such as penicillins, cephalosporins, NSAIDs, and ACE inhibitors may cause anaphylaxis.

NCLEX-RN® REVIEW QUESTIONS

1 The client in shock is prescribed an infusion of lactated Ringer's. The nurse recognizes the function of this fluid in the treatment of shock is to:

1. Replace fluid and promote urine output.
2. Draw water into cells.
3. Draw water from cells to blood vessels.
4. Maintain vascular volume.

2 The nurse evaluates the effectiveness of dopamine therapy for a client in shock. Which of the following may indicate treatment is successful? (Select all that apply.)

1. Improved urine output
2. Increased blood pressure
3. Creatinine, 4.6 mg/dl
4. BUN, 32 mg/dl
5. Hypotension

3 Dobutamine (Dobutrex) is used to treat a client experiencing cardiogenic shock. Nursing intervention includes:

1. Monitoring for fluid overload.
2. Monitoring for cardiac dysrhythmias.
3. Monitoring respiratory status.
4. Monitoring for hypotension.

4 Teaching for a client receiving plasma protein fraction (Plasmanate) should include reporting which of the following possible adverse reactions?

1. Unusual bleeding
2. Hyperglycemia
3. Anaphylactic reaction
4. Hypotension

5 Nursing assessment of a client receiving normal serum albumin for treatment of shock should include:

1. Assessing breath sounds.
2. Monitoring glucose.
3. Monitoring potassium level.
4. Monitoring hemoglobin and hematocrit.

CRITICAL THINKING QUESTIONS

1. A client is on a norepinephrine (Levophed) drip for cardiogenic shock with a blood pressure of 84/40 mm Hg. Why is this client on this medication? What nursing assessments should occur? When and how should the norepinephrine drip be discontinued?

2. The healthcare provider orders 3 L of 0.9% normal saline (NS) for a 22-year-old client with vomiting and diarrhea, and a heart rate of 122 bpm and blood pressure of 102/54 mm Hg. Is this an appropriate IV solution for this client? Why or why not?

3. A client with a severe head injury has been put on an IV drip of dextrose 5% water running at 150 ml/h. The nurse receives this transfer client and is reviewing the healthcare provider's orders. Is the IV solution appropriate for this client? Why or why not?

See Appendix D for answers and rationales for all activities.

EXPLORE
MediaLink

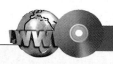 www.prenhall.com/adams

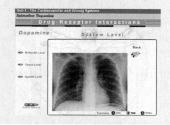

NCLEX-RN® review, case studies, and other interactive resources for this chapter can be found on the companion website at www.prenhall.com/adams. Click on "Chapter 29" to select the activities for this chapter. For animations, more NCLEX-RN® review questions, and an audio glossary, access the accompanying Prentice Hall Nursing MediaLink DVD-ROM in this textbook.

PRENTICE HALL NURSING MEDIALINK DVD-ROM

- **Animations**
  Mechanism in Action: Dopamine (*Dopastat*)
  Mechanism in Action: Epinephrine (*Adrenalin*)
- **Audio Glossary**
- **NCLEX-RN® Review**

COMPANION WEBSITE

- **NCLEX-RN® Review**
- **Dosage Calculations**
- **Case Study:** Client with shock
- **Care Plan:** Client with congestive heart failure treated with dopamine

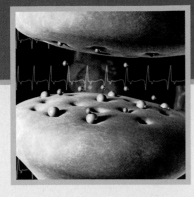

CHAPTER 30

Diuretic Therapy and Drugs for Renal Failure

DRUGS AT A GLANCE

LOOP (HIGH-CEILING) DIURETICS
THIAZIDE AND THIAZIDELIKE DIURETICS
    ⬥ *chlorothiazide (Diuril)*
POTASSIUM-SPARING DIURETICS
    ⬥ *spironolactone (Aldactone)*
MISCELLANEOUS AGENTS
Carbonic Anhydrase Inhibitors
Osmotic Diuretics

OBJECTIVES

After reading this chapter, the student should be able to:

1. Explain the role of the urinary system in maintaining fluid, electrolyte, and acid–base balance.
2. Explain the processes that change the composition of filtrate as it travels through the nephron.
3. Describe the adjustments in pharmacotherapy that must be considered in clients with renal failure.
4. Identify indications for diuretics.
5. Describe the general side effects of diuretic pharmacotherapy.
6. Compare and contrast the loop, thiazide, and potassium-sparing diuretics.
7. Describe the nurse's role in the pharmacological management of renal failure, and in diuretic therapy.
8. For each of the classes shown in Drugs at a Glance, know representative drugs, and explain the mechanism of drug action, primary actions, and important adverse effects.
9. Categorize diuretics and drugs used in the treatment of renal failure based on their classification and mechanism of action.
10. Use the Nursing Process to care for clients who are receiving drug therapy for renal failure, and diuretic therapy.

MediaLink

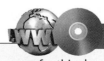

KEY TERMS

carbonic anhydrase   *page 433*
diuretic   *page 427*
filtrate   *page 424*
nephron   *page 424*
reabsorption   *page 425*
renal failure   *page 425*
secretion   *page 425*
urinalysis   *page 425*

The kidneys serve an amazing role in maintaining homeostasis. By filtering a volume equivalent to all the body's extracellular fluid every 100 minutes, the kidneys are able to make immediate adjustments to fluid volume, electrolyte composition, and acid–base balance. This chapter examines diuretics, agents that increase urine output, and other drugs used to treat kidney failure. Chapter 31 ∞ will present additional agents for treating fluid, electrolyte, and acid–base imbalances.

30.1 Functions of the Kidneys

When most people think of the kidneys, they think of excretion. Although this is certainly true, the kidneys have many other homeostatic functions. The kidneys are the primary organs for regulating fluid balance, electrolyte composition, and acid–base balance of body fluids. They also secrete the enzyme renin, which helps regulate blood pressure (Chapter 23 ∞) and erythropoietin, a hormone that stimulates red blood cell production (Chapter 28 ∞). In addition, the kidneys are responsible for the production of calcitriol, the active form of vitamin D, which helps maintain bone homeostasis (Chapter 47 ∞). It is not surprising that our overall health is strongly dependent on proper functioning of the kidneys.

The urinary system consists of two kidneys, two ureters, one urinary bladder, and a urethra. Each kidney contains more than 1 million **nephrons,** the functional units of the kidney. Blood enters the nephron through the large renal arteries and is filtered through a semipermeable membrane known as the glomerulus. Water and other small molecules readily pass through the glomerulus and enter *Bowman's capsule,* the first section of the nephron, and then the proximal tubule. Once in the nephron, the fluid is called **filtrate.** After leaving the proximal tubule, the filtrate travels through the loop of Henle and, subsequently, the distal tubule. Nephrons empty their filtrate into common collecting ducts, and then into larger and larger collecting structures inside the kidney. Fluid leaving the collecting ducts and entering subsequent portions of the kidney is called *urine*. Parts of the nephron are illustrated in ● Figure 30.1.

Many drugs are small enough to pass through the pores of the glomerulus and enter the filtrate. If the drug is bound to plasma proteins, however, it will be too large, and will continue circulating in the blood.

30.2 Renal Reabsorption and Secretion

When filtrate enters Bowman's capsule, its composition is very similar to that of plasma. Plasma proteins such as albumin, however, are too large to pass through the filter and will not be present in the filtrate or in the urine of healthy clients.

PharmFacts

Renal Disorders

- More than 12,000 kidney transplants are performed annually.
- More than 47,000 people are on a waiting list for kidney transplants.
- One of every 750 people is born with a single kidney. A single kidney is larger and more vulnerable to injury from heavy contact sports.
- Urinary tract infection (UTI) is more common in women: 20% to 30% of females experience recurrent infections.
- About 260,000 Americans suffer from chronic kidney failure, and 50,000 die annually from causes related to the disease.
- Type 2 diabetes is the leading cause of chronic kidney failure, accounting for 30% to 40% of all new cases each year.
- Hypertension is the second leading cause of chronic kidney failure, accounting for about 25% of all new cases each year.

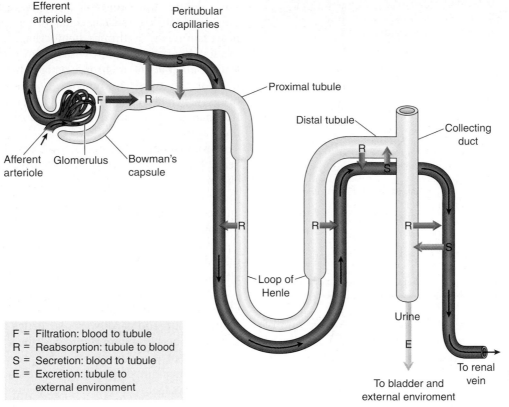

Efferent arteriole
Peritubular capillaries
Proximal tubule
Distal tubule
Collecting duct
Afferent arteriole
Glomerulus
Bowman's capsule
Loop of Henle
Urine
To bladder and external enviroment
To renal vein

F = Filtration: blood to tubule
R = Reabsorption: tubule to blood
S = Secretion: blood to tubule
E = Excretion: tubule to external environment

● **Figure 30.1** The nephron

If these proteins *do* appear in urine, it means they were able to pass through the filter owing to kidney pathology.

As filtrate travels through the nephron, its composition changes dramatically. Some substances in the filtrate cross the walls of the nephron to reenter the blood, a process known as tubular **reabsorption.** Water is the most important molecule reabsorbed in the tubule. For every 180 L of water entering the filtrate each day, approximately 178.5 L is reabsorbed, leaving only 1.5 L to be excreted in the urine. Glucose, amino acids, and essential ions such as sodium, chloride, calcium, and bicarbonate are also reabsorbed.

Certain ions and molecules too large to pass through Bowman's capsule may still enter the urine by crossing from the blood to the filtrate in a process called tubular **secretion.** Potassium, phosphate, hydrogen, and ammonium ions enter the filtrate through active secretion. Acidic drugs secreted in the proximal tubule include penicillin G, ampicillin, sulfisoxazole, nonsteroidal anti-inflammatory drugs (NSAIDs), and furosemide: basic drugs include procainamide, epinephrine, dopamine, neostigmine, and trimethoprim.

Reabsorption and secretion are critical to the pharmacokinetics of drugs. Some drugs are reabsorbed, whereas others are secreted into the filtrate. For example, approximately 90% of a dose of penicillin G enters the urine through secretion. When the kidney is damaged, reabsorption and secretion mechanisms are impaired and serum drug levels may be dramatically affected. The processes of reabsorption and secretion are shown in Figure 30.1.

RENAL FAILURE

Renal failure is a decrease in the kidneys' ability to maintain electrolyte and fluid balance and excrete waste products. Renal failure may result from disorders of other body systems or be intrinsic to the kidney itself. The primary treatment goals are to maintain blood flow through the kidney and adequate urine output.

30.3 Diagnosis and Pharmacotherapy of Renal Failure

Before pharmacotherapy may be considered in a client with renal failure, an assessment of the degree of kidney impairment is necessary. The basic diagnostic test is a **urinalysis,** which examines urine for the presence of blood cells, proteins, pH, specific gravity, ketones, glucose, and microorganisms. The urinalysis can detect proteinuria and albuminuria, which are the primary measures of structural kidney damage. Although it is easy to perform, the urinalysis is nonspecific: Many diseases can cause abnormal urinalysis values. Serum creatinine is an additional measure for detecting kidney disease. To provide a more definitive diagnosis, diagnostic imaging such as computed tomography, sonography, or magnetic resonance imaging may be necessary. Renal biopsy may be performed to obtain a more specific diagnosis.

The best marker for estimating kidney function is the *glomerular filtration rate (GFR),* which is the volume of water filtered through Bowman capsules per minute. The

TABLE 30.1   Nephrotoxic Drugs

Drug or Class	Indication
aminoglycosides	antibiotics
amphotericin B	systemic antifungal
angiotensin-converting enzyme (ACE) inhibitors	hypertension, heart failure
cisplatin/carboplatin	antineoplastic
cyclosporine/tacrolimus	immunosuppressant
foscarnet	antiviral
nonsteroidal anti-inflammatory drugs (NSAIDs)	inflammation
pentamidine	anti-infective (Pneumocystis)
radiographic contrast agents	diagnosis of kidney and vascular disorders

GFR can be used to predict the onset and progression of kidney failure, and provides an indication of the ability of the kidneys to excrete drugs from the body. A progressive decline in GFR indicates a decline in the number of functioning nephrons. As nephrons "die," however, the remaining healthy nephrons have the ability to compensate by increasing their filtration capacity. Thus, clients with significant kidney damage may show no symptoms until 50% or more of the nephrons have "died" and the GFR falls to less than half its normal value.

Renal failure is classified as acute or chronic, depending on its onset. Acute renal failure requires immediate treatment because retention of nitrogenous waste products in the body such as urea and creatinine can result in death if untreated. The most common cause of acute renal failure is renal hypoperfusion: lack of sufficient blood flow through the kidneys. Hypoperfusion can lead to permanent destruction to kidney cells and nephrons. To correct this type of renal failure, the cause of the hypoperfusion must be quickly identified and corrected. Potential causes include heart failure, dysrhythmias, hemorrhage, toxins, and dehydration. Pharmacotherapy with nephrotoxic drugs can also lead to either acute or chronic renal failure. It is good practice for the nurse to remember common nephrotoxic drugs, which are listed in Table 30.1, so that kidney function may be continuously monitored during therapy with these agents.

Chronic renal failure occurs over a period of months or years. More than half the cases of chronic renal failure occur in clients with long-standing hypertension or diabetes mellitus. Owing to the long, gradual development period and nonspecific symptoms, chronic renal failure may go undiagnosed for many years, until the impairment becomes irreversible. In end-stage renal disease (ESRD), dialysis and kidney transplantation become treatment alternatives.

Pharmacotherapy of renal failure attempts to cure the cause of the dysfunction. Diuretics are given to increase urine output, and cardiovascular drugs are administered to treat underlying hypertension or heart failure. Dietary management is often necessary to prevent worsening of renal impairment. Depending on the stage of the disease, dietary management may include protein restriction and reduction of sodium, potassium, phosphorus, and magnesium intake. For diabetic clients, control of blood glucose through intensive insulin therapy may reduce the risk of renal damage. Selected pharmacological agents used to prevent and treat kidney failure are summarized in Table 30.2.

The nurse serves a key role in recognizing and responding to renal failure. Once a diagnosis is established, all nephrotoxic medications should be either discontinued or used with extreme caution. Because the kidneys excrete most drugs or their metabolites, medications will require a significant dosage reduction in clients with moderate to severe renal failure. The importance of this

TABLE 30.2   Pharmacological Management of Renal Failure

Complication	Pathogenesis	Treatment
anemia	Kidneys are unable to synthesize enough erythropoietin for red blood cell production.	epoetin alfa (Procrit, Epogen)
hypocalcemia	Hyperphosphatemia leads to loss of calcium.	usually corrected by reversing the hyperphosphatemia, but additional calcium supplements may be necessary
hyperkalemia	Kidneys are unable to adequately excrete potassium.	dietary restriction of potassium; polystyrene sulfate (Kayexalate) with sorbitol
hyperphosphatemia	Kidneys are unable to adequately excrete phosphate.	dietary restriction of phosphate; phosphate binders such as calcium carbonate (Os-Cal 500, others), calcium acetate (Calphron, PhosLo), lanthanum carbonate (Fosrenol), or sevelamer (Renagel)
hypervolemia	Kidneys are unable to excrete sufficient sodium and water, leading to water retention.	dietary restriction of sodium; loop diuretics in acute conditions, thiazide diuretics in mild conditions
metabolic acidosis	Kidneys are unable to adequately excrete metabolic acids.	sodium bicarbonate or sodium citrate

cannot be overemphasized: *Administering the "average" dose to a client in severe renal failure can have mortal consequences.*

DIURETICS

Diuretics are drugs that adjust the volume and/or composition of body fluids. They are indicated for the treatment of renal failure, hypertension, and the removal of edema fluid.

30.4 Mechanism of Action of Diuretics

A **diuretic** is a drug that increases the rate of urine flow. The goal of most diuretic therapy is reduction of extracellular fluid volume, to reverse abnormal fluid retention by the body. Excretion of excess fluid in the body is particularly desirable in the following conditions:

- Hypertension
- Heart failure
- Kidney failure
- Liver failure or cirrhosis
- Pulmonary edema

The most common mechanism by which diuretics act is by blocking sodium (Na^+) reabsorption in the nephron, thus sending more Na^+ to the urine. Chloride ions (Cl^-) follow sodium. Because water molecules also travel with sodium ions, blocking the reabsorption of Na^+ will increase the volume of urination, or diuresis. Diuretics may affect the renal excretion of other ions, including magnesium, potassium, phosphate, calcium, and bicarbonate ions.

Diuretics are classified into three major groups, and one miscellaneous group, based on differences in their chemical structures and mechanism of action. Some drugs, such as furosemide (Lasix), act by preventing the reabsorption of sodium in the loop of Henle; thus, they are called *loop* diuretics. Because of the abundance of sodium in the filtrate within the loop of Henle, drugs in this class are capable of producing large increases in urine output. Other drugs, such as the *thiazides,* act by blocking sodium in the distal tubule. Because most Na^+ has already been reabsorbed from the filtrate by the time it reaches the distal tubule, the thiazides produce less diuresis than furosemide and other loop diuretics. The third major class is named *potassium-sparing,* because these diuretics have minimal effect on K^+ excretion. Miscellaneous agents include the osmotic diuretics and carbonic anhydrase inhibitors. The sites in the nephron at

PHARMACOTHERAPY ILLUSTRATED

30.1   Mechanisms of Action of Diuretics

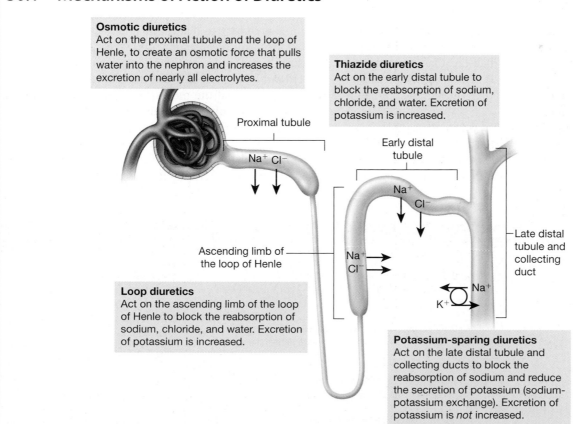

Osmotic diuretics
Act on the proximal tubule and the loop of Henle, to create an osmotic force that pulls water into the nephron and increases the excretion of nearly all electrolytes.

Thiazide diuretics
Act on the early distal tubule to block the reabsorption of sodium, chloride, and water. Excretion of potassium is increased.

Proximal tubule

Early distal tubule

Na^+ Cl^-

Na^+
Cl^-

Late distal tubule and collecting duct

Ascending limb of the loop of Henle

Na^+
Cl^-

Na^+

K^+

Loop diuretics
Act on the ascending limb of the loop of Henle to block the reabsorption of sodium, chloride, and water. Excretion of potassium is increased.

Potassium-sparing diuretics
Act on the late distal tubule and collecting ducts to block the reabsorption of sodium and reduce the secretion of potassium (sodium-potassium exchange). Excretion of potassium is *not* increased.

which the various diuretics act are shown in Pharmacotherapy Illustrated 30.1.

It is common practice to combine two or more drugs in the pharmacotherapy of hypertension and fluid retention disorders. The primary rationales for combination therapy are that the incidence of side effects is decreased and the pharmacological effect may be enhanced. For client convenience, some of these drugs are combined in single-tablet formulations. Examples of single-tablet diuretic combinations include the following:

- Aldactazide: hydrochlorothiazide and spironolactone
- Apresazide: hydrochlorothiazide and hydralazine
- Dyazide: hydrochlorothiazide and triamterene

30.5 Pharmacotherapy With Loop Diuretics

The most effective diuretics are called *loop* or *high-ceiling* diuretics. Drugs in this class act by blocking the reabsorption of sodium and chloride in the loop of Henle. When given IV, they have the ability to cause large amounts of fluid to be excreted by the kidney in a very short time. Loop diuretics are used to reduce the edema associated with heart failure, hepatic cirrhosis, or chronic renal failure. Furosemide and torsemide are also approved for hypertension. The loop diuretics are listed in Table 30.3.

Furosemide is the most commonly prescribed loop diuretic. A drug profile for furosemide was given in Chapter 24 ∞. Unlike the thiazide diuretics, furosemide is able to increase urine output even when blood flow to the kidneys is diminished, which makes it of particular value in clients with renal failure. Torsemide has a longer half-life than furosemide, which offers the advantage of once-a-day dosing. Bumetanide (Bumex) is 40 times more potent than furosemide but has a shorter duration of action.

The rapid excretion of large amounts of fluid has the potential to produce serious adverse effects such as dehydration and electrolyte imbalances. Signs of dehydration include thirst, dry mouth, weight loss, and headache. Hypotension, dizziness,

and fainting can result from the rapid fluid loss. Potassium depletion can be serious and result in dysrhythmias; potassium supplements may be prescribed to prevent hypokalemia. Potassium loss is of particular concern to clients who are also taking digoxin (Lanoxin). Although rare, ototoxicity is possible, and other ototoxic drugs such as the aminoglycoside antibiotics should be avoided during loop diuretic therapy. Because of the potential for serious side effects, the loop diuretics are normally reserved for clients with moderate to severe fluid retention, or when other diuretics have failed to achieve therapeutic goals.

NURSING CONSIDERATIONS

The role of the nurse in loop diuretic therapy for edema associated with congestive heart failure, pulmonary edema, hepatic disease, and nephrotic syndrome involves careful monitoring of a client's condition and providing education as it relates to the prescribed drug treatment. Interview the client for a medical history to determine the presence of diabetes mellitus; severe renal disease; use of digoxin, lithium, or other antihypertensives; a history of gout; and current pregnancy or lactation. Use loop diuretics cautiously in clients with these histories.

Obtain baseline lab values and current level of urine output. It is critical to measure electrolyte levels, especially potassium, sodium, and chloride, prior to loop diuretic therapy. Monitor the client's blood urea nitrogen (BUN), serum creatinine, uric acid, and blood glucose levels. Check serum potassium levels to determine whether potassium supplements are needed.

Careful monitoring of intake and output and daily weight is necessary to determine an effective response. Assessment of skin turgor, moisture, vital signs (check blood pressure lying, sitting, and standing), breath sounds, and presence of edema will also indicate the effectiveness of the loop diuretic. Hold the medication and notify the healthcare provider if your assessment indicates hypotension, serious dehydration or hypokalemia.

Adverse effects may be experienced with loop diuretic use. Assess for circulatory collapse (due to loss of fluid), dysrhythmias, hearing loss, renal failure, and anemia. Orthostatic

TABLE 30.3 Loop Diuretics		
Drug	**Route and Adult Dose (max dose where indicated)**	**Adverse Effects**
bumetanide (Bumex)	PO: 0.5–2 mg/day, may repeat at 4- to 5-h intervals if needed (max: 10 mg/day); IV/IM: 0.5–1 mg over 1–2 min, repeated q2–3h PRN (max: 10 mg/day)	*Minor hypokalemia, postural hypotension, tinnitus, nausea, diarrhea, dizziness, fatigue*
ethacrynic acid (Edecrin)	PO: 50–100 mg 1–2 times/day, may increase by 25–50 mg PRN up to 400 mg/day; IV: 0.5–1 mg/kg or 50 mg up to 100 mg, may repeat if necessary	<u>Serious hypokalemia, blood dyscrasias, dehydration, ototoxicity, electrolyte imbalances, circulatory collapse</u>
furosemide (Lasix) (see page 336 for the Prototype Drug box ∞)	PO: 20–80 mg in single or divided doses (max: 600 mg/day) IV/IM: 20–40 mg in single or divided doses up to 600 mg/day	
torsemide (Demadex)	PO/IV: 10–20 mg/day (max: 200 mg/day)	

Italics indicate common adverse effects; <u>underlining</u> indicates serious adverse effects.

hypotension, hypokalemia, hyponatremia, and polyuria are additional common side effects. Observe for a rash or pruritis, which can indicate hypersensitivity to loop diuretics.

Lifespan Considerations. Use loop diuretics with caution in elderly clients, because they are more susceptible to dehydration and electrolyte imbalances from the drugs. Diuretics can cause frequent urination, which can be inconvenient and increase the incidence of incontinence. This may cause embarrassment, and the older adult may opt for less participation in activities, leading to social isolation. Incontinent clients require meticulous skin care to reduce the risk of skin breakdown. Use these drugs with caution in pregnant or lactating women. Use is restricted in neonates and infants because the drug effects on their immature cardiovascular system may be exaggerated.

Client Teaching. Client education as it relates to loop diuretics should include the goals of therapy, the reasons for obtaining baseline data such as vital signs and the existence of underlying cardiac, renal, and electrolyte disorders, and the possible drug side effects. Include the following points when teaching clients about loop diuretics:

- Expect increased urine output.
- Take medication in the morning to avoid nighttime urination that could result in increased risk of injury.
- Immediately report signs and symptoms such as muscle weakness or cramps and pulse changes, because these may indicate hypokalemia.
- Take potassium supplements, if ordered, and eat potassium-rich foods.

- Monitor blood pressure weekly and report substantial changes.
- Change positions slowly to avoid dizziness.
- Avoid foods high in sodium content such as canned foods, "fast" foods, and frozen dinners.
- Check weight daily, and report a weight gain of 2 lb or greater in 24 hours, shortness of breath, or swelling of ankles.
- Keep all scheduled laboratory visits for electrolyte status testing.
- If diabetic, monitor glucose levels closely, because diabetic therapy may need to be adjusted.
- Report any tenderness or pain in joints, which may indicate gout.
- Report any change in hearing.

30.6 Pharmacotherapy With Thiazide Diuretics

The thiazides constitute the largest, most commonly prescribed class of diuretics. These drugs act on the distal tubule to block Na^+ reabsorption and increase potassium and water excretion. Their primary use is for the treatment of mild to moderate hypertension; however, they are also indicated for edema due to mild to moderate heart failure, liver failure, and renal failure. They are less efficacious than the loop diuretics and are not effective in clients with severe renal failure. The thiazide diuretics are listed in Table 30.4.

TABLE 30.4 Thiazide and Thiazide-like Diuretics

Drug	Route and Adult Dose (max dose where indicated)	Adverse Effects
SHORT ACTING		
chlorothiazide (Diuril)	PO; 250 mg–1 g/day in single or 2 divided doses; IV; 250 mg–1 g/day in single or 2 divided doses	*Minor hypokalemia, fatigue*
hydrochlorothiazide (HydroDIURIL, HCTZ) (see page 311 for the Prototype Drug box ∞)	PO; 25–100 mg daily in single or 2 divided doses	<u>Serious hypokalemia, electrolyte depletion, dehydration, hypotension, hyponatremia, hyperglycemia, coma, blood dyscrasias</u>
INTERMEDIATE ACTING		
bendroflumethiazide (Naturetin)	PO; 2.5–20 mg/day in single or 2 divided doses	
benzthiazide (Aquatag, Exna, Hydrex)	PO; 25–200 mg/day or every other day	
hydroflumethiazide (Diucardin, Saluron)	PO; 25 mg–200 mg/day in single or 2 divided doses	
metolazone (Zaroxolyn, Mykrox)	PO; 5–20 mg/day	
quinethazone (Hydromox)	PO; 50–100 mg/day	
LONG ACTING		
chlorthalidone (Hygroton)	PO; 50–100 mg/day	
indapamide (Lozol)	PO; 2.5–5 mg/day	
methyclothiazide (Aquatensen, Enduron)	PO; 2.5–10 mg/day	
polythiazide (Renese)	PO; 1–4 mg/day	
trichlormethiazide (Metahydrin, Naqua, Niazide, Diurese)	PO; 1–4 mg 1–2 times/day	

Italics indicate common adverse effects; <u>underlining</u> indicates serious adverse effects.

Pr PROTOTYPE DRUG | Chlorothiazide *(Diuril)* | Thiazide Diuretic

ACTIONS AND USES

The most common indication for chlorothiazide is mild to moderate hypertension. It may be combined with other antihypertensives in the multidrug therapy of severe hypertension. It is also prescribed to treat fluid retention due to heart failure, liver disease, and corticosteroid or estrogen therapy. When the drug is given orally, it may take as long as 4 weeks to obtain the *optimum* therapeutic effect.

ADMINISTRATION ALERTS

- Give oral doses in the morning to prevent interrupted sleep due to nocturia.
- Give IV at a rate of 0.5 g over 5 min when administering intermittently.
- When administering IV, take special care to avoid extravasation, because this drug is highly irritating to tissues.
- Pregnancy category C.

PHARMACOKINETICS

Onset: 2 h PO; 15 min IV

Peak: 3–6 h PO; 30 min IV

Half-life: 45–120 min

Duration: 6–12 h PO; 2 h IV

ADVERSE EFFECTS

Excess loss of water and electrolytes can occur during chlorothiazide pharmacotherapy. Symptoms include thirst, weakness, lethargy, muscle cramping, hypotension, and tachycardia. Because of the potentially serious consequences of hypokalemia, clients concurrently taking digoxin should be carefully monitored. The intake of potassium-rich foods should be increased, and potassium supplements may be indicated.

Contraindications: This drug is contraindicated in patients with anuria, hypokalemia, severe hepatic or renal impairment, and hypersensitivity to sulfonamides.

INTERACTIONS

Drug–Drug: When chlorothiazide is administered with amphotericin B or corticosteroids, hypokalemic effects are increased. Antidiabetic medications such as sulfonylureas and insulin may be less effective when taken with chlorothiazide. Cholestyramine and colestipol decrease the absorption of chlorothiazide. Concurrent administration with digoxin may cause toxicity owing to increased potassium and magnesium loss. Alcohol potentiates the hypotensive action of some thiazide diuretics, and caffeine may increase diuresis.

Lab Tests: May increase serum amylase values and sulfobromophthalein (SBP) retention. May decrease protein-bound iodine (PBI) values and interfere with urine steroid determination.

Herbal/Food: Absorption of the diuretic is increased when taken with food. Licorice, in large amounts, may create an additive effect of hypokalemia. Aloe may increase potassium loss.

Treatment of Overdose: Treatment is supportive and may include agents to replace fluid and electrolytes lost through diuresis, and drugs to raise blood pressure.

 See the Companion Website for a Nursing Process Focus specific to this drug.

All the thiazide diuretics are available by the oral route and have equivalent efficacy and safety profiles. They differ, however, in their potency and duration of action. Four drugs—chlorthalidone (Hygroton), indapamide (Lozol), metolazone (Mykrox, Zaroxolyn), and quinethazone (Hydromox)—are not true thiazides, although they are included with this drug class because they have similar mechanisms of action and side effects.

The side effects of thiazides are similar to those of the loop diuretics, though their frequency is less, and they do not cause ototoxicity. Dehydration and excessive loss of sodium, potassium, or chloride ions may occur with overtreatment. Concurrent therapy with digoxin requires careful monitoring to present dysthythmias caused by excessive potassium loss. Potassium supplements may be indicated during thiazide therapy to prevent hypokalemia. Diabetic clients should be aware that thiazide diuretics sometimes raise blood glucose levels.

NURSING CONSIDERATIONS

The role of the nurse in thiazide diuretic therapy for hypertension, edema associated with congestive heart failure, hepatic disease, and renal disease involves careful monitoring of a client's condition and providing education as it relates to the prescribed drug treatment. With initial use, thiazide diuretics may cause a decrease in cardiac output because the circulatory blood volume will be decreased. This decrease will stabilize as the therapy is continued.

Obtain a medical history to determine the presence of diabetes mellitus; severe renal disease; use of digoxin, lithium, or other antihypertensives; and current pregnancy or lactation. Thiazide diuretics should be used with caution in these clients. Obtain baseline lab values and current level of urine output. It is critical to measure electrolyte levels, especially sodium, chloride, and potassium levels prior to thiazide therapy. Monitor BUN, serum creatinine, uric acid, and blood glucose levels. Carefully record intake and output, daily weight, and the presence of pain, swelling, and redness of any joints to determine an effective response. Assess skin turgor, moisture, vital signs (check blood pressure lying, sitting, and standing), breath sounds, and the presence of edema to determine the effectiveness of the thiazide diuretic.

Assess for adverse effects, which may include orthostatic hypotension, hyponatremia, hypokalemia, and blood volume depletion. Other effects may include hyperglycemia, hyperuricemia, anorexia, and pancreatitis. Increased potassium loss may occur when used concurrently with digoxin.

TABLE 30.5 Potassium-sparing Diuretics		
Drug	**Route and Adult Dose (max dose where indicated)**	**Adverse Effects**
amiloride hydrochloride (Midamor)	PO; 5 mg/day (max: 20 mg/day)	*Minor hyperkalemia, headache, fatigue, gynecomastia*
eplerenone (Inspra)	PO; 50 mg/day (max: 100 mg/day)	
spironolactone (Aldactone)	PO; 25–400 mg 1–2 times/day	<u>Dysrhythmias (from hyperkalemia), dehydration, hyponatremia, agranulocytosis and other blood dyscrasias</u>
triamterene (Dyrenium)	PO; 100 mg bid (max: 300 mg/day)	

Italics indicate common adverse effects; <u>underlining</u> indicates serious adverse effects.

Clients taking lithium have an increased risk of toxicity when taking thiazide diuretics. Hypersensitivity reactions may occur more frequently in clients who are allergic to sulfa-based medications. These reactions often present as rashes.

Lifespan Considerations.   Use thiazide diuretics with caution in elderly clients because these drugs may cause dehydration and electrolyte imbalances. Provide meticulous skin care to incontinent clients to reduce the risk of skin breakdown. Use with caution in pregnant women. Do not administer thiazide diuretics to lactating women. Research continues on the safe use of some drugs in this class in children.

Client Teaching.   Client education as it relates to thiazide diuretics should include the goals of therapy, the reasons for obtaining baseline data such as vital signs and the existence of underlying cardiac, hepatic, and renal disorders, and the possible drug side effects. Include the following points when teaching clients about thiazide diuretics:

- When in direct sunlight, wear protective clothing and use sunscreen to prevent photosensitivity.
- Expect increased urine output.
- Take drug in the morning because nighttime urination increases the risk of injury.
- Immediately report signs and symptoms such as muscle weakness or cramps and pulse changes, as these may indicate hypokalemia.
- Take potassium supplements, if ordered, and consume potassium-rich foods.
- Monitor blood pressure weekly and report substantial changes.
- Change positions slowly to avoid dizziness.
- Avoid foods high in sodium content such as canned foods, "fast" foods, and frozen dinners.
- Check weight daily, and report a weight gain of 2 lb or more in 24 hours, shortness of breath, or swelling of ankles.
- Keep all scheduled laboratory visits for electrolyte status testing.
- If diabetic, monitor glucose levels closely, because adjustments in diabetic therapy may be necessary.
- Report any tenderness or pain in joints, which may indicate gout.

30.7 Pharmacotherapy With Potassium-sparing Diuretics

Hypokalemia is one of the most serious adverse effects of the thiazide and loop diuretics. The therapeutic advantage of the potassium-sparing diuretics is that increased diuresis can be obtained without affecting blood potassium levels. The potassium-sparing diuretics are listed in Table 30.5. There are two distinct mechanisms by which these drugs act.

Normally, sodium and potassium are exchanged in the distal tubule; Na^+ is reabsorbed back into the blood, and K^+ is secreted into the distal tubule. Triamterene and amiloride block this exchange, causing sodium to stay in the tubule and ultimately leave through the urine. When sodium is blocked, the body retains more potassium. Because most of the sodium has already been removed before the filtrate reaches the distal tubule, these potassium-sparing diuretics produce only a mild diuresis. Their primary use is in combination with thiazide or loop diuretics to minimize potassium loss.

The third potassium-sparing diuretic, spironolactone, acts by blocking the actions of the hormone aldosterone. It is sometimes called an *aldosterone antagonist*, and may be used to treat hyperaldosteronism. Blocking aldosterone enhances the *excretion* of sodium and the *retention* of potassium. Like the other two drugs in this diuretic class, spironolactone produces only a weak diuresis. Unlike the other two, spironolactone has been found to significantly reduce mortality in clients with heart failure (see Chapter 24 ∞). Eplerenone (Inspra) is a newly approved aldosterone antagonist that exhibits fewer side effects than spironolactone.

Clients taking potassium-sparing diuretics should *not* take potassium supplements or be advised to add potassium-rich foods to their diet. Intake of excess potassium when taking these medications may lead to hyperkalemia.

NURSING CONSIDERATIONS

The role of the nurse in potassium-sparing diuretic therapy for edema associated with congestive heart failure, diuretic-induced hypokalemia, cirrhosis, nephrotic syndrome, and hypertension involves careful monitoring of a client's condition and providing education as it relates to the prescribed drug treatment. The advantage of these medications is that the client will not experience hypokalemia.

Pr PROTOTYPE DRUG | Spironolactone *(Aldactone)* | Potassium-sparing Diuretic

ACTIONS AND USES

Spironolactone acts by inhibiting aldosterone, the hormone secreted by the adrenal cortex that is responsible for increasing the renal reabsorption of sodium in exchange for potassium, thus causing water retention. When aldosterone is blocked by spironolactone, sodium and water excretion is increased and the body retains more potassium. Spironolactone may also be used to treat primary hyperaldosteronism. It is available in tablet form, and as a fixed-dose combination with hydrochlorothiazide.

ADMINISTRATION ALERTS

- Give with food to increase absorption of drug.
- Do not give potassium supplements.
- Pregnancy category D.

PHARMACOKINETICS

Onset: 1–2 days

Peak: 2–3 days

Half-life: 12–24 h

Duration: 2–3 days or more

ADVERSE EFFECTS

Spironolactone does such an efficient job of retaining potassium that hyperkalemia may develop. The probability of hyperkalemia is increased if the client takes potassium supplements or is concurrently taking ACE inhibitors. Signs and symptoms of hyperkalemia include muscle weakness, ventricular tachycardia, or fibrillation. When serum potassium levels are monitored carefully and maintained within normal values, side effects from spironolactone are uncommon.

Contraindications: This drug is contraindicated in clients with anuria, significant impairment of renal function, or hyperkalemia. It is also contraindicated in pregnancy.

INTERACTIONS

Drug–Drug: When spironolactone is combined with ammonium chloride, acidosis may occur. Aspirin and other salicylates may decrease the diuretic effect of the medication. Concurrent use with digoxin may decrease the effects of digoxin. When taken with potassium supplements, ACE inhibitors, and ARBs, hyperkalemia may result. Concurrent use with antihypertensives will result in an additive hypotensive effect.

Lab Tests: May increase plasma cortisol values. May interfere with serum glucose determination.

Herbal/Food: Unknown.

Treatment of Overdose: Treatment is supportive and may include agents to replace fluid and electrolytes lost through diuresis, and drugs to raise blood pressure.

 See the Companion Website for a Nursing Process Focus specific to this drug.

Obtain a medical history to determine the presence of severe renal disease; use of digoxin, lithium, or other antihypertensives; and current pregnancy or lactation, because potassium-sparing diuretics should be used cautiously in such clients. Obtain baseline lab values and current level of urine output. It is critical to assess electrolytes, especially potassium and sodium levels, prior to administering potassium-sparing diuretics. Monitor the client's BUN and serum creatinine. Assessment of intake and output, skin turgor and moisture, vital signs (check blood pressure lying, sitting, and standing), breath sounds, and the presence of edema will indicate the effectiveness of the potassium-sparing diuretic.

Be alert for adverse effects, which may include hyperkalemia and GI bleeding. Other side effects may include confusion, dizziness, muscle weakness, blurred vision, impotence, amenorrhea, or gynecomastia. Spironolactone may also decrease the effectiveness of anticoagulants. Patients taking digoxin or lithium may be at increased risk for toxicity when taking a potassium-sparing diuretic. Watch for hypersensitivity reactions that may manifest as a rash or daily fever.

Lifespan Considerations. Use potassium-sparing diuretics cautiously in elderly clients, because these drugs may cause confusion, dehydration, and electrolyte imbalances. Provide meticulous skin care to incontinent clients to reduce the risk of skin breakdown. Use of spironolactone is strongly discouraged during pregnancy. Use with other potassium-sparing diuretics is cautioned in pregnancy. Do not use triameterene in lactating women; use all other drugs in this class with caution in such clients.

Client Teaching. Client education as it relates to potassium-sparing diuretics should include the goals of therapy, the reasons for obtaining baseline data such as vital signs and the existence of underlying cardiac, hepatic, and renal disorders, and possible drug side effects. Include the following points when teaching clients about potassium-sparing diuretics:

- Immediately report signs and symptoms of hyperkalemia, such as irritability, anxiety, abdominal cramping, or irregular heartbeat.
- Avoid use of potassium-based salt substitutes.
- When in direct sunlight, use sunscreen to decrease photosensitivity.
- Avoid performing tasks that require mental alertness until the effects of the medication are known.
- Do not eat excess amounts of foods high in potassium.

TABLE 30.6 Miscellaneous Diuretics		
Drug	**Route and Adult Dose (max dose where indicated)**	**Adverse Effects**
CARBONIC ANHYDRASE INHIBITORS		
acetazolamide (Diamox)	PO; 250–375 mg/day	*Electrolyte imbalances, fatigue, nausea, vomiting, dizziness*
dichlorphenamide (Daranide, Oratrol)	PO; 25–50 mg 1–3 times/day	
methazolamide (Neptazane)	PO; 50–100 mg bid–tid	<u>Dehydration, blood dyscrasias, pancytopenia, flaccid paralysis, hemolytic anemia, aplastic anemia</u>
OSMOTIC		
mannitol (Osmitrol)	IV; 100 g infused over 2–6 h	*Electrolyte imbalances, fatigue, nausea, vomiting, dizziness*
urea (Ureaphil)	IV; 1.0–1.5 g/kg over 1–2.5 h	<u>Hyponatremia, edema, convulsions, tachycardia</u>

Italics indicate common adverse effects, <u>underlining</u> indicates serious adverse effects.

- Take drug in the morning, because nighttime urination increases the risk of injury.
- Monitor blood pressure and report substantial changes.
- Change positions slowly to prevent dizziness.
- Keep all scheduled follow-up visits for blood tests and cardiac monitoring (ECG).

30.8 Miscellaneous Diuretics for Specific Indications

A few diuretics, listed in Table 30.6, cannot be classified as loop, thiazide, or potassium-sparing agents. These diuretics have limited and specific indications. Three of these drugs inhibit **carbonic anhydrase,** an enzyme that affects acid–base balance by its ability to form carbonic acid from water and carbon dioxide. For example, acetazolamide (Diamox) is a carbonic anhydrase inhibitor used to decrease intraocular fluid pressure in clients with open-angle glaucoma (see Chapter 49 ∞). In addition

HOME & COMMUNITY CONSIDERATIONS

Nutritional Therapy for Clients Needing Diuretic Therapy
The client requiring diuretic therapy at home needs detailed nutritional teaching. The nurse should share teaching with family members or caregivers who are involved with food shopping and preparation. Depending on the diuretic prescribed, the focus may be on foods high or low in sodium and potassium. Additional teaching is needed regarding reading and interpreting food labels. There may be added sodium and potassium in processed foods, beverages (sports drinks), and salt substitutes. Education will help with food shopping to ensure that electrolyte levels remain normal during diuretic therapy.

NATURAL THERAPIES

Cranberry for Urinary Tract Infections
Since the mid-1800s, cranberry has been used for the prevention of urinary tract infections. Cranberry increases urine acidity, which discourages the growth of pathogenic microorganisms. In addition, a substance in cranberries inhibits bacteria from adhering to bladder walls (Howell et al., 2005; Jepson, Mihaljevic & Gaig 2006). The only reported adverse effect from cranberry is increased diarrhea when large quantities are ingested. If a juice form is used, unsweetened juices are preferred over sweetened. Sugarless cranberry extracts are available in capsule or tablet form.

to its diuretic effect, acetazolamide also has applications as an anticonvulsant and in treating motion sickness. It has also been used to treat acute mountain sickness in patients at very high altitudes. The carbonic anhydrase inhibitors are not commonly used as diuretics, because they produce weak diuresis and can contribute to metabolic acidosis.

The osmotic diuretics also have very specific applications and are rarely first-choice diuretics. For example, mannitol is used to maintain urine flow in clients with acute renal failure or during prolonged surgery. Since this agent is not reabsorbed in the tubule, it is able to maintain the flow of filtrate even in cases with severe renal hypoperfusion. Mannitol can also be used to lower intraocular pressure in certain types of glaucoma, although it is used for this purpose only when safer agents have failed to produce an effect. It is a highly potent diuretic that is given only by the IV route. Unlike other diuretics that draw excess fluid away from tissue spaces, mannitol can worsen edema and thus must be used with caution in clients with preexisting heart failure or pulmonary edema. The exception is the brain: Mannitol and urea can reduce intracranial pressure due to cerebral edema.

NURSING PROCESS FOCUS Clients Receiving Diuretic Therapy

Assessment	Potential Nursing Diagnoses
Prior to administration: ■ Obtain a complete health history (mental and physical), including data on recent surgeries or trauma. ■ Obtain vital signs; assess in context of client's baseline values. ■ Obtain client's medication history, including nicotine and alcohol consumption and use of herbal supplements or alternative therapies to determine possible drug allergies and/or interactions. ■ Obtain blood and urine specimens for laboratory analysis.	■ Fluid Volume, Excess ■ Fluid Volume, Deficient, Risk for ■ Urinary Elimination, Impaired, related to diuretic use

Planning: Client Goals and Expected Outcomes

The client will:
■ Exhibit normal fluid balance and maintain electrolyte levels within normal limits during drug therapy.
■ Demonstrate an understanding of the drug's actions by accurately describing drug side effects and precautions.
■ Immediately report symptoms of hyperkalemia or hypokalemia and hypersensitivity.

Implementation

Interventions and (Rationales)	Client Education/Discharge Planning
■ Monitor for fluid overload by measuring intake, output, and daily weights. (Intake, output, and daily body weight are indications of the effectiveness of diuretic therapy.)	Instruct client to: ■ Immediately report any severe shortness of breath, frothy sputum, profound fatigue, edema in extremities, potential signs of heart failure, or pulmonary edema. ■ Accurately measure intake, output, and body weight and report weight gain of 2 lb or more within 2 days or decrease in output. ■ Avoid excessive heat, which contributes to fluid loss through perspiration. ■ Consume adequate amounts of *plain water*.
■ Monitor laboratory values, especially potassium and sodium. (Diuretics can cause electrolyte imbalances.)	■ Instruct client to inform laboratory personnel of diuretic therapy when providing blood or urine samples.
■ Monitor vital signs, especially blood pressure. (Diuretics reduce blood volume, resulting in lowered blood pressure.)	Instruct client to: ■ Monitor blood pressure as specified by the healthcare provider and ensure proper use of home equipment. ■ Stop medication if severe hypotension exists, as specified by the healthcare provider (e.g., "hold for levels below 88/50 mm Hg").
■ Observe for changes in level of consciousness, dizziness, fatigue, and postural hypotension. (Reduction in blood volume due to diuretic therapy may produce changes in level of consciousness or syncope.)	Instruct client to: ■ Immediately report any change in consciousness, especially feeling faint. ■ Change positions slowly. ■ Obtain blood pressure readings in sitting, standing, and lying positions.
■ Monitor potassium intake. (Potassium is vital to maintaining proper electrolyte balance and can become depleted with thiazide or loop diuretics.)	Instruct clients: ■ Receiving *loop* or *thiazide diuretics* to eat foods high in potassium. ■ Receiving *potassium-sparing diuretics* to avoid foods high in potassium. ■ To consult with healthcare provider before using vitamin/mineral supplements or electrolyte-fortified sports drinks.
■ Observe for signs of hypersensitivity reaction. (Allergic responses may be life threatening.)	Instruct client or caregiver to report: ■ Difficulty breathing, throat tightness, hives or rash, or bleeding. ■ Flulike symptoms: shortness of breath, fever, sore throat, malaise, joint pain, profound fatigue.
■ Monitor hearing and vision. (Loop diuretics are ototoxic. Thiazide diuretics increase serum digoxin levels; elevated levels produce visual changes.)	■ Instruct client to report any changes in hearing or vision such as ringing or buzzing in the ears, becoming "hard of hearing" or experiencing dimness of sight, seeing halos, or having "yellow vision."

NURSING PROCESS FOCUS Clients Receiving Diuretic Therapy *(Continued)*	
Implementation	
Interventions and (Rationales)	**Client Education/Discharge Planning**
▪ Monitor reactivity to light exposure. (Some diuretics cause photosensitivity.)	Instruct client to: ▪ Limit exposure to the sun. ▪ Wear dark glasses and light-colored loose-fitting clothes when outdoors.
Evaluation of Outcome Criteria	
Evaluate the effectiveness of drug therapy by confirming that patient goals and expected outcomes have been met (see "Planning"). ▪ The client maintains fluid balance and normal electrolyte levels. ▪ The client demonstrates an understanding of the drug's actions by accurately describing drug side effects and precautions. ▪ The client verbalizes signs and symptoms of hyperkalemia and hypersensitivity and the importance of reporting these. ∞ *See Tables 30.1 through 30.4 for lists of drugs to which these nursing actions apply.*	

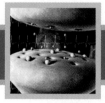

CHAPTER REVIEW

KEY CONCEPTS

The numbered key concepts provide a succinct summary of the important points from the corresponding numbered section within the chapter. If any of these points are not clear, refer to the numbered section within the chapter for review.

30.1 The kidneys regulate fluid volume, electrolytes, and acid–base balance.

30.2 The three major processes of urine formation are filtration, reabsorption, and secretion. As filtrate travels through the nephron, its composition changes dramatically as a result of the processes of reabsorption and secretion.

30.3 The dosage levels for most medications must be adjusted in clients with renal failure. Diuretics may be used to maintain urine output while the cause of the renal impairment is treated.

30.4 Diuretics are drugs that increase urine output, usually by blocking sodium reabsorption. The three primary classes are loop, thiazide, and potassium-sparing diuretics.

30.5 The most efficacious diuretics are the loop or high-ceiling agents, which block the reabsorption of sodium in the loop of Henle.

30.6 The thiazides act by blocking sodium reabsorption in the distal tubule of the nephron, and are the most widely prescribed class of diuretics.

30.7 Though less effective than the loop diuretics, potassium-sparing diuretics are used in combination with other agents, and help prevent hypokalemia.

30.8 Several less commonly prescribed classes such as the osmotic diuretics and the carbonic anhydrase inhibitors have specific indications in reducing intraocular fluid pressure (acetazolamide) or reversing severe renal hypoperfusion (mannitol).

NCLEX-RN® REVIEW QUESTIONS

1 Which of the following actions by the nurse is most important when caring for a client with renal disease?

1. Identify medications that have the potential for nephrotoxicity.
2. Check the specific gravity of the urine daily.
3. Eliminate potassium-rich foods from the diet.
4. Encourage the client to void every 4 hours.

2 The client admitted for congestive heart failure (CHF) is receiving digoxin (Lanoxin) and furosemide (Lasix). Which of the following laboratory levels should the nurse carefully monitor?

1. Potassium
2. Creatinine
3. Calcium
4. Sodium

3 Which of the following clinical manifestations may indicate the client is experiencing hypokalemia?

1. Hypertension
2. Polydipsia
3. Cardiac dysrhythmias
4. Diarrhea

4 Which of the following medications must be used with caution in clients with a history of CHF?

1. acetazolamide (Diamox)
2. mannitol (Osmitrol)
3. bumetanide (Bumex)
4. ethacrynic acid (Edecrin)

5 The nurse recognizes which of the disorders as a cause of chronic renal failure? (Select all that apply.)

1. Chronic urinary tract infections
2. Diabetes mellitus
3. Congential malformation
4. Hypertension
5. Hypotension

CRITICAL THINKING QUESTIONS

1. A 43-year-old man is diagnosed with hypertension following an annual physical examination. The client is thin and states that he engages in fairly regular exercise, but he describes his job as highly stressful. He also has a positive family history for hypertension and stroke. The healthcare provider initiates therapy with losartan (Cozaar). After 2 months, the client has noted no appreciable difference in blood pressure values. The healthcare provider switches the client to combination losartan and hydrochlorothiazide (Hyzaar), which proves to be very effective. Why is the new therapy more effective?

2. A 78-year-old woman is admitted to the intensive care unit with a diagnosis of heart failure. The nurse administers furosemide (Lasix) 40 mg IV push. What assessments should the nurse make to determine the effectiveness of this therapy?

3. A 17-year-old male client is admitted to the ICU following a car–train collision. The client sustained a depressed skull fracture and is on a ventilator. Two days after surgery, there are obvious signs of increasing intracranial pressure. The nurse administers 32 g of a 15% solution of mannitol (Osmitrol) per IV over 30 minutes. The client's mother asks the nurse to explain why her son needs this drug. What explanation should the nurse offer?

See Appendix D for answers and rationales for all activities.

EXPLORE MediaLink

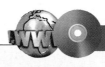 www.prenhall.com/adams

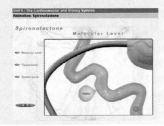

NCLEX-RN® review, case studies, and other interactive resources for this chapter can be found on the companion website at www.prenhall.com/adams. Click on "Chapter 30" to select the activities for this chapter. For animations, more NCLEX-RN® review questions, and an audio glossary, access the accompanying Prentice Hall Nursing MediaLink DVD-ROM in this textbook.

PRENTICE HALL NURSING MEDIALINK DVD-ROM

- **Animation**
  Mechanism in Action: Spironolactone (*Aldactone*)
  Basic Function of the Kidney
- **Audio Glossary**
- **NCLEX-RN® Review**

 COMPANION WEBSITE

- **NCLEX-RN® Review**
- **Dosage Calculations**
- **Case Study:** Client taking diuretics
- **Care Plan:** Client with congestive heart failure treated with furosemide and digoxin

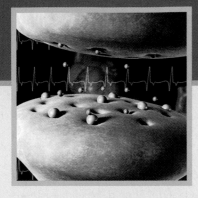

CHAPTER 31

Drugs for Fluid Balance, Electrolyte, and Acid–Base Disorders

DRUGS AT A GLANCE

FLUID REPLACEMENT AGENTS
Colloids
- 🔊 *dextran 40 (Gentran 40, Hyskon, 10% LMD, Rheo macrodex)*

Crystalloids
ELECTROLYTES
- 🔊 *sodium chloride*
- 🔊 *potassium chloride*

ACID–BASE AGENTS
- 🔊 *sodium bicarbonate*
- 🔊 *ammonium chloride*

OBJECTIVES

After reading this chapter, the student should be able to:

1. Describe conditions for which IV fluid therapy may be indicated.
2. Explain how changes in the osmolality or tonicity of a fluid can cause water to move to a different compartment.
3. Compare and contrast the use of colloids and crystalloids in IV therapy.
4. Explain the importance of electrolyte balance in the body.
5. Explain the pharmacotherapy of sodium and potassium imbalances.
6. Discuss common causes of alkalosis and acidosis and the medications used to treat these disorders.
7. Describe the nurse's role in the pharmacological management of fluid balance, electrolyte, and acid–base disorders.
8. For each of the classes listed in Drugs at a Glance, know representative drugs, and explain the mechanism of drug action, primary actions, and important adverse effects.
9. Categorize drugs used in the treatment of fluid balance, electrolyte, and acid–base disorders based on their classification and mechanism of action.
10. Use the Nursing Process to care for clients who are receiving drug therapy for fluid balance, electrolyte, and acid–base disorders.

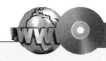

MediaLink

www.prenhall.com/adams

NCLEX-RN® review, case studies, and other interactive resources for this chapter can be found on the companion website at www.prenhall.com/adams. Click on "Chapter 31" to select the activities for this chapter. For animations, more NCLEX-RN® review questions, and an audio glossary, access the accompanying Prentice Hall Nursing MediaLink DVD-ROM in this textbook.

KEY TERMS

acidosis *page 447*

alkalosis *page 449*

anion *page 442*

buffer *page 446*

cation *page 442*

colloids *page 440*

crystalloids *page 440*

electrolytes *page 442*

extracellular fluid (ECF) compartment
page 438

hyperkalemia *page 445*

hypernatremia *page 443*

hypokalemia *page 445*

hyponatremia *page 443*

intracellular fluid (ICF) compartment
page 438

osmolality *page 439*

osmosis *page 439*

pH *page 446*

tonicity *page 439*

The volume and composition of fluids in the body must be maintained within narrow limits. Excess fluid volume can lead to hypertension, congestive heart failure, or peripheral edema, whereas depletion results in dehydration. Body fluids must also contain specific amounts of essential ions or electrolytes, and be maintained at particular pH values. Imbalances in electrolytes may have fatal consequences. In addition, accumulation of excess acids or bases can change the pH of body fluids and rapidly result in death if left untreated. This chapter will examine drugs used to reverse fluid balance, electrolyte, or acid–base disorders.

FLUID BALANCE

Body fluids travel between compartments, which are separated by semipermeable membranes. Control of water balance in the various compartments is essential to homeostasis. Fluid imbalances are frequent indications for pharmacotherapy.

31.1 Body Fluid Compartments

The greatest bulk of body fluid consists of water, which serves as the universal solvent in which most nutrients, electrolytes, and minerals are dissolved. Water alone is responsible for about 60% of the total body weight in a middle-age adult. A newborn may contain 80% water, whereas an elderly person may contain only 40%.

In a simple model, water in the body can be located in one of two places, or compartments. The **intracellular fluid (ICF) compartment,** which contains water that is *inside* cells, accounts for about two thirds of the total body water. The remaining one third of body fluid resides *outside* cells in the **extracellular fluid (ECF) compartment.** The ECF compartment is further divided into two parts: fluid in the *plasma,* or *intravascular space,* and fluid in the *interstitial spaces* between cells. The relationship between these fluid compartments is illustrated in ● Figure 31.1.

A continuous exchange and mixing of fluids occurs between the various compartments, which are separated by membranes. For example, the plasma membranes of cells separate the ICF from the ECF. The capillary membranes separate plasma from the interstitial fluid. Although water travels freely among the compartments, the movement of large molecules and those with electrical charges is governed by processes of diffusion and active transport. Movement

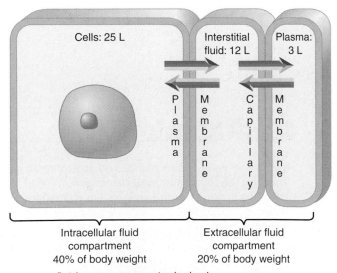

● **Figure 31.1** Major fluid compartments in the body

of ions and drugs across membranes is a primary concern of pharmacokinetics (Chapter 5 ∞).

31.2 Osmolality, Tonicity, and the Movement of Body Fluids

Osmolality and tonicity are two related terms central to understanding fluid balance in the body. Large changes in the osmolality or tonicity of a body fluid can cause significant shifts in water balance between compartments. The nurse will often administer IV fluids to compensate for these changes.

The **osmolality** of a fluid is determined by the number of dissolved particles, or solutes, in 1 kg (1 L) of water. In most body fluids, three solutes determine the osmolality: sodium, glucose, and urea. Sodium is the greatest contributor to osmolality owing to its abundance in most body fluids. The normal osmolality of body fluids ranges from 275 to 295 milliosmols per kilogram (mOsm/kg).

The term **tonicity** is sometimes used interchangeably with osmolality, although they are somewhat different. Tonicity is the ability of a solution to cause a change in water movement across a membrane due to osmotic forces. Whereas osmolality is a laboratory value that can be precisely measured, tonicity is a general term used to describe the *relative* concentration of IV fluids. The tonicity of the plasma is used as the reference point when administering IV solutions: Normal plasma is considered isotonic. Solutions that are isotonic have the same concentration of solutes (same osmolality) as plasma. *Hypertonic* solutions contain a greater concentration of solutes than plasma, whereas *hypotonic* solutions have a lesser concentration of solutes than plasma.

Through **osmosis,** water moves from areas of low solute concentration (low osmolality), to areas of high solute concentration (high osmolality). If a hypertonic (hyperosmolar) IV solution is administered, the plasma gains more solutes than the interstitial fluid. Water will move, by osmosis, from the interstitial fluid compartment to the plasma compartment. Water will move in the opposite direction, from plasma to interstitial fluid, if a hypotonic solution is administered. Isotonic solutions will produce no net fluid shift. These movements are illustrated in ● Figure 31.2.

31.3 Regulation of Fluid Intake and Output

The average adult has a water *intake* of approximately 2500 ml/day, most of which comes from food and beverages. Water *output* is achieved through the kidneys, lungs, skin, feces, and sweat. To maintain water balance, water intake must equal water output. Net gains or losses of water can be estimated by changes in total body weight.

The most important physiological regulator of fluid intake is the thirst mechanism. The sensation of thirst occurs when osmoreceptors in the hypothalamus sense that the ECF has become hypertonic. Saliva secretion diminishes and the mouth dries, driving the individual to drink liquids.

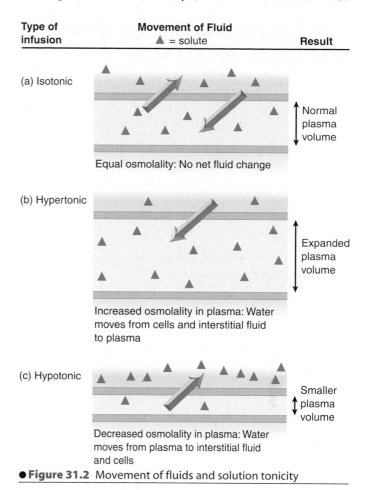

Type of infusion	Movement of Fluid ▲ = solute	Result

(a) Isotonic — Equal osmolality: No net fluid change — ↕ Normal plasma volume

(b) Hypertonic — Increased osmolality in plasma: Water moves from cells and interstitial fluid to plasma — ↕ Expanded plasma volume

(c) Hypotonic — Decreased osmolality in plasma: Water moves from plasma to interstitial fluid and cells — ↕ Smaller plasma volume

● **Figure 31.2** Movement of fluids and solution tonicity

As the ingested water is absorbed, the osmolality of the ECF falls and the thirst center in the hypothalamus is no longer stimulated.

The kidneys are the primary regulators of fluid output. Through the renin–angiotensin system (Chapter 23 ∞), the hormone aldosterone is secreted by the adrenal cortex. Aldosterone causes the kidneys to retain additional sodium and water in the body, thus increasing the osmolality of the ECF. A second hormone, antidiuretic hormone (ADH), is released during periods of high plasma osmolality. ADH acts directly on the distal tubules of the kidney to increase water reabsorption.

Failure to maintain proper balance between intake and output can result in fluid balance disorders that are indications for pharmacological intervention. Fluid *deficit* disorders can cause dehydration or shock, which are treated by administering oral or intravenous (IV) fluids. Fluid *excess* disorders are treated with diuretics (Chapter 30 ∞). In the treatment of fluid imbalances, the ultimate goal is to diagnose and correct the *cause* of the disorder while administering supporting fluids and medications to stabilize the client.

FLUID REPLACEMENT AGENTS

Net loss of fluids from the body can result in dehydration and shock. IV fluid therapy is used to maintain blood volume and support blood pressure.

31.4 Intravenous Therapy With Crystalloids and Colloids

When fluid output exceeds fluid intake, volume deficits may result. Shock, dehydration, or electrolyte loss may occur; large deficits are fatal, unless treated. The following are some common reasons for fluid depletion.

- Loss of GI fluids due to vomiting, diarrhea, chronic laxative use, or GI suctioning
- Excessive sweating during hot weather, athletic activity, or prolonged fever
- Severe burns
- Hemorrhage
- Excessive diuresis due to diuretic therapy or uncontrolled diabetic ketoacidosis

The immediate goal in treating a volume deficit disorder is to replace the depleted fluid. In nonacute circumstances, this may be achieved by drinking more liquids or by administering fluids via a feeding tube. In acute situations, IV fluid therapy is indicated. Regardless of the route, careful attention must be paid to restoring normal levels of blood elements and electrolytes, as well as fluid volume.

Intravenous replacement fluids are of two basic types: crystalloids and colloids. **Crystalloids** are IV solutions that contain electrolytes and other agents that closely mimic the body's extracellular fluid. They may be used to replace depleted fluids, and to promote urine output. Crystalloid solutions are capable of quickly diffusing across membranes, leaving the plasma and entering the interstitial fluid and ICF. It is estimated that two thirds of infused crystalloids are distributed in the interstitial space. Isotonic, hypotonic, and hypertonic solutions are available. Sodium is the most common crystalloid added to solutions. Some crystalloids contain dextrose, a form of glucose, commonly in concentrations of 2.5%, 5%, or 10%. Dextrose is added to provide nutritional value: 1 L of 5% dextrose supplies 170 calories. In addition, water is formed during the metabolism of dextrose, adding to the rehydration of the client. When dextrose is infused, it is metabolized, and the solution becomes hypotonic. Selected crystalloids are listed in Table 31.1.

Infusion of crystalloids will increase total fluid volume in the body, but the *compartment* that is most expanded depends on the solute (sodium) concentration of the fluid administered. *Isotonic* crystalloids can expand the circulating *intravascular* fluid volume without causing major fluid shifts between compartments. Isotonic crystalloids such as normal saline are often used to treat fluid loss due to vomiting, diarrhea, or surgical procedures, especially when the blood pressure is low. Because isotonic fluids can rapidly expand circulating blood volume, care must be taken not to create fluid overload.

Infusion of *hypertonic* crystalloids expands plasma volume by drawing water away from the cells and tissues. These agents may be used to relieve cellular edema, especially cerebral edema. When clients are dehydrated and have hypertonic plasma, hypertonic fluids (i.e., D5 1/2NS) match

TABLE 31.1	Selected Crystalloid IV Solutions
Drug	Tonicity
normal saline (0.9% NaCl)	isotonic
hypertonic saline (3% NaCl)	hypertonic
hypotonic saline (0.45% NaCl)	hypotonic
lactated Ringer's	isotonic
plasma-lyte 148	isotonic
plasma-lyte 56	hypotonic
DEXTROSE SOLUTIONS	
5% dextrose in water (D5W)	isotonic*
5% dextrose in normal saline	hypertonic
5% dextrose in 0.2% saline	hypertonic
5% dextrose in lactated Ringer's	hypertonic
5% dextrose in plasma-lyte 56	hypertonic

*Because dextrose is metabolized quickly, the solution is sometimes considered hypotonic.

the tonicity of the plasma as it is infused, but the dextrose is subsequently metabolized and the solution becomes hypotonic. This hypotonic solution then shifts into the intracellular space, relieving the dehydration within the cells. Overtreatment with hypertonic crystalloids (3% normal saline) can lead to excessive expansion of the intravascular compartment, and hypertension.

Hypotonic crystalloids will cause water to move out of the plasma to the tissues and cells in the *intracellular* compartment; thus, these solutions are not considered efficient plasma volume expanders. Hypotonic crystalloids are indicated for clients with hypernatremia and dehydration. Care must be taken not to cause depletion of the intravascular compartment (hypotension) or too much expansion of the intracellular compartment (peripheral edema). Clients who are dehydrated with *low* blood pressure should be given normal saline; clients who are dehydrated with *normal* blood pressure should be given a hypotonic solution.

Colloids are proteins, starches, or other large molecules that remain in the blood for a long time because they are too large to easily cross the capillary membranes. While circulating they have the same effect as hypertonic solutions, drawing water molecules from the cells and tissues into the plasma

TABLE 31.2	Selected Colloid IV Solutions (Plasma Volume Expanders)	
Drug	Tonicity	
5% albumin	isotonic	
dextran 40 in normal saline	isotonic	
dextran 40 in D5W	isotonic	
dextran 70 in normal saline	isotonic	
hetastarch 6% in normal saline	isotonic	
plasma protein fraction	isotonic	

Pr PROTOTYPE DRUG | Dextran 40 *(Gentran, others)* | Colloid/Plasma Volume Expander

ACTIONS AND USES

Dextran 40 is a polysaccharide that is too large to pass through capillary walls. It is similar to dextran 70, except dextran 40 has a lower molecular weight. Dextran 40 acts by raising the oncotic pressure of the blood, thereby causing fluid to move from the interstitial spaces of the tissues to the intravascular space (blood). Given as an IV infusion, it has the capability of expanding plasma volume within minutes after administration. Cardiovascular responses include increased blood pressure, increased cardiac output, and improved venous return to the heart. Dextran 40 is excreted rapidly by the kidneys. Indications include fluid replacement for clients experiencing hypovolemic shock due to hemorrhage, surgery, or severe burns. When given for acute shock it is infused as rapidly as possible until blood volume is restored.

Dextran 40 also reduces platelet adhesiveness, and improves blood flow, through its ability to reduce blood viscosity. These properties have led to its use in preventing deep vein thromboses and pulmonary emboli.

ADMINISTRATION ALERTS

- Emergency administration may be given 1.2 to 2.4 g/min.
- Nonemergency administration should be infused no faster than 240 mg/min.
- Discard unused portions once opened because dextran contains no preservatives.
- Pregnancy category C.

PHARMACOKINETICS

Onset: Several minutes

Peak: Unknown

Half-life: Unknown

Duration: 12 h

ADVERSE EFFECTS

Vital signs should be monitored continuously during dextran 40 infusions to prevent hypertension caused by plasma volume expansion. Signs of fluid overload include tachycardia, peripheral edema, distended neck veins, dyspnea, or cough. A small percentage of clients are allergic to dextran 40, with urticaria being the most common sign.

Contraindications: Dextran 40 is contraindicated in clients with renal failure or severe dehydration. Other contraindications include severe CHF and hypervolemic disorders.

INTERACTIONS

Drug–Drug: There are no clinically significant interactions.

Lab Tests: May prolong bleeding time.

Herbal/Food: Unknown.

Treatment of Overdose: For clients with normal renal function, discontinuation of the infusion will result in reduction of adverse effects. Clients with renal impairment may benefit from the administration of an osmotic diuretic.

 See the Companion Website for a Nursing Process Focus specific to this drug.

through their ability to increase plasma osmolality and oncotic pressure. These agents are sometimes called *plasma volume expanders,* and are particularly important in treating hypovolemic shock due to burns, hemorrhage, or surgery.

The most commonly used colloid is normal serum albumin, which is featured as a prototype drug for shock in Chapter 29 ∞. Several colloid products contain dextran, a synthetic polysaccharide. Dextran infusions can double the plasma volume within a few minutes, though its effects last only about 12 hours. Plasma protein fraction is a natural volume expander that contains 83% albumin and 17% plasma globulins. Plasma protein fraction and albumin are also indicated in clients with hypoproteinemia. Hetastarch is a synthetic colloid with properties similar to those of 5% albumin, but with an extended duration of action. Selected colloid solutions are listed in Table 31.2.

NURSING CONSIDERATIONS

The role of the nurse in colloidal solution therapy involves careful monitoring of a client's condition and providing education as it relates to the prescribed drug treatment. Colloidal solutions are used as plasma expanders, so first obtain a complete health history, drug history, and a physical examination. Obtain lab tests, including CBC, serum electrolytes, blood urea nitrogen (BUN), and creatinine levels. Because administration of colloidal solutions to dehydrated clients can lead to renal failure, evaluate the client's fluid balance before initiating therapy. Some colloidal solutions decrease platelet adhesion and lead to decreased coagulation. Plasma expanders lower hematocrit and hemoglobin levels because of increased intravascular volume. Report a hematocrit below 30% to the physician immediately.

Colloidal solutions are contraindicated in clients with renal failure, hypervolemic conditions, severe HF, thrombocytopenia, and those with clotting abnormalities. Use with caution in clients with active hemorrhage, severe dehydration, chronic liver disease, or impaired renal function. Carefully monitor vital signs and observe the client for the first 30 minutes of the infusion for hypersensitivity reactions. Stop the infusion at the first sign of hypersensitivity.

The primary nursing responsibility when caring for the client receiving plasma volume expanders is monitoring fluid volume status. Monitor closely for both fluid volume deficit and fluid volume excess. Assess vital signs and hemodynamic monitoring frequently during the infusion, until the client's condition stabilizes. Closely assess neurological status and urinary output, because these two systems are critically dependent on proper fluid balance. The infusion of the solutions can create a multitude of medical challenges for the critically ill client.

These medications are most often used to treat shock, so the client may not be alert. However, provide emotional support to caregivers, including updates about the client's condition and psychosocial support.

Client Teaching. Client education as it relates to colloidal solutions should include the goals of therapy, the reasons for obtaining baseline data such as vital signs and lab tests, and possible drug side effects. Include the following points when teaching clients colloidal solutions:

- Immediately report signs of bleeding such as easy bruising, blood in the urine, or dark, tarry stools.

- Immediately report flushing, shortness of breath, or itching, which could indicate hypersensitivity to the medication.

- Immediately report shortness of breath, cough, chest congestion, or heart palpitations, which could indicate circulatory overload.

ELECTROLYTES

Electrolytes are small charged molecules essential to homeostasis. Too little or too much of an electrolyte may result in serious complications and must be quickly corrected. Table 31.3 lists inorganic substances and their electrolytes that are important to human physiology.

31.5 Normal Functions of Electrolytes

Minerals are inorganic substances needed in very small amounts to maintain homeostasis (Chapter 42 ∞). In body fluids, some of these minerals, such as sodium, potassium, and

TABLE 31.3	Electrolytes Important to Human Physiology		
Compound	Formula	Cation	Anion
calcium chloride	$CaCl_2$	Ca^{+2}	$2Cl^-$
disodium phosphate	Na_2HPO_4	$2Na^+$	HPO_4^{-2}
potassium chloride	KCl	K^+	Cl^-
sodium bicarbonate	$NaHCO_3$	Na^+	HCO_3^-
sodium chloride	NaCl	Na^+	Cl^-
sodium sulfate	Na_2SO_4	$2Na^+$	SO_4^{-2}

calcium, become ions and possess a charge. Small inorganic molecules possessing a positive or negative charge are called **electrolytes**. Positively charged electrolytes are called **cations**; those with a negative charge are **anions**.

Inorganic compounds are held together by ionic bonds. When the compounds are placed in water, these bonds break and the compound undergoes dissociation or ionization. The resulting ions have charges and are able to conduct electricity, hence the name *electrolyte*. Electrolyte levels are measured in units of milliequivalents per liter (mEq/L).

Electrolytes are essential to many body functions, including nerve conduction, membrane permeability, muscle contraction, water balance, and bone growth and remodeling. Levels of electrolytes in body fluids are maintained within very narrow ranges, primarily by the kidneys and GI tract. As electrolytes are lost in normal excretory functions, they must be replaced by adequate intake, otherwise electrolyte imbalances will result. Although imbalances can occur with any ion, sodium, potassium, and calcium are of greatest importance. The major body electrolyte imbalance states are listed in Table 31.4. Calcium, phosphorous, and magnesium

TABLE 31.4	Electrolyte Imbalances		
Ion	Condition	Abnormal Serum Value (mEq/L)	Supportive Treatment*
calcium	hypercalcemia	>11	hypotonic fluid or calcitonin
	hypocalcemia	<4	calcium supplements or vitamin D
chloride	hyperchloremia	>112	hypotonic fluid
	hypochloremia	<95	hypertonic salt solution
magnesium	hypermagnesemia	>4	hypotonic fluid
	hypomagnesemia	<0.8	magnesium supplements
phosphate	hyperphosphatemia	>6	dietary phosphate restriction
	hypophosphatemia	<1	phosphate supplements
potassium	hyperkalemia	>5	hypotonic fluid, buffers, or dietary potassium restriction
	hypokalemia	<3.5	potassium supplements
sodium	hypernatremia	>145	hypotonic fluid or dietary sodium restriction
	hyponatremia	<135	hypertonic salt solution or sodium supplement

*For all electrolyte imbalances, the primary therapeutic goal is to identify and correct the *cause* of the imbalance.

imbalances are discussed in Chapter 42; the role of calcium in bone homeostasis is presented in Chapter 47 ∞.

31.6 Pharmacotherapy of Sodium Imbalances

Sodium is the major electrolyte in extracellular fluid. Because of sodium's central roles in neuromuscular physiology, acid–base balance, and overall fluid distribution, sodium imbalances can have serious consequences. Although definite sodium monitors or sensors have yet to be discovered in the body, the regulation of sodium balance is well understood.

Sodium balance and water balance are intimately connected. As sodium levels increase in a body fluid, solute particles accumulate, and the osmolality increases. Water will move toward this area of relatively high osmolality. In simplest terms, water travels toward or with sodium. The physiological consequences of this relationship cannot be overstated: As the sodium and water content of plasma increases, so does blood volume and blood pressure. Thus, sodium movement provides an important link between water retention, blood volume, and blood pressure.

In healthy individuals, sodium *intake* is equal to sodium *output,* which is regulated by the kidneys. High levels of aldosterone secreted by the adrenal cortex promote sodium and water retention by the kidneys, as well as potassium excretion. Inhibition of aldosterone promotes sodium and water excretion. When a client ingests high amounts of sodium, aldosterone secretion decreases, thus allowing excess sodium into the urine. This relationship is illustrated in ● Figure 31.3.

Sodium excess, or **hypernatremia,** occurs when the serum sodium level rises above 145 mEq/L. The most common cause of hypernatremia is decreased sodium excretion, due to kidney pathology. Hypernatremia may also be caused by excessive intake of sodium, either through dietary consumption or by overtreatment with IV fluids containing sodium chloride or sodium bicarbonate. Another cause of hypernatremia is high net water losses, such as occur from inadequate water intake, watery diarrhea, fever, or burns. High doses of glucocorticoids or estrogens also promote sodium retention.

A high serum sodium level increases the osmolality of the plasma, drawing fluid from interstitial spaces and cells, thus causing cellular dehydration. Manifestations of hypernatremia include thirst, fatigue, weakness, muscle twitching, convulsions, altered mental status, and a decreased level of consciousness. For minor hypernatremia, a low-salt diet may be effective in returning serum sodium to normal levels. In clients with acute hypernatremia, however, the treatment goal is to rapidly return the osmolality of the plasma to normal. If the client is hypovolemic, infusing hypotonic fluids such as 5% dextrose or 0.45% NaCl will increase plasma volume while at the same time reducing plasma osmolality. If the client is hypervolemic, diuretics may be used to remove sodium and fluid from the body.

Sodium deficiency, or **hyponatremia,** is a serum sodium level less than 135 mEq/L. Hyponatremia may occur through *excessive dilution* of the plasma, caused by excessive ADH

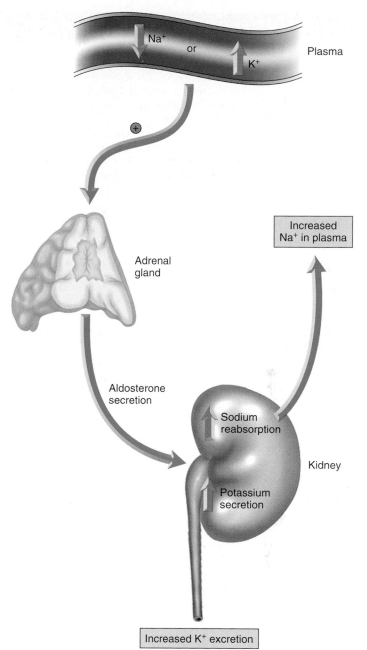

● **Figure 31.3** Renal regulation of sodium and potassium balance

secretion or administration of hypotonic IV solutions. Hyponatremia may also result from *increased sodium loss* due to disorders of the skin, GI tract, or kidneys. Significant loss of sodium by the skin may occur in burn clients, and in those experiencing excessive sweating or prolonged fever. Gastrointestinal sodium losses may occur from vomiting, diarrhea, or GI suctioning, and renal sodium loss may occur with diuretic use and in certain advanced kidney disorders. Early symptoms of hyponatremia include nausea, vomiting, anorexia, and abdominal cramping. Later signs include altered neurological function such as confusion, lethargy, convulsions, coma, and muscle twitching or tremors. Hyponatremia caused by excessive dilution is treated with loop diuretics (Chapter 30 ∞). These drugs will cause an isotonic diuresis, thus removing the fluid overload that caused the hyponatremia. Hyponatremia

Pr PROTOTYPE DRUG | Sodium Chloride (NaCl) | Electrolyte/Sodium Supplement

ACTIONS AND USES

Sodium chloride is administered for hyponatremia when serum levels fall below 130 mEq/L. The drug is available in several concentrations; the decision about which NaCl concentration to administer is driven by the severity of the sodium deficiency. Normal saline consists of 0.9% NaCl, and is used to treat mild hyponatremia. When serum sodium falls below 115 mEq/L, a highly concentrated 3% NaCl solution may be infused. Other concentrations include 0.45% and 0.22%, and both hypotonic and isotonic solutions are available. For less severe hyponatremia, 1-g tablets are available. Ophthalmic solutions of NaCl may be used to treat corneal edema, and an OTC nasal spray is available to relieve dry, inflamed nasal membranes. In conjunction with oxytocin, 20% NaCl may be used as an abortifacient late in pregnancy when instilled into the amniotic sac.

ADMINISTRATION ALERTS

- Pregnancy category C.

PHARMACOKINETICS

Because sodium chloride is a natural substance, pharmacokinetic data are difficult to obtain.

ADVERSE EFFECTS

Clients receiving NaCl infusions must be monitored frequently to prevent symptoms of hypernatremia, which include lethargy, confusion, muscle tremor or rigidity, hypotension, and restlessness. Because some of these symptoms are also common to hyponatremia, periodic lab assessments must be taken to be certain sodium values lie within the normal range. When infusing 3% NaCl solutions, the nurse should continuously check for signs of pulmonary edema.

Contraindications: This drug should not be administered to clients with hypernatremia, congestive heart failure, or impaired renal function.

INTERACTIONS

Drug–Drug: There are no clinically significant drug interactions.

Lab Tests: Increases serum sodium level.

Herbal/Food: Unknown.

Treatment of Overdose: If fluid accumulation occurs due to excess sodium, diuretics may be administered to reduce pulmonary or peripheral edema.

 See the Companion Website for a Nursing Process Focus specific to this drug.

---

caused by sodium loss may be treated with oral or parenteral sodium chloride, or with IV fluids containing salt, such as normal saline or lactated Ringer's.

NURSING CONSIDERATIONS

The role of the nurse in sodium replacement therapy involves careful monitoring of a client's condition and providing education as it relates to the prescribed drug treatment. Sodium replacement therapy is given to replace sodium and maintain blood volume, so assess fluid balance and blood pressure. Hyponatremia is seldom caused by inadequate dietary intake; however, in rare instances, hyponatremia may occur in individuals following sodium-restricted diets or receiving diuretic therapy. In most cases, infusion of 0.45% or 0.9% sodium solutions are used to restore extracellular fluid balance.

Prior to and during administration of sodium solutions, assess sodium and electrolyte balance. When assessing for hyponatremia, observe for signs of nausea, vomiting, muscle cramps, tachycardia, headache, irritability, confusion, seizures, and coma. Be alert for signs indicating hypernatremia, such as weakness, restlessness, hypertension, tachycardia, fluid accumulation, pulmonary edema, and respiratory arrest.

Monitor serum sodium levels, urine specific gravity, and serum and urine osmolarity closely when administering hypertonic solutions. Assess for symptoms that may relate to fluid overload during infusion of hypertonic saline solutions, such as shortness of breath, palpitation, headache, and restlessness.

Client Teaching. Client education as it relates to sodium replacement should include the goals of therapy, the reasons for obtaining baseline data such as vital signs and the existence of underlying cardiac sand renal disorders, and

possible drug side effects. Include the following points when teaching clients regarding sodium replacements:

- Avoid taking sodium chloride (salt) tablets to replace sodium lost through perspiration.
- Drink adequate amounts of water or balanced sports drinks to replenish lost fluids and electrolytes.
- Immediately report symptoms of low sodium such as nausea, vomiting, muscle cramps, rapid heart rate, irritability, seizures, and headache.
- Immediately report symptoms of high sodium such as weakness, restlessness, hypertension, and fluid retention.

31.7 Pharmacotherapy of Potassium Imbalances

Potassium, the most abundant intracellular cation, serves important roles in regulating intracellular osmolality and in maintaining acid–base balance. Potassium levels must be carefully balanced between adequate dietary intake and renal excretion. Like sodium excretion, potassium excretion is

HOME & COMMUNITY CONSIDERATIONS

Hypernatremia in Athletes

Side effects of sodium chloride when given as an electrolyte replacement are rare. Some clients self-induce hypernatremia by taking salt tablets, believing they will replace sodium lost due to sweating. Those who sweat profusely due to working outdoors or exercising can avoid heat-related problems by consuming adequate amounts of water or balanced electrolyte solutions contained in sports drinks. The client should consume salt tablets only when instructed by the healthcare provider.

influenced by the actions of aldosterone on the kidney. In fact, the renal excretion of sodium and potassium ions is closely linked—for every sodium ion that is *reabsorbed*, one potassium ion is *secreted* into the renal tubules. Serum potassium levels must be maintained within narrow limits; excess or deficiency states can be serious or fatal.

Hyperkalemia is a serum potassium level greater than 5 mEq/L, which may be caused by high consumption of potassium-rich foods or dietary supplements, particularly when clients are taking potassium-sparing diuretics such as spironolactone (Chapter 30 ∞). Excess potassium may also accumulate when renal excretion is diminished due to kidney pathology. The most serious consequences of hyperkalemia are related to cardiac function: dysrhythmias and heart block. Other symptoms are muscle twitching, fatigue, paresthesias, dyspnea, cramping, and diarrhea.

In mild cases of hyperkalemia, potassium levels may be returned to normal by restricting primary dietary sources of potassium such as bananas, citrus and dried fruits, peanut butter, broccoli, and green leafy vegetables. If the client is taking a potassium-sparing diuretic, the dose must be lowered, or a thiazide or loop diuretic substituted. In severe cases, serum potassium levels may be temporarily lowered by administering glucose and insulin, which cause potassium to leave the extracellular fluid and enter cells. Calcium gluconate or calcium chloride may be administered to counteract potassium toxicity to the heart. Sodium bicarbonate is sometimes infused to correct any acidosis that may be concurrent with the hyperkalemia. Excess potassium may be eliminated by giving polystyrene sulfonate (Kayexalate) orally or rectally. This agent, which exchanges sodium ion for potassium ion in the intestine, is given concurrently with a laxative such as sorbitol to promote rapid evacuation of the potassium.

Hypokalemia occurs when serum potassium level falls below 3.5 mEq/L. Hypokalemia is a relatively common adverse effect resulting from high doses of loop diuretics such as furosemide (Lasix). In addition, strenuous muscular activity and severe vomiting or diarrhea can result in significant potassium loss. Because the body does not have large stores of potassium, adequate daily intake is necessary.

Neurons and muscle fibers are most sensitive to potassium loss, and muscle weakness, lethargy, anorexia, dysrhythmias, and cardiac arrest are possible consequences. Mild hypokalemia is treated by increasing the dietary intake of potassium-rich foods, whereas more severe deficiencies require doses of oral or parenteral potassium supplements.

NURSING CONSIDERATIONS

The role of the nurse in potassium supplement therapy involves careful monitoring of a client's condition and providing education as it relates to the prescribed drug treatment. Potassium supplements are given as replacement therapy, so assess serum potassium level prior to administration. Quick recognition of potassium imbalance can prevent life-threatening complications such as dysrhythmias, heart blocks, and cardiac arrest.

Potassium supplements are contraindicated in conditions that predispose the client to hyperkalemia, such as severe renal impairment and use of potassium-sparing diuretics. Potassium supplements are also contraindicated in acute dehydration, heat cramps, and clients with digoxin intoxication with AV node disturbance. Use cautiously in clients with kidney impairment, cardiac disease, and systemic acidosis.

Oral potassium administration is used for the prevention and treatment of mild deficiency. Oral forms, especially tablets and capsules that can produce high local concentrations of potassium, are irritating to the GI tract and may cause peptic ulcers. This side effect is less likely with the use of tablets and capsules that contain microencapsulated particles. To minimize GI irritation, instruct the client to administer oral forms with meals. Check for the most recent serum potassium level before administering any form of potassium. Too much potassium can be just as dangerous for the client as too little potassium; in either case, the consequences can be fatal.

Intravenous potassium administration is used for clients with severe deficiency or those who cannot tolerate oral forms. Monitor serum potassium levels throughout treatment to reduce the risk of hyperkalemia. Assess renal function prior to and during treatment, and if renal failure develops, stop the infusion immediately. Monitor for ECG changes, which can be an early indication of developing hyperkalemia. Clients who experience potassium imbalances must be taught to avoid the underlying causes, comply with medication regimen, and use dietary interventions to correct and maintain normal electrolyte balance.

Client Teaching. Client education as it relates to potassium replacement should include the goals of therapy, the reasons for obtaining baseline data such as vital signs and the existence of underlying cardiac and renal disorders, and possible drug side effects. Include the following points when teaching clients regarding potassium replacements:

- Report symptoms of hypokalemia such as weakness, fatigue, lethargy, or anorexia.
- Report symptoms of hyperkalemia such as nausea, abdominal cramping, weakness, changes in heart rate, and numbness or tingling of arms or legs.

SPECIAL CONSIDERATIONS

Laxatives and Fluid–Electrolyte Balance

With aging, peristalsis slows, food intake diminishes, and physical activity declines; and these factors can change bowel movement regularity. Many older adults believe they must have a bowel movement every day and take daily laxatives. Chronic use of laxatives can result in fluid depletion and hypokalemia. Stimulant laxatives, the most frequently prescribed class of laxatives, alter electrolyte transport in the intestinal mucosa. The elderly are especially susceptible to fluid and electrolyte depletion due to chronic laxative use. The nurse should teach the client that drinking plenty of fluids is important when taking a laxative, that overuse of laxatives can result in adverse side effects, and that these agents should be used only as directed by their healthcare practitioner. The nurse should recommend that older clients increase exercise (as tolerated) and add insoluble fiber to the diet to maintain elimination regularity.

Pr PROTOTYPE DRUG | Potassium Chloride (KCl) | Electrolyte/Potassium Supplement

ACTIONS AND USES

Potassium chloride is a drug of choice for preventing or treating hypokalemia. It is also used to treat mild forms of alkalosis. Oral formulations include tablets, powders, and liquids, usually heavily flavored owing to potassium chloride's unpleasant taste. Because potassium supplements can cause peptic ulcers, the drug should be diluted with plenty of water. When given IV, potassium must be administered slowly, since bolus injections can overload the heart and cause cardiac arrest. Because pharmacotherapy with loop or thiazide diuretics is the most common cause of potassium depletion, clients taking these drugs are usually prescribed oral potassium supplements to prevent hypokalemia.

ADMINISTRATION ALERTS

- Always give oral medication while client is upright to prevent esophagitis.
- Do not crush or allow client to chew tablets.
- Dilute liquid forms before giving through a nasogastric tube.
- Never administer IV push or in concentrated amounts, and do not exceed an IV rate of 10 mEq/h.
- Be extremely careful to avoid extravasation and infiltration.
- Pregnancy category A.

PHARMACOKINETICS

Because potassium chloride is a natural substance, pharmacokinetic data are difficult to obtain.

ADVERSE EFFECTS

Nausea and vomiting are common, because potassium chloride irritates the GI mucosa. The drug may be taken with meals or antacids to lessen gastric distress. The most serious side effects of potassium chloride are related to the possible accumulation of excess potassium. Hyperkalemia may occur if the client takes potassium supplements concurrently with potassium-sparing diuretics. Because the kidneys perform more than 90% of the body's potassium excretion, reduced renal function can rapidly lead to hyperkalemia, particularly in clients taking potassium supplements.

Contraindications: Potassium chloride is contraindicated in clients with hyperkalemia, chronic renal failure, systemic acidosis, severe dehydration, extensive tissue breakdown as in severe burns, adrenal insufficiency, or the administration of a potassium-sparing diuretic.

INTERACTIONS

Drug–Drug: Potassium supplements interact with potassium-sparing diuretics and ACE inhibitors to increase the risk for hyperkalemia.

Lab Tests: Increases serum potassium level.

Herbal/Food: Unknown.

Treatment of Overdose: Potassium-sparing diuretics and all foods and medications containing significant amounts of potassium should be withheld. Treatment includes IV administration of 10% dextrose solution containing 10–20 units of crystalline insulin. Sodium bicarbonate may be infused to correct acidosis.

 See the Companion Website for a Nursing Process Focus specific to this drug.

- Report decreased urinary output, because this can lead to hyperkalemia.
- Keep all scheduled laboratory visits to assess serum potassium levels.
- If taking a potassium supplement, avoid potassium-rich foods and potassium-based salt substitutes.
- Take potassium supplements with food to decrease GI distress. Dilute potassium elixirs in juice to prevent esophageal irritation.

ACID–BASE BALANCE

Acidosis (excess acid) and alkalosis (excess base) are not diseases but are symptoms of an underlying disorder. Acidic and basic agents may be administered to rapidly correct pH imbalances in body fluids, supporting the client's vital functions while the underlying disease is being treated.

31.8 Buffers and the Maintenance of Body pH

The degree of acidity or alkalinity of a solution is measured by its **pH**. A pH of 7.0 is defined as neutral, above 7.0 as basic or alkaline, and below 7.0 as acidic. To maintain homeostasis, the pH of plasma and most body fluids must be kept within the narrow range of 7.35 to 7.45. Nearly all proteins and enzymes in the body function optimally within this narrow range of pH values. A few enzymes, most notably those in the digestive tract, require pH values outside the 7.35 to 7.45 range to function properly. The correction of acid–base imbalance is illustrated in ● Figure 31.4.

The body generates significant amounts of acid during normal metabolic processes. Without sophisticated means of neutralizing these metabolic acids, the overall pH of body fluids would quickly fall below the normal range. **Buffers** are chemicals that help maintain normal body pH by neutralizing strong acids and bases. The two primary buffers in the body are bicarbonate ions and phosphate ions.

The body uses two mechanisms to remove acid. The carbon dioxide (CO_2) produced during body metabolism is an acid efficiently removed by the lungs during exhalation. The kidneys remove excess acid in the form of hydrogen ion (H^+) by excreting it in the urine. If retained in the body, CO_2 and/or H^+ would lower body pH. Thus, the lung and the kidneys collaborate in the removal of acids to maintain normal acid–base balance.

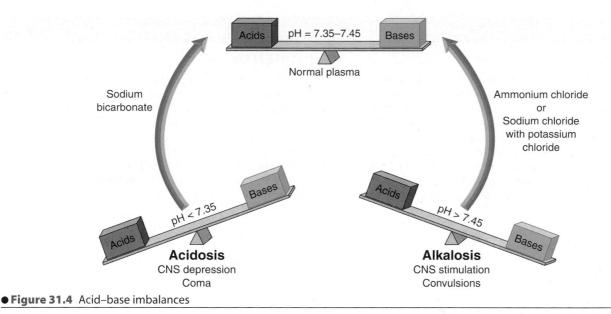

● **Figure 31.4** Acid–base imbalances

31.9 Pharmacotherapy of Acidosis

Acidosis occurs when the pH of the plasma falls below 7.35, which is confirmed by measuring arterial pH, partial pressure of carbon dioxide (P_{CO_2}), and plasma bicarbonate levels. Diagnosis must differentiate between respiratory etiology and metabolic (renal) etiology. Occasionally, the cause has mixed respiratory and metabolic components. The most profound symptoms of acidosis affect the central nervous system, and include lethargy, confusion, and CNS depression leading to coma. A deep, rapid respiration rate indicates an attempt by the lungs to rid the body of excess acid. Common causes of acidosis are listed in Table 31.5.

In clients with acidosis, the therapeutic goal is to quickly reverse the effects of excess acids in the blood. The treatment of choice for acute acidosis is to administer infusions of sodium bicarbonate. Bicarbonate ion acts as a base to quickly neutralize acids in the blood and other body fluids. The client must be carefully monitored during infusions because this drug can "overcorrect" the acidosis, causing blood pH to turn alkaline.

NATURAL THERAPIES

Sea Vegetables for Acidosis

Sea vegetables, or seaweeds, are a form of marine algae that grow in the upper levels of the ocean, where sunlight can penetrate. Examples of these edible seaweeds include spirulina, kelp, chlorella, arame, and nori, many of which are used in Asian cooking. Sea vegetables are found in coastal locations throughout the world. Kelp, or Laminaria, is found in the cold waters of the North Atlantic and Pacific Oceans.

Sea vegetables contain a multitude of vitamins, as well as protein. Their most notable nutritional aspect, however, is their mineral content. Plants from the sea contain more minerals than most other food sources, including calcium, magnesium, phosphoros, iron, potassium, and all essential trace elements. Because they are so rich in minerals, seaweeds act as alkalizers for the blood, helping to rid the body of acid conditions (acidosis). Spirulina, kelp, and chlorella are available in capsule or tablet form.

NURSING CONSIDERATIONS

The role of the nurse in sodium bicarbonate therapy involves careful monitoring of a client's condition and providing education as it relates to the prescribed treatment. Sodium bicarbonate is given to neutralize acidotic states, so

TABLE 31.5 Causes of Alkalosis and Acidosis	
Acidosis	**Alkalosis**
Respiratory origins of acidosis	**Respiratory origins of alkalosis**
hypoventilation or shallow breathing airway constriction	hyperventilation due to asthma, anxiety, or high altitude
damage to respiratory center in medulla	
Metabolic origins of acidosis	**Metabolic origins of alkalosis**
severe diarrhea	constipation for prolonged periods
kidney failure	ingestion of excess sodium bicarbonate
diabetes mellitus	diuretics that cause potassium depletion
excess alcohol ingestion	severe vomiting
starvation	

Pr PROTOTYPE DRUG | Sodium Bicarbonate | Electrolyte/Alkaline Agent

ACTIONS AND USES

Sodium bicarbonate is a drug of choice for correcting metabolic acidosis. After dissociation, the bicarbonate ion directly raises the pH of body fluids. Sodium bicarbonate may be given orally, if acidosis is mild, or IV in cases of acute disease. IV concentrations range from 4.2% to 8.4%. Although sodium bicarbonate also neutralizes gastric acid, it is rarely used to treat peptic ulcers due to its tendency to cause uncomfortable gastric distension. After absorption, sodium bicarbonate makes the urine more basic, which aids in the renal excretion of acidic drugs such as barbiturates and salicylates. The oral preparation of sodium bicarbonate is known as *baking soda*.

ADMINISTRATION ALERTS

- Do not add oral preparation to calcium-containing solutions.
- Give oral sodium bicarbonate 2 to 3 hours before or after meals and other medications.
- Pregnancy category C.

PHARMACOKINETICS

Onset: 15 min PO; immediate IV

Peak: 2 h PO; unknown IV

Half-life: Unknown

Duration: 1–3 h PO; 8–10 min IV

ADVERSE EFFECTS

Most of the side effects of sodium bicarbonate therapy are the result of metabolic alkalosis caused by receiving *too much* bicarbonate ion. Symptoms may include confusion, irritability, slow respiration rate, and vomiting. Simply discontinuing the sodium bicarbonate infusion often reverses these symptoms; however, potassium chloride or ammonium chloride may be administered to reverse acute alkalosis. During sodium bicarbonate infusions, serum electrolytes should be carefully monitored, as sodium levels may give rise to hypernatremia and fluid retention. In addition, high levels of bicarbonate ion passing through the kidney tubules increase potassium secretion, and hypokalemia is possible.

Contraindications: Sodium bicarbonate is contraindicated in clients with hypertension, renal impairment, peptic ulcers, excessive chloride loss due to GI suctioning, diarrhea, or vomiting.

INTERACTIONS

Drug–Drug: Sodium bicarbonate may decrease the absorption of ketoconazole, and may decrease elimination of dextroamphetamine, ephedrine, pseudoephedrine, and quinidine. The elimination of lithium, salicylates, and tetracyclines may be increased.

Lab Tests: Urinary and serum pH increase. Urinary urobilinogen levels may increase.

Herbal/Food: Chronic use with milk or calcium supplements may cause milk–alkali syndrome, a condition characterized by serious hypercalcemia and possible kidney failure.

Treatment of Overdose: Overdose results in metabolic alkalosis, which is treated by administering acidic agents (see Section 31.10).

 See the Companion Website for a Nursing Process Focus specific to this drug.

---

first analyze the arterial blood gas reports of pH, carbon dioxide levels (P_{CO_2}), bicarbonate levels (HCO^-_3), and oxygenation status (P_{O_2} and O_2 saturation). Assess the client for symptoms associated with acidosis such as sleepiness, coma, disorientation, dizziness, headache, seizures, and hypoventilation. Also, assess the client for causative factors that could produce acidosis such as diabetes mellitus, shock, and diarrhea. Acidosis is frequently corrected when the underlying disease condition is successfully managed.

The client receiving sodium bicarbonate is prone to alkalosis, especially if an excessive amount has been administered. Monitor the client for symptoms of alkalosis such as irritability, confusion, cyanosis, slow respirations, irregular pulse, and muscle weakness. These symptoms would warrant withholding the medication and notifying the healthcare provider.

There are several contraindications and precautions related to the administration of sodium bicarbonate. Clients who are vomiting or have continuous GI suctioning will lose acid and chloride and may be in a state of metabolic alkalosis; therefore, they should not receive sodium bicarbonate, because it may worsen alkalosis. Because of the sodium content of this drug, use it judiciously in clients with cardiac disease and renal impairment.

Sodium bicarbonate may also be used to alkalinize the urine and speed the excretion of acidic substances. This process is useful in the treatment of overdoses of certain acidic medications such as aspirin and phenobarbital, and as adjunctive therapy for certain chemotherapeutic drugs such as methotrexate. Sodium bicarbonate is also used in chronic renal failure to neutralize the metabolic acidosis that occurs when the kidneys cannot excrete hydrogen ion. When IV sodium bicarbonate is given, it causes the urine to become more alkaline. Less acid is reabsorbed in the renal tubules, so more acid and acidic medicine is excreted. This process is known as *ion trapping*. Monitor the client's acid–base status closely and report symptoms of imbalance to the healthcare provider. Provide care directed toward supporting critical body functions such as cardiovascular, respiratory, and neurological status that may be impaired secondary to the drug overdose.

Sodium bicarbonate (baking soda) is used as a home remedy to neutralize gastric acid, relieving heartburn, or sour stomach. Although occasional use is acceptable, be aware that clients may misinterpret cardiac symptoms as heartburn or may overuse sodium bicarbonate, leading to systemic alkalosis.

Client Teaching.   Client education as it relates to sodium bicarbonate should include the goals of therapy, the reasons for obtaining baseline data such as vital signs and electrolyte levels, and possible drug side effects. Include the following points when teaching clients regarding sodium bicarbonate:

- Immediately contact a healthcare provider if gastric discomfort continues, or is accompanied by chest pain, dyspnea, or diaphoresis.
- Use nonsodium antacids to prevent the absorption of excess sodium or bicarbonate into the systemic circulation.
- Do not use any antacid, including sodium bicarbonate, for longer than 2 weeks without consulting your healthcare provider.

31.10 Pharmacotherapy of Alkalosis

At plasma pH values above 7.45, **alkalosis** develops. Like acidosis, alkalosis may have either respiratory or metabolic causes, as listed in Table 31.5. Also as with acidosis, the central nervous system is greatly affected. Symptoms of CNS stimulation occur including nervousness, hyperactive reflexes, and convulsions. In metabolic alkalosis, slow, shallow breathing indicates that the body is attempting to compensate by retaining acid and lowering internal pH.

In mild cases, alkalosis may be corrected by administering sodium chloride concurrently with potassium chloride. This combination increases the renal excretion of bicarbonate ion, which indirectly increases the acidity of the blood. More severe alkalosis may be treated with infusions of an acidic drug such as ammonium chloride.

NURSING CONSIDERATIONS

The role of the nurse in ammonium chloride therapy involves careful monitoring of a client's condition and providing education as it relates to the prescribed treatment. Ammonium chloride is given for severe metabolic alkalosis, so assess the pH in arterial blood gas reports prior to administration. The major treatment for both metabolic alkalosis and respiratory alkalosis is to first attempt to correct the underlying disease condition creating the imbalance. The administration of ammonium chloride is used in clinical practice only when the alkalosis is so severe that the pH must be restored quickly to prevent life-threatening consequences. This drug is contraindicated in the presence of liver disease because its acidifying action depends on proper liver functioning to convert ammonium ions to urea.

During the IV infusion of ammonium chloride, continually assess for metabolic acidosis and ammonium toxicity. Symptoms of toxic levels of ammonium include pallor, sweating, irregular breathing, retching, bradycardia, twitching, and convulsions. If the client exhibits any of these symptoms, immediately stop the infusion and contact the healthcare provider.

Also, closely monitor the client's renal status during the administration of ammonium chloride, because the excretion of this drug depends on normal kidney function. Monitor intake and output ratios, body weight, electrolyte status, and renal function studies for any sign of renal impairment.

When ammonium chloride is administered IV, closely monitor the IV infusion site, because this drug is extremely irritating to veins and may cause severe inflammation. Infuse the drug slowly, no more than 5 ml/min, to prevent ammonia toxicity.

Like sodium bicarbonate, ammonium chloride is used as an ionic trapping agent in the treatment of drug overdoses.

Pr PROTOTYPE DRUG | Ammonium Chloride | Acidic Agent

ACTIONS AND USES

Severe metabolic alkalosis may be reversed by the administration of acidic agents such as ammonium chloride. During the hepatic conversion of ammonium chloride to urea, Cl^- and H^+ are formed, and the pH of body fluids decreases. Ammonium chloride acidifies the urine, which is beneficial in treating certain urinary tract infections. Historically, ammonium chloride has been used as a diuretic, though safer and more efficacious agents have made its use obsolete. By acidifying the urine, ammonium chloride promotes the excretion of alkaline drugs such as amphetamines. Oral and IV forms are available; when given for acidosis, the IV route is preferred.

ADMINISTRATION ALERTS

- IV solution should be infused slowly (no more than 5 ml/min) to prevent ammonia toxicity.
- Pregnancy category B.

PHARMACOKINETICS

Pharmacokinetic information for this drug is not available.

ADVERSE EFFECTS

Ammonium chloride is generally infused slowly, to minimize the potential for producing acidosis. The nurse should observe for signs of CNS depression, which is characteristic of acidosis.

Contraindications: Ammonium chloride should not be administered to clients with serious hepatic or renal impairment, or respiratory acidosis.

INTERACTIONS

Drug–Drug: Ammonium chloride may cause crystalluria when taken with aminosalicylic acid. Ammonium chloride reduces levels of amphetamines, flecainide, mexiletine, methadone, ephedrine, and pseudoephedrine. Urinary excretion of sulfonylureas and salicylates is decreased.

Lab Tests: Serum ammonia and AST levels are increased. Serum magnesium values may decrease.

Herbal/Food: Unknown.

Treatment of Overdose: Overdose results in metabolic acidosis, which is treated by administering alkaline agents (see Section 31.9).

 See the Companion Website for a Nursing Process Focus specific to this drug.

AVOIDING MEDICATION ERRORS

A physician orders digoxin (Lanoxin) 1.25 mg, but meant to write 0.125. The student nurse gives digoxin 1.25 mg. Who is responsible? The physician? The primary nurse? The nursing instructor? The nurse manager?
See Appendix D for the suggested answer.

Ammonium chloride acidifies urine, which increases the excretion of alkaline substances such as amphetamines, phencyclidine (PCP/angel dust), and other basic substances. Overdoses of alkaline substances can greatly compromise the cardiovascular, respiratory, and neurological status. The nursing role for this type of client is directed toward monitoring the client's acid–base status and supporting critical body functions.

Client Teaching.   Client education as it relates to ammonium chloride should include the goals of therapy, the reasons for obtaining baseline data such as vital signs and the existence of underlying renal disorders, and possible drug side effects. Include the following points when teaching clients and families about ammonium chloride:

- Report pain at IV site.
- If medication is taken orally, report anorexia, nausea, vomiting, and thirst.
- If medication is given parenterally, report rash, headache, bradycardia, drowsiness, confusion, depression, and excitement alternating with coma.
- Take ammonium chloride tablets for no longer than 6 days.
- Report severe GI upset, fever, chills, and changes in urine or stool color.
- Take medication after meals or use enteric-coated tablets to decrease GI upset; swallow tablets whole.

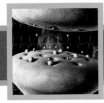

CHAPTER REVIEW

KEY CONCEPTS

The numbered key concepts provide a succinct summary of the important points from the corresponding numbered section within the chapter. If any of these points are not clear, refer to the numbered section within the chapter for review.

31.1   There is a continuous exchange of fluids across membranes separating the intracellular and extracellular fluid compartments. Large molecules and those that are ionized are less able to cross membranes.

31.2   Osmolality refers to the number of dissolved solutes (usually sodium, glucose, or urea) in a body fluid. Changes in the osmolality of body fluids can cause water to move to different compartments.

31.3   Overall fluid balance is achieved through complex mechanisms that regulate fluid intake and output. The greatest contributor to osmolality is sodium, which is controlled by the hormone aldosterone.

31.4   Intravenous fluid therapy using crystalloids and colloids replaces lost fluids. Colloids are large molecules that stay in the intravascular space to rapidly expand plasma volume. Crystalloids contain electrolytes, and are distributed primarily to the interstitial spaces.

31.5   Electrolytes are charged inorganic molecules that are essential to nerve conduction, membrane permeability, water balance, and other critical body functions. Imbalances may lead to serious abnormalities.

31.6   Sodium is essential to maintaining osmolality, water balance, and acid–base balance. Hypernatremia may be corrected with hypotonic IV fluids or diuretics, and hyponatremia may be treated with infusions of sodium chloride. Dilutional hyponatremia is treated with diuretics.

31.7   Potassium is essential for proper nerve and muscle function, as well as for maintaining acid–base balance.Hyperkalemia may be treated with glucose and insulin, or by administration of polystyrene sulfonate. Hypokalemia is corrected with oral or IV potassium supplements.

31.8   Buffers in the body maintain overall pH within narrow limits. The kidneys and lungs work together to remove excess metabolic acid.

31.9   Pharmacotherapy of acidosis, a plasma pH below 7.35, includes the administration of sodium bicarbonate.

31.10   Pharmacotherapy of alkalosis, a plasma pH above 7.45, includes the administration of ammonium chloride, or sodium chloride with potassium chloride.

NCLEX-RN® REVIEW QUESTIONS

1 Which of the following mechanisms is the most important regulator of fluid intake?

1. Thirst
2. Electrolytes
3. Renin–angiotensin
4. Kidneys

2 Which of the following nursing interventions is most important when caring for a client receiving a plasma volume expander?

1. Assess the client for deep vein thrombosis.
2. Observe for signs of fluid overload.
3. Encourage fluid intake.
4. Monitor arterial blood gases.

3 The client's serum sodium value is 149 mEq/L. Which of the following nursing interventions is most appropriate for this client? (Select all that apply.)

1. Encourage the client to eat a low-salt diet.
2. Administer a 0.45% NaCl IV solution.
3. Hold all doses of glucocorticoids.
4. Notify the healthcare provider.
5. Have client drink as much water as possible.

4 The client complains of muscle cramping in the calves, paresthesia of the toes, and the sensation of the heart skipping a beat. These symptoms can be symptoms of which of the following imbalances?

1. Hypernatremia
2. Hypercalcemia
3. Hypoglycemia
4. Hyperkalemia

5 The client's arterial blood gases reveal metabolic acidosis. What medication would the nurse anticipate being ordered?

1. Sodium chloride
2. Ammonium chloride
3. Sodium bicarbonate
4. Potassium chloride

CRITICAL THINKING QUESTIONS

1. A 72-year-old man with a history of heart failure presents to the emergency department complaining of weakness and palpitations. The client has been taking furosemide (Lasix) and digoxin (Lanoxin) at home. His current ECG reveals atrial fibrillation, and serum electrolyte testing reveals a potassium level of 2.5 mEq/L. The physician orders an IV solution of 1,000 ml of Ringer's lactate with 40 mEq KCl to infuse over 8 hours. What are the issues the nurse must consider to safely administer this drug?

2. An 18-year-old woman is admitted to the labor and delivery unit for observation with a blood pressure of 186/108 mm Hg. She has 3–4$^+$ pitting edema of the lower extremities and states that her hands and face are "swollen." The CBC reveals an elevated hemoglobin and hematocrit. The certified nurse midwife diagnoses the client with pregnancy-induced hypertension and orders an IV of D5LR. In addition, she requests that the nurse "push oral fluids." The nurse considers whether the midwife's order should be questioned. Discuss the appropriateness of this order.

3. An 84-year-old woman has recently returned home after being admitted to the hospital for persistent nausea and vomiting and dehydration. Her past medical history includes gastric reflux, hiatal hernia, GI bleeding, anemia, and coronary artery disease. Her current medication regimen is metoprolol (Lopressor), 50 mg PO bid; pantoprazole (Protonix), 40 mg PO daily; furosemide (Lasix), 20 mg PO daily; and lactulose, 20 g/30 ml PO at bedtime. Although this client's nausea and vomiting has resolved, she is still at risk for fluid and electrolyte imbalances secondary to her medication regimen. Which drug in particular places her at risk for fluid volume deficit, and which electrolyte must be monitored? What assessments should the nurse include?

See Appendix D for answers and rationales for all activities.

EXPLORE
MediaLink

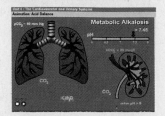

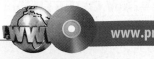
www.prenhall.com/adams

NCLEX-RN® review, case studies, and other interactive resources for this chapter can be found on the companion website at www.prenhall.com/adams. Click on "Chapter 31" to select the activities for this chapter. For animations, more NCLEX-RN® review questions, and an audio glossary, access the accompanying Prentice Hall Nursing MediaLink DVD-ROM in this textbook.

 PRENTICE HALL NURSING MEDIALINK DVD-ROM

- **Animations**
  Fluid Balance
  Acids
- **Audio Glossary**
- **NCLEX-RN® Review**

 COMPANION WEBSITE

- **NCLEX-RN® Review**
- **Dosage Calculations**
- **Case Study:** Client with fluid loss
- **Care Plan:** Client with potential hypokalemia secondary to routine furosemide use

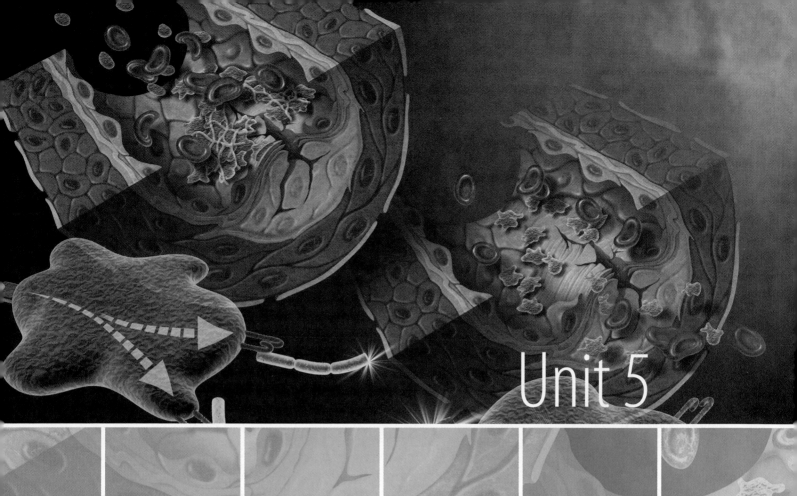

Unit 5

The Immune System

CHAPTER 32   Drugs for Immune System Modulation

CHAPTER 33   Drugs for Inflammation and Fever

CHAPTER 34   Drugs for Bacterial Infections

CHAPTER 35   Drugs for Fungal, Protozoal, and Helminthic Infections

CHAPTER 36   Drugs for Viral Infections

CHAPTER 37   Drugs for Neoplasia

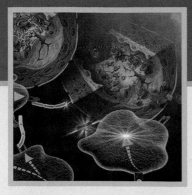

CHAPTER 32

Drugs for Immune System Modulation

DRUGS AT A GLANCE

IMMUNIZATION AGENTS
Vaccines
- *hepatitis B vaccine (Engerix-B, Recombivax HB)*

Immune Globulin Preparations
IMMUNOSTIMULANTS
Interferons
- *interferon alfa-2a (Roferon-A)*

Interleukins
IMMUNOSUPPRESSANTS
Antibodies
Antimetabolites and Cytotoxic Agents
Calcineurin Inhibitors
- *cyclosporine (Neoral, Sandimmune)*

Glucocorticoids

OBJECTIVES

After reading this chapter, the student should be able to:

1. Compare and contrast specific and nonspecific body defenses.
2. Compare and contrast the humoral and cell-mediated immune responses.
3. Explain why immunosuppressant medications are necessary following organ transplants.
4. Identify the types of agents used as immunosuppressants.
5. Compare and contrast active immunity and passive immunity.
6. Describe the nurse's role in the pharmacological management of immune disorders.
7. For each of the drug classes listed in Drugs at a Glance, know representative drugs, and explain their mechanism of drug action, primary actions related to the immune system, and important adverse effects.
8. Categorize drugs used in the treatment of immune disorders based on their classification and mechanism of action.
9. For each of the major vaccines, give the recommended dosage schedule.
10. Use the Nursing Process to care for clients receiving drug therapy for immune disorders.

MediaLink

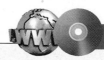

www.prenhall.com/adams

NCLEX-RN® review, case studies, and other interactive resources for this chapter can be found on the companion website at www.prenhall.com/adams. Click on "Chapter 32" to select the activities for this chapter. For animations, more NCLEX-RN® review questions, and an audio glossary, access the accompanying Prentice Hall Nursing MediaLink DVD-ROM in this textbook.

KEY TERMS

active immunity *page 457*

antibody *page 456*

antigen *page 455*

B cell *page 456*

biologic response modifiers *page 461*

calcineurin *page 466*

cytokine *page 459*

cytotoxic T cell *page 459*

helper T cell *page 459*

humoral immunity *page 456*

immune response *page 455*

immunosuppressant *page 463*

interferon *page 461*

interleukin *page 462*

nonspecific defenses *page 455*

passive immunity *page 457*

plasma cell *page 456*

T cell *page 459*

titer *page 457*

toxoid *page 456*

transplant rejection *page 463*

vaccination/immunization *page 457*

vaccine *page 456*

The body is under continuous attack from a host of foreign invaders that include viruses, bacteria, fungi, and even single-celled animals. Our extensive body defenses are capable of mounting a rapid and effective response against many of these pathogens. In some cases, pharmacotherapy can be used to stimulate body defenses so that microbes can be more readily attacked and disease prevented. On other occasions, it is desirable to dampen the immune response to allow a transplanted organ to survive. The purpose of this chapter is to examine the pharmacotherapy of agents affecting the body's response to disease.

32.1 Nonspecific Body Defenses and the Immune Response

The lymphatic system consists of lymphoid cells, tissues, and organs such as the spleen, thymus, tonsils, and lymph nodes. The overall purpose of the lymphatic system is to protect the body from pathogens.

The first line of protection from pathogens is **nonspecific defenses,** which serve as barriers to microbes or environmental hazards. The nonspecific defenses are unable to distinguish one type of threat from another; the response or protection is the same regardless of the pathogen. Nonspecific defenses include physical barriers such as the epithelial lining of the skin, and the respiratory and gastrointestinal mucous membranes that are potential entry points for pathogens. Other nonspecific defenses are phagocytes, natural killer (NK) cells, the complement system, fever, and interferons. From a pharmacological perspective, one of the most important nonspecific defenses is inflammation. Because of its significance, inflammation is discussed separately, in Chapter 33 ∞.

The body also has the capability to mount a *second* line of defense that is particular to certain threats. For example, a specific defense may act against only a single species of bacteria and be ineffective against all others. This type of defense is known as the **immune response.** Foreign agents that elicit an immune response are called **antigens.** Foreign proteins, such as those present on the surfaces of pollen grains, bacteria, nonhuman cells, and viruses, are the strongest antigens. The primary cell of the immune response that interacts with antigens is the *lymphocyte.*

The immune response is extremely complex. Basic steps involve recognition of the antigen, communication and coordination with other defense cells, and destruction or suppression of the antigen. A large number of chemical messengers and interactions are involved in the immune response, many of which have yet to be discovered. The two primary divisions of the immune response are

PHARMFACTS

Vaccines and Organ Transplants

- Vaccines have eradicated smallpox from the world, and the poliovirus from the Western Hemisphere.
- Vaccines lowered the number of diphtheria cases in the United States from 175,000 in 1922 to only 1 case annually.
- Vaccines lowered the number of measles cases in the United States from more than 503,000 in 1962 to only about 100 cases annually.
- Of the vaccine-preventable diseases, pneumococcal pneumonia is the most lethal, with 40,000 deaths annually in the United States.
- More than 79,000 clients are waiting organ transplants, with 3,000 added to the list every month.
- Because of lack of available transplants, many clients die every year, including approximately 2,000 kidney clients, 1,300 liver clients, 450 heart clients, and 361 lung clients.
- The most common transplanted organs are kidney, liver, and heart.

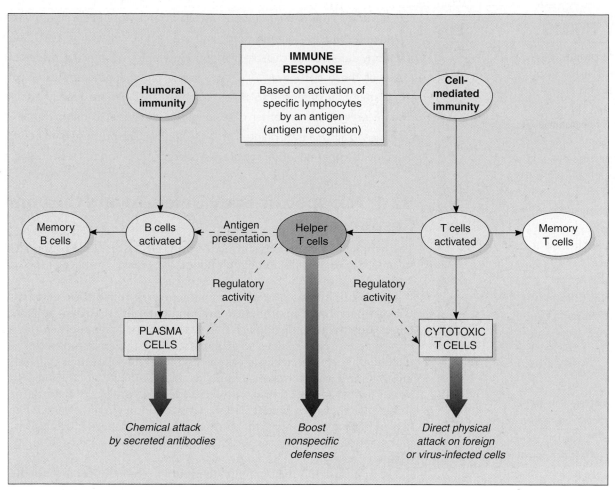

● **Figure 32.1** Steps in the humoral immune response   *Source:* Audesirk, Teresa; Audesirk, Gerald; Byers, Bruce, *Life on Earth,* 4th ed, © 2006, p. 435. Reprinted by permission of Pearson Education, Inc., Upper Saddle River, NJ.

antibody-mediated (humoral) immunity and cell-mediated immunity. These are shown in ● Figure 32.1.

32.2 Humoral Immunity and Antibodies

Humoral immunity is initiated when an antigen encounters a type of lymphocyte known as a **B cell.** The activated B cell divides rapidly to form clones of itself. Most cells in this clone are called **plasma cells** whose primary function is to secrete **antibodies** specific to the antigen that initiated the challenge. Circulating through the body, antibodies, also known as *immunoglobulins,* physically interact with the antigen to neutralize it or mark the foreign agent for destruction by other cells of the immune response. Peak production of antibodies occurs about 10 days after an initial antigen challenge. The important functions of antibodies are illustrated in ● Figure 32.2

Some B cells, called *memory B cells,* remember the initial antigen interaction. Should the body be exposed to the same antigen in the future, the immune system will be able to manufacture even higher levels of antibodies in a shorter period, approximately 2 to 3 days. For some antigens, such as those for measles, mumps, or chicken pox, memory can

be retained for an entire lifetime. Vaccines are sometimes administered to produce these memory cells in advance of exposure to the antigen, so that when the body is exposed to the actual organism it can mount a fast, effective response.

VACCINES

Vaccines are biological agents used to stimulate the immune system. The goal of vaccine administration is to prevent serious infections by life-threatening pathogens.

32.3 Administration of Vaccines

Lymphocytes attack antigens by recognizing certain foreign proteins on their surface. Sometimes they recognize a toxin or secretion produced by the pathogen. Pharmacologists have used this knowledge to create biological products that prevent disease, called vaccines, which consist of suspensions of one of the following:

- Microbes that have been killed
- Microbes that are alive but weakened (attenuated) so they are unable to produce disease
- Bacterial toxins, called **toxoids,** that have been modified to remove their hazardous properties

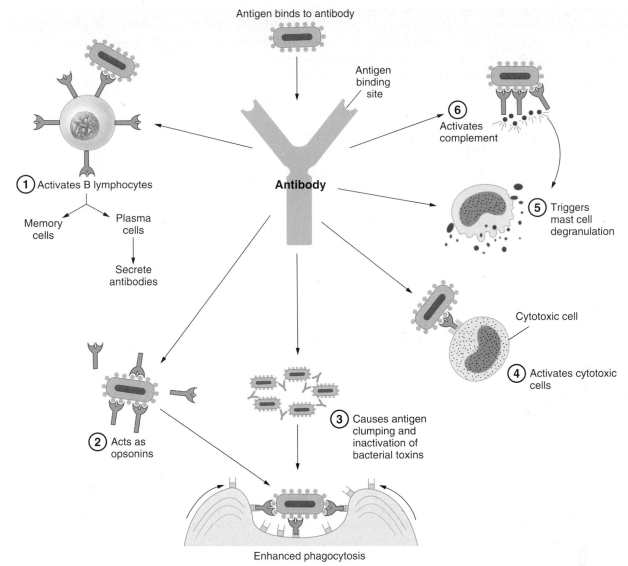

Antigen binds to antibody

Antigen binding site

Antibody

① Activates B lymphocytes

Memory cells

Plasma cells

Secrete antibodies

② Acts as opsonins

③ Causes antigen clumping and inactivation of bacterial toxins

⑥ Activates complement

⑤ Triggers mast cell degranulation

Cytotoxic cell

④ Activates cytotoxic cells

Enhanced phagocytosis

● **Figure 32.2** Functions of antibodies *Source:* Silverthorn, *Human Physiology: An Integrated Approach*, 2nd ed, © 2001, p. 700. Reprinted by permission of Pearson Education, Inc., Upper Saddle River, NJ.

Vaccination, or **immunization,** administers a modified, harmless microorganism or its toxoid to the client so that an immune response occurs in the following weeks or months. As a result of the vaccination, memory B cells are formed. When later exposed to the actual infectious organism, these cells will react quickly by producing large quantities of antibodies. Whereas some immunizations are needed only once, most require follow-up vaccinations, called *boosters,* to provide sustained protection. The effectiveness of most vaccines can be assessed by measuring the amount of antibody produced after the vaccine has been administered, a quantity called **titer.** If the titer falls below a specified protective level over time, a booster is indicated.

The type of immunity achieved through the administration of a vaccine is called **active immunity.** In active immunity, the client's immune system is stimulated to produce antibodies by exposure to the antigen or a vaccine. The active immunity induced by vaccines closely resembles that caused by natural exposure to the antigen, including the generation of memory cells.

Passive immunity occurs when preformed antibodies are transferred from one person to another. For example, maternal antibodies cross the placenta and provide protection for the fetus and newborn. Agents infused to provide passive immunity include immune globulin following exposure to hepatitis, antivenins for snakebites, and sera used to treat botulism, tetanus, and rabies. Drugs for passive immunity are administered when the client has already been exposed to a virulent pathogen, or is at very high risk to exposure, and there is not sufficient time to develop active immunity. Clients who are immunosuppressed may receive these agents to *prevent* infections. Because these drugs do not stimulate the client's immune system, no memory cells are produced, and protective effects last only 2 to 3 weeks. Table 32.1 lists selected immune globulin preparations. Pharmacotherapy Illustrated 32.1 shows the development of immunity through vaccines or the administration of antibodies.

TABLE 32.1 Immune Globulin Preparations

Drug	Route and Adult Dose (max dose where indicated)	Adverse Effects
cytomegalovirus immune globulin (CytoGam)	IV; 150 mg/kg within 72 h of transplantation; then 100 mg/kg for 2, 4, 6, and 8 wk posttransplant; then 50 mg/kg for 12 and 16 wk posttransplant	*Local reactions at injection site (pain, erythema, myalgia), influenza-like symptoms (malaise, fever, chills), headache*
hepatitis B immune globulin (BayHep B, HyperHep, H-BIG)	IM; 0.06 ml/kg as soon as possible after exposure, preferably within 24 h, but no later than 7 days; repeat 28–30 days after exposure	Anaphylaxis
immune globulin intramuscular (Gamastan)	IM; 0.02–0.06 ml/kg as soon as possible after exposure if H-BIG is unavailable	
immune globulin intravenous (Gamimune N, Gammagard, Gammar-P, IGIV, Iveegam, Sandoglobulin, Venoglobulin-S)	IV; 100–200 mg/kg/mo IM; 1.2 ml/kg followed by 0.6 ml/kg q2–4 wk	
rabies immune globulin (BayRab, Imogam Rabies-HT, Hyperab)	IM; (gluteal) 20 units/kg	
Rh$_0$(D) immune globulin (BayRho-D, WinRho SDF, MICRhoGAM, RhoGAM)	IM/IV; one vial or 300 mcg at approximately 28 wk; followed by one vial of minidose or 120 mcg within 72 h of delivery if infant is Rh-positive	
tetanus immune globulin (BayTet, HyperTet)	IM; 250 units	

Italics indicate common adverse effects; underlining indicates serious adverse effects.

Most vaccines are administered with the goal of *preventing* illness. Common vaccines include those used to prevent clients from acquiring measles, influenza, diphtheria, polio, whooping cough, tetanus, and hepatitis B. Anthrax vaccine has been used to immunize people who are at high risk for exposure to anthrax from a potential bioterrorism incident (Chapter 3 ∞). Current research is focusing on anticancer vaccines that may provide protection from specific cancers. In the case of infection by the human immunodeficiency virus (HIV), however, experimental HIV vaccines are given *after* infection has occurred for the purpose of enhancing the immune system, rather than preventing the disease. Unlike other vaccines, experimental vaccines for HIV have thus far been unable to prevent AIDS. Pharmacotherapy of HIV is discussed in Chapter 36 ∞.

Vaccines are not without adverse effects. Common side effects include redness and discomfort at the site of injection, and fever. Although severe reactions are uncommon, anaphylaxis is possible. Vaccinations are contraindicated for clients who have a weakened immune system or who are currently experiencing symptoms such as diarrhea, vomiting, or fever.

Effective vaccines have been produced for a number of debilitating diseases, and their widespread use has prevented serious illness in millions of clients, particularly children. One disease, smallpox, has been completely eliminated from the planet through immunization, and others such as polio have diminished to extremely low levels. The nurse plays a key role in encouraging clients to be vaccinated according to established guidelines. Table 32.2 lists selected vaccines and their recommended schedules.

Although vaccinations have proved to be a resounding success in children, many adults die of diseases that could be prevented by vaccination. Most mortality from vaccine-preventable disease in adults is from influenza and pneumococcal disease. Recent studies have shown that only 67% of adults older than age 65 had received influenza vaccine in the past 12 months, and only 56% had ever received pneumococcal vaccine. In 2002, the CDC published an adult immunization schedule that contained both age-based and risk-based recommendations (see www.cdc.gov). Risk-based considerations include pregnancy, diabetes, heart disease, renal failure, and various other serious and debilitating conditions.

NURSING CONSIDERATIONS

The role of the nurse in immunization to stimulate the immune system involves careful monitoring of a client's condition and providing education as it relates to the prescribed drug treatment. Prior to administration, assess for any risk-based precautions such as pregnancy, diabetes, heart disease, renal failure, and various other serious and debilitating conditions, and provide education on the importance of receiving vaccinations. Assess recent laboratory blood tests because vaccines are contraindicated in immunosuppressed clients. Answer all questions and concerns clients and family members may have regarding the risks and benefits of vaccines. Instruct clients and family on the recommended immunization schedule and the importance of any recommended follow-up vaccines.

Assess for common side effects such as redness and discomfort at the site of injection, and fever. Monitor the client carefully for signs of anaphylaxis.

Client Teaching. Client education as it relates to immunization therapy should include the goals of therapy; the reasons for obtaining baseline data such as vital signs and the

32.1 Mechanisms of Active and Passive Immunity

Booster Vaccine
Administered months or years after the inital vaccine, booster vaccines stimulate the immune system to maintian enough memory cells to mount a rapid response to an antigen.

Antibodies neutralize or destroy antigens

Memory cells provide long-lived protection.

Active immunity
Administration of vaccine or exposure to an antigen stimulates the body to produce **antibodies** and **memory cells**.

Antigen exposure

Passive immunity
Administration of immunoglobulins (antibodies) gives passive immunity which has a fast onset, but lasts only 3 to 6 months.

Plasma cell exposed to antigen or vaccine

Immunoglobulins

Response from antibodies (rapid but short-lived)

TABLE 32.2   Selected Vaccines and Their Schedules

Vaccine	Schedule and Age
diphtheria, tetanus, and pertussis (DPT, Tri-Immunol, Tripedia, Acel-Imune, Infanrix, Certiva)	IM; 0.5 ml at ages 2, 4, 6, and 18 mo
haemophilus type B conjugate (HibTITER, ActHIB, PedvaxHIB)	IM; 0.5 ml at ages 2, 4, 6, and 15 mo; children aged 12–14 mo who have not been vaccinated receive a single dose
hepatitis B (Recombivax HB, Engerix-B)	Children: 2.5–5 mcg at birth; then 0.5 ml at 1–4 mo and 6–18 mo Adults: 0.5 ml in 3 doses, with the second dose 30 days after the first, and the final dose 6 mo after the first
influenza vaccine (Fluzone, FluShield, Fluvirin)	Children: IM 2 doses 1 mo apart; then annual dose Adults: IM single annual dose
measles, mumps, and rubella (MMR II)	Subcutaneous; 0.5 ml single dose at age 15 mo to puberty
pneumococcal, polyvalent (Pneumovax 23, Pnu-Immune 23), or 7-valent (Prevnar)	Adults (Pneumovax 23 or Pnu-Immune 23): subcutaneous or IM; 0.5 ml as a single dose Children (Prenvar): IM 4 doses at ages 2 mo, 4 mo, 6 mo, and 12–15 mo
poliovirus, inactivated (IPOL)	Children: subcutaneous; 0.5 ml at ages 4–8 wk, 2–4 mo, and 6–12 mo
varicella zoster/chicken pox (Varivax)	Clients 12 mo and older: subcutaneous; 0.5 ml, 2 doses given 4–8 wk apart Younger than 12 mo: 0.5 ml as a single dose.

existence of underlying disorders such as diabetes, heart disease, or renal failure; and possible drug side effects. Include the following points when teaching clients about vaccines:

- Practice reliable contraception for 3 months after administration of vaccines.

- Maintain immunization records and bring to healthcare appointments during visits for immunizations.

- Keep all scheduled appointments for additional vaccinations.

- Realize that side effects may include pain at injection site, fever, and soreness.

- Immediately report shortness of breath or allergic reactions.

32.4 Cell-mediated Immunity and Cytokines

A second branch of the immune response involves lymphocytes called **T cells.** Two major types of T cells are called **helper T cells** and **cytotoxic T cells.** These cells are sometimes named after a protein receptor on their plasma membrane; the helper T cells have a CD4 receptor, and the cytotoxic T cells have a CD8 receptor. The helper T cells are particularly important because they are responsible for activating most other immune cells, including B cells. Cytotoxic T cells travel throughout the body, directly killing certain bacteria, parasites, virus-infected cells, and cancer cells.

Activated or sensitized T cells rapidly form clones after they encounter their specific antigen. Unlike B cells, however, T cells do not produce antibodies. Instead, activated T cells produce huge amounts of **cytokines**—hormonelike proteins that regulate the intensity and duration of the immune response and mediate cell-to-cell communication. Some cytokines kill foreign organisms directly, whereas others induce inflammation or enhance the killing power of macrophages. Specific cytokines released by activated T cells include interleukins, gamma interferon, and perforin. Some cytokines are used therapeutically to stimulate the immune system, as discussed in Section 32.5. In addition to T lymphocytes, certain macrophages, B lymphocytes, mast cells, endothelial cells, and stromal cells of the spleen, thymus, and bone marrow also secrete small amounts of cytokines.

Like B cells, some sensitized T cells become memory cells. If the person then encounters the same antigen in the future, the memory T cells assist in mounting a more rapid immune response.

Pr PROTOTYPE DRUG | Hepatitis B Vaccine *(Recombivax HB, Engerix-B)* | Vaccine

ACTIONS AND USES

Hepatitis B vaccine (Recombivax) is used to provide active immunity in individuals who are at risk for exposure to hepatitis B virus (HBV). It is indicated for infants born to HBV-positive mothers, and those at high risk for exposure to HBV-infected blood, including nurses, physicians, dentists, dental hygienists, morticians, and paramedics. Because HBV infection is extremely difficult to treat, it is prudent for all healthcare workers to receive HBV vaccine before beginning their clinical education, unless contraindicated. HBV vaccine does *not* provide protection against exposure to other (non-B) hepatitis viruses.

HBV vaccine is produced by splicing the gene for HBV surface antigen into yeast, and harvesting the protein product. It is prepared from recombinant yeast cultures rather than from human blood.

Vaccination requires three IM injections; the second dose is given 1 month after the first, and the third dose 6 months after the first dose.

ADMINISTRATION ALERTS

- In adults, use the deltoid muscle for the injection site, unless contraindicated.
- Epinephrine (1:1,000) should be immediately available to treat a possible anaphylactic reaction.
- Pregnancy category C.

PHARMACOKINETICS

Onset: 2 wk

Peak: 6 mo

Half-life: Unknown

Duration: At least 3 y

ADVERSE EFFECTS

HBV vaccine is well tolerated, and few serious adverse reactions have been reported. Pain and inflammation at the injection site is the most common side effect. Some clients experience transient fever or fatigue. Hypersensitivity reactions such as urticaria or anaphylaxis are possible.

Contraindications: This vaccine is contraindicated in clients with hypersensitivity to yeast or HBV vaccine. The drug should be administered with caution in clients with fever or active infections, or those with compromised cardiopulmonary status.

INTERACTIONS

Drug–Drug: Unknown.

Lab Tests: Unknown.

Herbal/Food: Unknown.

Treatment of Overdose: Overdoses have not been recorded.

 See the Companion Website for a Nursing Process Focus specific to this drug.

TABLE 32.3   Immunostimulants

Drug	Route and Adult Dose (max dose where indicated)	Adverse Effects
aldesleukin (Proleukin): interleukin-2	IV; 600,000 units/kg (0.037 mg/kg) q8h by a 15-min IV infusion for a total of 14 doses	*Flulike symptoms (fever, chills, malaise), rash, anemia, nausea, vomiting, diarrhea, confusion, dyspnea* Cardiac arrest, hypotension, tachycardia, thrombocytopenia, oliguria, anuria, pulmonary edema
Bacillus Calmette-Guérin (BCG) vaccine (Tice, TheraCys)	Interdermal (Tice); 0.1 ml as vaccine Intravesical (TheraCys); bladder instillation for bladder carcinoma	*Flulike symptoms (fever, chills, malaise), dysuria, hematuria, anemia* Thrombocytopenia, cystitis, UTI
levamisole (Ergamisol)	Initial: 50 mg q8h for 3 days; Maintenance: 50 mg q8h for 3 days q2 wk	*Nausea, vomiting, diarrhea, stomatitis, dermatitis, alopecia, fatigue* Leukopenia, anaphylaxis
INTERFERONS		
interferon alfa-2a (Roferon-A)	IM/subcutaneous; hairy cell leukemia: 3 million units/day for 16–24 wk, then reduced to 3 times/wk Kaposi's sarcoma: 36 million units/day for 10–12 wk, then reduced to 3 times/wk Hepatitis: 1–3 million units/day for 1 wk, then reduced to 3 times/wk for 48–52 wk	*Flulike symptoms, myalgia, fatigue, headache, anorexia, diarrhea* Myelosuppression, thrombocytopenia, suicide ideation, seizures (interferon beta)
interferon alfa-2b (Intron-A)	IM/subcutaneous; hairy cell leukemia: 2 million units/m^2 3 times/wk Kaposi's sarcoma: 30 million units/m^2 3 times/wk Hepatitis: 3 million units/m^2 3 times/wk for 18–24 mo	
interferon beta-1a (Avonex, Rebif)	IM (Avonex); 30 mcg/wk Subcutaneous (Rebif); 44 mcg 3 times/wk	
interferon beta-1b (Betaseron)	Subcutaneous; 0.25 mg (8 million units) every other day	
peginterferon alfa-2a (Pegasys)	Subcutaneous; 180 mcg/wk for 48 wk	

Italics indicate common adverse effects; underlining indicates serious adverse effects.

Cultural Effects on Immunizations

Although childhood immunizations have proved to be some of the most effective means of preventing and controlling the spread of infectious and communicable diseases, thousands of preschool children are not being properly immunized. Immunization levels are lower among African American, Hispanic, and American Indian/Alaska Native children. According to CDC statistics, 76% of White 2-year-old children compared with 68% of African American and Hispanics 2-year-old children were fully vaccinated in accordance with immunization guidelines. Children are not the only age group lacking sufficient immunization. In 1999, Hispanics and African Americans aged 65 years and older were less likely than Whites to report having received influenza and pneumococcal vaccines. Limited access to preventive services and client skepticism, attitudes, and cultural beliefs about health care may contribute to these statistics.

Community outreach programs have proved effective at reaching underserved ethnic groups. One of the goals of Healthy People 2010, a set of health objectives for the nation to achieve in the first decade of the 21st century, is eliminating racial and ethnic disparities in health. Racial and Ethnic Approaches to Community Health (REACH) 2010 serves as one of the Centers for Disease Control and Prevention's (CDC's) efforts to eliminate the disparities. Launched in 1999, REACH funds community coalitions designed to implement unique community-driven strategies. Government-funded health programs, such as the Children's Health Initiative Program (CHIP), were also initiated in the 1990s to promote preventive health care for America's children.

IMMUNOSTIMULANTS

Despite attempts over many decades to develop effective drugs that stimulate the immune system to fight disease, only a few such drugs have been approved. These agents include interferons and interleukins produced by recombinant DNA technology. Immunostimulants are listed in Table 32.3.

32.5 Pharmacotherapy With Biologic Response Modifiers

When challenged by specific antigens, certain cells in the immune system secrete cytokines that help defend against the invading organism. These natural cytokines have been identified, and through recombinant DNA technology, sufficient quantities have been produced to treat certain disorders. Sometimes called **biologic response modifiers,** some of these agents boost specific functions of the immune system. Biologic response modifiers that enhance hematopoiesis, such as colony-stimulating factors, epoetin alfa, and oprelvekin (Neumega), were presented in Chapter 28 ∞.

Interferons (IFNs) are cytokines secreted by lymphocytes and macrophages that have been infected with a virus.

NATURAL THERAPIES

Echinacea for Boosting the Immune System

Echinacea purpurea, or purple coneflower, is a popular medicinal botanical native to the midwestern United States and central Canada. The flowers, leaves, and stems of this plant are harvested and dried. Preparations include dried powder, tincture, fluid extracts, and teas. No single ingredient seems to be responsible for the herb's activity; a large number of potentially active chemicals have been identified from the extracts.

Echinacea was used by Native Americans to treat various wounds and injuries. Echinacea is claimed to boost the immune system by increasing phagocytosis and inhibiting the bacterial enzyme hyaluronidase. Some substances in echinacea appear to have antiviral activity; thus, the herb is sometimes taken to treat the common cold and influenza—an indication for which it has received official approval in Germany. In general, echinacea is used as a supportive treatment for any disease involving inflammation and to enhance the immune system. Side effects are rare; however, it may interfere with drugs that have immunosuppressant effects.

After secretion, interferons attach to uninfected cells and signal them to secrete antiviral proteins. Part of the nonspecific defense system, IFNs slow the spread of viral infections and enhance the activity of existing leukocytes. These agents have antiviral, anticancer, and anti-inflammatory properties. The actions of interferons include modulation of immune functions such as increasing phagocytosis and enhancing the cytotoxic activity of T cells.

The class of IFNs having the greatest clinical utility is the alpha interferons, for which six different formulations are available. These include IFN alfa-2a, IFN alfa-2b, IFN alfa-n3, IFN alfa-n1, pegIFN alfa-2a, and pegIFN alfa-2b (note that when used as medications, the spelling is changed from alpha to alfa). In the two peg formulations the inert molecule polyethylene glycol is attached to the interferon. This addition extends the half-life of the drug to allow for once-weekly dosing. Indications for IFN alfa therapy include hairy cell leukemia, AIDS-related Kaposi's sarcoma, chronic myelogenous leukemia (alfa-2a), and chronic hepatitis B or C (alfa-2b). The use of IFN alfa in the pharmacotherapy of hepatitis is presented in Chapter 36 ∞.

Interferon beta consists of two different formulations, beta-1a and beta-1b, which are primarily reserved for the treatment of severe multiple sclerosis. A third drug in this class, IFN gamma-1b has limited clinical application in the treatment of chronic granulomatous disease and severe osteopetrosis.

Interleukins (ILs) are another class of cytokines, synthesized primarily by lymphocytes, monocytes, and macrophages that enhance the capabilities of the immune system. The ILs have widespread effects on immune function including stimulation of cytotoxic T-cell activity against tumor cells, increased B-cell and plasma cell production, and promotion of inflammation. At least 20 different ILs have been identified, though only a few are available as medications. Interleukin-2, derived from T helper lymphocytes, promotes the proliferation of both T lymphocytes and activated B lymphocytes. It is available as aldesleukin (Proleukin), which is approved for the treatment of metastatic renal carcinoma. Aldesleukin must be administered in multiple, brief IV infusions because of its short half-life. Therapy is sometimes limited by capillary leak syndrome, a serious condition in which plasma proteins and other substances leave the blood and enter the interstitial spaces because of "leaky" capillaries. Interleukin-11, derived from bone marrow cells, is a growth factor with multiple hematopoietic effects. It is marketed as oprelvekin (Neumega) for its ability to stimulate platelet production in immunosuppressed clients (Chapter 28 ∞).

In addition to interferons and interleukins, a few additional biologic response modifiers are available to enhance the immune system. Levamisole (Ergamisole) is used to stimulate the production of B cells, T cells, and macrophages in clients with colon cancer. Bacillus Calmette–Guérin (BCG) vaccine (Tice, TheraCys) is an attenuated strain of *Mycobacterium bovis* used for the pharmacotherapy of certain types of bladder cancer.

NURSING CONSIDERATIONS

The role of the nurse in immunostimulant therapy involves careful monitoring of a client's condition and providing education as it relates to the prescribed drug treatment. Immunostimulants are powerful drugs that not only affect target cells but may also seriously affect other body systems. Prior to starting a client on these drugs, conduct a thorough assessment including a complete health history, present signs and symptoms, and allergy and medical history. Assess for the presence and/or history of the following diseases or disorders: chronic hepatitis, hairy cell leukemia, malignant melanoma, condylomata acuminata, AIDS-related Kaposi's sarcoma, and renal disorders including cancer. Assessment of infections and cancer verifies the need for these drugs. Immunostimulants are contraindicated for clients with renal or liver disease and pregnancy. Before starting therapy, obtain the results of lab tests including a complete blood count, electrolytes, renal function, and liver enzymes to provide baseline data. Measure vital signs and body weight at the initial assessment and throughout the treatment regimen to monitor progress.

Use interferon alfa-2b (Intron A) with caution in clients with hepatitis other than hepatitis C, leukopenia, and pulmonary disease. Interferon alfa-2a (Roferon-A) should be used with caution in clients with cardiac disease, herpes zoster, and recent exposure to chicken pox.

Keep the client well hydrated during pharmacotherapy. Use of immunostimulants can lead to the development of encephalopathy; therefore, assess for changes in mental status. Be especially vigilant for signs and symptoms of depression and suicidal ideation. Interferon alfa-2b (Intron A) may promote development of leukemia because of bone marrow suppression; therefore, periodically monitor blood tests.

Client Teaching. Client education as it relates to immunostimulant drugs should include the goals of therapy; the reasons for obtaining baseline data such as vital signs and the existence of underlying disorders such as leukemia,

Pr **PROTOTYPE DRUG** | Interferon alfa-2A *(Roferon-A)* | Biologic Response Modifer/Interferon

ACTIONS AND USES

Interferon alfa-2a is a biological response modifier that has the same actions and indications as interferon alfa-2b (Intron A). Interferon alfa-2a is a natural protein that is produced by human lymphocytes 4 to 6 hours after viral exposure. As a drug, it is prepared through recombinant DNA technology and is available as single-use prefilled syringes, administered by the subcutaneous or IM routes.

Interferon alfa-2a affects cancer cells by two mechanisms. First, it enhances or stimulates the immune system to remove antigens. Second, the drug suppresses the growth of cancer cells. As expected from its origin, interferon alfa-2a also has antiviral activity.

Indications for interferon alfa-2a include hairy cell leukemia, chronic hepatitis C infection, and malignant melanoma. Off-label uses include hepatitis B and AIDS-related Kaposi's sarcoma.

ADMINISTRATION ALERTS

- The drug should be administered under the careful guidance of a qualified healthcare provider.
- Subcutaneous administration is recommended for clients at risk for bleeding.
- Pregnancy category C.

PHARMACOKINETICS

Onset: Unknown

Peak: 1.8 h (IM)

Half-life: 5.1 h

Duration: Unknown

ADVERSE EFFECTS

A flulike syndrome of fever, chills, dizziness, and fatigue occurs in 50% or clients, although this usually diminishes as therapy progresses. Headache, nausea, vomiting, diarrhea, and anorexia are relatively common. Depression and suicidal ideation have been reported. With prolonged therapy, serious toxicity such as immunosuppression, hepatotoxicity, and neurotoxicity may be observed.

Contraindications: Contraindications include hypersensitivity to interferons, autoimmune hepatitis, or hepatic decompensation. Neonates and infants should not receive this drug because it contains benzyl alcohol, which is associated with an increased incidence of neurological and other serious complications in these age groups.

INTERACTIONS

Drug–Drug: Interferon alfa-2a may increase theophylline levels. There is additive myelosuppression with antineoplastics. Zidovudine may increase hematologic toxicity.

Lab Tests: May elevate triglyceride levels and may decrease hematocrit, leukocyte, and platelet counts.

Herbal/Food: Unknown.

Treatment of Overdose: There is no specific therapy for overdose.

 See the Companion Website for a Nursing Process Focus specific to this drug.

MediaLink Mechanism of Action: Interferon alfa

---

infection, leukopenia, and encephalopathy; and possible drug side effects. Include the following points when teaching clients about immunostimulant drugs:

- Practice reliable contraception and notify your healthcare provider if pregnancy is planned or suspected.
- Avoid the use of corticosteroids, because these hormones reduce the drug's antitumor effects.
- Liver, endocrine, or neurological adverse effects that occur during therapy may be permanent.
- Avoid alcohol use, because it may induce a disulfiram (Antabuse) reaction.
- Keep all scheduled appointments and laboratory visits for testing.
- Immediately report symptoms of nausea or stomatitis.
- Use nonalcoholic mouthwashes to treat stomatitis.
- Immediately report hematuria, petechiae, tarry stools, bruising, fever, sore throat, jaundice, dark-colored urine, clay-colored stools, feelings of sadness, and nervousness.

IMMUNOSUPPRESSANTS

Drugs used to inhibit the immune response are called *immunosuppressants.* They are used for clients receiving transplanted tissues or organs. These agents are listed in Table 32.4.

32.6 Immunosuppressants to Prevent Transplant Rejection and to Treat Autoimmune Disorders

The immune response is normally viewed as a lifesaver that protects individuals from a host of pathogens in the environment. For those receiving organ or tissue transplants, however, the immune response is the enemy. Transplanted organs from donors always contain antigens that trigger the immune response. This response, called **transplant rejection,** is often acute; antibodies sometimes destroy the transplanted tissue within a few days. The cell-mediated branch of the immune system responds more slowly to the transplant, attacking it about 2 weeks following surgery. Even if the organ survives these challenges, chronic rejection of the transplant may occur months or even years after surgery.

Immunosuppressants are drugs given to dampen the immune response. Transplantation would be impossible without the use of effective immunosuppressant drugs. In addition, these agents may be prescribed for severe cases of rheumatoid arthritis or other autoimmune diseases. Although the mechanisms of action of the immunosuppressant drugs differ, all suppress some aspect of T-cell function. Some act nonselectively by inhibiting all aspects of the immune system. Other, newer drugs are more specific, suppressing only

NURSING PROCESS FOCUS Clients Receiving Immunostimulant Therapy

Assessment	Potential Nursing Diagnoses
▪ Obtain a health history including allergies, drug history, and possible drug interactions. ▪ Assess a history of cytomegalovirus and any malignancies to verify need. ▪ Obtain laboratory work including complete blood count (CBC), electrolytes, and liver enzymes. ▪ Obtain weight and vital signs, especially blood pressure. ▪ Assess mental alertness.	▪ Injury, Risk for, related to side effects of drug ▪ Nutrition, Imbalanced: Less than Body Requirements, related to gastrointestinal upset secondary to drug ▪ Infection, Risk for, related to bone marrow suppression secondary to drug

Planning: Client Goals and Expected Outcomes

The client will:
▪ Experience increased immune system function.
▪ Demonstrate an understanding of the drug's action by accurately describing drug side effects and precautions.
▪ Immediately report effects such as fever, chills, sore throat, unusual bleeding, chest pain, palpitations, dizziness, or change in mental status.
▪ Demonstrate the ability to self-administer IM or subcutaneous injection.

Implementation

Interventions and (Rationales)	Client Education/Discharge Planning
▪ Monitor for leukopenia, neutropenia, thrombocytopenia, anemia, and increased liver enzymes. (Drugs can cause bone marrow suppression and liver damage.)	Instruct client to: ▪ Comply with all ordered laboratory tests. ▪ Immediately report any unusual bleeding or jaundice. ▪ Avoid crowds and people with infections. ▪ Avoid activities that can cause bleeding or impairment of skin integrity.
▪ Ensure that the drug is properly administered. (Client education of proper administration helps prevent injury and promotes optimal effectiveness of drug.)	▪ Instruct client in proper technique for self-administration of IM or subcutaneous injection.
▪ Monitor vital signs. (Loss of vascular tone leading to extravasation of plasma proteins and fluids into extravascular spaces may cause hypotension and dysrhythmias.)	Instruct client to: ▪ Monitor blood pressure and pulse every day and report any reading outside normal limits. ▪ Report any palpitations immediately.
▪ Monitor for common side effects such as muscle aches, fever, weight loss, anorexia, nausea or vomiting, and arthralgia. (Monitoring provides data for possible medical intervention.)	Instruct client to: ▪ Take medication at bedtime to reduce side effects. ▪ Perform frequent mouth care and eat small frequent meals to reduce gastrointestinal disturbances. ▪ Take acetaminophen for flulike symptoms.
▪ Monitor blood glucose levels. (Blood glucose may increase in clients with pancreatitis.)	▪ Instruct client to have blood glucose level checked at regular intervals.
▪ Monitor for changes in mental status such as depression, confusion, fatigue, visual disturbances, or numbness. (Alfa interferons cause or aggravate neuropsychiatric disorders.)	▪ Instruct client to report any mental changes, particularly depression or thoughts of suicide.

Evaluation of Outcome Criteria

Evaluate the effectiveness of drug therapy by confirming that client goals and expected outcomes have been met (see "Planning").
▪ The client's laboratory studies reveal improvement in immune system status.
▪ The client demonstrates an understanding of the drug's action by accurately describing drug side effects and precautions.
▪ The client verbalizes potential side effects that should be reported to the healthcare provider.
▪ The client demonstrates correct procedure for self-administering IM and subcutaneous injections.

∞ *See Table 32.3 for a list of drugs to which these nursing actions apply.*

TABLE 32.4 Immunosuppressants

Drug	Route and Adult Dose (max dose where indicated)	Adverse Effects
ANTIBODIES		
adalimumab (Humira)	Subcutaneous, 40 mg every other wk, or 40 mg/wk if used with methotrexate	*Local reactions at injection site (pain, erythema, myalgia), influenza-like symptoms (malaise, fever, chills), headache, dizziness*
basiliximab (Simulect)	IV; 20 mg times 2 doses (first dose 2 h before surgery; second dose 4 days after transplant)	
daclizumab (Zenapax)	IV; 1 mg/kg start first dose no more than 24 h prior to transplant, then repeat q 14 days for 4 more doses	Anaphylaxis, hypertension, infections (may occur in many different body systems), renal impairment (basiliximab), pulmonary edema (muromonab-CD3 and lymphocyte immune globulin), herpes simplex or cytomegalovirus infections (muromonab-CD3)
infliximab (Remicade)	IV; 3 mg/kg infused over at least 2 h, followed by 2 mg/kg on Weeks 2 and 6, then 2 mg/kg q8wk	
lymphocyte immune globulin (Antithymocyte Globulin)	IV; 10–30 mg/kg/day	
muromonab-CD3 (Orthoclone OKT3)	IV; 5 mg/day administered in <1 min for 10–14 days	
ANTIMETABOLITES AND CYTOTOXIC AGENTS		
anakinra (Kineret)	Subcutaneous; 100 mg/day	*Local reactions at injection site (pain, erythema, myalgia), headache* Infections
azathioprine (Imuran)	PO: 3–5 mg/kg/day initially; may be able to reduce to 1–3 mg/kg/day IV: 3–5 mg/kg/day initially; may be able to reduce to 1–3 mg/kg/day	*Nausea, vomiting, anorexia* Severe nausea and vomiting, bone marrow suppression, thrombocytopenia, infections
cyclophosphamide (Cytoxan) (see page 560 for the Prototype Drug box ∞)	PO; Initial: 1–5 mg/kg/day; Maintenance: 1–5 mg/kg q7–10 days IV; Initial: 40–50 mg/kg in divided doses over 2–5 days up to 100 mg/kg Maintenance: 10–15 mg/kg q7–10 days or 3–5 mg twice weekly	*Nausea, vomiting, anorexia, neutropenia, alopecia* Anaphylaxis, leukopenia, pulmonary emboli, interstitial pulmonary fibrosis, toxic epidermal necrolysis, Stevens–Johnson syndrome, hemorrhagic cystitis
etanercept (Enbrel)	Subcutaneous; 25 mg twice/wk or 0.08 mg/kg or 50 mg once/wk	*Local reactions at injection site (pain, erythema, myalgia), abdominal pain, vomiting, headache* Infections, pancytopenia, MI, heart failure
methotrexate (Amethopterin, Folex, Mexate, Rheumatrex) (see page 562 for the Prototype Drug box ∞)	PO: 15–30 mg/day for 5 days; repeat q12wk for 3 courses IM/IV: 15–30 mg/day for 5 days; repeat q12wk for 3–5 courses	*Headache, glossitis, gingivitis, mild leukopenia, nausea* Ulcerative stomatitis, myelosuppression, aplastic anemia, hepatic cirrhosis, nephrotoxicity, sudden death, pulmonary fibrosis
mycophenolate mofetil (CellCept)	PO/IV; start within 24 h of transplant, 1 g bid in combination with corticosteroids and cyclosporine	*Peripheral edema, diarrhea, headache, tremor, dyspepsia, abdominal pain* UTI, leukopenia, anemia, thrombocytopenia, sepsis, hypertension
sirolimus (Rapamune)	PO; 6-mg loading dose immediately after transplant, then 2 mg/day	*Hypercholesterolemia, rash, arthralgia, diarrhea, nausea, vomiting, asthenia, back pain, weight gain* Hypertension, leukopenia, anemia, thrombocytopenia, sepsis, secondary infections
thalidomide (Thalomid)	PO; 100–300 mg/day (max: 400 mg/day) times at least 2 wk	*Rash, mild leukopenia, fever, dizziness, diarrhea, malaise, drowsiness* Toxic epidermal necrolysis, birth defects (pregnancy category X), orthostatic hypotension

(Continued)

TABLE 32.4 Immunosuppressants *(Continued)*		
Drug	Route and Adult Dose (max dose where indicated)	Adverse Effects
CALCINEURIN INHIBITORS		
cyclosporine (Sandimmune, Neoral)	PO; 250 mg q12h for 2 wk; may increase to 500 mg q12h (max: 1g/day)	*Hirsutism, tremor, vomiting* Hypertension, MI, nephrotoxicity, hyperkalemia
tacrolimus (Prograf)	PO: 0.15–0.3 mg/kg/day in 2 divided doses q12h; start no sooner than 6 h after transplant; give first oral dose 8–12 h after discontinuing IV therapy IV: 0.05–0.1 mg/kg/day as continuous infusion; start no sooner than 6 h after transplant and continue until client can take oral therapy	*Oliguria, nausea, constipation, diarrhea, headache, abdominal pain, insomnia, peripheral edema, fever* Infections, hypertension, nephrotoxicity, neurotoxicity (tremors, paresthesia, psychosis), hyperkalemia, anemia, hyperglycemia
GLUCOCORTICOIDS		
(see Chapter 39 for individual doses ∞)		

Italics indicate common adverse effects; underlining indicates serious adverse effects.

MediaLink   Xenotransplants

specific aspects of the immune response. Obviously, the non-selective agents will provide more widespread immunosuppression, but with greater risk of side effects.

Many of the immunosuppressants are toxic to bone marrow and produce significant adverse effects. Because the immune system is suppressed, infections are common, and the client must be protected from situations in which exposure to pathogens is likely. Prophylactic therapy with anti-infectives may become necessary if immune function becomes excessively suppressed. Certain tumors such as lymphomas occur more frequently in transplant recipients than in the general population.

Immunosuppressants include glucocorticoids, antimetabolites, antibodies, and calcineurin inhibitors. The glucocorticoids are potent inhibitors of inflammation and are discussed in detail in Chapters 33 and 43 ∞. They are often drugs of choice in the short-term therapy of severe inflammation. Antimetabolites such as sirolimus (Rapamune) and azathioprine (Imuran) inhibit aspects of lymphocyte replication. By binding to the intracellular messenger **calcineurin,** cyclosporine (Sandimmune, Neoral) and tacrolimus (Prograf) disrupt T-cell function. The calcineurin inhibitors are of value in treating psoriasis, an inflammatory disorder of the skin (Chapter 48 ∞).

Pr PROTOTYPE DRUG | Cyclosporine *(Sandimmune, Neoral)* | Immunosuppressant

ACTIONS AND USES

Cyclosporine is a complex chemical obtained from a soil fungus. Its primary mechanism of action is to inhibit helper T cells. Unlike some of the more cytotoxic immunosuppressants, cyclosporine is less toxic to bone marrow cells. When prescribed for transplant recipients, it is used primarily in combination with high doses of a glucocorticoid such as prednisone.

ADMINISTRATION ALERTS

- Neoral (microemulsion) and Sandimmune are not bioequivalent and cannot be used interchangeably without healthcare provider supervision.
- Pregnancy category C.

PHARMACOKINETICS (Subcutaneous)

Onset: 7–14 days

Peak: Unknown

Half-life: 4–13 h

Duration: Unknown

ADVERSE EFFECTS

The primary adverse effect of cyclosporine occurs in the kidneys, with up to 75% of clients experiencing reduction in urine flow. Other common side effects are tremor, hypertension, and elevated hepatic enzymes. Although infections are common during cyclosporine therapy, they are fewer than with some of the other immunosuppressants. Periodic blood counts are necessary to ensure that WBCs do not fall below 4,000, or platelets below 75,000.

Contraindications: The only contraindication is prior hypersensitivity to the drug.

INTERACTIONS

Drug–Drug: Drugs that decrease cyclosporine levels include phenytoin, phenobarbital, carbamazepine, and rifampin. Certain antifungal drugs and macrolide antibiotics may increase cyclosporine levels.

Lab Tests: Unknown.

Herbal/Food: Grapefruit juice can raise cyclosporine levels by 50% to 200%. Use with caution with herbal supplements; for example, the immune-stimulating effects of astragalus and echinacea may interfere with immunosuppressants.

Treatment of Overdose: There is no specific treatment for overdose.

 See the Companion Website for a Nursing Process Focus specific to this drug.

NURSING PROCESS FOCUS Clients Receiving Immunosuppressant Therapy

Assessment	Potential Nursing Diagnoses
▪ Obtain a health history including allergies, drug history, and possible drug interactions. ▪ Assess for presence of metastatic cancer, active infection, renal or liver disease, and pregnancy. ▪ Assess skin integrity; specifically look for lesions and skin color. ▪ Obtain results of laboratory work including complete blood count (CBC), electrolytes, and liver enzymes. ▪ Obtain vital signs, especially temperature and blood pressure.	▪ Infection, Risk for, related to depressed immune response secondary to drug ▪ Injury, Risk for, related to thrombocytopenia secondary to drug

Planning: Client Goals and Expected Outcomes

The client will:

▪ Experience no symptoms of organ or allograft rejection.

▪ Immediately report elevated temperature, unusual bleeding, sore throat, mouth ulcers, and fatigue to healthcare provider.

▪ Demonstrate an understanding of the drug's action by accurately describing drug side effects and precautions.

Implementation

Interventions and (Rationales)	Client Education/Discharge Planning
▪ Assess renal function. (Drugs cause nephrotoxicity in many clients because of physiological changes in the kidneys such as microcalcifications and interstitial fibrosis.)	Advise client to: ▪ Keep accurate record of urine output. ▪ Report significant reduction in urine flow.
▪ Monitor liver function tests. (Drugs increase the risk for liver toxicity.)	▪ Instruct client about the importance of regular laboratory testing.
▪ Watch for signs and symptoms of infection, including elevated temperature. (There is an increased risk of infection owing to immune suppression.)	Instruct client to: ▪ Wash hands thoroughly and frequently. ▪ Avoid crowds and people with infection.
▪ Monitor vital signs, especially temperature and blood pressure. (Drugs may cause hypertension, especially in clients with kidney transplants.)	Teach client to: ▪ Monitor blood pressure and temperature, ensuring proper use of home equipment. ▪ Keep all appointments with healthcare provider.
▪ Monitor for hirsutism, leukopenia, gingival hyperplasia, gynecomastia, sinusitis, and hyperkalemia. (These are common side effects.)	Advise client to: ▪ See a dentist on a regular basis. ▪ Comply with regular laboratory assessments (CBC, electrolytes, and hormone levels).
▪ Avoid permitting client to ingest grapefruit juice. (Grapefruit juice increases cyclosporine levels 50% to 200%.)	Instruct client to: ▪ Avoid drinking grapefruit juice. ▪ Take medication with food to decrease GI upset.
▪ Assess nutritional status. (Drugs may cause weight gain.)	▪ Instruct client regarding a healthy diet that avoids excessive fats and sugars.

Evaluation of Outcome Criteria

Evaluate the effectiveness of drug therapy by confirming that client goals and expected outcomes have been met (see "Planning"):

▪ The client is free of signs of infecton or organ rejection.

▪ The client accurately states signs and symptoms to be reported to the healthcare provider.

▪ The client demonstrates an understanding of the drug's action by accurately describing drug side effects and precautions.

∞ *See Table 32.4 for a list of drugs to which these nursing actions apply.*

Recall from Section 32.2 that antibodies are proteins produced by the immune system to defend against microbes. In fact, Section 32.3 discussed how infusion of antibodies can provide passive immunity. It may seem puzzling, then, to learn that certain antibodies may be administered to clients to *suppress* the immune response. How is this possible?

When animals such as mice are injected with human T cells or T-cell protein receptors, the animal recognizes these as foreign and produces antibodies against the human T cells. When purified and injected into humans, these mouse antibodies will attack T cells (or T-cell receptors). Four of these antibodies are used as immunosuppressants. For example, muromonab-CD3 (Orthoclone OKT3) is administered to prevent rejection of kidney, heart, and liver transplants, and to deplete the bone marrow of T cells prior to marrow transplant. Basiliximab (Simulect) and daclizumab (Zenapax) are given to prevent acute rejection of kidney transplants. Infliximab (Remicade) is used to suppress the severe inflammation that often accompanies autoimmune disorders such as Crohn's disease and rheumatoid arthritis. Note that the suffix "ab" in the generic name refers to antibody. Because some drugs in the monoclonal antibody class are used as antineoplastics, the student should refer to Chapter 37 ∞.

NURSING CONSIDERATIONS

The role of the nurse in immunosuppressant therapy involves careful monitoring of a client's condition and providing education as it relates to the prescribed drug treatment. When providing care for clients taking immunosuppressants, complete a through health assessment, including the presence or history of organ transplant or grafting, and verify the need for these drugs. Immunosuppressants are contraindicated in clients with leukemia, metastatic cancer, active infection, renal or liver disease, or pregnancy. These drugs should be used with caution in clients who have pancreatic or bowel dysfunction, hyperkalemia, hypertension, and infection. Obtain vital signs and results of lab testing, including a complete blood count (CBC), electrolytes, and liver profile, to provide baseline data and reveal any abnormalities.

Many immunosuppressants act on T lymphocytes, suppressing the normal cell-mediated immune reaction. Because of their dampening effect on the immune system, a superimposed infection may occur, causing an increase in white blood cell count. Monitor vital signs, especially temperature, and blood testing for indications of infection. Carefully monitor the degree of bone marrow suppression (thrombocytopenia and leukopenia), because these adverse effects may be life threatening. Monitor clients who are taking azathioprine (Imuran) for the development of secondary malignancies; also inform clients of this possible adverse effect.

Client Teaching. Client education as it relates to immunosuppressant drugs should include the goals of therapy, the reasons for obtaining baseline data such as vital signs and the existence of underlying disorders such as infection and leukopenia, and possible drug side effects. Include the following points when teaching clients about immunosuppressants:

- Avoid exposure to individuals who have infections and other situations in which there is high risk for infection.
- Take any antibiotics prescribed by your physician to prevent infection.
- Immediately report signs of infection.
- Keep all scheduled laboratory visits for hematology studies.
- Practice reliable contraception and notify you healthcare provider if pregnancy is planned or suspected.
- Immediately report alopecia, increased pigmentation, arthralgia, respiratory distress, edema, nausea, vomiting, paresthesia, fever, blood in the urine, black stools, and feelings of sadness.

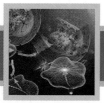

CHAPTER REVIEW

KEY CONCEPTS

The numbered key concepts provide a succinct summary of the important points from the corresponding numbered section within each chapter. If any of these points are not clear, refer to the numbered section within the chapter for review.

32.1 Nonspecific defenses deny entrance of pathogens to the body by providing general responses that are not specific to a particular threat. Specific body defenses are activated by specific antigens, and each is effective against one particular microbe species.

32.2 Antibody-mediated, or humoral, immunity involves the production of antibodies by plasma cells, which neutralize the foreign agent or mark it for destruction by other defense cells.

32.3 Vaccines are biological agents used to prevent illness by boosting antibody production and producing active immunity. Passive immunity is obtained through the administration of antibodies.

32.4 Cell-mediated immunity involves the activation of specific T cells and the secretion of cytokines such as interferons and interleukins that enhance the immune response and rid the body of the foreign agent.

32.5 Immunostimulants are biological response modifiers, including interferons and interleukins, that boost the client's immune system. They are used to treat certain viral infections, immunodeficiencies, and specific cancers.

32.6 Immunosuppressants inhibit the client's immune system and are used to treat severe autoimmune disease and to prevent tissue rejection following organ transplantation.

NCLEX-RN® REVIEW QUESTIONS

1 A 55-year-old female client is receiving cyclosporine (Neoral, Sandimmune) after a heart transplant. The client exhibits a white blood cell count of 12,000 cells/mm³, a sore throat, fatigue, and a low-grade fever. The nurse suspects:

1. Transplant rejection.
2. Heart failure.
3. Dehydration.
4. Infection.

2 Which of the following statements by a client taking cyclosporine (Neoral, Sandimmune) would indicate the need for more teaching by the nurse?

1. "I will report any reduction in urine output to my physician."
2. "I will wash my hands frequently."
3. "I will take my blood pressure at home every day."
4. "I will take my cyclosporine at breakfast with a glass of grapefruit juice."

3 The nurse should monitor a transplant client for the major adverse effect of cyclosporine (Neoral, Sandimmune) therapy by assessing which lab test?

1. CBC
2. Serum creatinine
3. Liver enzymes
4. Electrolytes

4 The nurse would question an order for immunostimulant therapy if the client had which of the following conditions? (Select all that apply.)

1. Pregnancy
2. Renal disease
3. Infection
4. Liver disease
5. Metastatic cancer

5 The type of immunity achieved through the administration of a vaccine is called:

1. Active immunity.
2. Passive immunity.
3. Titer.
4. Vaccine.

CRITICAL THINKING QUESTIONS

1. A client is taking sirolimus (Rapamune) following a liver transplant. On the most recent CBC, the nurse notes a marked 50% decrease in platelets and leukocytes. During the physical assessment, what signs and symptoms should the nurse look for? What are appropriate nursing interventions?

2. A client has been exposed to hepatitis A and has been referred for an injection of gamma globulin. The client is hesitant to get a "shot" and says that his immune system is fine. How should the nurse respond?

3. A client had a renal transplant 6 months ago and is taking cyclosporine (Neoral, Sandimmune) daily. Identify three precautions that the nurse should be aware of when caring for this client.

See Appendix D for answers and rationales for all activities.

EXPLORE
MediaLink

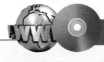
www.prenhall.com/adams

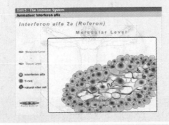

NCLEX-RN® review, case studies, and other interactive resources for this chapter can be found on the companion website at www.prenhall.com/adams. Click on "Chapter 32" to select the activities for this chapter. For animations, more NCLEX-RN® review questions, and an audio glossary, access the accompanying Prentice Hall Nursing MediaLink DVD-ROM in this textbook.

PRENTICE HALL NURSING MEDIALINK DVD-ROM

- **Animation**
  Mechanism in Action: Interferon alfa-2A (*Roferon-A*)
- **Audio Glossary**
- **NCLEX-RN® Review**

 COMPANION WEBSITE

- **NCLEX-RN® Review**
- **Dosage Calculations**
- **Case Study:** Client taking immunostimulants
- **Care Plan:** Client with chronic hepatitis B treated with interferon alfa-2a

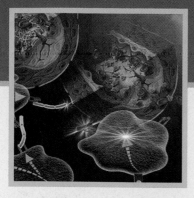

CHAPTER 33

Drugs for Inflammation and Fever

DRUGS AT A GLANCE

ANTI-INFLAMMATORY DRUGS

Nonsteroidal Anti-inflammatory Drugs (NSAIDs)

ibuprofen (Advil, Motrin, others)

Systemic Glucocorticoids

prednisone (Meticorten, others)

ANTIPYRETICS

acetaminophen (Tylenol)

OBJECTIVES

After reading this chapter, the student should be able to:

1. Identify common signs and symptoms of inflammation.
2. Outline the basic steps in the acute inflammatory response.
3. Explain the role of histamine in the inflammatory response.
4. Compare and contrast the actions and side effects of the nonsteroidal anti-inflammatory drugs (NSAIDs): aspirin, ibuprofen, and celecoxib.
5. Explain the role of systemic glucocorticoids in the pharmacological management of inflammation.
6. Describe the nurse's role in the pharmacological management of inflammation and fever.
7. For each of the classes listed in Drugs at a Glance, know representative drugs, and explain their mechanisms of drug action, primary actions related to inflammation, and/or allergies and important adverse effects.
8. Categorize drugs used in the treatment of inflammation and fever based on their classification and mechanism of action.
9. Use the Nursing Process to care for clients receiving drug therapy for inflammation and fever.

MediaLink

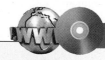

www.prenhall.com/adams

KEY TERMS

anaphylaxis *page 473*

antipyretic *page 478*

Cushing's syndrome *page 477*

cyclooxygenase (COX-1 and COX-2) *page 474*

H₁ receptor *page 473*

H₂ receptor *page 473*

histamine *page 472*

inflammation *page 471*

mast cell *page 472*

prostaglandins *page 474*

Reye's syndrome *page 475*

salicylism *page 474*

The pain and redness of inflammation following minor abrasions and cuts is something everyone has experienced. Although there is discomfort from such scrapes, inflammation is a normal and expected part of our body's defense against injury. For some diseases, however, inflammation can rage out of control, producing severe pain, fever, and other distressing symptoms. It is these sorts of conditions in which pharmacotherapy may be needed.

INFLAMMATION

Inflammation is a nonspecific defense system of the body. Through the process of inflammation a large number of potentially damaging chemicals and microorganisms may be neutralized.

33.1 The Function of Inflammation

The human body has developed many complex ways to defend against injury and invasion by microorganisms. Inflammation is one of these defense mechanisms. **Inflammation** occurs in response to many different stimuli, including physical injury, exposure to toxic chemicals, extreme heat, invading microorganisms, or death of cells. It is considered a *nonspecific* defense mechanism because inflammation proceeds in the same manner, regardless of the cause. The *specific* immune defenses of the body were presented in Chapter 32 ∞.

The central purpose of inflammation is to contain the injury or destroy the microorganism. By neutralizing the foreign agent and removing cellular debris and dead cells, repair of the injured area can proceed at a faster pace. Signs of inflammation include swelling, pain, warmth, and redness of the affected area.

Inflammation may be classified as *acute* or *chronic*. During acute inflammation, such as that caused by minor physical injury, 8 to 10 days are normally needed for the symptoms to resolve and for repair to begin. If the body cannot contain or neutralize the damaging agent, inflammation may continue for long periods and become chronic. In chronic autoimmune disorders such as lupus and rheumatoid arthritis, inflammation may persist for years, with symptoms becoming progressively worse over time. Other disorders such as seasonal allergy arise at predictable times during each year, and inflammation may produce only minor, annoying symptoms.

The pharmacotherapy of inflammation includes drugs that decrease the natural inflammatory response. Most anti-inflammatory drugs are nonspecific; that is, whether the cause of the inflammation is injury, autoimmune disease, or allergy, the drug will exhibit the same inhibitory actions. A few anti-inflammatory drugs are specific to certain diseases, such as those used to treat gout (Chapter 47 ∞). Following are some common diseases that have an inflammatory component that may benefit from anti-inflammatory pharmacotherapy:

- Allergic rhinitis
- Anaphylaxis

PHARMFACTS

Inflammatory Disorders

- Arthritis, the most common inflammatory disorder, is the leading cause of disability in the United States.
- Inflammatory bowel disease affects 300,000 to 500,000 Americans each year.
- More than 80 million prescriptions are written for NSAIDs each year, accounting for about 4.5% of all prescriptions written in the United States.
- More than 1% of the U.S. population uses NSAIDs on a daily basis.
- Worldwide, more than 30 million people consume NSAIDs daily, and of these, 40% are older than 60 years.

TABLE 33.1	Chemical Mediators of Inflammation
Mediator	**Description**
bradykinin	present in an inactive form in plasma and mast cells; vasodilator that causes pain; effects are similar to those of histamine
complement	series of at least 20 proteins that combine in a cascade fashion to neutralize or destroy an antigen
histamine	stored and released by mast cells; causes dilation of blood vessels, smooth-muscle constriction, tissue swelling, and itching
leukotrienes	stored and released by mast cells; effects are similar to those of histamine
prostaglandins	present in most tissues and stored and released by mast cells; increase capillary permeability, attract white blood cells to site of inflammation, and cause pain

- Ankylosing spondylitis
- Contact dermatitis
- Crohn's disease
- Glomerulonephritis
- Hashimoto's thyroiditis
- Peptic ulcers
- Rheumatoid arthritis
- Systemic lupus erythematosus
- Ulcerative colitis

33.2 The Role of Histamine in Inflammation

Whether the injury is due to pathogens, chemicals, or physical trauma, the damaged tissue releases a number of chemical mediators that act as "alarms" to notify the surrounding area of the injury. Chemical mediators of inflammation include histamine, leukotrienes, bradykinin, complement, and prostaglandins. Table 33.1 lists the sources and actions of these mediators.

Histamine is a key chemical mediator of inflammation. It is stored primarily within **mast cells** located in tissue spaces under epithelial membranes such as the skin, bronchial tree, digestive tract, and along blood vessels. Mast cells detect foreign agents or injury and respond by releasing histamine, which initiates the inflammatory response within seconds. In addition to its role in inflammation, histamine also directly stimulates pain receptors, and is a primary agent responsible for the symptoms of seasonal allergies (Chapter 38 ∞).

When released at an injury site, histamine dilates nearby blood vessels, causing capillaries to become more permeable. Plasma, complement proteins, and phagocytes can then enter the area to neutralize foreign agents. The affected area may become congested with blood, which can lead to significant swelling and pain. ● Figure 33.1 illustrates the fundamental steps in acute inflammation.

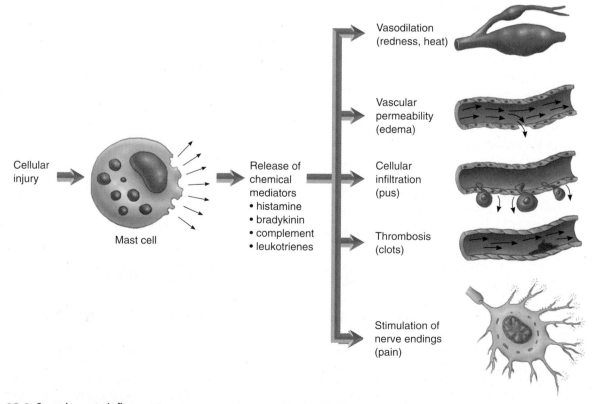

● **Figure 33.1** Steps in acute inflammation *Source: Pearson Education/PM College.*

TABLE 33.2 Selected Nonsteroidal Anti-inflammatory Drugs

Drug	Route and Adult Dose (max dose where indicated)	Adverse Effects
aspirin (ASA and others) (see page 235 for the Prototype Drug box ∞)	PO; 350–650 mg q4h (max: 4 g/day)	*Abdominal cramps, heartburn, nausea, vomiting, tinnitus* GI bleeding, bronchospasm, anaphylaxis, hemolytic anemia, Reye's syndrome in children
SELECTIVE COX-2 INHIBITOR		
celecoxib (Celebrex)	PO; 100–200 mg bid (max: 400 mg/day)	*Diarrhea, dyspepsia, headache, pharyngitis* No serious adverse effects, but cardiovascular risk is being investigated
IBUPROFEN AND SIMILAR AGENTS		
diclofenac (Voltaren, Cataflam)	PO; 50 mg bid–qid (max: 200 mg/day)	*Nausea, diarrhea, vomiting, abdominal cramping, dyspepsia, dizziness* Renal failure, GI bleeding, anaphylaxis, metabolic acidosis, hepatic impairment
diflunisal (Dolobid)	PO; 250–500 mg bid (max: 1,500 mg/day)	
etodolac (Lodine)	PO; 200–400 mg tid–qid (max: 1,200 mg/day)	
fenoprofen (Nalfon)	PO; 300–600 mg tid–qid (max: 3,200 mg/day)	
flurbiprofen (Ansaid)	PO; 50–100 mg tid–qid (max: 300 mg/day)	
ibuprofen (Motrin, Advil, others)	PO; 400–800 mg tid–qid (max: 3,200 mg/day)	
indomethacin (Indocin)	PO; 25–50 mg bid or tid (max: 200 mg/day) or 75 mg sustained-release 1–2 times/day	
ketoprofen (Actron, Orudis, Oruvail)	PO; 75 mg tid or 50 mg qid (max: 300 mg/day)	
meloxicam (Mobic)	PO; 7.5–15 mg once daily	
nabumetone (Relafen)	PO; 1,000 mg/day (max: 2,000 mg/day)	
naproxen (Naprosyn, others)	PO; 250–500 mg bid (max: 1,000 mg/day)	
naproxen sodium (Aleve, Anaprox, others)	PO; 275 mg bid (max: 1,100 mg/day)	
oxaprozin (Daypro)	PO; 600–1,200 mg/day (max: 1,800 mg/day)	
piroxicam (Feldene)	PO; 10–20 mg 1–2 times/day (max: 20 mg/day)	
tolmetin (Tolectin)	PO; 400 mg tid (max: 2 g/day)	

Italics indicate common adverse effects; underlining indicates serious adverse effects.

Rapid release of the chemical mediators of inflammation on a large scale throughout the body is responsible for **anaphylaxis,** a life-threatening allergic response that may result in shock and death. A number of chemicals, insect stings, foods, and some therapeutic drugs can cause this widespread release of histamine from mast cells if the person has an allergy to these substances. The pharmacotherapy of anaphylaxis was presented in Chapter 29 ∞.

33.3 Histamine Receptors

There are two different receptors with which histamine interacts to elicit a response. **H₁-receptors** are present in the smooth muscle of the vascular system, the bronchial tree, and the digestive tract. Stimulation of these receptors results in itching, pain, edema, vasodilation, bronchoconstriction, and the characteristic symptoms of inflammation and allergy. In contrast, **H₂-receptors** are present primarily in the stomach, and their stimulation results in the secretion of large amounts of hydrochloric acid.

Drugs that act as specific antagonists for H_1 and H_2 receptors are in widespread therapeutic use. H_1-receptor antagonists, used to treat allergies and inflammation, are discussed in Chapter 38 ∞. H_2-receptor antagonists are used to treat peptic ulcers and are discussed in Chapter 40 ∞.

NONSTEROIDAL ANTI-INFLAMMATORY DRUGS

Nonsteroidal anti-inflammatory drugs (NSAIDs) such as aspirin and ibuprofen have analgesic, antipyretic, and anti-inflammatory properties. They are widely prescribed for mild to moderate inflammation. These agents are listed in Table 33.2.

33.4 Treating Inflammation With NSAIDs

Because of their high safety margin and availability as over-the-counter (OTC) drugs, the NSAIDs are drugs of choice for the treatment of mild to moderate inflammation. The NSAID class includes some of the most commonly used drugs in medicine, including aspirin, ibuprofen, and the newer COX-2 inhibitors. All NSAIDs have approximately the same efficacy, although the side-effect profiles vary among the different drugs. The NSAIDs also exhibit analgesic and antipyretic actions. Although acetaminophen shares the analgesic and antipyretic properties of these other drugs, it has no anti-inflammatory action and is not classified as an NSAID.

NSAIDs act by inhibiting the synthesis of prostaglandins. **Prostaglandins** are lipids found in all tissues that have potent physiological effects, in addition to promoting inflammation, depending on the tissue in which they are found. The NSAIDs block inflammation by inhibiting **cyclooxygenase (COX),** the key enzyme in the biosynthesis of prostaglandins.

There are two forms of COX, cyclooxygenase-1 (COX-1) and cyclooxygenase-2 (COX-2). COX-1 is present is all tissues and serves *protective* functions such as reducing gastric acid secretion, promoting renal blood flow, and regulating smooth muscle tone in blood vessels and the bronchial tree. COX-2, on the other hand, is present only after tissue injury and serves to promote inflammation. Thus, two nearly identical enzymes serve very different functions. The two forms of cyclooxygenase are compared in Table 33.3.

First-generation NSAIDs such as aspirin and ibuprofen block both COX-1 and COX-2. Although this inhibition reduces inflammation, the inhibition of COX-1 results in *undesirable* effects such as bleeding, gastric upset, and reduced kidney function. Most of the side effects of aspirin and ibuprofen are due to inhibition of COX-1, the protective form of the enzyme.

Aspirin binds to both COX-1 and COX-2 enzymes, changing their structures and preventing them from forming inflammatory prostaglandins. This inhibition of cyclooxygenase is particularly prolonged in platelets, where a single dose of aspirin may cause total inhibition for the entire 8- to 11-day lifespan of the platelet. Because it is readily available, inexpensive, and efficacious, aspirin is often a drug of choice for treating mild inflammation. Aspirin also has a protective effect on the cardiovascular system and is taken daily in small doses by millions of clients to prevent abnormal clot formation and strokes. The fundamental pharmacology and a drug prototype for aspirin are presented in Chapter 18 ∞.

Unfortunately, the large doses of aspirin that are needed to suppress severe inflammation may result in a high incidence of adverse effects, especially on the digestive system. By increasing gastric acid secretion and irritating the stomach lining, aspirin may cause epigastric pain, heartburn, and even bleeding due to ulceration. Some aspirin formulations are buffered or given an enteric coating to minimize GI side effects. Because aspirin also has a potent anticoagulant effect, the potential for bleeding must be carefully monitored. High doses may produce **salicylism,** a syndrome that includes symptoms such as tinnitus (ringing in the ears), dizziness, headache, and excessive sweating.

Ibuprofen (Motrin, Advil) and a large number of ibuprofen-like drugs are first-generation NSAIDs developed as alternatives to aspirin. Like aspirin, they exhibit their effects through inhibition of both COX-1 and COX-2, although the inhibition by these drugs is reversible. Sharing the same mechanism of action, all drugs in this class have similar efficacy for treating pain, fever, and inflammation. For some clients, the choice of NSAID is based on cost and availability: aspirin, ibuprofen, and naproxen (Aleve) are the only NSAIDs sold over the counter. NSAIDs differ in their duration of action, which may be important when clients are taking these drugs on an ongoing basis. Although drugs in this class have similar *overall* efficacy, there is variability in response to NSAIDs, with some clients responding better to a particular drug. The choice of prescription NSAID is often based on the personal experiences and preference of the prescriber.

Most ibuprofen-like NSAIDs share a low incidence of adverse effects. The most common side effects are nausea and vomiting. These agents have the potential to cause gastric ulceration and bleeding; however, the incidence is less than that of aspirin. Kidney toxicity is possible, and renal assessments should be conducted periodically. Clients with significant preexisting renal impairment usually receive acetaminophen for pain or fever, rather than an NSAID. Ibuprofen-like NSAIDs affect platelet function and increase the potential for bleeding, although this risk is lower than from aspirin.

The newest, and most controversial, class of NSAIDs selectively inhibits COX-2. Inhibition of COX-2 produces the analgesic, anti-inflammatory, and antipyretic effects without causing most of the serious adverse effects of the older NSAIDs. Because they do not inhibit COX-1, these drugs do not produce adverse effects on the digestive system, as aspirin does. Because of their low GI toxicity and lack of effect on blood coagulation, selective COX-2 inhibitors quickly became the treatment of choice for moderate to severe inflammation.

However, in 2004, postmarketing data revealed that rofecoxib (Vioxx) doubled the risk of heart attack and stroke in

TABLE 33.3	**Forms of Cyclooxygenase**	
	Cyclooxygenase-1	Cyclooxygenase-2
location	present in all tissues	present at sites of tissue injury
functions	protects gastric mucosa, supports kidney function, promotes platelet aggregation	mediates inflammation, sensitizes pain receptors, mediates fever in the brain
inhibition by medications	undesirable: increases risk of gastric bleeding and kidney failure	desirable: results in suppression of inflammation

Pr PROTOTYPE DRUG | Ibuprofen *(Motrin, Advil)* | Nonsteroidal Anti-inflammatory Drug

ACTIONS AND USES

Ibuprofen is an older drug with an efficacy at relieving pain, fever, and inflammation similar to that of other NSAIDs. Its actions are due to inhibition of prostaglandin synthesis. Common indications include musculoskeletal disorders such as rheumatoid and osteoarthritis, mild to moderate pain, reduction of fever, and primary dysmenorrhea. It is available as tablets and as oral suspension for children.

ADMINISTRATION ALERTS

- Give drug on an empty stomach as tolerated. If nausea, vomiting, or abdominal pain occurs, give with food.
- Pregnancy category B.

PHARMACOKINETICS

Onset: 30–60 min

Peak: 1–2 h

Half-life: 2–4 h

Duration: 4–6 h

ADVERSE EFFECTS

Side effects of ibuprofen are generally mild and include nausea, heartburn, epigastric pain, and dizziness. GI ulceration with occult or gross bleeding may occur, especially in clients taking high doses for prolonged periods. Clients with active peptic ulcers should not take ibuprofen.

Contraindications: This drug is contraindicated in clients with significant renal or hepatic impairment and in those who have a syndrome of nasal polyps, angioedema, or bronchospasm due to aspirin or other NSAID use.

INTERACTIONS

Drug-Drug: Because ibuprofen can affect platelet function, its use should be avoided when taking anticoagulants. Aspirin use can decrease the anti-inflammatory action of ibuprofen. Ibuprofen may increase plasma levels of lithium, causing lithium toxicity. The actions of certain diuretics may be diminished when taken concurrently with ibuprofen.

Lab Tests: May increase bleeding time.

Herbal/Food: Feverfew, garlic, ginger, or ginkgo may increase the risk of bleeding.

Treatment of Overdose: There is no specific treatment for overdose. Administration of an alkaline drug may increase the urinary excretion of ibuprofen.

See the Companion Website for a Nursing Process Focus specific to this drug.

clients taking the drug for extended periods. At that time, more than 84 million people had used rofecoxib since its approval in 1999. Based on the data, the drug manufacturer voluntarily removed the drug from the market. Shortly afterward, a second COX-2 inhibitor, valdecoxib (Bextra) was also voluntarily withdrawn, leaving celecoxib (Celebrex) the sole drug in this class. Other selective COX-2 inhibitors are still available outside the United States. In addition to its anti-inflammatory indications, celecoxib also is used to reduce the number of c.olorectal polyps in adults with familial adenomatous polyposis (FAP). Clients with FAP have an inherited mutation in a gene that results in hundreds of polyps and an almost 100% risk of colon cancer.

NURSING CONSIDERATIONS

The role of the nurse in NSAID therapy involves careful monitoring a client's condition and providing education as it relates to the prescribed drug treatment. The group of drugs known as NSAIDs may be used for their analgesic, antipyretic, or anti-inflammatory properties. The primary uses are for rheumatoid and osteoarthritis, pain, and dysmenorrhea. NSAIDs are primarily metabolized by the liver; therefore, they should not be given to clients with liver dysfunction because, doing so could lead to toxic levels of metabolites that could cause hepatic failure. Assess clients for bleeding disorders, peptic ulcer disease, congestive heart failure, fluid retention, hypertension, renal disease, and use of diuretics, lithium, anticoagulants, herbal

supplements, alcohol, and cigarettes. NSAIDs may be contraindicated in these clients.

Prior to initiation of NSAID therapy, obtain baseline kidney and liver function tests and a CBC. Monitor bleeding time with long-term administration. Assess for changes in pain (intensity, frequency, and type) and reduction in temperature and inflammation to determine effectiveness. Assess for gastrointestinal bleeding, hepatitis, nephrotoxicity, hemolytic anemia, and salicylate toxicity. Other common side effects may include tinnitus, abdominal cramping, and heartburn. Hypersensitivity to NSAIDs may be exhibited as a rash or bronchospasm in asthmatic clients with nasal polyps.

Lifespan Considerations.   Use NSAIDs cautiously in elderly clients because of the potential for increased bleeding. Use may be cautioned in pregnancy and lactation, depending on the specific drug. Use ibuprofen with caution in infants younger than 6 months, and naproxen with caution in children younger than 2 years. Aspirin is generally contraindicated in pediatric clients younger than age 18. This is especially critical if the child has varicella or influenza infections because of the possibility of developing **Reye's syndrome.** Reye's syndrome is a rare, though serious, disorder characterized by an acute increase in intracranial pressure and massive accumulations of lipids in the liver.

Client Teaching.   Client education as it relates to NSAID therapy should include the goals of therapy, the reasons for obtaining baseline data such as vital signs and the existence of underlying liver disorders, and possible drug side effects.

TABLE 33.4	Selected Glucocorticoids for Severe Inflammation	
Drug	**Route and Adult Dose (max dose where indicated)**	**Adverse Effects**
betamethasone (Celestone, Betacort, others)	PO; 0.6–7.2 mg/day	*Mood swings, weight gain, acne, facial flushing, nausea, insomnia, sodium and fluid retention, impaired wound healing, menstrual abnormalities*
cortisone (Cortistan, Cortone)	PO; 20–300 mg/day in divided doses	
dexamethasone (Decadron, others)	PO; 0.25–4 mg bid–qid	
hydrocortisone (Cortef, others) (see page 676 for the Prototype Drug box ∞)	PO; 10–320 mg/day in 3–4 divided doses; IV/IM; 15–800 mg/day in 3–4 divided doses (max: 2 g/day)	Peptic ulcer, hypocalcemia, osteoporosis with possible bone fractures, loss of muscle mass, decreased growth in children, possible masking of infections
methylprednisolone (Depo-Medrol, Medrol, others)	PO; 2–60 mg/day in divided doses	
prednisolone (Delta-Cortef, Hydeltrasol, Key-Pred, others)	PO; 5–60 mg 1–4 times/day	
prednisone (Meticorten, others)	PO; 5–60 mg 1–4 times/day	
triamcinolone (Aristocort, Atolone, Kenacort, Kenalog)	PO; 4–48 mg 1–4 times/day	

Italics indicate common adverse effects; <u>underlining</u> indicates serious adverse effects.

Include the following points when teaching clients about NSAIDs:

- Take NSAIDs with food or milk to decrease gastric upset.
- Read labels of OTC drugs carefully, because many contain aspirin or other salicylates (for example: Excedrin and Pepto-Bismol).
- Avoid alcohol use.
- Report signs of bleeding such as prolonged bleeding from an injury, gingival bleeding, dark stools or urine, and an increase in severity or frequency of bruising.
- Do not take aspirin and other NSAIDs together, because the NSAID effect may be decreased.
- Optimal effects from NSAID therapy may not be experienced for 1 to 3 weeks.

See "Nursing Process Focus: Clients Receiving NSAID Therapy," page 236 in Chapter 18 ∞ for additional teaching points.

NATURAL THERAPIES

Fish Oils for Inflammation

Fish oils, also known as marine oils, are lipids found primarily in coldwater fish. These oils are rich sources of long-chain polyunsaturated fatty acids of the omega-3 type. The two most studied fatty acids found in fish oils are EPA (eicosapentaenoic acid) and DHA (docosahexaenoic acid). These fatty acids are known for their triglyceride-lowering activity, and they also have anti-inflammatory actions (Oh, 2005).

Several mechanisms are believed to account for the anti-inflammatory activity of EPA and DHA. The two competitively inhibit the conversion of arachidonic acid to the proinflammatory prostaglandins, thus reducing their synthesis.

Interactions may occur between fish oil supplements and aspirin and other NSAIDs. Although rare, such interactions might be manifested by increased susceptibility to bruising, nosebleeds, hemoptysis, hematuria, and blood in the stool.

SYSTEMIC GLUCOCORTICOIDS (CORTICOSTEROIDS)

Glucocorticoids have wide therapeutic application. One of their most useful properties is a potent anti-inflammatory action that can suppress severe cases of inflammation. Because of potentially serious adverse effects, however, systemic glucocorticoids are reserved for the short-term treatment of severe disease. These agents are listed in Table 33.4.

33.5 Treating Acute or Severe Inflammation With Systemic Glucocorticoids

Glucocorticoids are natural hormones released by the adrenal cortex that have powerful effects on nearly every cell in the body. When used as drugs to treat inflammatory disorders, the doses are many times higher than the amount naturally present in the blood. The uses of glucocorticoids include the treatment of neoplasia (Chapter 37 ∞), asthma (Chapter 39 ∞), arthritis (Chapter 47 ∞), and corticosteroid deficiency (Chapter 43 ∞).

Like the NSAIDs, glucocorticoids inhibit the biosynthesis of prostaglandins. Glucocorticoids, however, affect inflammation by additional mechanisms. They have the ability to suppress histamine release and can inhibit certain functions of phagocytes and lymphocytes. These multiple actions markedly reduce inflammation, making glucocorticoids the most efficacious medications available for the treatment of severe inflammatory disorders.

When given by the oral or parenteral routes, glucocorticoids have a number of serious adverse effects that limit their therapeutic utility. These include suppression of the normal functions of the adrenal gland (adrenal insufficiency), hyperglycemia, mood changes, cataracts, peptic ulcers, electrolyte imbalances, and osteoporosis. Because of their effectiveness at reducing the signs and symptoms of inflammation,

Pr PROTOTYPE DRUG | Prednisone *(Meticorten, Others)* | Anti-inflammatory Agent/Glucocorticoid

ACTIONS AND USES

Prednisone is a synthetic glucocorticoid. Its actions are the result of being metabolized to an active form, which is also available as a drug called prednisolone (Delta-Cortef, others). When used for inflammation, duration of therapy is commonly 4 to 10 days. For long-term therapy, alternate-day dosing is used. Prednisone is occasionally used to terminate acute bronchospasm in clients with asthma and as an antineoplastic agent for clients with certain cancers such as Hodgkin's disease, acute leukemia, and lymphomas.

ADMINISTRATION ALERTS

- Administer IM injections deep into the muscle mass to avoid atrophy or abscesses.
- Do not use if signs of a systemic infection are present.
- Do not discontinue drug abruptly.
- Pregnancy category C.

PHARMACOKINETICS

Onset: Unknown

Peak: 1–2 h

Half-life: 3.5 h

Duration: 24–36 h

ADVERSE EFFECTS

When used for short-term therapy, prednisone has few serious adverse effects. Long-term therapy may result in Cushing's syndrome, a condition that includes hyperglycemia, fat redistribution to the shoulders and face, muscle weakness, bruising, and bones that easily fracture. Because gastric ulcers may occur with long-term therapy, an antiulcer medication may be prescribed prophylactically. Use with caution in clients with peptic ulcer, ulcerative colitis, or diverticulitis.

Contraindications: Clients with active viral, bacterial, fungal, or protozoan infections should not take prednisone.

INTERACTIONS

Drug–Drug: Because barbiturates, phenytoin, and rifampin increase prednisone metabolism, increased doses may be required. Concurrent use with amphotericin B or diuretics increases potassium loss, which may be serious for clients taking digoxin. Because prednisone can raise blood glucose levels, diabetic clients may require an adjustment in insulin dose.

Lab Tests: Prednisone may inhibit antibody response to toxoids and vaccines and may increase blood glucose. Serum calcium, potassium, and thyroxine may decrease.

Herbal/Food: Herbal supplements such as aloe, buckthorn, and senna may increase potassium loss. Licorice may potentiate the effect of glucocorticoids.

Treatment of Overdose: There is no specific treatment for overdose.

 See the Companion Website for a Nursing Process Focus specific to this drug.

glucocorticoids can mask infections that may be present in the client. This combination of masking signs of infection and suppressing the immune response creates a potential for existing infections to grow rapidly and undetected. An active infection is usually a contraindication for glucocorticoid therapy.

Because the appearance of these adverse effects is a function of the dose and duration of therapy, treatment is often limited to the short-term control of acute disease. When longer therapy is indicated, doses are kept as low as possible and alternate-day therapy is sometimes implemented; the medication is taken every other day to encourage the client's adrenal gland to function on the days when no drug is given. During long-term therapy, the nurse must be alert for signs of excess glucocorticoids, a condition known as **Cushing's syndrome.** Because the body becomes accustomed to high doses of glucocorticoids, clients must discontinue these drugs gradually; abrupt withdrawal can result in acute lack of adrenal function.

NURSING CONSIDERATIONS

The role of the nurse in glucocorticoid therapy for inflammation involves careful monitoring of a client's condition and providing education as it relates to the prescribed drug treatment. Systemic glucocorticoids are primarily used on a short-term basis for the treatment of severe inflammation.

Glucocorticoids are contraindicated in clients with systemic fungal infections. Use glucocorticoids with great caution in clients who are immunocompromised, for instance, those with cancer, HIV, or tuberculosis. These clients are prone to infection, and use of these drugs may mask the early signs of infection. Keep in mind that these clients may have a systemic infection by the time it is determined that they have acquired another illness. Prior to administration of these drus, assess clients for current drug therapy, gastrointestinal ulcers, renal disease, hypertension, osteoporosis, varicella, diabetes mellitus, heart failure, and mental instability. Use cautiously in such clients.

Systemic glucocorticoids interact with many other drugs. For long-term use (longer than 1 month), an alternate-day therapy plan may be advised. Adverse effects may include Cushing's syndrome (adrenocortical excess). Signs include moon face, protruding abdomen, atrophied extremities, hirsutism, and acne. Other adverse effects may include severe depression, increased serum glucose levels, increased sodium and water retention, increased potassium secretion, and suppression of signs and symptoms of infection. Other effects may include mental status changes, impaired wound healing, increased susceptibility to fractures, weight gain, and exacerbation of symptoms of myasthenia gravis. Use of these drugs increases the risk of respiratory failure and may trigger mania in bipolar clients. Monitor the client for serum glucose levels, body weight, blood pressure, CBC, and electrolytes (especially sodium and potassium). A therapeutic response when used for asthma may be ease of respirations (decreased rate and effort) and clear lung sounds. A decrease in inflammation also indicates therapeutic response.

Lifespan Considerations. Use cautiously in pregnant or lactating women. In general, systemic glucocorticoids are not recommended for use in children younger than 2 years old.

Client Teaching. Client education as it relates to systemic glucocorticoids should include the goals of therapy, the reasons for obtaining baseline data such as vital signs and the existence of underlying infections, and possible drug side effects. Include the following points when teaching clients about glucocorticoids:

- Take with food or milk to decrease the risk of gastric ulcers.
- Take medication at the same time each day.
- Do not stop taking the drug suddenly, because adrenal crisis may occur.
- Avoid others who have active infections, and report symptoms of infection, such as sore throat, fever, or cough.
- Avoid use of alcohol, cigarettes, caffeine, or aspirin.
- Immediately report difficulty breathing; heartburn; chest, abdominal, or joint and bone pain; nose bleed; bloody cough, vomitus, urine, or stools; fever; chills; red streaks from wounds or any other sign of infection; increased thirst or urination; fruity breath odor (or significantly elevated daily serum glucose); falls or other accidents (deep lacerations may require antibiotic therapy); and mood swings.

See "Nursing Process Focus: Clients Receiving Systemic Glucocorticoid Therapy," page 676 in Chapter 43 ∞, for additional teaching points.

FEVER

Like inflammation, fever is a natural defense mechanism for neutralizing foreign organisms. Many species of bacteria are killed by high fever. Often, the healthcare provider must determine whether the fever needs to be dealt with aggressively or allowed to run its course. Drugs used to treat fever are called **antipyretics.**

33.6 Treating Fever With Antipyretics

In most clients, fever is more of a discomfort than a life-threatening problem. Prolonged, high fever, however, can become dangerous, especially in young children in whom fever can stimulate febrile seizures. In adults, excessively high fever can break down body tissues, reduce mental acuity, and lead to delirium or coma, particularly among elderly clients. In rare instances, an elevated body temperature may be fatal.

The goal of antipyretic therapy is to lower body temperature while treating the underlying cause of the fever, usually an infection. Aspirin, ibuprofen, and acetaminophen

are safe, inexpensive, and effective drugs for reducing fever. Many of these drugs are marketed for different age groups, including special, flavored brands for infants and children. For fast delivery and effectiveness, drugs may come in various forms including gels, caplets, enteric-coated tablets, and suspensions. Aspirin and acetaminophen are also available as suppositories. The antipyretics come in various dosages and concentrations, including extra strength.

Although most fevers are caused by infectious processes, drugs themselves may be the cause. When the etiology of fever cannot be diagnosed, the nurse should consider drugs as a possible source. In many cases, withdrawal of the agent causing the drug-induced fever will quickly return body temperature to normal. In rare cases, drug-induced fever may be lethal. It is important for the nurse to recognize drugs that are most likely to cause drug-induced fever, including those in the following list:

- *Anti-infectives:* Anti-infectives, especially those derived from microorganisms such as amphotericin B or penicillin G, may be seen as foreign by the body and produce fever. When antibiotics kill microorganisms, fever-producing chemicals known as *pyrogens* may be released. Anti-infectives are the most common drugs known to induce fever.
- *Selective serotonin reuptake inhibitors (SSRIs):* Use of SSRIs such as paroxetine (Paxil) for depression or other mood disorders can result in a high fever accompanied by serious mental status and cardiovascular changes, known as *serotonin syndrome* (see Chapter 16 ∞).
- *Conventional antipsychotic drugs:* Drugs such as chlorpromazine (Thorazine) may produce an elevated temperature with serious cardiovascular and respiratory distress, called *neuroleptic malignant syndrome (NMS)* (see Chapter 17 ∞).
- *Volatile anesthetics and depolarizing neuromuscular blockers:* Agents such as succinylcholine can cause life-threatening *malignant hyperthermia* (see Chapter 19 ∞).
- *Immunomodulators:* Interferons and monoclonal antibodies such as muromonab-CD3 may cause a flulike syndrome because they cause the release of fever-producing cytokines (see Chapter 32 ∞).
- *Cytotoxic drugs:* Agents such as those used in cancer chemotherapy and to prevent transplant rejection profoundly dampen the immune response and result in fevers due to secondary infections.
- *Neutropenic agents:* Drugs such as NSAIDs, phenothiazines, antithyroid drugs, and antipsychotic agents can cause neutropenia and a subsequent fever.
- *Other drugs:* Systemic hypersensitivity reactions can result in high fever and anaphylaxis.

NURSING CONSIDERATIONS

The role of the nurse in antipyretic therapy for an elevated temperature involves careful monitoring of a client's condition and providing education as it relates to the prescribed

Pr PROTOTYPE DRUG | Acetaminophen *(Tylenol, others)* | Antipyretic/Analgesic

ACTIONS AND USES

Acetaminophen reduces fever by direct action at the level of the hypothalamus and dilation of peripheral blood vessels, which enables sweating and dissipation of heat. Acetaminophen, ibuprofen, and aspirin have equal efficacy in relieving pain and reducing fever.

Acetaminophen has no anti-inflammatory properties; therefore, it is not effective in treating arthritis or pain caused by tissue swelling following injury. The primary therapeutic usefulness of acetaminophen is for the treatment of fever in children and for relief of mild to moderate pain when aspirin is contraindicated. It is available as tablets, caplets, solutions, and suppositories.

ADMINISTRATION ALERT

- Liquid forms are available in varying concentrations. Use the appropriate strength product in children to avoid toxicity.
- Do not administer with a high-carbohydrate meal, because absorption may be diminished.
- Pregnancy category B.

PHARMACOKINETICS

Onset: 30–60 min

Peak: 0.5–2 h

Half-life: 1–3 h

Duration: 3–4 h

ADVERSE EFFECTS

Acetaminophen is generally safe, and adverse effects are uncommon at therapeutic doses. Acetaminophen causes less gastric irritation than aspirin, and does not affect blood coagulation. It is not recommended in clients who are malnourished. In such cases, acute toxicity may result, leading to renal failure, which can be fatal. Other signs of acute toxicity include nausea, vomiting, chills, abdominal discomfort, and fatal hepatic necrosis.

Contraindications: Contraindications include hypersensitivity to acetaminophen or phenacetin and chronic alcoholism.

INTERACTIONS

Drug–Drug: Acetaminophen inhibits warfarin metabolism, causing the anticoagulant to accumulate to toxic levels. High-dose or long-term acetaminophen use may result in elevated warfarin levels and bleeding. Ingestion of this drug with alcohol, or other hepatotoxic drugs such as phenytoin or barbiturates, is not recommended because of the possibility of liver failure from hepatic necrosis.

Lab Tests: May increase hepatic function test values such as serum bilirubin, aspartate aminotransferase (AST), and alanine aminotranferease (ALT). May increase urinary 5-hydroxyindole acetic acid (5-HIAA) and serum uric acid.

Herbal/Food: The client should avoid taking herbs that have the potential for liver toxicity, including comfrey, coltsfoot, and chaparral.

Treatment of Overdose: The specific treatment for overdose is the oral or IV administration of *N*-acetylcysteine (Acetadote) as soon as possible after the overdose. This drug protects the liver from toxic metabolites of acetaminophen.

 See the Companion Website for a Nursing Process Focus specific to this drug.

MediaLink — Mechanism in Action: Acetaminophen

---

drug treatment. Prior to administering an antipyretic, obtain the client's vital signs, especially temperature. Assess the client's developmental status, the origin of the fever, and associated symptoms to determine the appropriate formulation or route for the antipyretic. For example, clients who are vomiting should receive an antipyretic by suppository, and very young children are generally given flavored elixirs.

Baseline laboratory data are necessary to assess the client's kidney and liver status; antipyretics may cause toxicity

HOME & COMMUNITY CONSIDERATIONS

Aspirin for Cardiovascular Event Risk Reduction

Current practice related to cardiovascular and neurovascular event prevention and treatment may include the use of aspirin therapy. This NSAID is the only one that has the additional property of decreasing the development of blood clots. The blood's clotting action is slowed by the administration of aspirin. This therapy has been recommended for men older than 40 years, postmenopausal women, and men younger than 40 years and premenopausal women who have high cholesterol, hypertension, diabetes, history of a clot-related stroke or transient ischemic attack, or a history of cigarette smoking. Even though the frequently used dose for this therapy—81 mg—is available over the counter, clients should be advised to consult their healthcare providers before initiating self-medication with aspirin.

in clients with diminished organ function. Acetaminophen is contraindicated in clients with significant liver disease, including viral hepatitis, cirrhosis, and alcoholism, because the drug is metabolized by the liver and can greatly increase the risk of hepatotoxicity. Acetaminophen also inhibits warfarin (Coumadin) metabolism, and may produce toxic accumulation of this drug, resulting in serious bleeding. NSAIDs may be contraindicated with warfarin as well, because they also promote bleeding. A therapeutic response may be determined by the reduction of fever. Adverse effects and general side effects may be experienced with antipyretic use. These effects are the same as those of NSAIDs.

Lifespan Considerations. Until the 1980s, aspirin was the most common therapy for fever in children; however, aspirin has been implicated in the development of Reye's syndrome. Aspirin and other salicylates are now contraindicated for pediatric clients younger than 18 years with fever. Because of the potential for Reye's syndrome, some healthcare practitioners advise against administering any NSAID to children. Therefore, acetaminophen has become the antipyretic of choice to treat most fevers. Use cautiously in pregnant and lactating women.

Client Teaching. Client education as it relates to antipyretics should include the goals of therapy, the reasons for obtaining baseline data such as vital signs and the existence of underlying hepatic and renal disorders, and possible drug side effects. Include the following points when teaching clients about antipyretics:

- Liquid forms of acetaminophen or ibuprofen come in different strengths; all children's liquid formulations are not the same.
- Give children younger than 1 year "infant drops" rather than "children's liquid" to decrease the amount of fluid to be consumed.
- Immediately report signs of acetaminophen toxicity such as nausea, vomiting, or abdominal pain.
- Notify healthcare provider if fever does not resolve within 3 days.

SPECIAL CONSIDERATIONS

Ethnic Considerations in Acetaminophen Metabolism

Certain ethnic populations, including Asians, African Americans, and Saudis, have higher rates of an enzyme deficiency that affects how they metabolize certain drugs. More than 200 million people worldwide are believed to have a hereditary deficiency of this enzyme, glucose-6-phosphate dehydrogenase (G6PD). Clients with G6PD deficiency are at risk for developing hemolysis after ingestion of certain drugs, including acetaminophen. Conflicting data exist on whether therapeutic dosages of acetaminophen can cause hemolysis in these clients. However, because acetaminophen is one of the most common drugs ingested in intentional overdoses, healthcare providers should recommend that clients with G6PD deficiency avoid this drug.

NURSING PROCESS FOCUS Clients Receiving Antipyretic Therapy

Assessment	Potential Nursing Diagnoses
Prior to administration: • Obtain a complete health history (mental and physical), including data on origin of fever, recent surgeries, or trauma. • Obtain vital signs; assess in context of client's baseline values. • Obtain client's complete medication history, including nicotine and alcohol consumption, herbal supplement use, and use of alternative therapies, to determine possible drug allergies and/or interactions.	• Pain • Hyperthermia • Injury, Risk for (hepatic toxicity), related to adverse effects of drug therapy

Planning: Client Goals and Expected Outcomes

The client will:
- Experience a reduction in body temperature.
- Demonstrate an understanding of the drug's action by accurately describing drug side effects and precautions.

Implementation

Interventions and (Rationales)	Client Education/Discharge Planning
• Assess for intolerance to ASA for possible cross-hypersensitivity to other NSAIDs or acetaminophen. (Allergies should always be assessed prior to drug administration.)	• Inform client to immediately report difficulty breathing, itching, or skin rash.
• Monitor hepatic and renal function. • (Antipyretics are metabolized in the liver and excreted by the kidneys.)	Instruct client: • To report signs of liver toxicity: nausea, vomiting, anorexia, bleeding, severe upper or lower abdominal pain, heartburn, jaundice, or a change in the color or character of stools. • To adhere to laboratory testing regimen for serum blood tests as directed.
• Use with caution in clients with a history of excessive alcohol consumption. (Alcohol increases the risk of liver damage associated with acetaminophen or NSAID administration.)	• Advise client to abstain from alcohol while taking this medication.
• Use with caution in clients with diabetes. (Hypoglycemia may occur with acetaminophen use.)	Instruct client to immediately report: • Excessive thirst. • Large increase or decrease in urine output. Advise clients with diabetes mellitus that: • Acetaminophen may cause low blood sugar and require insulin dose adjustments.

Evaluation of Outcome Criteria

Evaluate the effectiveness of drug therapy by confirming that client goals and expected outcomes have been met (see "Planning").
- The client's temperature is within normal limits.
- The client demonstrates an understanding of the drug's action by accurately describing drug side effects and precautions.

∞ See Table 33.2 for a list of the drugs to which these nursing actions apply. Acetaminophen is also covered in this Nursing Process Focus chart.

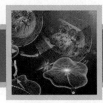

CHAPTER REVIEW

KEY CONCEPTS

The numbered key concepts provide a succinct summary of the important points from the corresponding numbered section within the chapter. If any of these points are not clear, refer to the numbered section within the chapter for review.

33.1 Inflammation is a natural, nonspecific body defense that limits the spread of invading microorganisms or injury. Acute inflammation occurs over several days, whereas chronic inflammation may continue for months or years.

33.2 Histamine is a key chemical mediator in inflammation. Release of histamine produces vasodilation, allowing capillaries to become leaky, thus causing tissue swelling.

33.3 Histamine can produce its effects by interacting with two different receptors. H_1 receptors are found in vascular smooth muscle, in the bronchi, and on sensory nerves, whereas the H_2 receptors are located in the GI tract.

33.4 Nonsteroidal anti-inflammatory drugs (NSAIDs) are the primary drugs for the treatment of simple inflammation. All drugs in this class have similar efficacy in treating inflammation. The newer selective COX-2 inhibitors cause less GI distress but have significant cardiovascular side effects.

33.5 Systemic glucocorticoids are effective in treating acute or severe inflammation. Overtreatment with these drugs can cause a serious condition called Cushing's syndrome; thus, therapy for inflammation is generally short term.

33.6 Acetaminophen and NSAIDs are the primary agents used to treat fever. Certain medications may cause drug-induced fever, which may range from mild to life threatening.

NCLEX-RN® REVIEW QUESTIONS

1 On discharge of the client, the nurse discusses types of over-the-counter NSAID medications that are available. The nurse states that an OTC medication that is not classified as an NSAID is:

1. Aspirin.
2. Ibuprofen.
3. Acetaminophen.
4. Motrin.

2 The client has been taking aspirin for several days for headache. During the assessment, the nurse discovers the client is experiencing ringing in the ears and dizziness. The most appropriate action by the nurse is:

1. To question the client about history of sinus infections.
2. To determine if the client has mixed the aspirin with other medications.
3. To tell the client not to take any more aspirin.
4. To tell the client to take the aspirin with food or milk.

3 While educating the client about glucocorticoids, the nurse would instruct the client to contact the physician immediately if:

1. There is an increase of 5 lb in weight.
2. There is any swelling in the ankles.
3. There is any diarrhea.
4. There is any difficulty breathing.

4 The nurse is admitting a client with rheumatoid arthritis. The client has been taking glucocorticoids for an extended period of time. During the assessment the nurse observes that the client has a very round moon-shaped face, bruising, and an abnormal contour of the shoulders. The nurse concludes that:

1. These are normal reactions with the illness.
2. These are probably birth defects.
3. These are symptoms of myasthenia gravis.
4. These are symptoms of Cushing's syndrome.

5 The client has had a high fever for the last 3 days. The nurse would assess for which of the following? (Select all that apply.)

1. Coma
2. Changes in level of consciousness
3. Delirium
4. Bleeding tendencies
5. GI distress

CRITICAL THINKING QUESTIONS

1. A 64-year-old diabetic client is on prednisone for rheumatoid arthritis. The client has recently been admitted to the hospital for stabilization of hyperglycemia. What are the nurse's primary concerns when caring for this client?

2. A 44-year-old client is requesting medication for a painful tendinitis of the elbow. This client has mild hypertension, a history of alcohol abuse, and nutritional deficits. This client has orders for acetaminophen (Tylenol), ibuprofen (Motrin), and celecoxib (Celebrex). Which one would the nurse give and why?

3. The mother of a 7-year-old child calls the physician's office stating that her daughter has a temperature of 101 °F. She states the child is also complaining of being tired and "achy" all over. The mother asks how much aspirin she can giver her daughter for her temperature. How should the nurse respond?

See Appendix D for answers and rationales for all activities.

EXPLORE MediaLink

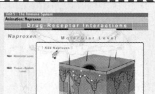

 www.prenhall.com/adams

NCLEX-RN® review, case studies, and other interactive resources for this chapter can be found on the companion website at www.prenhall.com/adams. Click on "Chapter 33" to select the activities for this chapter. For animations, more NCLEX-RN® review questions, and an audio glossary, access the accompanying Prentice Hall Nursing MediaLink DVD-ROM in this textbook.

PRENTICE HALL NURSING MEDIALINK DVD-ROM

- **Animation**
  Mechanism in Action: Acetaminophen (*Tylenol*)
- **Audio Glossary**
- **NCLEX-RN® Review**

COMPANION WEBSITE

- **NCLEX-RN® Review**
- **Dosage Calculations**
- **Case Study:** Client taking anti-inflammatory drugs
- **Care Plan:** Client with osteoarthritis being treated with celecoxib

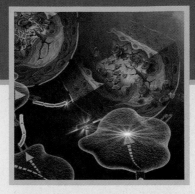

CHAPTER 34

Drugs for Bacterial Infections

DRUGS AT A GLANCE

PENICILLINS
- penicillin G (Pentids)

CEPHALOSPORINS
- cefotaxime (Claforan)

TETRACYCLINES
- tetracycline HCl (Achromycin, others)

MACROLIDES
- erythromycin (E-Mycin, Erythrocin)

AMINOGLYCOSIDES
- gentamicin (Garamycin)

FLUOROQUINOLONES
- ciprofloxacin (Cipro)

SULFONAMIDES
- trimethoprim–sulfamethoxazole (Bactrim, Septra)

ANTITUBERCULAR AGENTS
- isoniazid (INH)

OBJECTIVES

After reading this chapter, the student should be able to:

1. Compare and contrast the terms pathogenicity and virulence.
2. Explain how bacteria are described and classified.
3. Compare and contrast the terms bacteriostatic and bacteriocidal.
4. Using a specific example, explain how resistance can develop to an anti-infective drug.
5. Describe the nurse's role in the pharmacological management of bacterial infections.
6. Explain the importance of culture and sensitivity testing to anti-infective chemotherapy.
7. Identify the mechanism of development and symptoms of superinfections caused by anti-infective therapy.
8. For each of the drug classes listed in Drugs at a Glance, know representative drug examples, and explain their mechanism of action, primary actions, and important adverse effects.
9. Categorize antibacterial drugs based on their classification and mechanism of action.
10. Explain how the pharmacotherapy of tuberculosis differs from that of other infections.
11. Use the Nursing Process to care for clients who are receiving drug therapy for bacterial infections.

MediaLink

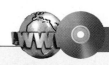

www.prenhall.com/adams

NCLEX-RN® review, case studies, and other interactive resources for this chapter can be found on the companion website at www.prenhall.com/adams. Click on "Chapter 34" to select the activities for this chapter. For animations, more NCLEX-RN® review questions, and an audio glossary, access the accompanying Prentice Hall Nursing MediaLink DVD-ROM in this textbook.

KEY TERMS

acquired resistance *page 487*

aerobic *page 485*

anaerobic *page 485*

antibiotic *page 486*

anti-infective *page 486*

bacteriocidal *page 486*

bacteriostatic *page 486*

beta-lactam ring *page 490*

beta-lactamase/penicillinase *page 490*

broad-spectrum antibiotic *page 487*

culture and sensitivity test *page 488*

folic acid *page 501*

gram-negative *page 485*

gram-positive *page 485*

host flora *page 488*

mutations *page 487*

narrow-spectrum antibiotic *page 487*

nosocomial infections *page 487*

pathogen *page 484*

pathogenicity *page 484*

penicillin-binding protein *page 490*

plasmid *page 487*

red-man syndrome *page 506*

superinfection *page 488*

tubercles *page 506*

virulence *page 484*

The human body has adapted quite well to living in a world teeming with microorganisms. Present in the air, water, food, and soil, microbes are an essential component of life on the planet. In some cases, such as with microorganisms in the colon, microbes play a beneficial role in human health. When in an unnatural environment or when present in unusually high numbers, however, microorganisms can cause a variety of ailments ranging from mildly annoying to fatal. The development of the first anti-infective drugs in the mid-1900s was a milestone in the field of medicine. In the last 50 years, pharmacologists have attempted to keep pace with microbes that rapidly become resistant to therapeutic agents. This chapter examines two groups of anti-infectives, the antibacterial agents and the specialized drugs used to treat tuberculosis.

34.1 Pathogenicity and Virulence

An organism that can cause disease is called a **pathogen.** Human pathogens include viruses, bacteria, fungi, unicellular organisms, and multicellular animals. To infect humans, pathogens must bypass a number of elaborate body defenses, such as those described in Chapters 32 and 33 ∞. Pathogens may enter through broken skin, or by ingestion, inhalation, or contact with a mucous membrane such as the nasal, urinary, or vaginal mucosa.

The ability of an organism to cause infection, or **pathogenicity,** depends on an organism's ability to evade or overcome body defenses. Fortunately for us, only a few dozen pathogens commonly cause disease in humans. Another common word used to describe a pathogen is **virulence.** A highly virulent microbe is one that can produce disease when present in minute numbers.

After gaining entry, pathogens generally cause disease by one of two basic mechanisms. Some pathogens grow rapidly and cause disease by their sheer numbers, overcoming body defenses and disrupting normal cellular function. A second mechanism is the production of toxins. Even very small amounts of some bacterial toxins may disrupt normal cellular activity and, in extreme cases, result in death.

PHARMFACTS

Bacterial Infections

- Infectious diseases are the third most common cause of death in the United States, and first in the world.
- Food-borne illness is responsible for 76,000,000 illnesses; 300,000 hospitalizations; and 5,000 deaths each year.
- Urinary tract infections (UTIs) are the most common infection acquired in hospitals, and nearly all are associated with the insertion of a urinary catheter. Hospital-acquired UTIs add an average of 3.8 days to a hospital stay and can cost more than $3,800 per infection.
- More than 2 million nosocomial infections are acquired each year. These infections add 1 day for UTIs, 7 to 8 days for surgical site infections, and 6 to 30 days for pneumonia.
- Pneumococcal infections are the most common invasive bacterial infections in children younger than age of 5, accounting for 1,400 cases of meningitis; 17,000 bloodstream infections; and 71,000 pneumonia infections.
- Up to 30% of all *S. pneumoniae* found in some areas of the United States are resistant to penicillin.
- Nearly all strains of *S. aureus* in the United States are resistant to penicillin.
- About 73,000 cases of *E. coli* poisoning are reported annually in the United States, with the most common source being ground beef.

34.2 Describing and Classifying Bacteria

Because of the enormous number of different bacterial species, several descriptive systems have been developed to simplify their study. It is important for nurses to learn these classification schemes, because drugs that are effective against one organism in a class are likely to be effective against other pathogens in the same class. Common bacterial pathogens and the types of diseases that they cause are listed in Table 34.1.

One of the simplest methods of classifying bacteria is to examine them microscopically after a crystal violet Gram stain is applied. Some bacteria contain a thick cell wall and retain a purple color after staining. These are called **gram-positive** bacteria and include staphylococci, streptococci, and enterococci. Bacteria that have thinner cell walls will lose the violet stain and are called **gram-negative.** Examples of gram-negative bacteria include bacteroides,

Escherichia coli, klebsiella, pseudomonas, and salmonella. The distinction between gram-positive and gram-negative bacteria is a profound one that reflects important biochemical and physiological differences between the two groups. Some antibacterial agents are effective only against gram-positive bacteria, whereas others are used to treat gram-negative bacteria.

A second descriptive method is based on cellular shape. Bacteria assume several basic shapes that can be readily determined microscopically. Rod shapes are called *bacilli*, spherical shapes are called *cocci*, and spirals are called *spirilla.*

A third factor used to classify bacteria is based on their ability to use oxygen. Those that thrive in an oxygen-rich environment are called **aerobic;** those that grow best without oxygen are called **anaerobic.** Some organisms have the ability to change their metabolism and survive in *either* aerobic or anaerobic conditions, depending on their external environment. Antibacterial drugs differ in

TABLE 34.1   Common Bacterial Pathogens and Disorders

Name of Organism	Disease(s)	Description
Borrelia burgdorferi	Lyme disease	acquired from tick bites
Chlamydia trachomatis	venereal disease	most common cause of sexually transmitted diseases in the United States
Escherichia coli	traveler's diarrhea, UTI, bacteremia	part of host flora in GI tract
Haemophilus	pneumonia, meningitis in children, bacteremia, otitis media, sinusitis	some *Haemophilus* species are normal host flora in the upper respiratory tract
Klebsiella	pneumonia, UTI	usually infects immunosuppressed clients
Mycobacterium leprae	leprosy	most cases in the United States occur in immigrants from Africa or Asia
Mycobacterium tuberculosis	tuberculosis	incidence very high in HIV-infected clients
Mycoplasma pneumoniae	pneumonia	most common cause of pneumonia in clients age 5–35
Neisseria gonorrhoeae	gonorrhea and other sexually transmitted diseases, endometriosis, neonatal eye infection	some *Neisseria* species are normal host flora
Neisseria meningitidis	meningitis in children	some *Neisseria* species are normal host flora
Pneumococci	pneumonia, otitis media, meningitis, bacteremia, endocarditis	part of normal host flora in upper respiratory tract
Proteus mirabilis	UTI, skin infections	part of normal host flora in GI tract
Pseudomonas aeruginosa	UTI, skin infections, septicemia	usually infects immunosuppressed clients
Rickettsia rickettsii	Rocky Mountain spotted fever	acquired from tick bites
Salmonella enteritidis	food poisoning	acquired from infected animal products; raw eggs, undercooked meat or chicken
Salmonella typhi	typhoid fever	acquired from inadequately treated food or water supplies
Staphylococcus aureus	pneumonia, food poisoning, impetigo, abscesses, bacteremia, endocarditis, toxic shock syndrome	some *Staphylococci* species are normal host flora
Streptococcus	pharyngitis, pneumonia, skin infections, septicemia, endocarditis	some *Streptococci* species are normal host flora
Vibrio cholerae	cholera	acquired from inadequately treated food or water supplies

their effectiveness in treating aerobic versus anaerobic bacteria.

34.3 Classification of Anti-infective Drugs

Anti-infective is a general term for any medication that is effective against pathogens. Although **antibiotic** is more frequently used, this term technically refers only to *natural* substances produced by microorganisms that can kill other microorganisms. In current practice, the terms *antibacterial, anti-infective, antimicrobial,* and *antibiotic* are often used interchangeably, as they are in this textbook.

With more than 300 anti-infectives available, it is useful to group these drugs into classes that have similar therapeutic properties. Chemical classes are widely used. Names such as *aminoglycoside, fluoroquinolone,* and *sulfonamide* refer to the fundamental chemical structure of a group of anti-infectives. Anti-infectives belonging to the same chemical class share similar antimicrobial properties and side effects.

Another method of classifying anti-infectives is by mechanism of action (pharmacological class). Examples include cell wall inhibitors, protein synthesis inhibitors,

folic acid inhibitors, and reverse transcriptase inhibitors. These classifications are used in this textbook, where appropriate.

34.4 Actions of Anti-infective Drugs

The primary goal of antimicrobial therapy is to assist the body's defenses in eliminating the pathogen. Medications that accomplish this goal by *killing* bacteria are called **bacteriocidal.** Some drugs do not kill the bacteria but instead slow their growth, depending on the body's natural defenses to dispose of the microorganisms. These *growth-slowing* drugs are called **bacteriostatic.**

Bacterial cells are quite different from human cells. Bacteria have cell walls, use different biochemical pathways, and contain certain enzymes that human cells lack. Antibiotics exert *selective toxicity* on bacterial cells by targeting these unique differences. Thus, bacteria can be killed or their growth severely hampered without major effects on human cells. Of course, there are limits to this selective toxicity, depending on the specific antibiotic and the dose employed, and side effects can be expected from all anti-infectives. The basic mechanisms of action of antimicrobial drugs are shown in ● Figure 34.1.

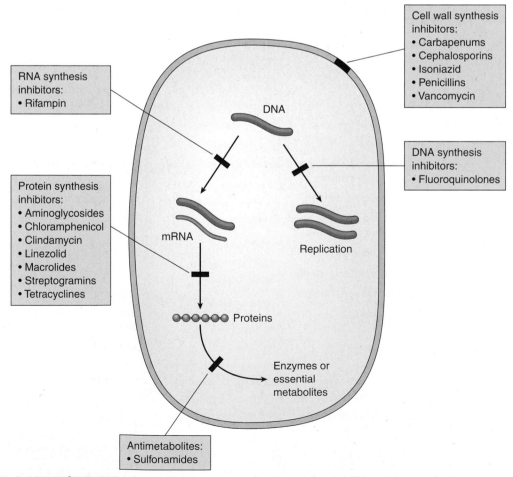

● **Figure 34.1** Mechanisms of action of antimicrobial drugs

34.5 Acquired Resistance

Microorganisms have the ability to replicate extremely rapidly. During cell division, bacteria make frequent errors in duplicating their genetic code. These **mutations,** or errors in the genetic code, occur spontaneously and randomly throughout the bacterial chromosome. Although most mutations are harmful to the organism, mutations occasionally result in a bacterial cell that has reproductive advantages over its neighbors. The mutated bacterium may be able to survive in harsher conditions or perhaps grow faster than other cells. Mutations that are of particular importance to medicine are those that confer drug resistance to a microorganism.

Antibiotics help promote the development of drug-resistant bacterial strains. Killing populations of bacteria that are sensitive to the drug leaves behind those microbes that possess mutations that made them insensitive to the effects of the antibiotic. These drug-resistant bacteria are then free to grow, unrestrained by their neighbors that were killed by the antibiotic, and the client develops an infection that is resistant to conventional drug therapy. This phenomenon, **acquired resistance,** is illustrated in ● Figure 34.2. Bacteria may pass the resistance gene to other bacteria through *conjugation,* the transfer of small pieces of circular DNA called **plasmids.**

It is important to understand that the antibiotic did not *create* the mutation that caused bacteria to become resistant. The mutation occurred randomly. The role that the antibiotic plays in resistance is to kill the surrounding cells that were susceptible to the drug, leaving the mutated ones plenty of room to divide and infect. It is the bacteria that have become resistant, not the client. An individual with an infection that is resistant to certain antibacterial agents can transmit the resistant bacteria to others.

The widespread and sometimes unwarranted use of antibiotics has led to a large number of resistant bacterial strains. At least 60% of *Staphylococcus aureus* infections are now resistant to penicillin, and resistant strains of *Enterococcus faecalis, Enterococcus faecium,* and *Pseudomonas aeruginosa* are becoming major clinical problems. The longer an antibiotic is used in the population and the more often it is prescribed, the larger the percentage of resistant strains. Infections acquired in a hospital or other healthcare setting, called **nosocomial infections,** are often resistant to common antibiotics. Resistant nosocomial infections are especially troublesome in critical care units, where seriously ill clients are treated with high amounts of antibiotics. Healthcare practitioners can play an important role in delaying the emergence of resistance by restricting the use of antibiotics to those conditions deemed medically necessary. Prescribing antibiotics when they are not needed, such as for the common cold virus, contributes greatly to the emergence of resistant strains of organisms.

In most cases, antibiotics are given when there is clear evidence of bacterial infection. Some clients, however, receive antibiotics to *prevent* an infection, a practice called *prophylactic* use, or *chemoprophylaxis.* Examples of clients who might receive prophylactic antibiotics include those who have a suppressed immune system, those who have experienced deep puncture wounds such as from dog bites, or those who have prosthetic heart valves and are about to have medical or dental surgery.

It is not uncommon for clients to discontinue taking their antibiotic once they begin feeling better. However, prematurely stopping antibiotic therapy allows some pathogens to survive, thus promoting the appearance of resistant strains. The nurse should instruct the client that many microorganisms still remain, even after the symptoms disappear. The importance of taking the entire drug regimen must be stressed.

34.6 Selection of an Effective Antibiotic

Some antibacterials are effective against many different species of pathogens. These are called **broad-spectrum antibiotics. Narrow-spectrum antibiotics** are effective against only one or a restricted group of microorganisms.

The selection of an antibiotic that will be effective against a specific pathogen is an important task of the healthcare practitioner. Selecting an incorrect drug will delay proper

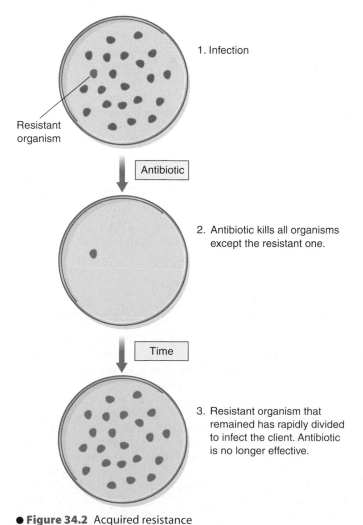

1. Infection

Resistant organism

Antibiotic

2. Antibiotic kills all organisms except the resistant one.

Time

3. Resistant organism that remained has rapidly divided to infect the client. Antibiotic is no longer effective.

● **Figure 34.2** Acquired resistance

MediaLink   Veterinary Antibiotics and Human Health

treatment, thus giving the microorganism more time to infect. Prescribing ineffective antibiotics also promotes the development of resistance and may cause unnecessary side effects in the client.

Ideally, laboratory tests should be conducted to identify the specific pathogen *prior to* beginning anti-infective therapy. Lab tests may include examination of urine, stool, spinal fluid, sputum, blood, or purulent drainage for microorganisms. Organisms isolated from the specimens may be grown in the laboratory and identified. After identification, the laboratory may test several different antibiotics to determine which is most effective against the infecting microorganism. This process of growing the pathogen and identifying the most effective antibiotic is called **culture and sensitivity testing.** Because antibiotic therapy alters the composition of infected fluids, samples should be collected prior to starting pharmacotherapy. Laboratory identification is not always necessary; some infections are mild, and skilled healthcare practitioners are often able to make an accurate diagnosis based on client signs and symptoms.

Proper laboratory testing and identification of bacteria may take several days or, in the case of viruses, several weeks. Some organisms cannot be cultured at all. If the infection is severe, therapy will likely be started immediately with a broad-spectrum antibiotic. After the results of the culture and sensitivity tests are obtained, therapy may be changed to include the antibiotic found to be most effective against the pathogen.

In most cases, antibacterial therapy is conducted using a single drug. Combining two antibiotics may actually decrease each drug's efficacy, a phenomenon known as *antagonism*. If incorrect combinations are prescribed, the use of multiple antibiotics also has the potential to promote resistance. Multidrug therapy is warranted, however, if several different organisms are causing the client's infection or if the infection is so severe that therapy must be started before laboratory tests have been completed. Multidrug therapy is clearly warranted in the treatment of tuberculosis or in clients infected with HIV.

One common side effect of anti-infective therapy is the appearance of secondary infections, known as **superinfections,** which occur when microorganisms normally present in the body are destroyed. These normal microorganisms, or **host flora,** inhabit the skin and the upper respiratory, genitourinary, and intestinal tracts. Some of these organisms serve a useful purpose by producing antibacterial substances and by competing with pathogenic organisms for space and nutrients. Removal of host flora by an antibiotic gives the remaining microorganisms an opportunity to grow, allowing for overgrowth of pathogenic microbes. Host flora themselves can cause disease if allowed to proliferate without control, or if they establish colonies in abnormal locations. For example *E. coli* is part of the host flora in the colon but can become a serious pathogen if it enters the urinary tract. Host flora may also become pathogenic if the client's immune system becomes suppressed. Microbes that become pathogenic

when the immune system is suppressed are called *opportunistic* organisms.

Superinfection should be suspected if a new infection appears while the client is receiving anti-infective therapy. Signs and symptoms of a superinfection commonly include diarrhea, bladder pain, painful urination, or abnormal vaginal discharges. Broad-spectrum antibiotics are more likely to cause superinfections because they kill so many different species of microorganisms.

34.7 Host Factors

The most important factor in selecting an appropriate antibiotic is to be certain that the microbe is sensitive to the effects of the drug. However, the nurse must also take into account certain host factors that can influence the success of antibacterial chemotherapy.

The primary goal of antibiotic therapy is to kill enough bacteria, or to slow the growth of the infection, so that natural body defenses can overcome the invading agent. Unless an infection is highly localized, the antibiotic alone may not be enough: the client's immune system and phagocytic cells will be needed to completely rid the body of the infectious agent. Clients with suppressed immune systems may require aggressive antibiotic therapy with bacteriocidal agents. These clients include those with AIDS and those being treated with immunosuppressive or antineoplastic drugs. Because therapy is more successful when the number of microbes is small, antibiotics may be given on a prophylactic basis to clients whose white blood cell (WBC) count is extremely low.

Local conditions at the infection site should be considered when selecting an antibiotic because factors that hinder the drug from reaching microbes will limit therapeutic success. Infections of the central nervous system are particularly difficult to treat because many drugs cannot cross the blood–brain barrier. Injury or inflammation can cause tissues to become acidic or anaerobic and to have poor circulation. Excessive pus formation or hematomas can block drugs from reaching their targets. Although most bacteria are extracellular in nature, pathogens such as *Mycobacterium*

SPECIAL CONSIDERATIONS

Hispanic Cultural Beliefs and Antibacterials
Certain ethnic groups such as Hispanics, believe that illness is caused by an imbalance in hot and cold. In a healthy individual, hot and cold are in balance; when an imbalance occurs, disease results.

Illnesses are classified as either hot or cold as well. For example, sore throat and diarrhea are considered hot diseases; colds, upper respiratory infections, arthritis, and rheumatism are considered cold diseases. Traditional treatment in such cultures is to restore the body's balance through the addition or subtraction of herbs, foods, or medications that are classified as either hot or cold. To treat a hot disease, medications or herbs considered cold are used. For example, penicillin is considered a hot medicine, but amoxicillin is less hot. Using acetaminophen with amoxicillin makes it cooler.

tuberculosis, salmonella, toxoplasma, and listeria may reside intracellularly and thus be resistant to antibacterial action. Consideration of these factors may necessitate a change in the route of drug administration or the selection of a more effective antibiotic specific for the local conditions.

Severe allergic reactions to antibiotics, while not common, may be fatal. The nurse's assessment must include a thorough drug history; a previous acute allergic incident is highly predictive of future hypersensitivity. If severe allergy to a medication is established, it is best to avoid all drugs in the same chemical class. Because the client may have been exposed to an antibiotic unknowingly, through food products or molds, allergic reactions can occur without previous incident. Penicillins are the class of antibacterials having the highest incidence of allergic reactions; between 0.7% and 4% of all clients who receive them exhibit hypersensitivity. The pharmacotherapy of anaphylaxis is presented in Chapter 29 ∞.

Other host factors to be considered are age, pregnancy status, and genetics. The very young and the very old are often unable to readily metabolize or excrete antibiotics; thus, doses are generally lowered. Some antibiotics cross the placenta. For example, tetracyclines taken by the mother can cause teeth discoloration in the newborn; aminoglycosides can affect the infant's hearing. The ben-efits of antibiotic use in pregnant or lactating women must be carefully weighed against the potential risks to the fetus and neonate. Lastly, some clients have a genetic absence of certain enzymes used to metabolize antibi-otics. For example, clients with a deficiency of the enzyme glucose-6-phosphate dehydrogenase should not receive sulfonamides, chloramphenicol, or nalidixic acid because their erythrocytes may rupture.

ANTIBACTERIAL AGENTS

Antibacterial agents form a large number of chemical classes. Although drugs within a class have similarities in their mechanisms and spectrum of activity, each is slightly different, and learning the differences and therapeutic ap-plications among antibacterial agents can be challenging. Basic nursing assessments and interventions apply to all an-tibiotic therapies; however, the nurse should individualize the plan of care based on the client's condition, the infec-tion, and the antibacterial agent prescribed.

PENICILLINS

Although not the first anti-infective discovered, penicillin was the first mass-produced antibiotic. Isolated from the fungus *Penicillium* in 1941, the drug quickly became a mir-acle product by preventing thousands of deaths from infec-tions. The penicillins are listed in Table 34.2.

TABLE 34.2 Penicillins		
Drug	**Route and Adult Dose (max dose where indicated)**	**Adverse Effects**
NARROW-SPECTRUM/PENICILLINASE SENSITIVE		
penicillin G benzathine (Bicillin)	IM; 1.2 million units as a single dose	*Rash, pruritus, diarrhea, nausea, fever*
penicillin G procaine (Crysticillin, Wycillin)	IM; 600,000–1.2 million units/day	
penicillin G sodium/potassium (Pentids)	PO; 400,000–800,000 units/day	Anaphylaxis symptoms, including angioedema, circulatory collapse and cardiac arrest; nephrotoxicity
penicillin V (Pen-Vee K, Veetids, Betapen)	PO; 125–250 mg qid	
PENICILLINASE RESISTANT		
cloxacillin (Tegopen)	PO; 250–500 mg bid	
dicloxacillin (Dynapen)	PO; 125–500 mg qid	
nafcillin (Nafcil, Unipen)	PO; 250 mg–1 g qid (max: 12 g/day)	
oxacillin (Prostaphlin, Bactocill)	PO; 250 mg–1 g qid (max: 12 g/day)	
BROAD-SPECTRUM (AMINOPENICILLINS)		
amoxicillin (Amoxil, Trimox, Wymox)	PO; 250–500 mg tid	
amoxicillin–clavulanate (Augmentin)	PO; 250 or 500 mg tablet (each with 125 mg clavulanic acid) q8–12h	
ampicillin (Polycillin, Omnipen)	PO; 250–500 mg bid	
bacampicillin (Spectrobid)	PO; 400–800 mg bid	
EXTENDED-SPECTRUM (ANTIPSEUDOMONAL)		
carbenicillin (Geocillin, Geopen)	PO; 382–764 mg qid	
piperacillin sodium (Pipracil)	IM; 2–4 g tid–qid (max: 24 g/day)	
piperacillin tazobactam (Zosyn)	IV; 3.375 g qid over 30 min	
ticarcillin (Ticar)	IM; 1–2 g qid (max: 40 g/day)	

Italics indicate common adverse effects; underlining indicates serious adverse effects.

34.8 Pharmacotherapy With Penicillins

Penicillins kill bacteria by disrupting their cell walls. Many bacterial cell walls contain a substance called **penicillin-binding protein** that serves as a receptor for penicillin. Penicillin weakens the cell wall and allows water to enter, thus killing the organism. Human cells do not contain cell walls; therefore, the actions of the penicillins are specific to bacterial cells. Gram-positive bacteria are the most commonly affected by the penicillins, including streptococci and staphylococci. Penicillins are indicated for the treatment of pneumonia; meningitis; skin, bone, and joint infections; stomach infections; blood and valve infections; gas gangrene; tetanus; anthrax; and sickle-cell anemia in infants.

The portion of the chemical structure of penicillin that is responsible for its antibacterial activity is called the **beta-lactam ring.** Some bacteria secrete an enzyme, called **beta-lactamase** or **penicillinase,** which splits the beta-lactam ring. This structural change allows these bacteria to become resistant to the effects of most penicillins. Since their discovery, large numbers of resistant bacterial strains have emerged that limit the therapeutic usefulness of the penicillins. The action of penicillinase is illustrated in ● Figure 34.3. Other classes of antibiotics also contain the beta-lactam ring, including the cephalosporins, carbapenems, and monobactams.

Chemical modifications to the original penicillin molecule produced drugs offering several advantages. Oxacillin (Prostaphlin, others) and cloxacillin (Tegopen) are effective against penicillinase-producing bacteria and are called *penicillinase-resistant* penicillins. The aminopenicillins such as ampicillin (Polycillin, others) and amoxicillin (Amoxil,

others) are effective against a wider range of microorganisms and are called *broad-spectrum* penicillins. The *extended-spectrum* penicillins, such as carbenicillin (Geocillin, Geopen) and piperacillin (Pipracil), are effective against even more microbial species, including pseudomonas, enterobacter, klebsiella, and *Bacteroides fragilis*.

Several drugs are available that inhibit bacterial beta-lactamase. When combined with a penicillin, these agents protect the penicillin molecule from destruction, extending its spectrum of activity. The three beta-lactamase inhibitors, clavulanate, sulbactam, and tazobactam, are available only in fixed-dose combinations with specific penicillins. These include Augmentin (amoxicillin plus clavulanate), Timentin (ticarcillin plus clavulanate), Unasyn (ampicillin plus sulbactam), and Zosyn (piperacillin plus tazobactam).

In general, the adverse effects of penicillins are minor; they are one of the safest classes of antibiotics. This has contributed to their widespread use for more than 60 years. Allergy to penicillin is the most common adverse effect. Common symptoms of penicillin allergy include rash, pruritus, and fever. Incidence of anaphylaxis ranges from 0.04% to 2%. Allergy to one penicillin increases the risk of allergy to other drugs in the same class. Other less common side effects of the penicillins include skin rashes and lowered red blood cell (RBC), WBC, or platelet counts.

NURSING CONSIDERATIONS

The role of the nurse in drug therapy with penicillins involves careful monitoring of a client's condition and providing education as it relates to the prescribed drug treatment. Because allergies occur more frequently with penicillins than with any other antibiotic class, assess previous

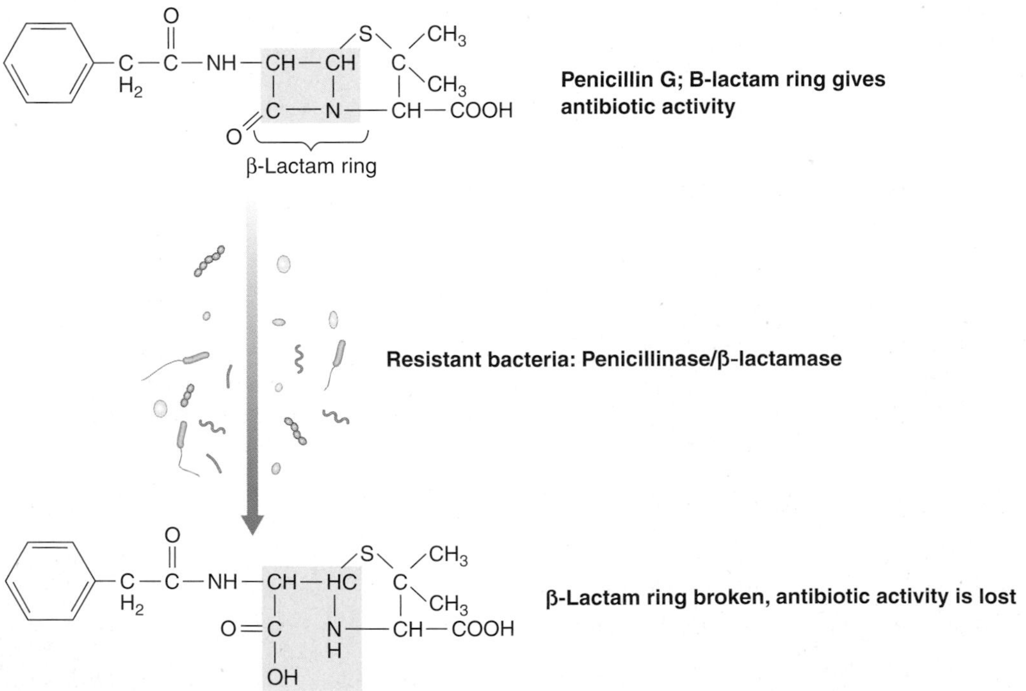

β-Lactam ring

Penicillin G; B-lactam ring gives antibiotic activity

Resistant bacteria: Penicillinase/β-lactamase

β-Lactam ring broken, antibiotic activity is lost

● **Figure 34.3** Action of penicillinase

drug reactions to penicillin prior to administration. If the client has a history of a severe penicillin allergic reaction, also avoid cephalosporins because of the risk of cross-hypersensitivity. Obtain specimens for culture and sensitivity prior to the start of antibiotic therapy.

Assess vital signs, electrolytes, and renal function tests prior to and during therapy. Because some penicillin preparations contain high levels of sodium and potassium salts, monitor for hyperkalemia and hypernatremia prior to and during therapy. Because of the possibility of worsening existing heart failure related to the increased sodium intake, monitor cardiac status, including ECG changes. Additionally, monitor for indications of response to therapy, including reduced fever, normal WBC count, improved appetite, and absence of symptoms such as cough.

After parenteral administration of penicillins, observe the client for possible allergic reactions for 30 minutes, especially with the first dose. Sensitivity may be immediate, accelerated, or delayed.

Because the majority of penicillin is excreted through the kidneys, clients with impaired renal function may require smaller doses. Penicillins should be used with caution during lactation because the drug enters breast milk. Monitor for possible bleeding in clients on anticoagulant therapy who are receiving high doses of parenteral carbenicillin (Geocillin), piperacillin (Pipracil), or ticarcillin (Ticar) because these drugs may interfere with platelet aggregation.

A small number of clients may develop a serious superinfection called *antibiotic-associated pseudomembranous colitis (AAPMC)*. In this condition, the organism *Clostridium difficile* secretes a toxin that causes severe inflammation of the bowel wall, followed by necrosis. This results in a potentially life-threatening infection. Clients with this condition have two to five semisolid or liquid stools per day. Antidiarrheal drugs should not be administered because these agents cause the toxin to be retained in the bowel. When AAPMC occurs, discontinue antibiotic therapy and replace fluids and electrolytes.

As with other antibiotics, penicillins may cause superinfections with symptoms such as abdominal cramping and diarrhea. Replacement of natural colon flora with probiotic supplements or cultured dairy products such as yogurt or buttermilk may help alleviate symptoms. Superinfections in elderly, debilitated, or immunosuppressed clients may be serious and require immediate interventions.

Client Teaching.   Client education as it relates to penicillins should include the goals of therapy, the reasons for obtaining baseline data such as vital signs and the existence of underlying disorders such as renal disease, and possible drug side effects. Include the following points when teaching clients about penicillins:

- Wear a medical alert bracelet if allergic to penicillins.
- Take penicillin V, amoxicillin, and amoxicillin–clavulanate with meals to decrease GI distress. Take all other penicillins with a full glass of water, 1 hour before or 2 hours after meals to increase absorption.

Pr PROTOTYPE DRUG | Penicillin G Potassium *(Pentids)* | Penicillin Antibiotic

ACTIONS AND USES

Similar to penicillin V, penicillin G is a drug of choice against streptococci, pneumococci, and staphylococci organisms that do not produce penicillinase. It is also a medication of choice for gonorrhea and syphilis caused by susceptible strains. Penicillin V is more acid stable; more than 70% is absorbed after an oral dose compared with 15% to 30% from penicillin G. Because of its low oral absorption, penicillin G is often given by the IV or IM routes. Penicillinase-producing organisms inactivate both penicillin G and penicillin V. Penicillin G benzathine (Bicillin) and penicillin G procaine (Wycillin) are longer acting parenteral salts of the drug.

ADMINISTRATION ALERTS

- After parenteral administration, observe for possible allergic reactions for 30 minutes, especially following the first dose.
- Do not mix penicillin and aminoglycosides in the same intravenous solution. Give IV medications 1 hour apart to prevent interactions.
- Pregnancy category B.

PHARMACOKINETICS

Onset: Rapid

Peak: 30–60 min PO; 15–20 min IM

Half-life: 30–60 min

Duration: 4–6 h

ADVERSE EFFECTS

Penicillin G has few side effects. Diarrhea, nausea, and vomiting are the most common adverse effects and can cause serious complications in certain populations, such as children and older adults. Pain at the injection site may occur, and superinfections are possible. Anaphylaxis is the most serious adverse effect.

Contraindications: The only contraindication is hypersensitivity to a drug in the penicillin class. Because penicillin G is excreted extensively by the kidneys, the drug should be used with caution in clients with severe renal disease.

INTERACTIONS

Drug–Drug: Penicillin G may decrease the efficacy of oral contraceptives. Colestipol taken with this medication will decrease the absorption of penicillin. Potassium-sparing diuretics may cause hyperkalemia when administered with penicillin G potassium.

Lab Tests: Unknown.

Herbal/Food: Unknown.

Treatment of Overdose: There is no specific treatment for overdose.

 See the Companion Website for a Nursing Process Focus specific to this drug.

- Take oral penicillin G with water because acidic fruit juice can inactivate the drug's antibacterial activity.
- Complete the full cause of treatment.
- Avoid use of penicillins while breast-feeding.
- Consult with your healthcare provider about taking pro- biotic supplements and/or cultured dairy products dur- ing antibiotic therapy.
- Immediately report rash, severe abdominal or stomach cramps, abdominal tenderness, convulsions, decreased urine output, and severe watery diarrhea or bloody diarrhea.

See "Nursing Process Focus: Clients Receiving Antibacte- rial Therapy" on page 504 for the Nursing Process applied to all antibacterials.

CEPHALOSPORINS

Isolated shortly after the penicillins, the four generations of cephalosporins (Table 34.3) constitute the largest antibiotic class. This class contains drugs with similar-sounding names, and it is often difficult for students to remember differ- ences among the various cephalosporins. The cephalosporins act by essentially the same mechanism as the penicillins and have similar pharmacological properties.

34.9 Pharmacotherapy With Cephalosporins

Like the penicillins, the cephalosporins contain a beta-lactam ring that is mostly responsible for their antimicrobial activity. The cephalosporins are bacteriocidal and act by attaching

TABLE 34.3 Cephalosporins		
Drug	**Route and Adult Dose (max dose where indicated)**	**Adverse Effects**
FIRST-GENERATION		
cefadroxil (Duricef)	PO; 500 mg–1 g 1–2 times/day (max: 2 g/day)	*Diarrhea, abdominal cramping, nausea, fatigue, rash, pruritus, pain at injection sites, oral or vaginal Candidiasis*
cefazolin (Kefzol, others)	IM; 250 mg–2 g tid (max: 12 g/day)	
cephalexin (Keflex, others)	PO; 250–500 mg qid	
cephapirin (Cefadyl)	IM/IV; 500 mg–1 g q4–6h (max: 12 g/day)	Pseudomembranous colitis, nephrotoxicity, anaphylaxis
cephradine (Velosef)	PO; 250–500 mg q6h or 500 mg–1 g q12h (max: 4 g/day)	
SECOND-GENERATION		
cefaclor (Ceclor)	PO; 250–500 mg tid	
cefmetazole (Zefazone)	IV; 1–2 g q6–12h	
cefonicid (Monocid)	IM; 1 g daily (max: 2 g/day)	
cefotetan (Cefotan)	IV/IM; 1–2 g q12h	
cefoxitin (Mefoxin)	IV/IM; 1–2 g q6–8h (max: 12 g/day)	
cefprozil (Cefzil)	PO; 250–500 mg 1–2 times/day	
cefuroxime (Ceftin, Kefurox, Zinacef)	PO; 250–500 mg bid	
loracarbef (Lorabid)	PO; 200–400 mg q12h taken 1 h before or 2 h after meals	
THIRD-GENERATION		
cefdinir (Omnicef)	PO; 300 mg bid	
cefditoren pivoxil (Spectracef)	PO; 400 mg bid for 10 days	
cefixime (Suprax)	PO; 400 mg/day or 200 mg bid	
cefoperazone (Cefobid)	IV/IM; 1–2 g q12h; 16 g/day in 2–4 divided doses	
cefotaxime (Claforan)	IM; 1–2 g bid–tid (max: 12 g/day)	
cefpodoxime (Vantin)	PO; 200 mg q12h for 10 days	
ceftazidime (Fortaz, others)	IV/IM; 1–2 mg q8–12h, up to 2 g q6h	
ceftibuten (Cedax)	PO; 400 mg/day for 10 days	
ceftizoxime (Cefizox)	IV/IM; 1–2 g q8–12h, up to 2 g q4h	
ceftriaxone (Rocephin)	IV/IM; 1–2 g q12–24h (max: 4 g/day)	
FOURTH-GENERATION		
cefepime (Maxipime)	IV/IM; 0.5–1.0 g q12h for 7–10 days	

Italics indicate common adverse effects; underlining indicates serious adverse effects.

to penicillin-binding proteins to inhibit bacterial cell-wall synthesis.

More than 20 cephalosporins are available and classified by their "generation," but there are not always clear distinctions among the generations. For example, cefdinir is considered either a third- or a fourth-generation drug, depending on the reference source. Following are the major distinctions among the generations:

- First-generation cephalosporins are most effective against gram-positive organisms; bacteria that produce beta-lactamase will usually be resistant to these agents.

- Second-generation cephalosporins are more potent, are more resistant to beta-lactamase, and exhibit a broader spectrum against gram-negative organisms than the first-generation drugs.

- Third-generation cephalosporins generally have a longer duration of action than second-generation agents, and an even broader spectrum against gram-negative organisms, and are resistant to beta-lactamase. Third-generation cephalosporins are sometimes the drugs of choice against infections by pseudomonas, klebsiella, neisseria, salmonella, proteus, and *Haemophilus influenza*.

- Fourth-generation cephalosporins are effective against organisms that have developed resistance to earlier cephalosporins. Third- and fourth-generation agents are capable of entering the cerebrospinal fluid (CSF) to treat CNS infections.

The primary therapeutic use of the cephalosporins as a class is for gram-negative infections and for clients who cannot tolerate the less expensive penicillins. Side effects are similar to those of the penicillins, with allergic reactions being the most common adverse effect. Skin rashes are a common sign of allergy, and may appear several days following the initiation of therapy. The nurse must be aware that 5% to 10% of the clients who are allergic to penicillin are also allergic to the cephalosporins. Cephalosporins are contraindicated for clients who have previously experienced a severe allergic reaction to a penicillin. Despite this incidence of cross-hypersensitivity, the cephalosporins offer a reasonable alternative for many clients who are unable to take penicillin. Earlier generation cephalosporins caused kidney toxicity, but this adverse effect is diminished with the newer drugs in this class.

NURSING CONSIDERATIONS

The role of the nurse in cephalosporin therapy involves careful monitoring of a client's condition and providing education as it relates to the prescribed drug treatment. As with all antibiotics, culture and sensitivity testing should be performed before and during therapy. Assess for the presence or history of bleeding disorders, because cephalosporins may reduce prothrombin levels through interference with vitamin K metabolism. Assess renal and hepatic function, because most cephalosporins are eliminated by the kidney, and liver function is important in vitamin K production. If

---

Pr PROTOTYPE DRUG | Cefotaxime *(Claforan)* | Cephalosporin Antibiotic

ACTIONS AND USES

Cefotaxime is a third-generation cephalosporin with a broad spectrum of activity against gram-negative organisms. It is effective against many bacterial species that have developed resistance to earlier generation cephalosporins and to other classes of anti-infectives. Cefotaxime exhibits bacteriocidal activity by inhibiting cell-wall synthesis. It is prescribed for serious infections of the lower respiratory tract, central nervous system, genitourinary system, bones, and joints. It may also be used for blood infections such as bacteremia or septicemia. Like many other cephalosporins, cefotaxime is not absorbed from the GI tract and must be given by the IM or IV route.

ADMINISTRATION ALERTS

- Administer IM injections deep into a large muscle mass to prevent injury to surrounding tissues.
- Pregnancy category B.

PHARMACOKINETICS

Onset: 30 min

Peak: Unknown

Half-life: 1 h

Duration: Unknown

ADVERSE EFFECTS

For most clients, cefotaxime and the other cephalosporins are safe medications. Hypersensitivity is the most common adverse effect, although symptoms may include only a minor rash and itching. Anaphylaxis is possible. GI-related side effects such as diarrhea, vomiting, and nausea may occur. Some clients experience considerable pain at the injection site.

Contraindications: The only contraindication is hypersensitivity to a drug in the cephalosporin class. Because cefotaxime is excreted extensively by the kidneys, the drug should be used with caution in clients with severe renal disease.

INTERACTIONS

Drug–Drug: Probenecid causes decreased renal elimination of cefotaxime and may result in cephalosporin toxicity. Alcohol interacts with cefotaxime to produce a disulfiram–like reaction. Cefotaxime interacts with NSAIDs to cause an increase in platelet inhibition.

Lab Tests: Liver function test values may be increased; may give a positive Coomb's test and false elevations of serum or urinary creatinine levels.

Herbal/Food: Unknown.

Treatment of Overdose: There is no specific treatment for overdose.

 See the Companion Website for a Nursing Process Focus specific to this drug.

TABLE 34.4 Tetracyclines

Drug	Route and Adult Dose (max dose where indicated)	Adverse Effects
demeclocycline (Declomycin)	PO; 150 mg q6h or 300 mg q12h (max: 2.4 g/day)	*Nausea, vomiting, abdominal cramping, flatulence, diarrhea, mild phototoxicity, rash, dizziness, stinging/burning with topical applications*
doxycycline (Vibramycin, others)	PO; 100 mg bid on Day 1, then 100 mg/day (max: 200 mg/day)	
methacycline (Rondomycin)	PO; 600 mg/day in 2–4 divided doses	
minocycline (Minocin, others)	PO; 200 mg as single dose followed by 100 mg bid	<u>Anaphylaxis, secondary infections, hepatotoxicity, exfoliative dermatitis</u>
ⓟ tetracycline (Achromycin, others)	PO; 250–500 mg bid–qid (max: 2 g/day)	
tigecycline (Tygacil)	IV; 100 mg, followed by 50 mg q12h	

Italics indicate common adverse effects; <u>underlining</u> indicates serious adverse effects.

the client is concurrently taking NSAIDs, monitor blood coagulation studies, because cephalosporins increase the effect of platelet inhibition.

Because cephalosporins are eliminated through the kidneys, monitor intake and output, blood urea nitrogen (BUN), and serum creatinine. Use cephalosporins with caution in pregnant or lactating clients because the drugs can be transferred to the fetus or infant. Adjust doses appropriately in clients with impaired renal or hepatic function. Certain cephalosporins cause a disulfiram (Antabuse)–like reaction when alcoholic beverages are consumed. Typical symptoms of this reaction include severe vomiting, weakness, blurred vision, and profound hypotension.

Cephalosporins may predispose clients to pseudomembranous colitis, especially if GI pathology preexists. Less severe superinfections may also occur. Eating cultured dairy products such as yogurt or kefir may suppress GI-related superinfections.

Client Teaching. Client education as it relates to cephalosporins should include the goals of therapy, the reasons for obtaining baseline data such as vital signs and the existence of underlying disorders such as renal and hepatic disorders, and possible drug side effects. Include the following points when teaching clients about cephalosporins:

- Avoid alcohol use.
- Eat cultured dairy products to help discourage superinfections.
- Complete the full course of treatment.
- Immediately report diarrhea, onset of flulike symptoms, blistering or peeling of skin, seizures, decreased urine output, hearing loss, skin rash, breathing difficulty, or unusual tiredness or weakness.

See "Nursing Process Focus: Clients Receiving Antibacterial Therapy" on page 504 for the Nursing Process applied to all antibacterials.

TETRACYCLINES

The first tetracyclines were extracted from *Streptomyces* soil microorganisms in 1948. The six tetracyclines are effective against a large number of different gram-negative and gram-positive organisms and have one of the broadest spectrums of any class of antibiotics. The tetracyclines are listed in Table 34.4.

34.10 Pharmacotherapy With Tetracyclines

Tetracyclines act by inhibiting bacterial protein synthesis. By binding to the bacterial ribosome, which differs in structure from a human ribosome, the tetracyclines slow microbial growth and exert a bacteriostatic effect. All tetracyclines have the same spectrum of activity and show similar side effects. Doxycycline (Vibramycin) and minocycline (Minocin) have longer durations of actions and are more lipid soluble, permitting them to enter the CSF.

The widespread use of tetracyclines in the 1950s and 1960s resulted in a large number of resistant bacterial strains that now limit the drugs' therapeutic utility. They are drugs of choice for only a few diseases: Rocky Mountain spotted fever, typhus, cholera, Lyme disease, peptic ulcers caused by *Helicobacter pylori,* and chlamydial infections.

Tetracyclines exhibit few serious adverse effects, but several side effects may limit therapy with these agents. Nausea, vomiting, and diarrhea are common. Calcium and iron bind with tetracycline, decreasing the drug's absorption by as much as 50%. Direct exposure to sunlight can result in severe photosensitivity during therapy. Unless suffering from a life-threatening infection, clients younger than 8 years of age are not given tetracyclines because these drugs may cause permanent yellow-brown discoloration of teeth in young children. Tetracyclines are pregnancy category D agents; therefore, they should be avoided during pregnancy. Because of the drugs' broad spectrum, the risk for superinfection is relatively high and the nurse should be observant for signs of a secondary infection.

NURSING CONSIDERATIONS

The role of the nurse in tetracycline therapy involves careful monitoring of a client's condition and providing education as it relates to the prescribed drug treatment. Prior to administration, assess for a history of hypersensitivity to tetracyclines. If possible, obtain culture and sensitivity results before therapy is initiated. Assess for the presence or history of acne vulgaris, actinomycosis, anthrax, malaria, syphilis, urinary tract infection (UTI), rickettsial infection, and Lyme disease. Tetracyclines can treat all these disorders. Perform CBC and kidney and liver function studies. Monitor the client's body temperature, WBC count, and

Pr PROTOTYPE DRUG | Tetracycline *(Achromycin, others)* | Tetracycline Antibiotic

ACTIONS AND USES

Tetracycline is effective against a broad range of gram-positive and gram-negative organisms, including chlamydiae, rickettsiae, and mycoplasma. Tetracycline is given orally, though it has a short half-life that may require administration four times per day. Topical and oral preparations are available for treating acne. An IM preparation is available; injections may cause local irritation and be extremely painful.

ADMINISTRATION ALERTS

- Administer oral drug with full glass of water to decrease esophageal and GI irritation.
- Administer antacids and tetracycline 1 to 3 hours apart.
- Administer antilipidemic agents at least 2 hours before or after tetracycline.
- Pregnancy category D.

PHARMACOKINETICS

Onset: 1–2 h

Peak: 2–4 h

Half-life: 6–12 h

Duration: 12 h

ADVERSE EFFECTS

Being a broad-spectrum antibiotic, tetracycline has a tendency to affect vaginal, oral, and intestinal flora and cause superinfections. Tetracycline irritates the GI mucosa and may cause nausea, vomiting, epigastric burning, and diarrhea. Diarrhea may be severe enough to cause discontinuation of therapy. Other common side effects include discoloration of the teeth and photosensitivity.

Contraindications: Tetracycline is contraindicated in clients with hypersensitivity to drugs in this class. The drug should not be used during the second half of pregnancy, in children 8 years or younger, and in clients with severe renal or hepatic impairment.

INTERACTIONS

Drug–Drug: Milk products, iron supplements, magnesium-containing laxatives, and antacids reduce the absorption and serum levels of tetracyclines. Tetracyline binds with certain lipid-lowering drugs (colestipol and cholestyramine), thereby decreasing the antibiotic's absorption. This drug decreases the effectiveness of oral contraceptives.

Lab Tests: May increase the following lab values: blood urea nitrogen (BUN), aspartate aminotransferase (AST), alanine aminotransferase (ALT), amylase, bilirubin, alkaline phosphatase.

Herbal/Food: Dairy products interfere with tetracycline absorption.

Treatment of Overdose: There is no specific treatment for overdose.

 See the Companion Website for a Nursing Process Focus specific to this drug.

---

culture/sensitivity results to determine the effectiveness of the treatment, and observe for superinfections.

Oral and perineal hygiene care is extremely important to decrease the risk of superinfections due to *Candida*. Tetracyclines cause photosensitivity, which may lead to tingling and burning of the skin, similar to sunburn. Photosensitivity reaction may appear within a few minutes to hours to sun exposure and may persist for several days after pharmacotherapy is completed. Use with caution in clients with impaired kidney or liver function.

Lifespan Considerations. Tetracyclines are contraindicated in pregnancy or lactation because of the drug's effect on linear skeletal growth of the fetus and child. They are also contraindicated in children less than 8 years of age because of the drug's ability to cause permanent mottling and discoloration of the teeth. Tetracyclines decrease the effectiveness of oral contraceptives, so advise female clients to use an alternative method of birth control while taking the medication.

Client Teaching. Client education as it relates to tetracyclines should include goals of therapy; the reasons for obtaining baseline data such as vital signs, tests for culture and sensitivity, and the existence of underlying disorders such as renal and hepatic disorders; and possible drug side effects. Include the following points when teaching clients about tetracyclines:

- Do not save medication, because toxic effects may occur if it is taken past the expiration date.

- Do not take these medications with milk products, iron supplements, magnesium-containing laxatives, or antacids.

- Wait 1 to 3 hours after taking tetracyclines before taking antacids.

- Wait at least 2 hours before or after taking tetracyclines before taking lipid-lowering drugs such as colestipol (Colestid) and cholestyramine (Questran).

- Complete the full course of treatment.

- Immediately report abdominal pain, loss of appetite, nausea and vomiting, visual changes, and yellowing of skin.

- Avoid exposure to direct sunlight; use sunscreen and protective clothing to decrease the effects of photosensitivity.

See "Nursing Process Focus: Clients Receiving Antibacterial Therapy" on page 504 for the Nursing Process applied to all antibacterials.

MACROLIDES

Erythromycin, the first macrolide antibiotic, was isolated from *Streptomyces* in a soil sample in 1952. Macrolides are considered safe alternatives to penicillin, although they are drugs of first choice for relatively few infections.

34.11 Pharmacotherapy With Macrolides

The macrolides inhibit protein synthesis by binding to the bacterial ribosome. At low doses this inhibition produces a bacteriostatic effect. At higher doses, and in susceptible species, macrolides may be bacteriocidal. Macrolides are effective against most gram-positive bacteria and many gram-negative species. Common uses include the treatment of whooping cough, Legionnaires' disease, and infections by streptococcus, *H. influenza, and Mycoplasma pneumoniae*. Drugs in this class are used against bacteria residing *inside* host cells, such as *Listeria, Chlamydia, Neisseria,* and *Legionella*. The macrolides are listed in Table 34.5.

The newer macrolides were synthesized from erythromycin. Although their spectrums are similar, the newer agents have a longer half-life and cause less gastric irritation than erythromycin. For example, azithromycin (Zithromax) has such an extended half-life that it is administered for only 3 to 4 days, rather than the 10 days required for most antibiotics. The shorter duration of therapy is thought to increase client compliance.

The macrolides exhibit almost no serious side effects. Mild GI upset, diarrhea, and abdominal pain are the most common side effects. Because macrolides are broad-spectrum agents, superinfections may occur. Other than prior allergic reactions to macrolides, there are no contraindications to therapy.

NURSING CONSIDERATIONS

The role of the nurse in macrolide therapy involves careful monitoring of a client's condition and providing education as it relates to the prescribed drug treatment. Because macrolides are indicated for the pharmacological treatment of respiratory disorders, assess for the presence of respiratory infection. Also assess for GI tract infection, skin and soft-tissue infections, otitis media, gonorrhea, nongonococcal urethritis, and *H. pylori*. Examine the client for history of cardiac disorders, because macrolides may exacerbate existing heart disease. Due to possible toxic effects on the liver, monitor hepatic enzymes with certain macrolides such as erythromycin estolate.

Assess for a history of hypersensitivity to macrolides. Report rashes or other signs of hypersensitivity immediately. Obtain culture and sensitivity testing before initiating macrolide therapy.

Do not administer macrolides to clients with serious hepatic impairment, because the liver metabolizes these drugs. Use cautiously in pregnant or breast-feeding women to avoid harm to the fetus or newborn.

Many drug–drug interactions occur with macrolides. Certain anesthetic agents (alfentanil) and anticonvulsant drugs (carbamazepine) may interact with macrolides to cause serum drug levels to rise and result in toxicity. Macrolides should be used cautiously in clients receiving cyclosporine (Sandimmune), and drug levels must be monitored because of the risk for nephrotoxicity. Closely monitor clients receiving warfarin (Coumadin) because macrolides may decrease warfarin metabolism and excretion. Perform coagulation laboratory studies, such as international normalized ratio (INR), more frequently, because dosage adjustments may be required. Administer clarithromycin (Biaxin) and zidovudine (AZT) at least 4 hours apart to avoid interaction, which results in a delayed time for peak concentration of AZT.

Client Teaching. Client education as it relates to macrolides should include the goals of therapy; the reasons for obtaining baseline data such as vital signs, culture and sensitivity tests, and the existence of underlying respiratory disorders; and possible drug side effects. Include the following points when teaching clients about macrolides:

- Complete the full course of treatment.
- Do not take macrolides with fruit juices.
- Do not take other prescription drugs or OTC medications, herbal remedies, or vitamins and minerals without notifying your healthcare provider, because macrolides interact with many substances.

TABLE 34.5 Macrolides		
Drug	**Route and Adult Dose (max dose where indicated)**	**Adverse Effects**
azithromycin (Zithromax)	PO; 500 mg as single dose, then 250 mg/day for 4 days	*Nausea, vomiting, diarrhea, abdominal cramping, dry skin or burning (topical route)*
clarithromycin (Biaxin)	PO; 250–500 mg bid	
dirithromycin (Dynabac)	PO; 500 mg/day	
erythromycin (E-Mycin, Erythrocin)	PO; 250–500 mg bid or 333 mg tid	Anaphylaxis, ototoxicity, hepatotoxicity, superinfections
troleandomycin (Tao)	PO; 250–500 mg q6h	

Italics indicate common adverse effects; <u>underlining</u> indicates serious adverse effects.

Pr **PROTOTYPE DRUG** | Erythromycin *(E-Mycin, Erythrocin)* | Macrolide Antibiotic

ACTIONS AND USES

Erythromycin is inactivated by stomach acid and is thus formulated as coated, acid-resistant tablets or capsules that dissolve in the small intestine. Its main application is for clients who are unable to tolerate penicillins or who may have a penicillin-resistant infection. It has a spectrum similar to that of the penicillins and is effective against most gram-positive bacteria. It is often a preferred drug for infections by *Bordetella pertussis* (whooping cough) and *Corynebacterium diphtheriae*.

ADMINISTRATION ALERTS

- Administer oral drug on an empty stomach with a full glass of water.
- For suspensions, shake the bottle thoroughly to ensure the drug is well mixed.
- Do not give with or immediately before or after fruit juices.
- Pregnancy category B.

PHARMACOKINETICS

Onset: 1 h

Peak: 1–4 h

Half-life: 1.5–2 h

Duration: Unknown

ADVERSE EFFECTS

The most common side effects from erythromycin are nausea, abdominal cramping, and vomiting, although these are rarely serious enough to cause discontinuation of therapy. Concurrent administration with food reduces these side effects. The most severe adverse effect is hepatotoxicity caused by the estolate salt (Ilosone) of the drug.

Contraindications: Erythromycin is contraindicated in clients with hypersensitivity to drugs in the macrolide class, and for those taking terfenadine, astemizole, or cisapride.

INTERACTIONS

Drug–Drug: Anesthetics and anticonvulsants may interact to cause serum drug levels of erythromycin to rise and result in toxicity. This drug interacts with cyclosporine, increasing the risk for nephrotoxicity. It may increase the effects of warfarin. Erythromycin may interact with medications containing xanthine, to cause an increase in theophylline levels.

Lab Tests: Erythromycin may interfere with AST and give false urinary catecholamine values.

Herbal/Food: Unknown.

Treatment of Overdose: There is no specific treatment for overdose.

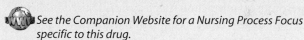 *See the Companion Website for a Nursing Process Focus specific to this drug.*

- Immediately report severe skin rash, itching, or hives; difficulty breathing or swallowing; yellowing of skin or eyes; dark urine; or pale stools.

See "Nursing Process Focus: Clients Receiving Antibacterial Therapy" on page 504 for the Nursing Process applied to all antibacterials.

AMINOGLYCOSIDES

The first aminoglycoside, streptomycin, was named after *Streptomyces griseus*, the soil organism from which it was isolated in 1942. Once widely used, streptomycin is now usually restricted to the treatment of tuberculosis because of the emergence of a large number of strains resistant to the antibiotic. Although more toxic than other antibiotic classes, aminoglycosides have important therapeutic applications for the treatment of aerobic gram-negative bacteria, mycobacteria, and some protozoans. The aminoglycosides are listed in Table 34.6.

34.12 Pharmacotherapy With Aminoglycosides

Aminoglycosides are bacteriocidal and act by inhibiting bacterial protein synthesis and causing the synthesis of abnormal proteins. They are normally reserved for serious systemic infections caused by aerobic gram-negative organisms, including those caused by *E. coli*, serratia, proteus, klebsiella, and pseudomonas. They are sometimes administered concurrently with a penicillin, cephalosporin, or vancomycin for treatment of enterococci infections. When used for systemic bacterial infections, aminoglycosides are given parenterally because they are poorly absorbed from the GI tract. They are occasionally given orally for their local effect on the GI tract to sterilize the bowel prior to intestinal surgery. Neomycin (Mycifradin, others) is available for topical infections of the skin, eyes, and ears. Paromomycin (Humatin) is given orally for the treatment of parasitic infections. The nurse should note the differences in spelling of some drugs—mycin versus-micin—which reflect the different organisms from which the drugs were originally isolated.

The aminoglycosides are capable of causing serious adverse effects in certain clients. Of greatest concern are their effects on the inner ear and the kidneys. Damage to the inner ear, or ototoxicity, is recognized by hearing impairment, dizziness, loss of balance, persistent headache, and ringing in the ears. Because ototoxicity may be irreversible, aminoglycosides are usually discontinued when these symptoms are first reported. Nephrotoxicity is recognized by abnormal urinary function tests, such as elevated serum creatinine or BUN. Nephrotoxicity is usually reversible.

NURSING CONSIDERATIONS

The role of the nurse in aminoglycoside therapy involves careful monitoring of a client's condition and providing education as it relates to the prescribed drug treatment. Assess the client for a history of previous allergic reaction to aminoglycosides. These anti-infectives are most noted for their toxic effects on the kidneys and inner ear; therefore, monitor for ototoxicity and nephrotoxicity during the

TABLE 34.6   Aminoglycosides

Drug	Route and Adult Dose (max dose where indicated)	Adverse Effects
amikacin (Amikin)	IM; 5.0–7.5 mg/kg as a loading dose, then 7.5 mg/kg bid	*Pain or inflammation at injection site, rash, fever, nausea, diarrhea, dizziness, tinnitus*
gentamicin (Garamycin, others)	IM; 1.5–2.0 mg/kg as a loading dose, then 1–2 mg/kg bid–tid	
kanamycin (Kantrex)	IM; 5.0–7.5 mg/kg bid–tid	<u>Anaphylaxis, nephrotoxicity, irreversible ototoxicity, superinfections</u>
neomycin (Mycifradin)	IM; 1.3–2.6 mg/kg qid	
netilmicin (Netromycin)	IM; 1.3–2.2 mg/kg tid or 2.0–3.25 mg/kg bid	
paromomycin (Humatin)	PO; 7.5–12.5 mg/kg tid	
streptomycin	IM; 15 mg/kg up to 1 g as a single dose	
tobramycin (Nebcin)	IM; 1 mg/kg tid (max: 5 mg/kg/day)	

Italics indicate common adverse effects; <u>underlining</u> indicates serious adverse effects.

course of therapy. Assess baseline audiometry and vestibular function prior to the initial administration of aminoglycosides and throughout therapy. Hearing loss may occur after therapy has been completed. Assess baseline renal function and obtain results of urinalysis (for microproteinuria) prior to initiation of therapy and throughout therapy, because renal impairment may increase the risk of toxicity.

Neuromuscular function may also be impaired in clients receiving aminoglycosides. Clients with neuromuscular diseases, such as myasthenia gravis and Parkinson's disease, may experi-

ence greater muscle weakness due to neuromuscular blockade caused by aminoglycosides. Use these antibiotics with caution in clients receiving anesthetics because of possible interactions that can cause neuromuscular blockade.

Use with caution in neonates, infants, and elderly clients. Infants may experience neuromuscular blockade from aminoglycosides because of their immature neurological systems. Elderly clients are at a higher risk of nephrotoxicity and ototoxicity because of reduced renal function, and may require lower doses. Instruct clients to increase fluid

Pr PROTOTYPE DRUG | Gentamicin *(Garamycin)* | Aminoglycoside Antibiotic

ACTIONS AND USES

Gentamicin is a broad-spectrum, bacteriocidal antibiotic usually prescribed for serious urinary, respiratory, nervous, or GI infections when less toxic antibiotics are contraindicated. It is often used in combination with other antibiotics or when drugs from other classes have proved ineffective. It is used parenterally, or as drops (Genoptic) for eye infections.

ADMINISTRATION ALERTS

- For IM administration, give deep into a large muscle.
- Use only IM and IV drug solutions that are clear and colorless or slightly yellow. Discard discolored solutions or those that contain particulate matter.
- Withhold the drug if the peak serum level lies above the normal range of 5–10 mcg/mL.
- Pregnancy category C.

PHARMACOKINETICS

Onset: Rapid

Peak: 1–2 h

Half-life: 2 h

Duration: 8–12 h

ADVERSE EFFECTS

As with other aminoglycosides, adverse effects from gentamicin may be severe. Ototoxicity can produce a loss of hearing or balance, which may become permanent with continued use. Frequent hearing tests should be conducted so that gentamicin may be discontinued if early signs of ototoxicity are detected.

Gentamicin is excreted unchanged, primarily by the kidneys. The nurse must be alert for signs of reduced kidney function, including proteinuria, and elevated BUN and creatinine levels. Nephrotoxicity is of particular concern to clients with preexisting kidney disease, and may limit pharmacotherapy. Resistance to gentamicin is increasing, and some cross-resistance among aminoglycosides has been reported.

Contraindications: Gentamicin is contraindicated in clients with hypersensitivity to drugs in the aminoglycoside class.

INTERACTIONS

Drug–Drug: The risk of ototoxicity increases if the client is currently taking amphotericin B, furosemide, aspirin, Bumex, Edecrin, cisplatin, or Humatin. Concurrent use with amphotericin B, capreomycin, cisplatin, polymyxin B, or vancomycin increases the risk of nephrotoxicity.

Lab Tests: May increase values of the following: serum bilirubin, serum creatinine, serum lactate dehydrogenase (LDH), BUN, AST, or ALT; may decrease values for the following: serum calcium, sodium, or potassium.

Herbal/Food: Unknown.

Treatment of Overdose: There is no specific treatment for overdose.

 See the Companion Website for a Nursing Process Focus specific to this drug.

TABLE 34.7 Fluoroquinolones		
Drug	**Route and Adult Dose (max dose where indicated)**	**Adverse Effects**
FIRST-GENERATION		
nalidixic acid (NeoGram)	PO; Acute therapy: 1 g qid; PO; Chronic therapy: 500 mg qid	*Nausea, diarrhea, vomiting, rash, restlessness, pain and inflammation at injection site, local burning, stinging and corneal irritation (ophthalmic)*
SECOND-GENERATION		
ciprofloxacin (Cipro, Septra)	PO; 250–750 mg bid	
lomefloxacin (Maxaquin)	PO; 400 mg/day	<u>Anaphylaxis, tendon rupture, superinfections, photosensitivity, pseudomembranous colitis</u>
norfloxacin (Noroxin)	PO; 400 mg bid	
ofloxacin (Floxin)	PO; 200–400 mg bid	
THIRD-GENERATION		
gatifloxacin (Tequin)	PO; 400 mg tid	
levofloxacin (Levaquin)	PO; 250–500 mg/day	
FOURTH-GENERATION		
gemifloxacin (Factive)	PO; 320 mg/day	
moxifloxacin (Avelox)	PO; 400 mg/day	
trovafloxacin mesylate (Trovan)	PO; 100–300 mg/day	

Italics indicate common adverse effects; <u>underlining</u> indicates serious adverse effects.

intake, unless otherwise contraindicated, to promote excretion of the medication. Superinfection is a side effect of aminoglycoside therapy; monitor clients carefully for diarrhea, vaginal discharge, stomatitis, and glossitis.

Client Teaching.   Client education as it relates to aminoglycosides should include goals of therapy, the reasons for obtaining baseline data such as vestibular function tests and the existence of underlying renal disorders, and possible drug side effects. Include the following points when teaching clients about aminoglycosides:

- Increase fluid intake.
- Complete the full course of treatment.
- Immediately report tinnitus, high-frequency hearing loss, persistent headache, nausea, or vertigo.

See "Nursing Process Focus: Clients Receiving Antibacterial therapy" on page 504 for the Nursing Process applied to all antibacterials.

FLUOROQUINOLONES

Fluoroquinolones were once reserved only for UTIs because of their toxicity, but development of safer drugs in this class began in the late 1980s and has continued to the present day. Newer fluoroquinolones have a broad spectrum of activity and are used for a variety of infections. The fluoroquinolones are listed in Table 34.7.

34.13 Pharmacotherapy With Fluoroquinolones

Although the first drug in this class, nalidixic acid (NegGram), was approved in 1962, it had a narrow spectrum of activity, and its use was restricted to UTIs. Since then, four generations of fluoroquinolones have become available. All fluoroquinolones have activity against gram-negative pathogens; the newer ones are significantly more effective against gram-positive microbes, such as staphylococci, streptococci, and enterococci.

The fluoroquinolones are bacteriocidal and affect DNA synthesis by inhibiting two bacterial enzymes: DNA gyrase and topoisomerase IV. Agents in this class are infrequently first-line drugs, although they are extensively used as alternatives to other antibiotics. Clinical applications include infections of the respiratory, GI, and genitourinary tracts, and some skin and soft-tissue infections. The most widely used drug in this class, ciprofloxacin (Cipro), is an agent of choice for postexposure prophylaxis of *Bacillus anthracis*. Two newer agents, moxifloxacin (Avelox) and trovafloxacin (Trovan), are highly effective against anaerobes. Recent studies suggest that some fluoroquinolones may be effective against *M. tuberculosis*.

A major advantage of the fluoroquinolones is that most are well absorbed orally and may be administered either once or twice a day. Although they may be taken with food, they should not be taken concurrently with multivitamins or mineral supplements because calcium, magnesium, iron, or zinc ions can reduce absorption of some fluoroquinolones by as much as 90%.

Fluoroquinolones are safe for most clients, with nausea, vomiting, and diarrhea being the most common side effects. The most serious adverse effects are dysrhythmias (gatifloxacin and moxifloxacin) and liver failure (trovafloxacin). Central nervous system effects such as dizziness, headache, and sleep disturbances affect 1% to 8% of clients. Because animal studies have suggested that fluoroquinolones affect cartilage development, use in children must be monitored carefully. Use in pregnancy or in lactating clients should be avoided.

Pr PROTOTYPE DRUG | Ciprofloxacin *(Cipro)* | Fluoroquinolone Antibiotic

ACTIONS AND USES

Ciprofloxacin, a second-generation fluoroquinolone, was approved in 1987 and is the most widely used drug in this class. By inhibiting bacterial DNA gyrase, ciprofloxacin affects bacterial replication and DNA repair. More effective against gram-negative than gram-positive organisms, it is pre-scribed for respiratory infections, bone and joint infections, GI infections, ophthalmic infections, sinusitis, and prostatitis. The drug is rapidly absorbed after oral administration and is distributed to most body tissues. Oral, intra-venous, ophthalmic, and otic formulations are available.

ADMINISTRATION ALERTS

- Administer at least 4 hours before antacids and ferrous sulfate.
- Pregnancy category C.

PHARMACOKINETICS

Onset: Rapid

Peak: 1–2 h

Half-life: 3–5 h

Duration: 12 h

ADVERSE EFFECTS

Ciprofloxacin is well tolerated by most clients, and serious adverse effects are uncommon. GI side effects, such as nausea, vomiting, and diarrhea, may occur in as many as 20% of clients. Ciprofloxacin may be administered with food to diminish adverse GI effects. The client should not, however, take this drug with antacids or mineral supplements, since drug absorption will be diminished. Some clients report phototoxicity, headache, and dizziness.

Contraindications: Ciprofloxacin is contraindicated in clients with hyper-sensitivity to drugs in the fluoroquinolone class. The drug should be discon-tinued if the client experiences pain or inflammation of a tendon, as tendon ruptures have been reported.

INTERACTIONS

Drug–Drug: Concurrent administration with warfarin may increase antico-agulant effects. This drug may increase theophylline levels 15% to 30%. Antacids, ferrous sulfate, and sucralfate decrease the absorption of ciprofloxacin. Caffeine should be restricted to prevent excessive nervous-ness, anxiety, or tachycardia.

Lab Tests: May increase values of ALT, AST, serum creatinine, and BUN.

Herbal/Food: Unknown.

Treatment of Overdose: There is no specific treatment for overdose.

 See the Companion Website for a Nursing Process Focus specific to this drug.

NURSING CONSIDERATIONS

The role of the nurse in fluoroquinolone therapy involves careful monitoring of a client's condition and providing education as it relates to the prescribed drug treatment. Assess for allergic reactions to fluoroquinolones before beginning therapy. Because these agents may decrease leukocytes, monitor the WBC count. When possible, obtain culture and sensitivity testing before beginning therapy.

These drugs are contraindicated in clients with a history of hypersensitivity to fluoroquinolones. Use with caution in clients with epilepsy, cerebral arteriosclerosis, or alcoholism because of a potential drug interaction that increases the risk of CNS toxicity. Carefully monitor clients with liver and renal dysfunction, because the drug is metabolized by the liver and excreted by the kidneys.

Give enoxacin (Penetrex) and norfloxacin (Noroxin) on an empty stomach. Antacids and ferrous sulfate may decrease the absorption of fluoroquinolones, reducing antibiotic effectiveness. Administer fluoroquinolones at least 2 hours before these drugs. Frequently monitor co-agulation studies if these antibiotics are administered concurrently with warfarin (Coumadin) because of in-teractions that may lead to increased anticoagulation effects.

Monitor urine output and report quantities of less than 1,000 ml in 24 hours. Encourage clients to drink eight or more glasses of water per day to decrease the risk of crystalluria, which irritates the kidneys. Advise clients to discontinue the drug and notify the healthcare provider if signs of hypersensitivity occur.

Inform the client that these drugs may cause dizziness and light-headedness, and advise against driving or performing hazardous tasks during drug therapy. Use with caution during pregnancy or breast-feeding because of the untoward effects caused by the passage of antimicrobials to the newborn. Safety for use by children under 18 has not been established.

Inform clients receiving norfloxacin (Noroxin) that pho-tophobia is possible. Some fluoroquinolones, such as ciprofloxacin (Cipro), may affect tendons, especially in chil-dren. Advise the client to refrain from physical exercise if calf, ankle, or Achilles pain occurs.

Client Teaching. Client education as it relates to fluoro-quinolones should include the goals of therapy; the reasons for obtaining baseline data such as lab tests, culture and sen-sitivity tests, and the existence of underlying disorders such as epilepsy; and possible drug side effects. Include the following points when teaching clients about fluoroquinolones:

- Wear sunglasses; avoid exposure to bright lights and direct sunlight when taking norfloxacin (Noroxin).
- Complete the full course of treatment.
- Immediately report signs of tendon pain or inflammation.
- Immediately report dizziness, restlessness, stomach distress, diarrhea, psychosis, confusion, or irregular or fast heart rate.

TABLE 34.8   Sulfonamides

Drug	Route and Adult Dose (max dose where indicated)	Adverse Effects
sulfacetamide (Cetamide, others)	Ophthalmic; 1–3 drops of 10%, 15%, or 30% solution into lower conjunctival sac q2–3h; may increase interval as client responds or use 1.5–2.5 cm (0.5–1.0 inch) of 10% ointment q6h and at bedtime	*Nausea, vomiting, anorexia, rash, crystalluria*
sulfadiazine (Microsulfon)	PO; Loading dose: 2–4 g; Maintenance dose: 2–4 g/day in 4–6 divided doses	<u>Anaphylaxis, Stevens–Johnson syndrome, blood dyscrasias, fulminant hepatic necrosis</u>
sulfadoxine–pyrimethamine (Fansidar)	PO; 1 tablet weekly (500 mg sulfadoxine, 25 mg pyrimethamine)	
sulfamethizole	PO; 2–4 g initially, followed by 1–2 g qid	
sulfamethoxazole (Gantanol)	PO; 2 g initially, followed by 1 g bid–tid	
sulfisoxazole (Gantrisin)	PO; 2–4 g initially, followed by 1–2 g qid	
trimethoprim–sulfamethoxazole (Bactrim, Septra)	PO; 160 mg TMP, 800 mg SMZ bid	

Italics indicate common adverse effects; <u>underlining</u> indicates serious adverse effects.

See "Nursing Process Focus: Clients Receiving Antibacterial Therapy" on page 504 for the Nursing Process applied to all antibacterials.

SULFONAMIDES

Sulfonamides are older drugs that have been prescribed for a variety of infections over the past 70 years. Although their use has declined, sulfonamides are still useful in treating susceptible UTIs. The sulfonamides are listed in Table 34.8.

34.14 Pharmacotherapy With Sulfonamides

The discovery of the sulfonamides in the 1930s heralded a new era in the treatment of infectious disease. With their wide spectrum of activity against both gram-positive and gram-negative bacteria, the sulfonamides significantly reduced mortality from susceptible microbes and earned their discoverer a Nobel Prize in Medicine in 1938. Sulfonamides suppress bacterial growth by inhibiting synthesis of the essential B-complex vitamin **folic acid** that is essential for cellular growth. These drugs are sometimes referred to as *folic acid inhibitors*. Sulfonamides are bacteriostatic and active against a broad spectrum of microorganisms.

Several factors led to a significant decline in the use of sulfonamides. Their widespread use over many decades produced a substantial number of resistant strains. The discovery of the penicillins, cephalosporins, and macrolides gave physicians greater choices of safer agents. Approval of the combination antibiotic sulfamethoxazole–trimethoprim (Bactrim, Septra) marked a resurgence in the use of sulfonamides in treating UTIs. Agents in this drug class are also prescribed for treatment of *Pneumocystis carinii* pneumonia and shigella infections of the small bowel. Sulfasalazine (Azulfidine) is a sulfonamide with anti-inflammatory properties that is prescribed for rheumatoid arthritis and ulcerative colitis.

Sulfonamides are classified by their route of administration: systemic or topical. Systemic agents, such as sulfisoxazole (Gantrisin) and sulfamethoxazole, are readily absorbed when given orally and excreted rapidly by the kidneys. Other sulfonamides, including sulfadiazine (Microsulfon), are used only for topical infections. The topical sulfonamides are not considered first-choice drugs because many clients are allergic to substances containing sulfur. One drug in this class, sulfadoxine (Fansidar) has an exceptionally long half-life and is occasionally prescribed for malarial prophylaxis.

In general, the sulfonamides are safe drugs; however, some adverse effects may be serious. Adverse effects include the formation of crystals in the urine, hypersensitivity reactions, nausea, and vomiting. Although not common, potentially fatal blood abnormalities, such as aplastic anemia, acute hemolytic anemia, and agranulocytosis, can occur.

NURSING CONSIDERATIONS

The role of the nurse in sulfonamide therapy involves careful monitoring of a client's condition and providing education as it relates to the prescribed drug treatment. Assess for anemia or other hematologic disorders, because sulfonamides may cause hemolytic anemia and blood dyscrasias owing to a genetically determined deficiency in some clients' RBCs. Assess renal function, because sulfonamides may increase the risk for crystalluria. Obtain culture and sensitivity results before initiating sulfonamide therapy. Also obtain CBC and urinalysis during therapy.

Sulfonamides are contraindicated during pregnancy and lactation and for infants younger than 2 months because of the drug's ability to promote jaundice. Use agents in this class cautiously in clients with renal impairment. Sulfonamides have a low solubility, which may cause crystals to form in the urine and obstruct the kidneys or ureters. Encourage clients to drink 3,000 ml of fluids per day to achieve a urinary output of 1,500 ml every 24 hours to decrease the possibility of crystalluria.

Cross-hypersensitivity exists with diuretics, such as acetazolamide and the thiazides, and with sulfonylurea antidiabetic agents. Avoid administering these agents in clients with a history of hypersensitivity to sulfonamides because this can induce a skin abnormality called Stevens–Johnson syndrome. Instruct the client to stop taking the drug and contact a healthcare provider if rash occurs.

Client Teaching. Client education as it relates to sulfonamides should include the goals of therapy, the reasons for obtaining baseline data such as culture and sensitivity tests and the existence of underlying renal disorders, and possible drug side effects. Include the following points when teaching clients about sulfonamides:

- Avoid exposure to direct sunlight; use sunscreen and protective clothing to decrease the effects of photosensitivity.
- Take oral medications with a full glass of water.
- Increase fluid intake to 1,500 to 3,000 ml per day unless otherwise contraindicated.
- Complete the full course of treatment.
- Immediately report abdominal or stomach cramps or pain, blood in urine, rash, confusion, difficulty breathing, and fever.

See "Nursing Process Focus: Clients Receiving Antibacterial Therapy" on page 504 for the Nursing Process applied to all antibacterials.

34.15 Miscellaneous Antibacterials

Some anti-infectives cannot be grouped into classes, or the class is too small to warrant separate discussion. That is not to diminish their importance in medicine, because some of the miscellaneous anti-infectives are critical drugs for specific infections. The miscellaneous antibiotics are listed in Table 34.9.

Clindamycin (Cleocin) is effective against gram-positive and gram-negative bacteria and is considered to be appropriate treatment when less toxic alternatives are not effective options. Susceptible bacteria include fusobacterium and *Clostridium perfringens*. Clindamycin is sometimes the drug of choice for oral infections caused by bacteroides. It is contraindicated in clients with a history of hypersensitivity to clindamycin or lincomycin, regional enteritis, or ulcerative colitis. Clindamycin is limited in use because it is associated with pseudomembranous colitis (AAPMC), the most severe adverse effect of this drug. The client should report significant side effects to the healthcare provider immediately, including diarrhea, rashes, difficulty breathing, itching, or difficulty swallowing.

Pr PROTOTYPE DRUG | Trimethoprim-Sulfamethoxazole *(Bactrim, Septra)* | Sulfonamide Antibiotic

ACTIONS AND USES

The fixed dose combination of sulfamethoxazole (SMZ) with the anti-infective trimethoprim (TMP) is most commonly used in the pharmacotherapy of urinary tract infections. It is also approved for the treatment of *Pneumocystis carinii* pneumonia, shigella infections of the small bowel, and for acute episodes of chronic bronchitis. Oral and IV preparations are available.

Both SMZ and TMP are inhibitors of the bacterial metabolism of folic acid, or folate. Their action is synergistic: a greater bacterial kill is achieved by the fixed combination than would be achieved with either drug used separately. Because humans obtain the precursors of folate in their diets and can use preformed folate, these medications are selective for *bacterial* metabolism. Another advantage of the combination is that development of resistance is lower than is observed when either of the agents is used alone.

ADMINISTRATION ALERTS

- Administer oral dosages with a full glass of water.
- Pregnancy category C.

PHARMACOKINETICS

Onset: 30–60 min

Peak: 1–4 h

Half-life: 8–12 h

Duration: Unknown

ADVERSE EFFECTS

The most common side effect of TMP-SMZ involves skin rashes, which are characteristic of sulfonamides. Nausea and vomiting are not uncommon. This medication should be used cautiously in clients with preexisting kidney disease, since crystalluria, oliguria, and renal failure have been reported. Periodic laboratory evaluation of the blood is usually performed to identify early signs of agranulocytosis or thrombocytopenia.

Contraindications: TMP-SMZ is contraindicated in clients with hypersensitivity to drugs in the sulfonamide class. Clients with documented megaloblastic anemia due to folate deficiency should not receive this drug. Clients at term and nursing mothers should not take this drug because sulfonamides may cross the placenta and are excreted in milk and may cause kernicterus.

INTERACTIONS

Drug–Drug: TMP-SMZ may enhance the effects of oral anticoagulants. These drugs may also increase methotrexate toxicity. By decreasing the hepatic metabolism of phenytoin, TMP-SMZ may cause phenytoin toxicity.

Lab Tests: Unknown.

Herbal/Food: Unknown.

Treatment of Overdose: Acidification of the urine will increase the renal elimination of trimethoprim. If signs of bone marrow depression occur during high-dose therapy, 5 to 15 mg of leucovorin should be given daily.

 See the Companion Website for a Nursing Process Focus specific to this drug.

TABLE 34.9 Selected Miscellaneous Antibacterials

Drug	Route and Adult Dose (max dose where indicated)	Adverse Effects
aztreonam (Azactam)	IM; 0.5–2.0 g bid–qid (max: 8 g/day)	*Nausea, vomiting, diarrhea, rash, fever, insomnia, cough* Anaphylaxis, superinfections
chloramphenicol (Chlorofair, others)	PO; 12.5 mg/kg qid	*Nausea, vomiting, diarrhea* Anaphylaxis, superinfections, pancytopenia, bone marrow depression, aplastic anemia
clindamycin (Cleocin)	PO; 150–450 mg qid	*Nausea, vomiting, diarrhea, rash* Anaphylaxis, superinfections, cardiac arrest, pseudomembranous colitis, blood dyscrasias
daptomycin (Cubicin)	IV; 4 mg/kg once every 24 h for 7–14 days	*Nausea, diarrhea, constipation, headache* Anaphylaxis, superinfections, myopathy, pseudomembranous colitis
ertapenem (Invanz)	IV/IM; 1 g/day	*Nausea, diarrhea, headache* Anaphylaxis, superinfections, pseudomembranous colitis, seizures
fosfomycin (Monurol)	PO; 3-g sachet dissolved in 3–4 oz of water as a single dose	*Nausea, diarrhea, back pain, headache* Anaphylaxis, superinfections
imipenem-cilastatin (Primaxin)	IV; 250–500 mg tid–qid (max: 4 g/day)	*Nausea, vomiting, diarrhea, pain at injection site, headache* Anaphylaxis, superinfections, pseudomembranous colitis
lincomycin (Lincocin)	PO; 500 mg tid–qid (max: 8 g/day)	*Nausea, vomiting, diarrhea* Anaphylaxis, superinfections, cardiac arrest, pseudomembranous colitis, blood dyscrasias
linezolid (Zyvox)	PO; 600 mg bid	*Nausea, diarrhea, headache* Anaphylaxis, superinfections, pseudomembranous colitis, blood dyscrasias
meropenem (Merrem IV)	IV; 1–2 g tid	*Nausea, vomiting, diarrhea, pain at injection site, headache* Anaphylaxis, superinfections, pseudomembranous colitis, seizures
methenamine (Mandelamine, Hiprex, Urex)	PO; 1 g bid (Hiprex) or qid (Mandelamine)	*Nausea, vomiting, diarrhea, increased urinary urgency* Anaphylaxis, crystalluria
nitrofurantoin (Furadantin, Macrobid, Macrodantin)	PO; 50–100 mg qid	*Nausea, vomiting, anorexia, dark urine* Anaphylaxis, superinfections, hepatic necrosis, interstitial pneumonitis, Stevens–Johnson syndrome
quinupristin–dalfopristin (Synercid)	IV; 7.5 mg/kg infused over 60 min q8h	*Pain and inflammation at injection site, myalgia, arthralgia, diarrhea* Superinfections, pseudomembranous colitis

(Continued)

TABLE 34.9 Selected Miscellaneous Antibacterials *(Continued)*		
Drug	**Route and Adult Dose (max dose where indicated)**	**Adverse Effects**
telithromycin (Ketek)	PO; 800 mg/day	*Nausea, diarrhea, dizziness, headache* Superinfections, pseudomembranous colitis, hepato-toxicity, dysrhythmias
vancomycin (Vancocin, others)	IV; 500 mg qid or 1 g bid	*Nausea, vomiting* Anaphylaxis, superinfections, nephrotoxicity, ototoxicity, red-man syndrome

Italics indicate common adverse effects; underlining indicates serious adverse effects.

NURSING PROCESS FOCUS Clients Receiving Antibacterial Therapy

Assessment	Potential Nursing Diagnoses
Prior to administration: ▪ Obtain a complete health history including allergies, drug history, and possible drug interactions. ▪ Obtain specimens for culture and sensitivity before initiating therapy. ▪ Perform infection-focused physical examination including vital signs, WBC count, and sedimentation rate.	▪ Infection ▪ Injury, Risk for ▪ Knowledge, Deficient, related to disease process, transmission, and drug therapy ▪ Noncompliance, related to therapeutic regimen

Planning: Client Goals and Expected Outcomes

The client will:

▪ Report reduction in symptoms related to the diagnosed infection and have negative results for laboratory and diagnostic tests for the presenting infection.

▪ Demonstrate an understanding of the drug's action by accurately describing drug side effects and precautions.

▪ Immediately report rash, shortness of breath, swelling, fever, stomatitis, loose stools, vaginal discharge, or cough.

▪ Complete the full course of antibiotic therapy and comply with follow-up care.

Implementation

Interventions and (Rationales)	Client Education/Discharge Planning
▪ Monitor vital signs and symptoms of infection to determine antibacterial effectiveness. (Another drug or different dosage may be required.)	▪ Instruct client to notify healthcare provider if symptoms persist or worsen.
▪ Monitor for hypersensitivity reaction. (Immediate hypersensitivity reaction may occur within 2 to 30 minutes; accelerated occurs in 1 to 72 hours, and delayed after 72 hours.)	▪ Instruct client to discontinue the medication and inform healthcare provider if symptoms of hypersensitivity reaction develop, such as wheezing; shortness of breath; swelling of face, tongue, or hands; and itching or rash.
▪ Monitor for severe diarrhea. (The condition may occur owing to superinfection or the possible adverse effect of antibiotic-associated pseudomembranous colitis, or AAPMC.)	Instruct client to: ▪ Consult healthcare provider before taking antidiarrheal drugs, which could cause retention of harmful bacteria. ▪ Consume cultured dairy products with live active cultures, such as kefir, yogurt, or buttermilk, to help maintain normal intestinal flora.
▪ Administer drug around the clock. (Steady administration maintains effective blood levels.)	Instruct client to: ▪ Take medication on schedule. ▪ Complete the entire prescription even if feeling better, to prevent development of resistant bacteria.
▪ Monitor for superinfection, especially in elderly, debilitated, or immunosuppressed clients. (Increased risk for superinfections is due to elimination of normal flora.)	▪ Instruct client to report signs and symptoms of superinfection such as fever; black hairy tongue; stomatitis; loose, foul-smelling stools; vaginal discharge; or cough.
▪ Monitor intake of OTC products such as antacids, calcium supplements, iron products, and laxatives containing magnesium. (These products interfere with absorption of many antibiotics.)	▪ Advise client to consult with healthcare provider before using OTC medications or herbal products.

NURSING PROCESS FOCUS Clients Receiving Antibacterial Therapy *(Continued)*	
Implementation	
Interventions and (Rationales)	**Client Education/Discharge Planning**
▪ Monitor for photosensitivity. (Tetracyclines, fluoroquinolones, and sulfon-amides can increase client's sensitivity to ultraviolet light and increase risk of sunburn.)	Encourage client to: ▪ Avoid direct exposure to sunlight during and after therapy. ▪ Wear protective clothing, sunglasses, and sunscreen when in the sun.
▪ Determine the interactions of the prescribed antibiotics with various foods and beverages. (Certain food and beverages will interfere with the medication's effectiveness.)	Instruct client regarding foods and beverages that should be avoided with specific antibiotic therapies, including: ▪ No acidic fruit juices with penicillins. ▪ No alcohol intake with cephalosporins. ▪ No dairy/calcium products with tetracyclines.
▪ Monitor IV site for signs and symptoms of tissue irritation, severe pain, and extravasation. (These are signs of infiltration.)	▪ Instruct client to report pain or other symptoms of discomfort immediately during intravenous infusion.
▪ Monitor for side effects specific to various antibiotic therapies. (See "Nursing Considerations" for each antibiotic classification in this chapter.)	▪ Instruct client to report side effects specific to the prescribed antibiotic therapy.
▪ Monitor renal function such as intake and output ratios and urine color and consistency. Monitor lab work including serum creatinine and BUN. (Some antibiotics such as the aminoglycosides are nephrotoxic.)	▪ Explain the purpose of required laboratory tests and scheduled follow-up with healthcare provider. ▪ Instruct client to increase fluid intake to 2,000 to 3,000 ml/day.
▪ Monitor for symptoms of ototoxicity. (Some antibiotics, such as the aminogly-cosides and vancomycin, may cause vestibular or auditory nerve damage.)	Instruct client to notify healthcare provider of: ▪ Changes in hearing, ringing in ears, or full feeling in the ears. ▪ Nausea and vomiting with motion, ataxia, nystagmus, or dizziness.
▪ Monitor client for compliance with antibiotic therapy. (Adhering to prescribing guidelines increase drug's effectiveness.)	Instruct client about the importance of: ▪ Completing the prescription as ordered. ▪ Follow-up care after antibiotic therapy is completed.
Evaluation of Outcome Criteria	
Evaluate the effectiveness of drug therapy by confirming that client goals and expected outcomes have been met (see "Planning"). ▪ The client reports a reduction in symptoms and has improved laboratory results. ▪ The client demonstrates an understanding of the drug's action by accurately describing drug side effects and actions. ▪ The client accurately states signs and symptoms to be reported to the healthcare provider. ▪ The client completes the full course of therapy and complies with follow-up care.	
∞ *See Tables 34.2 through 34.9 for lists of drugs to which these nursing actions apply.*	

Metronidazole (Flagyl) is another older anti-infective that is effective against many anaerobes that are common causes of abscesses, gangrene, diabetic skin ulcers, and deep-wound infections. A relatively new use is for the treatment of *H. pylori* infections of the stomach associated with peptic ulcer disease (see Chapter 40 ∞). Metronidazole is one of only a few drugs that have dual activity against both bacteria and multicellular parasites; it is a prototype for the antiprotozoal medications in Chapter 35 ∞. When metronidazole is given orally, side effects are generally minor, the most common being nausea, dry mouth, and headache. High doses can produce neurotoxicity.

Quinupristin/dalfopristin (Synercid) is a combination drug that is the first in a new class of antibiotics called *streptogramins*. This drug is primarily indicated for treatment of vancomycin-resistant *Enterococcus faecium* infections. It is contraindicated in clients with hypersensitivity

to the drug and should be used cautiously in clients with renal or hepatic dysfunction. Hepatotoxicity is the most serious adverse effect of this drug. The client should report significant side effects to the healthcare provider immediately, including irritation, pain, or burning at the IV infusion site, joint and muscle pain, rash, diarrhea, or vomiting.

Linezolid (Zyvox) is significant as the first drug in a new class of antibiotics called the *oxazolidinones*. This drug is as effective as vancomycin against methicillin-resistant *S. aureus* (MRSA) infections. Linezolid is administered intravenously or orally. Most clients can be converted from IV to oral routes in about 5 days. Linezolid is contraindicated in clients with hypersensitivity to the drug and in pregnancy, and should be used with caution in clients who have hypertension. Cautious use is also necessary in clients taking MAOIs or serotonin reuptake inhibitors, because the drugs can interact, causing a hypertensive crisis. Linezolid can cause thrombocytopenia.

The client should report significant side effects to the healthcare provider immediately, including bleeding, diarrhea, headache, nausea, vomiting, rash, dizziness, or fever.

Vancomycin (Vancocin) is an antibiotic usually reserved for severe infections from gram-positive organisms such as *S. aureus* and *Streptococcus pneumoniae*. It is often used after bacteria have become resistant to other, safer antibiotics. Vancomycin is the most effective drug for treating MRSA infections. Because of the drug's ototoxicity, hearing must be evaluated frequently throughout the course of therapy. Vancomycin can also cause nephrotoxicity, leading to uremia. Peak and trough levels are drawn after three doses have been administered. A reaction that can occur with rapid IV administration is known as **red-man syndrome** and includes hypotension with flushing and a red rash on the face and upper body. Other significant side effects include superinfections, generalized tingling after IV administration, chills, fever, skin rash, hives, hearing loss, and nausea.

In September 2003, the cyclic lipopeptides, the first in a new class of antibiotics, were approved. Daptomycin (Cubicin) is approved for the treatment of serious skin and skin-structure infections such as major abscesses, postsurgical skin-wound infections, and infected ulcers caused by *S. aureus, Streptococcus pyogenes, Streptococcus agalactiae,* and *E. faecalis.* The most common side effects are GI distress, injection site reactions, fever, headache, dizziness, insomnia, and rash.

Imipenem (Primaxin), ertapenem (Invanz), and meropenem (Merrem IV) belong to a newer class of antibiotics called *carbapenems.* These drugs are bacteriocidal and have some of the broadest antimicrobial spectrums of any class of antibiotics. Of the three carbapenems, imipenem has the broadest antimicrobial spectrum and is the most widely used. Imipenem is always administered in a fixed-dose combination with cilastatin, which increases the serum levels of the antibiotic. Meropenem is approved only for peritonitis and bacterial meningitis. Ertapenem has a narrower spectrum but longer half-life than the other carbapenems. It is approved for the treatment of serious abdominopelvic and skin infections, community-acquired pneumonia, and complicated UTI. All the carbapenems exhibit a low incidence of adverse effects. Diarrhea, nausea, rashes, and thrombophlebitis at injection sites are the most common side effects.

In 2004, the FDA approved telithromycin (Ketek), the first in a novel class of antibiotics known as the *ketolides,* for respiratory infections. Its indications include acute bacterial exacerbation of chronic bronchitis, acute bacterial sinusitis, and community-acquired pneumonia due to *S. pneumoniae.* Telithromycin is an oral drug, and its most common side effects are diarrhea, nausea, and headache. Because of the drug's recent approval, resistance is not yet a clinical problem.

Another "first in class" antibiotic is tigecycline (Tygacil), belonging to a new group known as the *glycylcyclines.* Tigecycline is approved for drug-resistant intra-abdominal infections and complicated skin and skin-structure infections, especially those caused by MRSA. The glycylcyclines are structurally similar to tetracyclines and have some of the same side effects, including teeth discoloration in children. They do not, however, exhibit cross-resistance with the tetracyclines or any other class of antibiotics. Nausea and vomiting are the most common adverse effects. Tigecycline is available by IV infusion.

TUBERCULOSIS

Tuberculosis (TB), caused by *Mycobacterium tuberculosis,* is a major worldwide health challenge. The incidence is staggering: more than 1.8 billion people, or 32% of the world population, are believed to be infected. When active, tuberculosis is easily transmitted from person to person through coughing, sneezing, or contaminated sputum. It is treated with multiple anti-infectives for a prolonged period. The antitubercular agents are listed in Table 34.10.

34.16 Pharmacotherapy of Tuberculosis

Although *M. tuberculosis* typically invades the lung, it may travel to other body systems, particularly bone, via the blood or lymphatic system. *M. tuberculosis* activates the body's immune defenses, which attempt to isolate the pathogens by creating a wall around them. The slow-growing mycobacteria usually become dormant, existing inside cavities called **tubercles.** They may remain dormant during an entire lifetime, or become reactivated if the client's immune response becomes suppressed. Because of the immune suppression characteristic of AIDS, the incidence of TB greatly increased from 1985 to 1992; as many as 20% of all AIDS clients develop active tuberculosis infections. The overall incidence of TB, however, has been declining in the United States since 1992, owing to the improved pharmacotherapy of HIV-AIDS.

Drug therapy of TB differs from that of most other infections. Mycobacteria have a cell wall that is resistant to penetration by anti-infective drugs. For medications to reach the isolated microorganisms in the tubercles, therapy must continue for 6 to 12 months. Although the client may not be infectious this entire time and may have no symptoms, it is critical that therapy continue for the entire period. Some clients develop multidrug-resistant infections and require therapy for as long as 24 months.

A second difference in the pharmacotherapy of tuberculosis is that at least two, and sometimes four or more, antibiotics are administered concurrently. During the 6- to 24-month treatment period, different combinations of drugs may be used. Multiple drug therapy is necessary because the mycobacteria grow slowly, and resistance is common. Using multiple drugs in different combinations during the long treatment period lowers the potential for resistance and increases the success of the therapy. There are two broad categories of antitubercular agents. One category consists of primary, first-line drugs, which are

TABLE 34.10   Antituberculosis Drugs

Drug	Route and Adult Dose (max dose where indicated)	Adverse Effects
FIRST-LINE AGENTS		
ethambutol (Myambutol)	PO; 15–25 mg/kg/day	*Nausea, vomiting, headache, dizziness* Anaphylaxis, optic neuritis
ⓟ isoniazid (INH, others)	PO; 15 mg/kg/day	*Nausea, vomiting, diarrhea, epigastric pain* Anaphylaxis, peripheral neuropathy, optic neuritis, hepatotoxicity, blood dyscrasias
pyrazinamide (PZA)	PO; 5–15 mg/kg tid–qid (max: 2 g/day)	*Gouty arthritis, increase in serum uric acid, rash* Anaphylaxis, hepatotoxicity, fatal hemoptysis, hemolytic anemia
rifampin (Rifadin, Rimactane)	PO; 600 mg/day as a single dose	*Nausea, vomiting, heartburn, epigastric pain, anorexia, flatulence, diarrhea, cramping* Pseudomembranous colitis, acute renal failure, hepatotoxicity
rifapentine (Priftin)	PO; 600 mg twice a week for 2 mo; then once a week for 4 mo	*Nausea, vomiting, anorexia* Hyperuricemia, neutropenia, blood dyscrasias
Rifater: combination of pyrazinamide with isoniazid and rifampin	PO; 6 tablets/day (for clients weighing 121 lb or more)	(See individual drugs)
streptomycin	IM; 15 mg/kg up to 1.0 g/day as a single dose	*Nausea, vomiting, pain at injection site, drowsiness, headache* Anaphylaxis, ototoxicity, profound CNS depression in infants, respiratory depression, exfoliative dermatitis, nephrotoxicity
SECOND-LINE AGENTS		
amikacin (Amikin)	IM; 5–7.5 mg/kg as a loading dose; then 7.5 mg/kg bid	(See Table 34.6)
capreomycin (Capastat Sulfate)	IM; 1 g/day (not to exceed 20 mg/kg/day) for 60–120 days, then 1 g 2–3 times/wk	*Rash, pain and inflammation at injection site* Blood dyscrasias, nephrotoxicity, ototoxicity
ciprofloxacin (Cipro)	PO; 250–750 mg bid	(See Table 34.7)
cycloserine (Seromycin)	PO; 250 mg q12h for 2 wk; may increase to 500 mg q12h (max 1 g/day)	*Drowsiness, headache, lethargy* Convulsions, psychosis, confusion
ethionamide (Trecator-SC)	PO; 0.5–1.0 g/day divided q8–12h	*Nausea, vomiting, epigastric pain, diarrhea* Convulsions, hallucinations, mental depression
kanamycin (Kantrex)	IM; 5–7.5 mg/kg bid–tid	(See Table 34.6)
ofloxacin (Floxin)	PO; 200–400 mg bid	(See Table 34.7)

Italics indicate common adverse effects; underlining indicates serious adverse effects.

safer and generally the most effective. Secondary (second-line) drugs, more toxic and less effective than the first-line agents, are used when resistance develops. Infections due to multidrug-resistant *M. tuberculosis* can be rapidly fatal and can cause serious public health problems in some populations.

A third difference is that antitubercular drugs are extensively used for *preventing* the disease in addition to treating it. Chemoprophylaxis is initiated for close contacts of recently infected tuberculosis clients or for those who are susceptible to infections because they are immunosuppressed. Therapy usually begins immediately after a client receives a positive tuberculin test. Clients with immunosuppression, such as those with AIDS or those receiving immunosuppressant drugs, may receive chemoprophylaxis with antituberculosis drugs. A short-term therapy of 2 months, consisting of a combination treatment with isoniazid (INH) and pyrazinamide (PZA), is approved for tuberculosis prophylaxis in HIV-positive clients.

Two other types of mycobacteria infect humans. *Mycobacterium leprae* is responsible for leprosy, a disease very rare in the United States. *M. leprae* is treated with multiple drugs, usually beginning with rifampin. *Mycobacterium avium complex* (MAC) causes an infection of the lungs, most commonly observed in AIDS clients. The most effective drugs against MAC are the macrolides azithromycin (Zithromax) and clarithromycin (Biaxin).

NURSING CONSIDERATIONS

The role of the nurse in antituberculosis therapy involves careful monitoring of a client's condition and providing education as it relates to the prescribed drug treatment. Because these drugs are indicated for the tuberculosis bacilli, assess for the presence or history of a positive tuberculin skin test, a positive sputum culture, or a close contact with a person recently infected with TB. Perform a complete physical exam including vital signs. Assess the client for a history of alcohol abuse, AIDS, liver disease, or kidney disease, because many antituberculosis drugs are contraindicated in those conditions. Assess for concomitant use of immunosuppressant drugs.

Use caution in clients with renal dysfunction, pregnancy and lactation, or with a history of convulsive disorders. Also use with caution in clients having chronic liver disease or alcoholism because of the risk for hepatic injury due to the production of toxic levels of drug metabolites. Some antitubercular drugs may cause asymptomatic hyperuricemia because they can inhibit the renal excre-

---

Pr PROTOTYPE DRUG | Isoniazid *(INH)* | Antitubercular

ACTIONS AND USES

Isoniazid has been a drug of choice for the treatment of *M. tuberculosis* for many years. The drug acts by inhibiting the synthesis of mycoloic acids, which are essential components of mycobacterial cell walls. It is bacteriocidal for actively growing organisms but bacteriostatic for dormant mycobacteria. It is selective for *M. tuberculosis*. Isoniazid is used alone for chemoprophylaxis, or in combination with other antituberculosis drugs for treating active disease.

ADMINISTRATION ALERTS

- Give on an empty stomach, 1 hour after or 2 hours before meals.
- Give with meals if GI irritation occurs.
- For IM administration, administer deep IM, and rotate sites.
- Pregnancy category C.

PHARMACOKINETICS

Onset: 30 min

Peak: 1–2 h

Half-life: 1–4 h

Duration: 6–8 h

ADVERSE EFFECTS

The most common side effects of isoniazid are numbness of the hands and feet, rash, and fever. Although rare, liver toxicity is a serious and sometimes fatal adverse effect; thus, the nurse should be alert for signs of jaundice, fatigue, elevated hepatic enzymes, or loss of appetite. Liver enzyme tests are usually performed monthly during therapy to identify early hepatotoxicity. Hepatotoxicity usually appears in the first 1 to 3 months of therapy but may occur at any time during treatment.

Contraindications: Isoniazid is contraindicated in clients with hypersensitivity to the drug and in clients with severe hepatic impairment.

INTERACTIONS

Drug–Drug: Aluminum-containing antacids decrease the absorption of isoniazid. When disulfiram is taken with INH, lack of coordination or psychotic reactions may result. Drinking alcohol with INH increases the risk of hepatotoxicity. Isoniazid may increase serum levels of phenytoin.

Lab Tests: May increase values of AST and ALT.

Herbal/Food: Food interferes with the absorption of isoniazid. Foods containing tyramine may increase isoniazid toxicity.

Treatment of Overdose: Isoniazid overdose may be fatal. Treatment is mostly symptomatic. Pyridoxine (vitamin B_6) may be infused in a dose equal to that of the isoniazid overdose. The dose may be repeated several times until the client regains consciousness. Pyridoxine helps reduce seizure activity and correct metabolic acidosis.

 See the Companion Website for a Nursing Process Focus specific to this drug.

tion of uric acid, leading to gouty arthritis. Ethambutol (Myambutol) is contraindicated in clients with optic neuritis. Because some antituberculosis drugs interact with oral contraceptives and decrease their effectiveness, female clients with childbearing potential should use an alternative form of birth control while using these medications.

Client Teaching.   Client education as it relates to antitubercular drugs should include the goals of therapy, the reasons for obtaining baseline data such as vital signs and the existence of underlying disorders, and possible drug side effects. Include the following points when teaching clients about antitubercular drugs:

- Immediately report yellow eyes and skin, loss of appetite, dark urine, or unusual tiredness.
- Take supplemental vitamin B_6 as ordered to reduce risk of adverse effects.
- If taking isoniazid, avoid foods containing tyramine, such as aged cheese, smoked and pickled fish, beer and red wine, bananas, and chocolate.
- Complete the full course of treatment.
- Wash hands frequently and cover the mouth when coughing or sneezing. Properly dispose of soiled tissues.
- If taking oral contraceptives, use an alternative form of birth control during antitubercular drug therapy.

See "Nursing Process Focus: Clients Receiving Antituberculosis Agents" on page 509 for specific teaching points.

NURSING PROCESS FOCUS   Clients Receiving Antituberculosis Agents

Assessment	Potential Nursing Diagnoses

Prior to administration:
• Obtain a complete health history including allergies, drug history, and possible drug interactions.
• Perform a complete physical examination including vital signs.
• Assess for presence or history of the following:
  • positive tuberculin skin test
  • positive sputum culture or smear
  • close contact with person recently infected with tuberculosis
  • HIV infection or AIDS
  • immunosuppressant drug therapy
  • alcohol abuse
  • liver or kidney disease
• Assess cognitive ability to comply with long-term therapy.
	• Infection, Risk for
	• Injury, Risk for, related to side effects of medication
	• Knowledge, Deficient, related to drug therapy and spread of infection
	• Noncompliance, related to therapeutic regimen

Planning: Client Goals and Expected Outcomes

The client will:
- Report reduction in tuberculosis symptoms and have negative results for laboratory and diagnostic tests indicating TB infection.
- Demonstrate an understanding of the drug's action by accurately describing drug side effects and precautions.
- Immediately report visual changes, difficulty voiding, changes in hearing, or symptoms of liver or kidney impairment.
- Complete the full course of antitubercular therapy and comply with follow-up care.

(Continued)

NURSING PROCESS FOCUS Clients Receiving Antituberculosis Agents *(Continued)*

Implementation

Interventions and (Rationales)	Client Education/Discharge Planning
▪ Monitor for hepatic side effects. (Antituberculosis agents, such as isoniazid and rifampin, cause hepatic impairment.)	▪ Instruct client to report yellow eyes and skin, loss of appetite, dark urine, and unusual tiredness.
▪ Monitor for neurological side effects such as numbness and tingling of the extremities. (Antituberculosis agents, such as isoniazid, cause peripheral neuropathy and depletion of vitamin B_6.)	Instruct client to: ▪ Report numbness and tingling of extremities. ▪ Take supplemental vitamin B_6 as ordered to reduce risk of side effects.
▪ Collect sputum specimens as directed by healthcare provider. (This will determine the effectiveness of the antituberculosis agent.)	▪ Instruct client in the proper technique needed to collect a quality sputum specimen.
▪ Monitor for dietary compliance when client is taking isoniazid. (Foods high in tyramine can interact with the drug and cause palpitations, flushing, and hypertension.)	▪ Advise clients taking isoniazid to avoid foods containing tyramine, such as aged cheese, smoked and pickled fish, beer and red wine, bananas, and chocolate.
▪ Monitor for side effects specific to various antituberculosis drugs. (Side effects should be reported to healthcare provider.)	Instruct client to report side effects specific to antituberculosis therapy prescribed: ▪ Blurred vision or changes in color or vision field (ethambutol) ▪ Difficulty in voiding (pyrazinamide) ▪ Fever, yellowing of skin, weakness, and dark urine (isoniazid, rifampin) ▪ GI system disturbances (rifampin) ▪ Changes in hearing (streptomycin) ▪ Numbness and tingling of extremities (isoniazid) ▪ Red discoloration of body fluids (rifampin) ▪ Dark concentrated urine, weight gain, edema (streptomycin)
▪ Establish infection control measures based on extent of disease condition, and established protocol. (These measures help to prevent further spread of infection.)	▪ Instruct client in infectious control measures, such as frequent handwashing, covering the mouth when coughing or sneezing, and proper disposal of soiled tissues.
▪ Establish therapeutic environment to ensure adequate rest, nutrition, hydration, and relaxation. (Symptoms of tuberculosis are manifested when the immune system is suppressed.)	▪ Teach client to incorporate health-enhancing activities, such as adequate rest and sleep, intake of essential vitamins and nutrients, and intake of six to eight glasses of water per day.
▪ Monitor client's ability and motivation to comply with therapeutic regimen. (Treatment must continue for the full length of therapy to eliminate all *M. tuberculosis* organisms.)	Explain to client the importance of complying with the entire therapeutic plan, including: ▪ Taking all medications as directed by healthcare provider. ▪ Not discontinuing medication until instructed. ▪ Wearing a medical alert bracelet. ▪ Keeping all appointments for follow-up care.

Evaluation of Outcome Criteria

Evaluate the effectiveness of drug therapy by confirming that client goals and expected outcomes have been met (see "Planning").
▪ The client reports reduction in tuberculosis symptoms and has negative lab results.
▪ The client demonstrates or understanding of the drug's actions by accurately describing drug side effects and precautions.
▪ The client accurately states signs and symptoms to be reported to the healthcare provider.
▪ The client completes the full course of therapy and complies with follow-up care.

∞ *See Table 34.10 for a list of drugs to which these nursing actions apply.*

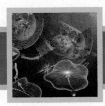

CHAPTER REVIEW

KEY CONCEPTS

The numbered key concepts provide a succinct summary of the important points from the corresponding numbered section within the chapter. If any of these points are not clear, refer to the numbered section within the chapter for review.

34.1 Pathogens are organisms that cause disease owing to their ability to divide rapidly or secrete toxins.

34.2 Bacteria are described by their shape (bacilli, cocci, or spirilla), their ability to utilize oxygen (aerobic or anaerobic), and by their staining characteristics (gram positive or gram negative).

34.3 Anti-infective drugs are classified by their chemical structures (e.g., aminoglycoside, fluoroquinolone) or by their mechanism of action (e.g., cell-wall inhibitor, folic acid inhibitor).

34.4 Anti-infective drugs act by affecting the target organism's unique structure, metabolism, or life cycle and may be bacteriocidal or bacteriostatic.

34.5 Acquired resistance occurs when a pathogen acquires a gene for bacterial resistance, either through mutation or from another microbe. Resistance results in loss of antibiotic effectiveness and is worsened by the overprescribing of these agents.

34.6 Careful selection of the correct antibiotic, through the use of culture and sensitivity testing, is essential for effective pharmacotherapy and to limit adverse effects. Superinfections may occur during antibiotic therapy if too many host flora are killed.

34.7 Host factors such as immune system status, local conditions at the infection site, allergic reactions, age, and genetics influence the choice of antibiotic.

34.8 Penicillins, which kill bacteria by disrupting the cell wall, are most effective against gram-positive bacteria. Allergies occur most frequently with the penicillins.

34.9 The cephalosporins are similar in structure and function to the penicillins and are one of the most widely prescribed anti-infective classes. Cross-sensitivity may exist with the penicillins in some clients.

34.10 Tetracyclines have some of the broadest spectrums of any antibiotic class. They are drugs of choice for Rocky Mountain spotted fever, typhus, cholera, Lyme disease, peptic ulcers caused by *Helicobacter pylori*, and chlamydial infections.

34.11 The macrolides are safe alternatives to penicillin. They are effective against most gram-positive bacteria and many gram-negative species.

34.12 The aminoglycosides are narrow-spectrum drugs, most commonly prescribed for infections by aerobic, gram-negative bacteria. They have the potential to cause serious adverse effects such as ototoxicity, nephrotoxicity, and neuromuscular blockade.

34.13 The use of fluoroquinolones has expanded far beyond their initial role in treating urinary tract infections. All fluoroquinolones have activity against gram-negative pathogens, and newer drugs in the class have activity against gram-positive microbes.

34.14 Resistance has limited the usefulness of once widely prescribed sulfonamides to urinary tract infections and a few other specific infections.

34.15 A number of miscellaneous antibacterials have specific indications, distinct antibacterial mechanisms, and related nursing care.

34.16 Multiple drug therapies are needed in the treatment of tuberculosis, since the complex microbes are slow growing and commonly develop drug resistance.

NCLEX-RN® REVIEW QUESTIONS

1 A client has been on an antibiotic for 2 weeks and has developed a superinfection. The client asks the nurse what a superinfection is. The nurse responds with:

1. "This is a secondary infection."
2. "The infection has developed an immunity to the current drug."
3. "The infection has become severe."
4. "The infection has a restricted group of microorganisms."

2 A client has been discharged with a prescription for penicillin. Discharge instructions include that:

1. Penicillins can be taken while breast-feeding.
2. The entire prescription must be finished.
3. All penicillins can be taken without regard to eating.
4. Some possible side effects include abdominal pain and constipation.

3 A client has been prescribed tetracycline. When providing information regarding this drug, the nurse would be correct in stating that tetracycline:

1. Is classified as a narrow-spectrum antibiotic.
2. Is used to treat a wide variety of disease processes.
3. Has been identified to be safe during pregnancy.
4. Is contraindicated in children younger than 8 years.

4 Important information to include in the client's education regarding taking aminoglycosides is that:

1. The drug can cause discoloration of teeth.
2. Fluid intake should be decreased to prevent urine retention.
3. This drug is primarily given orally because it is absorbed in the GI tract.
4. A serious side effect is hearing loss.

5 A client has been diagnosed with tuberculosis. While his medicine is being administered he asks questions regarding his treatment. What teaching should the nurse supply to this client? (Select all that apply.)

1. "It is critical to continue therapy for at least 6 to 12 months."
2. "Two or more drugs may be used to prevent resistance."
3. "These drugs may be used to prevent tuberculosis also."
4. "No special precautions are required."
5. "After 1 month of treatment, the medication will be discontinued."

CRITICAL THINKING QUESTIONS

1. An 18-year-old woman comes to a clinic for prenatal care. She is 8 weeks pregnant. She is healthy and takes no other medication other than low-dose tetracycline for acne. What is a priority of care for this client?

2. A 32-year-old client has a diagnosis of otitis external and the healthcare provider has ordered erythromycin PO. This client has a history of hepatitis B, allergies to sulfa and penicillin, and mild hypertension. Should the nurse give the erythromycin?

3. A 66-year-old hospitalized client has MRSA in a cellulitis of the lower extremity and is on gentamicin IV. What is a priority for the nurse to monitor in this client?

See Appendix D for answers and rationales for all activities.

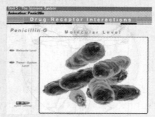

EXPLORE MediaLink

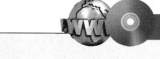

www.prenhall.com/adams

NCLEX-RN® review, case studies, and other interactive resources for this chapter can be found on the companion website at www.prenhall.com/adams. Click on "Chapter 34" to select the activities for this chapter. For animations, more NCLEX-RN® review questions, and an audio glossary, access the accompanying Prentice Hall Nursing MediaLink DVD-ROM in this textbook.

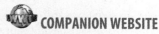

PRENTICE HALL NURSING MEDIALINK DVD-ROM

- **Animations**
  Mechanism in Action: Penicillin (*Pentids*)
  Mechanism in Action: Ciprofloxacin (*Cipro*)
- **Audio Glossary**
- **NCLEX-RN® Review**

COMPANION WEBSITE

- **NCLEX-RN® Review**
- **Dosage Calculations**
- **Case Study:** Client with tuberculosis
- **Care Plan:** Client with pneumonia treated with ceftriaxone

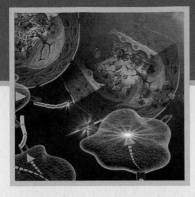

CHAPTER 35

Drugs for Fungal, Protozoal, and Helminthic Infections

DRUGS AT A GLANCE

ANTIFUNGAL DRUGS

Agents for Systemic Infections
- amphotericin B (Fungizone)
- fluconazole (Diflucan)

Agents for Superficial Infections
- nystatin (Mycostatin)

ANTIPROTOZOAL DRUGS

Antimalarial Agents
- chloroquine (Aralen)

Nonmalarial Antiprotozoal Agents
- metronidazole (Flagyl)

ANTIHELMINTHIC DRUGS
- mebendazole (Vermox)

OBJECTIVES

After reading this chapter, the student should be able to:

1. Compare and contrast the pharmacotherapy of superficial and systemic fungal infections.
2. Identify the types of clients who are at greatest risk for acquiring serious fungal infections.
3. Identify protozoal and helminthic infections that may benefit from pharmacotherapy.
4. Explain how an understanding of the *Plasmodium* life cycle is important to the effective pharmacotherapy of malaria.
5. Describe the nurse's role in the pharmacological management of fungal, protozoal, and helminthic infections.
6. For each of the classes shown in Drugs at a Glance, know representative examples, and explain their mechanism of drug action, primary actions, and important adverse effects.
7. Categorize drugs used in the treatment of fungal, protozoal, and helminthic infections based on their classification and mechanism of action.
8. Use the Nursing Process to care for clients receiving drug therapy for fungal, protozoal, and helminthic infections.

MediaLink

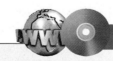

www.prenhall.com/adams

KEY TERMS

azole *page 517*

dermatophytic *page 515*

dysentery *page 526*

ergosterol *page 515*

erythrocytic stage *page 524*

fungi *page 514*

helminth *page 528*

malaria *page 524*

merozoites *page 524*

mycoses *page 515*

polyene *page 521*

protozoa *page 522*

yeast *page 514*

Fungi, protozoans, and multicellular parasites are more complex than bacteria. Because of structural and functional differences, most antibacterial drugs are ineffective against fungi. Although there are fewer drugs to treat these diseases, the available drugs are usually effective.

35.1 Characteristics of Fungi

Fungi are single-celled or multicellular organisms whose primary role on the planet is to serve as decomposers of dead plants and animals, returning their elements to the soil for recycling. Fungi include mushrooms, yeasts, and molds. Although 100,000 to 200,000 species exist in soil, air, and water, fewer than 300 are associated with disease in humans. A few species of fungi grow on skin and mucosal surfaces, as part of the normal host flora. **Yeasts,** which include the common pathogen *Candida albicans*, are unicellular fungi.

Most exposure to pathogenic fungi occurs through handling of contaminated soil or by inhalation of fungal spores. Thus, many fungal infections involve the skin, including the hair and nails, and respiratory tract. The lungs serve as a route for *invasive* fungi to enter the body and infect internal organs. An additional common source of fungal infections, especially of the mouth or vagina, is overgrowth of normal flora.

Unlike bacteria, which grow rapidly to overwhelm hosts' defenses, fungi grow slowly, and infections may progress for many months before symptoms develop. Fungi cause disease by replication; only a few secrete toxins like some bacterial species. With a few exceptions (such as athlete's foot), fungal infections are not readily transmitted through casual contact. In addition to causing infections, fungal spores may trigger a hypersensitivity response in susceptible clients, resulting in allergies to mold or mildew.

The human body is remarkably resistant to infection by these organisms, and clients with healthy immune systems experience few serious fungal diseases. Clients who have a suppressed immune system, however, such as those infected with HIV, may experience frequent fungal infections, some of which may require aggressive pharmacotherapy.

The species of pathogenic fungi that attack a host with a healthy immune system are somewhat distinct from those that infect clients who are immunocompromised. Clients with intact immune defenses are afflicted with *community-acquired* infections such as sporotrichosis, blastomycosis, histoplasmosis, and coccidioidomycosis. *Opportunistic* fungal infections acquired in a nosocomial setting are more likely to be candidiasis, aspergillosis, cryptococcosis, and mucormycosis. Table 35.1 lists the most common fungi that cause disease in humans.

PHARMFACTS

Fungal, Protozoal, and Helminthic Diseases

- Ninety percent of human fungal infections are caused by just a few dozen species.
- Of all human fungal infections, 86% are caused by *Candida albicans*. The second most common (1.3%) is caused by species of *Aspergillus*.
- Fungi cause 9% of nosocomial infections.
- Approximately 300 to 500 million cases of malaria occur worldwide each year, with an estimated 2.7 million deaths due to the disease.
- Chagas' disease, caused by *Trypanosoma cruzi*, is the most significant cause of heart disease in some South American countries. It infects 16 million people annually.
- *Ascaris lumbricoides* is the most common intestinal helminthic infection, affecting 1 billion people worldwide.

TABLE 35.1 Fungal Pathogens

Name of Fungus	Disease and Primary Organ System Affected
SYSTEMIC	
Aspergillus fumigatus, others	aspergillosis: opportunistic; most commonly affects lung but can spread to other organs
Blastomyces dermatitidis	blastomycosis: begins in the lungs and spreads to other organs
Candida albicans, others	candidiasis: most common opportunistic fungal infection; may affect nearly any organ
Coccidioides immitis	coccidioidomycosis: begins in the lungs and spreads to other organs
Cryptococcus neoformans	cryptococcosis: opportunistic; begins in the lungs but is the most common cause of meningitis in AIDS clients
Histoplasma capsulatum	histoplasmosis: begins in the lungs and spreads to other organs
Mucorales (various species)	mucormycosis: opportunistic; affects blood vessels, causes sinus infections, stomach ulcers, and others
Pneumocystis carinii (Pneumocystis jiroveci)	*Pneumocystis* pneumonia: opportunistic; primarily causes pneumonia of the lung but can spread to other organs*
SUPERFICIAL	
Candida albicans, others	candidiasis: affects skin, nails, oral cavity (thrush), vagina
Epidermophyton floccosum	athlete's foot (tinea pedis), jock itch (tinea cruris), and other skin disorders
Microsporum audouini, others	ringworm of scalp (tinea capitis)
Sporothrix schenckii	sporotrichosis: primarily affects skin and superficial lymph nodes
Trichophyton (various species)	affects scalp, skin, and nails

*Pneumocystis carinii was once believed to be a protozoan but has been reclassified as a fungus.

35.2 Classification of Mycoses

Fungal diseases are called **mycoses.** A simple and useful method of classifying mycoses is to consider them as either superficial or systemic.

Superficial mycoses affect the scalp, skin, nails, and mucous membranes such as the oral cavity and vagina. In most infections, the fungus invades only the surface layers of these regions. Mycoses of this type are often treated with topical drugs because the incidence of side effects is much lower using this route of administration. Superficial fungal infections are sometimes called **dermatophytic.**

Systemic mycoses are those affecting internal organs, typically the lungs, brain, and digestive organs. Although less common than superficial mycoses, systemic fungal infections affect multiple body systems and are sometimes fatal to clients with suppressed immune systems. Mycoses of this type often require aggressive oral or parenteral medications that produce more adverse effects than the topical agents.

Historically, the antifungal drugs used for superficial infections were clearly distinct from those prescribed for systemic infections. In recent years, this distinction has blurred, as some of the newer antifungal agents may be used for either superficial or systemic infections. Furthermore, some superficial infections may be treated with oral, rather than topical, agents. For example, nail infections are superficial, but are often treated with oral antifungal drugs. This therapeutic division between superficial and systemic mycoses is still useful, however, since it separates the pharmacotherapy of relatively benign infections (superficial) from those that may be life threatening (systemic).

35.3 Mechanism of Action of Antifungal Drugs

Biologically, fungi are classified as eukaryotes; their cellular structure and metabolic pathways are more similar to those of humans than to those of bacteria. Anti-infectives that are efficacious against bacteria are ineffective in treating mycoses because of these differences in physiology. Thus, an entirely different set of agents is needed to eliminate fungal infections.

One important difference between fungal cells and human cells is the steroid present in their plasma membranes. Whereas cholesterol is essential for animal cell membranes, **ergosterol** is present in fungi. This difference allows antifungal agents such as amphotericin B to be selective for *fungal* plasma membranes. The largest class of antifungals, the azoles, inhibits ergosterol synthesis, causing the fungal plasma membrane to become porous or leaky.

Some antifungals take advantage of enzymatic differences between fungi and humans. For example, in fungi, flucytosine (Ancobon) is converted to the toxic antimetabolite 5-fluorouracil, which inhibits both DNA and RNA synthesis in the pathogen. Humans do not have the enzyme necessary for this conversion. Indeed, 5-fluorouracil itself is a common antineoplastic drug (see Chapter 37 ∞).

DRUGS FOR SYSTEMIC ANTIFUNGAL INFECTIONS

Systemic or invasive fungal disease may require intensive pharmacotherapy for extended periods. Amphotericin B (Fungizone) and fluconazole (Diflucan) are drugs of choice. Selected systemic antifungal drugs are listed in Table 35.2.

TABLE 35.2   Drugs for Systemic Mycoses*

Drug	Route and Adult Dose (max dose where indicated)	Adverse Effects
amphotericin B (Fungizone, Abelcet, Amphotec, AmBisome)	IV; 0.25 mg/kg/day; may increase to 1 mg/kg/day or 1.5 mg/kg every other day (max: 1.5 mg/kg/ day)	*Hypokalemia, hypomagnesemia, rash, fever and chills, nausea and vomiting, anorexia, headache* Nephrotoxicity, liver failure, anaphylaxis, cardiac arrest, thrombocytopenia, leukopenia, agranulocytosis and anemia
anidulafungin (Eraxis)	IV; Loading dose 100 mg on Day 1 followed by 50 mg/day	*Minor allergic reactions such as rash, urticaria, flushing* Anaphylaxis
caspofungin acetate (Cancidas)	IV; Loading dose 70 mg infused over 1 h	*Fever, headache, infusion-related phlebitis and thrombophlebitis* Anaphylaxis
flucytosine (5-fluorocytosine, Ancobon)	PO; 50–150 mg/kg in divided doses	*Nausea, vomiting, headache* Blood dyscrasias, cardiac toxicity, renal failure, psychosis
micafungin (Mycamine)	IV; 150 mg/kg/day over 1 h for active *Candida* infection; 50 mg/kg/day IV over 1 h for *Candida* prophylaxis	*Headache, nausea, rash, phlebitis* Leukopenia, serious allergic reactions, delirium

*Azole antifungal drugs for systemic infections are included in Table 35.3.
Italics indicate common adverse effects; underlining indicates serious adverse effects.

35.4 Pharmacotherapy of Systemic Fungal Diseases

Because human immune defenses provide a formidable barrier to fungi, serious fungal infections are rarely encountered in persons with healthy body defenses. The AIDS epidemic, however, has resulted in the frequent clinical occurrence of previously rare mycoses, such as cryptococcosis and coccidioidomycosis. Opportunistic fungal disease in AIDS clients spurred the development of several new drugs for systemic fungal infections over the past 20 years. Others who may experience systemic mycoses include those clients receiving prolonged therapy with corticosteroids, experiencing extensive burns, receiving antineoplastic agents, having indwelling vascular catheters, or having recently received organ transplants. Systemic antifungal drugs have little or no antibacterial activity, and pharmacotherapy is sometimes continued for several months.

There are few drugs available for treating systemic mycoses. Amphotericin B (Fungizone) has been the drug of choice for systemic fungal infections for many years; however, this drug can cause a number of serious side effects. The newer azole drugs such as itraconazole have become drugs of choice for the treatment of less severe systemic infections. Although rarely used as monotherapy, flucytosine (Ancobon) is sometimes combined with amphotericin B in the pharmacotherapy of severe candidiasis. Flucytosine (Ancobon) can cause immunosuppression and liver toxicity, and resistance has become a major problem.

Recently, a new class of antifungals called *echinocandins* has been added to the treatments options for systemic mycoses. The first drug in this class, caspofungin, has become an important alternative to amphotericin B in the treatment of aspergillosis. Approved in 2006, anidulafungin (Eraxis) is approved for invasive candidiasis. The echinocandins are less nephrotoxic than amphotericin B and have few serious adverse effects.

NURSING CONSIDERATIONS

The role of the nurse in systemic antifungal therapy involves careful monitoring of a client's condition and providing education as it relates to the prescribed drug treatment. Prior to the initiation of therapy, obtain the client's health history. Systemic antifungal drugs are contraindicated in clients with known hypersensitivity to antifungal drugs and should be used cautiously in those with renal impairment, or severe bone marrow suppression, and in pregnancy. Obtain baseline culture and sensitivity tests prior to beginning therapy. Obtain baseline and periodic lab tests including blood urea nitrogen (BUN), creatinine, complete blood count (CBC), electrolytes, and liver function tests. Obtain vital signs, especially pulse and blood pressure, for baseline data, because clients with heart disease may develop fluid overload.

Because amphotericin B causes some degree of kidney damage in 80% of the clients who take it, closely monitor intake and output, as well as weight. Immediately report oliguria, changes in intake and output ratios, hematuria, or abnormal renal function tests to the primary care provider. Amphotericin B can cause ototoxicity: assess for hearing loss, vertigo, unsteady gait, or tinnitus.

Electrolyte imbalance is a significant side effect owing to excretion of the drug in the urine. Because hypokalemia may occur, monitor serum potassium levels and check for

Pr PROTOTYPE DRUG | Amphotericin B *(Fungizone)* | Systemic Antifungal

ACTIONS AND USES

Amphotericin B has a broad spectrum of activity that includes most of the fungi pathogenic to humans; thus, it is a drug of choice for most severe systemic mycoses. It may also be indicated as prophylactic antifungal therapy for clients with severe immunosuppression. It acts by binding to ergosterol in fungal cell membranes, causing them to become permeable or leaky. Because amphotericin B is not absorbed from the GI tract, it is normally given by IV infusion. Topical preparations are available for superficial mycoses. Treatment may continue for several months. Resistance to amphotericin B is not common.

To reduce toxicity, amphotericin B has been formulated with three lipid preparations: liposomal amphotericin B (AmBisome), amphotericin B lipid complex (Abelcet), and amphotericin B cholesteryl sulfate complex (Amphotec). The principal advantage of the lipid formulations is reduced nephrotoxicity and less infusion-related fever and chills. The lipid preparations are generally used only after therapy with other agents has failed, owing to their expense.

ADMINISTRATION ALERTS

- Infuse slowly, because cardiovascular collapse may result when the medication is infused too rapidly.
- Administer premedication to help decrease the chance of infusion reactions.
- Withhold drug if BUN exceeds 40 mg/dl or serum creatinine rises above 3 mg/dl.
- Pregnancy category B.

PHARMACOKINETICS (IV)

Onset: 1–2 h

Peak: 1–2 h

Half-life: 24–48 h

Duration: 20 h

ADVERSE EFFECTS

Amphotericin B can cause serious side effects. Many clients develop fever and chills, vomiting, and headache at the beginning of therapy, which subside as treatment continues. Phlebitis is common during IV therapy. Some degree of nephrotoxicity is observed in most clients. Electrolyte imbalances frequently occur. Cardiac arrest, hypotension, and dysrhythmias are possible.

Contraindications: The only contraindication is hypersensitivity to the drug. Caution must be observed when using amphotericin B in clients with severe renal impairment.

INTERACTIONS

Drug–Drug: Amphotericin B interacts with many drugs. Concurrent therapy with drugs that reduce renal function, such as aminoglycosides, vancomycin, or carboplatin is not recommended. Use with corticosteroids, skeletal muscle relaxants, and thiazole may potentiate hypokalemia. If hypokalemia is present, use with digoxin increases the risk of digoxin toxicity.

Lab Tests: May increase values of the following: serum creatinine, alkaline phosphatase, BUN, aspartate aminotransferase (AST), and alanine aminotransferase (ALT); may decrease values for serum potassium, calcium and magnesium.

Herbal/Food: Unknown.

Treatment for Overdose: There is no specific treatment for overdose.

---

symptoms of low potassium levels, including dysrhythmias. Evaluate all other medications taken by the client for compatibility with systemic antifungal medications. Concurrent therapy with medications that reduce liver or renal function is not recommended.

Lifespan Considerations. Because of changes in renal and liver function experienced by elderly clients, use extra caution when administering systemic antifungal drugs to this group. Check renal and liver function tests daily. Closely monitor client for changes in appetite, weight gain or loss, and changes in urine output.

Client Teaching. Client education as it relates to systemic antifungal medications should include the goals of therapy; the reasons for obtaining baseline data such as vital signs, weight, intake and output, and the existence of underlying renal or hepatic disorders; and possible drug side effects. Include the following points when teaching clients about systemic antifungal drugs:

- Complete the full course of treatment.
- Keep all scheduled appointments and laboratory visits for testing.
- Avoid alcohol use.

- Report changes in appetite, weight loss, or jaundice.
- Practice reliable contraception and notify your healthcare provider if pregnancy is planned or suspected.
- Monitor urine output and drink plenty of fluids.
- Immediately report any change in urine output, such as a decrease in frequency or amount of urine.

AZOLES

The **azole** drugs consist of two different chemical classes, the imidazoles and the triazoles. Azole antifungal drugs interfere with the biosynthesis of ergosterol, which is essential for fungal cell membranes. Depleting fungal cells of ergosterol impairs their growth. The azole drugs are listed in Table 35.3.

35.5 Pharmacotherapy With the Azole Antifungals

The azole class is the largest and most versatile group of antifungals. Drugs in this class have broad spectrums and may be used to treat nearly any fungal infection, systemic or superficial. Fluconazole (Diflucan), itraconazole (Sporanox), ketoconazole (Nizoral), and voriconazole (Vfend) are used

NURSING PROCESS FOCUS Clients Receiving Amphotericin B (*Fungizone, Abelcet*)

Assessment	Potential Nursing Diagnoses
Prior to administration: ▪ Obtain a complete health history including allergies, drug history, and possible drug interactions. ▪ Obtain a culture and sensitivity of suspected area of infection to determine need for therapy. ▪ Obtain baseline vital signs, especially pulse and blood pressure. ▪ Obtain renal function results including blood tests (CBC, chemistry panel, BUN, and creatinine).	▪ Injury, Risk for, related to adverse effects of drug ▪ Infection, Risk for, related to drug-induced leukopenia ▪ Knowledge, Deficient, related to lack of prior exposure to drug therapy ▪ Fluid Volume, Risk for Deficient, related to nausea and vomiting

Planning: Client Goals and Expected Outcomes

The client will:
- Report a reduction in symptoms related to the diagnosed infection and have negative results for laboratory and diagnostic tests for the presenting infection.
- Demonstrate an understanding of the drug's action by accurately describing drug side effects and precautions.
- Immediately report effects such as fever, chills, fluid retention, dizziness, or decrease in urine output.

Implementation

Interventions and (Rationales)	Client Education/Discharge Planning
▪ Monitor vital signs, especially pulse and blood pressure, frequently during and after infusion. (Cardiovascular collapse may result when the drug is infused too rapidly, causing the drug to bind to human cytoplasmic sterols.)	▪ Advise client to report dizziness, shortness of breath, heart palpitations, or faintness immediately.
▪ Monitor kidney function, including intake and output, urinalysis, electrolytes, BUN, creatinine and CBC. (Amphotericin B is nephrotoxic, is excreted in the urine, and causes significant renal electrolyte loss.)	Instruct client to: ▪ Keep all laboratory appointments for blood work for CBC, electrolytes every 2 weeks, and BUN and creatinine weekly. ▪ Keep an accurate record of intake and output. ▪ Drink at least 2.5 L of fluids daily. ▪ Report a decrease in urinary output, change in the appearance of urine, or weight gain or loss.
▪ Monitor for GI distress. (Symptoms may cause client to stop taking the drug and may indicate hepatotoxicity.)	Instruct client to: ▪ Take an antiemetic prior to drug therapy, if needed. ▪ Report GI distress such as anorexia, nausea, vomiting, extreme weight loss, and headache.
▪ Monitor for fluid overload and electrolyte imbalance especially hypokalemia. (Clients with cardiac disease are at high risk.)	▪ Advise clients with any form of cardiac disease to report any palpitations, chest pain, swelling of extremities, and shortness of breath.
▪ Monitor for signs/symptoms of toxicity and hypersensitivity. (Intolerance to the drug may necessitate discontinuation.)	Instruct client to report the following: ▪ IV: malaise, generalized pain, confusion, depression, hypotension, tachycardia, respiratory failure, evidence of otoxicity such as hearing loss, tinnitus, vertigo, and unsteady gait ▪ Topical: irritation, pruritus, dry skin, redness, burning, and itching
▪ Monitor IV site frequently for any signs of extravasation or thrombophlebitis. (Medication is irritating to the vein. Use a central line if possible.)	▪ Advise client to report any pain at the IV site.

Evaluation of Outcome Criteria

Evaluate the effectiveness of drug therapy by confirming that client goals and expected outcomes have been met (see "Planning").
- The client's laboratory values and symptoms indicate a decrease in fungal infection.
- The client demonstrates an understanding of the drug's action by accurately describing drug side effects and precautions.
- The client verbalizes signs and symptoms requiring notification of healthcare provider.

for both systemic and topical infections. The remainder of the azoles are prescribed for superficial infections. Ketoconazole is available only orally, and is the most hepatotoxic of the azoles. Itraconazole has begun to replace ketocona- zole in the therapy of systemic mycoses because it is less hepatotoxic and may be given either orally or intravenously. It also has a broader spectrum of activity than the other systemic azoles. Clotrimazole (Mycelex, others) is a drug of

TABLE 35.3 Azole Antifungals

Drug	Route and Adult Dose (max dose where indicated)	Adverse Effects
butoconazole (Femstat)	Topical: 1 applicator intravaginally at bedtime for 3 days	**Oral and parenteral routes:**
clotrimazole (FemCare, Gyne-Lotrimin, Mycelex, others)	Topical: apply bid for 4 wk; for vaginal mycoses, insert 1 applicator intravaginally at bedtime for 7 days	*Fever, chills, rash, dizziness, drowsiness, nausea, vomiting, diarrhea*
econazole (Spectazole)	Topical: apply bid for 4 wk	<u>Hepatotoxicity, anaphylaxis, blood dyscrasias</u>
fluconazole (Diflucan)	PO; 200–400 mg on Day 1, then 100–200 mg/day for 2–4 wk	
itraconazole (Sporanox)	PO; 200 mg/day; may increase to 200 mg bid (max: 400 mg/day)	
ketoconazole (Nizoral)	PO; 200–400 mg/day	
	Topical: apply once or twice daily to affected area	**Topical route:**
miconazole (Micatin, Monistat, Cruex, others)	Topical: apply bid for 2–4 wk	*Drying of skin, stinging sensation at application site, pruritus, urticaria, contact dermatitis*
oxiconazole (Oxistat)	Topical: apply daily in the evening for 2 mo	<u>No serious adverse effects</u>
sertaconazole (Ertaczo)	Topical; 2% cream bid for 4 wk	
sulconazole nitrate (Exelderm)	Topical: apply once or twice daily for 2–6 wk	
terconazole (Terazol)	Topical: 1 applicator intravaginally at bedtime for 3–7 wk	
tioconazole (Vagistat)	Topical: 1 applicator intravaginally at bedtime for 1 day	
voriconazole (Vfend)	IV; 6 mg/kg q12h on Day 1, then 4 mg/kg q12h; may reduce to 3 mg/kg q12h if not tolerated	

Italics indicate common adverse effects; <u>underlining</u> indicates serious adverse effects.

choice for superficial fungal infections of the skin, vagina, and mouth.

The *systemic* azole drugs have a spectrum of activity similar to that of amphotericin B, are considerably less toxic, and have the major advantage that they can be administered orally. Topical formulations are available for superficial mycoses, although they may also be given by the oral route for these infections.

The most common adverse effects of the systemic azoles are nausea and vomiting; severe nausea may require dose reduction or the concurrent administration of an antiemetic. Anaphylaxis and rash have been reported. Fatal drug-induced

---

Pr PROTOTYPE DRUG | Fluconazole *(Diflucan)* | Azole Antifungal

ACTIONS AND USES

Like other azoles, fluconazole acts by interfering with the synthesis of ergosterol. Fluconazole, however, offers several advantages over other systemic antifungals. It is rapidly and completely absorbed when given orally. Unlike itraconazole (Sporanox) and ketoconazole (Nizoral), fluconazole is able to penetrate most body membranes to reach infections in the CNS, bone, eye, urinary tract, and respiratory tract.

A major disadvantage of fluconazole is its relatively narrow spectrum of activity. Although it is effective against *Candida albicans,* it may not be effective against non–*albicans Candida* species, which account for a significant percentage of opportunistic fungal infections.

ADMINISTRATION ALERTS

- Do not mix IV fluconazole with other drugs.
- Pregnancy category C.

PHARMACOKINETICS

Onset: Unknown

Peak: 2 h

Half-life: 3–6 h

Duration: Unknown

ADVERSE EFFECTS

Fluconazole causes few serious side effects. Nausea, vomiting, and diarrhea are reported at high doses. Because most of the drug is excreted by the kidneys, it should be used cautiously in clients with preexisting kidney disease. Unlike with ketoconazole, hepatotoxicity with fluconazole is rare.

Contraindications: Fluconazole is contraindicated in clients with hypersensitivity to the drug. Coadministration with cisapride is contraindicated.

INTERACTIONS

Drug-Drug: Use of fluconazole with warfarin may cause increased risk for bleeding. Hypoglycemic reaction may be seen with oral sulfonylureas. Fluconazole levels may be decreased with concurrent rifampin or cimetidine use. The effects of fentanyl, alfentanil, or methadone may be prolonged with concurrent administration of fluconazole.

Lab Tests: Values for AST, ALT, and alkaline phosphatase may be increased.

Herbal/Food: Unknown.

Treatment of Overdose: There is no specific treatment for overdose. Dialysis can be used to lower serum drug level.

 See the Companion Website for a Nursing Process Focus specific to this drug.

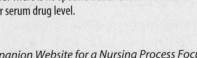

hepatitis has occurred with ketoconazole, though the incidence is rare and has not been reported with the other systemic azoles. Azoles may affect glycemic control in diabetic clients. Various reproductive abnormalities have been reported with systemic azoles, including menstrual irregularities, gynecomastia in men, and a decline in testosterone levels. Decreased libido and temporary sterility in men, are other potential side effects. The azoles should be used with caution in pregnant clients.

NURSING CONSIDERATIONS

The role of the nurse in azole therapy involves careful monitoring of a client's condition and providing education as it relates to the prescribed drug treatment. Prior to the initiation of pharmacotherapy, obtain a thorough health history. Azoles are contraindicated in clients with hypersensitivity to azole antifungals, and should be used with caution in clients with renal impairment. Obtain blood urea nitrogen (BUN), creatinine, and liver function tests before therapy begins and throughout the course of treatment. Do not give ketoconazole (Nizoral) to clients with chronic alcoholism, because additive hepatotoxicity may occur.

Because the azoles can cause GI side effects, assess for nausea, vomiting, abdominal pain, or diarrhea. Also monitor for signs and symptoms of hepatotoxicity, such as pruritus, jaundice, dark urine, and skin rash. Azoles may affect glycemic control in diabetic clients, so monitor blood sugar levels carefully in these clients. Evaluate all other medications taken by the client for compatibility with antifungal drugs. Concurrent therapy with drugs that reduce liver or renal function is not recommended. Monitor for alcohol use, because it increases the risk of side effects such as nausea and vomiting and increases blood pressure.

Client Teaching.   Client education as it relates to azole drugs should include the goals of therapy, the reasons for obtaining baseline data such as vital signs and the existence of underlying hepatic disorders, and possible drug side effects. Include the following points when teaching clients about azole drugs:

- Complete the full course of treatment.
- Report the use of any other prescription or OTC medications, herbal remedies or dietary supplements.
- Avoid alcohol use.
- Practice reliable contraception and notify your healthcare provider if pregnancy is planned or suspected.
- Monitor urine output and drink plenty of fluids.
- Immediately report increased GI distress, anorexia, weight loss, jaundice, yellow sclera, or dark urine.
- If diabetic, increase the frequency of blood glucose monitoring and report hypoglycemia.

DRUGS FOR SUPERFICIAL FUNGAL INFECTIONS

Superficial mycoses are generally not severe. If possible, superficial infections are treated with topical agents because they are safer than their systemic counterparts. Selected agents used to treat superficial mycoses are listed in Table 35.4.

35.6 Superficial Fungal Infections

Superficial fungal infections of the hair, scalp, nails, and the mucous membranes of the mouth and vagina are rarely medical emergencies. Infections of the nails and skin, for example, may be ongoing for months or even years before a client seeks treatment. Unlike systemic fungal infections, superficial infections may occur in any client, not just those who have suppressed immune systems. For example, about 75% of all adult women experience vulvovaginal candidiasis at least once in their lifetime. Athlete's foot (tinea pedis) and jock itch (tinea cruris) are two commonly experienced skin mycoses.

Superficial antifungal drugs are much safer than their systemic counterparts because penetration into the deeper layers of the skin or mucous membranes is poor, and only small amounts are absorbed into the circulation. Side effects are generally minor and limited to the region being

TABLE 35.4   Selected Drugs for Superficial Mycoses*

Drug	Route and Adult Dose (max dose where indicated)	Adverse Effects
butenafine (Mentax)	Topical: apply daily for 4 wk	*Drying of skin, stinging sensation at application site, pruritus, urticaria, contact dermatitis*
ciclopirox olamine (Loprox)	Topical: apply bid for 4 wk	
griseofulvin (Fulvicin)	PO; 500 mg microsize or 330–375 mg ultramicrosize daily	Granulocytopenia (griseofulvin), cholestatic hepatitis (oral terbinafine), neutropenia (oral terbinafine)
haloprogin (Halotex)	Topical: apply bid for 2–3 wk	
naftifine (Naftin)	Topical: apply cream daily or gel bid for 4 wk	
nystatin (Mycostatin, Nilstat, Nystex)	PO; 500,000–1,000,000 units tid; Intravaginal: 1–2 tablets daily for 2 wk	
terbinafine (Lamisil)	PO; 250 mg daily for 6–13 wk; Topical: apply once or twice daily for 7 wk	
tolnaftate (Aftate, Tinactin)	Topical: apply bid for 4–6 wk	
undecylenic acid (Fungi-Nail, Gordochom, others)	Topical: apply once or twice daily	

*Azole antifungal drugs for superficial infections are included in Table 35.3.
Italics indicate common adverse effects; underlining indicates serious adverse effects.

treated. Burning or stinging at the site of application, drying of the skin, rash, or contact dermatitis are the most frequent side effects from the topical agents.

Many agents for superficial mycoses are available as OTC creams, gels, powders, and ointments. If the infection has grown into the deeper skin layers, oral antifungal drugs may be indicated. Extensive superficial mycoses may be treated with both oral and topical antifungal agents to ensure that the infection is eliminated from deeper skin or mucous membrane layers.

Selection of a particular antifungal agent is based on the location of the infection and characteristics of the lesion. Griseofulvin (Fulvicin) is an inexpensive, older agent given by the oral route that is indicated for mycoses of the hair, skin, and nails that have not responded to conventional topical preparations. Itraconazole (Sporanox) and terbinafine (Lamisil) are oral preparations that have the advantage of accumulating in nail beds, allowing them to remain active many months after therapy is discontinued. Miconazole and clotrimazole are over-the-counter (OTC) drugs of choice for vulvovaginal candida infections, although several other drugs are equally effective. Some of the therapies for vulvovaginal candidiasis require only a single dose. Tolnaftate and undecyclenic acid are frequently used to treat athlete's foot and jock itch.

NURSING CONSIDERATIONS

The role of the nurse in superficial antifungal therapy involves careful monitoring of a client's condition and providing education as it relates to the prescribed drug treatment. Prior to the initiation of therapy with antifungals, obtain a thorough health history. Assess for signs of contact dermatitis; if this is present, withhold the drug and notify the primary healthcare provider.

Do not use superficial antifungals, such as nystatin (Mycostatin), intravaginally during pregnancy to treat infections caused by *Gardnerella vaginalis* or *Trichomonas* species. Use cautiously in clients who are lactating.

There are few side effects to antifungals used for superficial mycoses. The medications may be "swished and swallowed" when used to treat oral candidiasis. Monitor for side effects such as nausea, vomiting, and diarrhea when the client is taking high doses. If GI side effects are especially disturbing, advise client to spit out the medication rather than swallow it. Some orders will be to "swish only" and then to spit out the medication. Monitor for signs of improvement in the mouth and on the tongue to evaluate the effectiveness of the medication.

Client Teaching. Client education as it relates to superficial antifungal drugs should include the goals of therapy, the reasons for obtaining baseline data, and the possible drug side effects. Include the following points when teaching clients about superficial antifungal medications:

- Complete the full course of treatment; some infections require pharmacotherapy for several months.
- If self-treating with OTC preparations, follow the directions carefully and notify the healthcare provider if symptoms do not resolve in 7 to 10 days.

Pr **PROTOTYPE DRUG** | Nystatin *(Mycostatin)* | Superficial Antifungal

ACTIONS AND USES

Nystatin binds to sterols in the fungal cell membrane, causing leakage of intracellular contents as the membrane becomes weakened. Although it belongs to the same chemical class as amphotericin B, the **polyenes**, nystatin is available in a wider variety of formulations, including cream, ointment, powder, tablet, and lozenge. Too toxic for parenteral administration, nystatin is primarily used topically for candida infections of the vagina, skin, and mouth. It may also be used orally to treat candidiasis of the intestine, because it travels through the GI tract without being absorbed.

ADMINISTRATION ALERTS

- Apply with a swab to the affected area in infants and children, as swishing is difficult or impossible.
- For oral candidiasis, the drug should be swished in the mouth for at least 2 minutes.
- Pregnancy category C.

PHARMACOKINETICS

Onset: Unknown

Peak: Unknown

Half-life: Unknown

Duration: 6–12 h

ADVERSE EFFECTS

When given topically, nystatin produces few adverse effects other than minor skin irritation. There is a high incidence of contact dermatitis, related to the preservatives found in many of the formulations. When given orally, it may cause diarrhea, nausea, and vomiting.

Contraindications: The only contraindication is hypersensitivity to the drug.

INTERACTIONS

Drug–Drug: Unknown.

Lab Tests: Unknown.

Herbal/Food: Unknown.

Treatment of Overdose: There is no specific treatment for overdose.

 See the Companion Website for a Nursing Process Focus specific to this drug.

- Abstain from sexual intercourse until treatment for vaginal infection has been completed.
- For clients with vaginal candidiasis, use the correct method for administering vaginal suppositories, creams, and ointments.
- Perform oral hygiene before using oral lozenges or swish-and-swallow formulations.

PROTOZOAL INFECTIONS

Protozoa are single-celled animals. Although only a few of the more than 20,000 species cause disease in humans, they have a significant health impact in Africa, South America, and Asia. Travelers to these continents may acquire these infections overseas and bring them back to

NURSING PROCESS FOCUS Clients Receiving Pharmacotherapy for Superficial Fungal Infections

Assessment	Potential Nursing Diagnoses
Prior to administration: ▪ Obtain a complete health history including allergies, drug history, and possible drug interactions. ▪ Obtain a culture and sensitivity of suspected area of infection to determine need for therapy. ▪ Obtain baseline liver function tests.	▪ Injury, Risk for, rash related to side effect of drug ▪ Knowledge, Deficient, related to lack of experience with drug therapy ▪ Skin Integrity, Impaired

Planning: Client Goals and Expected Outcomes

The client will:
- Report a reduction in symptoms related to the diagnosed infection and have negative results for laboratory and diagnostic tests for the presenting infection.
- Demonstrates an understanding of the drug's action by accurately describing drug side effects and precautions.
- Immediately report hepatoxicity, GI distress, rash, or decreased urine output.
- Demonstrate correct technique for application of medication.

Implementation

Interventions and (Rationales)	Client Education/Discharge Planning
▪ Monitor for possible side effects or hypersensitivity. (Symptoms of hypersensitivity may require immediate interventions.)	Instruct client to report: ▪ Burning, stinging, dryness, itching, erythema, urticaria, angioedema, and local irritation to superficial drugs. ▪ Symptoms of hepatic toxicity—jaundice, dark urine, light-colored stools, and pruritus. ▪ Nausea, vomiting, and diarrhea. ▪ Signs and symptoms of hypoglycemia or hyperglycemia.
▪ Encourage compliance with instructions when taking oral antifungals. (Medication effectiveness increases.)	Instruct client to: ▪ Cleanse mouth by rinsing before inserting lozenge or solution. ▪ Swish the oral suspension to coat all mucous membranes, and then swallow medication. ▪ Spit out medication instead of swallowing if GI irritation occurs. ▪ Allow troche to dissolve completely, rather than chewing or swallowing; it may take 30 minutes for it to completely dissolve. ▪ Avoid food or drink for 30 minutes following administration. ▪ Remove dentures prior to using the oral suspension. ▪ Take ketoconazole with water, fruit juice, coffee, or tea to enhance dissolution and absorption.
▪ Monitor topical application and avoid occlusive dressings. (Dressings increase moisture in the infected areas and encourage development of additional yeast infections.)	Instruct client to: ▪ Cleanse the affected area with soap and water before applying medication. ▪ Avoid using the drug near open wounds and active lesions. ▪ Insert vaginal suppositories, creams, and tablets high into the vagina and remain recumbent for 1 to 15 minutes after insertion. ▪ Avoid wearing tight-fitting undergarments if using ointment in the vaginal or groin area.
▪ Monitor for contact dermatitis with topical formulations. (This side effect is related to the preservatives found in many of the formulations.)	▪ Instruct client to report any redness or skin rash.

NURSING PROCESS FOCUS Clients Receiving Pharmacotherapy for Superficial Fungal Infections *(Continued)*

Implementation

Interventions and (Rationales)	Client Education/Discharge Planning
▪ Encourage infection-control practices. (This prevents the spread of infections.)	Instruct client to: ▪ Clean affected area daily. ▪ Apply medication with a glove. ▪ Wash hands properly before and after application. ▪ Wear clean, dry socks, and change daily or more frequently if needed, if infection is on the feet.

Evaluation of Outcome Criteria

Evaluate the effectiveness of drug therapy by confirming that client goals and expected outcomes have been met (see "Planning").
▪ The client reports a reduction in symptoms and has improved laboratory results.
▪ The client demonstrates an understanding of the drug's action by accurately describing drug side effects and precautions.
▪ The client Verbalizes states effects that should be immediately reported.
▪ The client demonstrates correct application of lotion, creams, lozenges, and other topical drugs.

∞ *See Table 35.3, as well as the oral and topical systemic drugs in Table 35.2, for a list of drugs to which these nursing actions apply.*

the United States and Canada. These parasites often thrive in conditions where sanitation and personal hygiene are poor and population density is high. In addition, protozoal infections often occur in clients who are immunocompromised, such as those in the advanced stages of AIDS or who are receiving antineoplastic drugs. Agents for malarial infections are listed in Table 35.5.

TABLE 35.5 Selected Drugs for Malaria

Drug	Route and Adult Dose (max dose where indicated)	Adverse Effects
atovaquone and proguanil (Malarone)	PO; 1 tablet/day starting 1–2 days before travel, and continuing until 7 days after return	*Nausea, vomiting, abdominal pain, diarrhea, headache, myalgia* Neutropenia, hypotension
⊕ chloroquine hydrochloride (Aralen)	PO; 600 mg initial dose, then 300 mg/wk	*Nausea, vomiting and diarrhea; visual changes, including blurred vision, photophobia and difficulty focusing*
hydroxychloroquine sulfate (Plaquenil) (see page 748 for the Prototype Drug box ∞)	PO; 620 mg initial dose, then 310 mg/wk	Hemolytic anemia in clients with G6PD deficiency; irreversible retinal damage
mefloquine (Lariam)	PO; Prevention: begin 250 mg once a week for 4 wk, then 250 mg every other week Treatment: 1,250 mg as a single dose	*Vomiting, nausea, diarrhea, myalgia, dizziness, anorexia, abdominal pain* AV block, bradycardia, tachycardia, psychosis
primaquine phosphate	PO; 15 mg/day for 2 wk	*Vomiting, nausea, diarrhea, myalgia, headache, anorexia, abdominal pain* Hemolytic anemia in clients with G6PD deficiency
pyrimethamine (Daraprim)	PO; 25 mg once a week for 10 wk	*Vomiting, nausea, diarrhea, myalgia, abdominal pain* Megaloblastic anemia, leukopenia, thrombocytopenia
quinine (Quinamm)	PO; 260–650 mg tid for 3 day	*Vomiting, nausea, diarrhea* Cinchonism (tinnitus, ototoxicity, vertigo, fever, visual impairment), hypothermia, coma, cardiovascular collapse, agranulocytosis

Italics indicate common adverse effects; underlining indicates serious adverse effects.

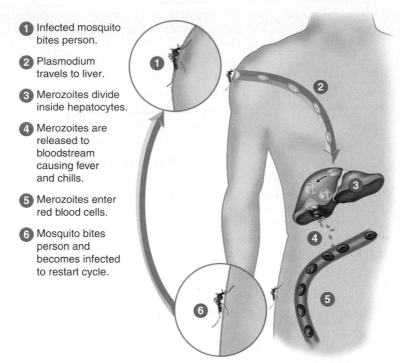

1. Infected mosquito bites person.

2. *Plasmodium* travels to liver.

3. Merozoites divide inside hepatocytes.

4. Merozoites are released to bloodstream causing fever and chills.

5. Merozoites enter red blood cells.

6. Mosquito bites person and becomes infected to restart cycle.

● **Figure 35.1** Life cycle of *Plasmodium*

35.7 Pharmacotherapy of Malaria

Drug therapy of protozoal infections is difficult because of the parasites' complicated life cycles, during which they may change form and travel to infect distant organs. When faced with adverse conditions, protozoans can form cysts that allow the pathogen to survive in harsh environments, and infect other hosts. When cysts occur inside the host, the parasite is often resistant to pharmacotherapy. With few exceptions, antibiotic, antifungal, and antiviral drugs are ineffective against protozoans.

Malaria is caused by four species of the protozoan *Plasmodium*. Although rare in the United States and Canada, malaria is the second most common fatal infectious disease in the world, with 300 to 500 million cases occurring annually.

Malaria begins with a bite from an infected female *Anopheles* mosquito, which is the *carrier* for the parasite. Once inside the human host, *Plasmodium* multiplies in the liver and transforms into progeny called **merozoites.** About 14 to 25 days after the initial infection, the merozoites are released into the blood. The merozoites infect red blood cells, which eventually rupture, releasing more merozoites, and causing severe fever and chills. This phase is called the **erythrocytic stage** of the infection. *Plasmodium* can remain in a latent state in body tissues for extended periods. Relapses may occur months, or even years, after the initial infection. The life cycle of *Plasmodium* is shown in ● Figure 35.1.

Pharmacotherapy of malaria attempts to interrupt the complex life cycle of *Plasmodium*. Although successful early in the course of the disease, therapy becomes increasingly difficult as the parasite enters different stages of its life cycle. Goals of antimalarial therapy include the following:

- *Prevention of the disease*: Prevention of malaria is the best therapeutic option, because the disease is very diffi-cult to treat after it has been acquired. The Centers for Disease Control and Prevention (CDC) recommends that travelers to infested areas receive prophylactic antimalarial drugs prior to and during their visit, and for 1 week after leaving. Proguanil (Paludrine) is the prototype antimalarial for prophylaxis.

- *Treatment of acute attacks:* Drugs are used to interrupt the erythrocytic stage and eliminate the merozoites from red blood cells. Treatment is most successful if begun immediately after symptoms are recognized. Chloroquine (Aralen) is the classic antimalarial for treating the acute stage, although resistance has become a major clinical problem in many regions of the world.

- *Prevention of relapse:* Drugs are given to eliminate the latent forms of *Plasmodium* residing in the liver. Primaquine phosphate is one of the few drugs able to effect a total cure.

NURSING CONSIDERATIONS

The role of the nurse in antimalarial therapy involves careful monitoring of the client's condition and providing education as it relates to the prescribed drug treatment. Prior to the initiation of drug therapy, obtain a thorough health history. Antimalarial drugs are contraindicated in clients with hematological disorders or severe skin disorders such as psoriasis, or during pregnancy. Use cautiously in clients with preexisting cardiovascular disease and those who are lactating.

Initial lab work includes a CBC, liver and renal function tests, and a test for G6PD deficiency (see Special Considerations, page 525). Chloroquine (Aralen) may precipitate anemia in clients with G6PD deficiency and may cause bone marrow depression. Obtain a baseline ECG because of potential cardiac complications associated with some

Pr PROTOTYPE DRUG | Chloroquine *(Aralen)* | Antimalarial

ACTIONS AND USES

Developed to counter the high incidence of malaria among American soldiers in the Pacific Islands during World War II, chloroquine has been the prototype medication for treating malaria for more than 60 years. It is effective in treating the erythrocytic stage, but has no activity against latent *Plasmodium*.

Chloroquine concentrates in the food vacuoles of *Plasmodium* residing in red blood cells. Once in the vacuoles, it is believed to prevent the metabolism of heme, which then builds to toxic levels within the parasite.

Chloroquine can reduce the high fever of clients in the acute stage in less than 48 hours. It also is used to *prevent* malaria by being administered 2 weeks before the client enters an endemic area and continuing 4 to 6 weeks after the client leaves. Although chloroquine is a drug of choice, many other agents are available, as resistance to chloroquine is common.

ADMINISTRATION ALERTS

- Pediatric dosage should be monitored closely, because children are susceptible to overdose.
- If administrating IM, inject into a deep muscle and aspirate prior to injecting medication because of its irritating effects to the tissues.
- Pregnancy category C.

PHARMACOKINETICS

Onset: 8–10 h

Peak: 3–4 h

Half-life: 1.5–2 days

Duration: Variable (several days to weeks)

ADVERSE EFFECTS

Chloroquine exhibits few serious side effects at low to moderate doses. Nausea and diarrhea may occur. At higher doses, CNS and cardiovascular toxicity may be observed. Symptoms include confusion, convulsions, reduced reflexes, hypotension, and dysrhythmias.

Contraindications: Because chloroquine can cause retinal toxicity, it is contraindicated in clients with preexisting retinal or visual field changes. It is also contraindicated in clients with renal impairment and in those with hypersensitivity to the drug.

INTERACTIONS

Drug–Drug: Antacids and laxatives containing aluminum and magnesium can decrease chloroquine absorption and must not be given within 4 hours of each other. Chloroquine may also interfere with the response to rabies vaccine.

Lab Tests: Unknown.

Herbal/Food: Unknown.

Treatment of Overdose: Overdose may be fatal. Symptomatic treatment may include anticonvulsants and vasopressors for shock. Ammonium chloride may be used to acidify the urine to hasten excretion of chloroquine.

 See the Companion Website for a Nursing Process Focus specific to this drug.

---

antimalarial drugs. Other baseline information includes vital signs, especially temperature and blood pressure, and hearing and vision testing. Evaluate all other medications taken by the client for compatibility with antimalarial medications, as drug–drug interactions are common.

During treatment, closely monitor all vital signs and obtain periodic ECGs and CBCs. Monitor for GI side effects such as vomiting, diarrhea, and abdominal pain; oral antimalarials can be given with food to reduce GI distress. Assess for signs of allergic reactions, such as flushing, rashes, edema, and pruritus. Monitor for signs of toxicity, which include tinnitus with quinine, and severe cardiac complications and/or CNS complications such as seizures and blurred vision with chloroquine.

Client Teaching. Client education as it relates to antimalarial drugs should include the goals of therapy, the reasons for obtaining baseline data such as vital signs and existence of underlying cardiac disorders, and possible drug side effects. Include the following points when teaching clients about antimalarial drugs:

- Complete the full course of treatment.
- Take the drug with food to decrease GI upset.
- Change positions slowly to avoid dizziness.
- Practice reliable contraception and notify your healthcare provider if pregnancy is planned or suspected.
- Avoid alcohol use.

- Use caution while performing hazardous activities.
- Immediately report flushing, rashes, edema, itching, ringing in the ears, blurred vision, or seizures.

35.8 Pharmacotherapy of Nonmalarial Protozoal Infections

Although infection by *Plasmodium* is the most significant protozoal disease worldwide, infections caused by other protozoans affect significant numbers of people in endemic areas. These infections include amebiasis, toxoplasmosis, giardiasis, cryptosporidiosis, trichomoniasis, trypanosomiasis, and leishmaniasis. Protozoans can invade nearly any tissue in the body. For example, *Plasmodia* prefer erythrocytes, *Giardia* the colon; and *Entamoeba* travels to the liver.

SPECIAL CONSIDERATIONS

G6PD Deficiency and Antimalarials

G6PD (glucose-6-phosphate dehydrogenase) deficiency is found in approximately 10% of African Americans and in 5% to 10% of Sephardic Jews, Greeks, Iranians, Filipinos, and Chinese. It is believed that people with this deficiency in their red blood cells may have some natural immunity to malaria. Without G6PD, chloroquine and other antimalarial drugs impair the metabolism of red blood cells and may cause acute intravascular hemolysis. If this deficiency is suspected, the client should be tested before treatment is initiated.

TABLE 35.6 Nonmalarial Protozoal Infections

Name of Protozoan	Disease and Primary Organ System Affected
Cryptosporidium (various species)	cryptosporidiosis: primarily a disease of the intestines; often seen in immunocompromised clients
Entamoeba histolytica	amebiasis: primarily a disease of the large intestine that may cause liver abscesses; rarely travels to other organs such as the brain, lungs, or kidneys
Giardia lamblia	giardiasis: primarily a disease of the intestines that may cause malabsorption, gas, and abdominal distension
Leishmania (various species)	leishmaniasis: affects various body systems including the skin, liver, spleen, or blood, depending on the species
Toxoplasma gondii	toxoplasmosis: causes a fatal encephalitis in immunocompromised clients
Trichomonas vaginalis	trichomoniasis: causes inflammation of the vagina and urethra and is spread through sexual contact
Trypanosoma brucei	trypanosomiasis: the African form, known as *sleeping sickness,* causes CNS depression in severe infections; the American form, known as *Chagas' disease,* invades cardiac tissue

Like *Plasmodium,* the nonmalarial protozoal infections occur more frequently in areas where public sanitation is poor and population density is high. Drinking water may not be disinfected before consumption and may be contaminated with pathogens from human waste. In regions with poor sanitation, infectious diseases are endemic and contribute significantly to mortality, especially in children, who are often more susceptible to the pathogens. Several of these infections occur in severely immunocompromised clients. Each of the organisms has unique differences in its distribution pattern and physiology. Descriptions of common nonmalarial protozoal infections are given in Table 35.6.

One such protozoal infection, amebiasis, affects more than 50 million people and causes 100,000 deaths worldwide. Caused by the protozoan *Entamoeba histolytica,* amebiasis is common in Africa, Latin America, and Asia. Although primarily a disease of the large intestine, where it causes ulcers, *E. histolytica* can invade the liver and create abscesses. The primary symptom of amebiasis is amebic **dysentery,** a severe form of diarrhea. Drugs used to treat amoebiasis include those that act directly on amoebas in the intestine and those that are administered for their systemic effects on the liver and other organs. Drugs for amebiasis and other nonmalarial protozoal infections are listed in Table 35.7.

TABLE 35.7 Selected Drugs for Nonmalarial Protozoal Infections

Drug	Route and Adult Dose (max dose where indicated)	Adverse Effects
iodoquinol (Yodoxin)	PO; 630–650 mg tid for 20 days (max: 2 g/day)	*Nausea, vomiting, headache, dizziness* Loss of vision, agranulocytosis, peripheral neuropathy
metronidazole (Flagyl)	PO; 250–750 mg tid	*Dizziness, headache, anorexia, abdominal pain, metallic taste, and nausea* Seizures, peripheral neuropathy, transient leukopenia
paromomycin (Humatin)	PO; 25–35 mg/kg in 3 divided doses for 5–10 days	*Nausea, vomiting, headache, diarrhea, abdominal cramps* Ototoxicity, nephrotoxicity
pentamidine (Pentam 300, Nebupent)	IV; 4 mg/kg/day for 14–21 days; infuse over 60 min	*Cough, bronchospasm, nausea, anorexia* Leukopenia, hypoglycemia, abscess or pain at injection site, hypotension, nephrotoxicity
sodium stibogluconate (Pentostam)	IM; 20 mg/kg/day	*Nausea, vomiting, diarrhea, anorexia, cough, substernal pain* ECG changes, pneumonia, blood dyscrasias
tinidazole (Tindamax)	PO; giardiasis: 50 mg/kg in single dose (max: 2 g); amebiasis: 2 g/day for 3–5 days	*Anorexia, metallic taste, and nausea* Seizures, peripheral neuropathy, transient leukopenia
trimetrexate (Neutrexin)	IV; 45 mg/m² daily	*Nausea, vomiting, stomatitis, rash* Bone marrow suppression, thrombocytopenia

Italics indicate common adverse effects; underlining indicates serious adverse effects.

Pr PROTOTYPE DRUG | Metronidazole (Flagyl) | Antiparasitic/Amebicide

ACTIONS AND USES

Metronidazole is the prototype drug for most forms of amebiasis, being effective against both the intestinal and hepatic stages of the disease. Resistant forms of *E. histolytica* have not yet emerged as a clinical problem with metronidazole. The drug is unique among antiprotozoal drugs in that it also has antibiotic activity against anaerobic bacteria and thus is used to treat a number of respiratory, bone, skin, and CNS infections. Metronidazole is a drug of choice for two other protozoal infections: giardiasis and trichomoniasis. Topical forms of this agent are used to treat rosacea, a disease characterized by skin reddening and hyperplasia of the sebaceous glands, particularly around the nose and face. Off-label uses include the pharmacotherapy of pseudomembranous colitis, Crohn's disease, and *H. pylori* infections of the stomach.

ADMINISTRATION ALERTS

- Extended-release form must be swallowed whole.
- Contraindicated during the first trimester of pregnancy.
- Pregnancy category B.

PHARMACOKINETICS (PO)

Onset: Rapid

Peak: 1–3 h

Half-life: 6–8 h

Duration: Unknown

ADVERSE EFFECTS

The most common side effects of metronidazole are anorexia, nausea, diarrhea, dizziness, and headache. Dryness of the mouth and an unpleasant metallic taste may be experienced. Although side effects are relatively common, most are not serious enough to cause discontinuation of therapy.

Contraindications: Metronidazole is contraindicated in clients with trichomoniasis during the first trimester of pregnancy and those with hypersensitivity to the drug. Metronidazole can cause bone marrow suppression; thus, it is contraindicated for clients with blood dyscrasias.

INTERACTIONS

Drug–Drug: Metronidazole interacts with oral anticoagulants to potentiate hypoprothrombinemia. In combination with alcohol, or other medications that may contain alcohol, metronidazole may elicit a disulfiram reaction. In clients taking lithium, the drug may elevate lithium levels.

Lab Tests: May decrease values for AST and ALT.

Herbal/Food: Unknown.

Treatment of Overdose: There is no specific treatment for overdose.

 See the Companion Website for a Nursing Process Focus specific to this drug.

Although several treatment options are available, metronidazole (Flagyl) has been the traditional drug of choice for nonmalarial protozoal infections. In 2005, tinidazole (Tindamax) was approved by the FDA for treatment of trichomoniasis, giardiasis, and amebiasis. This drug is very similar to metronidazole but has a longer duration of action that allows for less frequent dosing.

NURSING CONSIDERATIONS

The role of the nurse in nonmalarial antiprotozoal drug therapy involves careful monitoring of the client's condition and providing education as it relates to the prescribed drug treatment. Prior to initiating drug therapy, obtain a thorough health history. Antiprotozoal therapy is contraindicated in clients with blood dyscrasias or active organic disease of the CNS, and during the first month of pregnancy. These drugs are contraindicated in alcoholics; the medication is not administered until more than 24 hours after the client's last drink of alcohol. Used cautiously in clients with peripheral neuropathy or preexisting liver disease, and if there is a history of bone marrow depression, because the drugs may cause leukopenia. Safety and efficacy have not been established in children.

Obtain initial lab tests including a CBC and thyroid and liver function studies. Obtain baseline vital signs and evaluate all other drugs taken by the client for compatibility with antiprotozoal drugs. Closely monitor vital signs and thyroid function during therapy, because serum iodine may increase and cause thyroid enlargement with iodoquinol (Yodoxin).

Monitor for GI distress; oral medications can be given with food to decrease the incidence of nausea and vomiting. Clients taking metronidazole (Flagyl) may complain of a dry mouth and a metallic taste. Monitor for CNS toxicity such as seizures, paresthesia, and for allergic responses such as urticaria and pruritus.

Client Teaching. Client education as it relates to nonmalarial antiprotozoal drug therapy should include the goals of therapy, the reasons for obtaining baseline data and existence of underlying conditions such as thyroid and liver disorders, and possible drug side effects. Include the following points when teaching clients about antiprotozoal therapy:

- Complete the full course of treatment.
- Take the drug with food to decrease GI upset.

SPECIAL CONSIDERATIONS

Childhood Play Areas and Parasitic Infections

Pinworms and roundworms are more commonly seen in children because many of their hygiene and play habits contribute to the transmission and reinfestation of the worms. Instruct parents and family members about ways to prevent exposure to and spread of helminths. Teach children correct hand-washing techniques, emphasizing cleansing under the nails and washing before eating and after using the toilet. Discourage placing hands in mouth and biting nails. Do not allow child to scratch the anal area. Make sure that children wear shoes when playing outside. Avoid use of sandboxes, which can be accessed by dogs or cats; keep sandboxes covered when not in use. Cleanse all fruits and vegetables before eating. Change diapers frequently and dispose of properly (out of children's reach). Do not allow children to swim in pools that allow diapered children.

TABLE 35.8   Selected Drugs for Helminthic Infections

Drug	Route and Adult Dose (max dose where indicated)	Adverse Effects
albendazole (Albenza)	PO; 400 mg bid with meals (max: 800 mg/day)	*Abnormal liver function tests, abdominal pain, nausea, vomiting* Agranulocytosis, leukopenia
diethylcarbamazine (Hetrazan)	PO; 2–3 mg/kg tid	*Headache, arthralgia, malaise* Acute allergic or inflammatory response, loss of vision, swelling of face, and itching of eyes
ivermectin (Stromectol)	PO; 150–200 mcg/kg as single dose	*Fever, pruritus, dizziness, arthralgia, lymphadenopathy* Acute allergic or inflammatory response
Ⓟ mebendazole (Vermox)	PO; 100 mg as single dose, or 100 mg bid for 3 days	*Abdominal pain, diarrhea, rash* Angioedema, convulsions
praziquantel (Biltricide)	PO; 5 mg/kg as single dose, or 25 mg/kg tid	*Headache, dizziness, malaise, fever, abdominal pain* CSF reaction syndrome
pyrantel (Antiminth)	PO; 11 mg/kg as single dose (max: 1 g)	*Nausea, tenesmus, anorexia, diarrhea, fever* No serious adverse effects

Italics indicate common adverse effects; underlining indicates serious adverse effects.

- Practice reliable contraception and notify the healthcare provider if pregnancy is planned or suspected.
- Avoid using hepatotoxic drugs including alcohol to avoid a possible disulfiram-like reaction.
- Recognize that urine may turn reddish brown as an effect of the medication.
- Have any sexual partners treated concurrently to prevent reinfection.
- Immediately report seizures, numbness in limbs, nausea, vomiting, hives, or itching.

SPECIAL CONSIDERATIONS

Parasitic Infections in Children

Many parasitic infections are common among children, with the national rates highest among children less than 5 years of age. In public health labs, the most commonly diagnosed intestinal parasite is *Giardia*. Giardiasis cases are usually associated with water-related activities such as swimming, and possibly the presence of diapers.

Children adopted from Asian countries, central and South America, and Eastern Europe also have a high rate of parasitic infection. Up to 35% of foreign-born adopted children are reported to have *Giardia lamblia*. Environments in which these children have been living, particularly orphanages, often provide favorable conditions for infectious disease. The CDC recommends that internationally adopted children undergo examination of at least one stool sample, and three stool samples if GI symptoms are present. Unfortunately, evidence has shown that in communities where helminth infections are common, whether in the United States or overseas, poor nutritional status, anemia, and impaired growth and learning in children result.

DRUGS FOR HELMINTHIC INFECTIONS

Helminths consist of various species of parasitic worms, which have more complex anatomy, physiology, and life cycles than the protozoans. Diseases due to these pathogens affect more than 2 billion people worldwide, and are quite common in areas lacking high standards of sanitation. Helminthic infections in the United States and Canada are neither common nor fatal, although drug therapy may be indicated. Drugs used to treat these infections, the antihelminthics, are listed in Table 35.8.

35.9 Pharmacotherapy of Helminthic Infections

Helminths are classified as roundworms (nematodes), flukes (trematodes), or tapeworms (cestodes). The most common helminth disease worldwide is ascariasis, which is caused by the roundworm *Ascaris lumbricoides*. In the United States, this worm is most common in the Southeast, and primarily infects children aged 3 to 8 years, since this group is most likely to be exposed to contaminated soil without proper hand washing. Enteriobiasis, an infection by the pinworm *Enterobius vermicularis*, is the most common helminth infection in the United States.

Like protozoans, helminths have several stages in their life cycle, which include immature and mature forms. Typically, the immature forms of helminths enter the body through the skin or the digestive tract. Most attach to the human intestinal tract, although some species form cysts in skeletal muscle or in organs such as the liver.

Hepatoxicity With Long-term Drug Therapies

Many of the drug therapies presented in this chapter are taken for a prolonged period and so will be taken in the home setting. Since many of the drugs are hepatotoxic, clients need to understand the importance of avoiding alcohol and other hepatotoxic drugs. It is important to determine a client's typical intake of alcohol. Inform clients that many OTC products such as cough syrups and mouthwashes can contain significant amounts of alcohol and should be avoided as well. Assess clients' use of OTC analgesics and cough/cold/flu remedies. Instruct clients to avoid or strictly limit the use of acetaminophen, which can contribute to hepatotoxicity.

Not all helminthic infections require pharmacotherapy, because the adult parasites often die without reinfecting the host. When the infestation is severe or complications occur, pharmacotherapy is initiated. Complications caused by extensive infestations may include physical obstruction in the intestine, malabsorption, increased risk for secondary bacterial infections, and severe fatigue. Pharmacotherapy is targeted at killing the parasites locally in the intestine and systemically in the tissues and organs they have invaded. Some antihelminthics have a broad spectrum and are effective against multiple organisms, whereas others are specific for a certain species. Resistance has not yet become a clinical problem with antihelminthics.

NURSING CONSIDERATIONS

The role of the nurse in antihelminthic therapy involves careful monitoring of the client's condition and providing education as it relates to the prescribed drug treatment.

Prior to the initiation of drug therapy, obtain a thorough health history. Antihelminthic therapy should be used cautiously in clients who are pregnant or lactating, have preexisiting liver disease, or are younger than age 2.

Obtain baseline vital signs and lab tests, including a CBC and liver function studies. The specific worm must be identified before treatment is initiated, by analyzing samples of feces, urine, blood, sputum, or tissue. Evaluate all other medications taken by the client for compatibility with antihelminthic drugs.

Monitor lab results and vital signs closely during therapy. Cases of leukopenia, thrombocytopenia, and agranulocytosis have been associated with the use of albendazole (Albenza). The client needs to be educated on the nature of the worm infestation, including life cycle, transmission, and course of treatment. Inform the client that some types of worms will be expelled in stool as they are eradicated.

Tea Tree Oil for Fungal Infections

Of all the herbal products reported to have antifungal properties, tea tree oil is the most studied and has the most evidence of efficacy (Martin & Ernst, 2004). Tea tree oil is made from the Australian tea tree (Melaleuca alternifolia). All applications of this herbal oil are topical. Tea tree oil is used externally for fungal infections of the skin and nails; this oil is powerful and should be diluted with another oil such as olive oil. It is effective against vaginal yeast infections (Wilson, 2005). Over-the-counter vaginal suppositories are available to treat vaginal yeast infections. Tea tree oil has also been shown to be effective in treating dandruff (Satchell, Saurajen, Bell, & Barnetson, 2002). Many tea tree oil–infused shampoos are available for the treatment of dandruff.

When tea tree oil is used in the proper dilution, side effects are mild, and may include burning and redness of the area being treated.

Pr PROTOTYPE DRUG | Mebendazole *(Vermox)* | Antihelminthic

ACTIONS AND USES

Mebendazole is used in the treatment of a wide range of helminth infections, including those caused by roundworm (*Ascaris*) and pinworm (*Enterobiasis*). As a broad-spectrum drug, it is particularly valuable in mixed helminth infections, which are common in areas having poor sanitation. It is effective against both the adult and larval stages of these parasites. It is poorly absorbed after oral administration, which allows it to retain high concentrations in the intestine. For pinworm infections, a single dose is usually sufficient; other infections require 3 days of therapy.

ADMINISTRATION ALERTS

- Drug is most effective when chewed and taken with a fatty meal.
- Pregnancy category C.

PHARMACOKINETICS

Onset: Unknown

Peak: 1–7 h

Half-life: 3–9 h

Duration: Unknown

ADVERSE EFFECTS

Because so little of the drug is absorbed, mebendazole does not generally cause serious systemic side effects. As the worms die, some abdominal pain, distension, and diarrhea may be experienced.

Contraindications: The only contraindication is hypersensitivity to the drug.

INTERACTIONS

Drug–Drug: Carbamazepine and phenytoin can increase the metabolism of mebendazole.

Lab Tests: Unknown.

Herbal/Food: High-fat foods may increase the absorption of the drug.

Treatment of Overdose: There is no specific treatment for overdose.

 See the Companion Website for a Nursing Process Focus specific to this drug.

Instruct the client to take showers rather than baths, and to change undergarments, linens, and towels daily.

Assess the client for GI symptoms such as abdominal pain and distension and diarrhea, because these symptoms may occur as worms die. Such side effects are likely to occur more frequently in clients with Crohn's disease and ulcerative colitis because of the inflammatory process in the intestine. Monitor for CNS side effects, such as drowsiness with thiabendazole (Mintezol). Allergic responses include urticaria and pruritus.

Client Teaching. Client education as it relates to antihelminthic drug therapy should include the goals of therapy, the reasons for obtaining baseline data, and possible drug side effects. Include the following points when teaching clients about antihelminthic drugs:

- Complete the full course of treatment.
- Practice reliable contraception and notify your healthcare provider if pregnancy is planned or suspected.
- Have close personal contacts treated concurrently to prevent reinfestation.
- Report itching and hives, fatigue, fever, anorexia, dark urine, and abdominal pain.

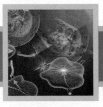

CHAPTER REVIEW

KEY CONCEPTS

The numbered key concepts provide a succinct summary of the important points from the corresponding numbered section within the chapter. If any of these points are not clear, refer to the numbered section within the chapter for review.

35.1 Fungi have more complex physiology than bacteria and are unaffected by most antibiotics. Most serious fungal infections occur in clients with suppressed immune defenses.

35.2 Fungal infections are classified as superficial (affecting hair, skin, nails, and mucous membranes) or systemic (affecting internal organs).

35.3 Antifungal medications act by disrupting aspects of growth or metabolism that are unique to these organisms.

35.4 Systemic mycoses affect internal organs and may require prolonged and aggressive drug therapy. Amphotericin B (Fungizone) is the traditional drug of choice for serious fungal infections.

35.5 The azole class of antifungal drugs has become widely used in the pharmacotherapy of both systemic and superficial mycoses owing to a favorable safety profile.

35.6 Antifungal drugs to treat superficial mycoses may be given topically or orally. They exhibit few serious side effects and are effective in treating infections of the skin, nails, and mucous membranes.

35.7 Malaria is the most common protozoal disease and requires multidrug therapy owing to the complicated life cycle of the parasite. Drugs may be administered for prophylaxis, and therapy for acute attacks and prevention of relapses.

35.8 Treatment of non-*Plasmodium* protozoal disease requires a different set of medications from those used for malaria. Other protozoal diseases that may be indications for pharmacotherapy include amebiasis, toxoplasmosis, giardiasis, cryptosporidiosis, trichomoniasis, trypanosomiasis, and leishmaniasis.

35.9 Helminths are parasitic worms that cause significant disease in certain regions of the world. The goals of pharmacotherapy are to kill the parasites locally and to disrupt their life cycle.

NCLEX-RN® REVIEW QUESTIONS

1 A client has been diagnosed with a systemic fungal infection. The physician has prescribed amphotericin B (Fungizone). The nurse will include which of the following in her client education?

1. Drug therapy will be for a very short time, probably 2 to 4 weeks.
2. Carefully inspect all intramuscular injection sites for bruising.
3. Notify the physician should you come down with symptoms of a bacterial infection.
4. Maintain a fluid intake of approximately 1,000 ml/day.

2 A client is taking quinine (Quinamm). Prior to beginning therapy, the client will need to:

1. Sign a consent form for taking this medicine.
2. Have an ECG done.
3. Stop all other medications for 24 hours.
4. Be admitted to an ICU for the first 24 hours of therapy.

3 A client has returned from South America, where malaria was contracted. The drug the nurse expects to see used is:

1. proguanil (Paludrine).
2. penicillin (Ampicillin).
3. rizatriptan (Maxalt).
4. chloroquine (Aralen).

4 The nurse is providing community education about pinworms and roundworms. Which of the following should be included in this teaching? (Select all that apply.)

1. Hand washing is very important in preventing the spread of pinworms and roundworms.
2. Play habits contribute to the transmission of pinworms and roundworms.
3. It is important that children wear shoes when playing outside.
4. Children should not be allowed to play in open sandboxes.
5. Once the child has had worms, reinfestation cannot occur.

5 Client teaching as it relates to the use of antihelminthic therapy should include:

1. Normal side effects include itching, fatigue, and abdominal pain.
2. Practicing reliable contraception is important.
3. Take medications until symptoms subside.
4. There is no potential for family members to become infected.

CRITICAL THINKING QUESTIONS

1. A nurse is caring for a severely immunosuppressed client who is on IV amphotericin B (Fungizone). The nurse understands that this medication is highly toxic to the client. What are three priority nursing assessment areas for clients on this medication?

2. A young female client recently diagnosed with insulin-dependent diabetes has been given a prescription for metronidazole (Flagyl) for a vaginal yeast infection. Identify priority teaching for this client.

3. A client is traveling to Africa for 3 months and is requesting a prescription for chloroquine (Aralen) to prevent malaria. What premedication assessment must be done for this client?

See Appendix D for answers and rationales for all activities.

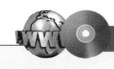

EXPLORE MediaLink

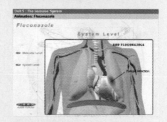

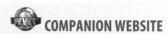

www.prenhall.com/adams

NCLEX-RN® review, case studies, and other interactive resources for this chapter can be found on the companion website at www.prenhall.com/adams. Click on "Chapter 35" to select the activities for this chapter. For animations, more NCLEX-RN® review questions, and an audio glossary, access the accompanying Prentice Hall Nursing MediaLink DVD-ROM in this textbook.

PRENTICE HALL NURSING MEDIALINK DVD-ROM

- **Animation**
  Mechanism in Action: Fluconazole (*Diflucan*)
- **Audio Glossary**
- **NCLEX-RN® Review**

COMPANION WEBSITE

- **NCLEX-RN® Review**
- **Dosage Calculations**
- **Care Plan:** Client with oropharyngeal candidiasis treated with fluconazole
- **Care Study:** Client with fungal, protozoal, and helminthic infections

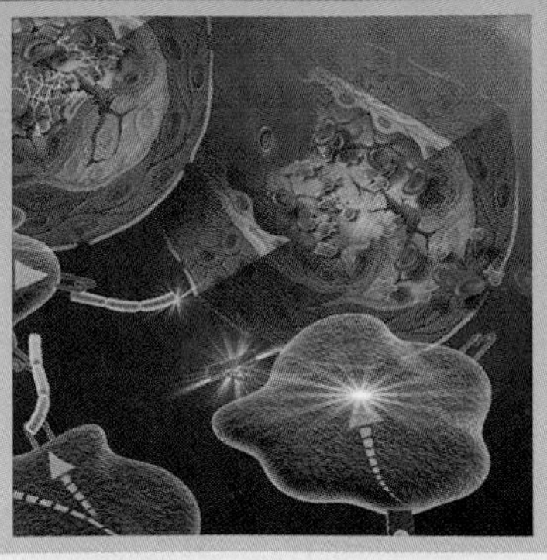

CHAPTER 36

Drugs for Viral Infections

DRUGS AT A GLANCE

AGENTS FOR HIV-AIDS

Nucleoside and Nucleotide Reverse Transcriptase Inhibitors

zidovudine (Retrovir, AZT)

Nonnucleoside Reverse Transcriptase Inhibitors

nevirapine (Viramune)

Protease Inhibitors

saquinavir mesylate (Fortovase, Invirase)

Fusion Inhibitors

AGENTS FOR HERPESVIRUSES

acyclovir (Zovirax)

AGENTS FOR INFLUENZA VIRUS

AGENTS FOR HEPATITIS VIRUS

Antivirals for Hepatitis

Interferons

OBJECTIVES

After reading this chapter, the student should be able to:

1. Describe the major structural components of viruses.
2. Identify viral infections that benefit from pharmacotherapy.
3. Explain the purpose and expected outcomes of HIV pharmacotherapy.
4. Explain the advantages of HAART in the pharmacotherapy of HIV infection.
5. Describe the nurse's role in the pharmacological management of clients receiving antiretroviral and antiviral drugs.
6. For each of the classes listed in Drugs at a Glance, know representative drugs, and explain the mechanism of drug action, primary actions, and important adverse effects.
7. Categorize drugs used in the treatment of viral infections based on their classification and mechanism of action.
8. Use the Nursing Process to care for clients receiving drug therapy for viral infections.

MediaLink www.prenhall.com/adams

NCLEX-RN® review, case studies, and other interactive resources for this chapter can be found on the companion website at www.prenhall.com/adams. Click on "Chapter 36" to select the activities for this chapter. For animations, more NCLEX-RN® review questions, and an audio glossary, access the accompanying Prentice Hall Nursing MediaLink DVD-ROM in this textbook.

KEY TERMS

acquired immune deficiency syndrome (AIDS) *page 534*

antiretroviral *page 534*

capsid *page 533*

CD4 receptor *page 534*

hepatitis *page 547*

highly active antiretroviral therapy (HAART) *page 536*

HIV-AIDS *page 534*

influenza *page 546*

intracellular parasite *page 534*

latent phase (of HIV infection) *page 535*

pegylation *page 549*

protease *page 534*

reverse transcriptase *page 534*

virion *page 533*

virus *page 533*

Viruses are tiny infectious agents capable of causing disease in humans and other organisms. After infecting an organism, viruses use host enzymes and cellular structures to replicate. Although the number of antiviral drugs has increased dramatically in recent years because of research into the AIDS epidemic, antivirals remain the least effective of all the anti-infective drug classes.

36.1 Characteristics of Viruses

Viruses are *nonliving* agents that infect bacteria, plants, and animals. Viruses contain none of the cellular organelles necessary for self-survival that are present in living organisms. In fact, the structure of viruses is quite primitive compared with that of even the simplest cell. Surrounded by a protective protein coat, or **capsid,** a virus possesses only a few dozen genes, either in the form of ribonucleic acid (RNA) or deoxyribonucleic acid (DNA), that contain the necessary information needed for viral replication. Some viruses also have a lipid envelope that surrounds the capsid. The viral envelope contains glycoprotein and protein "spikes" that are recognized as foreign by the host's immune system, and trigger body defenses to remove the invader. A mature infective particle is called a **virion.** ● Figure 36.1 shows the basic structure of the human immunodeficiency virus (HIV).

Although nonliving and structurally simple, viruses are capable of remarkable feats. They infect their host by locating and entering a target cell and then using the machinery inside that cell to replicate. Thus, viruses are **intracellular parasites:** They must be inside a host cell to cause infection. Virions do, however, bring along a few enzymes that assist the pathogen in duplicating its genetic material, inserting its genes into the host's chromosome, and assembling newly formed virions. These unique viral enzymes sometimes serve as important targets for antiviral drug action.

The viral host is often very specific; it may be a single species of plant, bacteria, or animal, or even a single type of cell within that species. Most often viruses infect only one species, although cases are documented in which viruses mutated and crossed species, as is likely the case for HIV.

Many viral infections, such as the rhinoviruses that cause the common cold, are self-limiting and require no medical intervention. Although symptoms may be annoying, they resolve in 7 to 10 days, and the virus causes no permanent effects if the client is otherwise healthy. Some viral infections, however, require

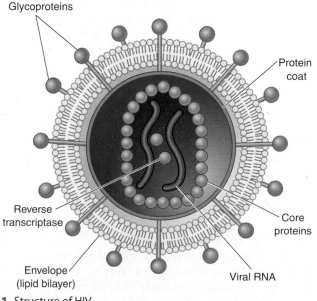

● **Figure 36.1** Structure of HIV

drug therapy to prevent the infection or to alleviate symptoms. For example, HIV is uniformly fatal if left untreated. The hepatitis B virus can cause permanent liver damage and increase a client's risk of hepatocellular carcinoma. Although not life threatening in most clients, herpesviruses can cause significant pain and, in the case of ocular herpes, permanent disability.

Antiviral pharmacotherapy can be extremely challenging because of the rapid mutation rate of viruses, which can quickly render drugs ineffective. Also complicating therapy is the intracellular nature of the virus, which makes it difficult to eliminate the pathogen without giving excessively high doses of drugs that injure normal cells. Antiviral drugs have narrow spectrums of activity, usually limited to one specific virus.

HIV-AIDS

Acquired immune deficiency syndrome (AIDS) is characterized by profound immunosuppression that leads to opportunistic infections and malignancies not commonly found in clients with healthy immune defenses. Antiretroviral drugs for **HIV-AIDS** slow the growth of the human immunodeficiency virus (HIV) by several different mechanisms. Resistance to these drugs is a major clinical problem, and a pharmacological cure for HIV-AIDS is not yet achievable.

36.2 Replication of HIV

Infection with HIV occurs by exposure to contaminated body fluids, most commonly blood or semen. Transmission may occur through sexual activity (oral, anal, or vaginal) or through contact of infected fluids with broken skin, mucous membranes, or needle sticks. Newborns can receive the virus during birth or from breast-feeding.

Shortly after entry into the body, the virus attaches to its preferred target—the **CD4 receptor** on T4 (helper) lymphocytes. During this early stage, structural proteins on the surface of HIV fuse with the CD4 receptor. The virus

uncoats, and the genetic material of HIV, single-stranded RNA, enters the cell. After entering the host cell, the RNA strands are converted to DNA by the viral enzyme **reverse transcriptase.** The viral DNA enters the nucleus of the T4 lymphocyte, where it becomes incorporated into the host's DNA. It may remain in the host's DNA for many years before it becomes activated to begin producing more viral particles. The new virions eventually bud from the host cell and enter the bloodstream. The new virions, however, are not yet infectious. As a final step, the viral enzyme **protease** cleaves some of the proteins associated with the HIV DNA, enabling the virion to infect other T4 lymphocytes. Once budding occurs, the immune system recognizes the cell is infected and kills the T4 lymphocyte. Unfortunately, it is too late; an HIV-infected client may produce as many as 10 billion new virions every day, and the client's devastated immune system is unable to remove them. Knowledge of the replication cycle of HIV is critical to understanding the pharmacotherapy of HIV-AIDS, as shown in ● Figure 36.2.

Only a few viruses such as HIV are able to construct DNA from RNA using reverse transcriptase; no bacteria, plants, or animals are able to perform this unique metabolic function. All living organisms make RNA from DNA. Because of their "backward" or reverse synthesis, these viruses are called retroviruses, and drugs used to treat HIV infections are called **antiretrovirals.** Progression of HIV to AIDS is characterized by gradual destruction of the immune system, as measured by the decline in the number of CD4 T-lymphocytes. Unfortunately, the CD4 T-lymphocyte is the primary cell coordinating the immune response. When the CD4 T-cell count falls below a certain level, the client begins to experience opportunistic bacterial, fungal, and viral diseases, and certain malignancies. A point is reached at which the client is unable to mount any immune defenses, and death ensues.

36.3 General Principles of HIV Pharmacotherapy

The widespread appearance of HIV infection in 1981 created enormous challenges for public health and an unprecedented need for the development of new antiviral drugs. HIV-AIDS is unlike any other infectious disease because it is sexually transmitted, is uniformly fatal, and demands a continuous supply of new drugs for client survival. The challenges of HIV-AIDS have resulted in the development of about 20 new antiretroviral drugs, and many others are in various stages of clinical trials. Unfortunately, the initial hopes of curing HIV-AIDS through antiretroviral therapy or vaccines have not been realized; none of these drugs produces a cure for this disease. Stopping antiretroviral therapy almost always results in a rapid rebound in HIV replication. HIV mutates extremely rapidly, and resistant strains develop so quickly that the creation of novel approaches to antiretroviral drug therapy must remain an ongoing process.

Although pharmacotherapy for HIV-AIDS has not produced a cure, it has resulted in a number of therapeutic

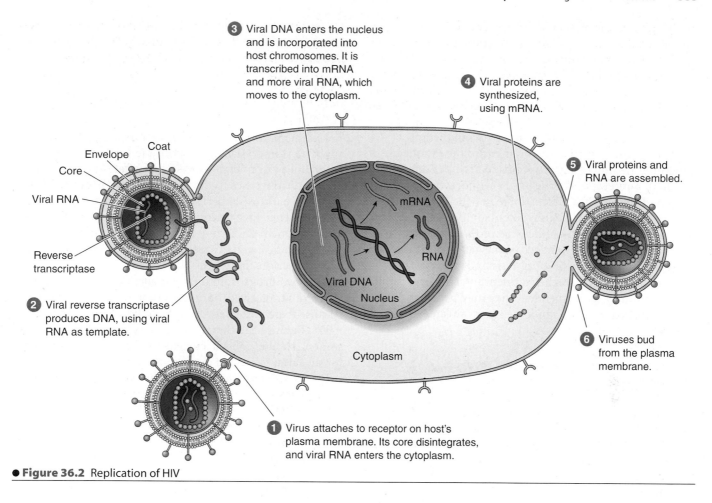

3 Viral DNA enters the nucleus and is incorporated into host chromosomes. It is transcribed into mRNA and more viral RNA, which moves to the cytoplasm.

4 Viral proteins are synthesized, using mRNA.

5 Viral proteins and RNA are assembled.

Envelope
Coat
Core
Viral RNA
Reverse transcriptase

mRNA
RNA
Viral DNA
Nucleus

2 Viral reverse transcriptase produces DNA, using viral RNA as template.

Cytoplasm

6 Viruses bud from the plasma membrane.

1 Virus attaches to receptor on host's plasma membrane. Its core disintegrates, and viral RNA enters the cytoplasm.

● **Figure 36.2** Replication of HIV

successes. For example, many clients with HIV infection are able to live symptom-free with the disease for a longer time because of medications. Furthermore, the transmission of the virus from an HIV-infected mother to her newborn has been reduced dramatically (see Section 36.7). Along with better client education and prevention, successes in pharmacotherapy have produced a 70% decline in the death rate due to HIV-AIDS in the United States. Unfortunately, this decline has not been observed in African countries, where antiviral drugs are not as readily available, largely because of their high cost. It is estimated that as many as 25 million Africans have HIV-AIDS, including more than one third of the entire adult population in several nations.

After HIV incorporates its viral DNA into the nucleus of the T4 lymphocyte, it may remain dormant for several months to many years. During this chronic **latent phase,** clients are asymptomatic and may not even realize they are infected. Once diagnosis is established, however, a decision must be made as to when to begin pharmacotherapy. The advantage of beginning during the asymptomatic stage is that the viral load or burden can be reduced. Presumably, early treatment will delay the onset of acute symptoms and the development of AIDS. Early therapy is especially critical for infants younger than 12 months, because the progression to AIDS can be rapidly fatal for these children.

Unfortunately, the decision to begin treatment during the asymptomatic phase has many negative consequences.

Drugs for HIV-AIDS are expensive; treatment with some of the newer agents costs more than $20,000 per year. These drugs produce a number of uncomfortable and potentially serious side effects that lower the quality of life for the client. Therapy over many years promotes viral resistance; thus, when the acute stage eventually develops, the drugs may no longer be effective. Because of these consequences, current protocols call for deferring treatment in adult asymptomatic clients who have CD4 T-cell counts greater than 350 cells/mcL.

The decision to begin therapy during the acute phase is much easier, because the severe symptoms of AIDS can rapidly lead to death. Thus, therapy is nearly always initiated during this phase when the CD4 T-cell count falls below 200 cells/mcL or AIDS-defining symptoms become apparent.

The therapeutic goals for the pharmacotherapy of HIV-AIDS include the following:

- Reduction of HIV RNA load in the blood to an undetectable level, or less than 50 copies/ml
- Increased lifespan
- Higher quality of life
- Decreased transmission from mother to child in HIV-infected pregnant clients

Two laboratory tests used to guide pharmacotherapy are absolute CD4 T-cell count and measurement of the amount of HIV RNA in the plasma. The number of CD4 T-cells is an important indicator of immune function and predicts the likelihood of opportunistic disease; however, it does not indicate how rapidly HIV is replicating. HIV RNA counts are better indicators of viral load and are considered more accurate measures of clinical outcome than CD4 T-cell counts. These tests are performed every 3 to 6 months to assess the degree of success of antiretroviral therapy.

At one point, physicians recommended the routine use of structured treatment interruptions (STIs): periods during which all antiretroviral drugs were withdrawn. This technique reduces adverse effects, increases the client's quality of life, and diminishes the potential for resistant HIV strains. Some research studies, however, have questioned the effectiveness of STIs; indeed, some data suggest that this strategy actually *promotes* drug resistance and hastens disease progression. Although treatment interruptions are no longer routinely recommended, they may be beneficial for certain clients, and the topic remains an area of active research.

36.4 Classification of Drugs for HIV-AIDS

Antiretroviral drugs target specific phases of the HIV replication cycle. The standard pharmacotherapy for HIV-AIDS includes aggressive treatment with multiple drugs concurrently, a regimen called **highly active antiretroviral therapy (HAART)**. The goal of HAART is to reduce the plasma HIV RNA to its lowest possible level. It must be understood, however, that HIV is harbored in locations other than the blood, such as lymph nodes; therefore, elimination of the virus from the blood is not a cure. The simultaneous use of drugs from several classes reduces the probability that HIV will become resistant to treatment. Antiretroviral therapy must be continued for the lifetime of the client. These drugs are listed in Table 36.1.

HIV-AIDS antiretrovirals are classified into the following groups, based on their mechanisms of action:

- Nucleoside reverse transcriptase inhibitor (NRTI)
- Nonnucleoside reverse transcriptase inhibitor (NNRTI)
- Protease inhibitor (PI)
- Nucleotide reverse transcriptase inhibitor (NtRTI)
- Fusion (entry) inhibitor

The last two classes include recently discovered agents that act by unique mechanisms. Tenofovir (Viread) is a nucleotide reverse transcriptase inhibitor that is structurally similar to adenosine monophosphate (AMP). After metabolism, tenofovir is incorporated into viral DNA in a manner similar to that of the NRTIs. Enfuvirtide (Fuzeon) blocks the fusion of the HIV virion to the CD4 receptor.

Research into HIV-AIDS is constantly evolving as clinicians strive to determine the most effective combinations of antiretroviral agents. Pharmacotherapeutic regimens are often different for clients who are receiving these drugs for the first time (treatment *naïve*) versus clients who have been taking antiretrovirals for months or years (treatment *experienced*). Current clinical guidelines suggest that treatment-naïve clients receive one of the following therapies:

1. A ritosnavir-boosted protease inhibitor plus two NRTIs or
2. A nonnucleoside reverse transcriptase inhibitor plus two NRTIs

Treatment failures are common with antiretroviral therapy. The primary factors responsible for treatment failure are inability to tolerate the adverse effects of the medications, nonadherence to the complex drug therapy regimen, emergence of resistant HIV strains, and genetic variability among clients. Pharmacological options available for clients with treatment failure are limited. Higher doses are generally not indicated, because they lead to an increased incidence of serious side effects. Ideally, the client is switched to at least two drugs from different chemical classes that they have not yet received, but this option is not always possible, because there are so few drug classes available to treat HIV-AIDS. Because the therapy of HIV is rapidly evolving, the student should consult current medical reference sources for the latest treatment guidelines.

Drug manufacturers have responded to the need for simpler treatment regimens by combining several medications into a single capsule or tablet. For example, one of the newer therapies combines three HIV-AIDS drugs, manufactured by two different companies. Atripla combines efavirenz, emtricitabine, and tenofovir into a fixed-dose tablet. Approved by the FDA in only 3 months, the once-daily tablet simplifies treatment and is expected to improve client compliance.

REVERSE TRANSCRIPTASE INHIBITORS (NRTIS, NNRTIS, AND NTRTIS)

Drugs in the reverse transcriptase inhibitor class are agents structurally similar to nucleosides, the building blocks of DNA. This class includes nonnucleoside reverse transcriptase inhibitors, which bind directly to the viral enzyme reverse transcriptase and inhibit its function, and nucleotide reverse transcriptase inhibitors.

36.5 Pharmacotherapy With Reverse Transcriptase Inhibitors

One of the early steps in HIV infection is the synthesis of viral DNA from the viral RNA inside the T4 lymphocyte by the enzyme reverse transcriptase. Because reverse transcriptase is a viral enzyme not found in human cells, it has been possible to design drugs able to selectively inhibit viral replication.

Viral DNA synthesis requires building blocks known as *nucleosides*. The NRTIs and NtRTIs chemically resemble naturally occurring nucleosides. Thus, as reverse transcriptase uses these drugs to build DNA, the viral DNA chain is prevented from lengthening. The "unfinished" viral DNA chain is unable to be inserted into the host chromosome.

A second mechanism for inhibiting reverse transcriptase affects the enzyme's function. Drugs in the NNRTI class act

TABLE 36.1 Antiretroviral Drugs for HIV-AIDS

Drug	Route and Adult Dose (max dose where indicated)	Adverse Effects
NONNUCLEOSIDE REVERSE TRANSCRIPTASE INHIBITORS		
delavirdine (Rescriptor)	PO; 400 mg tid	*Rash, fever, nausea, diarrhea, headache, stomatitis*
efavirenz (Sustiva)	PO; 600 mg/days	
nevirapine (Viramune)	PO; 200 mg/day for 14 days; then increase to bid	<u>Paresthesia, hepatotoxicity, Stevens–Johnson syndrome</u>
NUCLEOSIDE AND NUCLEOTIDE REVERSE TRANSCRIPTASE INHIBITORS		
abacavir (Ziagen)	PO; 300 mg bid	*Fatigue, generalized weakness, myalgia, nausea, headache, abdominal pain, vomiting, anorexia, rash*
didanosine (Videx, DDI)	PO; 125–300 mg bid	
emtricitabine (Emtriva)	PO; 200 mg/day	<u>Bone marrow suppression, neutropenia, anemia, granulocytopenia, lactic acidosis with steatorrhea, neurotoxicity, peripheral neuropathy (zalcitabine, stavudine), pancreatitis (lamivudine)</u>
lamivudine (Epivir, 3TC)	PO; 150 mg bid	
stavudine (Zerit, D4T)	PO; 40 mg bid	
tenofovir disoproxil fumarate (Viread)	PO; 300 mg/day	
zalcitabine (Hivid, DDC)	PO; 0.75 mg tid	
zidovudine (Retrovir, AZT)	PO; 200 mg q4h (1,200 mg/day); after 1 mo may reduce to 100 mg q4h (600 mg/day) IV; 1–2 mg/kg q4h (1,200 mg/day)	
PROTEASE INHIBITORS		
amprenavir (Agenerase)	PO; 1,200 mg bid	*Nausea, vomiting, diarrhea, abdominal pain, headache*
atazanavir (Reyataz)	PO; 400 mg/day	
darunavir (Prezista)	PO; 600 mg taken with ritonavir 100 mg bid	<u>Anemia, leukopenia, deep vein thrombosis, pancreatitis, lymphadenopathy, hemorrhagic colitis, nephrolithiasis (indinavir), cardiac arrest (atazanavir), thrombocytopenia (saquinavir), pancytopenia (saquinavir)</u>
fosamprenavir (Lexiva)	PO; 700–1,400 mg bid in combination with 100–200 mg ritonavir bid	
indinavir (Crixivan)	PO; 800 mg tid	
lopinavir/ritonavir (Kaletra)	PO; 400/100 mg (3 capsules or 5 ml of suspension) bid; increase dose to 533/133 mg (4 capsules or 6.5 ml) bid, with concurrent efavirenz or nevirapine	
nelfinavir (Viracept)	PO; 750 mg tid	
ritonavir (Norvir)	PO; 600 mg bid	
saquinavir (Invirase, Fortovase)	PO; 600 mg tid	
tipranavir (Aptivus)	PO; 500 mg taken with 200 mg of ritonavir bid	
FUSION INHIBITOR		
enfuvirtide (Fuzeon)	Subcutaneous; 90 mg bid	*Pain and inflammation at injection site, nausea, diarrhea, fatigue* <u>Hypersensitivity, neutropenia, thrombocytopenia, nephrotoxicity</u>

Italics indicate common adverse effects; <u>underlining</u> indicates serious adverse effects.

by binding near the active site, causing a structural change in the enzyme molecule. The enzyme can no longer bind nucleosides and is unable to construct viral DNA.

Although there are differences in their pharmacokinetic and toxicity profiles, no single NRTI or NNRTI offers a clear therapeutic advantage over any other. Choice of agent depends on client response and the experience of the clinician. Because some of these drugs, such as zidovudine (Retrovir, AZT), have been used consistently for more than 25 years, the potential for resistance must be considered when selecting the specific agent. There is a high degree of cross-resistance among the NRTIs. The NRTIs and NNRTIs are nearly always used in multidrug combinations in HAART.

As a class, the NRTIs are well tolerated, although nausea, vomiting, diarrhea, headache, and fatigue are common during the first few weeks of therapy. After prolonged therapy with NRTIs, inhibition of mitochondrial function can cause various organ abnormalities, blood disorders, lactic acidosis, and lipodystrophy, a disorder in which fat is redistributed in specific areas in the body. Areas such as the face, arms, and legs tend to lose fat, whereas the abdomen, breasts, and base of the neck (buffalo hump) develop excess fat.

Pr PROTOTYPE DRUG | Zidovudine *(Retrovir, AZT)* | Antiretroviral—NRTI

ACTIONS AND USES

Zidovudine was first discovered in the 1960s, and its antiviral activity was demonstrated prior to the AIDS epidemic. Structurally, it resembles thymidine, one of the four nucleoside building blocks of DNA. As the reverse transcriptase enzyme begins to synthesize viral DNA, it mistakenly uses zidovudine as one of the nucleosides, thus creating a defective DNA strand. Because of the drugs' widespread use since the beginning of the AIDS epidemic, resistant HIV strains have become common. Zidovudine is used in combination with other antiretrovirals for both symptomatic and asymptomatic HIV-infected clients, as well as for postexposure prophylaxis in HIV-exposed healthcare workers. An important indication is reduction of the transmission rate of HIV from an HIV-positive mother to her fetus.

ADMINISTRATION ALERTS

- Administer on an empty stomach, with water only.
- Avoid administering with fruit juice.
- Pregnancy category C.

PHARMACOKINETICS (PO)

Onset: Unknown

Peak: 1–2 h

Half-life: 1 h

Duration: Unknown

ADVERSE EFFECTS

Zidovudine can cause severe toxicity to blood cells at high doses; anemia and neutropenia are common and may limit therapy. Many clients experience anorexia, nausea, and diarrhea. Clients may report fatigue and generalized weakness.

Contraindications: Hypersensitivity to the drug is the only contraindication. It should be used with caution in clients with preexisting anemia or neutropenia.

INTERACTIONS

Drug-Drug: Zidovudine interacts with many drugs. Concurrent administration with other drugs that depress bone marrow function, such as ganciclovir, interferon alfa, dapsone, flucytosine, or vincristine should be avoided due to cumulative immunosuppression. The following drugs may increase the risk of AZT toxicity: atovaquone, amphotericin B, aspirin, doxorubicin, fluconazole, methadone, and valproic acid. Use with other antiretroviral agents may cause lactic acidosis and severe hepatomegaly with steatosis.

Lab Tests: Mean corpuscular volume may be increased during zidovudine therapy. WBC and Hgb may decrease due to neutropenia and anemia, respectively.

Herbal/Food: Use with caution with herbal supplements, such as St. John's wort, which may cause a decrease in antiretroviral activity.

Treatment of Overdose: There is no specific treatment for overdose.

 See the Companion Website for a Nursing Process Focus specific to this drug.

The NNRTIs are also generally well tolerated and exhibit few serious adverse effects. The side effects are different from those of the NRTIs. Rash is common with NNRTIs, and liver toxicity is possible, increasing the risk of drug–drug interactions. Efavirenz (Sustiva) exhibits a high incidence of CNS effects such as dizziness and fatigue, but these symptoms are rare in clients taking nevirapine. Unlike some other antiretrovirals that negatively affect lipid metabolism, nevirapine (Viramune) actually improves the lipid profiles of many clients by increasing HDL levels.

SPECIAL CONSIDERATIONS

Psychosocial Issues With Antiretroviral Drug Compliance

One key to success of an antiretroviral regimen is client compliance with the prescribed medication plan. Drug compliance is difficult for most people once they feel well; clients may be more prone to skip doses for various reasons. Many factors can enhance the probability that the client will adhere to treatment. For example, a multidisciplinary assessment can screen clients for depression, alcohol or drug abuse, or negative attitudes, and interventions can be initiated to minimize the impact on compliance. Education at an appropriate level is essential so the client can understand the disease process as well as the role the medications play in securing a positive outcome. Developing trust and open communication between the client and healthcare provider is essential to improving the chances of drug compliance and to reaching common therapeutic goals.

PROTEASE INHIBITORS

Drugs in the protease inhibitor class block the viral enzyme protease, which is responsible for the final assembly of the HIV virions.

36.6 Pharmacotherapy With Protease Inhibitors

Near the end of its replication cycle, HIV has assembled all the necessary molecular components to create new virions. HIV RNA has been synthesized using the metabolic machinery of the host cell, and the structural and regulatory proteins of HIV are ready to be packaged into a new virion.

As the newly formed virions bud from the host cell and are released into the surrounding extracellular fluid, one final step remains before the HIV is mature: a long polypeptide chain must be cleaved by the enzyme protease to produce the final HIV proteins. The protease inhibitors (PIs) attach to the active site of HIV protease, thus preventing the final maturation of the virions. Without this last step, the virions are noninfectious.

When combined with other antiretroviral drug classes, the PIs are capable of lowering plasma HIV RNA levels to below-detectable range. The PIs are metabolized in the liver and have the potential to interact with many different drugs. In general, they are well tolerated, with GI complaints being the most common side effects. Various

Pr PROTOTYPE DRUG | Nevirapine *(Viramune)* | Antiretroviral—NNRTI

ACTIONS AND USES

Nevirapine is an NNRTI that binds directly to reverse transcriptase, disrupting the enzyme's active site. This inhibition prevents viral DNA from being synthesized from HIV RNA. The drug is readily absorbed following an oral dose. Since resistance develops rapidly when nevirapine is used as monotherapy, it is always used in combination with other antivirals in treatment using HAART. Resistance to nevirapine usually extends to other NNRTIs.

ADMINISTRATION ALERTS

- Administer with food to minimize gastric distress.
- Pregnancy category C.

PHARMACOKINETICS

Onset: Rapid

Peak: 4 h

Half-life: 25–40 h

Duration: Unknown

ADVERSE EFFECTS

Nevirapine increases the levels of metabolic enzymes in the liver; thus, it has the potential to interact with drugs handled by this organ. GI-related effects such as nausea, diarrhea, and abdominal pain are experienced by some clients, and skin rashes, fever, and fatigue are frequent side effects. Rarely, some clients acquire Stevens–Johnson syndrome, a sometimes-fatal skin condition affecting mucous membranes and large areas of the body.

Contraindications: The only contraindication is hypersensitivity to the drug. Therapy should proceed with caution in clients with hepatic impairment, as the drug may accumulate to toxic levels in these clients.

INTERACTIONS

Drug–Drug: Nevirapine may decrease plasma concentrations of protease inhibitors and oral contraceptives. It may also decrease methadone levels, inducing opiate withdrawal.

Lab Tests: Nevirapine may increase values of the following: serum bilirubin, aspartate aminotransferase (AST), alanine aminotransferase (ALT), and gamma-glutamyltranspeptidase (GGT). Hemoglobin, platelet, and neutrophil values may decrease.

Herbal/Food: St. John's wort may cause a decrease in antiretroviral activity.

Treatment of Overdose: There is no specific treatment for overdose.

 See the Companion Website for a Nursing Process Focus specific to this drug.

---

lipid abnormalities have been reported, including elevated cholesterol and triglyceride levels, and abdominal obesity.

All PIs have equivalent efficacy and a similar range of adverse effects. Choice of PI is generally based on clinical response and the experience of the clinician. Cross-resistance among the various PIs has been reported. In 2006, a new PI was approved. Darunavir (Prezista) is to be coadministered with ritonavir when the client has not responded to other HIV-AIDS therapies.

NURSING CONSIDERATIONS

The following material discusses NRTIs, NNRTIs, and PIs. Because antiretrovirals are commonly prescribed for HIV infection, a Nursing Process Focus has been provided for them. See page 541 later in this section.

The role of the nurse in NRTI, NNRTI, and PI therapy involves careful monitoring of a client's condition and providing education as it relates to the prescribed drug treatment. Although NRTIs, NNRTIs, and PIs act by different mechanisms, the associated nursing care is similar. The nurse is instrumental in providing client education and psychosocial support, so it is vital that the nurse establish a trusting relationship with the client. The nurse's approach should be nonjudgmental toward the client and the client's lifestyle. Clients with HIV-AIDS will experience tremendous

emotional distress at various times during treatment. Denial and anger may be evident in clients' behavior as they attempt to cope with their diagnosis.

Assess the client's understanding of the HIV disease process. Although drug therapies may slow the progression of the virus, they are not a cure. Prior to the administration of antiretroviral drugs, assess for symptoms of HIV, any opportunistic infections, and the use of OTC and herbal supplements. Monitor plasma HIV RNA (viral load) assays, CD4 T-cell counts, complete blood count, liver and renal profiles, and blood glucose levels throughout antiretroviral therapy These diagnostic values will determine the effectiveness as well as the toxicity of the drugs employed.

Verify the ordered drug combinations to determine potential side effects and precautions. Serious adverse reactions of antiretroviral agents include bone marrow suppression, liver toxicity and Stevens–Johnson syndrome. Commonly, clients will experience fatigue, headache, and gastrointestinal (GI) disturbances such as nausea, vomiting, and diarrhea. Other side effects depend on the specific drugs used. Most antiretroviral agents are contraindicated during pregnancy and lactation.

Many of the side effects of antiretrovirals can dramatically influence activities of daily living. Some of these drugs may cause dizziness or other troublesome CNS effects. When such side effects occur, instruct the client to

---

Pr **PROTOTYPE DRUG** | Saquinavir *(Fortovase, Invirase)* | Antiretroviral—Protease Inhibitor

ACTIONS AND USES

Saquinavir was the first PI approved by the FDA in 1995. By effectively inhibiting HIV protease, the drug prevents the final step in the assembly of an infectious HIV virion. The first formulation of saquinavir (Invirase) was a hard gelatin capsule that was poorly absorbed. The newer formulation of saquinavir (Fortovase) is a soft gelatin capsule that has a significantly higher absorption rate, particularly when taken with a high-fat, high-calorie meal. Recently, an improved formulation of Invirase was developed, allowing for twice-daily dosing. Because of these changes to Invirase, the drug manufacturer has announced that Fortovase will be removed from the market. Combining Invirase with ritonavir boosting increases serum levels, making the drug more effective.

ADMINISTRATION ALERTS

- Administer with food to minimize gastric distress.
- Invirase and Fortovase are not equivalent and cannot be interchanged.
- Pregnancy category B.

PHARMACOKINETICS

Onset: Unknown

Peak: Unknown

Half-life: 7–12 h

Duration: Unknown

ADVERSE EFFECTS

Saquinavir is well tolerated by most clients, and the most frequently reported problems are GI related, such as nausea, vomiting, dyspepsia, and diarrhea. General fatigue and headache are possible. Reductions in platelets and erythrocytes have been reported, though not commonly. Resistance to saquinavir may develop with continued use, and may include cross-resistance with other protease inhibitors.

Contraindications: Use of Invirase with terfenadine, cisapride, astemizole, pimozide, triazolam, midazolam, or ergot derivatives is contraindicated because serious or life-threatening reactions such as cardiac dysrhythmias or profound sedation may result. Clients with severe hepatic impairment should not receive saquinavir.

INTERACTIONS

Drug–Drug: Rifampin, rifabutin, phenobarbital, phenytoin, and carbamazepine significantly decrease saquinavir levels. Conversely, ketoconazole and ritonavir may increase saquinavir levels. Saquinavir may increase the effects of calcium channel blockers.

Lab Tests: Saquinavir may decrease blood glucose and may affect serum CPK and amylase levels. Platelets and RBC values may decrease.

Herbal/Food: St. John's wort may cause a decrease in antiretroviral activity.

Treatment of Overdose: There is no specific treatment for overdose.

 See the Companion Website for a Nursing Process Focus specific to this drug.

---

take the medication just before sleep. Advise the client not to drive or perform hazardous activities until reactions to the medication are known. Be vigilant in assessing for side effects and assisting clients in managing their therapeutic regimen.

The list of diseases and conditions that necessitate close observation is extensive for the antiretrovirals. Typically, agents classified as NTRIs should be used cautiously in clients with pancreatitis, peripheral vascular disease, neuropathy, kidney disorders, liver disorders, cardiac disease, and alcohol abuse. NNTRI agents necessitate judicious use in clients with liver impairment and CNS diseases. PIs are potentially problematic in clients with sensitivity to sulfonamides, liver disorders, and renal insufficiency. However, in acute stages of AIDS, treatment may proceed despite relative contraindications.

Antiretroviral drugs vary in the way in which they should be taken. For example, NRTI drugs should be taken on an empty stomach. These drugs should always be taken with water only and never with fruit juice, because acidic fruit juices interact with them. On the other hand, nevirapine (Viramune) and saquinavir mesylate (Invirase, Fortovase) should be taken with food to minimize gastric distress. With all antiretroviral drugs, instruct the client to consult the healthcare provider before taking any OTC medication or herbal supplement to present drug interactions.

Client Teaching.   Client education as it relates to antiretroviral drugs should include the goals of therapy, the reasons for obtaining baseline data such as vital signs and the existence of underlying cardiac and renal disorders, and possible drug side effects. Include the following points when teaching clients about antiretroviral therapy:

- If taking NRTIs, report fever, skin rash, abdominal pain, nausea, vomiting, and numbness or burning of hands or feet.
- If taking NNRTIs, report fever, chills, rash, blistering or reddening of skin, or muscle or joint pain.
- If taking PIs, report rash, abdominal pain, headache, insomnia, fever, constipation, cough, fainting, and visual changes.
- Wash hands frequently and avoid crowds.
- Increase fluid intake, and empty the bladder frequently.
- To protect sexual partners, practice abstinence or use a barrier contraceptive device such as a condom during all sexual activity.
- Do not share needles.
- Take medication exactly as ordered.
- Get sufficient rest and sleep, and eat a healthy diet.
- Keep all scheduled appointments and laboratory visits for testing.

NURSING PROCESS FOCUS Clients Receiving Antiretroviral Agents

Assessment	Potential Nursing Diagnoses
Prior to administration: ■ Obtain a complete health history including allergies, drug history, and possible drug interactions. ■ Obtain a complete physical examination. ■ Assess for the presence or history of HIV infection. ■ Obtain the following laboratory studies: • HIV RNA assay/CD4 count • complete blood count (CBC) • liver function • renal function • blood glucose	■ Infection, Risk for , related to compromised immune system ■ Decisional Conflict, related to therapeutic regimen ■ Fear, related to HIV diagnosis ■ Injury, Risk for, related to side effects of drugs ■ Knowledge, Deficient, related to disease process, transmission, and drug therapy

Planning: Client Goals and Expected Outcomes

The client will:
■ Exhibit a decrease in viral load and an increase in CD4 counts.
■ Demonstrate knowledge of the disease process, transmission, and treatment.
■ Demonstrate an understanding of the drug's action by accurately describing drug side effects and precautions.
■ Complete the full course of therapy and comply with follow-up care.

Implementation

Interventions and (Rationales)	Client Education/Discharge Planning
■ Monitor for symptoms of hypersensitivity reactions. (Zalcitabine may cause anaphylactic reaction.)	■ Instruct client to discontinue the medication and inform the healthcare provider if symptoms of hypersensitivity reaction develop such as wheezing; shortness of breath; swelling of face, tongue, or hands; itching or rash.
■ Monitor vital signs, especially temperature, and for symptoms of infection. Monitor white blood cell (WBC) count. (Antiretroviral drugs such as delavirdine may cause neutropenia.)	Instruct client: ■ To report symptoms of infections such as fever, chills, sore throat, and cough. ■ About methods of minimizing exposure to infection such as frequent hand washing; avoiding crowds and people with colds, flu, and other infections; limiting exposure to children and animals; increasing fluid intake; emptying the bladder frequently; and coughing and deep breathing several times per day.
■ Monitor client for signs of stomatitis. (Immunosuppression may result in the proliferation of oral bacteria.)	■ Advise client to be alert for mouth ulcers and to report their appearance.
■ Monitor blood pressure. (Antiviral agents such as abacavir may cause a significant decrease in blood pressure.)	Instruct client to: ■ Rise slowly from a lying or sitting position to minimize effects of postural hypotension. ■ Report changes in blood pressure and symptoms of dizziness and light-headedness.
■ Monitor HIV RNA assay, CD4 counts, liver function, kidney function, CBC, blood glucose, and serum amylase and triglyceride levels. (These will determine effectiveness and toxicity of drug.)	Instruct client: ■ About the purpose of required laboratory tests and scheduled follow-ups with the healthcare provider. ■ To monitor weight and presence of swelling. ■ To keep all appointments for laboratory tests.

(Continued)

NURSING PROCESS FOCUS Clients Receiving Antiretroviral Agents (Continued)

Implementation

Interventions and (Rationales)	Client Education/Discharge Planning
■ Determine potential drug–drug and drug–food interactions. (Antiretroviral medications have multiple drug–drug interactions and must be taken as prescribed.)	Instruct client: ■ When to take the specific medication in relationship to food intake. ■ About foods or beverages to avoid when taking medication; some antiretrovirals should not be taken with acidic fruit juice. ■ To take medication exactly as directed and not to skip any doses. ■ To consult with the healthcare provider before taking any OTC medications or herbal supplements.
■ Monitor for symptoms of pancreatitis including severe abdominal pain, nausea, vomiting, and abdominal distention. (Antiretroviral agents such as didanosine may cause pancreatitis.)	■ Instruct client to report the following immediately: fever, severe abdominal pain, nausea/vomiting, and abdominal distention.
■ Monitor skin for rash; withhold medication and notify physician at first sign of rash. (Several antiretroviral drugs may cause Stevens–Johnson syndrome, which may be fatal.)	■ Advise client to check skin frequently and notify the healthcare provider at the first sign of any rash.
■ Establish a therapeutic environment to ensure adequate rest, nutrition, hydration, and relaxation. (Support of the immune system is essential in HIV clients to minimize opportunistic infections.)	Teach client to incorporate the following health-enhancing activities: ■ Adequate rest and sleep. ■ Proper nutrition that provides essential vitamins and nutrients. ■ Intake of 6 to 8 glasses of water per day.
■ Monitor blood glucose levels. (Antiretroviral drugs may cause hyperglycemia, especially in clients with type 1 diabetes.)	■ Instruct client to report excessive thirst, hunger, dizziness, and urination to the healthcare provider. ■ Instruct diabetic client to monitor blood glucose levels regularly.
■ Monitor for neurological side effects such as numbness and tingling of the extremities. (Many NRTI agents cause peripheral neuropathy.)	Instruct client to: ■ Report numbness and tingling of extremities. ■ Use caution when in contact with heat and cold owing to possible peripheral neuropathy.
■ Determine the effect of the prescribed antiretroviral agents on oral contraceptives. (Many agents reduce the effectiveness of oral contraceptives.)	■ Instruct client to practice reliable contraception while taking antiretroviral medications.
■ Provide resources for medical and emotional support. (Treatment requires a multidisciplinary approach.)	■ Advise client about community resources and support groups.
■ Assess client's knowledge level regarding use and effect of medication. (This discussion provides an opportunity to provide an additional education.)	Advise client: ■ That medication may decrease the level of HIV infection in the blood but will not prevent transmission of the disease. ■ To use barrier protection during sexual activity. ■ To avoid sharing needles. ■ Not to donate blood.

Evaluation of Outcome Criteria

Evaluate the effectiveness of drug therapy by confirming that client goals and expected outcomes have been met (see "Planning").

■ The client's laboratory values demonstrate a decrease in viral load and an increase in CD4 counts.

■ The client verbalizes an understanding of the disease process, transmission, and treatment modalities.

■ The client demonstrates an understanding of the drug's action by accurately describing drug side effects and precautions.

■ The client verbalizes the importance of taking medication as ordered and returning for follow-up care.

∞ See Table 36.1 for a list of drugs to which these nursing actions apply.

36.7 Prevention of HIV Infection

Early in the history of the AIDS epidemic, scientists were optimistic that the spread of HIV infection would be *prevented* by the development of an effective vaccine. After all, scientists had totally eradicated the smallpox virus as a human threat and have essentially controlled major viral infections such as measles and mumps. Such a vaccine could be given in childhood, offering lifetime protection against the fatal disease.

After decades of research, scientists are still far from developing a vaccine to prevent AIDS. A few HIV vaccines are currently in clinical trials, but none is expected to cause a major impact on the HIV epidemic. At best, the HIV vaccines produced thus far only boost the immune response; they are unable to prevent the infection or its fatal consequences. Although the immune response boost may help a client already infected with the virus to better control the disease, it does not prevent new infections.

PREVENTION OF PERINATAL TRANSMISSION OF HIV

One of the most tragic aspects of the AIDS epidemic is transmission of the virus from a mother to her child during pregnancy, delivery, or breast-feeding. Newborns with HIV may succumb to the infection within weeks, or symptoms may be delayed for months or years. The prognosis for these children is generally poor; thus, the best approach to dealing with HIV infections in neonates is prevention.

In 1994, clinical trials determined that perinatal transmission of HIV could be markedly reduced through pharmacotherapy. The probability of transmission may be reduced approximately 70% using the following regimen:

- Oral administration of zidovudine to the mother, beginning at week 14 and continuing to week 34 of gestation.
- Intravenous administration of zidovudine to the mother during labor.
- Oral administration of zidovudine to the newborn for 6 weeks following delivery. (HIV infection is established in infants by age 1 to 2 weeks; starting antiretroviral therapy more than 48 hours after birth is ineffective in preventing the infection.)

This original regimen to prevent perinatal transmission has been supported by subsequent research and remains essentially unchanged. To date, there does not appear to be an increased incidence of congenital abnormalities or malignancies among the children born to women receiving this regimen. If the HIV infection is diagnosed earlier than week 14 of pregnancy, the client is usually placed on HAART combination therapy, with zidovudine as one of the drugs in the regimen.

POSTEXPOSURE PROPHYLAXIS OF HIV INFECTION FOLLOWING OCCUPATIONAL EXPOSURE

Since the start of the AIDS epidemic, nurses and other healthcare professionals have been concerned about acquiring the infection from their HIV-AIDS clients. Fortunately, if proper precautions are observed, the disease is rarely transmitted from client to caregiver. Accidents have occurred, however, in which healthcare workers have acquired the infection by exposure to the blood or body fluids of an HIV-infected client. Approximately 56 cases of client-to-healthcare worker transmission have been documented in the United States following occupational exposure. Although the risk is very small, the question remains, Can HIV transmission be prevented *after* accidental occupational exposure to HIV? The answer is a qualified yes.

The success of postexposure prophylaxis (PEP) therapy following HIV exposure is difficult to assess because of the lack of controlled studies and the small number of cases. Enough data have been accumulated, however, to demonstrate that PEP is successful in certain circumstances. For prevention to be most successful, PEP should be started within 24 to 36 hours after exposure to a client who is *known* to be HIV positive. The healthcare professional should receive a baseline ELISA test as soon as possible after exposure and subsequent follow-up testing as recommended.

If the HIV status of the client is *unknown*, PEP is decided case by case, based on the type of exposure and the likelihood that the blood or body fluid contained HIV. In some cases, PEP is initiated for a few days, until the client can be tested. *PEP should be initiated only if the exposure was sufficiently severe and the source fluid is known, or strongly suspected, to contain HIV.* Using PEP outside established guidelines is both expensive and dangerous; the antiretrovirals used for PEP therapy produce side effects in more than half the clients.

Based on available data, current clinical guidelines recommend one of the following regimens, conducted over a 4-week period:

- Zidovudine (Retrovir, AZT) and lamivudine (Epivir, 3TC)
- Lamivudine and stavudine (Zerit, D4T), or
- Stavudine and didanosine (Videx, DDI)

If the accidental HIV exposure was particularly severe, a third drug may be added to the regimen, although this increases the risk for side effects and has not been proved to be more successful than a two-drug regimen.

HERPESVIRUSES

Herpes simplex viruses (HSVs) are a family of DNA viruses that cause repeated blisterlike lesions on the skin, genitals, and other mucosal surfaces. Antiviral drugs can lower the frequency of acute herpes episodes and diminish the intensity of acute disease. These drugs are listed in Table 36.2.

TABLE 36.2	Drugs for Herpesviruses	
Drug	**Route and Adult Dose (max dose where indicated)**	**Adverse Effects**
SYSTEMIC AGENTS		
acyclovir (Zovirax)	PO; 400 mg tid	*Nausea, vomiting, diarrhea, headache, pain and inflammation at injection sites (parenteral agents)*
cidofovir (Vistide)	IV; 5 mg/kg q1wk for 2 wk; then 5 mg/kg q2wk	
famciclovir (Famvir)	PO; 500 mg tid for 7 days	<u>Thrombocytopenic purpura/hemolytic uremic syndrome, nephrotoxicity, seizures (foscarnet), electrolyte imbalances (foscarnet), hematologic toxicity/bone marrow suppression (ganciclovir)</u>
foscarnet (Foscavir)	IV; 40–60 mg/kg infused over 1–2 h tid	
ganciclovir (Cytovene)	IV; 5 mg/kg infused over 1 h bid	
valacyclovir (Valtrex)	PO; 1.0 g tid	
TOPICAL AGENTS		
docosanol (Abreva)	Topical; 10% cream applied to cold sore up to 5 times/day for 10 days	*Burning, irritation, or stinging at site of application, headache*
idoxuridine (Herplex)	Topical; 1 drop in each eye q1h during the day and q2h at night	
penciclovir (Denavir)	Topical; apply q2h while awake for 4 days	<u>Photophobia, keratopathy, and edema of eyelids (ocular agents)</u>
trifluridine (Viroptic)	Topical; 1 drop in each eye q2h during waking hours (max: 9 drops/day)	
vidarabine (Vira-A)	Topical; 0.5 inch of ointment to each eye q3h not to exceed 5 applications/day	

Italics indicate common adverse effects; <u>underlining</u> indicates serious adverse effects.

36.8 Pharmacotherapy of Herpesvirus Infections

Herpesviruses are usually acquired through direct physical contact with an infected person, but they may also be transmitted from infected mothers to their newborns, sometimes resulting in severe CNS disease. The herpesvirus family includes the following:

- HSV-1 primarily causes infections of the eye, mouth, and lips, although the incidence of genital infections is increasing.
- HSV-2 causes genital infections.
- Cytomegalovirus (CMV) affects multiple body systems in immunosuppressed clients.
- Varicella-zoster virus (VZV) causes shingles (zoster) and chicken pox (varicella).
- Epstein–Barr virus (EBV) results in mononucleosis and a form of cancer known as Burkitt's lymphoma.
- Herpesvirus-6 causes roseola in children and hepatitis or encephalitis in immunosuppressed clients.

Following its initial entrance into the client, HSV may remain in a latent, asymptomatic state in ganglia for many years. Immunosuppression, physical challenges, or emotional stress can promote active replication of the virus and appearance of the characteristic lesions. Complications include secondary infections of nongenital tissues.

The pharmacological goals for the management of herpes infections are twofold: to *relieve acute symptoms* and to *prevent recurrences*. It should be noted that the antiviral drugs used to treat herpesviruses do not cure clients; the virus remains in clients for the remainder of their lives.

Initial HSV-1 and HSV-2 infections are usually treated with oral antiviral therapy for 5 to 10 days. The most commonly prescribed antivirals for HSV and VZV include acyclovir (Zovirax), famciclovir (Famvir), and valacyclovir (Valtrex). Topical forms of several antivirals are available for application to herpes lesions, although they are not as effective as the oral forms. In immunocompromised clients, IV acyclovir may be indicated.

SPECIAL CONSIDERATIONS

HIV in the Pediatric and Geriatric Populations

Children infected with the HIV virus appear to develop opportunistic conditions at a much more rapid rate than do adults. The younger age at which the child acquires the HIV virus, the poorer the prognosis tends to be. Although not all antiretroviral medications can be used in the treatment of HIV, with combination therapy is also used with children. Prophylactic treatment against *P. carinii* pneumonia is also started early in the treatment regimen, because respiratory infections are often a cause of death in young children. The caregivers of the child must be able to handle the intense medication regimen and also must be aware of the early symptoms of opportunistic diseases.

The diagnosis of the geriatric client may be delayed because HIV is often not suspected in this population. The geriatric client who has become infected with the HIV virus may be less than willing to disclose activities that are considered high-risk behaviors. The geriatric client's need for antiretroviral treatment depends on the CD4 count. The geriatric client may have greater difficulty handling the rigorous regimen of the treatment. The physiological changes associated with aging increase the possibility of drug toxicity in this population. The social factors must also be considered, because these clients may be living alone or even be the primary caretaker of a disabled spouse. The ability of a client to be sexually active is not determined by age; therefore, it is very important to stress sexual activity precautions to prevent spread of the HIV virus.

Pr PROTOTYPE DRUG | *Acyclovir (Zovirax)* | Antiviral

ACTIONS AND USES

Approved in 1982 as one of the first antiviral drugs, acyclovir is limited to pharmacotheraphy for herpesviruses, for which it is a drug of choice. It is most effective against HSV-1 and HSV-2, and effective only at high doses against CMV and varicella-zoster. Acyclovir acts by preventing viral DNA synthesis. Acyclovir decreases the duration and severity of herpes episodes. When given for prophylaxis, it may decrease the frequency of herpes appearance, but it does not cure the client. It is available as a 5% ointment for application to active lesions, in oral form for prophylaxis, and as an IV for severe episodes. Because of its short half-life, acyclovir is sometimes administered orally up to five times a day.

ADMINISTRATION ALERTS

- When given IV, the drug may cause painful inflammation of vessels at the site of infusion.
- Administer around the clock, even if sleep is interrupted.
- Administer with food.
- Pregnancy category C.

PHARMACOKINETICS (PO)

Onset: Unknown

Peak: 1.5–2 h

Half-life: 2.5–5 h

Duration: 4–8 h

ADVERSE EFFECTS

There are few adverse effects to acyclovir when it is administered topically or orally. Nephrotoxicity is possible when the medication is given IV. Resistance has developed to the drug, particularly in clients with HIV-AIDS.

Contraindications: Acyclovir is contraindicated in clients with hypersensitivity to drugs in this class.

INTERACTIONS

Drug–Drug: Concurrent use of acyclovir with nephrotoxic agents should be avoided. Probenecid decreases acyclovir elimination, and zidovudine may cause increased drowsiness and lethargy.

Lab Tests: Values for kidney function tests such as BUN and serum creatinine may increase.

Herbal/Food: Unknown.

Treatment of Overdose: There is no specific treatment for overdose.

 See the Companion Website for a Nursing Process Focus specific to this drug.

Recurrent herpes lesions are usually mild and often require no drug treatment. If drug therapy is initiated within 24 hours after recurrent symptoms first appear, the length of the acute episode may be shortened. Clients who experience particularly severe or frequent recurrences (more than six episodes per year) may benefit from low doses of prophylactic antiviral therapy. Prophylactic therapy may also be of benefit to immunocompromised clients, such as those undergoing antineoplastic therapy or those with AIDS.

Herpes of the eye is the most common infectious cause of corneal blindness in the United States. Ocular herpes causes a painful, inflamed lesion on the eyelid or surface of the eye. Prompt treatment with antiviral drugs prevents permanent tissue destruction. As with genital herpes, once clients acquire ocular herpes, they often experience recurrences, which may occur years after the initial symptoms. Ocular herpes is treated with local application of drops or ointment. Trifluridine (Viroptic), vidarabine (Vira-A), and idoxuridine (Herplex) are available in ophthalmic formulations. Oral acyclovir is used when topical drops or ointments are contraindicated. Uncomplicated ocular herpes usually resolves after 1 to 2 weeks of pharmacotherapy.

NURSING CONSIDERATIONS

The following material discusses nursing considerations for clients receiving antiviral medications not associated with HIV infections.

The role of the nurse in antiviral therapy involves careful monitoring of a client's condition and providing education as it relates to the prescribed drug treatment. Because many of these viral infections are systemic rather than localized, perform a complete physical assessment prior to drug administration. Once a baseline of assessment findings,

HOME & COMMUNITY CONSIDERATIONS

Viral Infections

Herpes zoster (shingles) is a viral infection that occurs most frequently in the older population. It is caused by varicella-zoster, the same virus that causes chicken pox. The first symptoms of this disease—itching, tingling, or pain_may occur a few days before the characteristic rash appears. This makes providing treatment to shorten the disease course difficult. Effective treatment with antivirals such as acyclovir (Zovirax) must be started within 48 hours after the first symptom develops. Clients may experience pain for many weeks and months after the skin rash disappears. It is important for clients to isolate themselves while the rash is present to prevent the spread of the varicella-zoster virus. The increased use of the varicella-zoster vaccine will, in time, dramatically decrease the number of cases of shingles.

Clients with HIV and AIDs must educate themselves on the disease process and understand the impact of the diagnosis on their lives. The nurse should recommend that these clients become involved in HIV/AIDs support and educational groups. The following websites may provide additional client support:

National Institutes of Health: http://www.nlm.nih.gov/medlineplus
National Institute on Drug Abuse: http://teens.drugabuse.gov

including vital signs, weight, and laboratory studies [complete blood count (CBC), viral cultures, and liver and kidney function] is completed, focus on the presenting symptoms of the viral infection. For clients with preexisting renal or hepatic disease, use antiviral drugs with extreme caution. Although many antiviral medications are listed as pregnancy categories B or C, judicious use is still warranted during pregnancy. Viruses that can be treated with antiviral drugs include herpes simplex, CMV infection, Epstein–Barr viral infection, varicella-zoster viral infection, respiratory syncytial viral infections, keratoconjunctivitis, and herpes zoster.

Depending on the specific antiviral drugs, these agents can be administered intravenously, orally, topically, and through inhalation. Instruct the client in the proper administration techniques. Additionally, emphasize compliance with antiviral therapy such as taking the exact amount around the clock even if sleep is interrupted. Although most antiviral drugs are well tolerated, some cause GI distress and should be taken with food. Severe adverse effects such as renal failure and thrombocytopenia have been noted but occur infrequently. Other more frequent adverse effects include headache, fatigue, and dizziness. Monitor for adverse effects throughout the course of the treatment, and assist the client with managing antiviral drug-related problems.

Client Teaching. Client education as it relates to antiviral drugs should include the goals of therapy, the reasons for obtaining baseline data such as vital signs and the existence of underlying cardiac and renal disorders, and possible drug side effects. Include the following points when teaching clients about antiviral therapy:

- Understand that medications do *not* prevent transmission of the virus to other individuals.
- Avoid activities that may transmit the virus.
- Immediately report blood in urine, bruising, yellowing of the skin, fever, chills, confusion, nervousness, dizziness, nausea, and vomiting.
- Complete the full course of treatment.
- Keep all scheduled appointments and laboratory visits for testing.
- Use caution while performing hazardous activities; some of these drugs may cause dizziness or drowsiness.
- Do not take other prescription drugs, OTC medications, herbal therapies, or vitamin supplements without notifying your healthcare provider.
- Apply topical preparations with an applicator or a glove to prevent the spread of the virus to other areas.
- Do not apply any other types of creams, ointments, or lotions to the infected sites.

INFLUENZA

Influenza is a viral infection characterized by acute symptoms that include sore throat, sneezing, coughing, fever, and chills. The infectious viral particles are easily spread via airborne droplets. In immunosuppressed clients, an influenza infection may be fatal. In 1919, a worldwide outbreak of influenza killed an estimated 20 million people. Influenza viruses are designated with the letters A, B, or C. Type A has been responsible for several serious pandemics throughout history. The RNA-containing influenza viruses should not be confused with *Haemophilus influenzae*, which is a bacterium that causes respiratory disease.

36.9 Pharmacotherapy of Influenza

The best approach to influenza infection is *prevention* through annual vaccination. Those who benefit greatly from vaccinations include residents of long-term care facilities, those with chronic cardiopulmonary disease, children ages 5 and younger, pregnant women in their second or third trimester during the peak flu season, and healthy adults older than age 65. Influenza vaccination is also recommended for healthcare workers who are involved in the direct care of clients at high risk for acquiring influenza, including HIV-infected clients. Depending on the stage of the disease, HIV-positive clients may also benefit from vaccination. Adequate immunity is achieved about 2 weeks after vaccination and lasts for several months up to a year. Additional details on vaccines are presented in Chapter 32 ∞.

Antivirals may be used to prevent influenza or decrease the severity of acute symptoms. Amantadine (Symmetrel) has been available to prevent and treat influenza for many years. Chemoprophylaxis with amantadine or rimantadine (Flumadine) is indicated for unvaccinated individuals during a confirmed outbreak of influenza type A. Therapy with these antivirals is sometimes started concurrently with vaccination; the antiviral offers protection during the 2 weeks before therapeutic antibody titers are achieved from the vaccine. Because of the expense and possible adverse effects of these drugs, they are generally reserved for clients who are at greatest risk for the severe complications of influenza. Antivirals for influenza are listed in Table 36.3.

A new class of drugs, the neuroaminidase inhibitors, was introduced in 1999 to treat *active* influenza infections. If given within 48 hours of the onset of symptoms, oseltamivir (Tamiflu) and zanamivir (Relenza) are reported to shorten the normal 7-day duration of influenza symptoms to 5 days. Oseltamivir is given orally, whereas zanamivir is inhaled. Because these agents are expensive and produce only modest results, prevention through vaccination remains the best alternative.

It is important to understand that these antivirals are not effective against the common cold virus. About 200 different viruses, including rhinoviruses, cause symptoms identified with the common cold. Despite considerable attempts to develop drugs to prevent this annoying infection, success has not yet been achieved. There are drugs, however, that may relieve symptoms of the common cold, and these are presented in Chapter 38 ∞.

TABLE 36.3	Drugs for Influenza	
Drug	**Route and Adult Dose (max dose where indicated)**	**Adverse Effects**
INFLUENZA PROPHYLAXIS		
amantadine (Symmetrel)	PO; 100 mg bid	*Nausea, dizziness, nervousness, difficulty concentrating, insomnia*
rimantadine (Flumadine)	PO; 100 mg bid	
		<u>Leukopenia, hallucinations, orthostatic hypotension, urinary retention</u>
INFLUENZA TREATMENT: NEUROAMINIDASE INHIBITORS		
oseltamivir (Tamiflu)	PO; 75 mg bid for 5 days	*Nausea, vomiting, diarrhea, dizziness*
zanamivir (Relenza)	Inhalation; 2 inhalations/day for 5 days	
		<u>Bronchitis</u>

Italics indicate common adverse effects; <u>underlining</u> indicates serious adverse effects.

VIRAL HEPATITIS

Viral **hepatitis** is a common infection caused by a number of different viruses. Although each virus has its own unique clinical features, all hepatitis viruses cause inflammation and necrosis of liver cells. Symptoms of hepatitis may be acute or chronic. Acute symptoms include fever, chills, fatigue, anorexia, nausea, and vomiting. Chronic hepatitis may result in prolonged fatigue, jaundice, liver cirrhosis, and ultimately hepatic failure.

36.9 Pharmacotherapy of Viral Hepatitis

HEPATITIS A

Hepatitis A (HAV) is spread by the oral–fecal route and causes epidemics in regions of the world having poor sanitation. Outbreaks in the United States, however, are most often sporadic events caused by contaminated food.

Although approximately 20% of HAV-infected clients require some hospitalization for symptoms related to the infection, most recover without pharmacotherapy and develop lifelong immunity to the virus. Fatalities due to chronic disease are rare, and only a small number of clients develop severe liver failure. Thus, HAV is normally considered an acute disease, having no significant chronic form. This makes HAV very different from hepatitis B or C.

Like all forms of hepatitis, the best treatment for HAV is prevention. HAV vaccine (Havrix, VAQTA) has been available since 1995. It is indicated for children living in communities or states with high infection rates, travelers to countries with high HAV infection rates, men who have sex with men, and illegal drug users. When a booster is given 6 to 12 months after the initial dose, close to 100% immunity is obtained. The average length of protection is approximately 5 to 8 years, although protection may last 20 years or longer in some clients. The availability of the HAV vaccine has led to a dramatic drop in the rate of this infection in the United States.

Prophylaxis or postexposure treatment for a client recently exposed to HAV includes hepatitis A immunoglobulins (HAIg), a concentrated solution of antibodies. HAIg is administered as prophylaxis for clients traveling to endemic areas and to close personal contacts of infected clients to prevent transmission of the virus. A single IM dose of HAIg can provide passive protection and prophylaxis for about 3 months. It is estimated that the immunoglobulins are 85% effective at preventing HAV in clients exposed to the virus.

Therapy for acute HAV infection is symptomatic. No specific drugs are indicated; in otherwise healthy adults, the infection is self-limiting.

HEPATITIS B

Although hepatitis B (HBV) in the United States is transmitted primarily through exposure to contaminated blood and body fluids, in many regions of the world the infection is transmitted by the perinatal route and from child to child. Major risk factors for HBV in the United States include injected drug abuse, sex with an HBV-infected partner, and sex between men. Healthcare workers are at risk because of accidental exposure to HBV-contaminated needles or body fluids.

Treatment of acute HBV infection is symptomatic, because no specific therapy is available. Ninety percent of acute HBV infections resolve with complete recovery and do not progress to chronic disease. Lifelong immunity to HBV is usually acquired following resolution of the infection.

Symptoms of chronic HBV may develop as long as 10 years following exposure. HBV has a much greater probability of progression to chronic hepatitis and a greater mortality rate than does HAV. The final stage of the infection is hepatic cirrhosis. In addition, chronic HBV infections are associated with an increased risk of hepatocellular carcinoma.

As with HAV, the best treatment for HBV infection is *prevention* through immunization. Traditionally, HBV vaccine (Recombivax HB, Engerix-B) has been indicated for healthcare workers and others routinely exposed to blood and body fluids. However, universal vaccination of all

TABLE 36.4 Drugs for Hepatitis

Drug	Route and Adult Dose (max dose where indicated)	Adverse Effects
INTERFERONS		
interferon alfacon-1 (Infergen)	Subcutaneous; 9 mcg 3 times/wk for 24 wk	*Flulike symptoms, myalgia, fatigue, headache, anorexia, diarrhea*
interferon alfa-n1 (Wellferon)	Subcutaneous/IM; 3 million units 3 times/wk for 48 wk	
interferon alfa-2a (Roferon-A) (see page 463 for the Prototype Drug box)	Subcutaneous/IM; 1–3 million units/day for 1 wk, then 3 times/wk for 48–52 wk	Myelosuppression, thrombocytopenia, suicide ideation
interferon alfa-2b (Intron A)	Subcutaneous/IM; 3 million units/m^2 3 times/wk	
peginterferon alfa-2a (Pegasys)	Subcutaneous; 180 mcg of 1wk for 48 wk	
peginterferon alfa-2b (PEG-Intron)	Subcutaneous; 1 mcg/kg/wk for monotherapy; 1.5 g/kg/wk when given with ribavirin	
NONINTERFERONS/COMBINATIONS		
adefovir dipivoxil (Hepsera)	PO; 10 mg/day	*Asthenia, headache, nausea, dizziness, fatigue, nasal disturbances (lamivudine)*
entecavir (Baraclude)	PO; 0.5 mg/day; 1 mg/day as a single dose for clients with history of lamivudine resistance	
lamivudine (Epivir HBV)	PO; 150 mg bid	Nephrotoxicity and lactic acidosis (adefovir), pancreatitis (lamivudine), hepatomegaly with steatorrhea (lamivudine, entecavir), cardiac arrest (ribavirin), hemolytic anemia (ribavirin), apnea (ribavirin)
ribavirin (Rebetrol)/interferon alfa-2b (Introl A): Combination is called Robetron	ribavirin: PO; 5–6, 200-mg capsules daily interferon alfa-2b: Subcutaneous; 3 million international units, 3 times/wk	

Italics indicate common adverse effects; underlining indicates serious adverse effects.

children is now recommended, and some states require HBV vaccination prior to entry into school. Three doses of the vaccine provide up to 90% of clients with protection against HBV following exposure to the virus. A combination vaccine is available that provides immunity to both HAV and HBV (Twinrix).

Postexposure prophylaxis of HBV includes hepatitis B immunoglobulins (HBIg). Indications for HBIg therapy include probable exposure to HBV through the perinatal, sexual, or parenteral routes, or exposure of an infant to a caregiver with HBV. HBIg is administered as soon as possible after suspected exposure to HBV.

Once chronic hepatitis becomes active, pharmacotherapy is indicated. Drugs for hepatitis are listed in Table 36.4. The two basic strategies for eliminating HBV are to give antivirals that stop viral replication, or to administer immunomodulators that boost body defenses. Three different therapies are approved for chronic HBV pharmacotherapy:

- Interferon alfa: 30% to 40% of clients respond to 4 months of therapy. Five to ten percent of these clients relapse after completion of therapy.

- Lamivudine (Epivir): 25% to 45% of clients respond to therapy, which lasts 1 year or longer. Emergence of resistant viral strains is becoming a clinical problem.

- Adefovir (Hespera): Approximately 50% of clients respond to 48 weeks of therapy. The drug is new, and long-term studies are in progress.

In 2005 the FDA approved entecavir (Baraclude), a new drug for chronic HBV. Early data suggest entecavir is as effective as or more effective than lamivudine. The role of entecavir in treating chronic HBV infection will be established as additional research becomes available.

NATURAL THERAPIES

Complementary and Alternative Medicine for HIV

With no cure available and a high incidence of adverse effects from current therapeutic drugs, it is not surprising that many clients infected with HIV turn to complementary and alternative medicine (CAM). It is estimated that as many as 70% of HIV-AIDS clients use CAM during the course of their illness. Most clients use CAM in addition to antiretroviral therapy, to control serious side effects, combat weight loss, and boost their immune system. Relieving stress and depression are also common reasons for seeking CAM. The most common herbal products reported by HIV-AIDS clients are garlic, ginseng, goldenseal, echinacea, St. John's wort, and aloe. Unfortunately, few controlled studies have examined the safety or efficacy of CAM in HIV-AIDS clients; CAM treatments that have been studied are discussed in the following paragraph.

The nurse should provide supportive education regarding the use of CAM. Although the use of these therapies should not be discouraged, clients must be strongly warned not to use CAM in place of conventional medical treatment. In addition, some herbs such as St. John's wort can increase the hepatic metabolism of antiretrovirals, resulting in an increased or decreased effect. Garlic coadministered with saquinavir has been shown to greatly reduce plasma levels of the antiretroviral (Mills, Montori, Perri, Phillips, & Koren, 2005). A study that evaluated the concurrent use of goldenseal root with indinavir found that clients can safely take goldenseal root concurrently with indinavir, and that interactions are unlikely (Sandhu, Prescilla, Simonelli & Edwards, 2003). The nurse should urge the client to obtain CAM information from reliable sources and always to report the use of CAM therapies to the healthcare provider.

HEPATITIS C AND OTHER HEPATITIS VIRUSES

The hepatitis C, D, E, and G viruses are sometimes referred to as non A–non B viruses. Of the non A–non B viruses, hepatitis C has the greatest clinical importance.

Transmitted primarily through exposure to infected blood or body fluids, hepatitis C (HCV) is more common than HBV. Approximately half of all HIV-AIDS clients are coinfected with HCV. About 70% of clients infected with HCV proceed to chronic hepatitis, and up to 30% may develop end-stage cirrhosis. HCV is the most common cause of liver transplants.

Unlike with HAV and HBV, no vaccine is available to prevent hepatitis C. In addition, postexposure prophylaxis of HAC with immunoglobulins is not recommended because its effectiveness has not been demonstrated.

Current pharmacotherapy for chronic HCV infection includes several types of interferon and the antiviral ribavirin. Combination therapy has been found to produce a more sustained viral suppression than monotherapy with either agent. Commercially available interferons for hepatitis include both the regular and pegylated formulations. **Pegylation** is a process that attaches polyethylene glycol (PEG) to an interferon to extend its duration of action, thus allowing it to be administered less frequently. Whereas standard interferon formulations must be administered three times per week, pegylated versions require only one dose per week. The PEG molecule is inert and does not influence antiviral activity. Additional information on interferons used for other indications may be found in Chapter 32 ∞.

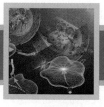

CHAPTER REVIEW

KEY CONCEPTS

The numbered key concepts provide a succinct summary of the important points from the corresponding numbered section within the chapter. If any of these points are not clear, refer to the numbered section within the chapter for review.

36.1 Viruses are nonliving intracellular parasites that require host organelles to replicate. Some viral infections are self-limiting, whereas others benefit from pharmacotherapy.

36.2 HIV targets the T4 lymphocyte, using reverse transcriptase to make viral DNA. The result is gradual destruction of the immune system.

36.3 Antiretroviral drugs used in the treatment of HIV-AIDS do not cure the disease, but they do help many clients live longer. Pharmacotherapy may be initiated in the acute (symptomatic) or chronic (asymptomatic) phase of HIV infection.

36.4 Drugs from five drug classes are used in various combinations in the pharmacotherapy of HIV-AIDS. The nucleotide reverse transcriptase inhibitors and the fusion inhibitors have recently been discovered.

36.5 The reverse transcriptase inhibitors block HIV replication at the level of the reverse transcriptase enzyme. These include the NRTIs, NNRTIs and the NtRTIs.

36.6 The protease inhibitors inhibit the final assembly of the HIV virion. They are always used in combination with other antiretrovirals.

36.7 Pharmacotherapy can lessen the severity of acute herpes simplex infections and prolong the latent period of the disease.

36.8 Drugs are available to prevent and to treat influenza infections. Vaccination is the best choice, as drugs are relatively ineffective once influenza symptoms appear.

36.9 Hepatitis A and B are best treated through immunization. Newer drugs for HBV and HBC have led to therapies for chronic hepatitis.

NCLEX-RN® REVIEW QUESTIONS

1 When the client is started on antiretroviral drugs for HIV, nursing education should include which of the following?

1. This drug will cure the disease over time.
2. This drug will not cure the disease but may extend the life expectancy.
3. This type of drug will be used prior to vaccines.
4. This drug is readily available all over the world for treatment.

2 The nurse understands that the laboratory tests that must be assessed while a client is on drug therapy for HIV-AIDS are: (Select all that apply.)

1. CBC.
2. Clotting factors.
3. HIV RNA.
4. CD4 lymphocyte count.
5. BUN.

3 When providing client and family education for the nucleoside reverse transcriptase inhibitor drugs for HIV-AIDS, the nurse would tell the client to take the medicine:

1. On an empty stomach.
2. On a full stomach.
3. With apple juice to decrease the taste.
4. With orange juice to increase absorption.

4 A client is concerned about contracting influenza. The best response by the nurse would be:

1. "After receiving the vaccination you will be protected in about 2 weeks."
2. "Once you are vaccinated, you will need a booster only every 2 years."
3. "You need to be vaccinated only if you are older than 50."
4. "The infectious particles are not easily spread, and you can wait to be vaccinated until there is an increase in the population."

5 A client wants to be vaccinated against hepatitis. The nurse would inform the client that the vaccine available is for:

1. Hepatitis B only.
2. Hepatitis A and B.
3. Hepatitis B and C.
4. Hepatitis A and C.

CRITICAL THINKING QUESTIONS

1. The client is a 72-year-old woman who lives in an assisted living community. The nurse advises the client of the importance of receiving an amantadine (Symmetrel) injection. What is the rationale supporting this recommendation? How could the nurse assist the client in complying with this recommendation?

2. A newly diagnosed HIV-positive client has been put on zidovudine (Retrovir). Identify priorities of nursing care for this client.

3. A healthcare provider has ordered acyclovir (Zovirax) as an IV bolus to be infused over 15 minutes. The client is seriously ill with a systemic herpesvirus infection, and the healthcare provider wants the client to have immediate access to the medication. What is the nurse's best response?

See Appendix D for answers and rationales for all activities.

EXPLORE MediaLink

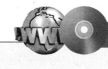

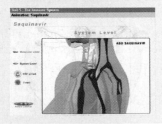

NCLEX-RN® review, case studies, and other interactive resources for this chapter can be found on the companion website at www.prenhall.com/adams. Click on "Chapter 36" to select the activities for this chapter. For animations, more NCLEX-RN® review questions, and an audio glossary, access the accompanying Prentice Hall Nursing MediaLink DVD-ROM in this textbook.

PRENTICE HALL NURSING MEDIALINK DVD-ROM

- **Animations**
  Mechanism in Action: Zidovudine (*Retrovir, AZT*)
  Mechanism in Action: Acyclovir (*Zovirax*)
  Mechanism in Action: Saquinavir Mesylate (*Fortovase, Invirase*)
- **Audio Glossary**
- **NCLEX-RN® Review**

COMPANION WEBSITE

- **NCLEX-RN® Review**
- **Dosage Calculations**
- **Case Study:** HIV pharmacotherapy
- **Care Plan:** Client with recurrent genital herpes treated with acyclovir

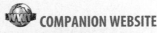
www.prenhall.com/adams

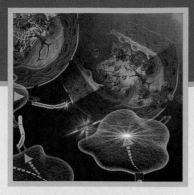

CHAPTER 37

Drugs for Neoplasia

DRUGS AT A GLANCE

ALKYLATING AGENTS
Nitrogen Mustards
   ◉ *cyclophosphamide (Cytoxan)*
Nitrosoureas
ANTIMETABOLITES
Folic Acid Antagonists
   ◉ *methotrexate (Folex, Mexate, others)*
Pyrimidine Analogs
Purine Analogs
ANTITUMOR ANTIBIOTICS
   ◉ *doxorubicin (Adriamycin)*
NATURAL PRODUCTS
Vinca Alkaloids
   ◉ *vincristine (Oncovin)*
Taxanes
Topoisomerase Inhibitors
Camptothecins
HORMONE AND HORMONE ANTAGONISTS
Glucocorticoids
Androgens and Androgen Antagonists
Estrogens and Estrogen Antagonists
   ◉ *tamoxifen (Nolvadex)*
Progestins
BIOLOGIC RESPONSE MODIFIERS AND IMMUNE THERAPIES

OBJECTIVES

After reading this chapter, the student should be able to:

1. Explain differences between normal cells and cancer cells.
2. Identify primary causes of cancer.
3. Describe lifestyle factors associated with a reduced risk of acquiring cancer.
4. Identify the three primary therapies for cancer.
5. Explain the significance of growth fraction and the cell cycle to the success of chemotherapy.
6. Describe the nurse's role in the pharmacological management of cancer.
7. Explain how combination therapy and special dosing protocols increase the effectiveness of chemotherapy.
8. List the general adverse effects of chemotherapeutic agents.
9. For each of the drug classes listed in Drugs at a Glance, know representative drugs, and explain their mechanism of drug action, primary actions, and important adverse effects.
10. Categorize anticancer drugs based on their classification and mechanism of action.
11. Use the Nursing Process to care for clients who are receiving antineoplastic medications as part of their treatment of cancer.

MediaLink 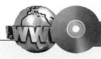 www.prenhall.com/adams

KEY TERMS

adjuvant chemotherapy *page 554*

alkylation *page 557*

alopecia *page 556*

aromatase inhibitor *page 569*

camptothecin *page 566*

cancer/carcinoma *page 552*

chemotherapy *page 554*

emetic potential *page 556*

growth fraction *page 555*

liposomes *page 564*

metastasis *page 552*

mucositis *page 556*

nadir *page 557*

neoplasm *page 552*

oncogenes *page 553*

palliation *page 554*

taxane *page 565*

topoisomerase I *page 566*

tumor *page 552*

vesicant *page 557*

vinca alkaloids *page 565*

Cancer is one of the most feared diseases in society for a number of valid reasons. It is often silent, producing no symptoms until it is far advanced. It sometimes requires painful and disfiguring surgery. It may strike at an early age, even during childhood, to deprive clients of a normal lifespan. Perhaps worst of all, the medical treatment of cancer often cannot offer a cure, and progression to death is sometimes slow, painful, and psychologically difficult for clients and their loved ones.

Despite its feared status, many successes have been made in the diagnosis, understanding, and treatment of cancer. Some types of cancer are now curable, and therapies may provide the client a longer, symptom-free life. This chapter examines the role of drugs in the treatment of cancer. Medications used to treat this disease are called *anticancer drugs, antineoplastics,* or *cancer chemotherapeutic agents.*

37.1 Characteristics of Cancer: Uncontrolled Cell Growth

Cancer, or **carcinoma,** is a disease characterized by abnormal, uncontrolled cell division. Cell division is a normal process occurring extensively in most body tissues from conception to late childhood. At some point in time, however, the suppressor genes responsible for cell growth stop this rapid division. This may result in a total lack of replication, in the case of muscle cells and perhaps brain cells. In other cells, genes controlling replication can be turned on when it becomes necessary to replace worn-out cells, as in the case of blood cells and the mucosa of the digestive tract.

Cancer is thought to result from damage to the genes controlling cell growth. Once damaged, the cell is no longer responsive to normal chemical signals checking its growth. The cancer cells lose their normal functions, divide rapidly, and invade surrounding cells. The abnormal cells often travel to distant sites where they populate new tumors, a process called **metastasis.** ● Figure 37.1 illustrates some characteristics of cancer cells.

Tumor is defined as a swelling, abnormal enlargement, or mass. The word **neoplasm** is often used interchangeably with tumor. Tumors may be solid masses, such as lung or breast cancer, or they may be widely disseminated in the blood, such as leukemia. Tumors are named according to their tissue of origin, generally with the suffix *-oma.* Table 37.1 lists examples of various types of tumors.

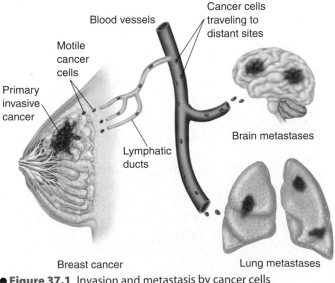

● Figure 37.1 Invasion and metastasis by cancer cells

TABLE 37.1 Classification and Naming of Tumors

Name	Description	Examples
benign tumor	slow growing; does not metastasize and rarely requires drug treatment	adenoma, papilloma and lipoma, osteoma, meningioma
carcinoma	cancer of epithelial tissue; most common type of malignant neoplasm; grows rapidly and metastasizes	malignant melanoma, renal cell carcinoma, adenocarcinoma, hepatocellular carcinoma
glioma	cancer of glial (interstitial) cells in the brain, spinal cord, pineal gland, posterior pituitary gland, or retina	telangiectatic glioma, brainstem glioma
leukemia	cancer of the blood-forming cells in bone marrow; may be acute or chronic	myelocytic leukemia, lymphocytic leukemia
lymphoma	cancer of lymphoid tissue	Hodgkin's disease, lymphoblastic lymphoma
malignant tumor	grows rapidly larger; becomes resistant to treatment and results in death if untreated	
sarcoma	cancer of connective tissue; grows extremely rapidly and metastasizes early in the progression of the disease	osteogenic sarcoma, fibrosarcoma, Kaposi's sarcoma, angiosarcoma

37.2 Causes of Cancer

Numerous factors have been found to cause cancer or to be associated with a higher risk for acquiring the disease. These factors are known as *carcinogens*.

Many chemical carcinogens have been identified. Chemicals in tobacco smoke are thought to be responsible for about one third of all cancer in the United States. Some chemicals, such as asbestos and benzene, have been associated with a higher incidence of cancer in the workplace. In some cases, the site of the cancer may be distant from the entry location, as with bladder cancer caused by the inhalation of certain industrial chemicals. Some known chemical carcinogens are listed in Table 37.2.

A number of physical factors are also associated with cancer. For example, exposure to large amounts of X-rays is associated with a higher risk of leukemia. Ultraviolet (UV) light from the sun is a known cause of skin cancer.

Viruses are associated with about 15% of all human cancers. Examples include herpes simplex types I and II, Epstein–Barr, papillomavirus, cytomegalovirus, and human T-lymphotrophic viruses. Factors that suppress the immune system, such as HIV or drugs given after transplant surgery, may encourage the growth of cancer cells.

Some cancers have a strong genetic component. The fact that close relatives may acquire the same type of cancer suggests that certain genes, called **oncogenes,** may predispose close relatives to the condition. These abnormal genes interact with chemical, physical, and biological agents to promote cancer formation. Other genes, called *tumor suppressor genes,* may inhibit the formation of tumors. If these suppressor genes are damaged, cancer may result. Damage to the suppressor gene p53 is associated with cancers of the breast, lung, brain, colon, and bone.

Although the formation of cancer has a genetic component, it also has strong environmental components. Adopting healthy lifestyle habits may reduce the risk of acquiring cancer. Following proper nutrition, avoiding chemical and physical risks, and maintaining a regular schedule of health checkups can help prevent cancer from developing into a fatal disease. The following are lifestyle factors regarding cancer prevention or diagnosis that should be used by the nurse when teaching clients about cancer prevention:

- Eliminate tobacco use and exposure to secondhand smoke.
- Limit or eliminate alcoholic beverage use.
- Reduce fat in the diet, particularly that from animal sources.
- Choose most foods from plant sources; increase fiber in the diet.
- Exercise regularly and keep body weight within recommended guidelines.
- Self-examine your body monthly for abnormal lumps and skin lesions.
- When exposed to direct sun, use skin lotions with the highest sun protection factor (SPF) value.

MediaLink CancerNet

PHARMFACTS

Cancer

- It is estimated that more than 1,368,000 new cancer cases occur each year, with more than 563,700 deaths (1,500 people each day).
- Cancer is the chief cause of death by disease in children younger than age 15.
- Leukemia is the most common childhood cancer and is responsible for one fourth of all cancers occurring before age 20.
- Lung cancer has the highest mortality rate: It is responsible for 28% of all cancer deaths.
- Prostate cancer is the second leading cause of cancer death in men.
- The highest 5-year survival rates are for cancers of the prostate, testis, and thyroid. The lowest survival rates are for pancreatic and liver cancers.
- Among ethnic groups, African Americans have the highest incidence rates in many types of cancers, including those of the lung, breasts, and prostate; since 1990, this gap has been narrowing.
- Although breast cancer is predominant in women (second in cancer deaths), about 1,500 men are diagnosed with the disease each year.

Source: Cancer Facts and Figures, American Cancer Society, 2006 (www.cancer.org)

TABLE 37.2	Agents Associated With an Increased Risk of Cancer
Agent	**Type of Cancer**
alcohol	liver
arsenic	skin and lung
asbestos	lung
benzene	leukemia
nickel	lung and nasal
polycyclic aromatic hydrocarbons	lung and skin
tobacco substances	lung; head and neck
vinyl chloride	liver

- Have periodic diagnostic testing performed at recommended intervals.
  - Women should have periodic mammograms, as directed by their healthcare provider.
  - Men should have a digital rectal prostate examination and a prostate-specific antigen (PSA) test annually after age 50.
  - Both should have a fecal occult blood test (FOBT) and flexible sigmoidoscopy performed at age 50 with FOBT annually after age 50.
  - Women who are sexually active or have reached age 18 should have an annual Pap test and pelvic examination.

37.3 Treatment of Cancer: Surgery, Radiation Therapy, and Chemotherapy

The possibility for cure is much greater if a cancer is treated in its early stages, when the tumor is small and localized to a single area. Once the cancer has spread to distant sites, cure is much more difficult; thus, it is important to diagnose the disease as early as possible. In an attempt to remove every cancer cell, three treatment approaches are utilized: surgery, radiation therapy, and drug therapy.

Surgery is performed to remove a tumor that is localized, or when the tumor is pressing on nerves, the airways, or other vital tissues. Surgery lowers the number of cancer cells in the body so that radiation therapy and pharmacotherapy can be more successful. Surgery is not an option for tumors of blood cells or when it would not be expected to extend a client's lifespan or to improve the quality of life.

Radiation therapy is an effective way to kill tumor cells through nonsurgical means; approximately 50% of clients with cancer receive radiation therapy as part of their treatment. Radiation therapy is most successful for cancers that are localized, when high doses of ionizing radiation can be aimed directly at the tumor and confined to this area. Radiation treatments may follow surgery to kill any cancer cells left behind following the operation. Radiation is sometimes given as **palliation** for inoperable cancers to shrink the size of a tumor that may be pressing on vital organs, and to relieve pain, difficulty breathing, or difficulty swallowing.

Pharmacotherapy of cancer is sometimes called **chemotherapy.** Because drugs are transported through the blood, they have the potential to reach cancer cells in virtually any location. Certain drugs are able to cross the blood–brain barrier to reach brain tumors. Others are instilled directly into body cavities such as the urinary bladder to bring the highest dose possible to the cancer cells without producing systemic side effects.

Antineoplastic drug therapy has three general purposes: cure, palliation, or prophylaxis. Anticancer drugs are sometimes given to attempt a total *cure* or complete eradication of tumor cells from the body. Examples of cancers in which chemotherapy may be used alone as a curative treatment include Hodgkin's lymphoma, certain leukemias, and choriocarcinoma. Antineoplastics may also be administered *after* surgery or radiation to effect a cure, a technique called **adjuvant chemotherapy.** In many cases, the cancer is too advanced to expect a cure, and antineoplastic agents are given for *palliation* to reduce the size of the tumor, thereby easing the severity of pain and possibly extending the client's lifespan or improving the quality of life. Examples of cancers for which palliatives are used for advanced tumors include osteosarcoma, pancreatic cancer, and Kaposi's sarcoma. In a few cases, drugs are given as *prophylaxis* with the goal of preventing cancer from occurring in clients at high risk for developing tumors. For example, some clients who have had a primary breast cancer removed may receive chemotherapy, even if there is no evidence of metastases, because there is a high likelihood that the disease will recur.

NATURAL THERAPIES

Selenium's Role in Cancer Prevention

Selenium is an essential trace element that is necessary to maintain healthy immune function. It is a vital antioxidant, especially when combined with vitamin E. It protects the immune system by preventing the formation of free radicals, which can damage the body.

Selenium can be found in meat and grains, Brazil nuts, brewer's yeast, broccoli, brown rice, dairy products, garlic, molasses, and onions. The amount of selenium in food, however, has a direct correlation to the selenium content of the soil. The soil of much American farmland is low in selenium, resulting in selenium-deficient produce. Low dietary intake of selenium is associated with increased incidence of several cancers, including lung, colorectal, skin, and prostate. Selenium supplementation has resulted in increased natural killer cell activity, and studies show its promise as protection against prostate and colorectal cancers, especially among smokers (Lee et al., 2006; Peters et al., 2006; Reid et al., 2006).

37.4 Growth Fraction and Success of Chemotherapy

Although cancers grow rapidly, not all cells in a tumor are replicating at any given time. Because antineoplastic agents are generally more effective against cells that are replicating, the percentage of tumor cells dividing at the time of chemotherapy is critical.

Both normal and cancerous cells go through a sequence of events known as the *cell cycle,* illustrated in ● Figure 37.2. Cells spend most of their lifetime in the G_0 phase. Although sometimes called the *resting stage,* the G_0 is the phase during which cells conduct their everyday activities such as metabolism, impulse conduction, contraction, or secretion. If the cell receives a signal to divide, it leaves G_0 and enters the G_1 phase, during which it synthesizes the RNA, proteins, and other components needed to duplicate its DNA during the S phase. Following duplication of its DNA, the cell enters the premitotic phase, or G_2. Following mitosis in the M phase, the cell reenters its resting G_0 phase, where it may remain for extended periods, depending on the specific tissue and surrounding cellular signals.

The actions of some antineoplastic agents are specific to certain phases of the cell cycle, whereas others are mostly independent of the cell cycle. For example, mitotic inhibitors such as vincristine (Oncovin) affect the M phase, which includes prophase, metaphase, anaphase, and telophase. Antimetabolites such as fluorouracil (Adrucil) are most effective during the S phase. The effects of alkylating agents such as cyclophosphamide (Cytoxan) are generally independent of the phases of the cell cycle. Some of these agents are shown in Figure 37.2.

The **growth fraction** is a measure of the number of cells undergoing mitosis in a tissue. It is a ratio of the number of *replicating* cells to the number of *resting* cells. Antineoplastic drugs are much more toxic to tissues and tumors with high growth fractions. For example, solid tumors such as breast and lung cancer generally have a *low* growth fraction; thus, they are less sensitive to antineoplastic agents. Certain leukemias and lymphomas have a *high* growth fraction and therefore have a greater antineoplastic success rate. Because certain normal tissues, such as hair follicles, bone marrow, and the gastrointestinal (GI) epithelium also have a high growth fraction, they are sensitive to the effects of the antineoplastics.

37.5 Achieving a Total Cancer Cure

To cure a client, it is believed that every single cancer cell in a tumor must be destroyed or removed from the body. Even one malignant cell could potentially produce enough offspring to kill a client. In contrast to the role of the immune system as an active partner in anti-infective therapy in eliminating massive numbers of microorganisms, when battling cancer the immune system is able to eliminate only a relatively small number of cancer cells.

As an example, consider that a small, 1-cm breast tumor may already contain 1 billion cancer cells before it can be detected on a manual examination. A drug that could kill 99% of these cells would be considered a very effective drug, indeed. Yet even with this fantastic achievement, 10 million cancer cells would remain, any one of which could potentially cause the tumor to return and kill the client. The relationship between cell kill and chemotherapy is shown in ● Figure 37.3. This example reinforces the need to diagnose and treat tumors at an *early* stage using several therapies such as drugs, radiation, and surgery when possible.

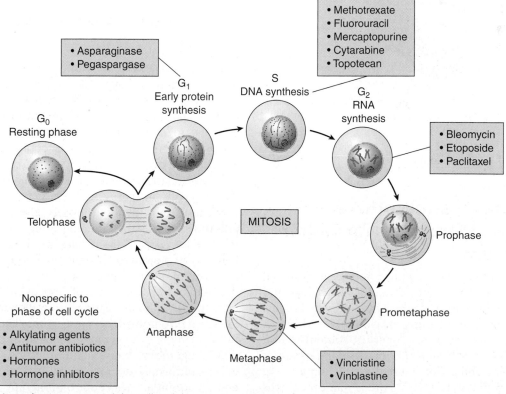

● **Figure 37.2** Antineoplastic agents and the cell cycle

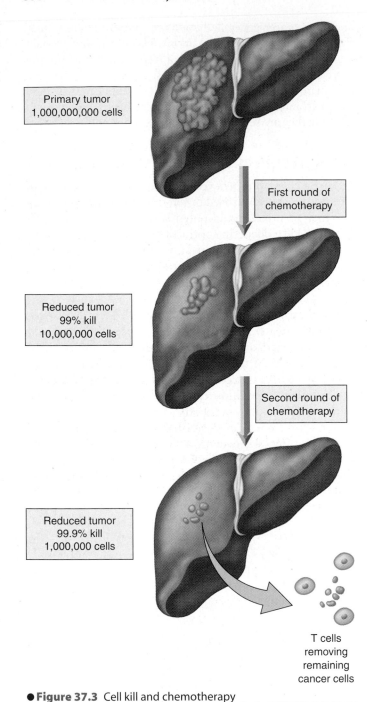

Primary tumor
1,000,000,000 cells

First round of
chemotherapy

Reduced tumor
99% kill
10,000,000 cells

Second round of
chemotherapy

Reduced tumor
99.9% kill
1,000,000 cells

T cells
removing
remaining
cancer cells

● **Figure 37.3** Cell kill and chemotherapy

37.6 Special Pharmacotherapy Protocols and Strategies for Cancer Chemotherapy

Because of their rapid cell division, tumor cells express a high mutation rate. This causes the tumor to change and become more heterogenous as it grows, essentially becoming a mass of hundreds of different clones with different growth rates and physiological properties. Administration of an antineoplastic drug may kill only a small portion of the tumor, leaving some clones unaffected. Complicating the chances for a pharmacological cure is that cancer cells often develop resistance to antineoplastic drugs. Thus a

therapy that was very successful in reducing the tumor mass at the start of chemotherapy may become less effective over time. The tumor becomes "refractory" to treatment.

A number of treatment strategies have been found to increase the effectiveness of anticancer drugs. In most cases, multiple drugs from different antineoplastic classes are given during a course of chemotherapy. The use of multiple drugs affects different stages of the cancer cell's life cycle, and attacks the various clones within the tumor via several mechanisms of action, thus increasing the percentage of cell kill. Combination chemotherapy also allows lower dosages of each individual agent, thus reducing toxicity and slowing the development of resistance. Examples of combination therapies include cyclophosphamide–methotrexate–fluorouracil (CMF) for breast cancer and cyclophosphamide–doxorubicin–vincristine (CDV) for lung cancer.

Specific dosing schedules, or protocols, have been found to increase the effectiveness of the antineoplastic agents. For example, some of the anticancer drugs are given as a single dose or perhaps several doses over a few days. A few weeks may pass before the next series of doses begins. This gives normal cells time to recover from the adverse effects of the drugs and allows tumor cells that may not have been replicating at the time of the first dose to begin dividing and become more sensitive to the next round of chemotherapy. Sometimes the optimum dosing schedule must be delayed until the client sufficiently recovers from the drug toxicities, especially bone marrow suppression. The specific combination of agents used and the dosing schedule chosen depend on the type of tumor, stage of the disease, and overall condition of the client.

37.7 Toxicity of Antineoplastic Agents

Although cancer cells are clearly abnormal in many ways, much of their physiology is identical with that of normal cells. Because it is difficult to kill cancer cells *selectively* without profoundly affecting normal cells, all anticancer drugs have the potential to cause serious toxicity. These drugs are often pushed to their maximum possible dosages, so that the greatest tumor kill can be obtained. Such high dosages always result in adverse effects in the client. Table 37.3 lists typical adverse effects of anticancer drugs.

Because these drugs primarily affect rapidly dividing cells, normal cells that are replicating are most susceptible to adverse effects. Hair follicles are damaged, resulting in hair loss or **alopecia.** The epithelial lining of the digestive tract commonly becomes inflamed, a condition known as **mucositis.** Consequences of mucositis include painful ulcerations, difficulty eating or swallowing, GI bleeding, intestinal infections, or severe diarrhea. The vomiting center in the medulla is triggered by many antineoplastics, resulting in significant nausea and vomiting. Because of this effect, antineoplastics are sometimes classified by their **emetic potential.** Before starting therapy with the highest emetic potential agents, clients may be pretreated with

TABLE 37.3 Adverse Effects of Anticancer Drugs

Changes to the Blood	Changes to the GI Tract	Other Effects
anemia (low red blood cell count)	anorexia	alopecia
leukopenia or neutropenia (low white blood cell count)	bleeding	fatigue
thrombocytopenia (low platelets)	diarrhea, extreme nausea and vomiting	fetal death/birth defects, opportunistic infections, ulceration and bleeding of the lips and gums

antiemetic drugs such as prochlorperazine (Compazine), metoclopramide (Reglan, others), or lorazepam (Ativan) (see Chapter 41 ∞).

Stem cells in the bone marrow may be destroyed by antineoplastics, causing anemia, leukopenia, and thrombocytopenia. These side effects are dose limiting and the ones that most often cause discontinuation or delays of chemotherapy. Severe bone marrow suppression is a contraindication to therapy with most antineoplastics. Efforts to minimize bone marrow toxicity may include bone marrow transplantation, platelet infusions, or therapy with growth factors such as epoetin alfa or granulocyte colony-stimulating factor (G-CSF), filgrastim (Neupogen), or sargramostim (Leukine) (see Chapter 28 ∞). The administration of G-CSFs often prevents or shortens the time period of neutropenia, thus lowering the risk of opportunistic infections and allowing the client to maintain an optimum dosing schedule.

Each antineoplastic drug has a documented **nadir,** the lowest point to which the neutrophil count is depressed by the chemotherapeutic agent. The nurse can calculate the absolute neutrophil count (ANC) by multiplying the white blood cell count by the percentage of neutrophils. This value can be obtained by reading the client's complete blood count (CBC) with differential. If the ANC falls below $500/mm^3$, the risk of infection increases. If a neutropenic client develops a fever, antibiotics are indicated.

When possible, antineoplastics are given locally by topical application or through direct instillation into a tumor site to minimize systemic toxicity. Most antineoplastics, however, are given intravenously. Many antineoplastics are classified as **vesicants,** agents that can cause serious tissue injury if they escape from an artery or vein during an infusion or injection. Extravasation from an injection site can produce severe tissue, and nerve damage, local infection, and even loss of a limb. Rapid treatment of extravasation is necessary to limit tissue damage, and certain antineoplastics have specific antidotes. For example, extravasation of carmustine (BiCNU, Gliadel) is treated with injections of equal parts of sodium bicarbonate and normal saline into the extravasation site. Before administering intravenous antineoplastic agents, the nurse should know the emergency treatment for extravasation. Antineoplastics with the strongest vesicant activity include busulfan, carmustine, dacarbazine, dactinomycin, daunorubicin, idarubicin, mechlorethamine, mitomycin, plicamycin, streptozocin, vinblastine, vincristine, and vinorelbine.

Cancer survivors face several possible long-term consequences from chemotherapy. Some antineoplastics, particularly the alkylating agents, affect the gonads and have been associated with infertility in both male and female clients. A second concern for long-term survivors is the induction of secondary malignancies caused by the antineoplastic agents. These secondary tumors may occur decades after the chemotherapy was administered. Although many different secondary malignancies have been reported, the most common is acute nonlymphocytic leukemia. In most cases, the immediate benefits of using antineoplastics to cure a cancer far outweigh the small risk of developing a secondary malignancy.

37.8 Classification of Antineoplastic Agents

Drugs used in cancer chemotherapy come from diverse pharmacological and chemical classes. Antineoplastics have been extracted from plants and bacteria, as well as created entirely in the laboratory. Some of the drug classes attack cellular macromolecules, such as DNA and proteins, whereas others poison vital metabolic pathways of rapidly growing cells. The common theme among all the antineoplastic agents is that they kill or at least stop the growth of cancer cells.

Classification of the various antineoplastics is quite variable because some of these drugs kill cancer cells by several different mechanisms and have characteristics from more than one class. Furthermore, the mechanisms by which some antineoplastics act are not completely understood. A simple method of classifying this complex group of drugs includes the following six categories:

- Alkylating agents
- Antimetabolites
- Antitumor antibiotics
- Hormones and hormone antagonists
- Natural products
- Biologic response modifiers and miscellaneous anticancer drugs

ALKYLATING AGENTS

The first alkylating agents, the nitrogen mustards, were developed in secrecy as chemical warfare agents during World War II. Although the drugs in this class have quite different chemical structures, all share the common characteristic of forming bonds or linkages with DNA, a process called **alkylation.** ● Figure 37.4 illustrates the process of alkylation.

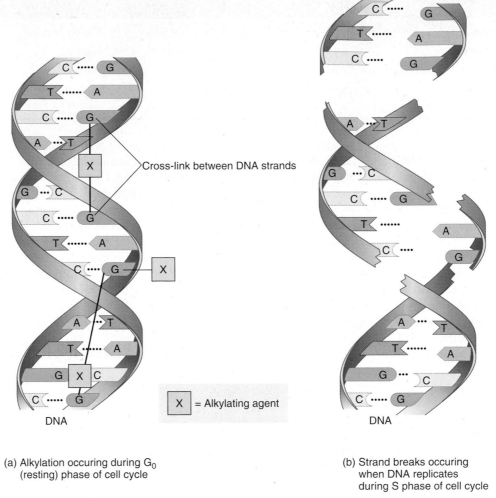

Cross-link between DNA strands

X = Alkylating agent

DNA

DNA

(a) Alkylation occuring during G₀
(resting) phase of cell cycle

(b) Strand breaks occuring
when DNA replicates
during S phase of cell cycle

● **Figure 37.4** Mechanism of action of the alkylating agents

37.9 Pharmacotherapy With Alkylating Agents

Alkylation changes the shape of the DNA double helix and prevents the nucleic acid from completing normal cell division. Each alkylating agent attaches to DNA in a different manner; however, collectively the alkylating agents have the effect of inducing cell death, or at least slowing the replication of tumor cells. Although the process of alkylation occurs independently of the cell cycle, the killing action does not occur until the affected cell divides. The alkylating agents have a broad spectrum and are used against many types of malignancies. They are some of the most widely used antineoplastic drugs. These agents are listed in Table 37.4.

Blood cells are particularly sensitive to alkylating agents, and bone marrow suppression is the primary dose-limiting adverse effect of drugs in this class. Within days after administration, the numbers of erythrocytes, leukocytes, and platelets begin to decline, reaching a nadir at 6 to 10 days. Epithelial cells lining the GI tract are also damaged with alkylating agents, causing nausea, vomiting, and diarrhea. Alopecia may be expected from most of the alkylating agents. The nitrosoureas and mechlorethamine are

strong vesicants. Approximately 5% of the clients treated with alkylating agents develop acute nonlymphocytic leukemia 4 years or more after chemotherapy has been completed.

NURSING CONSIDERATIONS

The role of the nurse in therapy with alkylating agents for cancer involves careful monitoring of a client's condition and providing education as it relates to the prescribed drug treatment. Because alkylating agents kill rapidly dividing cells, assess baseline vital signs, CBC with differential, and the client's overall health status, including renal and liver function, intake and output, and body weight. These drugs may be withheld if RBC, WBC, and platelet counts fall below a predetermined limit during therapy. Alkylating agents must be administered with caution to clients with hepatic or renal impairment, recent steroid therapy, leukopenia, or thrombocytopenia.

Hydrate clients with IV or oral fluids before starting chemotherapy. Increase fluids to 2 to 3 L/day. Assess for urinary frequency, dysuria, and hematuria.

Alkylating agents are highly toxic to tissues with a rapid growth rate. Bone marrow depression occurs because these

TABLE 37.4   Alkylating Agents

Drug	Route and Adult Dose (max dose where indicated)	Adverse Effects
NITROGEN MUSTARDS		
chlorambucil (Leukeran)	PO; Initial dose: 0.1–0.2 mg/kg/day; Maintenance dose 4–10 mg/day	*Nausea, vomiting, stomatitis, anorexia, rash, headache, alopecia*
cyclophosphamide (Cytoxan, Neosar)	PO; Initial dose 1–5 mg/day; Maintenance dose 1–5 mg/kg q 7–10 days	
estramustine (Emcyt)	PO; 14 mg/kg/day in 3–4 divided doses	Bone marrow suppression (neutropenia, anemia, thrombocytopenia), severe nausea, vomiting and diarrhea, Stevens–Johnson syndrome, hemorrhagic cystitis, pulmonary toxicity, neurotoxicity (carboplatin, cisplatin, oxaliplatin), ototoxicity (cisplatin), hypersensitivity reactions (including anaphylaxis)
ifosfamide (Ifex)	IV; 1.2 g/m^2/day for 5 consecutive days	
mechlorethamine (Mustargen)	IV; 6 mg/m^2 on Days 1 and 8 of a 28-day cycle	
melphalan (Alkeran)	PO; 6 mg/day for 2–3 wk	
NITROSOUREAS		
carmustine (BiCNU, Gliadel)	IV; 200 mg/m^2 q6wk	
lomustine (CeeNU, CCNU)	PO; 130 mg/m^2 as a single dose	
streptozocin (Zanosar)	IV; 500 mg/m^2 for 5 consecutive days	
MISCELLANEOUS ALKYLATING AGENTS		
altretamine (Hexalen)	PO; 65 mg/m^2/day	
busulfan (Myleran)	PO; 4–8 mg/day	
carboplatin (Paraplatin)	IV; 360 mg/m^2 once q4wk	
cisplatin (Platinol)	IV; 20 mg/m^2/day for 5 days	
dacarbazine (DTIC-Dome)	IV; 2–4.5 mg/kg/day for 10 days	
oxaliplatin (Eloxatin)	IV; 85 mg/m^2 for 2 h	
procarbazine (Matulane)	PO; 2–4 mg/kg/day	
temozolomide (Temodar)	PO; 150 mg/m^2/day for 5 consecutive days	
thiotepa (Thioplex, TSPA)	IV; 0.3–0.4 mg/kg q1–4wk	

Italics indicate common adverse effects; underlining indicates serious adverse effects.

agents kill normal hematopoietic cells. Advise clients to avoid crowds and those who have respiratory infections. Remain alert to the possible development of blood dyscrasias by observing the client for signs and symptoms such as bruising or bleeding and by closely monitoring the CBC with differential and platelet count. Secondary leukemias are frequently associated with this class of drugs.

Monitor nutritional intake. Assess for nausea and vomiting, because these drugs may cause injury to the GI mucosa, and administer antiemetic drugs, as necessary. Advise clients to eat small, frequent meals; to avoid high-purine foods such as organ meats, beans, and peas; and to avoid citric acid. Offer clients food and fluids (crackers, ginger ale) to reduce nausea. Also offer ice chips or ice pops to relieve mouth pain.

Assess skin integrity, because nitrogen mustards may cause skin eruptions such as blistering. Monitor for signs of hearing loss with platinum alkylating agents (for example, cisplatin), which may cause high-frequency hearing loss.

Alkylating agents may depress spermatogenesis and oocyte production, and clients of childbearing age should be informed of the potential adverse impact on fertility.

Counsel both women and men to abstain from coitus or to use reliable contraception during therapy and for 4 months thereafter. Assist the client in choosing an appropriate method for the client's cultural background, lifestyle, and health. Sterility and amenorrhea may occur in clients on mechlorethamine (Mustargen) or cyclophosphamide (Cytoxan) therapy, but these effects are reversible once therapy is discontinued. Cyclophosphamide also diminishes sex drive. Encourage clients to frankly discuss sexual issues with you, especially regarding options to preserve fertility. Alkylating agents range from pregnancy category C (streptozocin, cyclophosphamide) to category X (estramustine).

Client Teaching.   Client education as it relates to alkylating agents should include the goals of therapy; the reasons for obtaining baseline data such as vital signs, blood work, and the existence of underlying cardiac and renal disorders; and possible drug side effects. Include the following points when teaching clients about alkylating agents:

- Practice reliable contraception and notify your health-care provider if pregnancy is planned or suspected.
- Do not breast-feed during treatment.

Pr **PROTOTYPE DRUG** | Cyclophosphamide *(Cytoxan)* | Antineoplastic/Alkylating Agent

ACTIONS AND USES

Cyclophosphamide is a commonly prescribed nitrogen mustard. It is used alone, or in combination with other drugs, against a wide variety of cancers, including Hodgkin's disease, lymphoma, multiple myeloma, breast cancer, and ovarian cancer. Cyclophosphamide acts by attaching to DNA and disrupting replication, particularly in rapidly dividing cells. It is one of only a few anticancer drugs that are well absorbed when given orally. Because of its potent immunosuppressive properties, it has been used for nonneoplastic disorders such as prevention of transplant rejection and severe rheumatoid arthritis. PO and IV formulations are available.

ADMINISTRATION ALERTS

- Dilute prior to IV administration.
- Monitor platelet count prior to IM administration; if low, hold dose.
- To avoid GI upset, take with meals or divide doses.
- Pregnancy category C.

PHARMACOKINETICS (PO)

Onset: Unknown

Peak: 1 h

Half-life: 4–6 h

Duration: Unknown

ADVERSE EFFECTS

Cyclophosphamide exerts rapid and powerful immunosuppressant effects. Leukocyte counts often serve as a guide to dosage adjustments during therapy. Thrombocytopenia is common, though less severe than with many other alkylating agents. Nausea, vomiting, anorexia, and diarrhea are frequently experienced. Cyclophosphamide causes alopecia, although this effect is usually reversible. Several metabolites of cyclophosphamide may cause hemorrhagic cystitis if the urine becomes concentrated; clients should be advised to maintain high fluid intake during therapy. Unlike other nitrogen mustards, cyclophosphamide exhibits little neurotoxicity.

Contraindications: Cyclophosphamide is contraindicated in clients with hypersensitivity to the drug and for those who have active infections or severely suppressed bone marrow.

INTERACTIONS

Drug–Drug: Immunosuppressant agents used concurrently with cyclophosphamide may increase risk of infections and further development of neoplasms. There is an increased chance of bone marrow toxicity if cyclophosphamide is used concurrently with allopurinol. If anticoagulants are used concurrently, increased anticoagulant effects may occur, leading to hemorrhage.

If used concurrently with digoxin, decreased serum levels of digoxin occur. Use with insulin may lead to hypoglycemia. Phenobarbital, phenytoin, or glucocorticoids used concurrently may lead to an increased rate of cyclophosphamide metabolism by the liver. Thiazide diuretics increase the possibility of leukopenia.

Lab Tests: Serum uric acid levels may increase. Blood cell counts will diminish owing to bone marrow suppression. Positive reactions to *Candida*, mumps, and tuberculin skin tests (PPD) are suppressed. PAP smears may give false positives.

Herbal/Food: Use with caution with herbal supplements, such as echinacea, which is an immune stimulator and may interfere with the drug's immunosuppressant effects.

Treatment of Overdose: There is no specific treatment for overdose.

 See the Companion Website for a Nursing Process Focus specific to this drug.

- Obtain routine hearing screenings during therapy.
- Immediately report buzzing, ringing, or tingling sensation in the ears, or decreased hearing.
- Immediately report palpitations and dizziness or fainting when moving to an upright position; fever, chills, sore throat, dyspnea, and increased fatigue; gout and kidney stones; skin rashes; bleeding gums, petechiae, and bruises; blood in urine or stool.
- Avoid crowds or anyone with respiratory infection.
- Use good oral hygiene with a soft toothbrush.
- Know that hair loss may occur.
- Know that amenorrhea, menstrual irregularities, and sterility may occur in premenopausal women; impotence may occur in men.
- Avoid citric acid and foods high in purines (organ meats, beans, peas).
- Plan small, frequent meals.

Please refer to "Nursing Process Focus: Clients Receiving Antineoplastic Therapy" on page 572 for additional teaching points.

ANTIMETABOLITES

Antimetabolites are antineoplastic drugs chemically similar to essential building blocks of the cell. Because they resemble certain critical cell molecules, these drugs interfere with aspects of the nutrient or nucleic acid metabolism of rapidly growing tumor cells.

37.10 Pharmacotherapy With Antimetabolites

Rapidly growing cancer cells require large quantities of nutrients to construct proteins and nucleic acids. Antimetabolite drugs are structurally similar to these nutrients, but they do not perform the same functions as their natural counterparts. When cancer cells attempt to synthesize proteins, RNA, or DNA using the antimetabolites, metabolic pathways are disrupted and the cancer cells die or their growth is slowed. The three classes of antimetabolites are the folic acid analogs, the purine analogs, and the pyrimidine analogs. These agents are prescribed for leukemias and solid tumors and are listed in Table 37.5.

The purine and pyrimidine analogs are structurally similar to the natural building blocks of DNA and RNA. For example, the pyrimidine analog fluorouracil (Adrucil) is able to block the formation of thymidylate, an essential chemical needed to make DNA, and is used in treating various solid tumors. After becoming activated and incorporated into DNA, cytarabine (Cytosar) blocks DNA synthesis and is an important drug in treating acute myelocytic leukemia. Approved in 2005, azacitidine (Vidaza) is a pyrimidine analog that is the first drug approved to treat myelodysplastic syndrome, a bone marrow disorder characterized by the production of abnormal, immature cells. Another drug approved in 2005 was clofarabine (Clolar), a purine antimetabolite that is the first new drug approved for pediatric acute leukemia in over a decade. Methotraxate (Mexate, others) and the newly approved pemetrexed (Alimta) resemble folic acid, a natural B vitamin. ● Figure 37.5 illustrates the structural similarities of some of these antimetabolites to their natural counterparts.

Bone marrow toxicity is the principal dose-limiting adverse effect of many drugs in this class. Some also cause serious GI toxicity, including ulcerations of the mucosa. Mercaptopurine and thioguanine can cause hepatotoxicity, including cholestatic jaundice.

NURSING CONSIDERATIONS

The role of the nurse in antimetabolite therapy involves careful monitoring of a client's condition and providing education as it relates to the prescribed drug treatment. Because of bone marrow toxicity, assess baseline vital signs, CBC with differential, and platelet counts. Assess the client's overall health status, including renal and liver function, intake and output, and body weight before initiating chemotherapy. Assess temperature during therapy; fever may be a sign of infection.

Many antimetabolites are contraindicated in pregnancy; for example, methotrexate (Mexate) is a category X drug, and pregnancy should be avoided for 4 to 6 months following termination of therapy. Further contraindications include hepatic, cardiac, and renal insufficiency; myelosuppression; and blood dyscrasias. Antimetabolites cause many of the adverse effects common to other antineoplastics, including alopecia, fatigue, nausea, vomiting, diarrhea, bone marrow depression, and blood dyscrasias. These drugs may also cause photosensitivity and idiosyncratic pneumonitis.

Closely monitor clients with peptic ulcer disease, ulcerative colitis, or poor nutritional status. Assess for nausea and

TABLE 37.5 Antimetabolites

Drug	Route and Adult Dose (max dose where indicated)	Adverse Effects
FOLIC ACID ANTAGONISTS		
ⓟ methotrexate (Folex, Mexate, others)	PO; 10–30 mg/day for 5 days	*Nausea, vomiting, nausea, stomatitis, anorexia, rash, headache, alopecia*
pemetrexed (Alimta)	IV; 500mg/m^2 on Day 1 of each 21-day cycle	
PYRIMIDINE ANALOGS		
azacitidine (Vidaza)	Subcutaneous; 75 mg/m^2/day for 7 days q4wk	<u>Bone marrow suppression (neutropenia, anemia, thrombocytopenia), severe nausea, vomiting and diarrhea, hepatotoxicity, mucositis, pulmonary toxicity, hypersensitivity reactions (including anaphylaxis), neurotoxicity (cytarabine, fluorouracil, fludarabine, cladribine)</u>
capecitabine (Xeloda)	PO; 2,500 mg/m^2/day for 2 wk	
cytarabine (Cytosar-U, Tarabine, DepoCyt)	IV; 200 mg/m^2 as a continuous infusion over 24 h	
floxuridine (FUDR)	Intra-arterial: 0.1–0.6 mg/kg/day as a continuous infusion	
fluorouracil (5-FU, Adrucil, Efudex, Fluoroplex)	IV; 12 mg/kg/day for 4 consecutive days	
gemcitabine (Gemzar)	IV; 1,000 mg/m^2 q1wk for 7 wk	
PURINE ANALOGS		
cladribine (Leustatin)	IV; 0.09 mg/m^2/day as a continuous infusion	
fludarabine (Fludara)	IV; 25 mg/m^2/day for 5 consecutive days	
mercaptopurine (Purinethol)	PO; 2.5 mg/kg/day	
nelarabine (Arranon)	IV; 1500 mg/m^2 on Days 1, 3, and 5, repeated every 21 days	
pentostatin (Nipent)	IV; 4 mg/m^2 every other week	
thioguanine (Lanvis)	PO; 2 mg/kg/day	

Italics indicate common adverse effects; <u>underlining</u> indicates serious adverse effects.

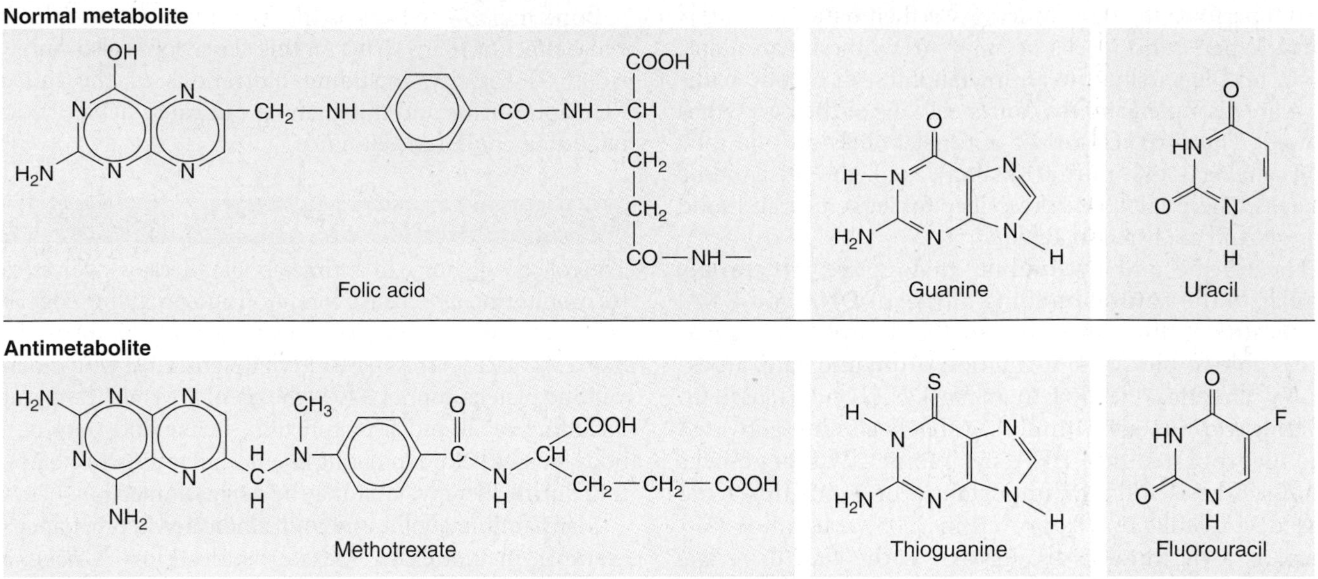

Normal metabolite

Folic acid

Guanine

Uracil

Antimetabolite

Methotrexate

Thioguanine

Fluorouracil

Figure 37.5 Structural similarities between antimetabolites and their natural counterparts

---

Pr PROTOTYPE DRUG | Methotrexate *(Folex, Mexate, others)* | Antineoplastic/Antimetabolite

ACTIONS AND USES

Methotrexate is an older drug; it was the first antineoplastic to cure a solid tumor (choriocarcinoma) in 1963. By blocking the synthesis of folic acid (vitamin B$_9$), methotrexate inhibits replication, particularly in rapidly dividing cells. It is prescribed alone or in combination with other drugs for choriocarcinoma, osteogenic sarcoma, leukemias, head and neck cancers, breast carcinoma, and lung carcinoma. It is occasionally used to treat non-neoplastic disorders such as severe psoriasis and rheumatoid arthritis that have not responded to other medications. Methotrexate may be administered by the oral, IM, or IV routes.

ADMINISTRATION ALERTS

- Avoid skin exposure to drug.
- Avoid inhaling drug particles.
- Dilute prior to IV administration.
- Pregnancy category X.

PHARMACOKINETICS

Onset: Unknown

Peak: 1–4 h PO; 0.5–2 h IM/IV

Half-life: 1–4 h

Duration: Unknown

ADVERSE EFFECTS

A potent immunosuppressant, methotrexate can result in fatal bone marrow toxicity at high doses. Hemorrhage and bruising are often observed owing to low platelet counts. Nausea, vomiting, and anorexia are common, and GI ulceration may result in serious intestinal bleeding. Although rare, serious pulmonary toxicity may develop.

Contraindications: Methotrexate is teratogenic and is contraindicated in pregnant clients. Clients with alcoholism or other chronic liver disease should not receive methotrexate. Immunodeficient clients or those with blood dyscrasias should not receive methotrexate.

INTERACTIONS

Drug–Drug: Bone marrow suppressants such as chemotherapy agents or radiation therapy may cause increased effects; the client will require a lower dose of methotrexate. Concurrent use with NSAIDs may lead to severe methotrexate toxicity. Aspirin may interfere with excretion of methotrexate, leading to increased serum levels and toxicity. Concurrent administration with live oral vaccine may result in decreased antibody response and increased adverse reactions to the vaccine.

Lab Tests: Serum uric acid levels may increase. Blood cell counts will diminish owing to bone marrow suppression.

Herbal/Food: Echinacea may interfere with the drug's immunosuppressant effects.

Treatment of Overdose: Leucovorin (folinic acid), a reduced form of folic acid, is sometimes administered with methotrexate to "rescue" normal cells, or to protect against severe bone marrow damage. It is most effective if administered as soon as possible after the overdose is discovered. In addition, the urine may be alkalinized to protect the kidneys from toxicity.

 See the Companion Website for a Nursing Process Focus specific to this drug.

vomiting, because these drugs may cause injury to the GI mucosa, and administer antiemetic drugs, as necessary. Offer client foods and fluids (crackers, ginger ale) that may decrease vomiting. Give ice chips or ice pops to reduce mouth pain. Advise clients to eat small, frequent meals, to avoid high-purine foods such as organ meats, beans, and peas, and to avoid citric acid.

Observe the client for signs and symptoms of respiratory infection, including shortness of breath, cough, fever, and especially rash or chest pain (pleurisy). Viral infections such as herpes/varicella strains can be especially virulent when experienced during antimetabolite therapy. Encourage clients to regularly practice deep breathing, if necessary, with the aid of an incentive spirometer.

Teach clients to use good oral hygiene and encourage mouth rinses every 2 hours with normal saline. Brush teeth with a soft toothbrush.

Monitor the IV site frequently for extravasation. Apply an ice pack and notify the healthcare provider if this occurs.

Client Teaching. Client education as it relates to antimetabolites should include the goals of therapy; the reasons for obtaining baseline data such as vital signs, weight, intake and output, CBC, and tests, and the existence of underlying immune, lung, and renal disorders; and possible drug side effects. Include the following points when teaching clients about antimetabolites:

- Practice reliable contraception and notify your healthcare provider if pregnancy is planned or suspected.
- Avoid pregnancy for 4 to 6 months after completing antineoplastic therapy.
- Do not breast-feed during treatment.
- Obtain routine hearing screenings during therapy.
- Immediately report buzzing, ringing, or tingling sensation in the ears, or decreased hearing.
- Immediately report palpitations and dizziness or fainting when moving to an upright position; fever, chills, sore throat, dyspnea, and increased fatigue; skin rashes; bleeding gums, petechiae, and bruises; blood in urine or stool.
- Avoid crowds or anyone with respiratory infection.
- Use good oral hygiene with a soft toothbrush.
- Know that hair loss may occur.
- Know that amenorrhea, menstrual irregularities, and sterility may occur in premenopausal women; impotence may occur in men.
- Avoid citric acid and foods high in purines (organ meats, beans, peas).
- Plan small, frequent meals.
- Regularly practice deep-breathing exercises.
- Eliminate or reduce respiratory irritants in the environment such as secondhand tobacco smoke or aerosol cosmetics (for example, hair spray or deodorants).

Please refer to "Nursing Process Focus: Clients Receiving Antineoplastic Therapy" on page 572 for additional teaching points.

ANTITUMOR ANTIBIOTICS

The antitumor antibiotics class contains substances obtained from bacteria that have the ability to kill cancer cells. Although not widely used, they are very effective against certain tumors.

37.11 Pharmacotherapy With Antitumor Antibiotics

Antitumor properties have been identified in a number of substances isolated from microorganisms. These chemicals are more cytotoxic than traditional antibiotics, and their use is restricted to treating a few specific types of cancer. For example, the only indication for idarubicin (Idamycin) is acute myelogenous leukemia. Testicular carcinoma is the only indication for plicamycin (Mithramycin). The antitumor antibiotics are listed in Table 37.6.

The antitumor antibiotics bind to DNA and affect its function by a mechanism similar to that of the alkylating agents. Thus, their general actions and side effects are similar to those of the alkylating agents. Unlike the alkylating agents, however, all the antitumor antibiotics must be administered intravenously or through direct instillation via a catheter into a body cavity.

As with other antineoplastics, a major dose-limiting adverse effect of drugs in this class is bone marrow suppression. Doxorubicin, daunorubicin, epirubicin, and idarubicin are all closely related in structure, and cardiac toxicity is a major limiting adverse effect. Cardiotoxicity may occur within minutes of administration, or be delayed for months or years after chemotherapy has been completed. Valrubicin is a newer antitumor antibiotic that is instilled into the bladder to treat bladder cancer; thus, its adverse effects are limited to that organ.

NURSING CONSIDERATIONS

The role of the nurse in antitumor antibiotic therapy involves careful monitoring of a client's condition and providing education as it relates to the prescribed drug treatment. Because of bone marrow and cardiac toxicity, assess CBC with differential, and platelet count weekly. The drug may be withheld if the RBC, WBC, and platelet counts fall below predetermined levels. Prophylactic antibiotics may be ordered to prevent infection. Assess the client's overall health status. Monitor renal and liver function, intake and output, and body weight before initiating chemotherapy. Interview the client regarding any history of allergy prior to initiating therapy. Assess vital signs—including auscultation of heart and chest sounds—and obtain a baseline ECG to rule out signs of cardiac abnormality or heart failure. Antitumor antibiotics can be damaging to the myocardium; thus, they should be used with extreme caution, if at all, for clients

TABLE 37.6 Antitumor Antibiotics

Drug	Route and Adult Dose (max dose where indicated)	Adverse Effects
bleomycin (Blenoxane)	IV; 0.25–0.5 unit/kg q4–7days	*Nausea, vomiting, stomatitis, anorexia, rash, headache, alopecia*
dactinomycin (Actinomycin-D, Cosmegen)	IV; 500 mcg/day for maximum of 5 days	
daunorubicin (Cerubidine)	IV; 30–60 mg/m^2/day for 3–5 days	Bone marrow suppression (neutropenia, anemia, thrombocytopenia), severe nausea, vomiting and diarrhea, cardiotoxicity, tissue necrosis due to extravasation, mucositis, pulmonary toxicity, hypersensitivity reactions (including anaphylaxis)
daunorubicin liposomal (DaunoXome)	IV; 40 mg/m^2 q2wk	
doxorubicin (Adriamycin, Rubex)	IV; 60–75 mg/m^2 as a single dose at 21-day intervals, or 30 mg/m^2 on each of 3 consecutive days (max: total cumulative dose 550 mg/m^2)	
doxorubicin liposomal (Doxil)	IV; 20 mg/m^2 q3wk	
epirubicin (Ellence)	IV; 100–120 mg/m^2 as a single dose	
idarubicin (Idamycin)	IV; 8–12 mg/m^2/day for 3 days	
mitomycin (Mutamycin)	IV; 2 mg/m^2 as a single dose	
mitoxantrone (Novantrone)	IV; 12 mg/m^2/day for 3 days	
plicamycin (Mithramycin, Mithracin)	IV; 25–30 mcg/kg/day for 8–10 days	
valrubicin (Valstar)	Intrabladder instillation; 800 mg q1wk for 6 wk	

Italics indicate common adverse effects; <u>underlining</u> indicates serious adverse effects.

Pr PROTOTYPE DRUG | Doxorubicin *(Adriamycin)* | Antitumor Antibiotic

ACTIONS AND USES

Doxorubicin attaches to DNA, distorting its double helical structure and preventing normal DNA and RNA synthesis. It is administered only by IV infusion. Doxorubicin is a broad-spectrum cytotoxic antibiotic, prescribed for solid tumors of the lung, breast, ovary, and bladder, and for various leukemias and lymphomas. It is structurally similar to daunorubicin.

A novel delivery method has been developed for both doxorubicin and daunorubicin. The drug is enclosed in small lipid sacs, or vesicles, called *liposomes*. The liposomal vesicle is designed to open and release the antitumor antibiotic when it reaches a cancer cell. The goal is to deliver a higher concentration of drug to the cancer cells, thus sparing normal cells. An additional advantage is that doxorubicin liposomal has a half-life of 50 to 60 hours, which is about twice that of regular doxorubicin. The primary indication for this delivery method is AIDS-related Kaposi's sarcoma.

ADMINISTRATION ALERTS

- Extravasation from an injection site can cause severe pain and extensive tissue damage.
- For infants and children, verify concentration and rate of IV infusion with healthcare provider.
- Avoid skin contact with drug. If exposure occurs, wash thoroughly with soap and water.
- Pregnancy category D.

PHARMACOKINETICS

Onset: Rapid

Peak: Unknown

Half-life: 17–32 h

Duration: Unknown

ADVERSE EFFECTS

The most serious dose-limiting adverse effect is cardiotoxicity. Acute effects include dysrhythmias; delayed effects may include irreversible heart failure. Like many of the anticancer drugs, doxorubicin may profoundly lower blood cell counts. Acute nausea and vomiting are common and often require antiemetic therapy. Complete, though reversible, hair loss occurs in most clients.

Contraindications: Doxorubicin is contraindicated in clients who are immunosuppressed or who have hypersensitivity to the drug.

INTERACTIONS

Drug–Drug: If digoxin is taken concurrently, client serum digoxin levels will decrease. Use with phenobarbital may lead to increased plasma clearance of doxorubicin and decreased effectiveness. Use with phenytoin may lead to decreased phenytoin level, and possible seizure activity. Hepatotoxicity may occur if mercaptopurine is taken concurrently. Use with verapamil may increase serum doxorubicin levels, leading to doxorubicin toxicity.

Lab Tests: Serum uric acid and aspartate aminotransferase (AST) levels may increase. Blood cell counts will diminish owing to bone marrow suppression.

Herbal/Food: Green tea may enhance the antitumor activity of doxorubicin.

Treatment of Overdose: The primary result of overdosage is immunosuppression. Treatment includes prophylactic antimicrobials, platelet transfusions, symptomatic treatment of mucositis, and possibly hemopoietic growth factor (G-CSF, GM-CSF).

 See the Companion Website for a Nursing Process Focus specific to this drug.

with cardiac disease. Monitor ECG throughout treatment, especially for T-wave flattening, ST depression, or voltage reduction. Assess for pregnancy and lactation, because antitumor antibiotics range from pregnancy category C (dactinomycin, plicamycin, and valrubicin) to category D (bleomycin, daunorubicin, all others).

Antitumor antibiotics require cautious use. These drugs produce the same general cytotoxic effects as other antineoplastics, including alopecia, fatigue, nausea, vomiting, diarrhea, bone marrow suppression, and blood dyscrasias. The risk of hypersensitivity reactions such as life-threatening angioedema exists as with other antibiotics. Doxorubicin (Adriamycin) should be used cautiously if the client has received cyclophosphamide, pelvic radiation, or radiotherapy to areas surrounding the heart, or has a history of atopic dermatitis. Other effects include hyperpigmentation of the mucosa and nail beds, particularly among African Americans, and changes in the rectal mucosa. For this reason, do not administer suppositories or take temperatures rectally.

Doxorubicin is easily absorbed through the skin and by inhalation and may cause fetal death or birth defects as well as liver disease. Therefore, wear protective clothing (gloves, mask, and apron) when preparing the drug.

Carefully monitor the IV site because doxorubicin is a severe vesicant. Give drug through a large-bore, quickly running IV. Apply an ice pack and notify the healthcare provider if extravasation occurs.

Assess for nausea and vomiting, because these drugs may cause injury to the GI mucosa. Be prepared to administer antiemetic drugs, as necessary. Offer client foods and fluids (crackers, ginger ale) that may decrease vomiting. Give ice chips or ice pops to reduce mouth pain. Advise clients to eat small, frequent meals, to avoid high-purine foods such as organ meats, beans, and peas, and to avoid citric acid.

Client Teaching.   Client education as it relates to antitumor antibiotics should include the goals of therapy; the reasons for obtaining baseline data such as vital signs, blood work, ECG, and the existence of underlying cardiac disorders; and possible drug side effects. Include the following points when teaching clients about antitumor antibiotics:

- Use good oral hygiene. Changes in the color of the mucosa can make it difficult to distinguish the degree of tissue oxygenation or the severity of mouth sores. Inform the dentist of antitumor antibiotic therapy.

- Do not take rectal temperatures, and avoid using OTC rectal suppositories.

- Immediate report signs of severe allergic reaction or possible heart attack, such as shortness of breath, thick tongue, throat tightness or facial swelling, rash, palpitations, and chest, arm, or back pain.

- Immediately report headache, dizziness, or rectal bleeding.

- Practice reliable contraception and notify your healthcare provider if pregnancy is planned or suspected.

- Avoid pregnancy for 4 months after completing antineoplastic therapy.

- Do not breast-feed during treatment.

- Avoid crowds or anyone with respiratory infection.

- Know that complete hair loss may occur with high doses.

- Know that amenorrhea, menstrual irregularities, and sterility may occur in premenopausal women; impotence may occur in men.

Please refer to "Nursing Process Focus: Clients Receiving Antineoplastic Therapy" on page 572 for additional teaching points.

NATURAL PRODUCTS (PLANT EXTRACTS AND ALKALOIDS)

Plants have been a valuable source for antineoplastic agents. These natural products act by preventing the division of cancer cells.

37.12 Pharmacotherapy With Natural Products

Agents with antineoplastic activity have been isolated from a number of plants, including the common periwinkle (*Vinca rosea*), Pacific yew (*Taxus baccata*), mandrake (May apple), and the shrub *Camptotheca acuminata*. Although structurally very different, medications in this class have the common ability to affect cell division; thus, some of them are called *mitotic inhibitors*. The plant extracts, or natural products, are listed in Table 37.7.

The **vinca alkaloids,** vincristine (Oncovin) and vinblastine (Velban), are two older drugs derived from more than 100 alkaloids isolated from the periwinkle plant. The medicinal properties of this plant were described in folklore in several regions of the world long before their antineoplastic properties were discovered. Despite being derived from the same plant, vincristine, vinblastine, and the semisynthetic vinorelbine (Navelbine) exhibit different effects and toxicity profiles. Vincristine is a common component of regimens for treating pediatric leukemias, lymphomas, and solid tumors. The use of vinblastine has declined because of the development of newer and more effective agents, but it has traditionally been used to treat Hodgkin's disease and testicular tumors.

The **taxanes,** which include paclitaxel (Taxol) and docetaxel (Taxotere), were originally isolated from the bark of the Pacific yew, an evergreen found in forests throughout the western United States. More than 19 different taxane alkaloids have been isolated from the tree, and several others are being investigated for potential antineoplastic activity. Like the vinca alkaloids, the taxanes are mitotic inhibitors. Paclitaxel is approved for metastatic ovarian and breast cancer and for Kaposi's sarcoma; however, off-label uses include many other cancers. A semisynthetic product of paclitaxel, docetaxel, is claimed to have greater antitumor

TABLE 37.7	Natural Products With Antineoplastic Activity	
Drug	**Route and Adult Dose (max dose where indicated)**	**Adverse Effects**
VINCA ALKALOIDS		
vinblastine sulfate (Velban)	IV; 3.7–18.5 mg/m^2 q1wk	*Nausea, vomiting, asthenia, stomatitis, anorexia, rash, alopecia*
vincristine sulfate (Oncovin)	IV; 1.4 mg/m^2 q1wk (max: 2 mg/m^2)	
vinorelbine tartrate (Navelbine)	IV; 30 mg/m^2 q1wk	
TAXANES		Bone marrow suppression (neutropenia, anemia, thrombocytopenia), severe nausea, vomiting and diarrhea, cardiotoxicity, mucositis, pulmonary toxicity, hypersensitivity reactions, (including anaphylaxis), neurotoxicity (docetaxel, vincristine), nephrotoxicity (vincristine)
docetaxel (Taxotere)	IV; 60–100 mg/m^2 q3wk	
paclitaxel (Taxol)	IV; 135–175 mg/m^2 q3wk	
TOPOISOMERASE INHIBITORS		
etoposide (VePesid)	IV; 50–100 mg/m^2/day for 5 days	
irinotecan hydrochloride (Camptosar)	IV; 125 mg/m^2 q1wk for 4 wk	
teniposide (Vumon)	IV; 165 mg/m^2 q3–4 days for 4 wk	
topotecan hydrochloride (Hycamtin)	IV; 1.5 mg/m^2/day for 5 days	

Italics indicate common adverse effects; underlining indicates serious adverse effects.

properties with lower toxicity. Bone marrow toxicity is usually the dose-limiting factor for the taxanes.

American Indians described uses of the May apple or wild mandrake (*Podophyllum peltatum*) long before pharmacologists isolated podophyllotoxin, the primary active ingredient in the plant. As a botanical, podophyllum has been used as an antidote for snakebites, as a cathartic, and as a topical treatment for warts. Teniposide (Vumon) and etoposide (VePesid) are semisynthetic products of podophyllotoxin. These agents act by inhibiting **topoisomerase I**, an enzyme that helps repair DNA damage. By binding in a complex with topoisomerase and DNA, these antineoplastics cause strand breaks that accumulate and permanently damage the tumor DNA. Etoposide is approved for refractory testicular carcinoma, small-cell carcinoma of the lung, and choriocarcinoma. Teniposide is approved only for refractory acute lymphoblastic leukemia in children. Bone marrow toxicity is the primary dose-limiting side effect.

More recently isolated topoisomerase I inhibitors include topotecan (Hycamtin) and irinotecan (Camptosar). These agents are called **camptothecins** because they were first isolated from *Camptotheca acuminata*, a tree native to China. The camptothecins are administered only intravenously, and their indications are limited. Topotecan is approved for metastatic ovarian cancer and small-cell lung cancer after failure of initial chemotherapy. Irinotecan is indicated for metastatic cancer of the colon or rectum. As with many other cytotoxic natural products, bone marrow suppression is the dose-limiting toxicity for the camptothecins.

NURSING CONSIDERATIONS

The role of the nurse in natural-product antineoplastic therapy involves careful monitoring of a client's condition and providing education as it relates to the prescribed drug treatment. Before initiating chemotherapy, assess baseline vital signs, CBC, and the client's overall health status, including renal and liver function, intake and output, and body weight.

Because natural-product extracts may produce allergic reactions in susceptible individuals, interview the client regarding any allergy to plants or flowers, including herbs or foods, which may provide clues to possible hypersensitivity to these drugs. Infusion hypersensitivity is an adverse reaction, which may be ameliorated by steroid therapy. Vincristine (Oncovin) may produce acute bronchospasm and skin rashes. Inquire if female clients are pregnant or breast-feeding, because many of these agents are contraindicated in pregnancy and lactation. Vincristine is contraindicated in clients with obstructive jaundice and those with demyelinating forms of Charcot–Marie–Tooth disease.

These drugs produce many of the same cytotoxic effects as other antineoplastics, including alopecia, fatigue, nausea, vomiting, diarrhea, bone marrow suppression, and blood dyscrasias. Natural product antineoplastics should also be used cautiously in many existing conditions, such as seizure disorders; vincristine may lower the seizure threshold. Vincristine should also be used cautiously in clients with leukopenia, neuromuscular disease, and hypertension. Natural products may cause muscle weakness, peripheral neuropathy (including nerve pain), and paralytic ileus. Emphasize the need to establish a nutritional plan to prevent constipation, including high fluid and fiber intake. Natural-product antineoplastics can affect blood pressure, causing either hypotension or hypertension. Observe clients for symptoms such as headache, dizziness, or syncope. These drugs may produce severe mental depression; thus, remain alert to the possibility of suicidal ideation. Offer referrals for spiritual or emotional care such as a chaplain, mental health nurse, or social worker.

Pr **PROTOTYPE DRUG** | Vincristine *(Oncovin)* | Antineoplastic/Vinca Alkaloid

ACTIONS AND USES

Vincristine is a cell-cycle-specific (M-phase) agent that kills cancer cells by preventing their ability to complete mitosis. It exerts this action by inhibiting microtubule formation in the mitotic spindle. Although vincristine must be given intravenously, its major advantage is that it causes minimal immunosuppression. It has a wider spectrum of clinical activity than vinblastine, and is usually prescribed in combination with other antineoplastics for the treatment of Hodgkin's and non-Hodgkin's lymphomas, leukemias, Kaposi's sarcoma, Wilms' tumor, bladder carcinoma, and breast carcinoma.

ADMINISTRATION ALERTS

- Extravasation may result in serious tissue damage. Stop injection immediately if extravasation occurs. Apply local heat and inject hyaluronidase as ordered. Observe site for sloughing.
- Avoid eye contact, which causes severe irritation and corneal changes.
- Pregnancy category D.

PHARMACOKINETICS

Onset: Unknown

Peak: Unknown

Half-life: 10–155 h

Duration: 7 days

ADVERSE EFFECTS

The most serious dose-limiting adverse effects of vincristine relate to nervous system toxicity. Children are particularly susceptible. Symptoms include numbness and tingling in the limbs, muscular weakness, loss of neural reflexes, and pain. Paralytic ileus may occur in young children. Severe constipation is common. Reversible alopecia occurs in most clients.

Contraindications: Vincristine is contraindicated during pregnancy and lactation. Caution should be used when treating clients with hepatic impairment or obstructive jaundice.

INTERACTIONS

Drug–Drug: Asparaginase used concurrently with or before vincristine may cause increased neurotoxicity secondary to decreased hepatic clearance of vincristine. Doxorubicin or prednisone may increase bone marrow depression. Calcium channel blockers may increase vincristine accumulation in cells. Concurrent use with digoxin may decrease digoxin levels. When vincristine is given with methotrexate, the client may need lower doses of methotrexate. Vincristine may decrease serum phenytoin levels, leading to increased seizure activity.

Lab Tests: Serum uric acid levels may increase.

Herbal/Food: Unknown.

Treatment of Overdose: Supportive treatment may include administration of leucovorin (folinic acid).

 See the Companion Website for a Nursing Process Focus specific to this drug.

Client Teaching.   Client education as it relates to natural-product antineoplastics should include the goals of therapy; the reasons for obtaining baseline data such as vital signs, blood work, and the existence of underlying renal or liver disorders; and possible drug side effects. Include the following points when teaching clients about natural-product antineoplastics:

- Immediately report signs of severe allergic reaction such as shortness of breath, thick tongue, throat tightness or difficulty swallowing, or rash.
- Immediately report severe convulsions or suicide risk, such as feelings of despair, verbalized suicide plan, or attempt.
- Immediately report muscle weakness; difficulty walking or talking; visual disturbances; stomach, bone, or joint pain; swelling, especially in the legs or ankles; rectal bleeding; or significant changes in bowel habits.
- Do not take rectal temperatures, and avoid using OTC rectal suppositories.
- Avoid activities requiring physical stamina until effects of the drug are known.
- Obtain assistance with walking if weakness or staggering gait is a problem.
- Maintain good bowel habits by increasing fluid and fiber intake.

Please refer to "Nursing Process Focus: Clients Receiving Antineoplastic Therapy" on page 572 for additional teaching points.

HORMONES AND HORMONE ANTAGONISTS

Hormones significantly affect the growth of some tumors. Use of hormones or their antagonists as antineoplastic agents is a strategy used to slow the growth of hormone-dependent tumors. As a group, they are the least toxic of the antineoplastic classes.

37.13 Pharmacotherapy With Hormones and Hormone Antagonists

A number of hormones are used in cancer chemotherapy, including glucocorticoids, progestins, estrogens, and androgens. In addition, several hormone antagonists have been found to exhibit antitumor activity. The mechanism of hormone antineoplastic activity is largely unknown. It is likely, however, that these antitumor properties are independent of their normal hormone mechanisms because the doses utilized in cancer chemotherapy are magnitudes larger than the amount normally present in the body. Only the antitumor properties of these hormones are discussed in this section; for other indications and actions, the student should

TABLE 37.8   Hormone and Hormone Antagonists Used for Neoplasia

Drug	Route and Adult Dose (max dose where indicated)	Adverse Effects
HORMONES		
dexamethasone (Decadron, others)	PO; 0.25 mg bid–qid	*Weight gain, insomnia, abdominal distension, sweating, flushing, diarrhea, nervousness, gynecomastia, hirsutism (testosterone, testolactone)*
diethylstilbestrol (DES, Stilbestrol)	PO; for treatment of prostate cancer, 500 mg tid; for palliation, 1–15 mg/day	
ethinyl estradiol (Estinyl, others)	PO; for treatment of breast cancer, 1 mg tid for 2–3 months; for palliation of prostate cancer, 0.15–3 mg/day	
fluoxymesterone (Halotestin)	PO; 10 mg tid	Thrombophlebitis, muscle wasting (pred-nisone, dexamethasone), osteoporosis, hepa-totoxicity (testosterone, testolactone)
medroxyprogesterone (Provera, Depo-Provera) (see page 710 for the Prototype Drug box ∞)	IM; 400–1,000 mg q1wk	
megestrol (Megace)	PO; 40–160 mg bid–qid	
prednisone (Deltasone, others) (see page 477 for the Prototype Drug box ∞)	PO; 20–100 mg/m^2/day	
testolactone (Teslac)	PO; 250 mg qid	
testosterone (Andro, Histerone, Testred, Delatest, others) (see page 721 for the Prototype Drug box ∞)	IM; 200–400 mg q2–4wk	
HORMONE ANTAGONISTS		
abarelix (Plenaxis)	IM; 100 mg on Days 1, 15, 29, and q4wk thereafter	*Hot flashes, insomnia, breast enlargement/pain, headache, diarrhea, asthe-nia, nausea*
aminoglutethimide (Cytadren)	PO; 250 mg bid–qid	
anastrozole (Arimidex)	PO; 1 mg/day	
bicalutamide (Casodex)	PO; 50 mg/day	Hypersensitivity reactions (including anaphy-laxis), thrombophlebitis, CHF (bicalutamide, goserelin), hepatotoxicity (flutamide), sexual dysfunction (goserelin, nilutamide, tamoxifen), ocular toxicity (toremifene)
exemestane (Aromasin)	PO; 25 mg/day after a meal	
flutamide (Eulexin)	PO; 250 mg tid	
fulvestrant (Faslodex)	IM; 250 mg once	
goserelin (Zoladex)	Subcutaneously; 3.6 mg q28days	
histrelin (Vantas)	Implant; 1 implant q12 mo (50 mg)	
letrozole (Femara)	PO; 2.5 mg/day	
leuprolide (Eligard, Lupron)	Subcutaneously; 1 mg/day	
nilutamide (Nilandron)	PO; 300 mg/day for 30 days; then 150 mg/day	
ⓟ tamoxifen citrate (Nolvadex)	PO; 10–20 mg 1–2 times/day (morning and evening)	
toremifene (Fareston)	PO; 60 mg/day	

Italics indicate common adverse effects; underlining indicates serious adverse effects.

refer to other chapters in this text. The antitumor hormones and hormone antagonists are listed in Table 37.8.

In general, the hormones and hormone antagonists act by blocking substances essential for tumor growth. Because these agents are not cytotoxic, they produce few of the debilitating adverse effects seen with other antineoplastics. They can, however, produce significant side effects when given at high doses for prolonged periods. Because they rarely produce cancer cures when used singly, these agents are normally given for palliation.

GLUCOCORTICOIDS

The primary glucocorticoids used in chemotherapy are dexamethasone and prednisone (Deltasone, others). Because of the natural ability of glucocorticoids to suppress cell division in lymphocytes, the principal value of these agents is in the treatment of lymphomas, Hodgkin's disease, and leukemias. They are sometimes given as adjuncts to chemotherapy to reduce nausea, weight loss, and tissue inflammation caused by other antineoplastics. Prolonged use can result in symptoms of Cushing's disease (see Chapter 43 ∞).

GONADAL HORMONES

Gonadal hormones are used to treat tumors that contain specific hormone receptors. Two androgens, fluoxymesterone (Halotestin) and testolactone (Teslac), are used for palliative therapy for advanced breast cancer in postmenopausal women. The estrogens ethinyl estradiol and diethylstilbestrol (DES) are used to treat metastatic breast cancer and prostate cancer. The progestins medroxyprogesterone and megestrol (Megace) are used to treat advanced endometrial cancer. Leuprolide (Lupron) and the newly approved abarelix (Plenaxis) are similar to gonadotropin releasing hormone (GnRH), and are used for advanced prostate cancer when other therapies have failed. Also similar to GnRH is histrelin (Vantas), a drug approved in 2006. Approved for advanced prostate cancer, histrelin is an implant that is inserted subcutaneously in the inner aspect of the upper arm to release the hormone over 12 months.

ANTIESTROGENS

The antiestrogens are used to treat tumors that are dependent on estrogen for their growth. Tamoxifen (Nolvadex), which is the most widely used drug for breast cancer, toremifene (Fareston), and raloxifene (Evista) are called selective estrogen-receptor modifiers (SERMs). These drugs *block* estrogen receptors on breast cancer cells but have an estrogen-*stimulating* effect on some nonbreast tissues. The progestogenic effects have positive actions on bone mineral density and improve lipid profiles (increase HDL and lower LDL).

The antiestrogen class also includes anastrozole (Arimidex), letrozole (Femara), and exemestane (Aromasin), which are called **aromatase inhibitors.** These antiestrogens block the enzyme aromatase, which normally converts adrenal androgen to estradiol. Aromatase inhibitors can reduce plasma estrogen levels by as much as 95% and are used in postmenopausal women with advanced breast cancer whose disease has progressed beyond tamoxifen therapy.

ANDROGEN ANTAGONISTS

Hormone inhibitors also include the antiandrogens bicalutamide (Casodex), nilutamide (Nilandron), and flutamide (Eulexin). These agents are prescribed for advanced prostate cancer, which is strongly dependent on androgens for growth.

NURSING CONSIDERATIONS

The role of the nurse in antitumor hormone and hormone antagonist therapy involves careful monitoring of a client's condition and providing education as it relates to the prescribed drug treatment. Because hormone antagonists are given to block the growth of hormone-dependent tumors, assess for pregnancy and breast-feeding, because both are contraindicated with the antitumor hormones and hormone antagonists. Before initiating chemotherapy, assess baseline vital signs, CBC, and the client's overall health status, including renal and liver function, intake and output, and body weight.

Therapy using hormones other than tamoxifen (Nolvadex) may be palliative rather than curative; it is important that both client and family understand this limitation before beginning chemotherapy. They must understand that although the client may appear to be improving, the cancer is likely continuing to worsen.

Pr PROTOTYPE DRUG | Tamoxifen *(Nolvadex)* | Antineoplastic/Antiestrogen

ACTIONS AND USES

Tamoxifen is a drug of choice for treating metastatic breast cancer. It is effective against breast tumor cells that require estrogen for their growth, which are known as estrogen receptor (ER) positive cells. Whereas it blocks estrogen receptors on breast cancer cells, tamoxifen actually activates estrogen receptors in other parts of the body, resulting in typical estrogen-like effects such as reduced LDL levels and increased mineral density of bone. The drug is unique among antineoplastics, because it is given not only to clients with breast cancer but also to high-risk clients to prevent the disease. Few if any other antineoplastics are given prophylactically, owing to their toxicity.

ADMINISTRATION ALERTS

- Give with food or fluids to decrease GI irritation.
- Do not crush or chew drug.
- Avoid antacids for 1–2 h following PO dosage of tamoxifen.
- Pregnancy category D.

PHARMACOKINETICS

Onset: Unknown

Peak: 3–6 h

Half-life: 7 days

Duration: Unknown

ADVERSE EFFECTS

Other than nausea and vomiting, tamoxifen produces little serious toxicity. Of concern, however, is the association of tamoxifen therapy with an increased risk of endometrial cancer and thromboembolic disease. Hot flashes, fluid retention, and vaginal discharges are relatively common. Tamoxifen causes initial "tumor flare"—an idiosyncratic increase in tumor size, but this is an expected therapeutic event.

Contraindications: Contraindications include hypersensitivity to the drug, those taking warfarin, and clients with a history of thromboembolic disease.

INTERACTIONS

Drug–Drug: Anticoagulants taken concurrently with tamoxifen may increase the risk of bleeding. Concurrent use with cytotoxic agents may increase the risk of thromboembolism. Estrogens will decrease the effectiveness of tamoxifen.

Lab Tests: Serum calcium levels may increase.

Herbal/Food: Unknown.

Treatment of Overdose: There is no specific treatment for overdose.

 See the Companion Website for a Nursing Process Focus specific to this drug.

One of the most common, yet distressing, side effects of sex hormone therapy is the development of cross-gender secondary sexual characteristics, such as gynecomastia in men and hirsutism in women. Fertility is sometimes affected. Discuss these effects frankly with the client and offer support and simple interventions to increase self-esteem. Discuss clothing options to disguise gynecomastia, or methods of facial hair removal, such as waxes or depilatories.

The use of glucocorticoids may increase the risk of sexually transmitted diseases and other infections, by suppressing the immune response. Glucocorticoid therapy may cause swelling, weight gain, redistribution of body fat (Cushing's syndrome), and hyperglycemia. Discuss body image concerns, and nutritional strategies to increase energy and limit weight gain. Weight gain remains a concern for a number of cancer clients—especially in the early phases of the disease. In some cases, cancer clients who are experiencing cachexia may benefit from glucocorticoid-induced weight gain. Glucocorticoids should be administered with caution to clients with diabetes mellitus. Obtain results of laboratory blood tests, including serum glucose, hormone levels, and electrolytes.

Client Teaching. Client education as it relates to hormone therapy for cancer should include the goals of therapy, the reasons for obtaining baseline data such as vital signs and the existence of underlying cardiac, renal and endocrine disorders, and possible drug side effects. client

SPECIAL CONSIDERATIONS

Chemotherapy in Elderly Patients

The elderly population has a higher incidence of most types of cancer as a result of a greater accumulation of carcinogenic effects over time and age-related reduction in immune system function. Studies show that hepatic drug enzyme activity (p450) is decreased by 30% in healthy older adults, resulting in decreased metabolism of drugs. The glomerular filtration rate also decreases, resulting in decreased excretion of drugs from the kidneys. Reduced hematopoietic stem cell mass and reduced ability to mobilize these cells from the bone marrow may slow recovery (Chatta et al., 1994). Myelosuppression is more common and more severe in the elderly client.

Include the following points when teaching elderly clients and their caregivers about chemotherapy:

- Elderly clients receiving chemotherapy drugs may experience toxicity from normal doses. Instruct client to monitor and report bleeding or bruising and to avoid aspirin products.

- To reduce neutropenia and prevent infection, instruct the client to monitor temperature daily and avoid taking antipyretics to reduce fever without asking the healthcare provider. Instruct the client to avoid crowds and people with respiratory infections, and to use frequent handwashing to prevent the transmission of pathogens.

- Because older adults often have deficient nutritional intake, teach the client and caregivers about healthy food choices, and assess the client's ability to swallow foods and medications.

- Constipation may occur owing to a decrease in elimination. Encourage the client to drink adequate fluids and to increase dietary fiber by using grains and leafy vegetables.

Include the following points when teaching clients about hormonal therapy for cancer:

- Immediately report fever, chills, sore throat, dyspnea, and increased fatigue; skin rashes; bleeding gums, petechiae, and bruises; blood in urine or stool.

- Avoid crowds or anyone with respiratory infection.

- Monitor serum glucose levels frequently, because antidiabetic medications may need to be adjusted.

- Use good oral hygiene with a soft toothbrush.

Please refer to "Nursing Process Focus: Clients Receiving Antineoplastic Therapy" on page 572 for additional teaching points.

BIOLOGIC RESPONSE MODIFIERS

Biologic response modifiers approach cancer treatment from a different perspective than other antineoplastics. Rather than being cytotoxic to cancer cells, they stimulate the client's own immune system to fight the cancer.

37.14 Pharmacotherapy With Biologic Response Modifiers, Immune Therapies, and Miscellaneous Antineoplastics

Biologic response modifiers and immune therapies are medications that stimulate the body's immune system to rid itself of tumor cells. The immunostimulants are less toxic than most other classes of antineoplastics. These agents, along with some miscellaneous antineoplastics, are listed in Table 37.9. Types of drugs within this subclass include the following:

- *Interferons:* natural proteins produced by T cells in response to viral infection and other biological stimuli. Interferons bind to specific receptors on cancer-cell membranes and suppress cell division, enhance the phagocytic activity of macrophages, and promote the cytotoxic activity of T lymphocytes. Interferon alfa-2a (Roferon-A) and interferon alfa-2b (Intron-A) are approved to treat hairy cell leukemia, chonic myelogenous leukemia, Kapsoi's sarcoma, and chronic hepatitis B or C.

- *Interleukin-2:* activates cytotoxic T lymphocytes and promotes other actions of the immune response. Marketed as aldesleukin (Proleukin), this drug is indicated only for metastatic renal cell carcinoma.

- *Monoclonal antibodies (MABs):* engineered to attack only one *specific* type of tumor cell, unlike interferons and interleukins, which are considered *general* immunostimulants. Once the MAB binds to its target cell, the cancer cell dies, or is marked for destruction by other cells of the immune response. For example, trastuzumab (Herceptin) binds to specific proteins on breast cancer cells (called *HER2* proteins) and induces cell death. Alemtuzumab (Campath) binds to a protein

TABLE 37.9 Biologic Response Modifiers and Miscellaneous Antineoplastics

Drug	Route and Adult Dose (max dose where indicated)	Adverse Effects
arsenic trioxide (Trisenox)	IV; 0.15 mg/kg/day (max: 60 doses)	*Nausea, vomiting, asthenia, stomatitis anorexia, rash, alopecia, hyperlipidemia (bexarotene)*
asparaginase (Elspar)	IV; 200 international units/kg/day	
bexarotene (Targretin)	PO; 100–400 mg/m^2/day; topical; 1% gel applied to lesion 1–4 times/day	
bortezomib (Velcade)	IV; 1.3 mg/m^3 as bolus twice weekly for 2 wk	Bone marrow suppression (neutropenia, anemia, thrombocytopenia), severe nausea, vomiting and diarrhea, pulmonary toxicity, hypersensitivity reactions, (including anaphylaxis), pancreatitis (asparaginase, bexarotene, gefitinib, pegaspargase), hypothyroidism (bexarotene), severe fluid retention (imatinib), hepatotoxicity (asparaginase, pegaspargase), brain damage (mitotane)
erlotinib (Tarceva)	PO; 150 mg/day	
gefitinib (Iressa)	PO; 250 mg/day	
hydroxyurea (Hydrea)	PO; 20–30 mg/kg/day	
imatinib mesylate (Gleevec)	PO; 400–600 mg/day	
interferon alfa-2 (Roferon-A, Intron A) (see page 463 for the Prototype Drug box ∞)	Subcutaneous /IM; 2–3 million units/day for leukemia; increase to 36 million units/day for Kaposi's sarcoma	
levamisole (Ergamisol)	PO; 50 mg tid for 3 days	
mitotane (Lysodren)	PO; 3–4 mg tid–qid	
pegaspargase (Oncaspar, PEG-L-asparaginase)	IV; 2,500 international units/m^2 q14days	
sorafenib (Nexavar)	PO; 400 mg bid	
zoledronic acid (Zometa)	IV; 4 mg over at least 15 min	
MONOCLONAL ANTIBODIES		
alemtuzumab (Campath)	IV; 3–30 mg/day	*Nausea, vomiting, asthenia, tremors (alemtuzumab), anorexia, rash, diarrhea, stomatitis, fever, chills*
bevacizumab (Avastin)	IV; 5 mg/kg q14days	
cetuximab (Erbitux)	IV; 400 mg/m^2 over 2 h; then continue with 250 mg/m^2 over 1 h weekly	
gemtuzumab ozogamicin (Mylotarg)	IV; 9 mg/m^2 for 2 h	Bone marrow suppression (neutropenia, anemia, thrombocytopenia), severe nausea, vomiting and diarrhea, pulmonary toxicity, pulmonary toxicity, CHF (bevacizumab, trastuzumab), hypersensitivity reactions (including anaphylaxis), dysrhythmias (rituximab)
ibritumomab tiuxetan (Zevalin)	IV; 250 mg/m^2 of rituximab is infused followed by 5 mCi of Zevalin in a 10-min IV push	
rituximab (Rituxan)	IV; 375 mg/m^2/day as a continuous infusion	
tositumomab (Bexxar)	IV; 450 mg over 60 min	
trastuzumab (Herceptin)	IV; 4 mg/kg as a single dose; then 2 mg/kg q1wk	

Italics indicate common adverse effects; <u>underlining</u> indicates serious adverse effects.

known as *CD52*, which is present on the surface of B and T lymphocytes, monocytes, and other white blood cells, and is used to treat chronic lymphocytic leukemia. The key point about MABs is that the tumor cells must posses the specific protein receptor; otherwise, the MAB will be ineffective. Cetuximab (Erbitux) and bevacizumab (Avastin) were both approved in 2006 to treat metastatic colorectal cancer.

When given concurrently with other antineoplastics, biologic response modifiers help limit the severe immunosuppressive effects caused by other agents. Additional information on the biologic response modifiers, a drug prototype for interferon alfa-2, and nursing considerations for this class of drugs can be found in Chapter 32 ∞.

Certain anticancer drugs act through mechanisms other than those previously described. For example, asparaginase (Elspar) deprives cancer cells of asparagine, an essential amino acid. It is used to treat acute lymphocytic leukemia. Mitotane (Lysodren), similar to the insecticide DDT, poisons cancer cells by forming links to proteins, and is used for advanced adrenocortical cancer. Two of the newer antineoplastics, imatinib (Gleevec) and sorafenib, inhibit the enzyme tyrosine kinase in tumor cells.

NURSING PROCESS FOCUS Clients Receiving Antineoplastic Therapy

Assessment	Potential Nursing Diagnoses
Prior to administration: ▪ Obtain a complete health history including lab values such as platelets, hematocrit (Hct), leukocyte count, liver and kidney function tests, and serum electrolytes. ▪ Obtain a drug history to determine possible drug interactions and allergies. ▪ Assess neurological status including mood and sensory impairment. ▪ Assess for history or presence of herpes zoster or chicken pox. (Immunosuppressive effects of cyclophosphamide and vincristine can cause life-threatening exacerbations.)	▪ Infection, Risk for, related to compromised immune system ▪ Fluid Volume, Deficient, Risk for related to decreased platelet count secondary to drug side effects ▪ Nutrition, Imbalanced, Less than Body Requirements, related to nausea, vomiting, diarrhea, anorexia secondary to drug side effects ▪ Skin Integrity, Impaired, related to extravasation ▪ Body Image, Disturbed, related to physical changes as a result of drug side effects ▪ Fatigue, related to decreased production of red blood cells (RBCs) secondary to drug therapy

Planning: Client Goals and Expected Outcomes

The client will:

▪ Experience a reduction in tumor mass or progression of abnormal cell growth.
▪ Maintain white blood cell (WBC) count higher than 4,000 and platelet count greater than 50,000.
▪ Demonstrate an understanding of the drug's action by accurately describing drug side effects and precautions.

Implementation

Interventions and (Rationales)	Client Education/Discharge Planning
▪ Monitor CBC and temperature. (Antineoplastics may cause blood dyscrasias and decreased immune function. Blood dyscrasias may indicate overdose.)	Instruct client to: ▪ Immediately report profound fatigue, fever, or sore throat. ▪ Avoid persons with active infections. ▪ Monitor vital signs (especially temperature) daily, ensuring proper use of home equipment. ▪ Anticipate fatigue, and balance daily activities to prevent exhaustion. ▪ Avoid activities requiring mental alertness and physical strength until effects of the drug are known.
▪ Collect stool samples for guaiac testing of occult blood. (Antineoplastics may cause GI bleeding.)	Instruct client to: ▪ Immediately report epigastric pain, coffee-grounds vomit, bruising, tarry stools, or frank bleeding. ▪ Avoid consuming aspirin.
▪ Monitor vital signs, cardiorespiratory status, including dyspnea, pitting edema, heart and chest sounds, and ECG, especially for T-wave flattening, ST depression, or voltage reduction. (Antineoplastics may cause cardiac and respiratory disorders. Cyclophosphamide may cause myopericarditis and lung fibrosis. Doxorubicin may cause sinus tachycardia, cardiac depression, and delayed-onset CHF.)	Instruct client to: ▪ Immediately report trouble breathing; chest, arm, neck, or back pain; tachycardia; cough; frothy sputum; swelling of extremities; or activity intolerance. ▪ Keep scheduled appointments for ECGs as advised by the healthcare provider because heart changes may be a sign of drug toxicity; HF may not appear for up to 6 months after completion of doxorubicin therapy.
▪ Monitor renal status, urine, intake and output, and daily weight. (Cyclophosphamide may cause renal toxicity and/or hemorrhagic cystitis. Vincristine and methotrexate increase uric acid levels, contributing to renal calculi and gout. Vincristine may also cause water retention and highly concentrated urine.)	Instruct client to: ▪ To immediately report changes in thirst; color, quantity, and character of urine (e.g., "cloudy," with odor or sediment); joint, abdominal, flank, or lower back pain; difficult urination; and weight gain. ▪ That doxorubicin will turn urine red-brown for 1–2 days after administration; blood in the urine may occur several months after cyclophosphamide has been discontinued. ▪ To consume 3 L of fluid on the day before treatment and daily for 72 h after (when client has no prescribed fluid restriction).

NURSING PROCESS FOCUS Clients Receiving Antineoplastic Therapy *(Continued)*

Implementation

Interventions and (Rationales)	Client Education/Discharge Planning
▪ Monitor GI status and nutrition, and administer antiemetics 30–45 minutes prior to antineoplastic administration or at the first sign of nausea. (Profound nausea, dry heaves, and/or vomiting are common with antineoplastic therapy. Dry mouth can also occur.)	Instruct client to: ▪ Report loss of appetite, nausea/vomiting, diarrhea, mouth redness, soreness, or ulcers. ▪ Consume frequent small meals, drink plenty of cold liquids, and avoid strong odors and spicy foods to control nausea. ▪ Examine mouth daily for changes. ▪ Use a soft toothbrush and avoid using toothpicks.
▪ Monitor for constipation. (Ileus or constipation and fecal impaction may occur with vincristine use, especially among elderly clients.)	Instruct client to: ▪ Report changes in bowel habits. ▪ Increase activity, fiber, and fluids to reduce constipation.
▪ Monitor neurological and sensory status. (Antineoplastics may cause peripheral neuropathy and mental depression. Vincristine may cause ataxia and hand/foot drop. Tamoxifen may cause photophobia and decreased vision. Such neurological changes may be irreversible.)	Instruct client to: ▪ Report changes in skin color, vision, hearing, numbness or tingling, staggering gait, or depressed mood; obtain no self-harm contract. ▪ Limit sun exposure; wear sunscreen, sunglasses, and long sleeves when outdoors.
▪ Monitor genitourinary status. (Antineoplastic agents, including hormones, and especially tamoxifen, may alter menstrual cycles in women and may produce impotence in men. Tamoxifen increases the risk of endometrial cancer.)	Instruct client: ▪ To report changes in menstruation, sexual functioning, or vaginal discharge. ▪ About the risk of endometrial cancer before giving tamoxifen.
▪ Monitor for hypersensitivity or other adverse reactions. (Hypersensitivity and adverse reactions require immediate healthcare provider notification.)	▪ Instruct client to immediately report chest or throat tightness, difficulty swallowing, swelling (especially facial), abdominal pain, headache, or dizziness.
▪ Monitor hair and skin status. (Alopecia is associated with most chemotherapy and may be a sign of overdosage. Methotrexate can cause a variety of skin eruptions.)	Instruct client to: ▪ Immediately report desquamation of skin on hands and feet, rash, pruritus, acne, or boils. ▪ Wear a cold gel cap during chemotherapy to minimize hair loss.
▪ Monitor for conjunctivitis. (Doxorubicin may cause conjunctivitis.)	▪ Instruct client or caregiver to immediately report eye redness, stickiness, or pain or weeping.
▪ Monitor liver function tests. (Antineoplastics are metabolized by the liver, increasing the risk of hepatotoxicity.)	Instruct client to: ▪ Report jaundice, abdominal pain, tenderness or bloating, or change in stool color. ▪ Adhere to laboratory testing regimen for serum blood level tests of liver enzymes as directed.
▪ Administer with caution to clients with diabetes mellitus. (Hypoglycemia may occur secondary to combination of cyclophosphamide and insulin; hyperglycemia may occur secondary to steroid use.)	Instruct client to: ▪ Report signs and symptoms of hypoglycemia (e.g., sudden weakness, tremors). ▪ Monitor blood glucose daily; consult the healthcare provider regarding reportable results (e.g., less than 70 mg/dl).

Evaluation of Outcome Criteria

Evaluate the effectiveness of drug therapy by confirming that client goals and expected outcomes have been met (see "Planning").

▪ The client exhibits a reduction in tumor mass or progression of abnormal cell growth.

▪ The client's WBC is greater than 4,000, and platelet count is greater than 50,000.

▪ The client demonstrates an understanding of the drug's actions by accurately describing drug side effects and precautions.

∞ *See Tables 37.2 through 37.8 for lists of drugs to which these nursing actions apply.*

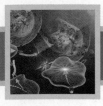

CHAPTER REVIEW

KEY CONCEPTS

The numbered key concepts provide a succinct summary of the important points from the corresponding numbered section within the chapter. If any of these points are not clear, refer to the numbered section within the chapter for review.

37.1 Cancer is characterized by rapid, uncontrolled growth of cells that eventually invade normal tissues and metastasize.

37.2 The causes of cancer may be chemical, physical, or biological. Many environmental and lifestyle factors are associated with a higher risk of cancer.

37.3 Cancer may be treated using surgery, radiation therapy, and drugs. Chemotherapy may be used for cure, palliation, or prophylaxis.

37.4 The growth fraction, the percentage of cancer cells undergoing mitosis at any given time, is a major factor determining success of chemotherapy. Antineoplastics are more effective against cells that are rapidly dividing.

37.5 To achieve a total cure, every malignant cell must be removed or killed through surgery, radiation, or drugs, or by the client's immune system.

37.6 Use of multiple drugs and special dosing protocols are strategies that allow for lower doses, fewer side effects, and greater success of chemotherapy.

37.7 Serious toxicity, including bone marrow suppression, severe nausea, vomiting, and diarrhea, limits therapy with most antineoplastic agents. Long-term consequences of chemotherapy include possible infertility and increased risk for secondary tumors.

37.8 Classes of antineoplastic drugs include alkylating agents, antimetabolites, hormones/hormone antagonists, natural products, biological response modifiers, and miscellaneous antineoplastics.

37.9 Alkylating agents have a broad spectrum of activity and act by changing the structure of DNA in cancer cells. Their use is limited because they can cause significant bone marrow suppression.

37.10 Antimetabolites act by disrupting critical pathways in cancer cells, such as folate metabolism or DNA synthesis. The three types of antimetabolites are purine analogs, pyrimidine analogs, and folate inhibitors.

37.11 Due to their cytotoxicity, a few antibiotics are used to treat cancer by inhibiting cell growth. They have a narrow spectrum of clinical activity.

37.12 Some plant extracts have been isolated that kill cancer cells by preventing cell division. These include the vinca alkaloids, taxanes, topoisomerase inhibitors, and camptothecins.

37.13 Some hormones and hormone antagonists are antineoplastic agents that are effective against reproductive-related tumors such as those of the breast, prostate, or uterus. They are less cytotoxic than other antineoplastics.

37.14 Biologic response modifiers and some additional antineoplastic drugs have been found to be effective against tumors by stimulating or assisting the client's immune system. These include interferons, interleukins, and monoclonal antibodies.

NCLEX-RN® REVIEW QUESTIONS

1 A client undergoing cancer chemotherapy asks the nurse why she is taking three different antineoplastics. The nurse's best response would be:

1. "Your cancer was very advanced and therefore requires more medications."
2. "Each drug attacks the cancer cells in a different way, increasing the effectiveness of the therapy."
3. "Several drugs are prescribed to find the right drug for your cancer."
4. "One drug will cancel out the side effects of the other."

2 The nurse understands the effective treatment method for the nausea and vomiting that accompany chemotherapy is to:

1. Administer an oral antiemetic when the client complains of nausea and vomiting.
2. Administer an antiemetic by IM injection when the client complains of nausea and vomiting.
3. Administer an antiemetic prior to the antineoplastic medication.
4. Push fluids prior to administering the antineoplastic medication.

3 Which of the following statements by a client undergoing antineoplastic therapy would be of concern to the nurse? (Select all that apply.)

1. "I have attended a meeting of a cancer support group."
2. "My husband and I are planning a short trip next week."
3. "I am eating six small meals plus two protein shakes a day."
4. "I am taking my 15-month-old granddaughter to the pediatrician next week for her baby shots."
5. "I am going to go shopping at the mall next week."

4 To monitor for the presence of bone marrow suppression, the nurse evaluates the results of the:

1. BUN and serum creatinine.
2. Serum electrolytes.
3. CBC.
4. Bone scan.

5 A 2-year-old client is receiving vincristine (Oncovin) for Wilms' tumor. Which of the following symptoms should be reported to the physician?

1. Diarrhea
2. Diminished bowel sounds
3. Stomatitis
4. Anorexia

CRITICAL THINKING QUESTIONS

1. A client is newly diagnosed with cancer and is about to start chemotherapy. Identify the teaching priorities for this client.

2. Chemotherapy medications often cause neutropenia in cancer clients. What would be a priority for the nurse to teach a client who is receiving chemotherapy at home?

3. A nurse is taking chemotherapy IV medication to a client's room and the IV bag suddenly leaks solution (approximately 50 ml) on the floor. What action should the nurse take?

See Appendix D for answers and rationales for all activities.

EXPLORE MediaLink

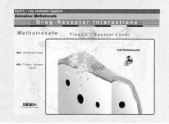

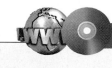

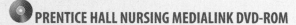

www.prenhall.com/adams

NCLEX-RN® review, case studies, and other interactive resources for this chapter can be found on the companion website at www.prenhall.com/adams. Click on "Chapter 37" to select the activities for this chapter. For animations, more NCLEX-RN® review questions, and an audio glossary, access the accompanying Prentice Hall Nursing MediaLink DVD-ROM in this textbook.

PRENTICE HALL NURSING MEDIALINK DVD-ROM

- **Animations**
  Mechanism in Action: Methotrexate (*Folex, Mexate, others*)
  Mechanism in Action: Cyclophosphamide (*Cytoxar, Neosar*)
- **Audio Glossary**
- **NCLEX-RN® Review**

 ### COMPANION WEBSITE

- **NCLEX-RN® Review**
- **Dosage Calculations**
- **Case Study:** Client taking antineoplastic agents
- **Care Plan:** Client with breast cancer and suspected bone metastasis treated with cyclophosphamide

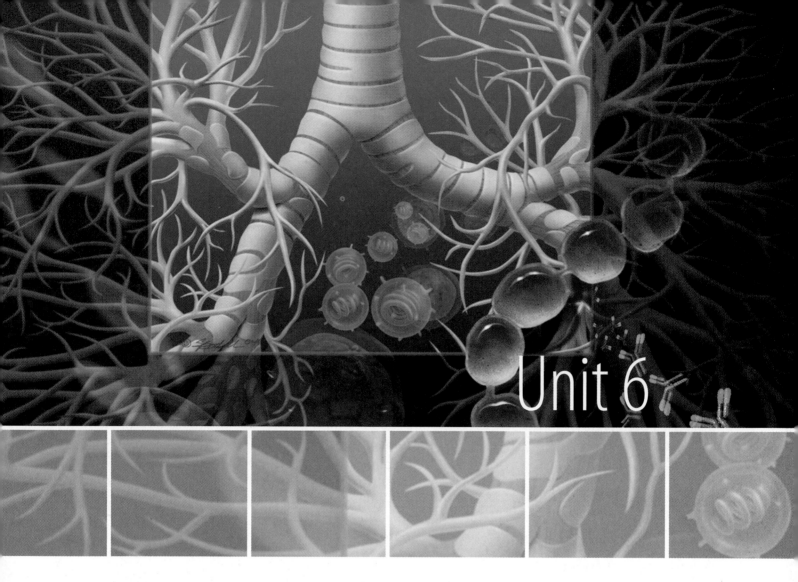

The Respiratory System

CHAPTER 38   Drugs for Allergic Rhinitis and the Common Cold

CHAPTER 39   Drugs for Asthma and Other Pulmonary Disorders

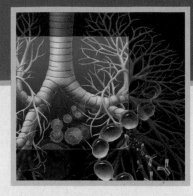

Drugs for Allergic Rhinitis and the Common Cold

DRUGS AT A GLANCE

H₁-RECEPTOR ANTAGONISTS (ANTIHISTAMINES)
- *diphenhydramine (Benadryl, others)*
- *fexofenadine (Allegra)*

INTRANASAL GLUCOCORTICOIDS
- *fluticasone (Flonase)*

MAST CELL STABILIZERS

DECONGESTANTS
- *oxymetazoline (Afrin, others)*

ANTITUSSIVES
- *dextromethorphan (Benylin, others)*

EXPECTORANTS AND MUCOLYTICS

OBJECTIVES

After reading this chapter, the student should be able to:

1. Identify major functions of the upper respiratory tract.
2. Describe common causes and symptoms of allergic rhinitis.
3. Differentiate between H_1 and H_2 histamine receptors.
4. Compare and contrast the oral and intranasal decongestants.
5. Discuss the pharmacotherapy of cough.
6. For each of the classes listed in Drugs at a Glance, know representative drugs, and explain their mechanism of drug action, primary actions on the respiratory system, and important adverse effects.
7. Categorize drugs used in the treatment of allergic rhinitis and the common cold based on their classification and mechanisms of action.
8. Use the Nursing Process to care for clients who are receiving pharmacotherapy for allergic rhinitis and the common cold.

MediaLink

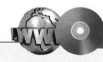

www.prenhall.com/adams

NCLEX-RN® review, case studies, and other interactive resources for this chapter can be found on the companion website at www.prenhall.com/adams. Click on "Chapter 38" to select the activities for this chapter. For animations, more NCLEX-RN® review questions, and an audio glossary, access the accompanying Prentice Hall Nursing MediaLink DVD-ROM in this textbook.

The respiratory system is one of the most important organ systems; a mere 5 to 6 minutes without breathing may result in death. When functioning properly, this system provides the body with the oxygen critical for all cells to carry on normal activities. The respiratory system also provides a means by which the body can rid itself of excess acids and bases, a topic that was presented in Chapter 31 ∞. This chapter examines drugs used for two conditions associated with the *upper* respiratory tract: allergic rhinitis, and nasal congestion and cough. Chapter 39 ∞ presents the pharmacotherapy of asthma and chronic obstructive pulmonary disease, conditions that affect the *lower* respiratory tract.

> ## KEY TERMS
>
> **allergen** *page 580*
> **allergic rhinitis** *page 580*
> **antitussives** *page 589*
> **expectorants** *page 591*
> **H₁-receptors** *page 581*
> **mucolytics** *page 591*
> **rebound congestion** *page 587*

38.1 Physiology of the Upper Respiratory Tract

Knowledge of the basic anatomy and physiology of the upper respiratory tract (URT) is necessary to understanding the pharmacotherapy of conditions affecting that region. The URT consist of the nose, nasal cavity, pharynx, and paranasal sinuses. These passageways warm, humidify, and clean the air before it enters the lungs. This process is sometimes referred to as the "air conditioning" function of the respiratory system. The basic structures of the upper respiratory system are shown in ● Figure 38.1.

The URT removes particulate matter and many pathogens before they reach the more delicate structures of the lungs, and before they are able to access the capillaries of the systemic circulation. The mucous membrane of the URT is lined with ciliated epithelium, which traps and "sweeps" the pathogens and particulate matter posteriorly, where it is swallowed when the person coughs or clears the throat.

The nasal mucosa is a dynamic structure, richly supplied with vascular tissue, under the control of the autonomic nervous system. For example, activation of the sympathetic nervous system constricts arterioles in the nose, reducing the thickness of the mucosal layer, and thus widens the airway to allow more air to enter. Parasympathetic activation has the opposite effect. This difference becomes important in drug therapy that affects the autonomic nervous system. For example,

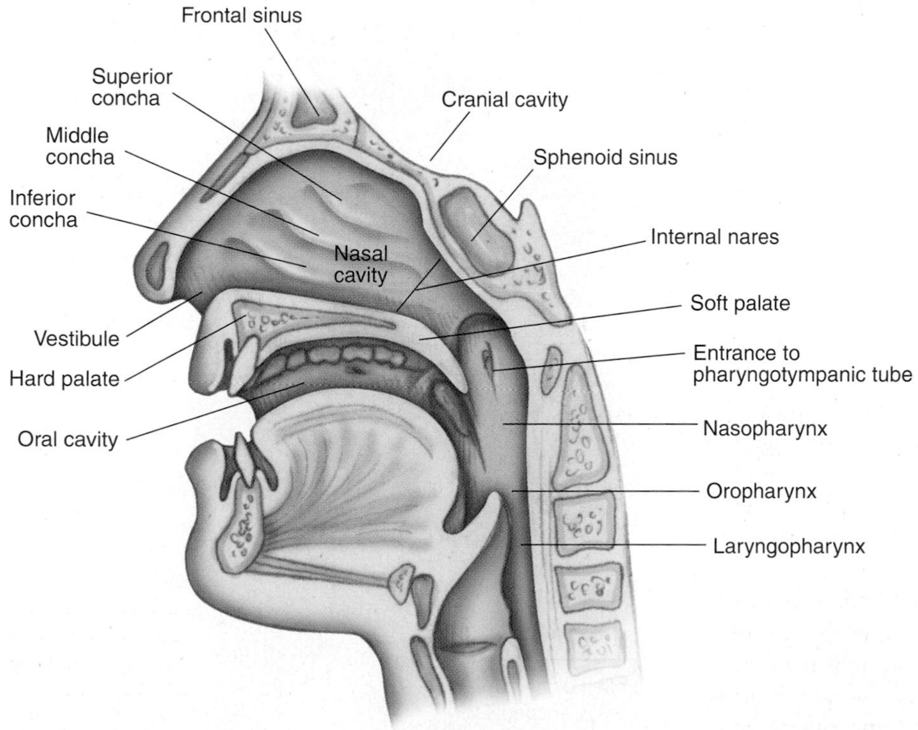

● **Figure 38.1** The respiratory system *Source: Rice, Jane, Medical Terminology with Human Anatomy, 5ᵗʰ ed., p. 292, © 2005. Reprinted by permission of Pearson Education, Inc., Upper Saddle River, NJ.*

administration of a sympathomimetic will shrink the nasal mucosa, relieving nasal stuffiness associated with the common cold (Section 38.5). Parasympathetic agents will cause increased blood flow to the nose, with increased nasal stuffiness and a runny nose as side effects.

The nasal mucosa is the first line of immunological defense. Up to a quart of nasal mucus is produced daily, and this fluid is rich that immunoglobulins that are able to neutralize airborne pathogens. The mucosa also contains various body defense cells that can activate complement or engulf microbes. Mast cells, which contain histamine, also line the nasal mucosa, and these play a major role in causing the symptoms of allergic rhinitis.

ALLERGIC RHINITIS

Allergic rhinitis is inflammation of the nasal mucosa due to exposure to allergens. Although not life threatening, allergic rhinitis is a disease affecting millions of clients, and pharmacotherapy is frequently necessary to control symptoms and to prevent secondary complications.

38.2 Pharmacotherapy of Allergic Rhinitis

Allergic rhinitis, or *hay fever*, is a common disorder with symptoms resembling those of the common cold: tearing eyes, sneezing, nasal congestion, postnasal drip, and itching of the throat. In addition to the acute symptoms, complications of allergic rhinitis may include loss of taste or smell, sinusitis, chronic cough, hoarseness, and middle ear infections in children.

As with other allergies, the cause of allergic rhinitis is exposure to an antigen. An antigen, also called an **allergen,** may be defined as anything that is recognized as foreign by the body's immune system. The specific allergen responsible for a client's allergic rhinitis is often difficult to pinpoint; however, the most common agents are pollens from weeds, grasses, and trees; mold spores; dust mites; certain foods; and animal dander. Chemical fumes, tobacco smoke, or air pollutants such as ozone are nonallergenic factors that may worsen symptoms. In addition, there is a strong genetic predisposition to allergic rhinitis.

Some clients experience symptoms of allergic rhinitis only at specific times of the year, when pollen is at high levels in their environment. These periods are typically in the spring and fall when plants and trees are blooming, thus the name *seasonal* allergic rhinitis. Obviously, the "blooming" season changes with geographic location, and with each species of plant. These clients may need pharmacotherapy for only a few months during the year.

Other clients, however, are afflicted with allergic rhinitis throughout the year because they are continuously exposed to indoor allergens, such as dust mites, animal dander, or mold. This variation is called *perennial* allergic rhinitis. These clients may require continuous pharmacotherapy.

The differences between seasonal and perennial allergic rhinitis are often not clear. Clients with seasonal allergies may also be sensitive to some of the perennial allergens. It is also common for one allergen to "sensitize" the client to another. For example, during ragweed season, a client may become hyperresponsive to other allergens such as mold spores or animal dander. The body's response and the symptoms of allergic rhinitis are the same, however, regardless of the specific allergen(s). Allergy testing can help pinpoint the particular allergens responsible for the symptoms.

The fundamental pathophysiology responsible for allergic rhinitis is inflammation of the mucous membranes in the nose, throat, and airways. The nasal mucosa is rich with mast cells and basophils, which recognize environmental agents as they try to enter the body. Clients with allergic rhinitis contain greater numbers of mast cells. An *immediate* hypersensitivity response releases histamine and other chemical mediators from the mast cells and basophils, producing sneezing, itchy nasal membranes, and watery eyes. A *delayed* hypersensitivity reaction also occurs 4 to 8 hours after the initial exposure, causing continuous inflammation of the mucosa and adding to the chronic nasal congestion experienced by these clients. Because histamine is released during an allergic response, many signs and symptoms of allergy are similar to those of inflammation (Chapter 33 ∞). The mechanism of allergic rhinitis is illustrated in ● Figure 38.2.

The therapeutic goals of treating allergic rhinitis are to prevent its occurrence and to relieve symptoms. Drugs used

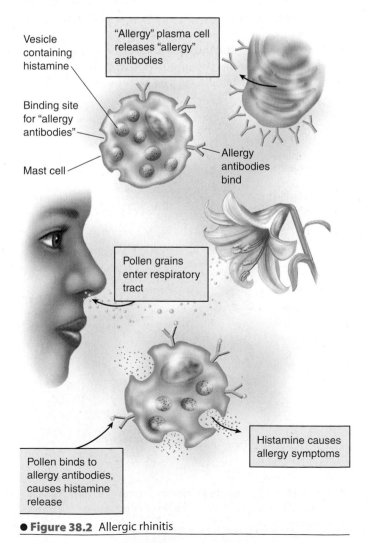

● Figure 38.2 Allergic rhinitis

to treat allergic rhinitis may thus be grouped into two basic categories: preventers and to relievers. *Preventers* are used for prophylaxis and include antihistamines, intranasal glucocorticoids, and mast cell stabilizers. *Relievers* are used to provide immediate, though temporary, relief for acute allergy symptoms once they have occurred. Relievers include the oral and intranasal decongestants, usually drugs from the sympathomimetic class. In addition to treating allergic rhinitis with drugs, the nurse should help clients identify sources of the allergy and recommend appropriate actions. These may include removing pets from the home environment, cleaning moldy surfaces, using microfilters on air conditioning units, and cleaning dust mites out of bedding, carpet, or couches.

H$_1$-RECEPTOR ANTAGONISTS/ANTIHISTAMINES

Antihistamines block the actions of histamine at the H$_1$-receptor. They are widely used as over-the-counter (OTC) remedies for relief of allergy symptoms, motion sickness, and insomnia. These agents are listed in Table 38.1.

38.3 Treating Allergic Rhinitis With H$_1$-receptor Antagonists

Histamine is a chemical mediator of the inflammatory response that is responsible for many of the symptoms of allergic rhinitis. When released from mast cells and basophils, histamine reaches its receptors to cause itching, increased mucus secretion, and runny nose. In more severe allergic states, histamine release may cause bronchoconstriction, edema, hypotension, and other symptoms of anaphylaxis. The receptors responsible for allergic symptoms are called **H$_1$-receptors**. The other major histamine receptor, H$_2$, is found in the gastric mucosa and is responsible for peptic ulcers (Chapter 40 ∞).

H$_1$-receptor antagonists, also called *antihistamines*, are drugs that block histamine from reaching its receptors, thus alleviating allergic symptoms. Because the term *antihistamine* is nonspecific and does not indicate which of the two histamine receptors are affected, H$_1$-receptor antagonist is a more accurate name. In clinical practice, as well as in this text, the two terms are used interchangeably.

The most frequent therapeutic use of H$_1$-receptor antagonists is for the treatment of allergies. These medications provide symptomatic relief from the characteristic sneezing, runny nose, and itching of the eyes, nose, and throat of allergic rhinitis. H$_1$-receptor antagonists are often combined with decongestants and antitussives in OTC cold and sinus medicines. Common OTC antihistamine combinations used to treat allergies are listed in Table 38.2. Antihistamines are most effective when taken prophylactically to *prevent* allergic symptoms; their effectiveness in *reversing* allergic symptoms is limited. Their effectiveness may diminish with long-term use.

MediaLink Pollen and Allergic Rhinitis

TABLE 38.1	H$_1$-receptor Antagonists	
Drug	**Route and Adult Dose (max dose where indicated)**	**Adverse Effects**
First-generation Agents		
azatadine (Optimine); Trinalin is a combination of azatadine and pseudoephedrine.	PO; 1–2 mg bid	*Dry mouth, headache, dizziness, urinary retention, thickening of bronchial secretions, nausea, vomiting*
azelastine (Astelin)	Intranasal; 2 sprays per nostril bid	
brompheniramine (Dimetapp, others)	PO; 4–8 mg tid–qid (max: 40 mg/day)	<u>Paradoxical excitation, sedation, hypersensitivity reactions, hypotension, extrapyramidal symptoms (promethazine), agranulocytosis (brompheniramine, promethazine)</u>
chlorpheniramine (Chlor-Trimeton, others)	PO; 2–4 mg tid–qid (max: 24 mg/day)	
clemastine (Tavist)	PO; 1.34 mg bid (max: 8.04 mg/day)	
cyproheptadine (Periactin)	PO; 4 mg tid or qid (max: 0.5 mg/kg/day)	
dexbrompheniramine (Drixoral)	PO; 6 mg bid	
dexchlorpheniramine (Dexchlor, Poladex, Polargen, Polaramine)	PO; 2 mg q4–6h (max: 12 mg/day)	
◯ diphenhydramine (Benadryl, others)	PO; 25–50 mg 3–4 times daily (max: 300 mg/day)	
promethazine (Phenergan, Anergan, Phenazine, others)	PO; 12.5 mg/day (max: 150 mg/day)	
tripelennamine (PBZ-SR, Pelamine)	PO; 25–50 mg q4–6h (max: 600 mg/day)	
triprolidine (Actifed, Actidil)	PO; 2.5 mg bid or tid	
Second-generation Agents		
cetirizine (Zyrtec)	PO; 5–10 mg/day	*Dry mouth, headache, dizziness, urinary retention, nausea*
desloratadine (Clarinex)	PO; 5 mg/day	
◯ fexofenadine (Allegra)	PO; 60 mg 1–2 times/day (max: 120 mg/day)	<u>Paradoxical excitation, hypersensitivity reactions, hypotension</u>
loratadine (Claritin)	PO; 10 mg/day	

Italics indicate common adverse effects; <u>underlining</u> indicates serious adverse effects.

TABLE 38.2   Selected Antihistamine Combinations Available OTC for Allergic Rhinitis

Brand Name	Antihistamine	Decongestant	Analgesic
Actifed Cold and Allergy tablets	chlorpheniramine	phenylephrine	————
Actifed Cold and Sinus caplets	chlorpheniramine	pseudoephedrine	acetaminophen
Benadryl Allergy/Cold caplets	diphenhydramine	phenylephrine	acetaminophen
Chlor-Trimeton Allergy/Decongestant tablets	chlorpheniramine	pseudoephedrine	————
Dimetapp Cold and Allergy Elixir	brompheniramine	phenylephrine	————
Drixoral Allergy and Sinus Extended Release tablets	dexobrompheniramine	pseudoephedrine	acetaminophen
Sinutab Sinus Allergy tablets	chlorpheniramine	pseudoephedrine	acetaminophen
Sudafed PE Nighttime	diphenhydramine	phenylephrine	————
Tavist Allergy 12-hour tablets	clemastine	————	————
Triaminic Cold/Allergy	chlorpheniramine	phenylephrine	————
Tylenol Allergy Sinus caplets	chlorpheniramine	phenylephrine	acetaminophen

In addition to producing their antihistamine effects, these drugs also block cholinergic receptors to cause typical anticholinergic effects. Anticholinergic effects are responsible for certain beneficial effects of the antihistamines, such as drying of mucous membranes, which results in less nasal congestion and tearing.

Although a large number of H_1-receptor antagonists are available, they are equally effective in treating allergic rhinitis and other mild allergies. Side effects are similar but differ in intensity among the various antihistamines. The older, first-generation drugs have the potential to cause significant drowsiness, which can be a limiting side effect in some clients. After a few doses tolerance generally develops to this sedative action. The newer, second-generation agents have less tendency to cause sedation. Alcohol and other CNS depressants should be used with caution when taking antihistamines, because their sedating effects may be additive, even for the second-generation agents. Some clients exhibit CNS *stimulation,* which can cause insomnia, nervousness, and tremors.

The second major side effect of antihistamines relates to their anticholinergic effects. Excessive drying of mucous membranes can lead to dry mouth, and urinary hesitancy may be troublesome for clients with prostatic hypertrophy. Some antihistamines produce more pronounced anticholinergic effects than others. Diphenhydramine and clemastine produce the greatest incidence of anticholinergic side effects, whereas the second-generation agents, loratadine, desloratadine, and fexofenadine, produce the least.

Although most antihistamines are given orally, azelastine (Astelin) was the first to be available by the intranasal route. Azelastine is as safe and effective as the oral antihistamines. Although a first-generation agent, azelastine causes less drowsiness than others in its class because it is applied locally to the nasal mucosa, and limited systemic absorption occurs.

H_1-receptor antagonists are effective in treating a number of other disorders. Motion sickness responds well to these drugs. They are also some of the few drugs available to treat vertigo, a form of dizziness that causes significant nausea. Some of the older antihistamines are marketed as OTC sleep aids, taking advantage of their ability to cause drowsiness.

NURSING CONSIDERATIONS

The role of the nurse in drug therapy with first- and second-generation H_1-receptor antagonists for the treatment of allergic rhinitis involves careful monitoring of a client's condition and providing education as it relates to the prescribed drug treatment. Before administering antihistamines, obtain baseline vital signs, including ECG in clients with a history of heart disease. These agents are contraindicated in clients with a history of dysrhythmias, heart failure, and hypertension because they can cause vasodilation due to H_1-receptor stimulation. Prior to initiation of therapy, assess for a history of allergy and identify the presence of symptoms, such as urticaria, angioedema, nausea, vomiting, motion sickness, conjunctivitis, or excess muus production.

First-generation H_1-receptor antagonists may cause CNS depression, so they may be contraindicated in clients with a history of depression or sleep disorders, such as narcolepsy or apnea. Because the anticholinergic effects of both first- and second-generation H_1-receptor antagonists can worsen symptoms of narrow-angle glaucoma, they are contraindicated in clients with this disorder. These anticholinergic effects also contraindicate the use of these drugs in clients who have asthma or who use nicotine. These effects may also cause problems for clients with preexisting urinary retention. Drugs in this class sometimes cause idiosyncratic CNS stimulation; therefore, they may be contraindicated in clients with seizure disorders. CNS stimulation, which is more common in children, may cause hyperactivity. These drugs are metabolized by the liver and excreted by the kidneys; therefore, they are contraindicated in clients with severe liver or renal impairment. Loratadine (Claritin) is most effective when given on an empty stomach.

Pr PROTOTYPE DRUG | Diphenhydramine *(Benadryl, others)* | H_1-receptor Antagonist (First-generation)

ACTIONS AND USES

Diphenhydramine is a first-generation H_1-receptor antagonist that is a component of some OTC drugs. Its primary use is to treat minor symptoms of allergy and the common cold such as sneezing, runny nose, and tearing of the eyes. OTC diphenhydramine is often combined with an analgesic, decongestant, or expectorant. Diphenhydramine is also used as a topical agent to treat rashes, and an IM form is available for severe allergic reactions. Other indications for diphenhydramine include Parkinson's disease, motion sickness, and insomnia.

ADMINISTRATION ALERTS

- There is an increased risk of anaphylactic shock when this drug is administered parenterally.
- When administering IV, inject at a rate of 25 mg/min to reduce the risk of shock.
- When administering IM, inject deep into the muscle to minimize tissue irritation.
- Pregnancy category C.

PHARMACOKINETICS

Onset: 15–30 min

Peak: 1–4 h

Half-life: 3–7 h

Duration: 4–7 h

ADVERSE EFFECTS

Older H_1-receptor antagonists such as diphenhydramine cause significant drowsiness, although this usually diminishes with long-term use. Occasionally, paradoxical CNS stimulation and excitability will be observed, rather than drowsiness. Anticholinergic effects such as dry mouth, tachycardia, and mild hypotension occur in some clients. Diphenhydramine may cause photosensitivity.

Contraindications: Hypersensitivity to the drug, prostatic hypertrophy, narrow-angle glaucoma, and GI obstruction are contraindications of use. The drug should be used cautiously in clients with asthma or hyperthyroidism.

INTERACTIONS

Drug–Drug: Use with CNS depressants such as alcohol or opioids will cause increased sedation. Other OTC cold preparations may increase anticholinergic side effects. MAO inhibitors may cause a hypertensive crisis.

Lab Tests: Drug should be discontinued at least 4 days prior to skin allergy tests; otherwise, false-negative tests may result.

Herbal/Food: Henbane may cause increased anticholinergic effects.

Treatment of Overdose: Overdose may cause either CNS depression or excitation. There is no specific treatment for overdose.

 See the Companion Website for a Nursing Process Focus specific to this drug.

Pr PROTOTYPE DRUG | Fexofenadine *(Allegra)* | H_1-receptor Antagonist (Second-generation)

ACTIONS AND USES

Fexofenadine is a second-generation H_1-receptor antagonist with efficacy equivalent to that of diphenhydramine. Its primary action is to block the effects of histamine at H_1-receptors. Most effective when taken *before* symptoms develop, fexofenadine reduces the severity of nasal congestion, sneezing, and tearing of the eyes. Its long half-life of over 14 hours offers the advantage of being administered once or twice daily. Fexofenadine is available only in oral form. Allegra-D combines fexofenadine with pseudoephedrine, a decongestant.

ADMINISTRATION ALERT

- Pregnancy category C.

PHARMACOKINETICS

Onset: 1 h

Peak: 2–3 h

Half-life: 14.4 h

Duration: 12 h

ADVERSE EFFECTS

The major advantage of fexofenadine over first-generation antihistamines is that it causes less drowsiness. Although less sedating than diphenhydramine, fexofenadine can still cause drowsiness in certain clients, at high doses and when combined with CNS depressants. Other side effects are usually minor and include headache and upset stomach.

Contraindications: The only contraindication to fexofenadine is hypersensitivity to the drug.

INTERACTIONS

Drug–Drug: Concurrent administration with ketoconazole or erythromycin increases the plasma concentrations of fexofenadine. Concurrent use with other antihistamines or CNS depressants may cause synergistic sedative effects.

Lab Tests: Skin allergy tests will read as false negative.

Herbal/Food: Absorption may be decreased when taken with food. Grapefruit, orange, or apple juice may reduce the bioavailability of fexofenadine.

Treatment of Overdose: Overdose may cause CNS depression. There is no specific treatment for overdose.

 See the Companion Website for a Nursing Process Focus specific to this drug.

Lifespan Considerations. Monitor elderly clients for profound sedation and altered consciousness, which may contribute to falls or other injuries. Use antihistamines with caution in elderly male clients with benign prostatic hypertrophy. Older clients experience a higher incidence of dizziness and confusion when taking these drugs. The agents should be used with caution during pregnancy (pregnancy category B or C). H_1-receptor antagonists are secreted in breast milk and should not be used by clients who are breast-feeding.

Client Teaching. Client education as it relates to first- and second-generation H_1-receptor antagonists should include the goals of therapy; the reasons for obtaining baseline data such as vital signs, ECG, and laboratory blood work, and the existence of underlying liver and renal disorders; and possible drug side effects. Include the following points when teaching clients about first- and second-generation H_1-receptor and antagonists.

- Take the medication exactly as prescribed.
- Immediately report difficulty urinating.
- Report fever, blurred vision, or eye pain.
- Avoid driving or performing hazardous activities until you know the effects of the drug.
- Avoid smoking or consuming large amounts of caffeinated beverages.
- Do not take OTC antihistamines or decongestants unless approved by your healthcare provider.
- Suck on sugar-free hard candy to relieve symptoms of dry mouth.

INTRANASAL GLUCOCORTICOIDS

Glucocorticoids, also known as *corticosteroids*, may be applied directly to the nasal mucosa to prevent symptoms of allergic rhinitis. They have begun to replace antihistamines

---

NURSING PROCESS FOCUS Clients Receiving Antihistamine Therapy

Assessment	Potential Nursing Diagnoses
Prior to administration: ■ Obtain a complete health history including data on anaphylaxis, asthma, or cardiac disease, plus allergies, drug history, and possible drug interactions. ■ Obtain ECG and vital signs; assess in context of client's baseline values. ■ Assess respiratory status, especially breathing pattern. ■ Assess neurological status and level of consciousness.	■ Airway Clearance, Ineffective ■ Breathing Pattern, Ineffective ■ Sleep Pattern, Disturbed, related to somnolence or agitation

Planning: Client Goals and Expected Outcomes

The client will:
■ Report relief from allergic symptoms such as congestion, itching, or postnasal drip.
■ Demonstrate an understanding of the drug's action by accurately describing drug side effects and precautions.

Implementation

Interventions and (Rationales)	Client Education/Discharge Planning
■ Auscultate breath sounds before administering. Use with extreme caution in clients with asthma or COPD. Keep resuscitative equipment accessible. (Anticholinergic effects of antihistamines may trigger bronchospasm.)	■ Instruct client to immediately report wheezing or difficulty breathing. ■ Advise asthmatics to consult the nurse regarding the use of injectable epinephrine in emergency situations.
■ Monitor vital signs (including ECG) before administering. Use with extreme caution in clients with a history of cardiovascular disease. (Anticholinergic effects can increase heart rate and lower blood pressure. Fatal dysrhythmias and cardiovascular collapse have been reported in some clients receiving antihistamines.)	Instruct client to: ■ Immediately report dizziness; palpitations; headache; or chest, arm, or back pain accompanied by nausea/vomiting and/or sweating. ■ Monitor vital signs daily, ensuring proper use of home equipment.
■ Monitor thyroid function. Use with caution in clients with a history of hyperthyroidism. (Antihistamines exacerbate CNS-stimulating effects of hyperthyroidism and may trigger thyroid storm.)	■ Instruct client to immediately report nervousness or restlessness, insomnia, fever, profuse sweating, thirst, or mood changes.
■ Monitor for vision changes. Use with caution in clients with narrow-angle glaucoma. (Antihistamines can increase intraocular pressure and cause photosensitivity.)	Instruct client to: ■ Immediately report head or eye pain and visual changes. ■ Wear dark glasses, use sunscreen, and avoid excessive sun exposure.
■ Monitor neurological status, especially LOC. Use with caution in clients with a history of seizure disorder. (Antihistamines lower the seizure threshold. The elderly are at increased risk of serious sedation and other anticholinergic effects.)	Instruct client to: ■ Immediately report seizure activity, including any changes in character and pattern of seizures. ■ Avoid driving or performing hazardous activities until effects of the drug are known.

NURSING PROCESS FOCUS Clients Receiving Antihistamine Therapy *(Continued)*

Implementation	
Interventions and (Rationales)	**Client Education/Discharge Planning**
▪ Observe for signs of renal toxicity. Measure intake and output. Use with caution in clients with a history of kidney or urinary tract disease. (Antihistamines promote urine retention.)	▪ Instruct client to immediately report flank pain, difficulty urinating, reduced urine output, or changes in the appearance of urine (cloudy, with sediment, odor, etc.).
▪ Use with caution in clients with diabetes mellitus. Monitor serum glucose levels with increased frequency (e.g., from daily to tid, ac). (Antihistamines decrease serum glucose levels.)	Instruct client to: ▪ Immediately report symptoms of hypoglycemia. ▪ Consult the healthcare provider regarding timing of glucose monitoring and reportable results (e.g., "less than 70 mg/dl").
▪ Monitor for GI side effects. Use with caution in clients with a history of GI disorders, especially peptic ulcers or liver disease. (Antihistamines block H_1 receptors, altering the mucosal lining of the stomach. These drugs are metabolized in the liver, increasing the risk of hepatotoxicity.)	Instruct client to: ▪ Immediately report nausea, vomiting, anorexia, bleeding, chest or abdominal pain, heartburn, jaundice, or a change in the color or character of stools. ▪ Avoid substances that irritate the stomach such as spicy foods, alcoholic beverages, and nicotine; take drug with food to avoid stomach upset.
▪ Monitor for side effects such as dry mouth; observe for signs of anticholinergic crisis. (Side effects may lead to patient noncompliance.)	Instruct client to: ▪ Immediately report fever or flushing accompanied by difficulty swallowing ("cotton mouth"), blurred vision, and confusion. ▪ Avoid mixing OTC antihistamines; always consult the healthcare provider before taking any OTC drugs or herbal supplements. ▪ Suck on sugar-free hard candy to relieve dry mouth, and maintain adequate fluid intake.

Evaluation of Outcome Criteria
Evaluate the effectiveness of drug therapy by confirming that client goals and expected outcomes have been met (see "Planning"). ▪ The client reports relief of allergic symptoms such as urticaria, congestion, and postnasal drip. ▪ The client demonstrates an understanding of the drug's action by accurately describing drug side effects and precautions.

∞ *See Table 33.6 for a list of drugs to which these nursing actions apply.*

as drugs of choice for the treatment of perennial allergic rhinitis. These drugs are listed in Table 38.3.

38.4 Treating Allergic Rhinitis With Intranasal Glucocorticoids

The importance of the glucocorticoids in treating severe inflammation was presented in Section 33.5. Although glucocorticoids are very effective, their use as *systemic* therapy is limited by potentially serious side effects. *Intranasal* glucocorticoids, however, produce virtually no serious adverse effects. Because of their effectiveness and safety, the intranasal glucocorticoids have joined antihistamines as first-line drugs in the treatment of allergic rhinitis.

When sprayed onto the nasal mucosa, these drugs act by multiple mechanisms. They decrease the secretion of inflammatory mediators, reduce tissue edema, and cause a mild vasoconstriction. All six agents are administered with a metered-spray device that delivers a consistent dose of drug per spray. All have equal effectiveness. Unlike with the sympathomimetics (Section 38.5), benefits are not immediate;

TABLE 38.3 Intranasal Glucocorticoids		
Drug	**Route and Adult Dose (max dose where indicated)**	**Adverse Effects**
beclomethasone (Beconase, Vancenase)	Intranasal; 1 spray bid–qid	*Transient nasal irritation, burning, sneezing, or dryness*
budesonide (Rhinocort)	Intranasal; 2 sprays bid	
flunisolide (Nasalide, Nasarel)	Intranasal; 2 sprays bid; may increase to tid if needed	<u>Hypercorticism (only if large amounts are swallowed)</u>
⊕ fluticasone propionate (Flonase)	Intranasal; 1 spray 1–2 times/day (max: 4 times daily)	
mometasone furoate (Nasonex)	Intranasal; 2 sprays/day	
triamcinolone acetonide (Nasacort AQ)	Intranasal; 2–4 sprays 4 times daily	

Italics indicate common adverse effects; <u>underlining</u> indicates serious adverse effects.

2 to 3 weeks may be required to achieve peak response. Because of this delayed effect, intranasal glucocorticoids must be taken in advance of the allergen exposure.

When these glucocorticoids are administered consistently, their action is limited to the nasal passages. The most frequently reported side effect is an intense burning sensation in the nose immediately after spraying. Excessive drying of the nasal mucosa may occur, leading to epistaxis.

For clients who do not respond to intranasal glucocorticoids, intranasal cromolyn (Nasalcrom) is an alternative. Because it inhibits the release of histamine from mast cells, cromolyn is called a *mast cell stabilizer*. Most effective when given prior to allergen exposure, cromolyn has few adverse effects, and was recently designated as an OTC drug for the treatment of allergy and cold symptoms. Further discussion on the mast cell stabilizers is presented in Chapter 39 ∞, because asthma is a second indication for drugs in this class.

NURSING CONSIDERATIONS

The role of the nurse in drug therapy with intranasal glucocorticoids for the treatment of allergic rhinitis involves careful monitoring of a client's condition and providing education as it relates to the prescribed drug treatment. Prior to administering glucocorticoid nasal spray, assess the nares for excoriation or bleeding. Broken mucous membranes allow direct access to the bloodstream, increasing the likelihood of systemic side effects. Examine the mouth and throat for signs of infection, because glucocorticoids may slow the healing process and mask infections. Monitor signs and symptoms of GI distress,

because swallowing large quantities of the drug may contribute to dyspepsia and systemic drug absorption. Monitor for signs of Cushing's syndrome. Intranasal glucocorticoids are contraindicated in clients who demonstrate hypersensitivity to any of the ingredients, including preservatives, in the nasal spray.

Client Teaching. Client education as it relates to intranasal glucocorticoids should include the goals of therapy; the reasons for obtaining baseline data such as vital signs, laboratory blood work, and the existence of underlying disorders such as acute infections; and possible drug side effects. Include the following points when teaching clients about intranasal glucocorticoids:

- Before the first dose, follow label instructions for priming the device to receive the entire dose of medication.
- Shake inhalers gently before spraying.
- Gently clear the nose before spraying. Avoid clearing the nose immediately after spraying.
- Avoid swallowing medication. Spit out the postnasal medication residue.
- If a nasal decongestant spray is prescribed with this medication, administer the decongestant spray first to clear the nasal passages. This allows the intranasal glucocorticoid to be most effective.
- Be aware that it may take 2 to 4 weeks to reach maximum effectiveness.
- Report nosebleeds, nasal burning, or irritation that lasts more than a few doses.
- Use a humidifier, preservative-free nasal saline spray, or petroleum jelly to ease nasal dryness.

Pr PROTOTYPE DRUG | Fluticasone *(Flonase, Flovent)* | Intranasal Glucocorticoid

ACTIONS AND USES

Fluticasone is typical of the intranasal glucocorticoids used to treat seasonal allergic rhinitis. Therapy usually begins with two sprays in each nostril, twice daily, and decreases to one dose per day. Fluticasone acts to decrease local inflammation in the nasal passages, thus reducing nasal stuffiness.

ADMINISTRATION ALERTS

- Instruct client to carefully follow the directions for use provided by the manufacturer.
- Pregnancy category C.

PHARMACOKINETICS

Onset: Unknown

Peak: Unknown

Half-life: 3 h

Duration: 12–24 h

ADVERSE EFFECTS

Side effects of fluticasone are rare. Swallowing large amounts increases the potential for systemic glucocorticoid side effects. Nasal irritation and epistaxis occur in a small number of clients.

Contraindications: The only contraindication to fluticasone is prior hypersensitivity to the drug. Because glucocorticoids can mask signs of infection, clients with known bacterial, viral, fungal or parasitic infections (especially of the respiratory tract) should not receive intranasal glucocorticoids.

INTERACTIONS

Drug–Drug: Concomitant use of an intranasal decongestant increases the risk of nasal irritation or bleeding. Use with ritonavir should be avoided, as this drug significantly increases plasma fluticasone levels.

Lab Tests: Unknown.

Herbal/Food: Use with caution with licorice, which may potentiate the effects of glucocorticoids.

Treatment of Overdose: There is no specific treatment for overdose.

 See the Companion Website for a Nursing Process Focus specific to this drug.

TABLE 38.4	Nasal Decongestants	
Drug	**Route and Adult Dose (max dose where indicated)**	**Adverse Effects**
SYMPATHOMIMETICS		
ephedrine (Pretz-D)	Intranasal (0.1%); 1–2 drops bid	*Intranasal: transient nasal irritation, burning, sneezing, or dryness, headache*
naphazoline (Privine)	Intranasal; 2 drops q3–6h	
oxymetazoline (Afrin 12 Hour, Neo-Synephrine 12 Hour, others)	Intranasal (0.05%); 2–3 sprays bid for up to 3–5 days	*PO: nervousness, insomnia, headache, dry mouth*
phenylephrine (Afrin 4–6 Hour, Neo-Synephrine 4–6 Hour, others)	Intranasal (0.1%); 2–3 drops or sprays q3–4h, as needed	<u>Intranasal: rebound congestion</u>
pseudoephedrine (Chlortrimeton, Drixoral, others)	PO; 60 mg 4–6h (max: 120 mg/day)	<u>PO: CNS excitation, tremors, dysrhythmias, tachycardia, difficulty in voiding</u>
tetrahydrozoline (Tyzine)	Intranasal; 2–4 drops or sprays q3h	
xylometazoline (Otrivin)	Intranasal (0.1%); 1–2 sprays bid (max: 3 doses/day)	
ANTICHOLINERGIC		
ipratropium bromide (Atrovent, Combivent)	Nasal spray; 2 sprays in each nostril 3–4 times/day up to 4 days	*Transient nasal irritation, burning, sneezing, or dryness, cough, headache* <u>Urinary retention, worsening of narrow-angle glaucoma</u>

Italics indicate common adverse effects; <u>underlining</u> indicates serious adverse effects.

DECONGESTANTS

Drugs affecting the autonomic nervous system are the most commonly used agents for relieving nasal congestion. Several sympathomimetics and one anticholinergic are administered orally or intranasally to dry the nasal mucosa. The nasal decongestants are listed in Table 38.4.

38.5 Treating Nasal Congestion With Decongestants

Sympathomimetics with alpha-adrenergic activity are effective at relieving the nasal congestion associated with the common cold or allergic rhinitis when given by either the oral or intranasal route. The intranasal preparations such as oxymetazoline (Afrin, others) are available OTC as sprays or drops, and produce an effective response within minutes.

Intranasal sympathomimetics produce few systemic effects because almost none of the drug is absorbed into the circulation. The most serious, limiting side effect of the intranasal preparations is **rebound congestion.** Prolonged

use causes hypersecretion of mucus, worsening nasal congestion once the drug effects wear off. This can lead to a cycle of increased drug use as the condition worsens. Because of this rebound congestion, intranasal sympathomimetics should be used for no longer than 3 to 5 days. Clients who develop dependence should be gradually switched to intranasal glucocorticoids.

When administered *orally*, sympathomimetics do not produce rebound congestion. Their onset of action by this route, however, is much slower than when administered intranasally, and they are less effective at relieving severe congestion. The possibility of systemic side effects is also greater with the oral drugs. Potential side effects include hypertension and CNS stimulation that may lead to insomnia and anxiety. Pseudoephedrine is a common sympathomimetic found in oral OTC cold and allergy medicines.

Because the sympathomimetics relieve only nasal congestion, they are often combined with antihistamines to control sneezing and tearing. It is interesting to note that some OTC drugs having the same basic name (Neo-Synephrine, Afrin, and Vicks) may contain different sympathomimetics. For example, Neo-Synephrine decongestants with 12-hour duration contain the drug oxymetazoline; Neo-Synephrine preparations that last 4 to 6 hours contain phenylephrine.

One anticholinergic, ipratropium (Atrovent), is indicated for symptoms associated with perennial allergic rhinitis and the common cold. Given by the intranasal route, ipratropium has no serious side effects. Its actions are limited to decreasing rhinorrhea; it does not stop the sneezing, postnasal drip, or itchy throat or eyes characteristic of allergic rhinitis or the common cold. A more common indication for ipratropium is in the pharmacotherapy of asthma, and a prototype feature for this drug may be found in Chapter 39 ∞.

Pr PROTOTYPE DRUG | Oxymetazoline *(Afrin, others)* | Decongestant/Sympathomimetic

ACTIONS AND USES

Oxymetazoline stimulates alpha-adrenergic receptors in the sympathetic nervous system. This causes arterioles in the nasal passages to constrict, thus drying the mucous membranes. Relief from nasal congestion occurs within minutes and lasts for 10 or more hours. Oxymetazoline is administered with a metered spray device or by nasal drops.

ADMINISTRATION ALERTS

- Wash hands carefully after administration to prevent anisocoria (blurred vision and inequality of pupil size).
- Pregnancy category C.

PHARMACOKINETICS

Onset: 5–10 min

Peak: Unknown

Half-life: Unknown

Duration: 6–10 h

ADVERSE EFFECTS

Rebound congestion is common when oxymetazoline is used for longer than 3 to 5 days. Minor stinging and dryness in the nasal mucosa may be experienced. Systemic side effects are unlikely, unless a large amount of the medicine is swallowed.

Contraindications: Clients with thyroid disorders, hypertension, diabetes, or heart disease should use sympathomimetics only on the direction of their healthcare provider.

INTERACTIONS

Drug–Drug: No clinically important interactions occur, because absorption of oxymetazoline is limited.

Lab Tests: Unknown.

Herbal/Food: Use with caution with herbal supplements such as St. John's wort that have properties of monoamine oxidase inhibitors.

Treatment of Overdose: There is no specific treatment for overdose.

 See the Companion Website for a Nursing Process Focus specific to this drug.

NURSING CONSIDERATIONS

The role of the nurse in drug therapy with sympathomimetics for nasal congestion involves careful monitoring of a client's condition and providing education as it relates to the prescribed drug treatment. Assess for the presence or history of nasal congestion. Also assess the nares for signs of excoriation or bleeding. Before and during pharmacotherapy, assess vital signs, especially pulse and blood pressure. Oral sympathomimetics are contraindicated in clients with hypertension due to vasoconstriction caused by stimulation of alpha-adrenergic receptors on systemic blood vessels.

Sympathomimetics (alpha-adrenergic agonists) should be used with caution in clients with prostatic enlargement, because these drugs increase smooth-muscle activity in the prostate gland and may diminish urinary outflow (Chapter 46 ∞). Clients with thyroid disorders and diabetes mellitus are at risk because sympathomimetics can increase serum glucose and body metabolism.

These agents should be used with caution in clients with psychiatric disorders because they may cause CNS stimulation and agitation in some clients. The CNS depression effect of these drugs can seriously exacerbate symptoms of clinical depression.

Client Teaching. Client education as it relates to sympathomimetics for nasal congestion should include the goals of therapy; the reasons for obtaining baseline data such as vital signs and tests for cardiac or metabolic disorders, and the existence of underlying disorders such as glaucoma and hypertension; and possible drug side effects. Include the following points when teaching clients about sympathomimetics:

- Limit use of intranasal preparations to 3 to 5 days to prevent rebound congestion.
- If taking a prescription decongestant, do not take other OTC cold or allergy preparations (especially those containing antihistamines), without notifying your healthcare provider because these agents may cause excessive drowsiness.
- Follow the manufacturer's directions for the use and care of nasal spray dispensers and proper administration technique.
- Immediately report palpitations or chest pain, dizziness or fainting, fever, visual changes, excessively dry mouth and confusion, numbness or tingling in the face or limbs, severe headache, insomnia, restlessness or nervousness, nosebleeds, or persistent intranasal pain or irritation.

HOME & COMMUNITY CONSIDERATIONS

Pseudoephedrine and Drug Abuse

Methamphetamine is a powerful CNS stimulant and is highly addictive. It is often produced in homes using easily available products. One of the ingredients is pseudoephedrine, a popular OTC decongestant. To address this problem, many states limit the amount of pseudoephedrine that can be purchased at any one time. These states also require that OTC drugs that contain pseudoephedrine be placed behind the counter. The consumer must then produce identification prior to purchasing the drug. The hope is that this restriction will decrease the manufacture of this illegal drug. Many manufacturers have replaced pseudoephedrine with phenylephrine as the active agent in OTC cold medications.

COMMON COLD

The common cold is a viral infection of the upper respiratory tract that produces a characteristic array of annoying symptoms. It is fortunate that the disorder is self-limiting, because there is no cure or effective prevention for colds. Therapies used to relieve symptoms include some of the same drugs classes used for allergic rhinitis, including antihistamines and decongestants. A few additional drugs, such as those that suppress cough and loosen bronchial secretions, are used for symptomatic cold treatment.

ANTITUSSIVES

Antitussives are drugs used to dampen the cough reflex. They are of value in treating coughs due to allergies or the common cold.

38.6 Pharmacotherapy With Antitussives

Cough is a natural reflex mechanism that serves to forcibly remove excess secretions and foreign material from the respiratory system. In diseases such as emphysema and bronchitis, or when liquids have been aspirated into the bronchi, it is not desirable to suppress the normal cough reflex. Dry, hacking, nonproductive cough, however, can be irritating to the membranes of the throat and can deprive a client of much-needed rest. It is these types of conditions in which therapy with medications that control cough, known as **antitussives,** may be warranted. Antitussives are classified as opioid or nonopioid and are listed in Table 38.5.

Opioids, the most efficacious antitussives, act by raising the cough threshold in the CNS. Codeine and hydrocodone are the most frequently used opioid antitussives. Doses needed to suppress the cough reflex are very low; thus, there is minimal potential for dependence. Most opioid cough mixtures are classified as Schedule III, IV, or V drugs, and are reserved for more serious cough conditions. Though not common, overdose from opioid cough remedies may cause significant respiratory depression. Care must be taken when using these medications in clients with asthma, because bronchoconstriction may occur. Opioids may be combined with other agents such as antihistamines, decongestants, and nonopioid antitussives in the therapy of severe cold or flu symptoms. Some of these combinations are listed in Table 38.6.

The most frequently used nonopioid antitussive is dextromethorphan, which is available in OTC cold and flu medications. Dextromethorphan is chemically similar to the opioids, and also acts on the CNS to raise the cough threshold. Though not as effective as codeine, dextromethorphan carries no risk of dependence.

Benzonatate (Tessalon) is a nonopioid antitussive that acts by a different mechanism. Chemically related to the local anesthetic tetracaine (Pontocaine), benzonatate suppresses the cough reflex by anesthetizing stretch receptors in the lungs. If chewed, the drug can cause the side effect of numbing the mouth and pharynx. Side effects are uncommon, but may include sedation, nausea, headache, and dizziness.

TABLE 38.5 Selected Antitussives and Expectorants

Drug	Route and Adult Dose (max dose where indicated)	Adverse Effects
ANTITUSSIVES: OPIOIDS		
codeine	PO; 10–20 mg q4–6h PRN (max: 120 mg/24 h)	*Nausea, vomiting, constipation, confusion, dizziness, sedation*
hydrocodone bitartrate (Hycodan, others)	PO; 5–10 mg q4–6h PRN (max: 15 mg/dose)	Hypotension, seizures, bradycardia, respiratory depression, severe somnolence
ANTITUSSIVES: NONOPIOIDS		
benzonatate (Tessalon)	PO; 100 mg tid PRN up to 600 mg/day	*Drowsiness, constipation, GI upset*
		Paradoxical excitation, tremors, euphoria, insomnia
dextromethorphan (Benylin, others)	PO; 10–20 mg q4h or 30 mg q6–8h (max: 120 mg/day)	*Drowsiness, headache, GI upset*
		CNS depression, paradoxical excitation
EXPECTORANT		
guaifenesin (Robitussin, others)	PO; 200–400 mg q4h (max: 2.4 g/day)	*Drowsiness, headache, GI upset*
		No serious adverse effects
MUCOLYTIC		
acetylcysteine (Mucomyst)	MDI; Inhalation: 1–10 ml of 20% solution q4–6h or 2–20 ml of 10% solution q4–6h	*Unpleasant odor, nausea*
		Severe nausea and vomiting

Italics indicate common adverse effects; underlining indicates serious adverse effects.

TABLE 38.6	Opioid Combination Drugs for Severe Cold Symptoms	
Trade Name	**Opioid**	**Nonopioid Ingredients**
Ambenyl Cough Syrup	codeine	bromodiphenhydramine
Calcidrine Syrup	codeine	calcium iodide
Cheracol Syrup	codeine	guaifenesin
Codiclear DH Syrup	hydrocodone	guaifenesin
Codimal DH	hydrocodone	phenylephrine, pyrilamine
Hycodan	hydrocodone	homatropine
Hycomine Compound	hydrocodone	phenylephrine, chlorpheniramine, acetaminophen
Hycotuss Expectorant	hydrocodone	guaifenesin
Novahistine DH	codeine	pseudoephedrine, chlorpheniramine
Phenergan with Codeine	codeine	promethazine
Robitussin A-C	codeine	guaifenesin
Tega-Tussin Syrup	hydrocodone	phenylephrine, chlorpheniramine
Triacin-C Cough Syrup	codeine	pseudoephedrine, triprolidine
Tussionex	hydrocodone	chlorpheniramine

NURSING CONSIDERATIONS

The role of the nurse in antitussive therapy for the treatment of cough involves careful monitoring of a client's condition and providing education as it relates to the prescribed drug treatment. The nursing care is dependent on the agent used. For all antitussive drugs, assess for a presence or history of persistent nonproductive cough, respiratory distress, shortness of breath, or productive cough.

When codeine or another opioid is prescribed, monitor the client for drowsiness. Cough is a protective mechanism used to cleanse the lungs of microbes; therefore, use antitussive drugs in moderation and only to treat cough when it interferes with activities of daily living, rest, or sleep. Extreme caution should be used in administering antitussive drugs to individuals with chronic lung conditions, because normal respiratory function is already impaired. Because cough may be a symptom of other serious pulmonary conditions, antitussive drugs should be used for only 3 days, unless otherwise approved by the healthcare provider.

Client Teaching.   Client education as it relates to antitussives should include the goals of therapy, the reasons for

---

Pr **PROTOTYPE DRUG** | Dextromethorphan *(Benylin, others)* | Antitussive

ACTIONS AND USES

Dextromethorphan is a component in most OTC severe cold and flu preparations. It is available in a large variety of formulations, including tablets, liquid-filled capsules, lozenges, and liquids. It has a rapid onset of action, usually within 15 to 30 minutes. Like codeine, it acts in the medulla, though it lacks the analgesic and euphoric effects of the opioids and does not produce dependence. Clients whose cough is not relieved by dextromethorphan after several days of therapy should see their healthcare provider.

ADMINISTRATION ALERTS

- Avoid pulmonary irritants, such as smoking or other fumes, because these agents may decrease drug effectiveness.
- Pregnancy category C.

PHARMACOKINETICS

Onset: 15–30 min

Peak: Unknown

Half-life: Unknown

Duration: 3–6 h

ADVERSE EFFECTS

Side effects due to dextromethorphan are rare. Dizziness, drowsiness, and GI upset occur in some clients.

Contraindications: Dextromethorphan is contraindicated in the treatment of chronic cough due to excessive bronchial secretions, such as in asthma, smoking, and emphysema. Suppressing the cough reflex is not desirable in these clients.

INTERACTIONS

Drug–Drug: Drug interactions with dextromethorphan include excitation, hypotension, and hyperpyrexia when used concurrently with MAO inhibitors. Use with alcohol, opioids, or other CNS depressants may result in sedation.

Lab Tests: Unknown.

Herbal/Food: Unknown.

Treatment of Overdose: There is no specific treatment for overdose.

 See the Companion Website for a Nursing Process Focus specific to this drug.

obtaining baseline data such as vital signs and tests for cardiac and renal disorders and the existence of underlying disorders such as COPD, and possible drug side effects. Include the following points when teaching clients regarding antitussives:

- Avoid driving or performing hazardous activities while taking opioid antitussives.
- Avoid alcohol use.
- Immediately report coughing up green- or yellow-tinged secretions, difficulty breathing, excessive drowsiness, constipation, and nausea or vomiting.
- Store opioid antitussives away from children.
- If taking a prescription antitussive, do not take OTC cough or cold preparations without notifying your healthcare provider because these agents can cause excessive drowsiness.
- Read label instructions carefully; do not take more than the recommended dose.

EXPECTORANTS AND MUCOLYTICS

Several drugs are available to control excess mucus production. Expectorants increase bronchial secretions, and mucolytics help loosen thick bronchial secretions. These agents are listed in Table 38.5.

38.7 Pharmacotherapy With Expectorants and Mucolytics

Expectorants reduce the thickness or viscosity of bronchial secretions, thus increasing mucus flow that can then be removed more easily by coughing. The most effective OTC expectorant is guaifenesin (Resyl, others). Like dextromethorphan, guaifenesin produces few adverse effects and is a common ingredient in many OTC cold and flu preparations.

Acetylcysteine (Mucomyst) is one of the few drugs available to *directly* loosen thick, viscous bronchial secretions. Drugs of this type, **mucolytics**, break down the chemical structure of mucus molecules. The mucus becomes thinner, and can be removed more easily by coughing. Acetylcysteine is delivered by the inhalation route and is not available OTC. It is used in clients who have cystic fibrosis, chronic bronchitis, or other diseases that produce large amounts of thick bronchial secretions. A second mucolytic, dornase alfa (Pulmozyme), is approved for maintenance therapy in the management of thick bronchial secretions. Dornase alfa breaks down DNA molecules in the mucus, causing it to become less viscous.

Acetylcysteine is also administered by the oral or IV route to clients who have received an overdose of acetaminophen. Its use in the pharmacotherapy of acetaminophen toxicity is presented in Chapter 33 ∞.

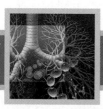

CHAPTER REVIEW

KEY CONCEPTS

The numbered key concepts provide a succinct summary of the important points from the corresponding numbered section within the chapter. If any of these points are not clear, refer to the numbered section within the chapter for review.

38.1 The upper respiratory tract humidifies and cleans incoming air. The nasal mucosa is richly supplied with vascular tissue and is the first line of immunological defense.

38.2 Allergic rhinitis is a disorder characterized by sneezing, watery eyes, and nasal congestion. Pharmacotherapy is targeted at preventing the disorder, or relieving its symptoms.

38.3 Antihistamines, or H_1-receptor antagonists, can provide relief from the symptoms of allergic rhinitis. Major side effects include drowsiness and anticholinergic effects such as dry mouth. Newer drugs in this class are nonsedating.

38.4 Intranasal glucocorticoids have become drugs of choice in treating allergic rhinitis owing to their high efficacy and

wide margin of safety. For maximum effectiveness, they must be administered 2–3 weeks prior to allergen exposure.

38.5 The most commonly used decongestants are oral and intranasal sympathomimetics that alleviate the nasal congestion associated with allergic rhinitis and the common cold. Intranasal drugs are more efficacious but should be used for only 3 to 5 days owing to rebound congestion.

38.6 Antitussives are effective at relieving cough due to the common cold. Opioids are used for severe cough. Nonopioids such as dextromethorphan are used for mild or moderate cough.

38.7 Expectorants promote mucus secretion, making it thinner and easier to remove by coughing. Mucolytics directly break down mucus molecules.

NCLEX-RN® REVIEW QUESTIONS

1 The client has been prescribed oxymetazoline (Afrin). The nurse understands:

1. The most serious side effect is rebound congestion.
2. The average use is for 10 days.
3. This drug should not be used in conjunction with antihistamines.
4. This is an OTC and may be used as needed for congestion.

2 A client is prescribed an intranasal glucocorticoid for allergic rhinitis. The nurse's teaching would include (select all that apply):

1. There are no known side effects.
2. The spray is a consistent dose.
3. It could take 2 to 4 weeks before improvement in symptoms is noticed.
4. It is contraindicated to use saline nasal sprays with this medicine.
5. The medication can be used any time symptoms increase.

3 The nurse assesses for which of the following findings in the history of a client that is related to taking a first-generation H_1-receptor antagonist?

1. A history of heart disease
2. Any recent weight gain
3. A history of respiratory illnesses
4. A history of peptic ulcer

4 When teaching clients how to self-administer intranasal corticorticoids, which of the following must be included? (Select all that apply.)

1. Prime device prior to initial use.
2. Clear nose before administration.
3. Clear nose after administration.
4. Swallow any excess that drains into the mouth.
5. Spit out any excess that drains into the mouth.

5 Prior to administration of antihistamines, the nurse assesses for:

1. Prostatic hypertrophy.
2. Itching.
3. Dry skin.
4. Increased restlessness.

CRITICAL THINKING QUESTIONS

1. A 74-year-old male client informs the nurse that he is taking diphendydramine (Benadryl) to reduce seasonal allergy symptoms. This client has a history of an enlarged prostate and mild glaucoma (controlled by medication). What is the nurse's response?

2. A 65-year-old client has bronchitis and has been coughing for several days. Which is the antitussive of choice for this client, dextromethorphan or codeine? Why?

3. A 67-year-old client has allergic rhinitis and always carries a handkerchief in his pocket because he has nasal discharge nearly every day. Sometimes his nose is stuffy and dry. The physician prescribes fluticasone (Flonase). He is to take one spray intranasally at bedtime. The client starts to take fluticasone and a week later calls the doctor's office and talks to the nurse. He says, "This Flonase is not helping me." What is the nurse's best response?

See Appendix D for answers and rationales for all activities.

EXPLORE MediaLink

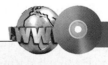
www.prenhall.com/adams

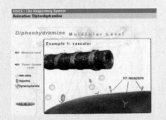

NCLEX-RN® review, case studies, and other interactive resources for this chapter can be found on the companion website at www.prenhall.com/adams. Click on "Chapter 38" to select the activities for this chapter. For animations, more NCLEX-RN® review questions, and an audio glossary, access the accompanying Prentice Hall Nursing MediaLink DVD-ROM in this textbook.

PRENTICE HALL NURSING MEDIALINK DVD-ROM

- **Animation**
  Mechanism in Action: Diphenhydramine (*Benadryl, others*)
- **Audio Glossary**
- **NCLEX-RN® Review**

 ### COMPANION WEBSITE

- **NCLEX-RN® Review**
- **Dosage Calculations**
- **Case Study:** Client with allergic rhinitis
- **Care Plan:** Client with allergic rhinitis treated with Sudafed

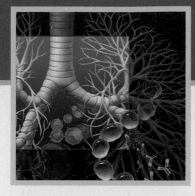

CHAPTER 39

Drugs for Asthma and Other Pulmonary Disorders

DRUGS AT A GLANCE

BRONCHODILATORS
Beta-adrenergic Agonists
   ⊕ *salmeterol (Serevent)*
Anticholinergics
   ⊕ *ipratropium (Atrovent)*
Methylxanthines
ANTI-INFLAMMATORY AGENTS
Glucocorticoids
   ⊕ *beclomethasone (Beclovent, Beconase, Vancenase, Vanceril)*
Leukotriene Modifiers
Mast Cell Stabilizers
   ⊕ *zafirlukast (Accolate)*

OBJECTIVES

After reading this chapter, the student should be able to:

1. Identify anatomical structures associated with the lower respiratory tract and their functions.
2. Explain how the autonomic nervous system controls airflow in the lower respiratory tract, and how this process can be modified with drugs.
3. Compare the advantages and disadvantages of using the inhalation route of drug administration for pulmonary drugs.
4. Describe the types of devices used to deliver aerosol therapies via the inhalation route.
5. Compare and contrast the pharmacotherapy of acute and chronic asthma.
6. Describe the nurse's role in the pharmacological treatment of lower respiratory tract disorders.
7. For each of the classes listed in Drugs at a Glance, know representative drugs, and explain their mechanism of drug action, primary actions on the respiratory system, and important adverse effects.
8. Categorize drugs used in the treatment of lower respiratory tract disorders based on their classification and mechanisms of action.
9. Use the Nursing Process to care for clients who are receiving pharmacotherapy for lower respiratory tract disorders.

MediaLink

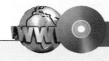 www.prenhall.com/adams

NCLEX-RN® review, case studies, and other interactive resources for this chapter can be found on the companion website at www.prenhall.com/adams. Click on "Chapter 39" to select the activities for this chapter. For animations, more NCLEX-RN® review questions, and an audio glossary, access the accompanying Prentice Hall Nursing MediaLink DVD-ROM in this textbook.

KEY TERMS

aerosol *page 595*

asthma *page 596*

bronchospasm *page 595*

chronic bronchitis *page 606*

chronic obstructive pulmonary disease (COPD) *page 605*

dry powder inhaler (DPI) *page 595*

emphysema *page 606*

leukotrienes *page 603*

metered dose inhaler (MDI) *page 595*

methylxanthine *page 600*

nebulizer *page 595*

perfusion *page 594*

status asthmaticus *page 596*

ventilation *page 594*

The airways that serve as essential passageways for gases in and out of the human body are dynamic and in constant flux. Minute-by-minute control of the airways is necessary to bring an abundant supply of essential gases to the pulmonary capillaries and to rid the body of some of its most toxic waste products. Any restriction in this dynamic flow, even for brief periods, may result in serious consequences. This chapter examines drugs used in the pharmacotherapy of two primary bronchoconstrictive disorders—asthma and chronic obstructive pulmonary disease.

39.1 Physiology of the Lower Respiratory Tract

The primary function of the respiratory system is to bring oxygen into the body and to remove carbon dioxide. The process by which gases are exchanged is called *respiration*. The basic structures of the lower respiratory tract are shown in ● Figure 39.1.

Ventilation is the process of moving air into and out of the lungs. As the diaphragm contracts and lowers in position, it creates a negative pressure that draws air into the lungs, and inspiration occurs. During expiration, the diaphragm relaxes and air leaves the lungs passively, with no energy expenditure required. Ventilation is a purely mechanical process that occurs approximately 12 to 18 times per minute in adults, a rate determined by neurons in the brainstem. This rate may be modified by a number of factors, including emotions, fever, stress, and the pH of the blood.

The bronchial tree ends in dilated sacs called *alveoli*, which have no smooth muscle but are abundantly rich in capillaries. An extremely thin membrane in the alveoli separates the airway from the pulmonary capillaries, allowing gases to readily move between the internal environment of the blood and the inspired air. As oxygen crosses this membrane, it is exchanged for carbon dioxide, a cellular waste product that travels from the blood to the air. The lung is richly supplied with blood. Blood flow through the lungs is called **perfusion.** The process of gas exchange is shown in Figure 39.1.

39.2 Bronchiolar Smooth Muscle

Bronchioles are muscular, elastic structures whose diameter, or lumen, varies with the metabolic demands of the body. Changes in the diameter of the bronchiolar lumen are made possible by smooth muscle controlled by the autonomic

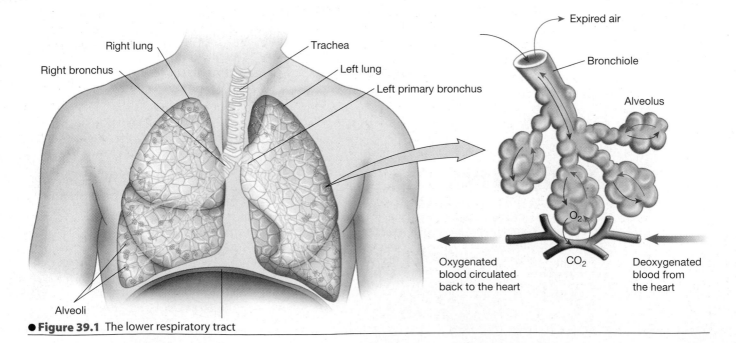

● **Figure 39.1** The lower respiratory tract

nervous system. During the fight-or-flight response, beta$_2$-adrenergic receptors of the sympathetic nervous system are stimulated, the bronchiolar smooth muscle relaxes, and bronchodilation occurs. This allows more air to enter the alveoli, thus increasing the oxygen supply to tissues during periods of stress or exercise. Sympathetic nervous system activation also increases the rate and depth of breathing. Drugs that stimulate beta$_2$-adrenergic receptors, commonly called *bronchodilators*, are some of the most commonly used drugs for treating pulmonary disorders.

When nerves from the parasympathetic nervous system are activated, bronchiolar smooth muscle contracts and the airway diameter narrows, resulting in bronchoconstriction. Bronchoconstriction increases airway resistance, causing breathing to be more labored and the client to become short of breath. Parasympathetic stimulation also has the effect of slowing the rate and depth of respiration.

39.3 Administration of Pulmonary Drugs via Inhalation

The respiratory system offers a rapid and efficient mechanism for delivering drugs. The enormous surface area of the bronchioles and alveoli, and the rich blood supply to these areas, results in an almost instantaneous onset of action for inhaled substances.

Medications are delivered to the respiratory system by aerosol therapy. An **aerosol** is a suspension of minute liquid droplets or fine solid particles suspended in a gas. The major advantage of aerosol therapy is that it delivers the drugs to their immediate site of action, thus reducing systemic side effects. To produce an equivalent therapeutic action, an oral drug would have to be given at higher doses, and be distributed to all body tissues. Aerosol therapy can give immediate relief for **bronchospasm**, a condition during which the bronchiolar smooth muscle rapidly contracts, leaving the client gasping for breath. Drugs may also be given to loosen viscous mucus in the bronchial tree.

It should be clearly understood that agents delivered by inhalation have the potential to produce *systemic* effects because of absorption across the pulmonary capillaries. For example, anesthetics such as nitrous oxide and halothane (Fluothane) are delivered via the inhalation route and are rapidly distributed to cause CNS depression (Chapter 19 ∞). Solvents such as paint thinners and glues are sometimes intentionally inhaled and can cause serious adverse effects on the nervous system and even death. In general, however, drugs administered by the inhalation route for respiratory conditions produce minimal systemic toxicity.

Several devices are used to deliver drugs via the inhalation route. **Nebulizers** are small machines that vaporize a liquid medication into a fine mist that can be inhaled, using a face mask or handheld device. If the drug is a solid, it may be administered using a **dry powder inhaler (DPI)**. A DPI is a small device that is activated by the process of inhalation to deliver a fine powder directly to the bronchial tree. Turbuhaler and Rotahaler are types of DPIs. **Metered dose inhalers (MDIs)** are a third type of device commonly used to deliver respiratory drugs. MDIs use a propellant to deliver a measured dose of drugs to the lungs during each breath. The client times the inhalation to the puffs of drug emitted from the MDI.

There are disadvantages to administering aerosol therapy. The precise dose received by the client is difficult to measure because it depends on the client's breathing pattern and the correct use of the aerosol device. Even under optimal conditions, only 10% to 50% of the drug actually reaches the lower respiratory tract. Clients must be carefully instructed on the correct use of these devices. Swallowing medication that has been deposited in the oral cavity may cause systemic side effects if the drug is absorbed in the GI tract. In addition, clients should rinse their mouth thoroughly following drug use to reduce the potential for absorption of the drug across the oral mucosa. Three devices used to deliver respiratory drugs are shown in ● Figure 39.2.

ASTHMA

Asthma is a chronic pulmonary disease with inflammatory and bronchospasm components. Drugs may be given to decrease the frequency of asthmatic attacks or to terminate attacks in progress.

MediaLink · Small-Volume Nebulizer

MediaLink · Dry Powder Inhaler

MediaLink · Metered Dose Inhaler

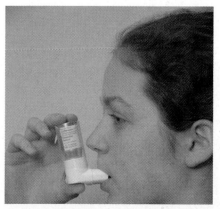 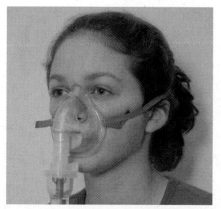 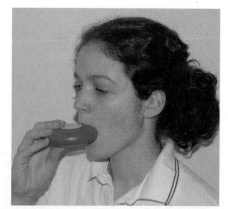

● **Figure 39.2** Devices used to deliver respiratory drugs: (a) metered-dose inhaler; (b) nebulizer with face mask; (c) dry-powder inhaler
Source: Pearson Education/PH College.

39.4 Pathophysiology of Asthma

Asthma is one of the most common chronic conditions in the United States, affecting almost 15 million Americans. Although the disorder can affect a client at any age, asthma is often considered a pediatric disease. Characterized by acute bronchospasm, asthma can cause intense breathlessness, coughing, and gasping for air. Along with bronchoconstriction, an acute inflammatory response stimulates histamine secretion, which increases mucus and edema in the airways. As in allergic rhinitis, the airway becomes hyperresponsive to allergens. Both bronchospasm and inflammation contribute to airway obstruction, illustrated in ● Figure 39.3.

The client with asthma can present with acute or chronic symptoms. Intervals between symptoms may vary from days to weeks to months. Some clients experience asthma when exposed to specific triggers, such as those listed in Table 39.1. Others experience the disorder on exertion, a condition called *exercise-induced asthma*. **Status asthmaticus** is a severe, prolonged form of asthma unresponsive to drug treatment that may lead to respiratory failure.

Because asthma has both a bronchoconstriction component and an inflammation component, pharmacotherapy of the disease focuses on one or both of these mechanisms. The goals of drug therapy are twofold: to *terminate* acute bronchospasms in progress and to *reduce the frequency* of asthma attacks. Different medications are needed to achieve each of these goals.

BETA-ADRENERGIC AGONISTS

Beta$_2$-agonists are effective bronchodilators for the management of asthma and other pulmonary diseases. They are some of the most frequently prescribed agents in pulmonary medicine. These drugs are listed in Table 39.2.

39.5 Treating Acute Asthma With Beta-adrenergic Agonists

Beta-adrenergic agonists are sympathomimetics that are drugs of choice in the treatment of *acute* bronchoconstriction. Some beta-agonists activate both beta$_1$- and beta$_2$-receptors,

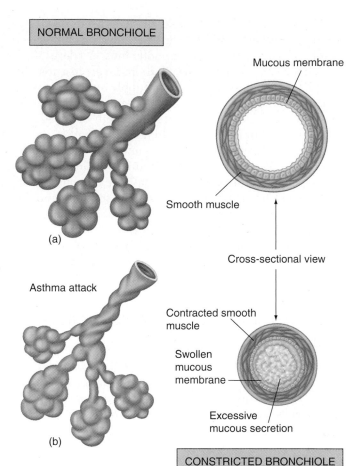

● **Figure 39.3** Changes in bronchioles during an asthma attack: (a) normal bronchiole; (b) in asthma attack

TABLE 39.1	Common Causes of Asthma
Cause	**Sources**
air pollutants	tobacco smoke
	ozone
	nitrous and sulfur oxides
	fumes from cleaning fluids or solvents
	burning leaves
allergens	pollen from trees, grasses, and weeds
	animal dander
	household dust
	mold
chemicals and food	drugs, including aspirin, ibuprofen, and beta-blockers
	sulfite preservatives
	food and condiments, including nuts, monosodium glutamate (MSG), shellfish, and dairy products
respiratory infections	bacterial, fungal, and viral
stress	emotional stress/anxiety
	exercise in dry, cold climates

TABLE 39.2   Bronchodilators for Asthma

Drug	Route and Adult Dose (max dose where indicated)	Adverse Effects
BETA-AGONISTS/SYMPATHOMIMETICS		
albuterol (Proventil, others)	PO; 2–4 mg tid–qid	*Headache, dizziness, tremor, nervousness, throat irritation, drug tolerance*
bitolterol mesylate (Tornalate)	MDI; 2 inhalations tid–qid	
epinephrine (Adrenalin, Bronkaid, Primatene) (see page 420 for the Prototype Drug box ∞)	Subcutaneous; 0.1–0.5 ml or 1:1000 q20 min–4h	Tachycardia, dysrhythmias, hypokalemia, hyperglycemia
formoterol fumarate (Foradil)	DPI; 12-mcg inhalation capsule q12h	
isoetharine HCl (Bronkosol, Bronkometer)	MDI; 1–2 inhalations q4h up to 5 days	
isoproterenol (Isuprel, Medihaler-Iso)	MDI; 1–2 inhalations q4h qid	
levalbuterol HCl (Xopenex)	Nebulizer; 0.63 mg tid–-qid	
metaproterenol sulfate (Alupent, Metaprel)	MDI; 2–3 inhalations q3–4h (max: 12 inhalations/day)	
pirbuterol acetate (Maxair)	MDI; 2 inhalations qid (max: 12 inhalations/day)	
salmeterol (Serevent)	MDI; 2 inhalations bid	
terbutaline sulfate (Brethaire, Brethine)	PO; 2.5–5 mg tid	
METHYLXANTHINES		
aminophylline (Truphylline)	PO; 0.25–0.75 mg/kg/h divided qid	*Nervousness, tremors, dizziness, headache*
theophylline (Theo-Dur, others)	PO; 0.4–0.6 mg/kg/h divided tid–qid	Tachycardia, dysrhythmias, hypotension, seizures, circulatory failure, respiratory arrest
ANTICHOLINERGICS		
ipratropium bromide (Atrovent, Combivent)	MDI; 2 inhalations qid (max: 12 inhalations/day)	*Headache, cough, dry mouth, nasal irritation*
tiotropium (Spiriva)	Handihaler device; 1 capsule inhaled/day	Worsening of narrow-angle glaucoma, sinusitis, pharyngitis, oropharyngeal candidiasis

Italics indicate common adverse effects; underlining indicates serious adverse effects.

whereas others activate *only* beta$_2$. Sympathomimetics selective for beta$_2$-receptors in the lung have largely replaced the older, nonselective agents such as epinephrine because they produce fewer cardiac side effects. Beta-agonists are commonly called *bronchodilators*, because this is their primary pharmacological action.

Bronchodilators relax bronchial smooth muscle, thus widening the airway and making breathing easier for the client. Although quite effective at relieving bronchospasm, beta-agonists have no anti-inflammatory properties; thus, other drug classes are required to control the inflammatory component of *chronic* asthma.

A practical method for classifying beta-adrenergic agonists for asthma is by their duration of action. The ultrashort-acting bronchodilators, including isoproterenol (Isuprel) and isoetharine (Bronkosol), act immediately, but their effects last only 2 to 3 hours. Short-acting agents, such as metaproterenol (Metaprel), terbutaline (Brethine), and pirbuterol (Maxair), also act quickly, but last 5 to 6 hours. Intermediate-acting beta-agonists such as albuterol (Proventil), levalbuterol (Xopenex), and bitolterol (Tornalate) last about 8 hours. The longest-acting agent, salmeterol (Serevent), has bronchodilation effects lasting as long as 12 hours. Formoterol (Foradil) is a newer beta$_2$-adrenergic agonist that combines a very rapid

onset of action (1 to 3 minutes) with 12 hours' duration. The specific drug chosen for pharmacotherapy is dependent on the pattern of symptoms experienced by the client.

The ultrashort-, short-, and intermediate-acting bronchodilators act quickly enough to terminate acute asthmatic episodes. The onset of action for salmeterol is too long for it to be indicated for asthma termination. The long-acting agents, however, are more convenient because they require less frequent dosing, and are especially useful for clients who are frequently awakened during the night with an asthma attack. The long-acting formulations are sometimes used concurrently with inhaled glucocorticoids to control persistent chronic asthma.

Inhaled beta-adrenergic agonists produce little systemic toxicity, because only small amounts of the drugs are absorbed. When these drugs are given orally, a longer duration of action is achieved, but systemic side effects such as tachycardia, dysrhythmias, and hyperglycemia are more frequently experienced; they are sometimes contraindicated for clients with dysrhythmias. With chronic use, tolerance may develop to the beta-agonist, and the duration of bronchodilator action will become shorter. Should this occur, the dose of beta-agonist may need to be increased, or a second drug such as a glucocorticoid may be added to the therapeutic regimen. Increased use of a beta-agonist over a period of hours or days is an indication that the client's condition is rapidly deteriorating, and medical attention should be sought immediately.

NURSING CONSIDERATIONS

The role of the nurse in beta-adrenergic agonist therapy for asthma involves careful monitoring of a client's condition and providing education as it relates to the prescribed drug treatment. Experiencing breathing difficulties can be distressing and greatly affect a client's quality of life. Controlling asthma is vital to a person's ability to perform normal activities of daily living. When beta-adrenergic agonists are used as bronchodilators, they help reduce acute respiratory distress. Some facilitate the expectoration of respiratory secretions.

Assess the client's vital signs, especially respiration and pulse rates, lung sounds, respiratory effort, skin color, and oxygen saturation level prior to administration of beta-adrenergic agonists. Assess for the presence and history of bradycardia, dysrhythmias, myocardial infarction (MI), hypothyroidism, decreased renal function, diabetes mellitus, glaucoma, benign prostatic hyperplasia, and tuberculosis. Beta-adrenergic agonists should not be used if the client has a history of dysrhythmia or MI. Use is limited in children younger than 6 years. Beta-adrenergic agonists are not recommended for use by women who are breast-feeding.

Drugs in this class may cause many undesirable side effects. Severe side effects include rebound bronchospasm, chest pain, or respiratory distress. Other common side effects include palpitations, tachycardia, dry mouth, nervousness, cough, or hyperglycemia.

Client Teaching. Client education as it relates to beta-adrenergic agonists should include the goals of therapy, the reasons for obtaining baseline data such as vital signs and the existence of underlying cardiac and renal disorders, and possible drug side effects. Include the following points when teaching clients about beta-adrenergic agonists:

- Limit the use of products that contain caffeine.
- Immediately report difficulty breathing, heart palpitations, tremors, vomiting, and nervousness, or vision changes.
- Follow the healthcare provider's instructions for the correct use of the inhaler, including the following:
  - Hold breath for 10 seconds after inhaling medication.
  - Wait 2 minutes before the second inhalation.
  - Rinse mouth after use.
- Be aware that saliva and sputum may be pink after inhaler use.
- Take medication as prescribed and do not increase, decrease, omit, or change intervals between doses.
- Report unsatisfactory relief of symptoms.

See "Nursing Process Focus: Clients Receiving Sympathomimetic Therapy," page 139 in Chapter 13 ∞, for the complete Nursing Process applied to caring for clients receiving beta-adrenergic agonists (sympathomimetics).

ANTICHOLINERGICS

Although beta-agonists are drugs of choice for treating acute asthma, anticholinergics are alternative bronchodilators. Only two anticholinergics are commonly used for pulmonary disease, and these agents are listed in Table 39.2.

Pr **PROTOTYPE DRUG** | Salmeterol *(Serevent)* | Bronchodilator/Beta₂-adrenergic Agonist

ACTIONS AND USES

Salmeterol acts by selectively binding to beta₂-adrenergic receptors in bronchial smooth muscle to cause bronchodilation. When taken 30 to 60 minutes prior to physical activity, it can prevent exercise-induced bronchospasm. Its 12-hour duration of action is longer than that of many other bronchodilators, thus making it best suited for the management of chronic asthma. Because salmeterol takes 15 to 25 minutes to act, it is not indicated for the termination of acute bronchospasm.

ADMINISTRATION ALERTS

- Proper use of the metered dose inhaler is important to effective delivery of drug. Observe and instruct client in proper use.
- Pregnancy category C.

PHARMACOKINETICS

Onset: 10–20 min

Peak: 2 h

Half-life: 3–4 h

Duration: Up to 12 h

ADVERSE EFFECTS

Serious adverse effects from salmeterol are uncommon. Some clients experience headaches, throat irritation, nervousness, and restlessness. Because of its potential to cause tachycardia, clients with heart disease should be monitored regularly.

Contraindications: The only contraindication to salmeterol use is hypersensitivity to the drug.

INTERACTIONS

Drug–Drug: Concurrent use with beta-blockers will inhibit the bronchodilation effect of salmeterol.

Lab Tests: May cause hypokalemia.

Herbal/Food: Unknown.

Treatment of Overdose: Overdose results in an exaggerated sympathetic activation, causing dysrhythmias, hypokalemia, and hyperglycemia. In severe cases, administration of a cardioselective beta-adrenergic antagonist may be necessary.

 See the Companion Website for a Nursing Process Focus specific to this drug.

Asthma Management in the Schools

Approximately 9 million children younger than age 18 have asthma. Researchers suggest that asthma accounts for 14 million missed school days each year and potential missed workdays for parents, making this disease condition one of the most common causes for school and work absenteeism. In a typical class of 30 children, two students suffer from asthmatic attacks each year while at school. Children cannot learn while experiencing wheezing, coughing, and shortness of breath.

Assisting schools to develop asthma management programs has become the focus of several federal agencies and dozens of professional and client advocacy groups. Many schools are adopting asthma management plans as part of a coordinated school health program. Schools with these programs have established "asthma-friendly" policies, such as allowing students to carry and administer quick-relief asthma medications. Additionally, the schools routinely maintain a copy of the student's asthma action plan from the caregiver or healthcare provider. The role of the school nurse is to review the plan, determine the student's specific needs, and be sure that the student has immediate access to quick-relief asthma medications. The optimal plan for each student is determined case by case, with input from the student, parents, healthcare provider, and school nurse. Typically, older students are permitted to carry the inhaler and self-administer as needed. The nurse often keeps a backup supply of the student's medication. For younger children, a supervised health assistant may be delegated to administer the medication.

cholinergic drugs would cause bronchodilation and have potential applications in the pharmacotherapy of asthma and other pulmonary diseases. For example, despite its many side effects, atropine was once widely used in asthma pharmacotherapy prior to the discovery of the inhaled beta-agonists.

Ipratropium (Atrovent) is the most common anticholinergic prescribed for the pharmacotherapy of chronic obstructive pulmonary disease (COPD) and asthma. It has a slower onset of action than most beta-agonists and produces a less intense bronchodilation. However, combining ipratropium with a beta-agonist produces a greater and more prolonged bronchodilation than using either drug separately. Taking advantage of this increased effect, Combivent is a mixture of ipratropium and albuterol in a single MDI canister. Tiotropium (Spiriva) is a newer anticholinergic related to ipratropium that has recently been approved for COPD.

The inhaled anticholinergics are safe medications. The wide range of anticholinergic side effects observed when drugs in this class are administered systemically rarely occur by inhalation. Dry mouth, gastrointestinal (GI) distress, headache, and anxiety are the most common client complaints.

39.6 Treating Chronic Asthma With Anticholinergics

Blocking the parasympathetic nervous system produces effects similar to those caused by activation of the sympathetic nervous system. It is predictable, then, that anti-

NURSING CONSIDERATIONS

The role of the nurse in anticholinergic therapy for asthma involves careful monitoring of a client's condition and providing education as it relates to the prescribed drug treatment. Drugs in this group are used for maintenance and not

---

Pr PROTOTYPE DRUG | Ipratropium Bromide *(Atrovent, Combivent)* | Bronchodilator/Anticholinergic

ACTIONS AND USES

Ipratropium is an anticholinergic (muscarinic antagonist) that causes bronchodilation by blocking cholinergic receptors in bronchial smooth muscle. It is administered via inhalation and can relieve acute bronchospasm within minutes after administration, although peak effects may take 1 to 2 hours. Effects may continue for up to 6 hours. Ipratropium is less effective than the beta$_2$-agonists but is sometimes combined with beta-agonists or glucocorticoids for their additive effects. It is also prescribed for chronic bronchitis and for the symptomatic relief of nasal congestion.

ADMINISTRATION ALERTS

- Proper use of the metered dose inhaler (MDI) is important to effective delivery of drug. Observe and instruct client in proper use.
- Wait 2–3 minutes between dosages.
- Avoid contact with eyes; otherwise, blurred vision may occur.
- Pregnancy category B.

PHARMACOKINETICS

Onset: 5–15 min

Peak: 1.5–2 h

Half-life: 1.5–2 h

Duration: 3–6 h

ADVERSE EFFECTS

Because it is not readily absorbed from the lungs, ipratropium produces few systemic side effects. Irritation of the upper respiratory tract may result in cough, drying of the nasal mucosa, or hoarseness. It produces a bitter taste, which may be relieved by rinsing the mouth after use.

Contraindications: Ipratropium is contraindicated in clients with hypersensitivity to soya lecithin or related food products such as soybean and peanut. Soya lecithin is used as a propellant in the inhaler.

INTERACTIONS

Drug–Drug: Use with other anticholinergics may lead to additive anticholinergic side effects.

Lab Tests: Unknown.

Herbal/Food: Unknown.

Treatment of Overdose: Overdose with ipratropium does not occur because very little of the drug is absorbed when given by aerosol.

 See the *Companion Website for a Nursing Process Focus specific to this drug.*

as first-response treatments in an acute respiratory episode. The effects of the drugs are delayed compared with those of the rapid-acting beta-adrenergic agonist drugs.

Assess respiratory rate before and after the first dose of a MDI, because the first dose may precipitate bronchospasm. Monitor vital signs, especially respiratory rate and pulse, respiratory effort, skin color, oxygen saturation level, and lung sounds. Assess for history of narrow-angle glaucoma, benign prostatic hyperplasia, renal disorders, and urinary bladder neck obstruction. Anticholinergics should be used with caution in clients with a history of any of these disorders and in elderly clients. Ipratropium is not recommended in children younger than 12 years, and tiotropium is not recommended for use in clients younger than 18 years. Anticholinergics are not recommended for women who are breast-feeding.

Anticholinergic drugs may cause undesirable side effects, although they are usually not severe. These include cough, sinusitis, upper respiratory tract infection, dry mouth, urine retention, nausea, vomiting, or constipation.

Client Teaching.   Client education as it relates to anticholinergics should include the goals of therapy, the reasons for obtaining baseline data such as vital signs and the existence of underlying bladder or renal disorders, and possible drug side effects. Include the following points when teaching clients about anticholinergics:

- Do not use this medication to terminate an acute asthma attack.
- Wait 5 minutes between using this and any other inhaled medication.
- Do not let medication contact eyes.
- Rinse mouth after inhaling medication to eliminate bitter taste.
- Correctly use inhaler.
- Report changes in urinary pattern, especially elderly clients.
- Report a change in color or amount of sputum.
- Report unsatisfactory relief of symptoms.

The complete Nursing Process applied to clients receiving anticholinergics is presented in "Nursing Process Focus: Clients Receiving Anticholinergic Therapy," on page 148 in Chapter 13 ∞.

For additional nursing considerations, please refer to "Nursing Process Focus: Clients Receiving Bronchodilator Therapy," on page 602.

METHYLXANTHINES

The methylxanthines are older, established drugs. They are alternative bronchodilators, prescribed for persistent, chronic asthma. These agents are shown in Table 39.2.

39.7 Treating Chronic Asthma With Methylxanthines

The **methylxanthines** comprise a group of bronchodilators chemically related to caffeine. Theophylline (Theo-Dur, others) and aminophylline (Somophyllin) were considered

drugs of choice for asthma 20 years ago. Theophylline, however, has a very narrow margin of safety and interacts with numerous other drugs. In addition, side effects such as nausea, vomiting, and CNS stimulation are relatively common, and dysrhythmias may be observed at high doses. Like caffeine, methylxanthines can cause nervousness and insomnia.

Methylxanthines are administered by the PO or IV routes, rather than by inhalation. Having been largely replaced by safer and more effective drugs, theophylline is currently used primarily for the long-term oral prophylaxis of asthma that is unresponsive to beta-agonists or inhaled glucocorticoids.

NURSING CONSIDERATIONS

The role of the nurse in methylxanthine therapy for asthma involves careful monitoring of a client's condition and providing education as it relates to the prescribed drug treatment. Methylxanthine use is limited because of CNS stimulation and the availability of other drugs that act more selectively on the respiratory system. The actions of the methylxanthines on the cardiovascular system are not as great as those of caffeine, but they do affect cardiac function.

Assess the client's vital signs, especially respiration and pulse rates, cardiac rhythm, lung sounds, respiratory effort, skin color, and oxygen saturation level prior to administration of methylxanthines. Assess for a history of coronary artery disease, angina pectoris, severe renal or liver disorders, peptic ulcer, benign prostatic hyperplasia, and diabetes mellitus. Methylxanthine use in clients with coronary artery disease or angina pectoris is contraindicated. Use is cautioned in elderly clients and children and not recommended in women who are breast-feeding.

Drugs in this class may cause many undesirable side effects. Severe adverse effects may include drug-induced seizures, circulatory failure, and respiratory arrest. Other common side effects may include tachycardia, irritability, restlessness, insomnia, dizziness, headache, palpitations, vomiting, and abdominal pain.

Client Teaching.   Client education as it relates to methylxanthines should include the goals of therapy, the reasons for obtaining baseline data such as vital signs and the existence of underlying cardiac or renal disorders, and possible drug side effects. Include the following points when teaching clients about methylxanthines:

- Limit the use of products that contain caffeine.
- Report early signs of toxicity, including anorexia, nausea, vomiting, dizziness, restlessness, hypotension, or seizures.
- Take medication as prescribed, and do not increase, decrease, omit, or change intervals between doses.
- Limit cigarette smoking because smoking reduces the therapeutic response from methylxanthine.
- Encourage fluid intake, if not restricted.

TABLE 39.3   Anti-inflammatory Drugs for Asthma

Drug	Route and Adult Dose (max dose where indicated)	Adverse Effects
INHALED GLUCOCORTICOIDS*		
beclomethasone (Beclovent, Vanceril, others)	MDI; 1–2 inhalations tid–qid (max: 20 inhalations/day)	*Hoarseness, dry mouth, cough, sore throat*
budesonide (Pulmicort Turbuhaler)	DPI; 1–2 inhalations (200 mcg/inhalation) qid (max: 800 mcg/day)	<u>Oropharyngeal candidiasis, hypercorticism, hypersensitivity reactions</u>
flunisolide (AeroBid)	MDI; 2–3 inhalations bid–tid (max: 12 inhalations/day)	
fluticasone (Flonase, Flovent) (see page 586 for the Prototype Drug box ∞)	MDI (44 mcg); 2 inhalations bid (max: 10 inhalations/day)	
triamcinolone (Azmacort)	MDI; 2 inhalations tid–qid (max: 16 inhalations/day)	
MAST CELL STABILIZERS		
cromolyn (Intal)	MDI; 1 inhalation qid	*Nausea, sneezing, nasal stinging, throat irritation, unpleasant taste*
nedocromil sodium (Tilade)	MDI; 2 inhalations qid	<u>Anaphylaxis, angioedema, bronchospasm</u>
LEUKOTRIENE MODIFIERS		
montelukast (Singulair)	PO; 10 mg/day in evening	*Headache, nausea, diarrhea*
zafirlukast (Accolate)	PO; 20 mg bid 1 h before or 2 h after meals	<u>No serious adverse effects</u>
zileuton (Zyflo)	PO; 600 mg qid	

*For doses of systemic glucocorticoids, refer to Chapter 43 ∞.
Italics indicate common adverse effects; <u>underlining</u> indicates serious adverse effects.

- Do not take any OTC cold medications without notifying your healthcare provider.
- Keep all scheduled appointments and laboratory visits for testing.
- Report unsatisfactory relief of symptoms.

GLUCOCORTICOIDS

Inhaled glucocorticoids are used for the long-term prevention of asthmatic attacks. Oral glucocorticoids may be used for the short-term management of acute severe asthma. The glucocorticoids are listed in Table 39.3.

39.8 Prophylaxis of Asthma With Glucocorticoids

Glucocorticoids are the most potent natural anti-inflammatory substances known. Because asthma has a major inflammatory component, it should not be surprising that drugs in this class play a major role in the management of this disorder. Glucocorticoids dampen the activation of inflammatory cells and increase the production of anti-inflammatory mediators. Mucus production and edema is diminished, thus reducing airway obstruction. Although glucocorticoids are not bronchodilators, they sensitize the bronchial smooth muscle to be more responsive to beta-agonist stimulation. In addition, they reduce the bronchial hyperresponsiveness to allergens that is responsible for triggering some asthma attacks. In the pharmacotherapy of asthma, glucocorticoids may be given systemically or by inhalation.

Inhaled glucocorticoids are the preferred therapy for *preventing* asthma attacks. When inhaled on a daily schedule, glucocorticoids suppress inflammation without producing major side effects. Although symptoms will improve in the first 1 to 2 weeks of therapy, 4 to 8 weeks may be required for maximum benefit. For clients with persistent asthma, a long-acting beta$_2$-adrenergic agonist may be prescribed along with the inhaled glucocorticoid to obtain an additive effect. Clients should be informed that inhaled glucocorticoids must be taken daily to produce their therapeutic effect and that these drugs are not effective at terminating acute asthmatic episodes in progress. Most clients with asthma carry an inhaler containing a rapid-acting beta-agonist to terminate acute attacks if they occur.

For severe, unstable asthma that is unresponsive to other treatments, systemic glucocorticoids such as oral prednisone may be prescribed. Treatment time is limited to the shortest length possible, usually 5 to 7 days. At the end of the brief treatment period, clients are switched to inhaled glucocorticoids for long-term management.

Inhaled glucocorticoids are absorbed into the circulation so slowly that systemic adverse effects are rarely observed. Local side effects include hoarseness and oropharyngeal candidiasis. If taken for longer than 10 days, *systemic* glucocorticoids can produce significant adverse effects, including adrenal gland atrophy, peptic ulcers, osteoporosis, and hyperglycemia. Because asthma most commonly occurs in children, growth retardation is a concern with the use of these drugs. Because these effects are all dose and time dependent, they can be avoided by limiting systemic therapy to less than 10 days. Other uses and adverse effects of glucocorticoids are presented in Chapters 33 and 43 ∞.

NURSING PROCESS FOCUS Clients Receiving Bronchodilator Therapy

Assessment	Potential Nursing Diagnoses
Prior to administration: ■ Obtain a complete health history including allergies, drug history, possible drug reactions, and use of complementary and herbal remedies. ■ Assess for symptoms related to respiratory deficiency such as dyspnea, orthopnea, cyanosis, nasal flaring, wheezing, and weakness. ■ Obtain vital signs. ■ Auscultate bilateral breath sounds for air movement and adventitious sounds (rales, rhonchi, wheezes). ■ Assess pulmonary function with pulse oximeter, peak expiratory flow meter, and/or arterial blood gases to establish baseline levels.	■ Gas Exchange, Impaired, related to bronchial constriction ■ Tissue Perfusion, Ineffective, related to adverse effects of drugs ■ Knowledge, Deficient, related to drug therapy ■ Anxiety, related to difficulty in breathing ■ Sleep Pattern, Disturbed, related to side effects of drugs ■ Activity Intolerance, related to ineffective drug therapy

Planning: Client Goals and Expected Outcomes

The client will:
■ Exhibit adequate oxygenation as evidenced by improved lung sounds and pulmonary function values.
■ Report a reduction in subjective symptoms of respiratory deficiency.
■ Demonstrate an understanding of the drug's action by accurately describing drug side effects and precautions.
■ Report at least 6 hours of uninterrupted sleep.

Implementation

Interventions and (Rationales)	Client Education/Discharge Planning
■ Monitor vital signs including pulse, blood pressure, and respiratory rate. (Baseline data is needed to monitor therapy.)	Instruct client to: ■ Use medication as directed even if asymptomatic. ■ Report difficulty with breathing.
■ Monitor pulmonary function with pulse oximeter, peak expiratory flow meter, and/or arterial blood gases. (Monitoring is necessary to assess drug effectiveness.)	■ Instruct client to report symptoms of deteriorating respiratory status such as increased dyspnea, breathlessness with speech, increased anxiety, and/or orthopnea.
■ Monitor the client's ability to use inhaler. (Proper use ensures correct dosage.)	Instruct client: ■ In proper use of metered dose inhaler. ■ To strictly use the medication as prescribed; do not "double up" on doses. ■ To rinse mouth thoroughly following use.
■ Observe for side effects specific to the medication used. (Dosage or medication changes may be needed.)	■ Instruct client to report specific drug side effects.
■ Maintain environment free of respiratory contaminants such as dust, dry air, flowers, and smoke. (These substances may exacerbate bronchial constriction.)	Instruct client to: ■ Avoid respiratory irritants. ■ Maintain "clean air environment." ■ Stop smoking and avoid secondhand smoke, if applicable.
■ Maintain dietary intake that is adequate in essential nutrients and vitamins, and ensure adequate hydration (3–4 L/day). (Dyspnea interferes with proper nutrition. Adequate hydration liquefies pulmonary secretions.)	Instruct client to: ■ Maintain nutrition with foods high in essential nutrients such as protein and carbohydrates. ■ Consume small frequent meals to prevent fatigue. ■ Consume 3–4 L of fluid per day if not contraindicated. ■ Avoid caffeine, because this increases CNS irritability.
■ Provide emotional and psychosocial support during periods of shortness of breath. (This may decrease anxiety, ease breathing effort, and improve gas exchange.)	■ Instruct client in relaxation techniques and controlled breathing techniques.
■ Monitor client compliance with pharmacotherapy. (Maintaining therapeutic drug levels is essential to effective therapy.)	■ Inform client of the importance of ongoing medication compliance and follow-up.

NURSING PROCESS FOCUS Clients Receiving Bronchodilator Therapy *(Continued)*

Evaluation of Outcome Criteria

Evaluate the effectiveness of drug therapy by confirming that client goals and expected outcomes have been met (see "Planning").

- The client's breath sounds and pulmonary function values demonstrate adequate oxygenation.
- The client reports a decrease in respiratory deficiency symptoms.
- The client demonstrates an understanding of the drug's actions by accurately describing drug side effects and precautions.
- The client reports having at least 6 hours of uninterrupted sleep.

∞ *See Table 39.2 for a list of drugs to which these nursing actions apply.*

NURSING CONSIDERATIONS

The role of the nurse in glucocorticoid therapy for asthma involves careful monitoring of a client's condition and providing education as it relates to the prescribed drug treatment. Assess the client for the presence and history of asthma, allergic rhinitis, hypertension, heart disease, blood clots, Cushing's syndrome, fungal infections, and diabetes mellitus. Monitor the client's vital signs, especially respiration and pulse rates, respiratory effort, lung sounds, skin color, oxygen saturation level, and body weight. Assess for signs and symptoms of infection. Steroid inhalers should be used cautiously in clients with hypertension, GI disease, congestive heart failure, and thromboembolic disease. Use of glucocorticoids is not recommended for pregnant or breast-feeding women.

Glucocorticoids may cause many undesirable side effects when given systemically. Severe adverse effects may include vertebral compression fractures, anaphylactoid reactions, and aggravation or masking of infections. Other common side effects may include sodium and fluid retention, nausea, acne, impaired wound healing, hyperglycemia, oral candidiasis, and Cushingoid features.

Because the primary purpose of inhaled glucocorticoids is to *prevent* respiratory distress, advise the client not to use this medication during an acute asthma attack. Additionally, alert the client to watch for signs and symptoms of simple infections, because glucocorticoids inhibit the inflammatory response and can mask the signs of infection. Advise the client to rinse the mouth after using steroid inhalers, because the drugs may promote fungal infections of the mouth and throat. Glucocorticoids also increase blood glucose levels and should be closely monitored in individuals with diabetes mellitus.

Client Teaching. Client education as it relates to glucocorticoids for asthma should include the goals of therapy, the reasons for obtaining baseline data such as vital signs and the existence of underlying cardiac and renal disorders, and possible drug side effects. Include the following points when teaching clients about glucocorticoids:

- Monitor temperature and blood pressure daily and report elevations.
- If diabetic, monitor blood glucose level closely and report unexplained or consistent elevations.
- Report tarry stools, edema, dizziness, or difficulty breathing.

- Do not use these medications to terminate acute asthma attacks.
- Monitor for signs of infection, such as poor wound healing, low-grade temperature, or general ill feeling.
- Rinse mouth after use.
- Monitor weight weekly and report unusual changes.
- Add potassium-rich foods to diet unless contraindicated, and monitor for hypokalemia.
- Take medication as prescribed and do not increase, decrease, omit, or change intervals between doses.
- Do not use aspirin without notifying your healthcare provider.
- Report increased incidence of asthma symptoms.

See "Nursing Process Focus: Clients Receiving Systemic Glucocorticoid Therapy," on page 676 in Chapter 43 ∞, for the complete Nursing Process applied to caring for clients receiving glucocorticoids.

LEUKOTRIENE MODIFIERS

The leukotriene modifiers are newer drugs, approved in the 1990s, used to reduce inflammation and ease bronchoconstriction. They modify the action of leukotrienes, which are mediators of the inflammatory response in asthmatic clients. These drugs are listed in Table 39.3.

39.9 Prophylaxis of Asthma With Leukotriene Modifiers

Leukotrienes are mediators of the immune response that are involved in allergic and asthmatic reactions. Although the prefix *leuko*-implies white blood cells, these mediators are synthesized by mast cells, as well as neutrophils, basophils, and eosinophils. When released in the airway, they promote edema, inflammation, and bronchoconstriction.

There are currently three drugs that modify leukotriene function. Zileuton (Zyflo) acts by blocking lipoxygenase, the enzyme that synthesizes leukotrienes. The remaining two agents in this class, zafirlukast (Accolate) and montelukast (Singulair), act by blocking leukotriene receptors. These drugs reduce inflammation. They are not considered bronchodilators like the beta$_2$-agonists, although they do reduce bronchoconstriction indirectly.

Pr PROTOTYPE DRUG | Beclomethasone *(Beclovent, Beconase, others)* | Inhaled Glucocorticoid

ACTIONS AND USES

Beclomethasone is a glucocorticoid available through aerosol inhalation (MDI) for asthma or as a nasal spray for allergic rhinitis. For asthma, two inhalations, two to three times per day, usually provide adequate prophylaxis. Beclomethasone acts by reducing inflammation, thus decreasing the frequency of asthma attacks. It is not a bronchodilator and should not be used to terminate asthma attacks in progress.

ADMINISTRATION ALERTS

- Do not use if the client is experiencing an acute asthma attack.
- Oral inhalation products and nasal spray products are not to be used interchangeably.
- Pregnancy category C.

PHARMACOKINETICS

Onset: Unknown

Peak: Unknown

Half-life: 15 h

Duration: Unknown

ADVERSE EFFECTS

Inhaled beclomethasone produces few systemic side effects. Because small amounts may be swallowed with each dose, the client should be observed for signs of glucocorticoid toxicity (hypercorticism) when taking the drug for prolonged periods. Local effects may include hoarseness.

As with all glucocorticoids, the anti-inflammatory properties of beclomethasone can mask signs of infections, and the drug is contraindicated if active infection is present. A large percentage of clients taking beclomethasone on a long-term basis will develop oropharyngeal candidiasis, a fungal infection in the throat, owing to the constant deposits of drug in the oral cavity.

Contraindications: The only contraindication to using beclomethasone is hypersensitivity to the drug.

INTERACTIONS

Drug–Drug: Unknown.

Lab Tests: Unknown.

Herbal/Food: Unknown.

Treatment of Overdose: Overdose does not occur when drug is given by the inhalation route.

See the Companion Website for a Nursing Process Focus specific to this drug.

The leukotriene modifiers are oral medications approved for the prophylaxis of chronic asthma. Because zileuton is taken four times a day, it is less convenient than montelukast or zafirlukast, which are taken every 12 hours. Zileuton has a more rapid onset of action (2 hours) than the other two leukotriene modifiers, which take as long as 1 week to produce optimum therapeutic benefit. Because of their delayed onset, leukotriene modifiers are ineffective in terminating acute asthma attacks. The current role of leukotriene modifiers in the management of asthma is for persistent asthma that cannot be controlled with other agents.

Few serious adverse effects are associated with the leukotriene modifiers. Headache, cough, nasal congestion, or GI upset may occur. Clients older than age 65 have been found to experience an increased frequency of infections when taking leukotriene modifiers. These agents may be contraindicated in clients with significant hepatic dysfunction or in chronic alcoholics, because they are extensively metabolized by the liver.

NURSING CONSIDERATIONS

The role of the nurse in leukotriene therapy for asthma involves careful monitoring of a client's condition and providing education as it relates to the prescribed drug treatment. Assess the client for the presence and history of asthma. Monitor vital signs, especially respiration and pulse rates, respiratory effort, lung sounds, skin color, and oxygen saturation level. Monitor CBC and periodic liver function tests. Closely monitor prothrombin time (PT) and international normalized ratio (INR) in clients concurrently taking warfarin (Coumadin). Closely monitor phenytoin level with

concurrent phenytoin therapy; reduce theophylline dose and closely monitor levels (zileuton) if client is using this therapy concurrently. Assess for signs and symptoms of infection, especially in clients older than 65 years. Closely monitor heart rate and blood pressure in clients concurrently taking propranolol (Inderal). Monitor effectiveness of montelukast in clients taking phenobarbital concurrently.

Because of the delayed onset of leukotriene modifiers, advise clients not to use them during an acute asthma attack. Additionally, alert clients to watch for signs and symptoms of liver toxicity and flulike symptoms, because these drugs are metabolized in the liver.

Lifespan Considerations. Leukotriene modifiers should be used cautiously in older adults, because they may increase the risk of infection. They should not be used in clients who abuse alcohol or in pregnant women (pregnancy category B). Safety in children younger than 2 years (zirflukast) is not established; montelukast should not be used in children younger than 1 year.

Client Teaching. Client education as it relates to leukotriene therapy for asthma should include the goals of therapy, the reasons for obtaining baseline data such as vital signs and the existence of underlying liver disorders, and possible drug side effects. Include the following points when teaching clients about leukotriene modifiers:

- Take drug as prescribed, even during symptom-free periods.
- Do not use these medications to terminate acute asthma attacks.
- Immediately report nausea, fatigue, lethargy, itching, abdominal pain, dark-colored urine, and flulike symptoms.

Pr PROTYPE DRUG | Zafirlukast *(Accolate)* | Leukotriene Modifier

ACTIONS AND USES

Zafirlukast is used for the prophylaxis of persistent, chronic asthma. It prevents airway edema and inflammation by blocking leukotriene receptors in the airways. An advantage of the drug is that it is given by the oral route. Its relatively long onset of action makes it unsuitable for termination of acute bronchospasm.

ADMINISTRATION ALERTS

- Do not use to terminate acute asthma attacks.
- Pregnancy category B.

PHARMACOKINETICS

Onset: 1 wk

Peak: 3 h

Half-life: 10 h

Duration: Unknown

ADVERSE EFFECTS

Zafirlukast produces few serious adverse effects. Headache is the most common complaint, and nausea and diarrhea are reported by some clients.

Contraindications: The only contraindication is hypersensitivity to the drug. Because a few rare cases of hepatic failure have been reported, clients with preexisting hepatic impairment should be treated with caution.

INTERACTIONS

Drug–Drug: Use with warfarin may increase prothrombin time. Erythromycin may decrease serum levels of zafirlukast.

Lab Tests: May increase serum ALT values.

Herbal/Food: Food can reduce the bioavailability; thus, the drug should be taken on an empty stomach.

Treatment of Overdose: There is no specific treatment for overdose.

 See the Companion Website for a Nursing Process Focus specific to this drug.

- Keep all scheduled appointments and laboratory visits for testing.
- Report unsatisfactory relief of symptoms.
- Do not breast-feed while taking these drugs.

MAST CELL STABILIZERS

Two mast cell stabilizers serve limited, though important, roles in the prophylaxis of asthma. These drugs act by inhibiting the release of histamine from mast cells, and are listed in Table 39.3.

39.10 Prophylaxis of Asthma With Mast Cell Stabilizers

Cromolyn (Intal) and nedocromil (Tilade) are classified as mast cell stabilizers because their action serves to inhibit mast cells from releasing histamine and other chemical mediators of inflammation. By reducing inflammation, they are able to prevent asthma attacks. As with the glucocorticoids, these agents should be taken on a daily basis because they are not effective for terminating acute attacks. Maximum therapeutic benefit may take several weeks. Both cromolyn and

nedocromil are pregnancy category B and exhibit no serious toxicity. The mast cell stabilizers are less effective in preventing chronic asthma than the inhaled glucocorticoids.

Cromolyn (Intal) was the first mast stabilizer discovered. The drug is administered via an MDI or a nebulizer, and an intranasal form (Nasalcrom) is used in the treatment of seasonal allergic rhinitis (Chapter 38 ∞). Side effects include stinging or burning of the nasal mucosa, irritation of the throat, and nasal congestion. Although not common, bronchospasm and anaphylaxis have been reported. Because of its short half-life (80 minutes), cromolyn must be inhaled four to six times per day.

Nedocromil (Tilade) is a newer mast cell stabilizer that has actions and uses similar to those of cromolyn. Administered with an MDI, the drug produces side effects similar to those of cromolyn, although the longer half-life of nedocromil allows less frequent dosing. Clients often experience a bitter, unpleasant taste, which is a common cause for discontinuation of therapy.

CHRONIC OBSTRUCTIVE PULMONARY DISEASE

Chronic obstructive pulmonary disease (COPD) is a general term used to describe several pulmonary conditions characterized by cough, mucus production, and impaired gas exchange. Drugs may be used to bring symptomatic relief, but they do not cure the disorders.

39.11 Pharmacotherapy of COPD

COPD is a major cause of death and disability. The three specific COPD conditions are asthma, chronic bronchitis, and emphysema. Chronic bronchitis and emphysema are

---

HOME & COMMUNITY CONSIDERATIONS

Helping Clients Manage Asthma

One noninvasive, inexpensive, and easy-to-use tool that can assist a client with managing asthma is the peak-flow meter. The meter measures lung capacity and gives a reading. The result can then be categorized on a chart to determine if the client is having any changes, even early breathing changes. This will allow the client to select which level of treatment, if any, may be needed prior to visiting the healthcare provider. It can give an early warning and possibly help the client avoid an acute attack with early intervention. The categories can be set up with the healthcare provider and be individualized for the client.

NATURAL THERAPIES

Fish Oil for COPD

The American Heart Association now recommends a diet that includes omega-3 fatty acids for heart disease prevention. New research shows that the omega-3 fatty acids may have similar benefits for COPD clients. Currently, no medication is able to stop the progressive inflammation that characterizes COPD. The anti-inflammatory effects of omega-3 fatty acids are well documented. Recent research showed a significant decrease in pulmonary inflammation in COPD clients when their diets were supplemented with omega-3 fatty acids (Matsuyama et al., 2005). Fish oil is the best source of omega-3 fatty acids, although they can also be obtained from flax seeds and walnuts. There are many fish oil supplements on the market today that have been molecularly distilled to remove any heavy metals (including mercury), making them safe from contamination that is now present in so many fish.

Interactions may occur between fish oil supplements and aspirin and other NSAIDs. Although rare, such interactions may be manifested by increased susceptibility to bruising, nosebleeds, hemoptysis, hematuria, and blood in the stool.

strongly associated with smoking tobacco products (cigarette smoking accounts for 85% to 90% of all cases of nonasthmatic COPD) and, secondarily, breathing air pollutants. In **chronic bronchitis,** excess mucus is produced in the lower respiratory tract owing to the inflammation and irritation from cigarette smoke or pollutants. The airway becomes partially obstructed with mucus, thus resulting in the classic signs of dyspnea and coughing. An early sign of bronchitis is often a productive cough on awakening. Gas exchange may be impaired; thus wheezing and decreased exercise tolerance are additional clinical signs. Microbes thrive in the mucus-rich environment, and pulmonary infections are common. Because most clients with COPD are lifelong tobacco users, they often have serious comorbid cardiovascular conditions such as heart failure and hypertension.

COPD is progressive, with the terminal stage being **emphysema.** After years of chronic inflammation, the bronchioles lose their elasticity, and the alveoli dilate to maximum size to allow more air into the lungs. The client suffers extreme dyspnea from even the slightest physical activity. The clinical distinction between chronic bronchitis and emphysema is sometimes unclear, because clients may exhibit symptoms of both conditions concurrently.

The goals of pharmacotherapy of COPD are to relieve symptoms and avoid complications of the condition. Various classes of drugs are used to treat infections, control cough, and relieve bronchospasm. Most clients receive bronchodilators such as ipratropium (Atrovent), beta2-agonists, or inhaled glucocorticoids. Both short-acting and long-acting bronchodilators are prescribed. Mucolytics and expectorants are sometimes used to reduce the viscosity of the bronchial mucus and to aid in its removal. Long-term oxygen therapy assists breathing and has been shown to decrease mortality in clients with advanced COPD. Antibiotics may be prescribed for clients who experience multiple bouts of pulmonary infections.

Clients with COPD should not receive drugs that have beta-adrenergic antagonist activity or otherwise cause bronchoconstriction. Respiratory depressants such as opioids and barbiturates should be avoided. It is important to note that none of the pharmacotherapies offer a cure for COPD; they only treat the symptoms of a progressively worsening disease. The most important teaching point for the nurse is to strongly encourage smoking cessation in these clients. Smoking cessation has been shown to slow the progression of COPD and to result in fewer respiratory symptoms.

SPECIAL CONSIDERATIONS

Respiratory Distress Syndrome

Respiratory distress syndrome (RDS) is a condition, primarily occurring in premature babies, in which the lungs are not producing surfactant. Surfactant forms a thin layer on the inner surface of the alveoli to raise the surface tension, thereby preventing the alveoli from collapsing during expiration. If birth occurs before the pneumocytes in the lung are mature enough to secrete surfactant, the alveoli collapse and RDS results.

Surfactant medications can be delivered to the newborn, either as prophylactic therapy or as rescue therapy after symptoms develop. The two natural surfactant agents used for RDS are calfactant (Infasurf) and beractant (Survanta). Calfactant is harvested from calf lungs, and beractant from mature cattle lungs. These drugs are administered intratracheally every 4 to 6 hours, until the client's condition improves. The only synthetic surfactant, colfosceril (Exosurf), is no longer used in the United States because it is less effective than the natural surfactants.

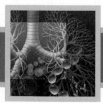

CHAPTER REVIEW

KEY CONCEPTS

The numbered key concepts provide a succinct summary of the important points from the corresponding numbered section within the chapter. If any of these points are not clear, refer to the numbered section within the chapter for review.

39.1 The physiology of the respiratory system involves two main processes. Ventilation moves air into and out of the lungs, and perfusion allows for gas exchange across capillaries.

39.2 Bronchioles are lined with smooth muscle that controls the amount of air entering the lungs. Dilation and constriction of the airways are controlled by the autonomic nervous system.

39.3 Inhalation is a common route of administration for pulmonary drugs because it delivers drugs directly to the sites of action. Nebulizers, MDIs, and DPIs are devices used for aerosol therapies.

39.4 Asthma is a chronic disease that has both inflammatory and bronchospasm components. Drugs are used to prevent asthmatic attacks and to terminate an attack in progress.

39.5 Beta-adrenergic agonists are the most effective drugs for relieving acute bronchospasm. These agents act by activating beta$_2$-receptors in bronchial smooth muscle to cause bronchodilation.

39.6 The anticholinergic ipratropium is a bronchodilator occasionally used as an alternative to the beta-agonists in asthma therapy.

39.7 Methylxanthines such as theophylline were once the mainstay of chronic asthma pharmacotherapy. They are less effective and produce more side effects than the beta-agonists.

39.8 Inhaled glucocorticoids are often drugs of choice for the long-term prophylaxis of asthma. Oral glucocorticoids are used for the short-term therapy of severe, acute asthma.

39.9 The leukotriene modifiers, primarily used for asthma prophylaxis, act by reducing the inflammatory component of asthma.

39.10 Mast cell stabilizers are safe drugs for the prophylaxis of asthma. They are less effective than the inhaled glucocorticoids and are ineffective at relieving acute bronchospasm.

39.11 Chronic obstructive pulmonary disease (COPD) is a progressive disorder treated with multiple pulmonary drugs. Bronchodilators, expectorants, mucolytics, antibiotics, and oxygen may offer symptomatic relief.

NCLEX-RN® REVIEW QUESTIONS

1 The client receives treatment for a respiratory condition through aerosol therapy. The nurse explains that the major advantage of this type if therapy is that:

1. It has no systemic side effects.
2. It delivers the medication to the site of action.
3. It requires no skill to use it.
4. It is safe for all clients.

2 The client is using a beta-adrenergic agonist for treatment of asthma. The nurse teaches that the action of this drug is:

1. Reducing mucus production.
2. Relaxing bronchiole smooth muscle, thereby causing bronchodilation.
3. Liquefying mucus.
4. Reducing cough.

3 Client teaching for clients on long-term therapy with beta-adrenergic agonists for treatment of asthma should include:

1. Discontinuing the drug if the heart rate increases.
2. Monitoring intake and output.
3. Reducing the dosage of the drug if insomnia occurs.
4. Notifying the physician if the drug no longer seems effective.

4 A 35-year-old woman is prescribed ipratropium (Atrovent) for the treatment of asthma. Appropriate nursing intervention includes:

1. Teaching the client to avoid caffeine in the diet.
2. Assessing for an enlarged liver.
3. Teaching the client to report inability to urinate.
4. Monitoring for development of diarrhea.

5 Nursing assessment for a client on long-term oral glucocorticoids would include (select all that apply):

1. Assessing liver function tests.
2. Assessing of cardiac dysrhythmias.
3. Assessing for signs of peptic ulcers.
4. Monitoring blood glucose for hyperglycemia.
5. Assessing for changes in level of consciousness.

CRITICAL THINKING QUESTIONS

1. A 72-year-old male client has recently been started on an ipratropium (Atrovent) inhaler. What teaching is important for the nurse to provide?

2. A 45-year-old client with chronic asthma is on glucocorticoids. What must be the nurse monitor when caring for this client?

3. A 7-year-old boy with a history of asthma goes to the health room at his elementary school and states he has increased shortness of breath and chest tightness. On assessment, the school nurse also notes scattered expiratory wheezes throughout his upper and middle lung fields and a decreased peak meter flow. Current therapeutic regimen for this child includes salmeterol (Serevent) 2 puffs q12h, montelukast (Singulair) 5 mg/day PO in the evening, triamcinolone (Azmacort) 2 puffs tid, and albuterol (Proventil) 2 puffs q4h PRN. After observing the child's technique in using the metered dose inhaler (MDI), the school nurse wishes to reinforce the child's education as it relates to the administration technique of his inhalants. What areas should be emphasized?

See Appendix D for answers and rationales for all activities.

EXPLORE
MediaLink

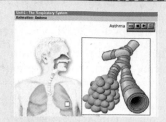

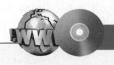

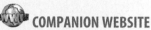

NCLEX-RN® review, case studies, and other interactive resources for this chapter can be found on the companion website at www.prenhall.com/adams. Click on "Chapter 39" to select the activities for this chapter. For animations, more NCLEX-RN® review questions, and an audio glossary, access the accompanying Prentice Hall Nursing MediaLink DVD-ROM in this textbook.

PRENTICE HALL NURSING MEDIALINK DVD-ROM

- **Animation**
  Mechanism in Action: Salmeterol (*Serevent*)
  Small-volume Nebulizer
  Metered Dose Inhaler (MDI)
  Dry Powder Inhaler (DPI)
- **Audio Glossary**
- **NCLEX-RN® Review**
- **Nursing in Action**
  Administering Medications by Inhaler

COMPANION WEBSITE

- **NCLEX-RN® Review**
- **Dosage Calculations**
- **Case Study:** Client with asthma
- **Care Plan:** Client with chronic pulmonary obstructive disease and benign prostatic hypertrophy treated with ipratropium

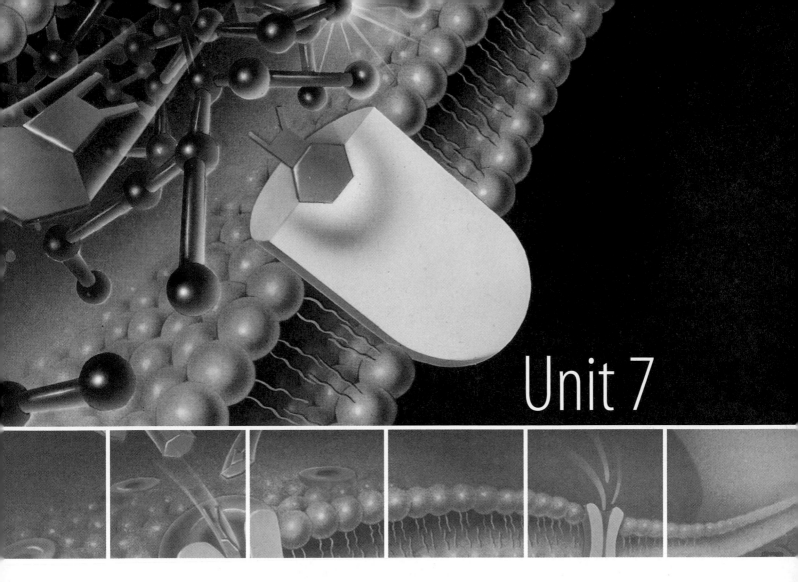

Unit 7

The Gastrointestinal System

CHAPTER 40   Drugs for Peptic Ulcer Disease
CHAPTER 41   Drugs for Bowel Disorders and Other Gastrointestinal Conditions
CHAPTER 42   Drugs for Nutritional Disorders

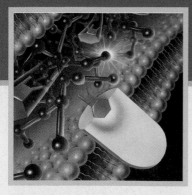

Drugs for Peptic Ulcer Disease

DRUGS AT A GLANCE

H₂-RECEPTOR ANTAGONISTS
- *ranitidine (Zantac)*

PROTON PUMP INHIBITORS
- *omeprazole (Prilosec)*

ANTACIDS
- *aluminum hydroxide (Amphojel, others)*

ANTIBIOTICS

OBJECTIVES

After reading this chapter, the student should be able to:

1. Describe major anatomical structures of the upper gastrointestinal tract.
2. Identify common causes, signs, and symptoms of peptic ulcer disease and gastroesophageal reflux disease.
3. Compare and contrast duodenal ulcers and gastric ulcers.
4. Describe treatment goals for the pharmacotherapy of gastroesophageal reflux disease.
5. Identify the classification of drugs used to treat peptic ulcer disease.
6. Explain the pharmacological strategies for eradicating *Helicobacter pylori*.
7. Describe the nurse's role in the pharmacological management of clients with peptic ulcer disease.
8. For each of the classes listed in Drugs at a Glance, know representative drugs, and explain their mechanism of drug action, describe primary actions, and identify important adverse effects.
9. Categorize drugs used in the treatment of peptic ulcer disease based on their classification and mechanism of action.
10. Use the Nursing Process to care for clients who are receiving drug therapy for peptic ulcer disease.

MediaLink 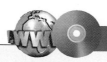 www.prenhall.com/adams

NCLEX-RN® review, case studies, and other interactive resources for this chapter can be found on the companion website at www.prenhall.com/adams. Click on "Chapter 40" to select the activities for this chapter. For animations, more NCLEX-RN® review questions, and an audio glossary, access the accompanying Prentice Hall Nursing MediaLink DVD-ROM in this textbook.

KEY TERMS

antiflatulent *page 619*

antacid *page 619*

chief cells *page 612*

esophageal reflux *page 611*

gastroesophageal reflux disease (GERD)
  page 613

H+, K+-ATPase *page 617*

H2-receptor antagonist *page 615*

Helicobacter pylori *page 613*

intrinsic factor *page 612*

mucosa layer *page 611*

parietal cells *page 612*

peptic ulcer *page 612*

peristalsis *page 611*

proton pump inhibitor *page 617*

Zollinger–Ellison syndrome *page 618*

Very little of the food we eat is directly available to body cells. Food must be broken down, absorbed, and chemically modified before it is in a form useful to cells. The digestive system performs these functions, and more. Some disorders of the digestive system are mechanical in nature, slowing or accelerating the transit of substances through the gastrointestinal tract. Others are metabolic, affecting the secretion of digestive enzymes and fluids, or the absorption of essential nutrients. Many signs and symptoms are nonspecific and may be caused by any number of different disorders. This chapter examines the pharmacotherapy of two common disorders of the upper digestive system: peptic ulcer disease (PUD) and gastroesophageal reflux disease (GERD).

40.1 Normal Digestive Processes

The digestive system consists of two basic anatomical divisions: the alimentary canal and the accessory organs. The alimentary canal, or gastrointestinal (GI) tract, is a long, continuous, hollow tube that extends from the mouth to the anus. The accessory organs of digestion include the salivary glands, liver, gallbladder, and pancreas. Major structures of the digestive system are illustrated in ● Figure 40.1.

The inner lining of the alimentary canal is the **mucosa layer,** which provides a surface area for the various acids, bases, mucus, and enzymes to break down food. In many parts of the alimentary canal, the mucosa is folded and contains deep grooves and pits. The small intestine is lined with tiny projections called *villi* and *microvilli,* which provide a huge surface area for the absorption of food and medications.

Substances are propelled along the GI tract by **peristalsis,** rhythmic contractions of layers of smooth muscle. The speed at which substances move through the GI tract is critical to the absorption of nutrients and water and for the removal of wastes. If peristalsis is too fast, nutrients and drugs will not have sufficient contact with the mucosa to be absorbed. In addition, the large intestine will not have enough time to absorb water, and diarrhea may result. Abnormally slow transit may result in constipation or even obstructions in the small or large intestine. Disorders of the lower digestive tract are discussed in Chapter 41 ∞.

To chemically break down ingested food, a large number of enzymes and other substances are required. Digestive enzymes are secreted by the salivary glands, stomach, small intestine, and pancreas. The liver makes bile, which is stored in the gallbladder, until needed for lipid digestion. Because these digestive substances are not common targets for drug therapy, their discussion in this chapter is limited, and the student should refer to anatomy and physiology texts for additional information.

40.2 Acid Production by the Stomach

Food passes from the esophagus to the stomach by traveling through the lower esophageal (cardiac) sphincter. This ring of smooth muscle usually prevents the stomach contents from moving backward, a condition known as **esophageal reflux.**

PHARMFACTS

Upper Gastrointestinal Tract Disorders

- Sixty to 70 million Americans are affected by a digestive disease.
- Approximately 10% of Americans will experience a peptic ulcer in their lifetime.
- More than 400,000 new cases of peptic ulcer disease are diagnosed each year.
- Peptic ulcers are responsible for about 40,000 surgeries annually.
- About 6,000 people die annually of peptic ulcer–related complications.
- Seven percent of Americans suffer from daily symptoms of GERD.

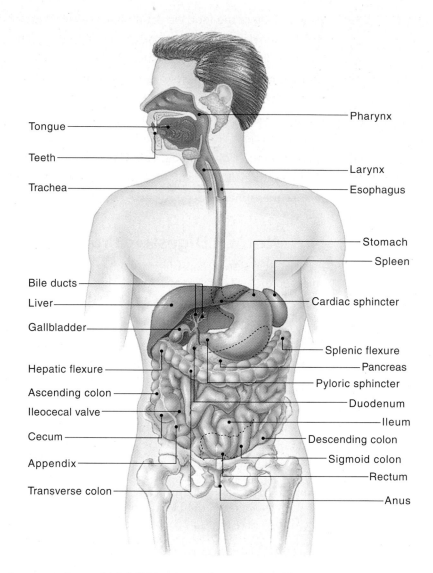

● Figure 40.1 The digestive system *Source: Mulvihill, Mary Lou; Zelman, Mark; Holdaway, Paul; Tompary, Elaine; Raymond, Jill, Human Diseases: A Systemic Approach, 6th edition, © 2006, p. 276. Reprinted by permission of Pearson Education, Inc., Upper Saddle River, NJ.*

A second ring of smooth muscle, the pyloric sphincter, is located at the entrance to the small intestine. This sphincter regulates the flow of substances leaving the stomach.

The stomach thoroughly mixes ingested food and secretes substances that promote the processes of chemical digestion. Gastric glands extending deep into the mucosa of the stomach contain several cell types critical to digestion and important to the pharmacotherapy of digestive disorders. **Chief cells** secrete pepsinogen, an inactive form of the enzyme pepsin that chemically breaks down proteins. **Parietal cells** secrete 1 to 3 L of hydrochloric acid each day. This strong acid helps break down food, activates pepsinogen, and kills microbes that may have been ingested. Parietal cells also secrete **intrinsic factor,** which is essential for the absorption of vitamin B_{12} (Chapter 42 ∞). Parietal cells are targets for the classes of antiulcer drugs that limit acid secretion.

The combined secretion of the chief and parietal cells, gastric juice, is the most acidic fluid in the body, having a pH of 1.5 to 3.5. A number of natural defenses protect the stomach mucosa against this extremely acidic fluid. Certain cells lining the surface of the stomach secrete a thick mucous layer and bicarbonate ion to neutralize the acid. These form such an effective protective layer that the pH at the mucosal surface is nearly neutral. Once they reach the duodenum, the stomach contents are further neutralized by bicarbonate from pancreatic and biliary secretions. These natural defenses are shown in ● Figure 40.2.

40.3 Pathogenesis of Peptic Ulcer Disease

An *ulcer* is an erosion of the mucosa layer of the GI tract, usually associated with acute inflammation. Although ulcers may occur in any portion of the alimentary canal, the duodenum is the most common site. The term **peptic ulcer** refers to a lesion located in either the stomach (gastric) or small intestine (duodenal). Peptic ulcer disease is associated with the following risk factors.

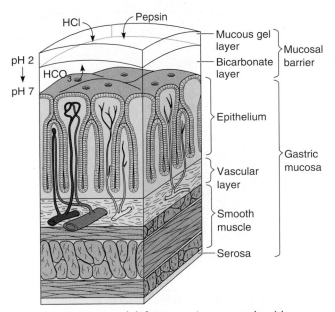

● **Figure 40.2** Natural defenses against stomach acid

- Close family history of PUD
- Blood group O
- Smoking tobacco
- Beverages and food containing caffeine
- Drugs, particularly glucocorticoids and nonsteroidal anti-inflammatory drugs (NSAIDs), including aspirin
- Excessive psychological stress
- Infection with *Helicobacter pylori*

The primary cause of PUD is infection by the gram-negative bacterium **Helicobacter pylori.** Approximately 50% of the population has *H. pylori* present in their stomach and proximal small intestine. In *noninfected* clients, the most common cause of PUD is drug therapy with NSAIDs. Secondary factors that *contribute* to the ulcer and its subsequent inflammation include secretion of excess gastric acid and hyposecretion of adequate mucous protection.

The characteristic symptom of *duodenal* ulcer is a gnawing or burning, upper abdominal pain that occurs 1 to 3 hours after a meal. The pain is worse when the stomach is empty and often disappears on ingestion of food. Nighttime pain, nausea, and vomiting are uncommon. If the erosion progresses deeper into the mucosa, bleeding occurs and may be evident as either bright red blood in vomit or black, tarry stools. Many duodenal ulcers heal spontaneously, although they frequently recur after months of remission. Long-term medical follow-up is usually not necessary.

Gastric ulcers are less common than the duodenal type and have different symptoms. Although relieved by food, pain may continue even after a meal. Loss of appetite, known as anorexia, as well as weight loss and vomiting are more common. Remissions may be infrequent or absent. Medical follow-up of gastric ulcers should continue for several years, because a small percentage of the erosions become cancerous. The most severe ulcers may penetrate the wall of the stomach and cause death. Whereas duodenal ulcers occur most frequently in the 30- to 50-year age group, gastric ulcers are more common over age 60.

Ulceration in the distal small intestine is known as *Crohn's disease,* and erosions in the large intestine are called *ulcerative colitis.* These diseases, together categorized as inflammatory bowel disease, are discussed in Chapter 41 ∞.

40.4 Pathogenesis of Gastroesophageal Reflux Disease

Gastroesophageal reflux disease (GERD) is a common condition in which the acidic contents of the stomach move upward into the esophagus. This causes an intense burning (heartburn) sometimes accompanied by belching. In severe cases, untreated GERD can lead to complications such as esophagitis, or esophageal ulcers or strictures. Although most often thought a disease of people older than age 40, GERD also occurs in a significant percentage of infants.

The cause of GERD is usually a weakening of the lower esophageal sphincter. The sphincter may no longer close tightly, allowing the contents of the stomach to move upward when the stomach contracts. GERD is associated with obesity, and losing weight may eliminate the symptoms. Other lifestyle changes that can improve GERD symptoms include elevating the head of the bed, avoiding fatty or acidic foods, eating smaller meals at least 3 hours before sleep, and eliminating tobacco and alcohol use.

Because clients often self-treat this disorder with OTC drugs, a good medication history may give clues to the presence of GERD. Many of the drugs prescribed for peptic ulcers are also used to treat GERD, with the primary goal being to reduce gastric acid secretion. Drug classes include antacids, H_2-receptor antagonists, and proton pump inhibitors. Because drugs provide only symptomatic relief, surgery may become necessary to eliminate the cause of GERD in clients with persistent disease.

40.5 Pharmacotherapy of Peptic Ulcer Disease

Before initiating pharmacotherapy, clients are usually advised to change lifestyle factors contributing to the severity of PUD or GERD. For example, eliminating tobacco and alcohol use and reducing stress often allow healing of the ulcer and cause it to go into remission. Avoiding certain foods and beverages can lessen the severity of symptoms.

The goals of PUD pharmacotherapy are to provide immediate relief from symptoms, promote healing of the ulcer, and prevent future recurrence of the disease. A wide variety of both prescription and OTC drugs are available. These drugs fall into four primary classes, plus one miscellaneous group. The mechanisms of action of the four major drug classes for PUD are shown in Pharmacotherapy Illustrated 40.1.

- H_2-receptor antagonists
- Proton pump inhibitors

PHARMACOTHERAPY ILLUSTRATED

40.1 Mechanisms of Action of Antiulcer Drugs

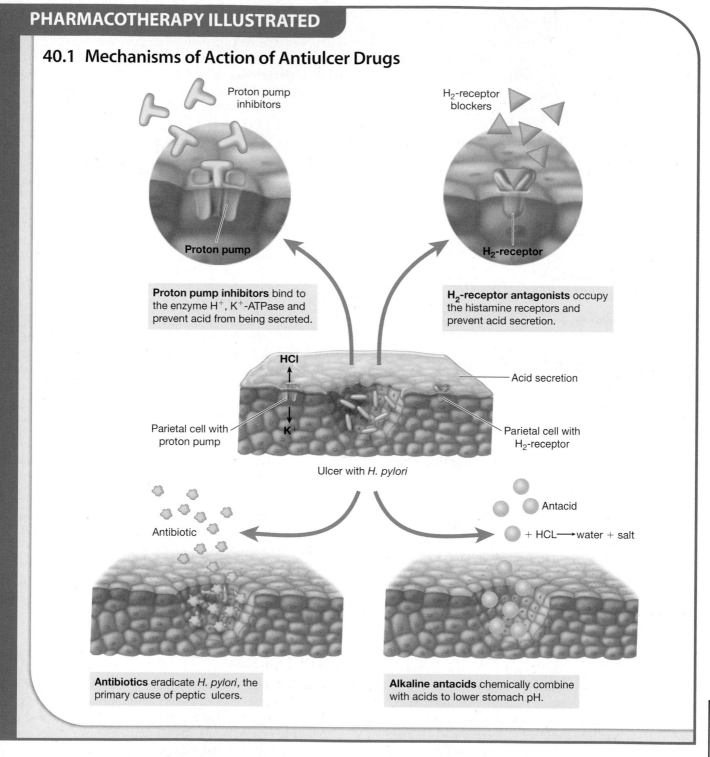

Proton pump inhibitors

H$_2$-receptor blockers

Proton pump

H$_2$-receptor

Proton pump inhibitors bind to the enzyme H$^+$, K$^+$-ATPase and prevent acid from being secreted.

H$_2$-receptor antagonists occupy the histamine receptors and prevent acid secretion.

HCl

Acid secretion

Parietal cell with proton pump

K$^+$

Parietal cell with H$_2$-receptor

Ulcer with *H. pylori*

Antibiotic

Antacid

+ HCL ⟶ water + salt

Antibiotics eradicate *H. pylori*, the primary cause of peptic ulcers.

Alkaline antacids chemically combine with acids to lower stomach pH.

- Antacids
- Antibiotics
- Miscellaneous drugs

For clients on NSAIDs, the initial approach to PUD is to switch the client to an alternative medication, such as acetaminophen or a selective COX-2 inhibitor. This is not always possible, because NSAIDs are drugs of choice for treating chronic arthritis and other disorders associated with pain and inflammation. If discontinuation of the NSAID is not possible, or if symptoms persist after the NSAID has been withdrawn, antiulcer medications are indicated.

For clients with *H. pylori* infection, eradication of the bacteria with antibiotics is the primary goal of pharmacotherapy (see Section 40.9). Treatment using only antiulcer drugs *without* eradicating *H. pylori* results in a very high recurrence rate of PUD.

TABLE 40.1 H$_2$-receptor Antagonists

Drug	Route and Adult Dose (max dose where indicated)	Adverse Effects
cimetidine (Tagamet)	PO; 300–400 mg 1 to 2 times/day or 800 mg at bedtime for active ulcers; 300 mg bid or 400 mg at bedtime for ulcer prophylaxis	*Diarrhea, constipation, headache, fatigue*
famotidine (Pepcid, Mylanta AP)	PO; 20 mg bid or 40 mg at bedtime for active ulcers; 20 mg at bedtime for ulcer prophylaxis	<u>Hepatitis, blood dyscrasias, anaphylaxis, dysrhythmias (nizatidine, cimetidine), confusion or psychoses (cimetidine)</u>
nizatidine (Axid)	PO; 300 mg at bedtime for active ulcers; 150 mg at bedtime for ulcer prophylaxis	
ⓟ ranitidine HCl (Zantac)	PO; 100–150 mg bid or 300 mg at bedtime for active ulcers; 150 mg at bedtime for ulcer prophylaxis	

Italics indicate common adverse effects; <u>underlining</u> indicates serious adverse effects.

H$_2$-RECEPTOR ANTAGONISTS

The discovery of the H$_2$-receptor antagonists in the 1970s marked a major breakthrough in the treatment of PUD. Since then, they have become available OTC and are often drugs of choice in the treatment of hyperacidity disorders of the GI tract. These agents are listed in Table 40.1.

40.6 Pharmacotherapy With H$_2$-receptor Antagonists

Histamine has two types of receptors: H$_1$ and H$_2$. Activation of H$_1$-receptors produces the classic symptoms of inflammation and allergy, whereas the H$_2$-receptors are responsible for increasing acid secretion in the stomach. Cimetidine (Tagamet), the first **H$_2$-receptor antagonist,** and other drugs in this class, are quite effective at suppressing the volume and acidity of parietal cell secretions. These drugs are used to treat the symptoms of both PUD and GERD, and several agents in this class are available OTC for the treatment of heartburn.

All drugs in this class have similar safety profiles: side effects are minor and rarely cause discontinuation of therapy. Clients taking high doses, or those with renal or hepatic disease may experience confusion, restlessness, hallucinations, or depression. Cimetidine is used less frequently than other H$_2$-receptor antagonists because of numerous drug–drug interactions (it inhibits hepatic drug-metabolizing enzymes) and because it must be taken up to four times a day. Antacids should not be taken at the same time as H$_2$-receptor antagonists, as the absorption will be diminished.

Ⓟ PROTOTYPE DRUG | Ranitidine HCl *(Zantac)* | H$_2$-receptor Antagonist

ACTIONS AND USES

Ranitidine acts by blocking H$_2$-receptors in the stomach to decrease acid production. It has a higher potency than cimetidine, which allows it to be administered once daily, usually at bedtime. Adequate healing of the ulcer takes approximately 4 to 8 weeks, although those at high risk for PUD may continue on drug maintenance for prolonged periods to prevent recurrence. Gastric ulcers heal more slowly than duodenal ulcers, and thus require longer therapy. IV and IM forms are available for the treatment of acute stress-induced bleeding ulcers. Tritec is a combination drug with ranitidine and bismuth citrate.

ADMINISTRATION ALERT

- Administer after meals and monitor liver function.
- Pregnancy category B.

PHARMACOKINETICS

Onset: Unknown

Peak: 2–3 h

Half-life: 2–3 h

Duration: 8–12 h

ADVERSE EFFECTS

Ranitidine does not cross the blood–brain barrier to any appreciable extent, so the confusion and CNS depression observed with cimetidine is not expected with ranitidine. Although rare, severe reductions in the number of red and white blood cells and platelets are possible; thus, periodic blood counts may be performed. High doses may result in impotence or loss of libido in men.

Contraindications: Contraindications include hypersensitivity to H$_2$-receptor antagonists, acute porphyria, and OTC administration in children less than 12 years of age.

INTERACTIONS

Drug–Drug: Ranitidine has fewer drug–drug interactions than cimetidine. Ranitidine may reduce the absorption of cefpodoxime, ketoconazole, and itraconazole. Smoking decreases the effectiveness of ranitidine.

Lab Tests: May increase values of serum creatinine, AST, ALT, LDH, alkaline phosphatase and bilirubin. May produce false positives for urine protein.

Herbal/Food: Unknown.

Treatment of Overdose: There is no specific treatment for overdose.

 See the Companion Website for a Nursing Process Focus specific to this drug.

MediaLink

Mechanism in Action: Ranitidine

NURSING PROCESS FOCUS Clients Receiving H₂-receptor Antagonist Therapy

Assessment	Potential Nursing Diagnoses
Prior to administration: ▪ Obtain a complete health history including allergies, drug history, and possible drug interactions. ▪ Assess client for signs of GI bleeding. ▪ Obtain vital signs. ▪ Assess level of consciousness. ▪ Obtain results of CBC, liver, and renal function tests.	▪ Falls, Risk for, related to adverse effect of drug ▪ Knowledge, Deficient, related to drug therapy ▪ Pain, Acute, related to gastric irritation from ineffective drug therapy ▪ Nutrition, Altered, Less than Body Requirements, related to adverse effects of drug

Planning: Client Goals and Expected Outcomes

The client will:
▪ Report episodes of drowsiness, dizziness.
▪ Report recurrence of abdominal pain or discomfort during drug therapy.
▪ Demonstrate an understanding of the drug's actions by accurately describing drug side effects and precautions.

Implementation

Interventions and (Rationales)	Client Education/Discharge Planning
▪ Monitor use of OTC drugs to avoid drug interactions, especially with cimetidine therapy. (Client should not use any OTC medications without consulting with healthcare provider.)	▪ Instruct client to consult with healthcare provider before taking other medications or herbal products.
▪ Monitor level of abdominal pain or discomfort to assess effectiveness of drug therapy. (Abdominal pain or discomfort should decrease with therapy.)	▪ Advise client that pain relief may not occur for several days after beginning therapy.
▪ Monitor client use of alcohol. (Alcohol can increase gastric irritation.)	▪ Instruct client to avoid alcohol use.
▪ Discuss possible drug interactions. (Antacids can decrease the effectiveness of other drugs taken concurrently.)	▪ Instruct client to take H₂-receptor antagonists and other medications at least 1 hour before antacids.
▪ Institute effective safety measures regarding falls. (Drugs may cause drowsiness or dizziness.)	▪ Instruct client to avoid driving or performing hazardous activities until drug effects are known.
▪ Explain need for lifestyle changes. (Smoking and certain foods increase gastric acid secretion.)	Encourage client to: ▪ Stop smoking; provide information on smoking cessation programs. ▪ Avoid foods that cause stomach discomfort.
▪ Observe client for signs of GI bleeding. (Ranitidine does not heal a peptic ulcer; it only decreases acid production; therefore, bleeding may occur from an ulcer.)	▪ Instruct client to immediately report episodes of blood in stool or vomitus or increase in abdominal discomfort.

Evaluation of Outcome Criteria

Evaluate the effectiveness of drug therapy by confirming that client goals and expected outcomes have been met (see "Planning").
▪ The client reports drowsiness and dizziness.
▪ The client reports a decrease in occurrence of abdominal pain or discomfort during drug therapy.
▪ The client demonstrates an understanding of the drug's actions by accurately describing drug side effects and precautions.

∞ *See Table 40.1 for a list of drugs to which these nursing actions apply.*

NURSING CONSIDERATIONS

The role of the nurse in H₂-receptor antagonist therapy for treatment of peptic ulcer disease involves careful monitoring of a client's condition and providing education as it relates to the prescribed drug treatment. Because some H₂-receptor blockers are available without prescription, assess the client's use of OTC formulations to avoid duplication of treatment. If using OTC formulations, clients should be advised to seek medical attention if symptoms persist or recur. Persistent epigastric pain or heartburn

may be symptoms of more serious disease that requires different medical treatment.

Intravenous preparations of H₂-receptor antagonists are occasionally utilized. Because dysrhythmias and hypotension have occurred with IV cimetidine, ranitidine (Zantac) or famotidine (Pepcid) are administered if the IV route is necessary.

Drugs in this class are usually well tolerated. CNS side effects such as dizziness, drowsiness, confusion, and headache are more likely to occur in elderly clients. Assess kidney and liver function. These drugs are mainly excreted

TABLE 40.2 Proton Pump Inhibitors

Drug	Route and Adult Dose (max dose where indicated)	Adverse Effects
esomeprazole (Nexium)	PO; 20–40 mg/day	*Headache, diarrhea, nausea, rash, dizziness*
lansoprazole (Prevacid)	PO; 15–60 mg/day	
omeprazole (Prilosec)	PO; 20–60 mg 1 to 2 times/day	<u>Serious adverse effects are rare</u>
pantoprazole (Protonix)	PO; 40 mg/day	
rabeprazole (Aciphex)	PO; 20 mg/day	

Italics indicate common adverse effects; <u>underlining</u> indicates serious adverse effects.

via the kidneys, and clients with diminished kidney function require smaller dosages and are more likely to experience adverse effects owing to the accumulation of the drug in the blood. These medications can cause hepatotoxicity, although rarely. Long-term use of H_2-receptor antagonists may lead to vitamin B_{12} deficiency because they decrease absorption of the vitamin. Iron supplements may be needed, as this mineral is best absorbed in an acidic environment. Evaluate the client's CBC for possible anemia during long-term use of these drugs. Safety during pregnancy and lactation for drugs in this class has not been established (pregnancy category B).

Client Teaching. Client education as it relates to H_2-receptor antagonists should include the goals of therapy; the reasons for obtaining baseline data such as vital signs, tests for cardiac and renal disorders, and the existence of underlying conditions such as pregnancy; and possible drug side effects. Include the following points when teaching clients about H_2-receptor antagonists.

- Keep all scheduled laboratory visits for liver and kidney function tests.
- Do not take other prescription drugs, OTC medications, herbal remedies, or vitamins or minerals without notifying your healthcare provider.
- Do not drink alcohol or smoke while taking this medication.
- Notify your healthcare provider if you are breast-feeding.

SPECIAL CONSIDERATIONS

H_2-receptors and Vitamin B_{12} in Older Adults

H_2-receptor blockers decrease the secretion of hydrochloric acid in the stomach. Unfortunately, gastric acid is essential for releasing vitamin B_{12} in food, which is bound in a protein matrix. By affecting stomach acidity, these drugs can affect the absorption of this essential vitamin.

H_2-receptor blockers are frequently prescribed for the elderly, who are more likely to have preexisting lower vitamin B_{12} reserves or even deficiencies. With aging, the ability to produce adequate amounts of hydrochloric acid, intrinsic factor, and digestive enzymes progressively diminishes. These losses can lead to lower absorption rates, depletion of reserves, and eventually B_{12} deficiency. The nurse must educate older adults taking these drugs as to the importance of including plenty of foods rich in vitamin B_{12} in their diets, including red meat, poultry, fish, and eggs.

- Immediately report fever or excessive bruising.
- Immediately report vomiting of blood or black-colored stools.

PROTON PUMP INHIBITORS

Proton pump inhibitors act by blocking the enzyme responsible for secreting hydrochloric acid in the stomach. They are widely used in the short-term therapy of PUD and GERD. These agents are listed in Table 40.2.

40.7 Pharmacotherapy With Proton Pump Inhibitors

Proton pump inhibitors reduce acid secretion in the stomach by binding irreversibly to the enzyme **H^+, K^+-ATPase**. In the parietal cells of the stomach, this enzyme acts as a pump to release acid (also called H^+, or protons) onto the surface of the GI mucosa. The proton pump inhibitors reduce acid secretion to a greater extent than the H_2-receptor antagonists and have a longer duration of action. All agents in this class have similar efficacy and side effects.

Several days of proton pump inhibitor therapy may be needed before clients gain relief from ulcer pain. Beneficial effects continue for 3 to 5 days after the drugs have been stopped. These drugs are used only for the short-term control of peptic ulcers and GERD: typical length of therapy is 4 weeks. Omeprazole and lansoprazole are used concurrently with antibiotics to eradicate *H. pylori*. The newer agents esomeprazole (Nexium) and pantoprazole (Protonix) offer the convenience of once-a-day dosing.

Side effects from proton pump inhibitors are uncommon. Headache, abdominal pain, diarrhea, nausea, and vomiting are the most commonly reported side effects.

NURSING CONSIDERATIONS

The role of the nurse in proton pump inhibitor therapy for PUD involves careful monitoring of a client's condition and providing education as it relates to prescribed drug treatment. Proton pump inhibitors are usually well tolerated for short-term use. With long-term use, liver function should be periodically monitored as well as serum gastrin, because oversecretion of gastrin occurs with constant acid suppression. Generally, proton pump inhibitors are not used during pregnancy and lactation; they range from

Pr PROTOTYPE DRUG | Omeprazole (Prilosec) | Proton Pump Inhibitor

ACTIONS AND USES

Omeprazole was the first proton pump inhibitor to be approved for PUD. It reduces acid secretion in the stomach by binding irreversibly to the enzyme H^+, K^+-ATPase. Although this agent can take 2 hours to reach therapeutic levels, its effects last up to 72 hours. It is used for the short-term, 4- to 8-week therapy of peptic ulcers and GERD. Most clients are symptom free after 2 weeks of therapy. It is used for longer periods in clients who have chronic hypersecretion of gastric acid, a condition known as **Zollinger–Ellison syndrome**. It is the most effective drug for this syndrome. Omeprazole is available only in oral form.

ADMINISTRATION ALERTS

- Administer before meals.
- Tablets should not be chewed, divided, or crushed.
- May be administered with antacids.
- Pregnancy category C.

PHARMACOKINETICS

Onset: 0.5–3.5 h

Peak: 5 days

Half-life: 0.5–1.5 h

Duration: 3–4 days

ADVERSE EFFECTS

Adverse effects are generally minor and include headache, nausea, diarrhea, rash, and abdominal pain. The main concern with proton pump inhibitors is that long-term use has been associated with an increased risk of gastric cancer in laboratory animals. Because of this possibility, therapy is generally limited to 2 months.

Contraindications: The only contraindication is hypersensitivity to the drug.

INTERACTIONS

Drug–Drug: Concurrent use with diazepam, phenytoin, and CNS depressants may cause increased blood levels of these drugs. Concurrent use with warfarin may increase the likelihood of bleeding.

Lab Tests: May increase values for ALT, AST, and serum alkaline phosphatase.

Herbal/Food: Unknown.

Treatment of Overdose: There is no specific treatment for overdose.

 See the Companion Website for a Nursing Process Focus specific to this drug.

---

pregnancy category B (rabeprazole) to C (omeprazole and lansoprazole). Assess for drug–drug interactions. Proton pump inhibitors will affect the absorption of medications, vitamins, and minerals that need an acidic environment in the stomach. Obtain the client's history of smoking, because smoking increases stomach acid production.

Administer these drugs 30 minutes prior to eating, usually before breakfast. Proton pump inhibitors are unstable in an acidic environment and are enteric coated to be absorbed in the small intestine. These drugs may be administered at the same time as antacids. Proton pump inhibitors are often administered in combination with clarithromycin (Biaxin) for the treatment of *H. pylori*.

Monitor for adverse effects such as diarrhea, headache, and dizziness. Proton pump inhibitors are a relatively new class of drug; therefore, the long-term effects have not been fully determined.

Client Teaching. Client education as it relates to proton pump inhibitors should include the goals of therapy; the reasons for obtaining baseline data such as vital signs, diagnostic procedures, and laboratory tests, and the existence of underlying disorders such as metabolic alkalosis and hypocalcemia; and possible drug side effects. Include the following points when teaching clients about proton pump inhibitors:

- Take medication before meals, preferably before breakfast.
- Report significant diarrhea.
- Do not crush, break, or chew medication.
- Avoid smoking, alcohol use, and foods that cause gastric discomfort.
- Immediately report GI bleeding, abdominal pain, and heartburn.
- Immediately report pain with urination or blood in urine.
- Do not breast-feed while taking this drug.
- Eat foods with beneficial bacteria, such as yogurt, or take acidophilus to replace "friendly" bacteria.
- If experiencing heart burn, sleep with a foam wedge or risers placed under the top of the bed frame to keep the head elevated 30°.

ANTACIDS

Antacids are alkaline substances that have been used to neutralize stomach acid for hundreds of years. These agents, listed in Table 40.3, are readily available as OTC drugs.

HOME & COMMUNITY CONSIDERATIONS

Over-the-counter Medications for GI Disorders

Many clients purchase OTC medications based on information obtained from the media. Both H_2-receptor agonists and a proton pump inhibitor are available as OTC medications. Although every OTC medication includes an information sheet, many people do not read them. Some don't read them because they feel that all OTC medications are safe, and others have difficulty reading the small print on the information sheets. Still others may not realize that they are taking an OTC that may interact with a prescribed medication. It is important to stress to clients that OTC medications may result in drug–drug interactions and produce adverse effects. Clients should also be instructed to check with their healthcare provider before taking any OTC medication.

TABLE 40.3 Antacids

Drug	Route and Adult Dose (max dose where indicated)	Adverse Effects
aluminum hydroxide (Amphojel, others)	PO; 600 mg tid–qid	*Constipation, nausea* Fecal impaction, hypophosphatemia
calcium carbonate (Titralac, Tums) calcium carbonate with magnesium hydroxide (Mylanta Gel-caps, Rolaids)	PO; 1–2 g bid–tid PO; 2–4 capsules or tablets PRN (max: 12 tablets/day)	*Constipation, flatulence* Fecal impaction, metabolic alkalosis, hypercalcemia, renal calculi
magnesium hydroxide (Milk of Magnesia) magnesium hydroxide and aluminum hydroxide (Maalox) magnesium hydroxide and aluminum hydroxide with simethicone (Mylanta, Maalox Plus, others) magaldrate (Riopan)	PO; 2.4–4.8 g (30–60 ml)/day in single dose or divided doses PO; 2–4 tablets PRN (max: 16 tablets/day) PO; 10–20 ml PRN (max: 120 ml/day) or 2–4 tablets PRN (max 24 tablets/day) PO; 480–1,080 mg (5–10 ml suspension or 1–2 tablets) daily (max: 20 tablets or 100 ml/day)	*Diarrhea, nausea, vomiting, abdominal cramping* Hypermagnesemia, dysrhythmias (when given parenterally)
sodium bicarbonate (Alka-Seltzer, baking soda) (see page 448 for the Prototype Drug box ∞)	PO; 0.3–2.0 g 1 to 4 times/day or 1/2 tsp of powder in glass of water	*Abdominal distention, belching* Metabolic alkalosis, fluid retention, edema, hypernatremia

Italics indicate common adverse effects; <u>underlining</u> indicates serious adverse effects.

40.8 Pharmacotherapy With Antacids

Prior to the development of H_2-receptor antagonists and proton pump inhibitors, **antacids** were the mainstays of peptic ulcer and GERD pharmacotherapy. Indeed, many clients still use these inexpensive and readily available OTC drugs. Although antacids may provide temporary relief from heartburn or indigestion, they are no longer recommended as the primary drug class for PUD. This is because antacids do not promote healing of the ulcer, nor do they help to eradicate *H. pylori*.

Antacids are alkaline, inorganic compounds of aluminum, magnesium, sodium, or calcium. Combinations of aluminum hydroxide and magnesium hydroxide, the most common type, are capable of rapidly neutralizing stomach acid. Chewable tablets and liquid formulations are available. A few products combine antacids and H_2-receptor blockers into a single tablet; for example, Pepcid Complete contains calcium carbonate, magnesium hydroxide, and famotidine.

Simethicone is sometimes added to antacid preparations, because it reduces gas bubbles that cause bloating and discomfort. For example, Mylanta contains simethicone, aluminum hydroxide, and magnesium hydroxide. Simethicone is classified as an **antiflatulent,** because it reduces gas. It also is available by itself in OTC products such as Gas-X and Mylanta Gas.

Self-medication with antacids is safe, unless they are taken in extremely large amounts. Although antacids act within 10 to 15 minutes, their duration of action is only 2 hours; thus, they must be taken often during the day. Antacids containing sodium, calcium, or magnesium can result in absorption of these minerals in the general circulation. Absorption of antacids is clinically unimportant unless the client is on a sodium-restricted diet or has diminished renal function that could result in accumulation of these minerals. In fact, some manufacturers advertise their calcium-based antacid products as mineral supplements. Clients should follow the label instructions carefully and keep within the recommended dosage range.

NURSING CONSIDERATIONS

The role of the nurse in antacid therapy for PUD involves careful monitoring of a client's condition and providing education as it relates to prescribed drug treatment. Antacids are for occasional use only, and clients should seek medical attention if symptoms persist or recur. Obtain a medical history, including the use of OTC and prescription drugs. Assess the client for signs of renal insufficiency; magnesium-containing antacids should be used with caution in these clients. Hypermagnesemia may occur in clients with renal impairment, because the kidneys are unable to excrete excess magnesium. Magnesium- and aluminum-based products may cause diarrhea, and those with calcium may cause constipation.

Client Teaching.   Client education as it relates to antacids should include the goals of therapy; the reasons for obtaining baseline data such as vital signs, and the existence of underlying cardiac, renal, or phosphate-deficiency disorders; and possible drug side effects. Include the following points when teaching clients about antacid therapy:

• Keep all scheduled laboratory visits for phosphorus and calcium levels.

Pr PROTOTYPE DRUG | Aluminum Hydroxide *(Amphojel, others)* | Antacid

ACTIONS AND USES

Aluminum hydroxide is an inorganic agent used alone or in combination with other antacids such as magnesium hydroxide. Unlike calcium-based antacids that can be absorbed and cause systemic effects, aluminum compounds are minimally absorbed. Their primary action is to neutralize stomach acid by raising the pH of the stomach contents. Unlike H$_2$-receptor antagonists and proton pump inhibitors, aluminum antacids do not reduce the volume of acid secretion. They are most effectively used in combination with other antiulcer agents for the symptomatic relief of heartburn due to PUD or GERD. Aluminum carbonate (Basaljel) and aluminum phosphate (Phosphaljel) are also available.

ADMINISTRATION ALERTS

- Administer aluminum antacids at least 2 hours before or after other drugs because absorption could be affected.
- Pregnancy category C.

PHARMACOKINETICS

Onset: 20–40 min

Peak: 30 min

Half-life: Unknown

Duration: 2 h when taken with food, 3 h when taken 1 h after food

ADVERSE EFFECTS

When given in high doses, aluminum antacids may interfere with phosphate metabolism and cause constipation. They are often combined with magnesium compounds, which counteract the constipation commonly experienced with aluminum antacids.

Contraindications: This drug should not be used in clients with suspected bowel obstruction.

INTERACTIONS

Drug–Drug: Aluminum compounds should not be taken with other medications, as they may interfere with their absorption. Use with sodium polystyrene sulfonate may cause systemic alkalosis.

Lab Tests: Values for serum gastrin and urinary pH may increase. Serum phosphate values may decrease.

Herbal/Food: Unknown.

Treatment of Overdose: There is no specific treatment for overdose.

 See the Companion Website for a Nursing Process Focus specific to this drug.

- Do not take antacids with magnesium if you have kidney disease.
- Do not take antacids with sodium if you have heart failure or high blood pressure.
- Take antacids at least 2 hours before other oral medications, because drug absorption may be affected.
- Note the number and consistency of stools, because antacids may alter bowel activity.
- Medication may make stools appear white.
- Shake liquid preparations thoroughly before dispensing.
- Thoroughly chew tablets until wet before swallowing.

ANTIBIOTICS FOR *H. PYLORI*

The gram-negative bacterium *H. pylori* is associated with 90% of clients with duodenal ulcers and 70% of those with gastric ulcers. It is also strongly associated with gastric cancer. To more rapidly and completely eliminate peptic ulcers, combination therapy with several antibiotics is used to eradicate this bacterium.

40.9 Pharmacotherapy With Combination Antibiotic Therapy

H. pylori has adapted well as a human pathogen by devising ways to neutralize the high acidity surrounding it and by making chemicals called *adhesins* that allow it to stick tightly to the GI mucosa. *H. pylori* infections can remain active for life, if not treated appropriately. Elimination of

this organism allows ulcers to heal more rapidly and remain in remission longer. The following antibiotics are commonly used for this purpose:

- amoxicillin (Amoxil, others)
- clarithromycin (Biaxin)
- metronidazole (Flagyl)
- tetracycline (Achromycin, others)
- bismuth subsalicylate (Pepto-Bismol) or ranitidine bismuth citrate (Tritec)

Two or more antibiotics are given concurrently to increase the effectiveness of therapy and to lower the potential for bacterial resistance. The antibiotics are also combined with a proton pump inhibitor or an H$_2$-receptor antagonist. Bismuth compounds (Pepto-Bismol, Tritec) are sometimes added to the antibiotic regimen. Although technically not antibiotics, bismuth compounds inhibit bacterial growth and prevent *H. pylori* from adhering to the gastric mucosa. Antibiotic therapy generally continues for 7 to 14 days. Additional information on anti-infectives can be found in Chapters 21 and 22 ∞.

40.10 Miscellaneous Drugs for Peptic Ulcer Disease

Several additional drugs are beneficial in treating PUD. Sucralfate (Carafate) consists of sucrose (a sugar) plus aluminum hydroxide (an antacid). The drug produces a thick, gel-like substance that coats the ulcer, protecting it against further erosion and promoting healing. It does not affect the secretion of gastric acid. Other than constipation, side effects are minimal, because little of the drug is absorbed from the GI tract. A major disadvantage of sucralfate is that it must be taken four times daily.

Misoprostol (Cytotec) inhibits gastric acid secretion and stimulates the production of protective mucus. Its primary use is for the prevention of peptic ulcers in clients taking high doses of NSAIDs or glucocorticoids. Diarrhea and abdominal cramping are relatively common. Classified as a pregnancy category X drug, misoprostol is contraindicated during pregnancy. In fact, misoprostol is sometimes used to terminate pregnancies, as discussed in Chapter 45 ∞.

Prior to the discovery of safer and more effective drugs, anticholinergics such as atropine were used to treat peptic ulcers. Pirenzepine (Gastozepine) is a cholinergic blocker (muscarinic) available in Canada that inhibits gastric acid secretion. Although the action of pirenzepine is somewhat selective to the stomach, other anticholinergic effects such as dry mouth and constipation are possible. Anticholinergics are now rarely used for PUD owing to the availability of safer, more effective drugs.

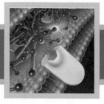

CHAPTER REVIEW

KEY CONCEPTS

The numbered key concepts provide a succinct summary of the important points from the corresponding numbered section within the chapter. If any of these points are not clear, refer to the numbered section within the chapter for review.

40.1 The digestive system is responsible for breaking down food, absorbing nutrients, and eliminating wastes.

40.2 The stomach secretes enzymes and hydrochloric acid that accelerate the process of chemical digestion. A thick mucus layer and bicarbonate ion protect the stomach mucosa from the damaging effects of the acid.

40.3 Peptic ulcer disease (PUD) is caused by an erosion of the mucosal layer of the stomach or duodenum. Gastric ulcers are more commonly associated with cancer and require longer follow-up.

40.4 Gastroesophageal reflux disease (GERD) results when acidic stomach contents enter the esophagus. GERD and PUD are treated with similar medications.

40.5 Peptic ulcer disease is best treated by a combination of lifestyle changes and pharmacotherapy. Treatment goals are to eliminate infection by *H. pylori*, promote ulcer healing, and prevent recurrence of symptoms.

40.6 H_2-receptor blockers slow acid secretion by the stomach and are often drugs of choice in treating PUD and GERD.

40.7 Proton pump inhibitors block the enzyme H^+, K^+-ATPase and are effective at reducing gastric acid secretion.

40.8 Antacids are effective at neutralizing stomach acid and are inexpensive OTC therapy for PUD and GERD. Although they relieve symptoms, antacids do not promote ulcer healing.

40.9 Combinations of antibiotics are administered to treat *H. pylori* infections of the GI tract, the cause of many peptic ulcers. A proton pump inhibitor and bismuth compounds are included in the regimen.

40.10 Several miscellaneous drugs, including sucralfate, misoprostol, and pirenzepine are also beneficial in treating PUD.

NCLEX-RN® REVIEW QUESTIONS

1 A woman has been using OTC antacids for relief of gastric upset. She is on renal dialysis three times a week. The nurse should carefully monitor the client for the development of what condition?

1. Hypomagnesemia
2. Hyperkalemia
3. Hypermagnesemia
4. Hyponatremia

2 In the treatment of *H. pylori*, the nurse must recognize that the use of two or more antibiotics is essential for what reason?

1. To lower the potential for bacterial resistance
2. To decrease the chances of development of duodenal ulcers
3. To increase the likelihood of eliminating redevelopment of gastric ulcers
4. To decrease the cost of future drug therapies

3 What natural therapy should the nurse encourage clients to use to strengthen the upper GI tract?

1. Ginger
2. Peppermint
3. Basil
4. Green tea

4 In addition to multiple antibiotics, what compound should the nurse anticipate will be added to the regimen treatment of *H. pylori*?

1. Antacids
2. H₂-receptor antagonists
3. Bismuth compounds
4. Vitamin E compounds

5 The nurse assesses for which of the following risk factors associated with PUD? (Select all that apply.)

1. Smoking tobacco
2. Blood group O
3. Excessive psychological stress levels
4. Type II diabetes mellitus
5. Caffeine use

CRITICAL THINKING QUESTIONS

1. A client with chronic hyperacidity of the stomach takes aluminum hydroxide (Amphojel) on a regular basis. The client presents to the clinic with complaints of increasing weakness. What may be the cause of this increasing weakness?

2. Identify why nurses who work at night are at higher risk for developing PUD.

3. A client who is on ranitidine (Zantac) for PUD smokes and drinks alcohol daily. What education will the nurse provide to this client?

See Appendix D for answers and rationales for all activities.

EXPLORE MediaLink

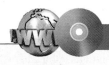

 www.prenhall.com/adams

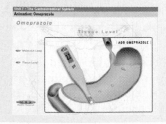

NCLEX-RN® review, case studies, and other interactive resources for this chapter can be found on the companion website at www.prenhall.com/adams. Click on "Chapter 40" to select the activities for this chapter. For animations, more NCLEX-RN® review questions, and an audio glossary, access the accompanying Prentice Hall Nursing MediaLink DVD-ROM in this textbook.

PRENTICE HALL NURSING MEDIALINK DVD-ROM

- **Animations**
  Mechanism in Action: Ranitidine (*Zantac*)
  Mechanism in Action: Omeprazole (*Prilosec*)
- **Audio Glossary**
- **NCLEX-RN® Review**

COMPANION WEBSITE

- **NCLEX-RN® Review**
- **Dosage Calculations**
- **Case Study:** Client with peptic ulcer disease
- **Care Plan:** Client with peptic ulcer disease who will begin ranitidine

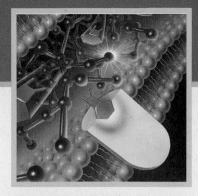

CHAPTER 41

Drugs for Bowel Disorders and Other Gastrointestinal Conditions

DRUGS AT A GLANCE

LAXATIVES
Bulk Forming
  ☞ *psyllium mucilloid (Metamucil, others)*
Stool Softener/Surfactant
Stimulant
Saline and Osmotic
ANTIDIARRHEALS
Opioids
  ☞ *diphenoxylate with atropine (Lomotil)*
DRUGS FOR INFLAMMATORY BOWEL DISEASE AND IRRITABLE BOWEL SYNDROME
  ☞ *tegaserod (Zelnorm)*
ANTIEMETICS
Anticholinergics
Antihistamines
Benzodiazepines
Cannabinoids
Glucocorticoids
Phenothiazines and Phenothiazine-like
  ☞ *prochlorperazine (Compazine)*
Serotonin-receptor Antagonists
APPETITE SUPPRESSANTS: ANOREXANTS
  ☞ *sibutramine (Meridia)*
PANCREATIC ENZYME REPLACEMENT
  ☞ *pancrelipase (Lipancreatin, Pancrease, Zymase)*

OBJECTIVES

After reading this chapter, the student should be able to:

1. Identify the major anatomical structures of the lower gastrointestinal tract.
2. Explain the pathogenesis of constipation and diarrhea.
3. Discuss conditions in which the pharmacotherapy of bowel disorders is indicated.
4. Explain conditions in which the pharmacotherapy of nausea and vomiting is indicated.
5. Describe the types of drugs used in the short-term management of obesity.
6. Describe the nurse's role in the pharmacological management of bowel disorders, nausea and vomiting, and other GI conditions.
7. Explain the use of pancreatic enzyme replacement in the pharmacotherapy of pancreatitis.
8. For each of the drug classes listed in Drugs at a Glance, know representative drugs, and explain the mechanism of drug action, describe primary actions, and identify important adverse effects.
9. Categorize drugs used in the treatment of bowel disorders, nausea, and vomiting based on their classification and mechanism of action.
10. Use the Nursing Process to care for clients who are receiving drug therapy for bowel disorders, nausea and vomiting, and other GI conditions.

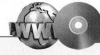

KEY TERMS

anorexiant *page 635*

antiemetic *page 633*

cathartic *page 626*

chemoreceptor trigger zone (CTZ)
   page 632

chyme *page 624*

constipation *page 625*

Crohn's disease *page 630*

defecation *page 626*

diarrhea *page 628*

dietary fiber *page 625*

emesis *page 632*

emetics *page 633*

emetogenic potential *page 633*

irritable bowel syndrome (IBS)
   page 630

laxative *page 625*

nausea *page 632*

steatorrhea *page 638*

ulcerative colitis *page 630*

vomiting center *page 632*

Bowel disorders, nausea, and vomiting are among the most common complaints for which clients seek medical consultation. These nonspecific symptoms may be caused by a large number of infectious, metabolic, inflammatory, neoplastic, or neuropsychological disorders. In addition, nausea, vomiting, constipation, and diarrhea are the most common side effects of oral medications. Although symptoms often resolve without the need for pharmacotherapy, when severe or prolonged, these conditions may lead to serious consequences unless drug therapy is initiated. This chapter examines the pharmacotherapy of these and other conditions associated with the gastrointestinal (GI) tract.

41.1 Normal Function of the Lower Digestive Tract

The lower portion of the GI tract consists of the small and large intestines, as shown in ● Figure 41.1. The first 10 inches of the small intestine, the duodenum, is the site where partially digested food from the stomach, known as **chyme,** mixes with bile from the gallbladder and digestive enzymes from the pancreas. It is sometimes considered part of the upper GI tract because of its close proximity to the stomach. The most common disorder of the duodenum, peptic ulcer, was discussed in Chapter 40 ∞.

The remainder of the small intestine consists of the jejunum and ileum. The jejunum is the site where most nutrient absorption occurs. The ileum empties its contents into the large intestine through the ileocecal valve. Peristalsis through the intestines is controlled by the autonomic nervous system. Activation of the parasympathetic division will increase peristalsis and speed materials through the intestine; the sympathetic division has the opposite effect. Travel time for chyme through the entire small intestine varies from 3 to 6 hours.

The large intestine, or colon, receives chyme from the ileum in a fluid state. The major functions of the colon are to reabsorb water from the waste material and to excrete the remaining fecal material from the body. The colon harbors a substantial number of bacteria and fungi, the host flora, which serve a useful purpose by synthesizing B-complex vitamins and vitamin K. Disruption of the host flora in the colon can lead to diarrhea. With few exceptions, little reabsorption of nutrients occurs during the 12- to 24-hour journey through the colon.

PHARMFACTS

Gastrointestinal Disorders

- Ulcerative colitis has a peak onset from ages 15 to 30 and another from ages 60 to 80.
- As many as 40% of those aged 65 and older report recurrent constipation.
- Approximately 140,000 new cases of colorectal cancer occur each year; it is the second leading cause of cancer deaths, killing more than 55,000 Americans.
- Irritable bowel syndrome affects 10% to 20% of adults.
- Americans spend more than $33 billion annually on weight-reduction products and services.
- The incidence of motion sickness peaks from ages 4 to 10, and then begins to decline.
- Gallstones account for 90% of all cases of acute pancreatitis, whereas alcohol consumption is associated with 70% of all chronic pancreatitits.
- About 25% of Americans (more than 1 million adults) who are using weight-loss supplements are not overweight.

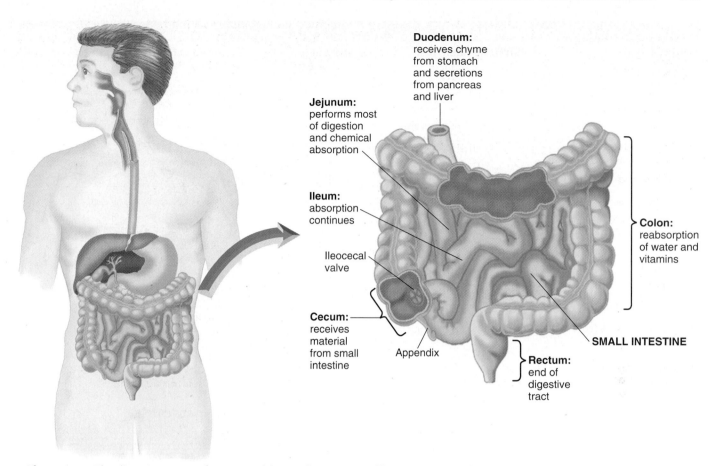

Duodenum:
receives chyme
from stomach
and secretions
from pancreas
and liver

Jejunum:
performs most
of digestion
and chemical
absorption

Ileum:
absorption
continues

Ileocecal
valve

Cecum:
receives
material
from small
intestine

Appendix

Colon:
reabsorption
of water and
vitamins

SMALL INTESTINE

Rectum:
end of
digestive
tract

● **Figure 41.1** The digestive system: functions of the small intestine and large intestine (colon) *Source: Pearson Education/PH College.*

CONSTIPATION

Constipation is defined as a decrease in the frequency or number and/or amount of bowel movements. Stools may become dry, hard, and difficult to evacuate from the rectum without straining.

41.2 Pathophysiology of Constipation

As waste material travels through the large intestine, water is reabsorbed. Reabsorption of the proper amount of water results in stools of a normal, soft-formed consistency. If the waste material remains in the colon for an extended period, however, too much water will be reabsorbed, leading to small, hard stools. Constipation may cause abdominal distention and discomfort, and flatulence.

Constipation is not a disease, but a symptom of an underlying disorder. The etiology of constipation may be related to a lack of exercise, insufficient food intake, especially insoluble **dietary fiber,** diminished fluid intake, or a medication regimen that includes drugs that reduce intestinal motility. Opioids, anticholinergics, antihistamines, certain antacids, and iron supplements are just some of the medications that promote constipation. Foods that can cause constipation include alcoholic beverages, products with a high content of refined white flour, dairy products, and chocolate. In addition, certain diseases such as hypothyroidism, diabetes, and irritable bowel syndrome (IBS) can cause constipation.

The normal frequency of bowel movements varies widely among individuals, from two to three per day, to as few as one per week. Clients should understand that variations in frequency are normal, and that a daily bowel movement is not a requirement for good health.

Occasional constipation is self-limiting and does not require drug therapy. Lifestyle modifications that incorporate increased dietary fiber and physical activity should be considered before drugs are utilized for constipation. Chronic, infrequent, and painful bowel movements, accompanied by severe straining, may justify initiation of treatment. In its most severe form, constipation can lead to a fecal impaction and complete obstruction of the bowel. Constipation occurs more frequently in older adults, because fecal transit time through the colon slows with aging; this population also exercises less and has a higher frequency of chronic disorders that cause constipation.

LAXATIVES

Laxatives are drugs that promote bowel movements. Many are available over the counter (OTC) for the self-treatment of simple constipation. Doses of laxatives are identified in Table 41.1.

TABLE 41.1   Laxatives and Cathartics

Drug	Route and Adult Dose (max dose where indicated)	Adverse Effects
BULK FORMING		
calcium polycarbophil (FiberCon, Fiberall, Mitrolan)	PO; 1 g/day PRN	*Abdominal fullness or cramping, fainting*
methylcellulose (Citrucel)	PO; 5–20 ml tid in 8–10 oz water	
ⓟ psyllium mucilloid (Metamucil, Naturacil, others)	PO; 1–2 tsp in 8 oz water daily PRN	Esophageal or GI obstruction if taken with insufficient fluid
SALINE AND OSMOTIC		
magnesium hydroxide (Milk of Magnesia)	PO; 20–60 ml/day PRN	*Diarrhea, abdominal cramping, diarrhea*
polyethylene glycol (MiraLax) sodium	PO; 17g in 8 oz of liquid daily for 2–4 days	
sodium biphosphate (Fleet Phospho-Soda)	PO; 15–30 ml mixed in water daily PRN	Hypermagnesemia with magnesium hydroxide (dysrhythmias, respiratory failure)
STIMULANT		
bisacodyl (Dulcolax)	PO; 10–15 mg/day PRN	*Abdominal cramping, nausea, fainting, diarrhea*
castor oil (Emulsoil, Neoloid, Purge)	PO; 15–60 ml/day PRN	
phenolphthalein (Ex-Lax, Feen-a-Mint, Correctol)	PO; 60–240 mg/day PRN	Fluid and electrolyte loss
STOOL SOFTENER/SURFACTANT		
docusate (Surfak, Dialose, Colace, others)	PO; 50–500 mg/day	*Abdominal cramping, diarrhea*
		No serious adverse effects
HERBAL AGENT		
Senna	PO; 8.6–17.2 mg/day	*Abdominal cramping, diarrhea*
		No serious adverse effects
MISCELLANEOUS AGENT		
mineral oil	PO; 15–30 ml bid	*Diarrhea, nausea*
lubiprostone (Amitiza)	PO; 24 mcg bid	Nutritional deficiencies (mineral oil), aspiration pneumonia (mineral oil)

Italics indicate common adverse effects; <u>underlining</u> indicates serious adverse effects.

41.3 Pharmacotherapy With Laxatives

Laxatives promote evacuation of bowel, or **defecation**, and are widely used to prevent and treat constipation. **Cathartic** is a related term that implies a stronger and more complete bowel emptying. A variety of prescription and OTC products are available, including tablet, liquid, and suppository formulations.

Prophylactic laxative pharmacotherapy is appropriate postoperatively. Such treatment is indicated to preclude straining or bearing down during defecation—a situation that has the potential to precipitate increased intra-abdominal, intraocular, or blood pressure. In addition, laxatives, in conjunction with enemas, are often given to cleanse the bowel prior to diagnostic or surgical procedures of the colon or genitourinary tract. Cathartics are usually the drug of choice preceding diagnostic procedures of the colon, such as colonoscopy or barium enema.

When taken in prescribed amounts, laxatives have few side effects. These drugs are often classified into five primary groups and a miscellaneous category.

- *Bulk-forming agents* absorb water, thus adding size to the fecal mass. These are agents of choice for the treatment and prevention of chronic constipation, and may be taken on a regular basis without ill effects.
- *Stool softeners* or *surfactants* cause more water and fat to be absorbed into the stools. They are ineffective at *treating* constipation but are most often used to *prevent* the condition, especially in clients who have undergone recent surgery.
- *Stimulants* irritate the bowel to increase peristalsis. They should not be used routinely because they may cause laxative dependence, abdominal cramping, and depletion of fluid and electrolytes.
- *Saline* or *osmotic laxatives* are not absorbed in the intestine; they pull water into the fecal mass to create a more watery stool. These agents can produce a bowel movement

Pr PROTOTYPE DRUG | Psyllium Mucilloid *(Metamucil, others)* | Bulk-forming Laxative

ACTIONS AND USES

Psyllium is derived from a natural product, the seeds of the plantain plant. Like other bulk-forming laxatives, psyllium is an insoluble fiber that is indigestible and not absorbed from the GI tract. When taken with a sufficient quantity of water, psyllium swells and increases the size of the fecal mass. The larger the size of the fecal mass, the more the defecation reflex will be stimulated, thus promoting the passage of stool. Several doses of psyllium may be needed over 1 to 3 days to produce a therapeutic effect. Frequent use of psyllium may effect a small reduction in blood cholesterol level.

ADMINISTRATION ALERTS

- Mix with 8 oz of water, fruit juice, or milk, and administer immediately. Follow each dose with an additional 8 oz of liquid.
- Observe elderly clients closely for possible aspiration.
- Pregnancy category C.

PHARMACOKINETICS

Onset: 12–24 h

Peak: 1–3 days

Half-life: Unknown

Duration: Unknown

ADVERSE EFFECTS

Psyllium rarely produces side effects. It causes less cramping than stimulant-type laxatives and results in a more natural bowel movement. If taken with insufficient water, it may cause obstructions in the esophagus or intestine.

Contraindications: Psyllium should not be administered to clients with undiagnosed abdominal pain, intestinal obstruction, or fecal impaction.

INTERACTIONS

Drug–Drug: Psyllium may decrease the absorption and effects of warfarin, digoxin, nitrofurantoin, antibiotics, and salicylates.

Lab Tests: May increase serum glucose level.

Herbal/Food: Unknown.

Treatment of Overdose: There is no specific treatment for overdose.

 See the Companion Website for a Nursing Process Focus specific to this drug

---

very quickly (1 to 6 hours) but should not be used on a regular basis because of the possibility of fluid and electrolyte depletion.

- *Herbal agents* are natural products available OTC that are widely used for self-treatment of constipation. The most commonly used herbal laxative is senna, a potent herb that irritates the bowel and increases peristalsis.

- *Miscellaneous agents* include mineral oil, which acts by lubricating the stool and the colon mucosa. The use of mineral oil should be discouraged, because it may interfere with the absorption of fat-soluble vitamins and can cause other potentially serious adverse effects. In 2006, lubiprostone (Amitza) was approved for chronic idiopathic constipation.

NURSING CONSIDERATIONS

The role of the nurse in laxative therapy for bowel evacuation involves careful monitoring of a client's condition and providing education as it relates to the prescribed drug treatment. Prior to pharmacotherapy with laxatives, assess the abdomen for distention, bowel sounds, and bowel patterns. If there is absence of bowel sounds, peristalsis must be restored prior to laxative therapy. Evaluate a client with a sudden, unexplained change in bowel patterns, because it could indicate a serious condition such as colon cancer. Also assess for esophageal obstruction, intestinal obstruction, fecal impaction, and undiagnosed abdominal pain. Laxatives are contraindicated in all these conditions because of the risk of bowel perforation. If diarrhea occurs,

discontinue laxative use. There are many products to prevent and treat constipation. Because most are OTC medications, there is a risk for misuse and overuse.

Bulk-forming laxatives are pregnancy category C and should be used with caution during pregnancy and lactation. Because fiber absorbs water and expands to provide "bulk," these agents must be taken with one to two glasses of water. Assess the client's ability to swallow, because obstruction can occur if the product does not clear the esophagus or if a stricture exists. Bulk-forming products may take 24 to 48 hours to be effective and may be taken on a regular basis to prevent constipation.

Stool softeners are generally prescribed for clients who have experienced a sudden change in lifestyle that puts them at risk for constipation, such as a surgery, injury, or conditions such as MI in which straining during defecation should be avoided. They are contraindicated during pregnancy and lactation (pregnancy category C). Assess for the development of diarrhea and cramping; if diarrhea develops, withhold the medication. Docusate is contraindicated in clients with abdominal pain accompanied by nausea and vomiting, fecal impaction, and in intestinal obstruction or perforation. Do not give docusate sodium (Colace) to clients on sodium restriction. Do not give docusate potassium (Dialose) to clients with renal impairment. Docusate increases systemic absorption of mineral oil, so these two medications should not be given concurrently. Docusate should not be taken with certain herbal products such as senna, cascara, rhubarb, or aloe, because it will increase their absorption and the risk of liver toxicity.

Stimulant laxatives act as irritants to the bowel and increase peristalsis. They are the quickest acting and most likely to cause diarrhea and cramping. Bowel rupture could occur if obstruction is present. Do not give stimulant laxatives to pregnant or lactating women (pregnancy category C). Because of the rapid and potent effects of stimulant laxatives, respond quickly to a client's request to use a bedpan or to get to the bathroom. These products are also used as "bowel prep" prior to bowel exams or surgeries, sometimes in combination with stimulant laxatives, osmotic laxatives, and enemas. Because the client will be NPO (nothing by mouth) prior to the procedure, assess for signs of dehydration and changes in vital signs. It may be necessary to initiate IV fluids. Herbal stimulant laxatives, such as cascara or senna, are common components of OTC weight-loss products, and clients taking them may experience rebound, severe constipation if these medications are abruptly withdrawn.

Saline or osmotic laxatives pull water into the GI tract. Most are pregnancy category B. Dehydration may result when these medications are taken frequently or in excess if the client has inadequate fluid intake. Osmotic laxatives are highly potent, work within hours, and are often a part of bowel prep.

Lifespan Considerations. Do not give laxatives and bowel softeners to pediatric clients without a physician's order. Pregnant women and mothers that are breast-feeding should avoid taking laxatives and stool softeners unless recommended by their physician. It is very important that the client education for pregnant and breast-feeding mothers include a reminder that any medication given to the mother has the potential to pass through the placenta into the fetus's bloodsteam or into breast milk.

Elderly clients frequently abuse laxatives and stool softeners. Many factors contribute to changes in bowel movement habits in elderly clients. Some medications, reduction in physical exercise, changes in dietary habits, and reduced fluid intake may result in chronic constipation and the abuse of laxatives and stool softeners.Assess for and educate clients about the proper use of laxatives and stool softeners.

Client Teaching. Client education as it relates to laxative therapy should include the goals of therapy; the reasons for obtaining baseline data such as vital signs and the existence of underlying disorders such as intestinal obstruction, nausea and vomiting, and undiagnosed abdominal pain; and possible drug side effects. Include the following points when teaching clients about laxatives:

- Follow instructions carefully and do not take more than the recommended dose.
- If changes in bowel patterns persist or become more severe, seek medical attention.
- Take bulk-forming agents at a different time than other medications to ensure proper absorption of other drugs.

DIARRHEA

Diarrhea is an increase in the frequency and fluidity of bowel movements. Like constipation, diarrhea is not a disease but a symptom of an underlying disorder.

41.4 Pathophysiology of Diarrhea

When the large intestine does not reabsorb enough water from the fecal mass, stools become watery. Like constipation, occasional diarrhea is often a self-limiting disorder that does not warrant drug therapy. Indeed, diarrhea may be considered a type of body defense, rapidly and completely eliminating the body of toxins and pathogens. When prolonged or severe, especially in children, diarrhea can result in significant loss of body fluids, and pharmacotherapy is then indicated. Prolonged diarrhea may lead to fluid, acid–base, or electrolyte disorders (Chapter 31∞).

Diarrhea may be caused by certain medications, infections of the bowel, and substances such as lactose. Antibiotics often cause diarrhea by killing normal intestinal flora, thus allowing an overgrowth of opportunistic pathogenic organisms. The primary goal in treating diarrhea is to assess and treat the underlying condition causing the diarrhea. Assessing the client's recent travels, dietary habits, immune system competence, and recent drug history may provide information about its etiology. Critically ill clients with a reduced immune response who are exposed to many antibiotics may have diarrhea related to pseudomembranous colitis, a condition that may lead to shock and death.

TABLE 41.2 Antidiarrheals		
Drug	**Route and Adult Dose (max dose where indicated)**	**Adverse Effects**
OPIOIDS		
camphorated opium tincture (Paregoric)	PO; 5–10 ml q2h–qid PRN	*Drowsiness, light-headedness, nausea, dizziness, dry mouth (from atropine), constipation*
difenoxin with atropine (Motofen)	PO; 1–2 mg after each diarrhea episode (max: 8 mg/day)	
diphenoxylate with atropine (Lomotil)	PO; 1–2 tabs or 5–10 ml tid–qid	<u>Paralytic ileus with toxic megacolon, respiratory depression, CNS depression</u>
loperamide (Imodium)	PO; 4 mg as a single dose, then 2 mg after each diarrhea episode (max: 16 mg/day)	
MISCELLANEOUS AGENTS		
bismuth salts (Pepto-Bismol)	PO; 2 tabs or 30 ml PRN	*Constipation, nausea*
furazolidone (Furoxone)	PO; 100 mg qid	<u>Agranulocytosis (Furoxone), disulfiram-like reaction (furazolidone)</u>

Italics indicate common adverse effects; <u>underlining</u> indicates serious adverse effects.

Acidophilus for Diarrhea

Lactobacillus acidophilus is a probiotic bacterium normally found in the human alimentary canal and vagina. It is considered to be protective flora, inhibiting the growth of potentially pathogenic species such as *Escherichia coli*, *Candida albicans*, *H. pylori*, and *Gardnerella vaginalis*. One mechanism used by *L. acidophilus* to limit the growth of other bacterial species is the generation of hydrogen peroxide, which is toxic to most cells.

The primary use of *L. acidophilus* is to restore the normal flora of the intestine following diarrhea, particularly from antibiotic therapy. It has also been shown to be effective at shortening episodes of acute infectious diarrhea (Teitelbaum, 2005). *L. acidophilus* may be obtained by drinking acidophilus milk or by eating yogurt or kefir containing live (or active) cultures. Those wishing to obtain *L. acidophilus* from yogurt should read the labels carefully, because not all products contain active cultures; frozen yogurt contains no active cultures. Supplements include capsules, tablets, and granules. Doses are not standardized, and tablet doses range from 50 to 500 mg.

ANTIDIARRHEALS

For mild diarrhea, OTC products are effective at returning elimination patterns to normal. For chronic or severe cases, the opioids are the most efficacious of the antidiarrheal agents. The antidiarrheals are listed in Table 41.2.

41.5 Pharmacotherapy With Antidiarrheals

Pharmacotherapy related to diarrhea depends on the severity of the condition and identifiable etiologic factors. If the cause is an infectious disease, then an antibiotic or antiparasitic drug is indicated. If the cause is inflammatory in nature, anti-inflammatory drugs are warranted. When the diarrhea appears to be a side effect of pharmacotherapy, the healthcare provider may discontinue the offending medication, lower the dose, or substitute an alternative drug.

The most effective drugs for the symptomatic treatment of diarrhea are the opioids, which can dramatically slow peristalsis in the colon. The most common opioid antidiarrheals are codeine and diphenoxylate with atropine (Lomotil). Diphenoxylate is a Schedule V agent that acts directly on the intestine to slow peristalsis, thereby allowing more fluid and electrolyte absorption in the large intestine. The opioids cause CNS depression at high doses, and are generally reserved for the short-term therapy of acute diarrhea because of the potential for dependence. Details on indications and adverse effects of opioids may be found in Chapter 18 ∞.

OTC drugs for diarrhea act by a number of different mechanisms. Loperamide (Imodium) is an analog of meperidine, although it has no narcotic effects and is not classified as a controlled substance. Low-dose loperamide is available OTC; higher doses are available by prescription. Other OTC treatments include bismuth subsalicylate (Pepto-Bismol), which acts by binding and absorbing toxins. Psyllium preparations may also slow diarrhea, because they absorb large amounts of fluid, which helps form bulkier stools. Probiotic supplements containing *Lactobacillus*, a normal inhabitant of the human gut and vagina, are sometimes taken to correct the altered GI flora following a serious diarrhea episode. A good source of healthy *Lactobacillus* is yogurt with active cultures, although a freeze-dried form of the bacteria is available in tablet form.

NURSING CONSIDERATIONS

The role of the nurse in antidiarrheal therapy involves careful monitoring of a client's condition and providing education as it relates to the prescribed drug treatment. Antidiarrheal drugs

---

Pr **PROTOTYPE DRUG** | Diphenoxylate With Atropine *(Lomotil)* | Antidiarrheal

ACTIONS AND USES

The primary antidiarrheal ingredient in Lomotil is diphenoxylate. Like other opioids, diphenoxylate slows peristalsis, allowing time for additional water reabsorption from the colon and more solid stools. It acts within 45 to 60 minutes. It is effective for moderate to severe diarrhea, but is not recommended for children. The atropine in Lomotil is not added for its anticholinergic effect, but to discourage clients from taking too much of the drug. At higher doses, the anticholinergic effects of atropine may be observed, which include drowsiness, dry mouth, and tachycardia.

ADMINISTRATION ALERT

- Pregnancy category C.

PHARMACOKINETICS

Onset: 45–60 min

Peak: 2 h

Half-life: 4.4 h

Duration: 3–4 h

ADVERSE EFFECTS

Unlike most opioids, diphenoxylate has no analgesic properties and has an extremely low potential for abuse. Some clients experience dizziness or drowsiness, and they should not drive or operate machinery until the effects of the drug are known.

Contraindications: Contraindications include hypersensitivity to the drug, severe liver disease, obstructive jaundice, and diarrhea associated with pseudomembranous colitis.

INTERACTIONS

Drug–Drug: Diphenoxylate with atropine interacts with other CNS depressants, including alcohol, to produce additive sedative effects. When taken with MAO inhibitors, diphenoxylate may cause hypertensive crisis.

Lab Tests: Unknown.

Herbal/Food: Unknown.

Treatment of Overdose: Overdose with Lomotil may be serious. Narcotic antagonists such as naloxone may be administered parenterally to reverse respiratory depression within minutes.

 See the Companion Website for a Nursing Process Focus specific to this drug.

should be given for symptomatic relief of diarrhea while the underlying etiology is treated. Because diarrhea can cause a loss of fluid and electrolytes, assess hydration status and serum potassium, magnesium, and bicarbonate. Also assess for blood in the stool. Antidiarrheals are contraindicated in clients with severe dehydration, electrolyte imbalance, liver and renal disorders, and glaucoma. Use opioid antidiarrheals with caution in clients with a history of drug abuse.

Antidiarrheals should not be used in pseudomembranous colitis or severe ulcerative colitis, because the drugs could worsen or mask these conditions. Toxic megacolon has occurred in clients with ulcerative colitis taking loperamide (Imodium).

Lifespan Considerations. Special care in the assessment of infants, children, and the elderly is extremely important, because diarrhea can quickly lead to dehydration and electrolyte imbalance. Adverse reactions occur more frequently in children, especially those with Down syndrome. Teach these clients to seek medical care for diarrhea that does not resolve within 2 days, if a fever develops, or if dehydration occurs. Infants, children, and the elderly are at greatest risk and may need medical attention sooner. Antidiarrheals are not generally used during pregnancy and lactation.

Carefully assess hepatic and renal function in elderly clients, because antidiarrheals are excreted by the liver and kidneys. Elderly clients are also at an increased risk for falls related to the drowsiness that may occur with opioids. Assess the client's ability to get out of bed safely.

Client Teaching. Client education as it relates to antidiarrheal therapy should include the goals of therapy, the reasons for obtaining baseline data such as vital signs and the existence of underlying disorders such as electrolyte imbalances and blood in stool, and possible drug side effects. Include the following points when teaching clients about antidiarrheals:

- Seek medical care for diarrhea that does not resolve within 2 days, if a fever develops, or if dehydration occurs.
- Discontinue medication as soon as frequent or watery stools have stopped.
- Seek medical care if blood is found in the stool.

SPECIAL CONSIDERATIONS

Cultural Remedies for Diarrhea

Because diarrhea is an age-old malady that affects all populations, different cultures have adopted tried-and-true symptomatic remedies for the condition. One preparation used by people in many regions of the world is cornstarch (a heaping teaspoonful) in a glass of tepid water. For centuries, mothers have boiled rice and given the diluted rice water to babies to treat diarrhea. The rationale behind these two therapies is that they work by absorbing excess water in the intestines, thus stopping the diarrhea. Although a rationale was not specified in earlier times, people of many cultures found that eating grated apple that had turned brown alleviated symptoms. These practices apparently evolved into what today is known as the ABC of diarrhea treatment: apples, bananas (just barely ripe), and carrots. The underlying principle is that the pectin present in these foods is oxidized, producing the same ingredient found in many OTC diarrhea medicines.

41.6 Pharmacotherapy of Inflammatory Bowel Disease and Irritable Bowel Syndrome

Ulceration in the distal portion of the small intestine is called **Crohn's disease,** and erosions in the large intestine are known as **ulcerative colitis.** Together these diseases are categorized as *inflammatory bowel disease (IBD)* and are treated with medications from several classifications. More than 1 million Americans are estimated to have inflammatory bowel disease.

Symptoms of IBD range from mild to acute, and the condition is often characterized by alternating periods of remission and exacerbation. The most common clinical presentation of ulcerative colitis is abdominal cramping with frequent bowel movements. Severe disease may result in weight loss, bloody diarrhea, high fever, and dehydration. The client with Crohn's disease also presents with abdominal pain, cramping and diarrhea, which may have been present for years before the client sought treatment. Symptoms of Crohn's are often similar to those of ulcerative colitis.

Mild-to-moderate IBD is treated with 5-aminosalicylic acid (5-ASA) agents. These include the sulfonamide sulfasalazine (Azulfidine), olsalazine (Dipentum), and mesalamine (Asacol, Pentasa, others). Corticosteroids such as prednisone, methylprednisolone, or hydrocortisone are used in more persistent cases. Particularly severe disease may require immunosuppressant drugs such as azathioprine (Imuran) or methotrexate (MTX). Infliximab (Remicade) is a monoclonal antibody approved for Crohn's disease and ulcerative colitis. A single infusion of infliximab can cause remission in 65% of clients with moderate-to-severe Crohn's disease that may last up to 12 weeks.

Irritable bowel syndrome (IBS), also known as *spastic colon* or *mucous colitis,* is a common disorder of the lower GI tract. Symptoms include abdominal pain, bloating, excessive gas, and colicky cramping. Bowel habits are altered, with diarrhea alternating with constipation, and there may be mucus in the stool. IBS is considered a functional bowel disorder, meaning that the normal operation of the digestive tract is impaired without the presence of detectable organic disease. It is not a precursor of more serious disease. Stress is often a precipitating factor along with dietary factors.

Treatment of IBS is supportive, with drug therapy targeted at symptomatic treatment, depending on whether constipation or diarrhea is the predominant symptom. Nonprescription bulk laxatives such as psyllium can bring relief to some clients. Dicyclomine (Bentyl) is an older anticholinergic drug used to reduce bowel spasms in clients with diarrhea-predominant IBS. Tegaserod (Zelnorm) is one of the few drugs approved for the short-term pharmacotherapy of IBS in women presenting with constipation as the primary complaint. It is classified as a serotonin agonist because it acts by binding to serotonin (5-HT) receptors in the GI tract, which stimulates the peristaltic reflex. Another serotonin agonist, alosetron, was removed from the U.S. market in 2000 because of severe GI adverse effects.

NURSING PROCESS FOCUS Clients Receiving Antidiarrheal Therapy

Assessment	Potential Nursing Diagnoses
Prior to administration: • Obtain a complete health history including allergies, drug history, and possible drug interactions. • Assess sodium, chloride, and potassium levels. • Evaluate results of stool culture. • Assess for presence of dehydration. • Obtain vital signs and ECG.	• Fluid Volume, Imbalanced, Risk for: Less than Body Requirements, related to fluid loss secondary to diarrhea • Injury (falls), Risk for, related to drowsiness secondary to drug therapy

Planning: Client Goals and Expected Outcomes

The client will:
• Report relief of diarrhea.
• Demonstrate an understanding of the drug's action by accurately describing drug side effects and precautions.
• Immediately report effects such as persistent diarrhea, constipation, abdominal pain, blood in stool, confusion, dizziness, or fever.

Implementation

Interventions and (Rationales)	Client Education/Discharge Planning
• Monitor frequency, volume, and consistency of stools. (This determines the effectiveness of drug therapy.)	Advise client to: • Record the frequency of stools. • Note if any blood is present in stools. • Report any abdominal pain or abdominal distention immediately.
• Minimize the risk of dehydration and electrolyte imbalance. (These adverse effects may occur secondary to diarrhea.)	• Instruct client to increase fluid intake and drink electrolyte-enriched fluids.
• Prevent accidental overdosage. (Overdosage can cause constipation.)	• Instruct client to use the dropper included in liquid medications, not household teaspoons, to measure liquid medication dosage.
• Monitor for dry mouth. (This is a side effect of medications.)	• Instruct client to suck on ice or sour candy, or chew gum, to relieve sensation of dry mouth.
• Initiate safety measures to prevent falls. (These medications may cause drowsiness.)	Instruct client to: • Refrain from driving or performing hazardous activities until the effects of drug are known. • Abstain from using alcohol or other CNS depressants.
• Monitor electrolyte levels. (With diarrhea, electrolyte imbalance may occur.)	Instruct client to: • Keep all laboratory appointments. • Report weakness and muscle cramping.

Evaluation of Outcome Criteria

Evaluate the effectiveness of drug therapy by confirming that the client goals and expected outcomes have been met (see "Planning").
• The client reports relief of diarrhea.
• The client demonstrates an understanding of the drug's action by accurately describing drug side effects and precautions.
• The client accurately states signs and symptoms to be reported to the healthcare provider.

∞ See Table 41.2 for a list of drugs to which these nursing actions apply.

NURSING CONSIDERATIONS

The role of the nurse in tegaserod (Zelnorm) therapy for IBD involves careful monitoring of a client's condition and providing education as it relates to the prescribed drug treatment. Prior to and during therapy, monitor liver and renal function. Monitor cardiovascular status, especially in clients with preexisting cardiovascular disease.

Tegaserod is contraindicated in severe hepatic or renal impairment, bowel obstruction, gallbladder disease, and abdominal pain.

Administer the drug just prior to a meal with a full glass of water. Tablets may be crushed. Do not give the drug to clients with frequent diarrhea because tegaserod accelerates gastric emptying. Monitor symptom relief and report frequent diarrhea or lack of relief. Side effects of tegaseod

Pr PROTYPE DRUG | Tegaserod (Zelnorm) | Agent for Irritable Bowel Syndrome

ACTIONS AND USES

Tegaserod is one of the few drugs specifically indicated for IBS. It is prescribed for clients who have the constipation-dominant form of the disease. The bowel is rich in serotonin (5-HT) receptors, which promote peristalsis and bowel movements. Tegaserod is a serotonin receptor agonist that activates these receptors, resulting in an increase in stool formation and the number of bowel movements. At this time it is approved only for women, for a maximum of 12 weeks of therapy. Effectiveness in men is being investigated, but has not been established. It is available in tablet form only.

ADMINISTRATION ALERTS

- Tegaserod is poorly absorbed, so it is best administered prior to a meal, with plenty of water.
- Pregnancy category B.

PHARMACOKINETICS

Onset: Unknown

Peak: 1 h

Half-life: 11 h

Duration: Unknown

ADVERSE EFFECTS

Tegaserod has no serious adverse effects. The most common side effect is diarrhea, which usually occurs as a single episode and resolves as therapy progresses.

Contraindications: Tegaserod is contraindicated in clients who have severe hepatic or renal impairment, a history of bowel obstruction, symptomatic gallbladder disease, abdominal adhesions, or a prior hypersensitivity to the drug.

INTERACTIONS

Drug–Drug: No clinically significant drug interactions have been reported.

Lab Tests: Unknown.

Herbal/Food: Food significantly inhibits the absorption of tegaserod.

Treatment of Overdose: There is no specific treatment for overdose.

 See the Companion Website for a Nursing Process Focus specific to this drug.

---

include leg pain, heachaches, abdominal pain, diarrhea, nausea and back pain.

Lifespan Considerations. It is not known whether tegaserod is distributed in breast milk. Safety has not been established in children.

Client Teaching. Client education as it relates to tegaserod therapy should include the goals of therapy, the reasons for obtaining baseline data such as vital signs and the existence of underlying hepatic and renal disorders, and possible drug side effects. Include the following points when teaching clients about tegaserod:

- Report lack of symptom relief after 4 weeks of therapy.
- Immediately report new or worsening abdominal pain.
- Do not breast-feed while taking this drug.

NAUSEA AND VOMITING

Nausea is an unpleasant, subjective sensation that is accompanied by weakness, diaphoresis, and hyperproduction of saliva. It is sometimes accompanied by dizziness. Intense nausea often leads to vomiting, or **emesis,** in which the stomach contents are forced upward into the esophagus and out of the mouth.

41.7 Pathophysiology of Nausea and Vomiting

Vomiting is a defense mechanism used by the body to rid itself of toxic substances. Vomiting is a reflex primarily controlled by a portion of the medulla of the brain, known as the **vomiting center,** which receives sensory signals from the digestive tract, the inner ear, and the **chemoreceptor trigger zone (CTZ)** in the cerebral cortex. Interestingly, the CTZ is not protected by the blood–brain barrier, as is the vast majority of the brain; thus, these neurons can directly sense the presence of toxic substances in the blood. Once the vomiting reflex is triggered, wavelike contractions of the stomach quickly propel its contents upward and out of the body.

Nausea and vomiting are common symptoms associated with a wide variety of conditions such as GI infections, food poisoning, nervousness, emotional imbalances, changes in body position (motion sickness), and extreme pain. Other conditions that promote nausea and vomiting are general anesthetic agents, migraine headache, trauma to the head or abdominal organs, inner ear disorders, and diabetes. Psychological factors play a significant role, as clients often become nauseated during periods of extreme stress or when confronted with unpleasant sights, smells, or sounds.

The nausea and vomiting experienced by many women during the first trimester of pregnancy is referred to as *morning sickness.* If this condition becomes acute, with continual vomiting, it may lead to *hyperemesis gravidarum,* a situation in which the health and safety of the mother and developing baby can become severely compromised. Pharmacotherapy is initiated after other antinausea measures have proved ineffective.

Many drugs, by their chemical nature, bring about nausea or vomiting as a side effect. In fact, nausea and vomiting are the most frequently listed side effects of oral medications. The nurse should remember that because the vomiting center lies in the brain, nausea and vomiting occur just as frequently with parenteral formulations as with oral drugs. The most extreme example of this phenomenon occurs with the antineoplastic drugs, most of which cause intense nausea and vomiting regardless of the route of administration. The capacity of a drug to cause vomiting is called its **emetogenic potential**. Severe nausea and vomiting is a common reason for client noncompliance and for discontinuation of drug therapy.

When large amounts of fluids are vomited, dehydration may occur. Because the contents lost from the stomach are strongly acidic, vomiting may cause a change in the pH of the blood, resulting in metabolic alkalosis. With excessive loss, severe acid–base disturbances can lead to vascular collapse, resulting in death if medical intervention is not initiated. Dehydration is especially dangerous for infants, small children, and elderly people, and is evidenced by dry mouth, sticky saliva, and reduced urine output that is dark yellow-orange to brown.

Nausea and vomiting may be prevented or alleviated with natural remedies or with drugs from several different classes. The treatment goal for nausea or vomiting should focus on removal of the cause, whenever feasible.

ANTIEMETICS

Drugs from at least eight different classes are used to prevent nausea and vomiting. Many of these act by inhibiting dopamine or serotonin receptors in the brain. The antiemetics are listed in Table 41.3.

41.8 Pharmacotherapy With Antiemetics

A large number of **antiemetics** are available to treat nausea and vomiting. Selection of a particular agent depends on the experience of the healthcare provider and the cause of the nausea and vomiting. Clients seeking self-treatment can find several options available OTC. For example, simple nausea and vomiting is sometimes relieved by antacids or diphenhydramine (Benadryl). Herbal options include peppermint and ginger, the most popular herbal therapy for nausea and vomiting. Relief of serious nausea or vomiting, however, requires prescription medications.

ANTIHISTAMINES AND ANTICHOLINERGIC AGENTS

These agents are effective for treating simple nausea, with some being available OTC. For example, nausea due to motion sickness is effectively treated with anticholinergics or antihistamines. Motion sickness is a disorder affecting a portion of the inner ear that is associated with significant nausea. The most common drug used for motion sickness is scopolamine (Transderm), which is usually administered as a transdermal patch. Antihistamines such as dimenhydrinate (Dramamine) and meclizine (Antivert) are also effective, but may cause significant drowsiness in some clients. Drugs used to treat motion sickness are most effective when taken 20 to 60 minutes before travel is expected.

PHENOTHIAZINES

The major indication for phenothiazines relates to treating psychoses (Chapter 17 ∞), but they are also very effective antiemetics. The serious nausea and vomiting associated with

antineoplastic therapy is often treated with the phenothiazines. To prevent loss of the antiemetic medication due to vomiting, some of these agents are available through the IM, IV, and/or suppository routes. Clients receiving antineoplastic drugs may receive three or more antiemetics concurrently to reduce the nausea and vomiting from chemotherapy. In fact, therapy with antineoplastic drugs is one of the most common reasons for prescribing antiemetic drugs.

GLUCOCORTICOIDS

Dexamethasone (Decadron) and methylprednisolone (Solu-Medrol) are used for chemotherapy-induced and postsurgical nausea and vomiting. They are reserved for acute cases because of the possibility of serious side effects.

SELECTIVE SEROTONIN REUPTAKE INHIBITORS (SSRIS)

These agents are often drugs of choice in the pharmacotherapy of serious nausea and vomiting due to antineoplastic therapy, radiation therapy, or surgical procedures. They are usually given prophylactically, just prior to antineoplastic therapy.

OTHER ANTIEMETICS

Aprepitant (Emend) is the first of a new class of antiemetics, the neurokinin receptor antagonists, used to prevent nausea and vomiting following antineoplastic therapy. The benzodiazepine lorazepam (Ativan) has the advantage of promoting relaxation along with having antiemetic properties. Cannabinoids are drugs that contain the same active ingredient as marijuana. Dronabinol (Marinol) and nabilone (Cesamet) are given orally to produce antiemetic effects and relaxation without the euphoria produced by marijuana.

On some occasions, it is desirable to *stimulate* the vomiting reflex with drugs called **emetics.** Indications for emetics include ingestion of poisons and overdoses of oral drugs. Ipecac syrup, given orally, or apomorphine, given subcutaneously, will induce vomiting in about 15 minutes.

NURSING CONSIDERATIONS

The role of the nurse in antiemetic therapy involves careful monitoring of a client's condition and providing education as it relates to the prescribed drug treatment. Assess symptoms that precipitated the vomiting or that are occurring concurrently. If a client becomes sedated and continues to vomit, a nasogastric tube with suction may be indicated. Antiemetics are contraindicated in clients who are hypersensitive to the drugs, have bone marrow depression, are comatose, or are experiencing vomiting of unknown etiology. These drugs are used with caution in clients with breast cancer. Client safety is a concern because drowsiness is a frequent side effect of antiemetics. Clients may be at risk for falls because of medication side effects and the sensation of weakness from vomiting. Orthostatic hypotension is a side effect of some antiemetics.

Drugs used to stimulate emesis should be used only in emergency situations under the direction of a healthcare provider. They are used only when the client is alert, because of the risk of aspiration. When the client is comatose, a

TABLE 41.3 Selected Antiemetics

Drug	Route and Adult Dose (max dose where indicated)	Adverse Effects
ANTICHOLINERGICS: ANTIHISTAMINES		
cyclizine hydrochloride (Marezine)	PO; 50 mg q4–6h (max: 200 mg/day)	*Drowsiness, dry mouth, blurred vision (scopolamine)*
dimenhydrinate (Dramamine, others)	PO; 50–100 mg q4–6h (max: 400 mg/day)	
diphenhydramine (Benadryl, others) (see page 583 for the Prototype Drug box ∞)	PO; 25–50 mg tid–qid (max: 300 mg/day)	Hypersensitivity reaction, sedation, tremors, seizures, hallucinations, paradoxical excitation (more common in children), hypotension
hydroxyzine (Atarax, Vistaril)	PO; 25–100 mg tid–qid	
meclizine (Antivert, Bonine, others)	PO; 25–50 mg/day, taken 1 h before travel	
scopolamine (Hyoscine, Transderm-Scop)	Transdermal; 0.5 mg q72h	
BENZODIAZEPINE		
lorazepam (Ativan) (see page 163 for the Prototype Drug box ∞)	IV; 1. 0–1.5 mg prior to chemotherapy	*Dizziness, drowsiness, ataxia, fatigue, slurred speech*
		Paradoxical excitation (more common in children), seizures (if abruptly discontinued), coma
CANNABINOIDS		
dronabinol (Marinol)	PO; 5 mg/m^2 1–3 h before administration of chemotherapy, then q2–4h after chemotherapy for a total of 4–6 doses; dose may be increased by 2.5 mg/m^2 (max: 15 mg/m^2)	*Dizziness, drowsiness, euphoria, confusion, ataxia, asthenia, increased sensory awareness*
nabilone (Cesamet)	PO; 1–2 mg bid	Paranoia, decreased motor coordination, hypotension
GLUCOCORTICOIDS		
dexamethasone (Decadron)	PO; 0. 25–4 mg bid–qid	*Mood swings, weight gain, acne, facial flushing, nausea, insomnia, sodium and fluid retention, impaired wound healing, menstrual abnormalities, insomnia*
methylprednisolone (Medrol, Solu-Medrol, others)	PO; 4–48 mg/day in divided doses	
		Peptic ulcer, hypocalcemia, osteoporosis with possible bone fractures, loss of muscle mass, decreased growth in children, possible masking of infections
NEUROKININ RECEPTOR ANTAGONIST		
aprepitant (Emend)	PO; 125 mg 1 h prior to chemotherapy	*Fatigue, constipation, diarrhea, anorexia, nausea, hiccup*
		Dehydration, peripheral neuropathy, blood dyscrasias, pneumonia
PHENOTHIAZINE AND PHENOTHIAZINE-LIKE		
metoclopramide (Reglan, others)	PO; 2 mg/kg 1 h prior to chemotherapy	*Dry eyes, blurred vision, dry mouth, constipation, drowsiness, photosensitivity*
perphenazine (Phenazine, Trilafon)	PO; 8–16 mg bid–qid	
℗ prochlorperazine (Compazine, others)	PO; 5–10 mg tid–qid	Extrapyramidal symptoms, neuroleptic malignant syndrome, agranulocytosis
promethazine (Phenergan, others)	PO; 12. 5–25 mg q4h–qid	
SEROTONIN RECEPTOR ANTAGONISTS		
dolasetron (Anzemet)	PO; 100 mg 1 h prior to chemotherapy	*Headache, drowsiness, fatigue, constipation, diarrhea*
granisetron (Kytril)	IV; 10 mcg/kg 30 min prior to chemotherapy	
ondansetron (Zofran)	PO; 4 mg tid PRN	Dysrhythmias, extrapyramidal symptoms
palonosetron (Aloxi)	IV; 0.25 mg 30 min prior to chemotherapy	

Italics indicate common adverse effects; <u>underlining</u> indicates serious adverse effects.

Pr PROTOTYPE DRUG | Prochlorperazine *(Compazine)* | Antiemetic

ACTIONS AND USES

Prochlorperazine is a phenothiazine, a class of drugs usually prescribed for psychoses. The phenothiazines are the largest group of drugs prescribed for severe nausea and vomiting, and prochlorperazine is the most frequently prescribed antiemetic in its class. Prochlorperazine acts by blocking dopamine receptors in the brain, which inhibits signals to the vomiting center in the medulla. As an antiemetic, it is frequently given by the rectal route, where absorption is rapid. It is also available in tablet, extended-release capsule, and IM formulations.

ADMINISTRATION ALERTS

- Administer 2 hours before or after antacids and antidiarrheals.
- Pregnancy category C.

PHARMACOKINETICS

Onset: 30–40 min PO; 60 min rectal

Peak: Unknown

Half-life: Unknown

Duration: 3–4 h PO or rectal

ADVERSE EFFECTS

Prochlorperazine produces dose-related anticholinergic side effects such as dry mouth, sedation, constipation, orthostatic hypotension, and tachycardia. When used for prolonged periods at higher doses, extrapyramidal symptoms resembling those of Parkinson's disease are a serious concern.

Contraindications: This drug should not be used in clients with hypersensitivity to phenothiazines, in comatose clients or in the presence of profound CNS depression. It is also contraindicated in children younger than age 2 or weighing less than 20 lb.

INTERACTIONS

Drug–Drug: Prochlorperazine interacts with alcohol and other CNS depressants to cause additive sedation. Antacids and antidiarrheals inhibit the absorption of prochlorperazine. When taken with phenobarbital, metabolism of prochlorperazine is increased. Use with tricyclic antidepressants may produce increased anticholinergic and hypotensive effects.

Lab Tests: Unknown.

Herbal/Food: Unknown.

Treatment of Overdose: Overdose may result in serious CNS depression and extrapyramidal signs. Clients may be treated with antiparkinsonism drugs (for extrapyramidal symptoms) and possibly a CNS stimulant such as dextroamphetamine.

 See the Companion Website for a Nursing Process Focus specific to this drug.

gastric lavage tube is placed and attached to suction to empty gastric contents.

Client Teaching. Client education as it relates to antiemetics should include the goals of therapy, the reasons for obtaining baseline data such as vital signs and the existence of underlying disorders such as renal disorders, and possible drug side effects. Include the following points when teaching clients about antiemetics:

- Change positions slowly to avoid dizziness.
- Avoid driving or performing hazardous tasks until the effects of the drug are known.
- Immediately report vomiting of blood, or if the vomiting is associated with severe abdominal pain.
- Do not use OTC antiemetics for prolonged periods; vomiting may be a symptom of a serious disorder that requires medical attention.
- Before inducing vomiting with an OTC emetic, check with your healthcare provider; some poisons and caustic chemicals should not be vomited.

HUNGER AND APPETITE

Hunger occurs when the hypothalamus recognizes the levels of certain chemicals (glucose) or hormones (insulin) in the blood. Hunger is a normal physiological response that drives people to seek nourishment. Appetite is somewhat different than hunger. Appetite is a *psychological* response that drives food intake based on associations and memory. For example, people often eat not because they are experiencing hunger but because it is a particular time of day, or because they find the act of eating pleasurable or social.

ANOREXIANTS

Anorexiants are drugs used to induce weight loss by suppressing appetite and hunger. Despite the public's desire for effective drugs to promote weight loss, however, there are few such drugs on the market. The approved agents produce only modest effects.

41.9 Pharmacotherapy of Obesity

Obesity may be defined as being more than 20% above the ideal body weight. Because of the prevalence of obesity in society and the difficulty most clients experience when following weight reduction plans for extended periods, drug manufacturers have long sought to develop safe drugs that induce weight loss. In the 1970s, amphetamine and dextroamphetamine (Dexedrine) were widely prescribed to reduce appetite; however, these drugs are addictive and rarely prescribed for this purpose today. In the 1990s, the combination of fenfluramine and phentermine (fen-phen) was widely prescribed, until fenfluramine was removed from the market for causing heart valve defects. An OTC appetite suppressant, phenylpropanolamine, was removed from the market in 2000 owing to an increased incidence of strokes and adverse cardiac events. Until 2004, natural alternative weight-loss products

PROTOTYPE DRUG | Sibutramine *(Meridia)* | Anorexiant

ACTIONS AND USES

Sibutramine (Meridia), a selective serotonin reuptake inhibitor (SSRI), is the most widely prescribed appetite suppressant for the short-term control of obesity. When combined with a reduced-calorie diet, sibutramine may produce a gradual weight loss of at least 10% of initial body weight, over a period of a year. Sibutramine therapy is not recommended for longer than 1 year.

ADMINISTRATION ALERTS

- Allow at least 2 weeks between discontinuing MAO inhibitors and starting sibutramine.
- Pregnancy category C.

PHARMACOKINETICS

Onset: Unknown

Peak: 1.2 h

Half-life: 14–16 h

Duration: Unknown

ADVERSE EFFECTS

Headache is the most common complaint reported during sibutramine therapy, although insomnia and dry mouth also occur. It should be used with great care in clients with cardiac disorders, as it may cause tachycardia and raise blood pressure. It is a Schedule IV drug with low potential for dependence.

Contraindications: Sibutramine is contraindicated in clients with eating disorders (anorexia nervosa or bulimia) and those taking MAO inhibitors.

INTERACTIONS

Drug–Drug: Use with decongestants, cough, and allergy medications may cause elevated blood pressure. Ketoconazole and erythromycin may inhibit the metabolism of sibutramine. Concurrent use with a monoamine oxidase inhibitor (MAOI) or selective serotonin reuptake inhibitor (SSRI) may cause serotonin syndrome.

Lab Tests: Unknown.

Herbal/Food: Unknown.

Treatment of Overdose: Tachycardia and hypertension may result from overdose. Beta-adrenergic blockers may be administered.

 See the Companion Website for a Nursing Process Focus specific to this drug.

contained ephedra alkaloids, but these have been removed from the market because of an increased incidence of adverse cardiovascular events. The quest to produce a "magic pill" to lose weight has indeed been elusive.

One strategy to reduce weight is to block the absorption of dietary fats. Attempts to produce drugs that promote weight loss resulted in orlistat (Xenical), which acts to block lipid absorption in the GI tract. Unfortunately, orlistat may also decrease absorption of other substances, including fat-soluble vitamins and warfarin (Coumadin). To avoid having severe GI effects such as flatus with discharge, oily stool, abdominal pain, and discomfort, clients should restrict their fat intake when taking this drug. GI effects often diminish after 4 weeks of therapy. This drug produces only a very small increase in weight reduction compared with placebos.

Another strategy to reduce weight is to block parts of the nervous system responsible for hunger and appetite. Sibutramine (Meridia), a selective serotonin reuptake inhibitor (SSRI), is the most widely prescribed appetite suppressant for the short-term control of obesity. Two other SSRIs, fluoxetine (Prozac) and sertraline (Zoloft), produce a similar loss in weight, although they are not FDA approved for this purpose. Phentermine, once part of the now-banned combination of fen-phen, is still available as monotherapy, although it produces only a small, transient weight loss.

All the anorexiants have the potential to produce serious side effects; thus, their use is limited to short-term therapy. Anorexiants are prescribed for clients with a body mass index (BMI) of at least 30 or greater, or a BMI of 27 or greater, with other risk factors for disease such as hypertension, hyperlipidemia, or diabetes.

NURSING CONSIDERATIONS

The role of the nurse in anorexiant therapy involves careful monitoring of a client's condition and providing education as it relates to the prescribed drug treatment. When administering anorexiants, focus on lifestyle changes that will have a greater effect on weight reduction in the long term. Drugs for weight loss have limited effectiveness and potentially serious side effects.

Orlistat (Xenical) is contraindicated in malabsorption syndrome, cholestasis, and obesity due to organic causes. It is used with caution in clients with frequent diarrhea and those with known deficiencies of fat-soluble vitamins. Monitor blood glucose levels in clients with diabetes mellitus.

Amphetamine and other stimulant-type anorexiants can be dangerous owing to cardiovascular side effects such as hypertension, tachycardia, and dysrhythmias, and because of their potential for dependence. Closely monitor use of these drugs. Sibutramine is contraindicated in clients with cardiac conditions such as dysrhythmias, coronary artery disease, heart failure, or poorly controlled hypertension. It should not be administered concurrently with other SSRIs such as fluoxetine. Use sibutramine with caution in clients with a history of hypertension, seizures, and narrow-angle glaucoma. Prior to and during administration, obtain liver function tests, bilirubin levels, alkaline phosphatase levels, and lipid profiles. Assess heart rate and blood pressure regularly, and report sustained increases immediately.

Lifespan Considerations. Orlistat is contraindicated in pregnancy and lactation (pregnancy category B). Amphetamine and other stimulant-type anorexiants can be dangerous during pregnancy and lactation (pregnancy category C) because of cardiovascular side effects such as hypertension, tachycardia, and dysrhythmias and their potential for dependence. Sibutramine should not be used during pregnancy or lactation (pregnancy category C).

Client Teaching. Client education as it relates to these drugs should include the goals of therapy, the reasons for obtaining baseline data such as vital signs and the existence of underlying cardiac disorders, and possible drug side effects. Include the following points when teaching clients about anorexiants:

- Lifestyle modifications are necessary for sustained weight loss to occur; seek support groups for long-term weight management.
- Keep all scheduled appointments when taking amphetamines.
- Do not take other prescribed drugs, OTC medications, or herbal therapies, or vitamin supplements without notifying your healthcare provider.
- If taking orlistat:
  - Take a multivitamin each day.
  - Omit a dose if there is no fat present in a meal or a meal is skipped.
  - Know that excessive flatus and fecal leaking may occur when a high-fat meal is consumed.

PANCREATIC ENZYMES

The pancreas secretes essential digestive enzymes. The enzymatic portion of pancreatic juice contains carboxypeptidase, chymotrypsin, and trypsin, which are converted to their active forms once they reach the small intestine. Three other pancreatic enzymes—lipase, amylase, and nuclease—are secreted in their active form but require the presence of bile for optimum activity. Because lack of secretion will result in malabsorption disorders, replacement therapy is sometimes warranted.

41.10 Pharmacotherapy of Pancreatitis

Pancreatitis results when amylase and lipase remain in the pancreas rather than being released into the duodenum. The enzymes escape into the surrounding tissue, causing inflammation in the pancreas, or pancreatitis. Pancreatitis can be either acute or chronic.

Acute pancreatis usually occurs in middle-aged adults and is often associated with gallstones in women and alcoholism in men. Symptoms of acute pancreatitis present suddenly, often after eating a fatty meal or consuming excessive amounts of alcohol. The most common symptom is a continuous severe pain in the epigastric area that often radiates to the back. The client usually recovers from the

---

Pr **PROTOTYPE DRUG** | Pancrelipase *(Cotazym, Pancrease, others)* | Pancreatic Enzyme

ACTIONS AND USES

Pancrelipase contains lipase, protease, and amylase of pork origin. This agent facilitates the breakdown and conversion of lipids into glycerol and fatty acids, starches into dextrin and sugars, and proteins into peptides. Given orally, it is not absorbed, acts locally in the GI tract, and is excreted in the feces. It is used as replacement therapy for clients with insufficient pancreatic exocrine secretions, including pancreatitis and cystic fibrosis. Pancrelipase is available in powder, tablet, and delayed-release capsule formulations.

On an equal-eight basis, pancrelipase is more potent than pancretin, with 12 times the enzyme activity. It also contains at least 4 times as much trypsin and amylase.

ADMINISTRATION ALERTS

- Do not crush or open enteric-coated tablets.
- Powder formulations may be sprinkled on food.
- Give the drug 1–2 h before or with meals, or as directed by the healthcare provider.
- Pregnancy category C.

PHARMACOKINETICS

Onset: Unknown

Peak: Unknown

Half-life: Unknown

Duration: Unknown

ADVERSE EFFECTS

Side effects of pancrelipase are uncommon, since the enzymes are not absorbed. The most common side effects are GI symptoms of nausea, vomiting, and/or diarrhea; it can also cause metabolic symptom of hyperuricosuria.

Contraindications: Pancrelipase is contraindicated in clients allergic to the drug or to pork products. The delayed-release products should not be given to clients with acute pancreatitis.

INTERACTIONS

Drug–Drug: Pancrelipase interacts with iron, which may result in decreased absorption of iron.

Lab Tests: May increase serum or urinary levels of uric acid.

Herbal/Food: Unknown.

Treatment of Overdose: High levels of uric acid may occur with overdose. Clients are treated symptomatically.

 See the Companion Website for a Nursing Process Focus specific to this drug.

illness and regains normal function of the pancreas. Some clients with acute pancreatitis have recurring attacks and progress to chronic pancreatitis.

Many clients with acute pancreatitis require only bed rest and withholding food and fluids by mouth for a few days for the symptoms to subside. For clients with acute pain, meperidine (Demerol) brings effective relief. To reduce or neutralize gastric secretions, H_2-receptor blockers such as cimetidine (Tagamet) or proton pump inhibitors such as omeprazole (Prilosec) may be prescribed. To decrease the amount of pancreatic enzymes secreted, carbonic anhydrase inhibitors such as acetazolamide (Diamox) or antispasmodics such as dicyclomine (Bentyl) may be used. In particularly severe cases, IV fluids and total parenteral nutrition may be necessary.

The majority of chronic pancreatitis is associated with alcoholism. Alcohol is thought to promote the formation of insoluble proteins that occlude the pancreatic duct. Pancreatic juice is prevented from flowing into the duodenum and remains in the pancreas to damage cells and cause inflammation. Symptoms include chronic epigastric or left upper quadrant pain, anorexia, nausea, vomiting, and weight loss. **Steatorrhea,** the passing of bulky, foul-smelling fatty stools, occurs late in the course of the disease. Chronic pancreatitis eventually leads to pancreatic insufficiency that may necessitate insulin therapy as well as replacement of pancreatic enzymes.

Drugs prescribed for the treatment of acute pancreatitis may also be prescribed in cases of chronic pancreatitis. In addition, the client with chronic pancreatitis may require insulin and is likely to need antiemetics and a pancreatic enzyme supplement such as pancrelipase (Cotazym, Pancrease, others) or pancreatin (Creon, Pankreon, other) to digest fats, proteins, and complex carbohydrates.

NURSING CONSIDERATIONS

The role of the nurse in pancreatic enzyme replacement therapy involves careful monitoring of a client's condition and providing education as it relates to the prescribed drug treatment. Assessment of the client with acute or chronic pancreatitis includes a complete physical exam, health history, psychosocial history, and lifestyle history, including history of alcohol, drug, and tobacco use. Assess dietary habits for use of foods that stimulate gastric and pancreatic secretions such as spicy foods, gas-forming foods, cola drinks, coffee, and tea.

Assess for and monitor the presence, amount, and type of pain. Breathing patterns may be rapid and shallow due to pain. Monitor blood gases for hypercapnia. Assess the symmetry of the chest wall and the movement of the chest and diaphragm. The client with pancreatitis is at risk for atelectasis and pleural effusion. Monitor for other abnormal findings such as elevated serum and urinary amylase and elevated serum bilirubin. Also monitor the client's nutritional and hydration status and for signs of infection, which may be impaired owing to nausea and vomiting. Contraindications include a history of allergy to pork protein or enzymes,

because the drug has a porcine (pork) origin. Safety in pregnancy and lactation has not been established.

Client Teaching. Client education as it relates to pancreatic enzymes should include the goals of therapy, the reasons for obtaining baseline data such as vital signs and existence of underlying cardiac and renal disorders, and possible drug side effects. Include the following points when teaching clients about pancreatic enzyme replacements:

- Avoid alcohol use, smoking, spicy foods, gas-forming foods, cola drinks, coffee, and tea.
- Take pancreatic enzymes with meals or snacks.
- Weigh self and report significant changes.
- Observe stools for color, frequency, and consistency, and report abnormalities.
- Restrict fat intake, and eat smaller and more frequent meals.
- Report episodes of nausea and vomiting.
- Immediately report pain and seek relief before intensity increases.
- Sitting up, leaning forward, or curling in fetal position may help decrease pain.

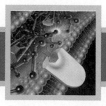

CHAPTER REVIEW

KEY CONCEPTS

The numbered key concepts provide a succinct summary of the important points from the corresponding numbered section within the chapter. If any of these points are not clear, refer to the numbered section within the chapter for review.

41.1 The small intestine is the location for most nutrient and drug absorption. The large intestine is responsible for the reabsorption of water.

41.2 Constipation, the infrequent passage of hard, small stools, is a common condition caused by insufficient dietary fiber and slow motility of waste material through the large intestine.

41.3 Laxatives and cathartics are drugs given to promote emptying of the large intestine by stimulating peristalsis, lubricating the fecal mass, or adding more bulk or water to the colon contents.

41.4 Diarrhea is an increase in the frequency and fluidity of bowel movements that occurs when the colon fails to reabsorb enough water.

41.5 For simple diarrhea, OTC medications such as loperamide or bismuth compounds are effective. Opioids are the most effective drugs for controlling severe diarrhea.

41.6 Inflammatory bowel disease includes ulcerative colitis and Crohn's disease. Treatment includes 5-aminosalicylic

acid (5-ASA) agents or glucocorticoids. Irritable bowel syndrome is often treated with tegaserod.

41.7 Vomiting is a defense mechanism used by the body to rid itself of toxic substances. Nausea is an uncomfortable feeling that may precede vomiting. Many drugs can cause nausea and vomiting as side effects.

41.8 Symptomatic treatment of nausea and vomiting includes drugs from many different classes, including phenothiazines, antihistamines, anticholinergics, cannabinoids, glucocorticoids, benzodiazepines, and serotonin receptor antagonists.

41.9 Anorexiants are drugs that affect hunger and/or appetite that are used for the short-term management of obesity. These drugs produce only modest effects.

41.10 Pancreatitis results when pancreatic enzymes are trapped in the pancreas and not released into the duodenum. Pharmacotherapy includes replacement enzymes and supportive drugs for reduction of pain and gastric acid secretion.

NCLEX-RN® REVIEW QUESTIONS

1 In a client with a prolonged episode of vomiting, the nurse must assess for the development of what problem?

1. Acid–base disturbances
2. Intractable diarrhea
3. Esophageal tears
4. Hypoventilation

2 The nurse should educate clients to take diphenhydrinate (Dramamine) how long before they board an airplane for a trip?

1. 20 to 60 minutes
2. 15 minutes
3. 2 hours
4. 6 hours

3 The nurse assesses for one of the major precipitating factors in the development IBS, which is:

1. Stress.
2. Peptic ulcers.
3. Gastroesophageal reflux disease (GERD).
4. *Helicobacter pylori.*

4 The client has been given a drug for treatment of nausea and vomiting and is now complaining of dry mouth, constipation, and a rapid heart rate. What drug would cause these side effects? (Select all that apply).

1. Loperamide (Immodium, Kaopectate)
2. Prochlorperazine (Compazine)
3. Peppermint
4. Diphenoxylate (Lomotil)
5. Promethazine hydrochloride (Phenergan)

5 The client has been prescribed sibutramine (Meridia) for obesity. The nurse assesses for what as a possible contraindication? (Select all that apply.)

1. Uncontrolled hypertension
2. Hepatic impairment
3. Renal impairment
4. Coronary artery disease (CAD)
5. Bowel obstruction

CRITICAL THINKING QUESTIONS

1. The client has been taking diphenoxylate (Lomotil) for diarrhea for the past 3 days. The client has had diarrhea five times today. Identify the priorities of nursing care.

2. The healthcare provider has ordered morphine and prochlorperazine (Compazine) for a client with postoperative pain. The client insists that she is "needle phobic" and wants all the medication in one syringe. What is the nurse's response?

3. A client comes to the clinic complaining of no bowel movement for 4 days (other than small amounts of liquid stool). The client has been taking psyllium mucilloid (Metamucil) for his constipation and wants to know why this is not working. What is the nurse's response?

See Appendix D for answers and rationales for all activities.

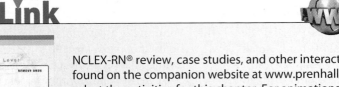

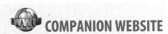

www.prenhall.com/adams

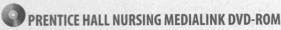

NCLEX-RN® review, case studies, and other interactive resources for this chapter can be found on the companion website at www.prenhall.com/adams. Click on "Chapter 41" to select the activities for this chapter. For animations, more NCLEX-RN® review questions, and an audio glossary, access the accompanying Prentice Hall Nursing MediaLink DVD-ROM in this textbook.

PRENTICE HALL NURSING MEDIALINK DVD-ROM

- **Animation**
  Mechanism of Action: Tegaserod (*Zelnorm*)
- **Audio Glossary**
- **NCLEX-RN® Review**

COMPANION WEBSITE

- **NCLEX-RN® Review**
- **Dosage Calculations**
- **Case Study:** Constipation and diarrhea
- **Care Plan:** Client with chronic diarrhea who has been prescribed loperamide

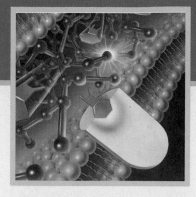

CHAPTER 42

Drugs for Nutritional Disorders

DRUGS AT A GLANCE

VITAMINS
Lipid Soluble
   💊 *vitamin A*
Water Soluble
   💊 *folic acid (Folacin, Folvite)*
MINERALS
Macrominerals
   💊 *magnesium sulfate*
Microminerals
NUTRITIONAL SUPPLEMENTS
Enteral Nutrition
Parenteral Nutrition

OBJECTIVES

After reading this chapter, the student should be able to:

1. Identify characteristics that differentiate vitamins from other nutrients.
2. Describe the functions of common vitamins and minerals.
3. Compare and contrast the properties of water-soluble and fat-soluble vitamins.
4. Identify diseases and conditions that may benefit from vitamin or mineral pharmacotherapy.
5. Describe the nurse's role in the pharmacological management of nutritional disorders.
6. Compare and contrast the properties of macrominerals and trace minerals.
7. Identify differences among oligomeric, polymeric, modular, and specialized formulations for enteral nutrition.
8. Compare and contrast enteral and parenteral methods of providing nutrition.
9. For each of the drug classes listed in Drug at a Glance, know representative drugs, and explain the mechanism of drug action, describe primary actions, and identify important adverse effects.
10. Use the Nursing Process to care for clients who are receiving drug therapy for nutritional disorders.

MediaLink

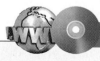

www.prenhall.com/adams

NCLEX-RN® review, case studies, and other interactive resources for this chapter can be found on the companion website at www.prenhall.com/adams. Click on "Chapter 42" to select the activities for this chapter. For animations, more NCLEX-RN® review questions, and an audio glossary, access the accompanying Prentice Hall Nursing MediaLink DVD-ROM in this textbook.

KEY TERMS

beriberi   *page 646*

carotene   *page 644*

enteral nutrition   *page 654*

ergocalciferol   *page 645*

hypervitaminosis   *page 644*

macromineral (major mineral)   *page 651*

micromineral (trace mineral)   *page 653*

pellagra   *page 646*

pernicious (megaloblastic) anemia   *page 647*

provitamins   *page 642*

Recommended Dietary Allowance (RDA)
   page 643

scurvy   *page 647*

tocopherol   *page 645*

total parenteral nutrition (TPN)   *page 655*

undernutrition   *page 654*

vitamins   *page 642*

The nutritional supplement business is a multibillion-dollar industry. Although clever marketing often leads clients to believe that vitamin and dietary supplements are essential to maintain health, most people obtain all the necessary nutrients through a balanced diet. Once the body has obtained the amounts of vitamins, minerals, or nutrients it needs to carry on metabolism, the excess is simply excreted or stored. In certain conditions, however, dietary supplementation is necessary and benefits the client's health. This chapter focuses on these conditions and explores the role of vitamins, minerals, and nutritional supplements in pharmacology.

VITAMINS

Vitamins are essential substances needed in very small amounts to maintain homeostasis. Clients having a low or unbalanced dietary intake, those who are pregnant, or those experiencing a chronic disease may benefit from vitamin therapy.

42.1 Role of Vitamins in Maintaining Health

Vitamins are organic compounds required by the body in small amounts for growth and for the maintenance of normal metabolic processes. Since the discovery of thiamine in 1911, more than a dozen vitamins have been identified. Because scientists did not know the chemical structures of the vitamins when they were discovered, they assigned letters and numbers such as A, B_{12}, and C. These names are still widely used today.

An important characteristic of vitamins is that, with the exception of vitamin D, human cells cannot synthesize them. They, or their precursors known as **provitamins,** must be supplied in the diet. A second important characteristic is that if the vitamin is not present in adequate amounts, then the body's metabolism will be disrupted and disease will result. However, the symptoms of the deficiency can be reversed by administering the missing vitamin.

Vitamins serve diverse and important roles. For example, the B-complex vitamins are coenzymes essential to many metabolic pathways. Vitamin A is a precursor of retinal, a pigment needed for vision. Calcium metabolism is regulated by a hormone that is derived from vitamin D. Without vitamin K, abnormal prothrombin is produced, and blood clotting is affected.

42.2 Classification of Vitamins

A simple way to classify vitamins is by their ability to mix with water. Those that dissolve easily in water are called *water-soluble* vitamins. Examples include vitamin C and the B vitamins. Those that dissolve in lipids are called *fat-* or *lipid-soluble* and include vitamins A, D, E, and K.

PHARMFACTS

Vitamins, Minerals, and Nutritional Supplements

- About 40% of Americans take vitamin supplements daily.
- There is no difference between the chemical structure of a natural vitamin and a synthetic vitamin, yet consumers pay much more for the natural type.
- Vitamin B_{12} is present only in animal products. Vegetarians may find adequate amounts in fortified cereals, nutritional supplements, or yeast.
- Administration of folic acid during pregnancy has been found to reduce birth defects in the nervous system of the baby.
- Clients who never go outside or never receive sun exposure may need vitamin D supplements.
- Vitamins technically cannot increase a client's energy level. Energy can be provided only by adding calories from carbohydrates, proteins, and lipids.
- Heavy menstrual periods may result in considerable iron loss.

The difference in solubility affects the way the vitamins are absorbed by the gastrointestinal (GI) tract and stored in the body. The water-soluble vitamins are absorbed with water in the digestive tract and readily dissolve in blood and body fluids. When excess water-soluble vitamins are absorbed, they cannot be stored for later use and are simply excreted in the urine. Because they are not stored to any significant degree, they must be ingested daily; otherwise, deficiencies will quickly develop.

Fat-soluble vitamins, on the other hand, cannot be absorbed in sufficient quantity in the small intestine unless they are ingested with other lipids. These vitamins can be stored in large quantities in the liver and adipose tissue. Should the client not ingest sufficient amounts, fat-soluble vitamins are removed from storage depots in the body, as needed. Unfortunately, storage may lead to dangerously high levels of these vitamins if they are taken in excessive amounts.

42.3 Recommended Dietary Allowances

Based on scientific research on humans and animals, the Food and Nutrition Board of the National Academy of Sciences has established levels for the dietary intake of vitamins and minerals called **Recommended Dietary Allowances (RDAs).** Canada publishes similar data called the Recommended Nutrient Intake (RNI). The RDA values represent the *minimum* amount of vitamin or mineral needed to prevent a deficiency in a healthy adult. The RDAs are revised periodically to reflect the latest scientific research. Current RDAs for vitamins are listed in Table 42.1.

The need for certain vitamins and minerals varies widely. Clients who are pregnant, have chronic disease, or exercise vigorously have different nutritional needs from those of the average adult. Recognizing and adjusting for these nutritional differences is essential to maintaining good health.

Vitamin, mineral, or herbal supplements should never substitute for a balanced diet. Sufficient intake of proteins, carbohydrates, and lipids is needed for proper health. Furthermore, although the label on a vitamin supplement may indicate that it contains 100% of the RDA for a particular vitamin, the body may absorb as little as 10% to 15% of the amount ingested. With the exception of vitamins A and D, it is not harmful for most clients to consume two to three times the recommended levels of vitamins.

TABLE 42.1   Vitamins

Vitamin	Function(s)	RDA Men	RDA Women	Common cause(s) of deficiency
A	visual pigments, epithelial cells	1,000 mg RE*	800 mg RE	prolonged dietary deprivation, particularly when rice is the main food source; pancreatic disease; cirrhosis
B complex: biotin	coenzyme in metabolic reactions	30 mcg	30 mcg	deficiencies are rare
cyanocobalamin (B$_{12}$)	coenzyme in nucleic acid metabolism	2 mcg	2 mcg	lack of intrinsic factor, inadequate intake of foods from animal origin
folate	coenzyme in amino acid and nucleic acid metabolism	200 mcg	160–180 mcg	pregnancy, alcoholism, cancer, oral contraceptive use
niacin (B$_3$)	coenzyme in oxidation–reduction reactions	15–20 mg	13–15 mg	prolonged dietary deprivation, particularly when Indian corn (maize) or millet is the main food source; chronic diarrhea; liver disease; alcoholism
pantothenic acid	coenzyme in metabolic reactions	5 mg	5 mg	deficiencies are rare
pyridoxine (B$_6$)	coenzyme in amino acid metabolism	2 mg	1.5–1.6 mg	alcoholism, oral contraceptive use, malabsorption diseases
riboflavin (B$_2$)	coenzyme in oxidation–reduction reactions	1.4–1.8 mg	1.2–1.3 mg	inadequate consumption of milk or animal products, chronic diarrhea, liver disease, alcoholism
thiamine (B$_1$)	coenzyme in metabolic reactions	1.2–1.5 mg	1.0–1.1 mg	prolonged dietary deprivation, particularly when rice is the main food source; hyperthyroidism; pregnancy; liver disease; alcoholism
C	coenzyme and antioxidant	60 mg	60 mg	inadequate intake of fruits and vegetables, pregnancy, chronic inflammatory disease, burns, diarrhea, alcoholism
D	calcium and phosphate metabolism	5–10 mg	5–10 mg	low dietary intake, inadequate exposure to sunlight
E	antioxidant	10 TE**	8 mg TE	prematurity, malabsorption diseases
K	cofactor in blood clotting	65–80 mcg	55–65 mcg	newborns, liver disease, long-term parenteral nutrition, certain drugs such as cephalosporins and salicylates

*RE = retinoid equivalents; **TE = alpha-tocopherol equivalents

42.4 Indications for Vitamin Pharmacotherapy

Most people who eat a normal, balanced diet obtain all the necessary nutrients without vitamin supplementation. Indeed, megavitamin therapy is not only expensive but also harmful to health if taken for long periods. **Hypervitaminosis,** or toxic levels of vitamins, has been reported for vitamins A, C, D, E, B_6, niacin, and folic acid. In the United States, it is actually more common to observe syndromes of vitamin *excess* than of vitamin *deficiency*.

Vitamin deficiencies follow certain patterns. The following are general characteristics of vitamin deficiency disorders:

- Clients more commonly present with *multiple* vitamin deficiencies than with a single vitamin deficiency.
- Symptoms of deficiency are *nonspecific,* and often do not appear until the deficiency has been present for a long period.
- Deficiencies in the United States are most often the result of poverty, fad diets, chronic alcohol or drug abuse, or prolonged parenteral feeding.

Certain clients and conditions require higher levels of vitamins. Infancy and childhood are times of potential deficiency owing to the high growth demands placed on the body. In addition, requirements for all nutrients are increased during pregnancy and lactation. With normal aging, the absorption of food diminishes and the quantity of ingested food is often reduced, leading to a higher risk of vitamin deficiencies in elderly clients. Vitamin deficiencies in clients with chronic liver and kidney disease are well documented.

Certain drugs have the potential to affect vitamin metabolism. Alcohol is known for its ability to inhibit the absorption of thiamine and folic acid: Alcohol abuse is the most common cause of thiamine deficiency in the United States. Folic acid levels may be reduced in clients taking phenothiazines, oral contraceptives, phenytoin (Dilantin), or barbiturates. Vitamin D deficiency can be caused by therapy with certain anticonvulsants. Inhibition of vitamin B_{12} absorption has been reported with a number of drugs, including trifluoperazine (Stelazine), alcohol, and oral contraceptives. The nurse must be aware of these drug interactions and recommend vitamin therapy when appropriate.

LIPID-SOLUBLE VITAMINS

The lipid- or fat-soluble vitamins are abundant in both plant and animal foods, and are relatively stable during cooking. Because the body stores them, it is not necessary to ingest the recommended amounts on a daily basis.

42.5 Pharmacotherapy With Lipid-soluble Vitamins

Lipid-soluble vitamins are absorbed from the intestine with dietary lipids and are stored primarily in the liver. When consumed in high amounts, these vitamins can accumulate to toxic levels and produce hypervitaminosis. Because these are OTC agents, clients must be strongly advised to carefully follow the instructions of the healthcare provider, or the label directions, for proper dosage. It is not unusual to find some over-the-counter (OTC) preparations that contain 200% to 400% of the RDA. Medications containing lipid-soluble vitamins, and their doses, are listed in Table 42.2.

Vitamin A, also known as *retinol,* is obtained from foods containing **carotenes,** precursors to vitamin A that are converted to retinol in the wall of the small intestine following absorption. The most abundant and biologically active carotene is beta-carotene. During metabolism, each molecule of beta-carotene yields two molecules of vitamin A. Good sources of dietary vitamin A include yellow and dark leafy vegetables, butter, eggs, whole milk, and liver.

TABLE 42.2 Lipid-soluble Vitamins for Treating Nutritional Disorders

Drug	Route and Adult Dose (max dose where indicated)	Adverse Effects
↻ vitamin A (Aquasol A)	PO; 500,000 units/day for 3 days, followed by 50,000 units/day for 2 wk; then 10,000–20,000 units/day for 2 mo IM; 100,000 units/day for 3 days followed by 50,000 units/day for 2 wk	*Side effects are uncommon at normal doses* High doses: nausea, vomiting, fatigue, irritability, night sweats, alopecia, dry skin
vitamin D: calcitriol (Calcijex, Rocaltrol)	PO; 0.25 mcg/day; may be increased by 0.25 mcg/day q4–8wk for dialysis clients or q2–4wk for hypoparathyroid clients, if necessary IV; 0.5 mcg 3 times/wk at the end of dialysis; may need up to 3 mcg 3 times/wk	*Side effects are uncommon at normal doses* High doses: nausea, vomiting, fatigue, headache, polyuria, weight loss, hallucinations, dysrhythmias
vitamin E: tocopherol (Aquasol E, Vita-Plus E, others)	PO/IM; 60–75 units /day	*Side effects are uncommon at normal doses* High doses: nausea, vomiting, fatigue, headache, blurred vision
vitamin K: phytonadione (AquaMEPHYTON)	PO/IM/subcutaneous; 2.5–10 mg (up to 25 mg), may be repeated after 6–8 h if needed	*Facial flushing, pain at injection site* IV route may result in dyspnea, hypotension, shock, cardiac arrest

Italics indicate common adverse effects; <u>underlining</u> indicates serious adverse effects.

Vitamin D is actually a group of chemicals sharing similar activity. Vitamin D_2, also known as **ergocalciferol,** is obtained from fortified milk, margarine, and other dairy products. Vitamin D_3 is formed in the skin by a chemical reaction requiring ultraviolet radiation. The pharmacology of the D vitamins and a drug prototype for the active form of vitamin D are detailed in Chapter 46 ∞.

Vitamin E consists of about eight chemicals, called **tocopherols,** having similar activity. Alpha-tocopherol constitutes 90% of the tocopherols, and is the only one of pharmacological importance. Dosage of vitamin E is sometimes reported as milligrams of alpha-tocopherol equivalents (TE). Vitamin E is found in plant-seed oils, whole-grain cereals, eggs, and certain organ meats such as liver, pancreas, and heart. It is considered a primary antioxidant, preventing the formation of free radicals that damage plasma membranes and other cellular structures. Deficiency in adults has been observed only with severe malabsorption disorders; however, deficiency in premature neonates may lead to hemolytic anemia. Clients often self-administer vitamin E because it is thought to be useful in preventing heart disease and increasing sexual prowess, although research has not always supported these claims. Unlike with most other vitamins, therapeutic doses of vitamin E have not been clearly established, although available OTC supplements suggest doses of 100 to 400 units per day. In addition to oral and IM preparations, a topical form is available to treat dry, cracked skin.

Vitamin K is also a mixture of several chemicals. Vitamin K_1 is found in plant sources, particularly green leafy vegetables, tomatoes, and cauliflower, an in egg yolks, liver, and cheeses. Vitamin K_2 is synthesized by microbial flora in the colon. Deficiency states, caused by inadequate intake or by antibiotic destruction of normal intestinal flora, may result in delayed hemostasis. The body does not have large stores of vitamin K, and a deficiency may occur in only 1 to 2 weeks. Certain clotting factors (II, VII, IX, and X) are dependent on vitamin K for their biosynthesis. Vitamin K is used as a treatment for clients with clotting disorders and is the antidote for warfarin (Coumadin) overdose. It is also given to infants at birth to promote blood clotting. Administration of vitamin K completely reverses deficiency symptoms.

SPECIAL CONSIDERATIONS

Vitamin Supplements and Client Communication

Product advertising promotes vitamin supplements as a means to maintain optimal health. If vitamins are taken in recommended dosages, toxicity is not a concern in healthy people; however, some vitamin supplements should be taken with caution because they can interact with prescribed medications. Some products are fortified with vitamins or minerals. For example, certain manufacturers claim that their cereals and juices have 100% of the RDA for particular vitamins and minerals. People who take supplements may not consider these fortified foods as vitamin sources, and accidental overdosage can result.

Healthcare providers should adopt a nonjudgmental attitude that promotes trust and honest communication with the client. In this way, the client will be open about the use of vitamin and nutritional supplements. Acceptance and understanding are necessary to help clients take vitamins in a responsible way that does not compromise clinical drug treatment.

Pr **PROTOTYPE DRUG** | Vitamin A *(Aquasol A)* | Lipid-soluble Vitamin

ACTIONS AND USES

Vitamin A is essential for general growth and development, particularly of the bones, teeth, and epithelial membranes. It is necessary for proper wound healing, is essential for the biosynthesis of steroids, and is one of the pigments required for night vision. Vitamin A is indicated in deficiency states and during periods of increased need such as pregnancy, lactation, or undernutrition. Night blindness and slow wound healing can be effectively treated with as little as 30,000 units of vitamin A given daily over a week. It is also prescribed for GI disorders, when absorption in the small intestine is diminished or absent. Topical forms are available for acne, psoriasis, and other skin disorders. Doses of vitamin A are sometimes measured in retinoid equivalents (RE). In severe deficiency states, up to 500,000 units may be given per day for 3 days, gradually tapering off to 10,000 to 20,000 units /day.

ADMINISTRATION ALERTS

- Pregnancy category A at low doses.
- Pregnancy category X at high doses.

PHARMACOKINETICS

Onset: Unknown

Peak: Unknown

Half-life: Unknown

Duration: Unknown

ADVERSE EFFECTS

Adverse effects are not observed with low doses of vitamin A. Acute ingestion produces serious CNS toxicity, including headache, irritability, drowsiness, delirium, and possible coma. Long-term ingestion of high amounts causes drying and scaling of the skin, alopecia, fatigue, anorexia, vomiting, and leukopenia.

Contraindications: Vitamin A in excess of the RDA is contraindicated in pregnant clients, or those who may become pregnant. Fetal harm may result.

INTERACTIONS

Drug–Drug: People taking vitamin A should avoid taking mineral oil and cholestyramine, because both may decrease the absorption of vitamin A. Concurrent use with isoretinoin may result in additive toxicity.

Lab Tests: Unknown.

Herbal/Food: Unknown.

Treatment of Overdose: There is no specific treatment for overdose.

 See the Companion Website for a Nursing Process Focus specific to this vitamin.

NURSING CONSIDERATIONS

The role of the nurse in drug therapy with fat-soluble vitamins involves careful monitoring of a client's condition and providing education as it relates to the prescribed drug treatment. The nurse is responsible for assessing, counseling, and monitoring clients taking fat-soluble vitamins. Because these vitamins are available OTC, clients consider them relatively harmless. Teach clients that excessive vitamin intake can be harmful.

For all fat-soluble vitamin therapy, begin with assessment for deficiency. The symptoms of inadequate supply or storage of fat-soluble vitamins are dependent on the specific nutrient. For example, clients deficient in vitamin A frequently report problems with night vision, skin lesions, or mucous membrane dysfunction. A baseline visual acuity exam should be performed. In severe vitamin D deficiency, clients experience skeletal abnormalities, such as rickets in children and osteomalacia in adults. Assess laboratory tests for serum levels of calcium, phosphorus, magnesium, alkaline phosphatase (ALP), and creatinine to determine electrolyte and mineral balance. An insufficient level of vitamin E has no obvious effects, but the vitamin is believed to protect cellular components from oxidation. Bleeding tendencies are characteristic of vitamin K deficiency. Assess clients for impaired liver function, because fat-soluble vitamins are stored in the liver, and for malabsorption disorders that could prevent the absorption of the vitamins.

Include a history of the client's dietary intake in your assessment. Instruct clients about foods that may supply the necessary fat-soluble vitamins essential for good health. When performing dietary counseling, consider the socioeconomic status and culture of the client. Recommend foods that both treat the deficiency and are affordable for and liked by the client.

Fat-soluble vitamins stored in the liver can accumulate to toxic levels, causing accidental hypervitaminosis. Chronic overdose affects many organs, including the liver. Excessive vitamin A intake during pregnancy can result in severe birth defects. Intravenous infusion of vitamin K is used only in emergency situations because it may cause bronchospasm, and respiratory and cardiac arrest. Large doses of vitamin E appear to be nontoxic; however, monitor clients who are concurrently taking warfarin (Coumadin) for increased risk of bleeding.

Client Teaching. Client education as it relates to fat-soluble vitamins should include the goals of therapy; the reasons for obtaining baseline data such as lab tests for liver function and CBC, and the existence of possible underlying disorders such as anemia; and possible drug side effects. Include the following points when teaching clients about fat-soluble vitamins:

- Keep all scheduled laboratory visits for testing.
- Take vitamins only as prescribed or as directed on the label. Do not double doses.
- If you are taking medications, notify your healthcare provider before adding an OTC medication, herbal therapy, or vitamin supplement.

- Immediately report nausea, vision difficulties, hair loss, diarrhea, and lethargy or malaise.
- Include vitamin-rich foods in your diet.

See the companion website for "Nursing Process Focus: Clients Receiving Vitamin A (Aquasol)."

WATER-SOLUBLE VITAMINS

The water-soluble vitamins consist of the B-complex vitamins and vitamin C. These vitamins must be consumed on a daily basis because they are not stored in the body.

42.6 Pharmacotherapy With Water-soluble Vitamins

The B-complex group of vitamins comprises of 12 different substances that are grouped together because they were originally derived from yeast and foods that counteracted the disease beriberi. They have very different chemical structures and serve different metabolic functions. The B vitamins are known by their chemical names as well as their vitamin number. For example, vitamin B_{12} is also called *cyanocobalamin*. Medications containing water-soluble vitamins, and their doses, are listed in Table 42.3.

Vitamin B_1, or *thiamine*, is a precursor of an enzyme responsible for several steps in the oxidation of carbohydrates. It is abundant in both plant and animal products, especially whole-grain foods, dried beans, and peanuts. Because of the vitamin's abundance, thiamine deficiency in the United States is not common, except in alcoholics and in clients with chronic liver disease. Thiamine deficiency, or **beriberi**, is characterized by neurological signs such as paresthesia, neuralgia, and progressive loss of feeling and reflexes. Chronic deficiency can result in heart failure. Severe deficiencies may require parenteral thiamine up to 100 mg/day. With pharmacotherapy, symptoms can be completely reversed in the early stages of the disease; however, permanent disability can result in clients with prolonged deficiency.

Vitamin B_2, or *riboflavin*, is a component of coenzymes that participate in a number of different oxidation–reduction reactions. Riboflavin is abundantly found in plant and meat products, including wheat germ, eggs, cheese, fish, nuts, and leafy vegetables. As with thiamine, deficiency of riboflavin is most commonly observed in alcoholics. Signs of deficiency include corneal vascularization and anemia, as well as skin abnormalities such as dermatitis and cheilosis. Most symptoms resolve by administering 25 to 100 mg/day of the vitamin until improvement is observed.

Vitamin B_3, or *niacin*, is a key component of coenzymes essential for oxidative metabolism. Niacin is synthesized from the amino acid tryptophan and is widely distributed in both animal and plant foodstuffs, including beans, wheat germ, meats, nuts, and whole-grain breads. Niacin deficiency, or **pellagra**, is most commonly seen in alcoholics, and in those areas of the world where corn is the primary food source. Early symptoms include fatigue, anorexia, and drying of the skin. Advanced symptoms include three classic signs: dermatitis, diarrhea, and dementia. Deficiency is treated with

TABLE 42.3   Water-soluble Vitamins for Treating Nutritional Disorders

Drug	Route and Adult Dose (max dose where indicated)	Adverse Effects
vitamin B_1: thiamine hydrochloride (Betalins, Biamine)	IV/IM; 50–100 mg tid	*Pain at injection site* IV route may result in angioedema, cyanosis, pulmonary edema, GI bleeding, and cardiovascular collapse
vitamin B_2: riboflavin	PO; 5–10 mg/day	*Side effects have not been reported*
vitamin B_3: niacin (Niac, Nicobid, Nicolar, others)	PO; 10–20 mg/day IV/IM/subcutaneous; 25–100 mg 2–5 times/day	*Side effects are uncommon at doses used for vitamin therapy* High doses: dysrhythmias
vitamin B_6: pyridoxine hydrochloride (Beesix, hexaBetalin, NesTrex)	PO/IM/IV; 2.5–10 mg/day for 3 wk; then may reduce to 2.5–5 mg/day	*Pain at injection site* High doses: neuropathy, ataxia, seizures
⊙ vitamin B_9: folic acid (Folacin, Folvite)	PO/IM/IV/subcutaneous; 0.4–1 mg/day	*Side effects are uncommon at normal doses* Parenteral routes: allergic hypersensitivity
vitamin B_{12}: cyanocobalamin (Betalin 12, Cobex, Cyanabin, others) (see page 403 for the Prototype Drug Box ∞)	IM/deep subcutaneous; 30 mcg/day for 5–10 day; then 100–200 mcg/mo	*Rash, diarrhea* High doses: thrombosis, hypokalemia, pulmonary edema, heart failure
vitamin C: ascorbic acid (Ascorbicap, Cebid, Vita-C, others)	PO/IV/IM/subcutaneous; 150–500 mg/day in 1–2 doses	*Side effects are uncommon at normal doses* High doses: deep vein thrombosis (IV route), crystalluria

Italics indicate common adverse effects; underlining indicates serious adverse effects.

niacin at dosages ranging from 10 to 25 mg/day. When used to treat hyperlipidemia, niacin is given as nicotinic acid, and doses are much higher—up to 3 g/day (Chapter 22).

Vitamin B_6, or *pyridoxine,* consists of several closely related compounds, including pyridoxine itself, pyridoxal, and pyridoxamine. Vitamin B_6 is essential for the synthesis of heme, and is a primary coenzyme involved in the metabolism of amino acids. Deficiency states can result from alcoholism, uremia, hypothyroidism, or heart failure. Certain drugs can also cause vitamin B_6 deficiency, including isoniazid (INH), cycloserine (Seromycin), hydralazine (Apresoline), oral contraceptives, and pyrazinamide (PZA). Clients receiving these drugs may routinely receive B_6 supplementation. Deficiency symptoms include skin abnormalities, cheilosis, fatigue, and irritability. Symptoms reverse after administration of about 10 to 20 mg/day for several weeks.

Vitamin B_9, more commonly known as *folate* or *folic acid,* is metabolized to tetrahydrofolate, which is essential for normal DNA synthesis and for erythropoiesis. Folic acid is widely distributed in plant products, especially green leafy vegetables and citrus fruits. This vitamin is highlighted as a drug prototype in this chapter.

Vitamin B_{12}, or cyanocobalamin, is a cobalt-containing vitamin that is a required coenzyme for a number of metabolic pathways. It also has important roles in cell replication, erythrocyte maturation, and myelin synthesis. Sources include lean meat, seafood, liver, and milk. Deficiency of vitamin

B_{12} results in **pernicious (megaloblastic) anemia.** This vitamin is featured as a prototype drug in Chapter 28 ∞.

Vitamin C, or *ascorbic acid,* is the most commonly purchased OTC vitamin. It is a potent antioxidant, and serves many functions including collagen synthesis, tissue healing, and maintenance of bone, teeth, and epithelial tissue. Many consumers purchase the vitamin for its ability to prevent the common cold, a function that has not been definitively proved. Deficiency of vitamin C, or **scurvy,** is caused by diets lacking fruits and vegetables. Alcoholics, cigarette smokers, cancer clients, and those with renal failure are at highest risk for vitamin C deficiency. Symptoms include fatigue, bleeding gums and other hemorrhages, gingivitis, and poor wound

NATURAL THERAPIES

Vitamin C and the Common Cold

Although there is a great deal of anecdotal evidence that vitamin C helps to fend off a cold, the claims are unsubstantiated; however, vitamin C may be useful as an immune stimulator and modulator in some circumstances. Several studies have shown that vitamin C can significantly reduce the duration and severity of colds in some people and reduce the incidence in others. It is thought that this effect is due, at least in part, to antihistamine activity of vitamin C. The best results were obtained with 2-g (or greater) daily doses. Preliminary evidence also suggests that vitamin C can be useful in improving respiratory infections. However, the most recent review of evidence shows that vitamin C fails to reduce the *incidence* of colds (Douglas, 2006).

Pr PROTOTYPE DRUG | Folic Acid *(Folacin, Folvite)* | Water-soluble Vitamin

ACTIONS AND USES

Folic acid is administered to reverse symptoms of deficiency, which most commonly occurs in clients with inadequate intake, such as with chronic alcohol abuse. Because this vitamin is destroyed at high temperatures, people who overcook their food may experience folate deficiency. Pregnancy markedly increases the need for dietary folic acid; folic acid is given during pregnancy to promote normal fetal growth. Because insufficient vitamin B_{12} creates a lack of activated folic acid, deficiency symptoms resemble those of vitamin B_{12} deficiency. The megaloblastic anemia observed in folate-deficient clients, however, does not include the severe nervous system symptoms seen in clients with B_{12} deficiency. Administration of 1 mg/day of oral folic acid often reverses the deficiency symptoms within 5 to 7 days.

ADMINISTRATION ALERTS

- Pregnancy category A.

PHARMACOKINETICS

Onset: Unknown

Peak: 30–60 min

Half-life: Unknown

Duration: Unknown

ADVERSE EFFECTS

Side effects during folic acid therapy are uncommon. Clients may feel flushed following IV injections. Allergic hypersensitivity to folic acid by the IV route is possible.

Contraindications: Folic acid is contraindicated in anemias other than those caused by folate deficiency.

INTERACTIONS

Drug–Drug: Phenytoin, trimethoprim–sulfasoxazole, and other medications may interfere with the absorption of folic acid. Chloramphenicol may antagonize effects of folate therapy. Oral contraceptives, alcohol, barbiturates, methotrexate, and primidone may cause folate deficiency.

Lab Tests: May decrease serum levels of vitamin B_{12}.

Herbal/Food: Unknown.

Treatment of Overdose: There is no specific treatment for overdose.

---

healing. Symptoms can normally be reversed by the administration of 300 to 1,000 mg/day of vitamin C for several weeks.

NURSING CONSIDERATIONS

The role of the nurse in water-soluble vitamin therapy involves careful monitoring of a client's condition and providing education as it relates to the prescribed drug treatment. Water-soluble vitamins are used for multiple reasons in health care. Determine the reason for the specific vitamin therapy being prescribed, and assess for the presence or absence of the associated symptoms.

Thiamine is often administered to hospitalized clients who have severe liver disease. If thiamine deficiency is not corrected in these clients, irreversible brain damage can occur. There are no known adverse effects from oral administration of thiamine, and parenteral administration rarely causes any type of adverse effect. Niacin may be administered in the treatment of niacin deficiency or as an adjunct in cholesterol-lowering therapy. Pyridoxine deficiency is also associated with poor nutritional status, chronic debilitating diseases, and alcohol abuse. Both niacin and pyridoxine may cause severe flushing. Inform the client that this is an expected reaction and will not cause permanent harm. Most clients tolerate therapy with B vitamins with few adverse effects.

Assess menstruating women for folic acid deficiency, especially prior to their attempting pregnancy and during pregnancy (see "Home/Community Considerations"). Recommend that adequate levels be obtained from a multivitamin to avoid overdose.

Vitamin C may cause diarrhea, nausea, vomiting, abdominal pain, and hyperuricemia in high doses. Caution clients with a history of kidney stones against using vitamin C, unless directed by a healthcare provider, because excessive intake may promote renal calculi formation. Advise clients taking vitamin C to increase fluid intake. Most clients are able to take vitamin C without experiencing serious side effects.

Client Teaching. Client education as it relates to water-soluble vitamins should include the goals of therapy; the reasons for obtaining baseline data such as lab tests for liver function and CBC, and the existence of underlying disorders such as kidney stones; and possible drug side effects. Include the following points when teaching clients about water-soluble vitamins:

- Keep all scheduled laboratory visits for hemoglobin and hematocrit tests.
- Niacin and pyridoxine may cause a feeling of warmth and flushing of skin, but this will diminish with continued therapy.

HOME & COMMUNITY CONSIDERATIONS

Vitamin B_9 and Neural Tube Defects

It has recently been determined that low vitamin B_9 (folic acid) levels in pregnant women may contribute to the formation of neural tube defects in the fetus. Women's healthcare providers are now suggesting that young women begin taking folic acid prior to attempting pregnancy. It has not been determined how long a woman must take folic acid prior to conception, but it is now being suggested that young women begin taking the supplement as soon as menstruation begins. To avoid possible overdoses, most healthcare providers recommend taking a daily multivitamin that contains folic acid.

NURSING PROCESS FOCUS   Clients Receiving Folic Acid

Assessment	Potential Nursing Diagnoses
Prior to administration: ■ Obtain a complete health history including allergies, drug history, and possible drug interactions. ■ Obtain a complete physical examination with special attention to symptoms related to anemic states such as pallor, fatigue, weakness, tachycardia, and shortness of breath. ■ Obtain the following laboratory studies: folic acid levels, hemoglobin (Hb), hematocrit (Hct), and reticulocyte counts. ■ Obtain a complete blood count (CBC) to determine the type of anemia present. (Folic acid is not beneficial in normocytic anemia, refractory anemia, and aplastic anemia.)	■ Nutrition, Imbalanced: Less than Body Requirements ■ Knowledge, Deficient, related to drug therapy ■ Noncompliance, related to dietary and drug treatment ■ Health Maintenance, Impaired, related to insufficient knowledge of actions and effects of prescribed drug therapy

Planning: Client Goals and Expected Outcomes

The client will:
■ Exhibit improvement in serum folic acid level.
■ Experience less fatigue and weakness.
■ Demonstrate an understanding of the drug's action by accurately describing drug side effects and precautions.
■ Verbalize potential complications related to drug use and when to notify the healthcare provider.

Implementation

Interventions and (Rationales)	Client Education/Discharge Planning
■ Monitor client's dietary intake of folic acid–containing foods. (Deficiency state may be caused by poor dietary habits.)	Instruct client to: ■ Eat foods high in folic acid such as vegetables, fruits, and organ meats. ■ Consult with the healthcare provider concerning amount of folic acid that should be in the diet.
■ Encourage client to conserve energy. (Anemia caused by folic acid deficiency may lead to weakness and fatigue.)	Advise client to: ■ Rest when tired and not overexert. ■ Plan activities to avoid fatigue.
■ Encourage client to take medication appropriately. (Taking medication as ordered increases its effectiveness.)	Instruct client to: ■ Avoid use of alcohol, because it increases folic acid requirements. ■ Take only the amount of drug prescribed.

Evaluation of Outcome Criteria

Evaluate the effectiveness of drug therapy by confirming that client goals and expected outcomes have been met (see "Planning").
■ The client's serum folic acid level improves.
■ The client reports less fatigue and weakness.
■ The client demonstrates an understanding of the drug's action by accurately describing drug side effects and precautions.
■ The client verbalizes potential complications related to drug use and when to notify the healthcare provider.

- Include vitamin-rich foods (whole grains, fresh vegetables, fresh fruits, lean meats, and dairy products) in the diet.

- If taking vitamin C, drink 6 to 8 large glasses of water every day.

- Immediately report severe back pain, vomiting, abdominal cramps, dizziness, or difficulty breathing.

- Be aware that water-soluble vitamins are not stored in the body and must be replenished daily.

- Take vitamins only as prescribed or as directed on the label. Do not double doses.

- If attempting pregnancy, be sure to get adequate folic acid. Discuss folic acid requirements with your healthcare provider, and take a multivitamin to ensure adequate intake.

MINERALS

Minerals are inorganic substances needed in small amounts to maintain homeostasis. Minerals are classified as macrominerals or microminerals; the macrominerals must be ingested in larger amounts. A normal, balanced diet will provide the proper amounts of the required minerals in most people. The primary minerals used in pharmacotherapy are listed in Table 42.4.

TABLE 42.4 Selected Minerals for Treating Nutritional and Electrolyte Disorders

Drug	Route and Adult Dose (max dose where indicated)	Adverse Effects
sodium bicarbonate (see page 448 for the Prototype Drug box ∞)	PO; 0.3–2.0 g/day–qid or 1 tsp of powder in glass of water	*Headache, weakness, belching, flatulence* Hypernatremia, hypertension, muscle twitching, dysrhythmias, pulmonary edema, peripheral edema
potassium chloride (K-Dur, Micro-K, Klor-Con, others) (see page 446 for the Prototype Drug box ∞)	PO; 10–100 mEq/h in divided doses IV; 10–40 mEq/h diluted to at least 10–20 mEq/100 ml of solution (max: 200–400 mEq/day)	*Nausea, vomiting, diarrhea, abdominal cramping* Hyperkalemia, hypotension, confusion, dysrhythmias
CALCIUM SALTS		
calcium carbonate (BioCal, Titralac, others)	PO; 1–2 g bid–tid	*Parenteral route: flushing, nausea, vomiting, pain at injection site*
calcium chloride (Calciject, Calcitrans, Solucalcine)	IV; 0.5–1.0 g/ q3days	
calcium citrate (Citracal)	PO; 1–2 g bid–tid	Hypercalcemia, hypotension, constipation, fatigue, anorexia, confusion, dysrhythmias
calcium glyceptate (Glu-calcium, Calcitrans)	IV; 1.1–4.4 g/day IM; 0.5–1.1 g/day	
calcium phosphate tribasic (Posture)	PO; 1–2 g bid–tid	
calcium gluconate (Kalcinate) (see page 736 for the Prototype Drug box ∞)	PO; 1–2 g bid–qid	
calcium lactate (Cal-Lac, Calcimax, others)	PO; 325 mg–1.3 g tid with meals	
IRON SALTS		
ferrous fumarate (Feco-T, Femiron, Feostat, others)	PO; 200 mg tid–qid	*Nausea, constipation or diarrhea, abdominal pain, leg cramps (iron sucrose)*
ferrous gluconate (Fergon, Simron)	PO; 325–600 mg qid; may be gradually increased to 650 mg qid as needed and tolerated	
ferrous sulfate (Feosol, Fer-Iron, others) (see page 404 for the Prototype Drug box ∞)	PO; 750–1,500 mg/day in single dose or 2–3 divided doses	Anaphylaxis (iron dextran), hypovolemia, hematemesis, hepatotoxicity, metabolic acidosis
iron dextran (Dexferrum, Imfed, Imferon)	IM/IV; dose is individualized and determined from a table of correlations between client's weight and hemoglobin (max: 100 mg (2 ml) of iron dextran within 24 h)	
iron sucrose injection (Venofer)	IV; 1 ml (20 mg) injected in dialysis line at rate of 1 ml/min up to 5 ml (100 mg), or infuse 100 mg in NS over 15 min 1–3 times/wk	
MAGNESIUM		
magnesium chloride (Chloromag, Slo-Mag)	PO; 270–400 mg/day	*Nausea, vomiting, diarrhea, flushing*
magnesium oxide (Mag-Ox, Maox, others)	PO; 400–1,200 mg/day in divided doses	
℗ magnesium sulfate (Epsom salts)	IV/IM; 0.5–3.0 g/day	Cardiotoxicity, respiratory failure, hypotension, deep tendon reflex reduction, facial paresthesias, weakness
PHOSPHORUS/PHOSPHATE		
monobasic potassium phosphate (K-Phos original)	PO; 1 g qid	*Nausea, vomiting, diarrhea*
monobasic potassium and sodium phosphates (K-Phos MF, K-Phos neutral)	PO; 250 mg qid (max: 2 g phosphorus/day)	Hyperphosphatemia, bone pain, fractures, muscle weakness, confusion
potassium phosphate (Neutra-Phos-K)	PO; 1.45 g qid; IV; 10 mmol phosphorus/day	
potassium and sodium phosphates (Neutra-Phos, Uro-KP neutral)	PO; 250 mg phosphorus qid	
ZINC		
zinc acetate (Galzin)	PO; 50 mg tid	*Side effects are uncommon at normal doses*
zinc gluconate	PO; 20–100 mg (20-mg lozenges may be taken to a max of six lozenges/day)	High doses: nausea, vomiting, fever, immunosuppression, anemia
zinc sulfate (Orazinc, Zincate, others)	PO; 15–220 mg/day	

Italics indicate common adverse effects; underlining indicates serious adverse effects.

42.7 Pharmacotherapy With Minerals

Minerals are essential substances that constitute about 4% of the body weight and serve many diverse functions. Some are essential ions or electrolytes in body fluids; others are bound to organic molecules such as hemoglobin, phospholipids, or metabolic enzymes. Those minerals that function as critical electrolytes in the body, most notably sodium and potassium, are covered in more detail in Chapter 31 ∞. Sodium chloride and potassium chloride are featured as drug prototypes in that chapter.

Because minerals are needed in very small amounts for human metabolism, a balanced diet will supply the necessary quantities for most clients. As with vitamins, excess amounts of minerals can lead to toxicity, and clients should be advised not to exceed recommended doses. Mineral supplements are, however, indicated for certain disorders. Iron-deficiency anemia is the most common nutritional deficiency in the world and is a common indication for iron supplements. Women at high risk for osteoporosis are advised to consume extra calcium, either in their diet or as a dietary supplement.

Certain drugs affect normal mineral metabolism. For example, loop or thiazide diuretics can cause significant urinary potassium loss. Corticosteroids and oral contraceptives are among several classes of drugs that can promote sodium retention. The uptake of iodine by the thyroid gland can be impaired by certain oral hypoglycemics and lithium carbonate (Eskalith). Oral contraceptives have been reported to lower the plasma levels of zinc and to increase those of copper. The nurse must be aware of drug-related mineral interactions, and recommend changes to mineral intake when appropriate.

42.8 Pharmacotherapy With Macrominerals

Macrominerals (major minerals) are inorganic substances that must be consumed daily in amounts of 100 mg or higher. The macrominerals include calcium, chlorine, magnesium, phosphorus, potassium, sodium, and sulfur. Approximately 75% of the total mineral content in the body consists of calcium and phosphorus salts in bony matrix. Recommended daily allowances have been established for each of the macrominerals except sulfur, as listed in Table 42.5.

Calcium is essential for nerve conduction, muscular contraction, construction of bony matrix, and hemostasis. Hypocalcemia occurs when serum calcium falls below 4.5 mEq/L and may be caused by inadequate intake of calcium-containing foods, lack of vitamin D, chronic diarrhea, or decreased secretion of parathyroid hormone. Symptoms of hypocalcemia involve the nervous and muscular systems. The client often becomes irritable and restless, and muscular twitches, cramps, spasms, and cardiac abnormalities are common. Prolonged hypocalcemia may lead to fractures. Pharmacotherapy includes calcium compounds, which are available in many oral salts such as calcium carbonate, calcium citrate, calcium gluconate, or calcium lactate. In severe cases, IV preparations are administered. Calcium gluconate is featured as a prototype drug for hypocalcemia and osteoporosis in Chapter 47 ∞.

Phosphorus is an essential mineral, 85% of which is bound to calcium in the form of calcium phosphate in bones. In addition to playing a role in bone structure, phosphorus is a component of proteins, adenosine triphosphate (ATP), and nucleic acids. Phosphate (PO_4^{3-}) is an important buffer in the blood. Because phosphorus is a primary component of phosphate, phosphorus balance is normally considered the same as phosphate balance. Hypophosphatemia is most often observed in clients with serious medical illnesses, especially those with kidney disorders that cause excess phosphorus loss in the urine. Because of its abundance in food, the client must be suffering from severe malnutrition or an intestinal malabsorption disorder to experience a dietary deficiency. Symptoms of hypophosphatemia include weakness, muscle tremor, anorexia, weak pulse, and bleeding abnormalities. When serum phosphorus levels fall below 1.5 mEq/L, phosphate supplements are usually administered. Sodium phosphate and potassium phosphate are available for treating phosphorus deficiencies.

Magnesium is the second most abundant intracellular cation. Like potassium, it is necessary for proper neuromuscular function. Magnesium also serves a metabolic role in activating certain enzymes in the breakdown of carbohydrates and proteins. Because it produces few symptoms until serum

TABLE 42.5	Macrominerals	
Mineral	**RDA**	**Function**
calcium	800–1,200 mg	forms bony matrix; regulates nerve conduction and muscle contraction
chloride	750 mg	major anion in body fluids; part of gastric acid secretion
magnesium	Men: 350–400 mg Women: 280–300 mg	cofactor for many enzymes; necessary for normal nerve conduction and muscle contraction
phosphorus	700 mg	forms bone matrix; part of ATP and nucleic acids
potassium	2.0 g	necessary for normal nerve conduction and muscle contraction; principal cation in intracellular fluid; essential for acid–base and electrolyte balance
sodium	500 mg	necessary for normal nerve conduction and muscle contraction; principal cation in extracellular fluid; essential for acid–base and electrolyte balance
sulfur	not established	component of proteins, B vitamins, and other critical molecules

levels fall below 1.0 mEq/L, hypomagnesemia is sometimes called the most common undiagnosed electrolyte abnormality. Clients may experience general weakness, dysrhythmias, hypertension, loss of deep tendon reflexes, and respiratory depression—signs and symptoms that are sometimes mistaken for hypokalemia. Pharmacotherapy with magnesium sulfate can quickly reverse symptoms of hypomagnesemia. Magnesium sulfate is a CNS depressant and is sometimes given to prevent or terminate seizures associated with eclampsia. Magnesium salts have additional applications as cathartics or antacids (magnesium citrate, magnesium hydroxide, and magnesium oxide) and as analgesics (magnesium salicylate).

NURSING CONSIDERATIONS

The role of the nurse in macromineral therapy for mineral deficiencies or eclampsia involves careful monitoring of a client's condition and providing education as it relates to the prescribed drug treatment. Macrominerals are used for multiple reasons in health care. Determine the reason for the specific macromineral therapy being prescribed, and assess for the presence, or absence of the associated symptoms.

Although minerals cause no harm in small amounts, larger doses can cause life-threatening adverse effects. Calcium is one of the most common minerals in use. To prevent and treat osteoporosis, it is recommended that adult women take 1,200 mg/day of calcium. Assess for common side effects, including GI distress and constipation. With prolonged therapy with calcium, assess for hypercalcemia, especially in clients with decreased liver and renal function. Symptoms of hypercalcemia include nausea, vomiting, constipation, frequent urination, lethargy, and depression. Calcium interacts with many drugs, including glucocorticoids, thiazide diuretics, and tetracyclines. Zinc-rich foods such as legumes, nuts, sprouts, and soy impair calcium absorption. Monitor serum calcium levels to determine success of pharmacotherapy.

Phosphorus is a mineral sometimes used as a dietary supplement. Teach clients who are on a sodium- or potassium-restricted not to use phosphorus supplements. Most adverse effects of excess phosphate are mild, and include GI distress, diarrhea, and dizziness. Phosphorus can promote seizures. Antacids may decrease serum phosphorus levels. Monitor serum phosphorus levels to determine success of pharmacotherapy.

Magnesium sulfate is given to correct hypomagnesemia, to evacuate the bowel in preparation for diagnostic examinations, and to treat seizures associated with eclampsia of pregnancy. The medication is given orally to replace magnesium, and by the IM or IV routes to prevent or terminate eclampsia seizure. When given IV, assess the neurological status of the client, because overdose can lead to reduced reflexes and muscle weakness. Monitor for LOC changes, deep tendon reflexes, thirst, and confusion. Because of its effects on muscles and the heart, magnesium sulfate is contraindicated in clients

---

Pr PROTOTYPE DRUG | Magnesium Sulfate | Mineral/Electrolyte

ACTIONS AND USES

Severe hypomagnesemia can be rapidly reversed by the administration of IM or IV magnesium sulfate. Hypomagnesemia has a number of causes, including loss of body fluids due to diarrhea, diuretics, or nasogastric suctioning, and prolonged parenteral feeding with magnesium-free solutions. After administration, magnesium sulfate is distributed throughout the body, and therapeutic effects are observed within 30 to 60 minutes. Oral forms of magnesium sulfate are used as cathartics, when complete evacuation of the colon is desired. Its action as a CNS depressant has led to its occasional use as an anticonvulsant.

ADMINISTRATION ALERTS

- Continuously monitor client during IV infusion for early signs of decreased cardiac function.
- Monitor serum magnesium levels q6h during parenteral infusion.
- When giving IV infusion, give required dose over 4 h.
- Pregnancy category A.

PHARMACOKINETICS

Onset: 1–2 h PO; 1 h IM

Peak: Unknown

Half-life: Unknown

Duration: 3–4 h PO; 30 min IV

ADVERSE EFFECTS

IV infusions of magnesium sulfate require careful observation to prevent toxicity. Early signs of magnesium overdose include flushing of the skin, sedation, confusion, intense thirst, and muscle weakness. Extreme levels cause neuromuscular blockade with resultant respiratory paralysis, heart block, and circulatory collapse. Plasma magnesium levels should be monitored frequently. Because of these potentially fatal adverse effects, the use of magnesium sulfate is restricted to severe magnesium deficiency: Mild-to-moderate hypomagnesemia is treated with oral forms of magnesium such as magnesium gluconate or magnesium hydroxide.

Contraindications: Magnesium is contraindicated in clients with serious cardiac disease. Oral administration is contraindicated in clients with undiagnosed abdominal pain, intestinal obstruction, or fecal impaction.

INTERACTIONS

Drug–Drug: Use with neuromuscular blockers may increase respiratory depression and apnea. Clients receiving CNS depressants may experience increased sedation. Magnesium salts may decrease the absorption of certain anti-infectives such as tetracycline.

Lab Tests: Unknown.

Herbal/Food: Unknown.

Treatment of Overdose: Serious respiratory and cardiac suppression may result from overdose. Calcium gluconate or gluceptate may be administered IV as an antidote.

 See the Companion Website for a Nursing Process Focus specific to this mineral.

with myocardial damage, heart block, and recent cardiac arrest. It has a laxative effect when given orally, so do not give to clients with abdominal pain, nausea, vomiting, or intestinal obstruction. Use magnesium sulfate with caution in clients with impaired kidney function and those on cardiac glycosides. Monitor serum magnesium levels to determine success of pharmacotherapy.

Client Teaching. Client education as it relates to macromineral therapy should include the goals of therapy; the reasons for obtaining baseline data such as lab tests for liver function and CBC, and the presence of underlying kidney or liver disorders; and possible drug side effects. Include the following points when teaching clients about minerals:

- Take minerals only as prescribed or as directed on the label. Overdose may lead to toxicity.
- Do not take other prescribed drug, OTC medications, herbal therapies, or vitamin supplements without notifying your healthcare provider.
- Eat a well-balanced diet to eliminate or reduce the need for mineral supplements.
- If prescribed calcium, inform the healthcare provider of the use of glucocorticoids, thiazide diuretics, and tetracyclines.
- If taking calcium, avoid eating exessive amounts of zinc-rich foods, such as legumes, nuts, sprouts, and soy, that impair calcium absorption.
- If prescribed phosphorus, inform your healthcare provider of a sodium- or potassium-restricted diet.
- If taking phosphorus, immediately report seizure activity and stop taking the drug.
- If taking phosphorus, avoid antacids.
- If taking magnesium sulfate, immediately report changes in consciousness, deep tendon reflexes, thirst, and confusion, and stop the drug.

See the companion website for "Nursing Process Focus: Clients Receiving Magnesium Sulfate."

42.9 Pharmacotherapy With Microminerals

The nine **microminerals,** commonly called *trace* minerals, are required daily in amounts of 20 mg or less. The fact that they are needed in such small amounts does not diminish their key role in human health; deficiencies in some of the trace minerals can result in profound illness. The functions of some of the trace minerals, such as iron and iodine, are well established; the role of others are less completely understood. The RDA for each of the microminerals is listed in Table 42.6.

Iron is an essential micromineral most commonly associated with hemoglobin. Excellent sources of dietary iron include meat, shellfish, nuts, and legumes. Excess iron in the body results in hemochromatosis, whereas lack of iron results in iron-deficiency anemia. The pharmacology of iron supplements is presented in Chapter 28 ∞, where ferrous sulfate is featured as a drug prototype for anemia.

Iodine is a trace mineral needed to synthesize thyroid hormone. The most common source of dietary iodine is iodized salt. When dietary intake of iodine is low, hypothyroidism occurs and enlargement of the thyroid gland (goiter) results. At high concentrations, iodine suppresses thyroid function. *Lugol's solution,* a mixture containing 5% elemental iodine and 10% potassium iodide, is given to hyperthyroid clients prior to thyroidectomy or during a thyrotoxic crisis. Sodium iodide acts by rapidly suppressing the secretion of thyroid hormone and is indicated for clients having an acute thyroid crisis. Radioactive iodine (I-131) is given to destroy overactive thyroid glands. Pharmacotherapeutic uses of iodine as a drug extend beyond the treatment of thyroid disease. Iodine is an effective topical antiseptic that can be found in creams, tinctures, and solutions. Iodine salts such as iothalamate and diatrizoate are very dense and serve as diagnostic contrast agents in radiological procedures of the urinary and cardiovascular systems. The role of potassium iodide in protecting the thyroid gland during acute radiation exposure is discussed in Chapter 3 ∞.

TABLE 42.6 Microminerals		
Trace Mineral	**RDA**	**Function**
chromium	0.05–2.0 mg	potentiates insulin and is necessary for proper glucose metabolism
cobalt	0.1 mcg	cofactor for vitamin B_{12} and several oxidative enzymes
copper	1.5–3.0 mg	cofactor for hemoglobin synthesis
fluorine	1.5–4.0 mg	influences tooth structure and possibly affects growth
iodine	150 mcg	component of thyroid hormones
iron	Men: 10–12 mg Women: 10–15 mg	component of hemoglobin and some enzymes of oxidative phosphorylation
manganese	2–5 mg	cofactor in some enzymes of lipid, carbohydrate, and protein metabolism
molybdenum	75–250 mg	cofactor for certain enzymes
selenium	Men: 50–70 mcg Women: 50–55 mcg	antioxidant cofactor for certain enzymes
zinc	12–15 mg	cofactor for certain enzymes, including carbonic anhydrase; needed for proper protein structure, normal growth, and wound healing

Fluorine is a trace mineral found abundantly in nature and is best known for its beneficial effects on bones and teeth. Research has validated that adding fluoride to the water supply in very small amounts (1 part per billion) can reduce the incidence of dental caries. This effect is more pronounced in children, because fluoride is incorporated into the enamel of growing teeth. Concentrated fluoride solutions can also be applied to the teeth topically by dental professionals. Sodium fluoride and stannous fluoride are components of most toothpastes and oral rinses. Because high amounts of fluoride can be quite toxic, the use of fluoride-containing products should be closely monitored in children.

Zinc is a component of at least 100 enzymes, including alcohol dehydrogenase, carbonic anhydrase, and alkaline phosphatase. This trace mineral has a regulatory function in enzymes controlling nucleic acid synthesis and is believed to have roles in wound healing, male fertility, bone formation, and cell-mediated immunity. Because symptoms of zinc deficiency are often nonspecific, diagnosis is usually confirmed by a serum zinc level of less than 70 mcg/dl. Zinc sulfate, zinc acetate, and zinc gluconate are available to prevent and treat deficiency states, at doses of 60 to 120 mg/day. In addition, lozenges containing zinc are available OTC for treating sore throats and symptoms of the common cold.

NUTRITIONAL SUPPLEMENTS

The nurse will encounter many clients who are undernourished. Major goals in resolving nutritional deficiencies are to identify the specific type of deficiency and supply the missing nutrients. Nutritional supplements may be needed for short-term therapy or for the remainder of the client's life.

42.10 Etiology of Undernutrition

When the client is ingesting or absorbing fewer nutrients than required for normal body growth and maintenance, **undernutrition** occurs. Successful pharmacotherapy relies on the skills of the nurse in identifying the symptoms and causes of the client's undernutrition.

Causes of undernutrition range from the simple to the complex, and include the following:

- Advanced age
- HIV-AIDS
- Alcoholism
- Burns
- Cancer
- Chronic inflammatory bowel disease (IBD)
- Eating disorders
- GI disorders
- Chronic neurological disease such as progressive dysphagia and multiple sclerosis
- Surgery
- Trauma

The most obvious cause for undernutrition is low dietary intake, although reasons for the inadequate intake must be assessed. Clients may have no resources to purchase food and may be suffering from starvation. Clinical depression leads many clients to shun food. Elderly clients may have poorly fitting dentures or difficulty chewing or swallowing after a stroke. In terminal disease, clients may be comatose or otherwise unable to take food orally. Although the etiologies differ, clients with insufficient intake exhibit a similar pattern of general weakness, muscle wasting, and loss of subcutaneous fat.

When the undernutrition is caused by lack of one specific nutrient, vitamin, or mineral, the disorder is more difficult to diagnose. Clients may be on a fad diet lacking only protein or fat in their intake. Certain digestive disorders may lead to malabsorption of specific nutrients or vitamins. Clients may simply avoid certain foods such as green leafy vegetables, dairy products, or meat products, which can lead to specific nutritional deficiencies. Proper pharmacotherapy requires the expert knowledge and assessment skills of the nurse, and sometimes a nutritional consult, so that the correct treatment can be administered.

42.11 Enteral Nutrition

Numerous nutritional supplements are available, and a common method of classifying these agents is by their *route of administration*. Products that are administered via the GI tract, either orally or through a feeding tube, are classified as **enteral nutrition.** Those that are administered by means of IV infusion are called parenteral nutrition.

When the client's condition permits, enteral nutrition is best provided by oral consumption. Oral feeding allows natural digestive processes to occur and requires less intense nursing care. It does, however, rely on client compliance, because it is not feasible for the healthcare provider to observe the client at every meal.

Tube feeding, or enteral tube alimentation, is necessary when the client has difficulty swallowing or is otherwise unable to take meals orally. An advantage of tube feeding is that the amount of enteral nutrition the client receives can be precisely measured and recorded. Various tube feeding routes are possible, including nasogastric (nose to stomach), nasoduodenal (nose to duodenum), nasojejunal (nose to jejunum), gastrostomy, or jejunostomy (tube is placed directly into the stomach or jejunum, respectively, through a surgical incision). A nasogastric tube may be inserted by a registered nurse or licensed practical nurse. The nasoduodenal and nasojejunal are usually inserted by a radiologist or other physician. The gastrostomy and jejunostomy tubes are placed by a surgeon or a gastroenterologist.

The particular enteral product is chosen to address the specific nutritional needs of the client. Because of the wide diversity in their formulations, it is difficult to categorize enteral products, and several different methods are used. A simple method is to classify enteral products as oligomeric, polymeric, modular, or specialized formulations.

- *Oligomeric* formulations are agents containing varying amounts of free amino acids and peptide combinations. Indications include partial bowel obstruction, irritable bowel syndrome, radiation enteritis, bowel fistulas, and short-bowel syndrome. Sample products include Vivonex® T.E.N., and Peptamen Liquid®.

- *Polymeric* formulations are the most common enteral preparations. These products contain various mixtures of proteins, carbohydrates, and lipids. Indications include general undernutrition, although the client must have a fully functioning GI tract. Sample products include Compleat® regular, Sustacal® Powder, and Ensure®-Plus.

- *Modular* formulations contain a single nutrient, protein, lipid, or carbohydrate. Indications include a single nutrient deficiency or specific nutrient needs, in which case the nutrient may be added to other formulations. Sample products include Casec®, Polycose®, Microlipid®, and MCT® Oil.

- *Specialized* formulations are products that contain a specific nutrient combination for a particular condition. Indications include a specific disease state such as hepatic failure, renal failure, or a specific genetic enzyme deficiency. Sample products include Amin-Aid®, Hepatic-Aid II®, and Pulmocare®.

NURSING CONSIDERATIONS

The role of the nurse in enteral feedings involves careful monitoring of a client's condition and providing education as it relates to the prescribed drug treatment. Prior to administration of each feeding, assess for tube placement by either aspirating gastric contents or injecting air into the tube to listen for stomach placement. Administer enteral feedings at regular intervals (bolus feedings) or in a continuous manner. At regular intervals, check for the presence of residual feedings. The frequency of this measurement varies according to institutional policy. Enteral feeding tubes are narrow in diameter and are easily clogged. All medications administered through these tubes should be liquid or be able to be finely crushed. Be sure to determine that the medications are compatible with the enteral formula or with the feeding tube itself. Certain medications, such as phenytoin (Dilantin), bind with the plastic in the feeding tube. Liberally flush the tube with water before and after administering this medication to ensure that the entire dose is obtained by the client and to prevent dehydration.

Clients sometimes exhibit GI intolerance to enteral nutrition, usually expressed as vomiting, nausea, or diarrhea. Therefore, start therapy slowly with small quantities so that side effects can be assessed. Be observant for drug interactions that occasionally occur when drugs are given along with enteral nutrition.

Client Teaching. Client education as it relates to enteral feedings should include the goals of therapy, the reasons for obtaining baseline data such as vital signs and the existence of underlying disorders, and possible drug side effects. Include the following points when teaching clients about enteral feedings:

- Sit upright while receiving an enteral feeding to avoid GI upset.

- If receiving enteral nutrition at home, be sure you (or your family) flush the tube before and after tube feeding with 30 ml of water.

- Report abdominal pain, constipation, or diarrhea to the healthcare provider.

- Monitor weight and report significant changes.

- Do not put any other medications in the feeding tube unless instructed to by the healthcare provider.

42.12 Total Parenteral Nutrition

When a client's metabolic needs are unable to be met through enteral nutrition, **total parenteral nutrition (TPN)**, or hyperalimentation, is indicated. For short-term therapy, peripheral vein TPN may be used. Because of the risk of phlebitis, however, long-term therapy often requires central vein TPN. Clients who have undergone major surgery or trauma and those who are severely undernourished are candidates for central vein TPN. Because the GI tract is not being utilized, clients with severe malabsorption disease may be treated successfully with TPN.

TPN is able to provide all of a client's nutritional needs in a hypertonic solution containing amino acids, lipid emulsions, carbohydrates (as dextrose), electrolytes, vitamins, and minerals. The particular formulation may be specific to the disease state, such as renal failure or hepatic failure. TPN is administered through an infusion pump, so that nutrition delivery can be precisely monitored. Clients in various settings such as acute care, long-term care, and home health care often benefit from TPN therapy.

NURSING CONSIDERATIONS

The role of the nurse in TPN involves careful monitoring of the client's condition and providing education as it relates to the prescribed drug treatment. While the client is receiving TPN, it is vital to assess vital signs and monitor electrolytes, glucose, and protein laboratory values. Also assess for fluid overload and signs and symptoms of infection. Change TPN solution, tubing, and dressings every 24 hours, and use sterile technique with each TPN dressing. TPN should never be administered in a peripheral line, but rather through a central line. Never administer other medications through the same line with the TPN solution.

Client Teaching. Client education as it relates to TPN feedings should include the goals of therapy, the reasons for obtaining baseline data such as vital signs and the existence of underlying disorders, and possible drug side effects. Include the following points when teaching clients about TPN feedings:

- If diabetic, check blood sugar levels frequently.

- Immediately report any signs of infection such as elevated temperature.

- Immediately report significant changes in weight.

- Follow specific instructions for changing the dressing around the IV to prevent infection.

- Keep all scheduled appointments with your healthcare provider.

MediaLink A.S.P.E.N.

NURSING PROCESS FOCUS Clients Receiving Total Parenteral Nutrition

Assessment	Potential Nursing Diagnoses
Prior to administration: ■ Obtain a complete health history including allergies, drug history, and possible drug interactions. ■ Obtain a complete physical examination. ■ Assess for the presence or history of nutritional deficits such as inadequate oral intake, GI disease, and increased metabolic need. ■ Obtain the following laboratory studies: total protein/albumin levels, creatinine/blood urea nitrogen (BUN), CBC electrolytes, lipid profile, and serum iron levels.	■ Infection, Risk for ■ Nutrition, Imbalanced: Less than Body Requirements ■ Fluid Volume, Imbalanced, Risk for ■ Knowledge, Deficient, related to drug therapy ■ Injury, Risk for

Planning: Client Goals and Expected Outcomes

The client will:
■ Exhibit improvement or stabilization of nutritional status.
■ Be free of infection or injury related to TPN.
■ Demonstrate an understanding of the drug's action by accurately describing drug side effects and precautions.
■ Immediately report side effects such as symptoms of hypoglycemia or hyperglycemia, fever, chills, cough, or malaise.

Implementation

Interventions and (Rationales)	Client Education/Discharge Planning
■ Monitor vital signs, observing for signs of infection such as elevated temperature. (Bacteria may grow in high-glucose and high-protein solutions.)	■ Instruct client to report fever, chills, soreness or drainage of the infusion site, cough, or malaise.
■ Use strict aseptic technique with IV tubing, dressing changes, and TPN solution, and refrigerate solution until 30 min before using. (Infusion site is at high risk for development of infection.)	■ Instruct client that infusion site has high risk for infection development; hence, sterile dressings and aseptic technique with solutions and tubing are needed.
■ Monitor blood glucose levels. Observe for signs of hyperglycemia or hypoglycemia and administer insulin as directed. (Blood glucose levels may be affected if TPN is turned off, if the rate is reduced, or if excess levels of insulin are added to the solution.)	Instruct client to report symptoms of: ■ Hyperglycemia (excessive thirst, copious urination, and insatiable hunger). ■ Hypoglycemia (nervousness, irritability, and dizziness).
■ Monitor for signs of fluid overload. (TPN is a hypertonic solution and can create intravascular shifting of extracellular fluid.)	■ Instruct client to report shortness of breath, heart palpitations, swelling, or decreased urine output.
■ Monitor renal status. (Intake and output ratio, daily weight, and laboratory studies such as serum creatinine and BUN are used to assess renal function.)	Instruct client to: ■ Weigh self daily. ■ Monitor intake and output. ■ Report sudden increases in weight or decreased urine output. ■ Keep all appointments for follow-up care and laboratory testing.
■ Maintain accurate infusion rate with infusion pump, make rate changes gradually, and never discontinue TPN abruptly. (Abrupt discontinuation may cause hypoglycemia, and a sudden change in flow rate can cause fluctuations in blood glucose levels.)	Instruct client: ■ About the importance of maintaining the prescribed rate of infusion. ■ Never to stop the TPN solution abruptly unless instructed by the healthcare provider.

Evaluation of Outcome Criteria

Evaluate the effectiveness of drug therapy by confirming that client goals and expected outcomes have been met (see "Planning").
■ The client demonstrates improved nutritional status.
■ The client is free of infection or injury related to the TPN.
■ The client demonstrates an understanding of the drug's action by accurately describing drug side effects and precautions.
■ The client verbalizes the importance of immediately reporting side effects such as symptoms of hypoglycemia, hyperglycemia, fever, chills, cough, or malaise.

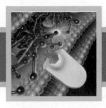

CHAPTER REVIEW

KEY CONCEPTS

The numbered key concepts provide a succinct summary of the important points from the corresponding numbered section within the chapter. If any of these points are not clear, refer to the numbered section within the chapter for review.

42.1 Vitamins are organic substances needed in small amounts to promote growth and maintain health. Deficiency of a vitamin will result in disease.

42.2 Vitamins are classified as lipid soluble (A, D, E, and K) or water soluble (C and B complex). Excess quantities of lipid-soluble vitamins are stored in the liver and adipose tissue.

42.3 Failure to meet the Recommended Dietary Allowances (RDAs) for vitamins may result in deficiency disorders. The RDA is the amount of a vitamin needed to prevent symptoms of deficiency.

42.4 Vitamin therapy is indicated for conditions such as poor nutritional intake, pregnancy, and chronic disease states. Symptoms of deficiency are usually nonspecific and occur over a prolonged period.

42.5 Deficiencies of vitamins A, D, E, or K are indications for pharmacotherapy with lipid-soluble vitamins.

42.6 Deficiencies of vitamins C, thiamine, niacin, riboflavin, folic acid, cyanocobalamin, or pyridoxine are indications for pharmacotherapy with water-soluble vitamins.

42.7 Minerals are inorganic substances needed in very small amounts to maintain normal body metabolism.

42.8 Pharmacotherapy with macrominerals includes agents containing calcium, magnesium, potassium, or phosphorus.

42.9 Pharmacotherapy with microminerals includes agents containing iron, iodine, fluorine, or zinc.

42.10 Undernutrition may be caused by low dietary intake, malabsorption disorders, fad diets, or wasting disorders such as cancer or AIDS.

42.11 Enteral nutrition, provided orally or through a feeding tube, is a means of meeting a client's complete nutritional needs.

42.12 Total parenteral nutrition (TPN) is a means of supplying nutrition to clients via a peripheral vein (short term) or central vein (long term).

NCLEX-RN® REVIEW QUESTIONS

1 A client has been diagnosed with hypothyroidism due to low iodide intake. The nurse should assess for which abnormality?

1. Enlargement of the thyroid gland, known as goiter
2. Atrophy of the thyroid gland
3. Increased metabolic rate, leading to rapid weight loss
4. Increased hair loss (alopecia)

2 The nurse is preparing to administer magnesium sulfate intravenously. The nurse should assess for which of the following side affects? (Select all that apply.)

1. Decreased liver function
2. Respiratory failure
3. Complete heart block
4. Circulatory collapse
5. Increase in peripheral edema

3 The nurse is assessing a client who is exhibiting generalized weakness, cardiac dysrhythmias, hypertension, loss of deep tendon reflexes, and respiratory distress. What could be the possible cause of these symptoms?

1. Hypocalcemia
2. Hypercalcemia
3. Hypomagnesemia
4. Hypermagnesemia

4 The client is a long-time alcoholic. The nurse understands that alcoholism is the most common cause of which vitamin deficiency?

1. Vitamin E
2. Vitamin A
3. Vitamin D
4. Thiamine

5 The client is a 12-year-old with hemophilia. The nurse is aware that this client will require administration of which vitamin to improve the function of clotting factors?

1. Folic acid
2. Riboflavin
3. Vitamin K
4. Vitamin A

CRITICAL THINKING QUESTIONS

1. A client has been self-medicating with vitamin B₃ (niacin) for an elevated cholesterol level. The client comes to the clinic with a severe case of redness and flushing and is concerned about an allergic reaction. What is the nurse's best response?

2. A client complains of a constant headache for the past several days. The only supplements the client has been taking are megadoses of vitamins A, C, and E. What would be a priority for the nurse with this client?

3. A client presents to the healthcare provider with complaints of severe flank pain. This client has a history of renal calculi. The only medication the client takes is a daily multivitamin as well as vitamin C. The nurse should assess for what potential problem?

See Appendix D for answers and rationales for all activities.

EXPLORE MediaLink

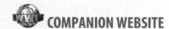

www.prenhall.com/adams

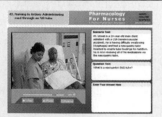

NCLEX-RN® review, case studies, and other interactive resources for this chapter can be found on the companion website at www.prenhall.com/adams. Click on "Chapter 42" to select the activities for this chapter. For animations, more NCLEX-RN® review questions, and an audio glossary, access the accompanying Prentice Hall Nursing MediaLink DVD-ROM in this textbook.

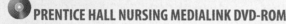

PRENTICE HALL NURSING MEDIALINK DVD-ROM

- **Audio Glossary**
- **NCLEX-RN® Review**
- **Nursing in Action**
  Administering Medications Through a Nasogastric Tube

COMPANION WEBSITE

- **NCLEX-RN® Review**
- **Dosage Calculations**
- **Case Study:** Vitamin pharmacotherapy
- **Care Plan:** Pregnant client prescribed vitamin A

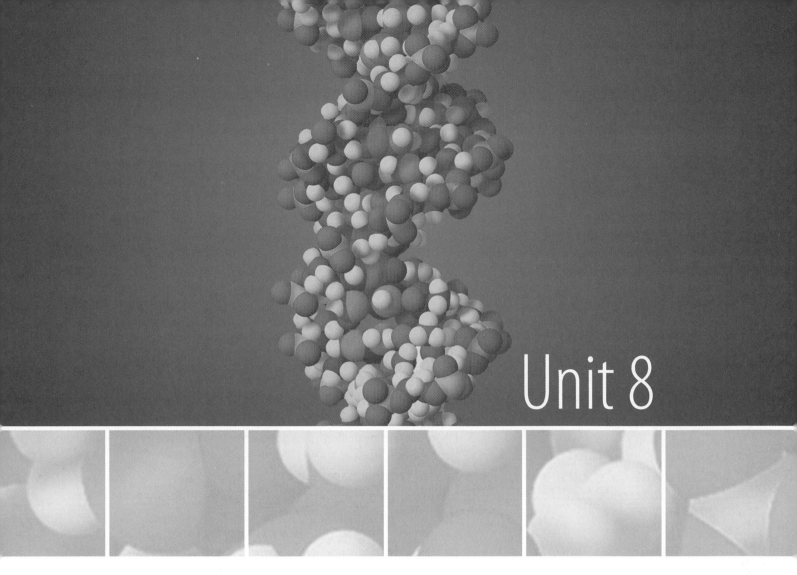

Unit 8

The Endocrine System

CHAPTER 43   Drugs for Pituitary, Thyroid, and Adrenal Disorders

CHAPTER 44   Drugs for Diabetes Mellitus

CHAPTER 45   Drugs for Disorders and Conditions of the Female Reproductive System

CHAPTER 46   Drugs for Disorders and Conditions of the Male Reproductive System

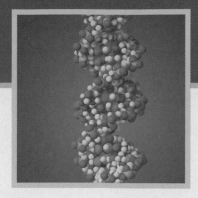

CHAPTER 43

Drugs for Pituitary, Thyroid, and Adrenal Disorders

DRUGS AT A GLANCE

HYPOTHALAMIC AND PITUITARY DRUGS
Hypothalamic Agents
Anterior Pituitary Agents
  ⊙ *vasopressin injection (Pitressin)*
THYROID DRUGS
Thyroid Agents
  ⊙ *levothyroxine (Synthroid)*
Antithyroid Agents
  ⊙ *propylthiouracil (PTU)*
ADRENAL DRUGS
Glucocorticoids
  ⊙ *hydrocortisone (Aeroseb-HC, Alphaderm, others)*
Antiadrenal Agents

OBJECTIVES

After reading this chapter, the student should be able to:

1. Describe the general structure and functions of the endocrine system.
2. Through the use of a specific example, explain the concept of negative feedback in the endocrine system.
3. Describe the clinical applications of the hypothalamic and pituitary hormones.
4. Explain the pharmacotherapy of diabetes insipidus.
5. Identify the signs and symptoms of hypothyroidism and hyperthyroidism.
6. Explain the pharmacotherapy of thyroid disorders.
7. Describe the signs and symptoms of Addison's disease and Cushing's syndrome.
8. Explain the pharmacotherapy of adrenal gland disorders.
9. Describe the nurse's role in the pharmacological management of pituitary, thyroid, and adrenal disorders.
10. For each of the classes listed in Drugs at a Glance, know representative drugs, and explain the mechanisms of drug action, primary actions, and important adverse effects.
11. Categorize drugs used in the treatment of endocrine disorders based on their classification and mechanism of action.
12. Use the Nursing Process to care for clients who are receiving drug therapy for pituitary, thyroid, and adrenal disorders.

MediaLink

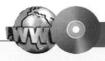

www.prenhall.com/adams

NCLEX-RN® review, case studies, and other interactive resources for this chapter can be found on the companion website at www.prenhall.com/adams. Click on "Chapter 43" to select the activities for this chapter. For animations, more NCLEX-RN® review questions, and an audio glossary, access the accompanying Prentice Hall Nursing MediaLink DVD-ROM in this textbook.

Like the nervous system, the endocrine system is a major controller of homeostasis. Whereas a nerve exerts instantaneous control over a single muscle fiber or gland, a hormone from the endocrine system may affect all body cells and take as long as several days to produce an optimum response. Hormonal balance is kept within a narrow range: too little or too much of a hormone may produce profound physiologic changes. This chapter examines common endocrine disorders and their pharmacotherapy. The reproductive hormones are covered in Chapters 45 and 46 ∞.

43.1 The Endocrine System and Homeostasis

The endocrine system consists of various glands that secrete **hormones,** chemical messengers released in response to a change in the body's internal environment. The role of hormones is to maintain the body in homeostasis. For example, when the level of glucose in the blood rises above normal, the pancreas secretes insulin to return glucose levels to normal. The various endocrine glands and their hormones are illustrated in ● Figure 43.1.

After secretion from an endocrine gland, hormones enter the blood and are transported throughout the body. Some, such as insulin and thyroid hormone,

KEY TERMS

Addison's disease *page 674*
adenohypophysis *page 662*
adrenocorticotropic hormone (ACTH) *page 673*
basal metabolic rate *page 666*
Cushing's syndrome *page 678*
diabetes insipidus *page 665*
follicular cells *page 666*
glucocorticoid *page 673*
Graves' disease *page 670*
hormone *page 661*
myxedema *page 667*
negative feedback *page 662*
neurohypophysis *page 662*
parafollicular cells *page 666*
releasing hormone *page 662*
somatostatin *page 665*
somatotropin *page 664*
thyrotoxic crisis (thyroid storm) *page 672*

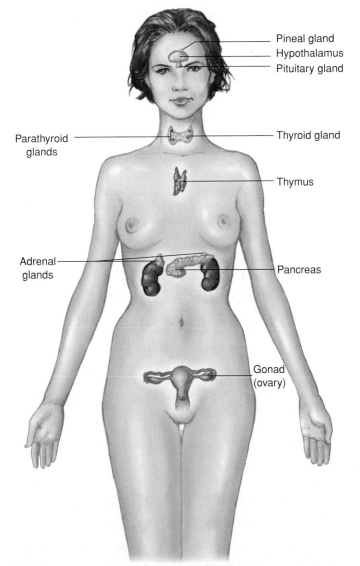

Pineal gland
Hypothalamus
Pituitary gland

Parathyroid glands

Thyroid gland

Thymus

Adrenal glands

Pancreas

Gonad (ovary)

● **Figure 43.1** The endocrine system *Source: Pearson Education/PH College.*

have receptors on nearly every cell in the body; thus, these hormones have widespread effects. Others, such as parathyroid hormone (PTH) and oxytocin, have receptors on only a few specific types of cells.

In the endocrine system, it is common for one hormone to control the secretion of another hormone. In addition, it is common for the last hormone or action in the pathway to provide feedback to turn off the secretion of the first hormone. For example, as serum calcium levels fall, PTH is released; PTH causes an increase in serum calcium, which provides feedback to the parathyroid glands to shut off PTH secretion. This characteristic feature of endocrine homeostasis is known as **negative feedback.**

43.2 The Hypothalamus and Pituitary Gland

Two endocrine structures in the brain, the hypothalamus and the pituitary gland, deserve special recognition because they control many other endocrine glands. The hypothalamus secretes **releasing hormones** that travel via blood vessels a short distance to the pituitary gland. These releasing hormones signal the pituitary which hormone is to be released. After secretion, the pituitary hormone travels to its target tissues to cause its effects. For example, the hypothalamus secretes thyrotropin-releasing hormone (TRH) that travels to the pituitary gland with the message to secrete thyroid-stimulating hormone (TSH). TSH then travels to its target organ, the thyroid gland, to stimulate the release of thyroid hormone. Although the pituitary is often called the master gland, the pituitary and hypothalamus are best visualized as an integrated unit.

The pituitary gland comprises two distinct regions. The anterior pituitary, or **adenohypophysis,** consists of *glandular tissue* and secretes adrenocorticotropic hormone (ACTH), thyroid-stimulating hormone (TSH), growth hormone, prolactin, follicle-stimulating hormone (FSH), and leuteinizing hormone (LH). The posterior pituitary, or **neurohypophysis,** contains *nervous tissue* rather than glandular tissue. Neurons in the posterior pituitary store antidiuretic hormone (ADH) and oxytocin, which are released in response to nerve impulses from the hypothalamus. Those hormones that affect the female reproductive tract are presented in Chapter 45 ∞ . Selected hormones associated with the hypothalamus and pituitary gland are shown in ● Figure 43.2.

43.3 Indications for Hormone Pharmacotherapy

The goals of hormone pharmacotherapy vary widely. In many cases, a hormone is administered as replacement therapy for clients who are unable to secrete sufficient quantities of their own endogenous hormones. Examples of replacement therapy include the administration of thyroid hormone after the thyroid gland has been surgically removed, or supplying insulin to clients whose pancreas is not functioning. Replacement therapy supplies the same physiological, low-level amounts of the hormone that would

AVOIDING MEDICATION ERRORS

A premature infant weighs 2,000 g. The order is for chloramphenicol (Chloromycetin) 25 mg/kg/day administered in two equally divided doses. The nurse administers 50 mg for the 10 A.M. dose. Is that the correct dose?
See Appendix D for the suggested answer.

normally be present in the body. Selected endocrine disorders and their drug therapy are summarized in Table 43.1.

Some hormones are used in cancer chemotherapy to shrink the size of hormone-sensitive tumors. Examples include testosterone for breast cancer and estrogen for testicular cancer. The antineoplastic mechanism of action of these hormones is not known. When hormones are used as antineoplastics, their doses far exceed physiological levels normally present in the body. Hormones are nearly always used in combination with other antineoplastic medications, as discussed in Chapter 37 ∞.

Another goal of hormonal pharmacotherapy may be to produce an *exaggerated response* that is part of the normal action of the hormone. Administering hydrocortisone to suppress inflammation takes advantage of the normal action of the glucocorticoids, but at higher amounts than would normally be present in the body. Supplying estrogen or progesterone at specific times during the menstrual cycle can prevent ovulation and pregnancy. In this example, the client is given natural hormones; however, they are taken at a time when levels in the body are normally low.

Endocrine pharmacotherapy also involves the use of "antihormones." These hormone antagonists block the actions of endogenous hormones. For example, propylthiouracil (PTU) is given to block the effects of an overactive thyroid gland (Section 43.7). Tamoxifen (Nolvadex) is given to block the actions of estrogen in estrogen-dependent breast cancers (Chapter 37 ∞).

DISORDERS OF THE HYPOTHALAMUS AND THE PITUITARY GLAND

Because of the critical role of the pituitary gland in controlling other endocrine tissues, lack of adequate pituitary secretion can have multiple, profound effects on body function. Hypopituitarism can be caused by various tumors of the pituitary and associated brain regions, trauma, autoimmune disorders, or stroke. Pharmacotherapy involves administration of the missing hormone, perhaps for the lifetime of the client.

43.4 Pharmacotherapy With Pituitary and Hypothalamic Hormones

Of the 15 different hormones secreted by the pituitary and the hypothalamus, only a few are used in pharmacotherapy, as listed in Table 43.2. There are valid reasons

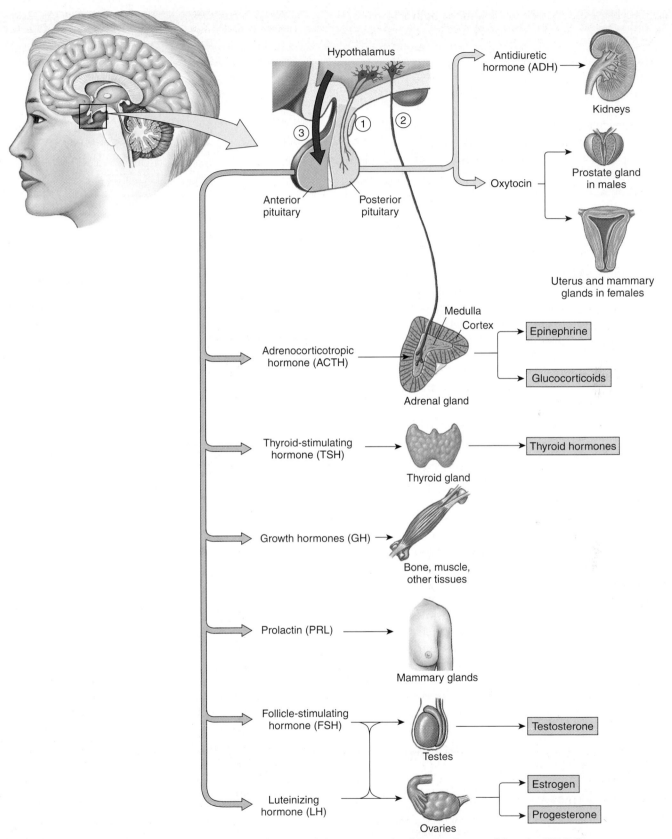

● **Figure 43.2** Hormones associated with the hypothalamus and the pituitary gland *Source: Pearson Education/PH College.*

TABLE 43.1 Selected Endocrine Disorders and Their Pharmacotherapy

Gland	Hormone(s)	Disorder	Drug Therapy
adrenal cortex	glucocorticoids	hypersecretion: Cushing's syndrome	antiadrenal agents
		hyposecretion: Addison's disease	glucocorticoids
pituitary	growth hormone	hyposecretion: small stature	somatrem (Protropin) and somatropin (Genotropin)
		hypersecretion: acromegaly (adults)	octreotide (Sandostatin)
	antidiuretic hormone	hyposecretion: diabetes insipidus	vasopressin, desmopressin, and lypressin
thyroid	thyroid hormone (T_3 and T_4)	hypersecretion: Graves' disease	propylthiouracil (PTU), methimazole (Tapazole), and I-131
		hyposecretion: myxedema (adults)	thyroid hormone, levothyroxine (T_4)

why they are not widely used. Some of these hormones can be obtained only from natural sources (human brains) and can be quite expensive when used in therapeutic quantities. Furthermore, it is usually more effective to give drugs that *directly* affect secretion at the target organs. Two pituitary hormones, prolactin and oxytocin, affect the female reproductive system and are discussed in Chapter 45 ∞. Corticotropin affects the adrenal gland, and is discussed later in this chapter. Of the remaining, growth hormone and antidiuretic hormone have the most clinical utility.

GROWTH HORMONE (GH)

Growth hormone, or **somatotropin,** stimulates the growth and metabolism of nearly every cell in the body. Deficiency of this hormone in children can cause short stature, a condition characterized by significantly decreased physical height compared with the norm of a specific age group. Severe deficiency results in dwarfism. Short stature is caused by many conditions other than GH deficiency, and often a specific cause cannot be identified.

TABLE 43.2 Selected Hypothalamic and Pituitary Agents*

Drug	Route and Adult Dose (max dose where indicated)	Adverse Effects
HYPOTHALAMIC AGENTS		
octreotide (Sandostatin)	Subcutaneous; 100–600 mcg/day in 2–4 divided doses; may switch to IM depot injection after 2 wk at 20 mg q4wk for 2 mo	*Nausea, vomiting, diarrhea, headache, pain at injection site, upper respiratory infection (pegvisomant)*
pegvisomant (Somavert)	Subcutaneous; 40–mg loading dose, then 10 mg/day (max: 30 mg/day)	
		Cholelithiasis, hypothyroidism, seizures, GI bleeding, hypertension/hypotension (protirelin)
protirelin (Thypinone)	IV; 500 mcg bolus over 15–30 sec	
ANTERIOR PITUITARY AGENTS		
corticotropin (ACTH, Acthar)	IV; 10–25 international units in 500 ml D5W infused over 8 h	*Sodium and water retention*
cosyntropin (Cortrosyn)	IM/IV; 0.25 mg injected over 2 min	
		Cushing's syndrome
somatrem (Protropin)	IM/subcutaneous (child); up to 0.1 mg/kg (0.2 international unit/kg) 3 times/wk with a minimum of 48 h between doses	*Otitis media, swelling at injection site, hypercalciuria*
somatropin (Genotropin, Humatrope, others)	Subcutaneous (child); Humatrope; 0.18 mg/kg/wk divided into equal doses on 3 alternate days	Allergic reactions, myalgia
thyrotropin (thyrogen, thyroid-stimulating hormone (TSH)	IM/subcutaneous; 10 international units/day for 1–3 days	*Nausea, headache, asthenia*
		No serious adverse reactions
POSTERIOR PITUITARY AGENTS		
desmopressin acetate (DDAVP, Stimate)	IV; 0.3mcg/kg, repeated as needed Intranasal; 0.1 ml (10 mcg) bid	*Pain at injection site, eructation, flatulence, circumoral pallor, nausea, vomiting, headache*
lypressin (Diapid)	Intranasal; 1–2 sprays (2–4 pressor units) in each nostril qid	
℗ vasopressin (Pitressin)	IM/subcutaneous; 5–10 international units aqueous solution bid–qid (5–60 international units/day) or 1.25–2.5 international units in oil q2–3 days	Cardiac arrest, anaphylaxis, hypertension, dysrhythmias, water intoxication

*Hypothalamic and pituitary agents used for conditions of the female reproductive system are presented in Chapter 45 ∞.
Italics indicate common adverse effects; underlining indicates serious adverse effects.

Prior to 1985, all GH was obtained by extracting the hormone from human pituitary glands, which severely limited the amount available for pharmacotherapy. Several preparations of human GH are now available in large quantities through recombinant DNA technology. For example, somatrem (Protropin) and somatropin (Humatrope, others) are preparations of human GH made by recombinant DNA techniques that are available as replacement therapy in children. If therapy is begun early in life, as much as 6 inches of growth may be achieved. GH therapy is contraindicated in clients after the epiphyses have closed. GH agents are usually well tolerated, although clients must undergo regular assessments of glucose tolerance and thyroid function during pharmacotherapy. All the growth hormone preparations are administered by the subcutaneous route.

Prior to 2003, growth hormone therapy was approved only for treating short stature in children who had deficiencies in GH. The FDA, however, has now approved growth hormone therapy to treat children with short stature who have *normal* levels of GH. The height criterion for treatment is defined as an expected adult height of less than 5 feet 3 inches for men and 4 feet 11 inches for women. GH therapy in children with normal growth hormone levels may add 1 to 3 inches in height to children after 4 to 6 years of pharmacotherapy. The annual cost of $30,000 to $40,000 may discourage many parents from seeking this therapy for their children.

Excess secretion of growth hormone in adults is known as *acromegaly*. A rare disease nearly always caused by a pituitary tumor, acromegaly sometimes requires pharmacotherapy.

Octreotide (Sandostatin) is a synthetic growth hormone *antagonist* structurally related to growth hormone–inhibiting hormone (**somatostatin**). In addition to inhibiting growth hormone, octreotide promotes fluid and electrolyte reabsorption from the GI tract and prolongs intestinal transit time. It has limited applications in treating acromegaly in adults and in treating the severe diarrhea sometimes associated with metastatic carcinoid tumors. Acromegaly may also be treated with pegvisomant (Somavert), a recently approved growth hormone–receptor antagonist.

ANTIDIURETIC HORMONE

As its name implies, antidiuretic hormone (ADH) conserves water in the body. ADH is secreted from the posterior pituitary gland when the hypothalamus senses that plasma volume has decreased, or that the osmolality of the blood has become too high. ADH acts on the collecting ducts in the kidneys to increase water reabsorption. ADH is also called *vasopressin*, because it has the capability to raise blood pressure, when secreted in large amounts. Vasopressin is available as a drug for the treatment of **diabetes insipidus,** a rare disease caused by a deficiency of ADH. Clients with this disorder have an intense thirst and produce very dilute urine owing to the large volume of water lost by the kidneys.

Desmopressin (DDAVP) is the most common form of antidiuretic hormone in use. It has a duration of action of up to 20 hours, whereas vasopressin (Pitressin) and lypressin (Diapid) have durations of only 2 to 8 hours. In addition, desmopressin is available as a nasal spray and is easily self-

---

ACTIONS AND USES

Three ADH preparations are available for the treatment of diabetes insipidus: vasopressin (Pitressin), desmopressin (DDAVP, Stimate), and lypressin (Diapid). Vasopressin is a synthetic hormone that has a structure identical with that of human ADH. It acts on the renal collecting tubules to increase their permeability to water, thus enhancing water reabsorption. Although it acts within minutes, vasopressin has a short half-life that requires it to be administered 3 to 4 times per day. Vasopressin tannate is formulated in peanut oil to increase its duration of action. Vasopressin is usually given IM or IV, although an intranasal form is available for mild diabetes insipidus.

ADMINISTRATION ALERTS

- Never administer vasopressin tannate IV, because it is an oil.
- Vasopressin aqueous injection may be given by continuous IV infusion after it is diluted in normal saline or D5W.
- Pregnancy category X.

PHARMACOKINETICS

Onset: 1–2 h (IM)

Peak: Unknown

Half-life: 10–20 min

Duration: 2–8 h IM; 30–60 Min IV

ADVERSE EFFECTS

Vasopressin has a strong vasoconstrictor action that is unrelated to its antidiuretic properties; thus, hypertension is possible. The drug can precipitate angina episodes and myocardial infarction in clients with coronary artery disease. Excessive fluid retention can cause water intoxication: Symptoms include headache, restlessness, confusion, drowsiness, and coma. Water intoxication can usually be avoided by teaching the client to decrease water intake during vasopressin therapy.

Contraindications: The only contraindication to ADH is hypersensitivity to the drug.

INTERACTIONS

Drug–Drug: Alcohol, epinephrine, heparin, lithium, and phenytoin may decrease the antidiuretic effects of vasopressin. Neostigmine may increase vasopressor actions. Carbamazepine, tricyclic antidepressants, and thiazide diuretics may increase antidiuretic activity.

Lab Tests: Unknown.

Herbal/Food: Unknown.

Treatment of Overdose: Overdose may cause severe water intoxication. Treatment includes water restriction and osmotic diuretics

 See the Companion Website for a Nursing Process Focus specific to this drug.

administered, whereas vasopressin must be administered IM or subcutaneously. The client may also more easily increase or decrease the dosage depending on urine output. Desmopressin is available in subcutaneous, intravenous, and oral forms, and is occasionally used by the intranasal route for enuresis, or bed-wetting. Desmopressin and lypressin do not have the intense vasoconstricting effects of vasopressin; thus, they produce fewer adverse effects.

NURSING CONSIDERATIONS

The role of the nurse in antidiuretic hormone therapy for ADH deficiency involves careful monitoring of a client's condition and providing education as it relates to the prescribed drug treatment. Assess for electrolyte imbalances, changes in specific gravity of urine, and fluid intake, because antidiuretic hormone causes water to be reabsorbed into the body. Monitoring of serum sodium and potassium levels is crucial to determining whether ADH treatment is therapeutic. A decreased urinary specific gravity indicates dilute urine in which ADH is deficient; therefore, routine urinalysis and monitoring of fluid intake and output is crucial to evaluating therapeutic response to the treatment regimen.

Assess vital signs, especially blood pressure and pulse, because fluid retention may raise blood pressure, and ADH is a potent vasoconstrictor. Vasopressin is contraindicated in clients with heart disease and should be used cautiously in elderly clients who might have undiagnosed heart disease. Monitor intake, output, and body weight, because these drugs may cause water retention, thus leading to peripheral edema and increased body weight. Assess neurological status, because water intoxication causes decreased sodium levels: Clients may display symptoms of headache and changes in mental status such as drowsiness and confusion.

Obtain a current list of the client's medications and lifestyle patterns, to determine whether any are contraindicated. Alcohol, epinephrine, heparin, lithium, and phenytoin may also decrease the therapeutic effects of ADH.

Lifespan Considerations. Desmopressin is administered to children age 6 and older for enuresis. The drug is most effective in children older than age 9. It is usually used as a second choice, when behavioral and motivational therapies have failed. It is sometimes used sporadically, when the child will be away from home for special events and there is added emotional stress. It does not cure bed-wetting, but it does decrease its incidence. After the drug is discontinued, relapse rates are high.

Client Teaching. Client education as it relates to antidiuretic therapy should include the goals of therapy, the reasons for obtaining baseline data such as vital signs and the existence of underlying cardiac disorders, and possible drug side effects. Include the following points when teaching clients about antidiuretic hormone therapy:

- Keep all scheduled laboratory visits for urinalysis and serum electrolyte tests.
- Monitor weight twice a week and report significant increases or decreases.
- Report headaches, changes in mental status, and increased swelling of the feet or ankles, which may indicate water retention and/or hypertension.
- Avoid alcohol use, because alcohol lowers the therapeutic effects of ADH.
- Do not take other prescription drugs, OTC medications, herbal remedies, or vitamins or minerals without notifying your healthcare provider.
- Immediately report episodes of angina.

43.5 Normal Function of the Thyroid Gland

The thyroid gland secretes hormones that affect nearly every cell in the body. By stimulating the enzymes involved with glucose oxidation, thyroid gland hormones regulate **basal metabolic rate,** the baseline speed at which cells perform their functions. By increasing cellular metabolism, thyroid hormone increases body temperature. The gland also helps maintain blood pressure and regulate growth and development.

The thyroid gland has two basic types of cells, which secrete different hormones. **Parafollicular cells** secrete calcitonin, a hormone that is involved with calcium homeostasis (Chapter 47 ∞). **Follicular cells** in the gland secrete thyroid hormone, which is actually a combination of two different hormones: thyroxine (T_4) and triiodothyronine (T_3). Iodine is essential for the synthesis of these hormones, and is provided through the dietary intake of common iodized salt. The names of these hormones refer to the number of bound iodine atoms in each molecule, either three (T_3) or four (T_4). Thyroxine is the major hormone secreted by the thyroid gland.

As it travels through the blood, thyroid hormone is attached to a carrier protein, thyroxine-binding globulin (TBG), which protects it from degradation. Because of the importance of TBG in transporting thyroid hormone to its active sites, deficiencies may result in thyroid dysfunction. At the target tissues thyroxine is converted to T_3 through the enzymatic cleavage of one iodine atom. T_3 then enters the target cells, where it binds to intracellular receptors within the nucleus.

Thyroid function is regulated through multiple levels of hormonal control. Falling thyroxine levels in the blood sig-

PHARMFACTS

Thyroid Disorders

- Hypothyroidism is 10 times more common in women; hyperthyroidism is 5 to 10 times more common in women.
- The two most common thyroid diseases, Graves' disease and Hashimoto's thyroiditis, are autoimmune diseases and may have a genetic link.
- One of every 4,000 babies is born without a working thyroid gland.
- About 15,000 new cases of thyroid cancer are diagnosed each year.
- One of every five women older than 75 years has Hashimoto's thyroiditis.
- Postpartum thyroiditis occurs in 5% to 9% of women and may recur in future pregnancies.
- Both hyperthyroidism and hypothyroidism can affect a woman's ability to become pregnant and can cause miscarriages.

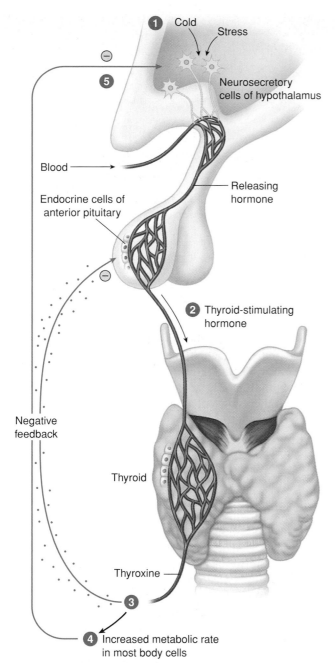

● **Figure 43.3** Feedback mechanisms of the thyroid gland: (1) stimulus; (2) release of TSH; (3) release of thyroid hormone; (4) increased BMR; (5) negative feedback

43.6 Pharmacotherapy of Hypothyroidism

Hypothyroidism may result from either a poorly functioning thyroid gland or low secretion of TSH by the pituitary gland. The most common cause of hypothyroidism in the United States is destruction of the thyroid gland due to chronic autoimmune thyroiditis, known as *Hashimoto's disease.* Early symptoms of hypothyroidism in adults, or **myxedema,** include general weakness, muscle cramps, and dry skin. More severe symptoms include slurred speech, bradycardia, weight gain, decreased sense of taste and smell, and intolerance to cold environments. Lab results generally reveal elevated TSH with diminished T_3 and T_4 levels. The etiology of myxedema may include autoimmune disease, surgical removal of the thyroid gland, or aggressive treatment with antithyroid drugs. At high doses, the antidysrhythmic drug amiodarone (Cordarone) can induce hypothyroidism in clients owing to its high iodine content. Enlargement of the

nal the hypothalamus to secrete thyroid-releasing hormone (TRH), or thyrotropin. TRH stimulates the pituitary gland to secrete TSH, which then stimulates the thyroid gland to release thyroid hormone. Rising levels of thyroid hormone in the blood trigger a negative feedback response to shut off secretion of TRH and TSH. The negative feedback mechanism for the thyroid gland is shown in ● Figure 43.3.

THYROID AGENTS

Thyroid disorders are common and drug therapy is often indicated. The correct dose of thyroid drug is highly individualized and requires careful, periodic adjustment. The medications used to treat thyroid disease are listed in Table 43.3.

TABLE 43.3 Thyroid and Antithyroid Drugs

Drug	Route and Adult Dose (max dose where indicated)	Adverse Effects
THYROID AGENTS		
levothyroxine (Levothroid, Synthroid, others)	PO; 100–400 mcg/day	*Weight loss, headache, tremors, nervousness, heat intolerance, insomnia, menstrual irregularities*
liothyronine (Cytomel, Triostat)	PO; 25–75 mcg/day	
liotrix (Euthroid, Thyrolar)	PO; 12.5–30 mcg/day	<u>Dysrhythmias, hypertension, palpitations</u>
thyroid (Thyrar, Thyroid USP)	PO; 60–100 mg/day	
ANTITHYROID AGENTS		
methimazole (Tapazole)	PO; 5–15 mg tid	*Nausea, rash, pruritus, weight gain, headache, fever, numbness in fingers, leukopenia, diarrhea*
potassium iodide and iodine (Lugol's Solution, Thyro-Block)	PO; 0.1–1.0 ml tid	
propylthiouracil (PTU)	PO; 100–150 mg tid	<u>Agranulocytosis, bradycardia, hepatotoxicity (methimazole)</u>
radioactive iodide (I-131, Iodotope)	PO; 0.8–150 mCi (Ci: curie, a unit of radioactivity)	

Italics indicate common adverse effects; <u>underlining</u> indicates serious adverse effects.

thyroid gland, or goiter, may be absent or present, depending on the cause of the disease.

Hypothyroidism usually responds well to pharmacotherapy with natural or synthetic thyroid agents. Choices include desiccated thyroid gland from beef, pork, or sheep sources (Thyroid USP), synthetic T_3, and synthetic T_4. Levothyroxine (T_4) is more stable than thyroid USP and eliminates the possibility of allergic reactions to animal protein. Because small changes in drug bioavailability can affect thyroid function, clients should avoid switching brands once their condition has stabilized. Liothyronine sodium is a short-acting synthetic form of the natural thyroid hormone that can be administered IV to individuals with myxedema coma. The short duration of action allows for a rapid response to critically ill clients.

NURSING CONSIDERATIONS

The role of the nurse in thyroid hormone therapy involves careful monitoring of a client's condition and providing education as it relates to the prescribed drug treatment. Obtain a current list of the client's medications, herbal therapies, dietary supplements, and OTC medications, because thyroid hormone interacts with many substances (see the Prototype Drug feature on page 669). Because the thyroid regulates basal metabolic rate, assess the client's weight and vital signs. Weight gain, decreased pulse, and hypotension are characteristic of decreased metabolic rate seen in hypothyroidism. Levothyroxine increases metabolic rate, which can cause cardiovascular collapse in clients with undiagnosed heart disease. Monitor pulse and blood pressure to assess for early signs of cardiovascular collapse. Desiccated thyroid can cause the same cardiovascular complications as levothyroxine. Assess tachycardia, irregular heart rate, and hypertension, which could indicate an overdose of thyroid hormone. Too much of the drug causes hyperthyroidism, in which the client displays nervousness, weight loss, diarrhea, and heat intolerance. Monitor clients with impaired renal function closely, because an increased metabolic rate increases the workload of the kidneys. Levothyroxine is contraindicated in those with adrenal insufficiency.

Lifespan Considerations. During the first 12 weeks of pregnancy, the thyroid gland of the fetus is not fully functional and the mother is the only source of thyroid hormone for the growing baby. If the mother is hypothyroid during this period, there is an increased risk of miscarriage, and the baby is at increased risk of developmental problems. For example, babies born to mothers with untreated hypothyroidism are almost four times more likely to have lower IQs and learning difficulties. For this reason, women who have a history of hypothyroidism should receive a consultation with an endocrinologist prior to becoming pregnant. The healthcare provider will evaluate T_3 and T_4 levels and adjust the thyroid replacement hormone dosage to therapeutic levels, thus preventing developmental complications. Most women can continue to take thyroid hormone during lactation, because only trace amounts of thyroid hormone are excreted in breast milk.

Client Teaching. Client education as it relates to thyroid hormone replacement therapy should include the goals of therapy, the reasons for obtaining baseline data such as vital signs and the existence of underlying disorders such as cardiac disease, and possible drug side effects. Include the following points when teaching clients about thyroid replacement therapy:

- Inform your healthcare provider if you have Addison's disease, diabetes mellitus, or diabetes insipidus, because thyroid replacement therapy may be contraindicated.
- Take thyroid medications on an empty stomach at the same time each day.
- Immediately report nervousness, palpitations, and heat intolerance, because these may indicate overdosage.
- Immediately report excess fatigue, slow speech, hoarseness or slow pulse, because these may indicate underdosage.
- Do not stop taking this medication without consulting your healthcare provider.

Pr PROTOTYPE DRUG | Levothyroxine *(Synthroid)* | Thyroid Hormone

ACTIONS AND USES

Levothyroxine, a synthetic form of thyroxine (T_4), is a drug of choice for replacement therapy in clients with low thyroid function. Actions are those of thyroid hormone, and include loss of weight, improved tolerance to environmental temperature, increased activity, and increased pulse rate. Doses are highly individualized. Therapy may take 3 weeks or longer before T_4 levels stabilize; Doses may require periodic adjustments for several months. Serum TSH levels are monitored to determine whether the client is receiving sufficient levothyroxine—high TSH levels usually indicate that the dosage of T_4 needs to be increased.

ADMINISTRATION ALERTS

- Administer medication at the same time every day, preferably in the morning to decrease incidence of drug-related insomnia.
- Pregnancy category A.

PHARMACOKINETICS

Onset: Unknown

Peak: 3–4 wk

Half-life: 6–7 days

Duration: 1–3 wk

ADVERSE EFFECTS

The difference between a therapeutic and a toxic dose of levothyroxine is narrow, and care must be taken to avoid overtreatment. Adverse effects are those of hyperthyroidism and include palpitations, dysrhythmias, anxiety, insomnia, weight loss, and heat intolerance. Menstrual irregularities may occur in females, and long-term use of levothyroxine has been associated with osteoporosis in women.

Contraindications: This drug is contraindicated in clients with known or suspected adrenal insufficiency, and in clients hypersensitive to the drug.

INTERACTIONS

Drug–Drug: Cholestyramine and colestipol decrease the absorption of levothyroxine. Concurrent administration of epinephrine and norepinephrine increases the risk of cardiac insufficiency. Use with oral anticoagulants may potentiate hypoprothrombinemia.

Lab Tests: Unknown.

Herbal/Food: Lemon balm may interfere with thyroid hormone action.

Treatment of Overdose: Overdose can cause serious thyrotoxicosis, which may not present until several days after the overdose. Treatment is symptomatic, usually targeted at preventing cardiac toxicity with beta-adrenergic antagonists such as propranolol.

 See the Companion Website for a Nursing Process Focus specific to this drug.

NURSING PROCESS FOCUS Clients Receiving Thyroid Hormone Replacement

Assessment	Potential Nursing Diagnoses
Prior to administration: - Obtain a complete health history including weight, allergies, drug history, and possible drug interactions. - Obtain a complete physical examination. - Assess for the presence and history of symptoms of hypothyroidism. - Obtain ECG and laboratory studies including T_4, T_3, and serum TSH levels.	- Activity Intolerance, related to disease process - Fatigue, related to impaired metabolic status - Knowledge, Deficient, related to drug therapy - Health Maintenance, Ineffective, related to side effects of drug

Planning: Client Goals and Expected Outcomes

The client will:
- Exhibit normal thyroid hormone levels.
- Report a decrease in hypothyroid symptoms.
- Experience no significant adverse effects from drug therapy.
- Demonstrate an understanding of the drug's action by accurately describing drug side effects and precautions.

Implementation

Interventions and (Rationales)	Client Education/Discharge Planning
- Monitor vital signs. (Changes in metabolic rate are manifested as changes in blood pressure, pulse, and body temperature.)	- Instruct client to report dizziness, palpitations, and intolerance to temperature changes.
- Monitor for decreasing symptoms related to hypothyroidism such as fatigue, constipation, cold intolerance, lethargy, depression, and menstrual irregularities. (Decreasing symptoms demonstrate that drug is achieving therapeutic affect.)	- Instruct client about the signs of hypothyroidism and to report symptoms.
- Monitor for symptoms related to hyperthyroidism such as nervousness, insomnia, tachycardia, dysrhythmias, heat intolerance, chest pain, and diarrhea. (Symptoms of hyperthyroidism indicate the drug is at a toxic level.)	- Instruct client about the signs of hyperthyroidism and to report symptoms.

(Continued)

NURSING PROCESS FOCUS Clients Receiving Thyroid Hormone Replacement *(Continued)*

Implementation	
Interventions and (Rationales)	**Client Education/Discharge Planning**
▪ Monitor T_3, T_4, and TSH levels. (These levels help determine the effectiveness of pharmacotherapy.)	Instruct client: ▪ About the importance of ongoing monitoring of thyroid hormone levels. ▪ To keep all laboratory appointments.
▪ Monitor blood glucose levels, especially in individuals with diabetes mellitus. (Thyroid hormone increases metabolic rate, and glucose utilization may be altered.)	Instruct the diabetic client: ▪ To monitor blood glucose levels. ▪ Adjust insulin doses as directed by the healthcare provider.
▪ Provide supportive nursing care to cope with symptoms of hypothyroidism such as constipation, cold intolerance, and fatigue until drug has achieved therapeutic effect. (Supportive nursing care decreases the client's anxiety, which will promote healing and compliance.)	Instruct client to: ▪ Increase fluid and fiber intake and activity to reduce constipation. ▪ Wear additional clothing and maintain a comfortable room environment for cold intolerance. ▪ Plan activities and include rest periods to avoid fatigue.
▪ Monitor weight at least weekly. (Weight loss is expected because of increased metabolic rate. Weight changes help determine the effectiveness of drug therapy.)	▪ Instruct client to weigh self weekly and to report significant changes.
▪ Monitor client for signs of decreased compliance with therapeutic regimen. (Decreased compliance requires early intervention and education about the medical regimen and the disease process.)	Instruct client about: ▪ The importance of lifelong therapy. ▪ The disease. ▪ The importance of follow-up care.

Evaluation of Outcome Criteria
Evaluate the effectiveness of drug therapy by confirming that client goals and expected outcomes have been met (see "Planning"). ▪ The client's thyroid hormone levels are normal. ▪ The client demonstrates decreased symptoms of hypothyroidism. ▪ The client is free from significant adverse effects from drug therapy. ▪ The client demonstrates an understanding of the drug's action by accurately describing drug side effects and precautions.

∞ *See Table 43.3, under the heading "Thyroid Agents," for a list of drugs to which these nursing actions apply.*

• Do not take other prescribed drugs, OTC medications, herbal therapies, or dietary supplements without notifying your healthcare provider.

• Keep all scheduled appointments and laboratory visits for testing.

ANTITHYROID AGENTS

Medications are often used to treat the cause of hyperthyroidism or to relieve its distressing symptoms. The goal of antithyroid therapy is to lower the activity of the thyroid gland.

43.7 Pharmacotherapy of Hyperthyroidism

Hypersecretion of thyroid hormone results in symptoms that are the opposite of those caused by hypothyroidism: increased body metabolism, tachycardia, weight loss, elevated body temperature, and anxiety. The most common type of hyperthyroidism is called **Graves' disease.** Considered an autoimmune disease in which the body develops antibodies against its own thyroid gland, Graves' disease is four to eight times more common in women, and most often occurs be-

tween the ages of 30 and 40. Other causes of hyperthyroidism are adenomas of the thyroid, pituitary tumors, and pregnancy. If the cause of the hypersecretion is found to be a tumor, or if the disease cannot be controlled through pharmacotherapy, surgical removal of the thyroid gland is indicated.

The two primary drugs for hyperthyroidism, propylthiouracil (PTU) and methimazole (Tapazole), are called thioamides. These agents act by inhibiting the incorporation of iodine atoms into T_3 and T_4. Methimazole has a much longer half-life that offers the advantage of less frequent dosing, although side effects can be more severe. Both thioamides are pregnancy category D agents, but methimazole crosses the placenta more readily than propylthiouracil and is contraindicated in pregnant clients.

A third antithyroid drug, sodium iodide-131 (Iodotope) is a radioactive isotope that destroys overactive thyroid glands with ionizing radiation. Shortly after oral administration, I-131 accumulates in the thyroid gland, where it destroys follicular cells. The goal of pharmacotherapy with I-131 is to destroy just enough of the thyroid gland so that levels of thyroid function return to normal. Full benefits may take several months. Although most clients require only a single dose, others need multiple treatments. Small diagnostic doses of

Pr PROTOTYPE DRUG | Propylthiouracil *(PTU)* | Antithyroid Agent

ACTIONS AND USES

Propylthiouracil is administered to clients with hyperthyroidism. It acts by interfering with the synthesis of T_3 and T_4 in the thyroid gland. It also prevents the conversion of T_4 to T_3 in the target tissues. Its action may be delayed from several days to as long as 6 to 12 weeks. Effects include a return to normal thyroid function: weight gain, reduction in anxiety, less insomnia, and slower pulse rate. Owing to its short half-life, PTU is usually administered several times a day.

ADMINISTRATION ALERTS

- Administer with meals to reduce GI distress.
- Pregnancy category D.

PHARMACOKINETICS

Onset: 30–40 min

Peak: 1–1.5 h

Half-life: 1–2 h

Duration: 2–4 h

ADVERSE EFFECTS

Overtreatment with propylthiouracil produces symptoms of hypothyroidism. Rash and transient leucopenia are the most common side effects. A small percentage of clients experience agranulocytosis, which is its most serious adverse effect. Periodic laboratory blood counts and TSH values are necessary to establish proper dosage.

Contraindications: Propylthiouracil should not be given during pregnancy or lactation or to clients with known or suspected hypothyroidism.

INTERACTIONS

Drug–Drug: Propylthiouracil can reverse the effects of drugs such as aminophylline, heparin, and digoxin. Drugs containing iodine may diminish the antithyroid effects of propylthiouracil.

Lab Tests: May increase prothrombin time and increase serum levels of aspartate aminotransferase (AST), alanine aminotransferase (ALT), and alkaline phosphatase (ALP).

Herbal/Food: Unknown.

Treatment of Overdose: Overdose will cause signs of hypothyroidism. Treatment includes a thyroid agent, atropine for bradycardia, and symptomatic treatment as necessary.

 See the Companion Website for a Nursing Process Focus specific to this drug.

NURSING PROCESS FOCUS   Clients Receiving Antithyroid Therapy

Assessment

Prior to administration:

- Obtain a complete health history including allergies, drug history, and possible drug interactions.
- Obtain a complete physical examination.
- Assess for the presence and history of hyperthyroidism.
- Obtain laboratory studies including T_3, T_4, and TSH levels, level, ECG, and complete blood count (CBC).

Potential Nursing Diagnoses

- Infection, Risk for, related to drug-induced agranulocytosis
- Injury, Risk for, related to side effects of drug therapy
- Health Maintenance, Ineffective, related to adverse GI effects
- Knowledge, Deficient, related to drug therapy

Planning: Client Goals and Expected Outcomes

The client will:

- Exhibit a decrease in the symptoms of hyperthyroidism.
- Exhibit normal thyroid hormone levels.
- Exhibit no drug adverse effects such as agranulocytosis or GI distress.
- Demonstrate an understanding of the drug's action by accurately describing drug side effects and precautions.

Implementation

Interventions and (Rationales)	Client Education/Discharge Planning
• Monitor vital signs. (Changes in metabolic rate is manifested as changes in blood pressure, pulse, and body temperature.)	Instruct client: • To count pulse for a full minute, record pulse with every dose, and report rates as ordered by the healthcare provider. • To report dizziness, palpitations, and intolerance to temperature changes.
• Monitor thyroid function tests. (Test results determine the effectiveness of the drug therapy.)	• Instruct client in the importance of follow-up care and to keep all laboratory appointments.
• Monitor for signs of infection, including CBC and white blood cell (WBC) count. (Antithyroid drug may cause agranulocytosis.)	Instruct client: • That antithyroid medication may affect the body's ability to defend against bacteria and viruses.

(Continued)

NURSING PROCESS FOCUS Clients Receiving Antithyroid Therapy *(Continued)*

Implementation

Interventions and (Rationales)	Client Education/Discharge Planning
	■ To report sore throat, fever, chills, malaise, and weakness. ■ Of the importance of proper hand-washing techniques to decrease the risk of developing an infection.
■ Monitor weight at least weekly. (As a result of slower metabolism, weight gain is expected.)	■ Instruct client to weigh weekly and to report significant changes.
■ Monitor for drowsiness. (Antithyroid medications may cause drowsiness.)	■ Instruct client that medication may cause drowsiness and to avoid hazardous activities until the effects of the drug are known.
■ Monitor for gastrointestinal distress. (Antithyroid medications may cause nausea and vomiting.)	■ Instruct client to take antithyroid medication with food.
■ Monitor for a decrease in symptoms related to hyperthyroidism such as nervousness, insomnia, tachycardia, dysrhythmias, heat intolerance, chest pain, and diarrhea. (These parameters help determine whether the drug is at a therapeutic level.)	■ Instruct client about the signs of hyperthyroidism and to report any to the healthcare provider.
■ Monitor for symptoms related to hypothyroidism such as fatigue, constipation, cold intolerance, lethargy, depression, and menstrual irregularities. (These symptoms indicate drug toxicity.)	■ Instruct client about the signs of hypothyroidism and to report any to the healthcare provider.
■ Monitor for activity intolerance. (Hyperthyroidism results in protein catabolism, overactivity, and increased metabolism leading to exhaustion.)	■ Instruct client to schedule rest periods while performing activities of daily living until medication has achieved therapeutic effect.
■ Monitor dietary intake. (Iodine increases the production of thyroid hormones, which is not desirable in these clients.)	■ Instruct client to avoid foods with high iodine content such as soy, tofu, turnips, iodized salt, and some breads as directed.
■ Monitor client's response to drug therapy. (Response determines effectiveness of drug therapy.)	■ Instruct client to keep a log of responses to medication including pulse, weight, mood status, and energy level and to be aware that stabilization of thyroid hormone levels may take several months.

Evaluation of Outcome Criteria

Evaluate the effectiveness of drug therapy by confirming that client goals and expected outcomes have been met (see "Planning").
■ The client demonstrates decreased symptoms of hyperthyroidism.
■ The client demonstrates normal serum thyroid levels.
■ The client is free of adverse effects such as agranulocytosis or GI distress.
■ The client demonstrates an understanding of the drug's action by accurately describing drug side effects and precautions.

∞ *See Table 43.3, under the heading "Antithyroid Agents," for a list of drugs to which these nursing actions apply.*

I-131 are used in nuclear medicine to determine the degree of iodide uptake in the various parts of the thyroid gland.

Nonradioactive iodine is also available to treat other thyroid conditions. Lugol's solution is a mixture of 5% elemental iodine and 10% potassium iodide that is used to suppress thyroid function 10 to 15 days prior to thyroidectomy. Sodium iodide is administered IV (along with propylthiouracil) to manage an acute, life-threatening form of hyperthyroidism known as **thyrotoxic crisis,** or **thyroid storm.** Potassium iodide (Thyro-Block, ThyroSafe) is administered to protect the thyroid from radiation damage following a nuclear bioterrorist act, as discussed in Chapter 3 ∞.

NURSING CONSIDERATIONS

The role of the nurse in hyperthyroidism therapy involves careful monitoring of a client's condition and providing education as it relates to the prescribed drug treatment. Assess for signs and symptoms of hypothyroidism such as weight gain, hypotension, bradycardia, fatigue, depression, sensitivity to cold environments, hair loss, and dry skin in those clients receiving antithyroid therapy. Assess for complications and adverse effects specific to the antithyroid medication prescribed for the client. For clients receiving propylthiouracil (PTU), monitor white blood cell (WBC) levels periodically, because PTU may cause agranulocytosis, which places the client at risk for infection. Assess for signs of jaundice and monitor liver enzymes, because PTU is metabolized by the liver. The administration of anticoagulants should be monitored carefully, because PTU causes an increase in bleeding. Methimazole (Tapazole) is similar to PTU but is more toxic. Assess for blood dyscrasias such as agranulocytosis and jaundice. These adverse effects usually disappear when the drug is discontinued.

Radioactive iodine (I-131) is used to permanently decrease thyroid function. Assess thyroid function tests, because this medication must be carefully calibrated to achieve a therapeutic dose that achieves a euthyroid state. Instruct the client on signs and symptoms of hypothyroidism. Because the client emits radiation after receiving this drug, children and pregnant women should be avoided for 1 week after administration and close physical contact with others should be limited for a few days.

Lifespan Considerations.   Radioactive iodine (I-131) is contraindicated in clients who are pregnant or breast-feeding. Women who are receiving this agent should take precautions to avoid pregnancy. If a woman suspects she is pregnant, she should contact her healthcare provider immediately. Women who will be receiving this treatment should stop breast-feeding for the duration of therapy and discuss alternative feeding methods with their healthcare provider.

Client Teaching.   Client education as it relates to antithyroid agents should include the goals of therapy, the reasons for obtaining baseline data such as vital signs and the existence of underlying cardiac and renal disorders, and possible drug side effects. Include the following points when teaching clients about antithyroid agents:

- Keep all scheduled laboratory visits for testing.
- Do not breast-feed.
- Practice reliable contraception and notify your healthcare provider if pregnancy is planned or suspected.
- Immediately report nervousness, palpitations, and heat intolerance, because these may indicate underdosage.
- Immediately report excess fatigue, slow speech, hoarseness or slow pulse, because these may indicate overdosage.
- Inform your healthcare provider if you are taking any of the following medications because they are contraindicated with antithyroid agents: aminophylline, heparin, or digoxin.

ADRENAL GLAND DISORDERS

Though small, the adrenal glands secrete hormones that affect every body tissue. Adrenal disorders include those resulting from *excess* hormone secretion and *deficient* hormone secretion. The specific pharmacotherapy depends on which portion of the adrenal gland is responsible for the abnormal secretion.

43.8 Normal Function of the Adrenal Gland

The adrenal glands secrete three essential classes of steroid hormones: the glucocorticoids, mineralocorticoids, and gonadocorticoids. Collectively, the glucocorticoids and mineralocorticoids are called *corticosteroids* or *adrenocortical hormones*. The terms *corticosteroid* and *glucocorticoid* are sometimes used interchangeably in clinical practice. However, it should be understood that the term corticosteroid implies a drug has both glucocorticoid *and* mineralocorticoid activity.

Gonadocorticoids The gonadocorticoids secreted by the adrenal cortex are mostly androgens (male sex hormones), though small amounts of estrogens are also produced. The amounts of these adrenal sex hormones are far less than the levels secreted by the testes or ovaries. It is believed that the adrenal gonadocorticoids contribute to the onset of puberty. The adrenal glands also are the primary source of endogenous estrogen in postmenopausal women. Hypersecretion of gonadocorticoids, such as that caused by a tumor of the adrenal cortex, results in hirsutism and masculinization, signs that are more noticeable in female clients. The physiologic effects of androgens are detailed in Chapter 46 ∞.

Mineralocorticoids Aldosterone accounts for more than 95% of the mineralocorticoids secreted by the adrenals. The primary function of aldosterone is to promote sodium reabsorption and potassium excretion by the renal tubule, thus regulating plasma volume. When plasma volume falls, the kidney secretes renin, which results in the production of angiotensin II. Angiotensin II then causes aldosterone secretion, which promotes sodium and water retention. Attempts to modify this pathway led to the development of the angiotensin-converting enzyme (ACE) inhibitor class of medications, which are often drugs of choice for cardiovascular disorders such as hypertension and heart failure (Chapters 23 and 24 ∞). Certain adrenal tumors cause excessive secretion of aldosterone, a condition known as *hyperaldosteronism*, which is characterized by hypertension and hypokalemia.

Glucocorticoids More than 30 **glucocorticoids** are secreted from the adrenal cortex, including cortisol, corticosterone, and cortisone. Cortisol, also called *hydrocortisone*, is secreted in the highest amount, and is the most important pharmacologically. Glucocorticoids affect the metabolism of nearly every cell and prepare the body for long-term stress. The effects of glucocorticoids are diverse, and include the following:

- Increasing the level of blood glucose (hyperglycemic effect) by inhibiting insulin secretion and promoting gluconeogenesis, the synthesis of carbohydrates from lipid and protein sources
- Increasing the breakdown of proteins and lipids and their utilization as energy sources
- Suppressing the inflammatory and immune responses (Chapters 32 and 33 ∞)
- Increasing the sensitivity of vascular smooth muscle to norepinephrine and angiotensin II
- Influencing the CNS by affecting mood and maintaining normal brain excitability

43.9 Control of Glucocorticoid Secretion

Control of glucocorticoid levels in the blood begins with corticotropin-releasing factor (CRF), secreted by the hypothalamus. CRF travels to the pituitary where it causes the release of **adrenocorticotropic hormone (ACTH).** ACTH then travels through the blood and reaches the adrenal cortex, causing it to release glucocorticoids. When the level of cortisol in the blood rises, it provides negative feedback to the hypothalamus and the pituitary to shut off further release of glucocorticoids. This negative feedback mechanism is shown in ● Figure 43.4.

ACTH, also known as *corticotropin*, is available as a medication in three different preparations: corticotropin

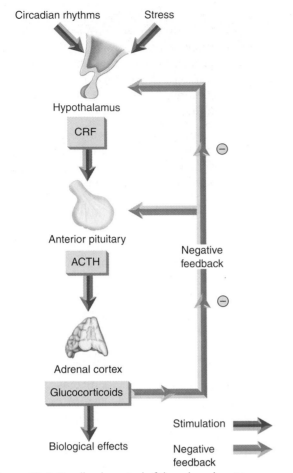

Circadian rhythms   Stress

Hypothalamus

CRF

Anterior pituitary

ACTH

Negative
feedback

Adrenal cortex

Glucocorticoids

Biological effects

Stimulation

Negative
feedback

● **Figure 43.4** Feedback control of the adrenal cortex

injection (Acthar, ACTH), repository corticotropin (H.P. Acthar, ACTH-40, ACTH-80), and corticotropin zinc hydroxide (Cortrophin-Zinc). A fourth drug, cosyntropin (Cortrosyn) closely resembles ACTH. Although these preparations stimulate the adrenal gland to produce glucocorticoids, they are rarely used to correct corticosteroid deficiency. The ACTH agents must be given parenterally, and they produce numerous side effects. The primary use of these agents is to diagnose adrenal disorders. After administration of cosyntropin, plasma levels of cortisol are measured to determine if the adrenal gland responded to the ACTH stimulation.

GLUCOCORTICOIDS

The glucocorticoids are used as replacement therapy for clients with adrenocortical insufficiency and to dampen inflammatory and immune responses. The glucocorticoids, listed in Table 43.4, are one of the most widely prescribed drug classes.

43.10 Pharmacotherapy With Glucocorticoids

Lack of adequate corticosteroid production, known as *adrenocortical insufficiency,* may be caused by either hyposecretion of the adrenal cortex or inadequate secretion of ACTH from the pituitary. Symptoms include hypoglycemia,

fatigue, hypotension, increased skin pigmentation, and GI disturbances such as anorexia, vomiting, and diarrhea. Low plasma cortisol, accompanied by high plasma ACTH levels, is diagnostic, because this indicates that the adrenal gland is not responding to ACTH stimulation. *Primary* adrenocortical insufficiency, known as **Addison's disease,** is quite rare and includes a deficiency of both glucocorticoids and mineralocorticoids. Autoimmune destruction of both adrenal glands is the most common cause of Addison's disease. *Secondary* adrenocortical insufficiency is more common and is associated with glucocorticoid pharmacotherapy.

Acute adrenocortical insufficiency may result when glucocorticoids are abruptly withdrawn from a client who has been on long-term therapy. When glucocorticoids are taken as medications for prolonged periods, they provide negative feedback to the pituitary to stop secreting ACTH. Without stimulation by ACTH, the adrenal cortex shrinks and stops secreting *endogenous* glucocorticoids, a condition known as *adrenal atrophy.* If the glucocorticoid medication is abruptly withdrawn, the shrunken adrenal glands will not be able to secrete sufficient glucocorticoids, and symptoms of acute adrenocortical insufficiency will appear. Symptoms include nausea, vomiting, lethargy, confusion, and coma. Immediate administration of IV therapy with hydrocortisone is essential, as shock may quickly result if symptoms remain untreated. Other possible causes of acute adrenocortical insufficiency include infection, trauma, and cancer.

For chronic corticosteroid insufficiency, replacement therapy with glucocorticoids is indicated. The goal of replacement therapy is to achieve the same physiological level of hormones in the blood that would be present if the adrenal glands were functioning properly. Clients requiring replacement therapy usually need to take glucocorticoids their entire lifetime. Clients with adrenal insufficiency may also need a mineralocorticoid, such as fludrocortisone (Florinef).

Glucocorticoids are prescribed for a large number of other disorders in addition to acute and chronic adrenal insufficiency. Their ability to quickly and effectively suppress the inflammatory and immune responses gives them tremendous therapeutic utility to treat a diverse set of conditions. Indeed, no other drug class is used for so many different indications. Following are the indications for pharmacotherapy with glucocorticoids:

- Adrenal insufficiency
- Allergies, including seasonal rhinitis (Chapter 38 ∞)
- Asthma and chronic obstructive pulmonary disease (Chapter 39 ∞)
- Chronic inflammatory bowel disease, including ulcerative colitis and Crohn's disease (Chapter 41 ∞)
- Hepatic, neurological, and renal disorders characterized by edema
- Neoplastic disease, including Hodgkin's disease, leukemias, and lymphomas (Chapter 37 ∞)
- Posttransplant surgery (Chapter 32 ∞)

Table 43.4	Selected Glucocorticoids	
Drug	**Route and Adult Dose (max dose where indicated)**	**Adverse Effects**
SHORT ACTING		
cortisone (Cortistan, Cortone)	PO; 20–300 mg/day daily	*Sodium/fluid retention, nausea, acne, anxiety, insomnia, mood swings, increased appetite, weight gain, facial flushing*
ⓟ hydrocortisone (Cortef, Hydrocortone, others)	PO; 2–80 mg tid–qid	
INTERMEDIATE ACTING		
methylprednisolone (Medrol, others)	PO; 2–60 mg 1–4 times/day	Impaired wound healing, masking of infections, adrenal atrophy, hypokalemia, peptic ulcers, glaucoma, osteoporosis, muscle wasting/weakness, CHF, edema, worsening of psychoses
prednisolone (Delta-Cortef, others)	PO; 5–60 mg 1–4 times/day	
prednisone (Deltasone, Meticorten, others) (see page 477 for the Prototype Drug box ∞)	PO; 5–60 mg 1–4 times/day	
triamcinolone (Aristocort, Kenacort, others)	PO; 4–48 mg 1–2 times/day	
LONG ACTING		
betamethasone (Celestone)	PO; 0.6–7.2 mg/day	
dexamethasone (Decadron, Dexasone, others)	PO; 0.25–4.0 mg bid–qid	

Italics indicate common adverse effects; underlining indicates serious adverse effects.

- Rheumatic disorders, including rheumatoid arthritis, ankylosing spondylitis, and bursitis (Chapter 47 ∞)
- Shock (Chapter 29 ∞)
- Skin disorders, including contact dermatitis and rashes (Chapter 48 ∞)

More than 20 glucocorticoids are available as medications, and choice of a particular agent depends primarily on the pharmacokinetic properties of the drug. The duration of action, which is often used to classify these agents, ranges from short to long acting. Some, such as hydrocortisone, have mineralocorticoid activity that causes sodium and fluid retention; others, such as prednisone, have no such effect. Some glucocorticoids are available by only one route: for example, topical for dermal conditions or intranasal for allergic rhinitis.

Glucocorticoids interact with many drugs. Their hyperglycemic effects may decrease the effectiveness of antidiabetic agents. Combining glucocorticoids with other ulcerogenic drugs such as aspirin and other NSAIDs markedly increases the risk of peptic ulcer disease. Administration with non-potassium-sparing diuretics may lead to hypocalcemia and hypokalemia.

The following strategies are used to limit the incidence of serious adverse effects from glucocorticoids.

- Keep doses to the lowest possible amount that will achieve a therapeutic effect.
- Administer glucocorticoids every other day (alternate-day dosing) to limit adrenal atrophy.
- For acute conditions, give clients large amounts for a few days and then gradually decrease the drug dose until it is discontinued.
- Give the drugs locally by inhalation, intra-articular injections, or topical applications to the skin, eyes, or ears, when feasible, to diminish the possibility of systemic effects.

NURSING CONSIDERATIONS

The role of the nurse in glucocorticoid therapy for adrenocortical insufficiency involves careful monitoring of a client's condition and providing education as it relates to the prescribed drug treatment. Assess vital signs for temperature and blood pressure elevations, because glucocorticoid therapy may predispose the client to infection and raises blood pressure. Monitor potassium, T_3, and T_4 levels, because they may be decreased when taking glucocorticoids. Monitor glucose levels, because glucocorticoids may cause hyperglycemia and immunosuppression, which delays wound healing. Monitor clients on long-term glucocorticoid therapy for osteoporosis and elevated serum cholesterol levels. Long-term administration of glucocorticoids may cause Cushing's syndrome. Assess for signs and symptoms of Cushing's syndrome, such as moonface, buffalo hump, and mood and personality disorders.

Individuals with medical conditions such as asthma, COPD, chronic renal failure, Crohn's disease, ulcerative colitis, rheumatoid arthritis, and lupus typically receive long-term glucocorticoid therapy in times of stress or exacerbations of their condition to suppress the inflammatory response. These individuals should be taught the importance of and rationale for adherence to the prescribed medication administration and the importance of gradual dosage reductions.

Lifespan Considerations.   Systemic glucocorticoid therapy is generally contraindicated for pregnant and lactating women. Animal studies have demonstrated that high doses of systemic glucocorticoids consistently cause cleft palate, although human data are less clear. Use of a systemic glucocorticoid during pregnancy must be carefully weighed against the severity of maternal disease. If pharmacotherapy is necessary, hydrocortisone, cortisone, prednisone, and methylprednisolone are suggested, since they are more

Pr PROTOTYPE DRUG | Hydrocortisone *(Cortef, Hydrocortone, others)* | Glucocorticoid

ACTIONS AND USES

Structurally identical with the natural hormone cortisol, hydrocortisone is a synthetic corticosteroid that is the drug of choice for treating adrenocortical insufficiency. When used for replacement therapy, it is given at physiological doses. Once proper dosing is achieved, its therapeutic effects should mimic those of endogenous corticosteroids. Hydrocortisone is also available for the treatment of inflammation, allergic disorders, and many other conditions. Intra-articular injections may be given to decrease severe inflammation in affected joints.

Hydrocortisone is available in six different formulations. Hydrocortisone base (Aeroseb-HC, Alphaderm, Cetacort, others) and hydrocortisone acetate (Anusol HC, Cortaid, Cortef Acetate) are available as oral preparations, creams, and ointments. Hydrocortisone cypionate (Cortef Fluid) is an oral suspension. Hydrocortisone sodium phosphate (Hydrocortone Phosphate) and hydrocortisone sodium succinate (A-Hydrocort, Solu-Cortef) are for parenteral use only. Hydrocortisone valerate (Westcort) is only for topical applications.

ADMINISTRATION ALERTS

- Administer exactly as prescribed and at the same time every day.
- Administer oral formulations with food.
- Pregnancy category C.

PHARMACOKINETICS

Onset: 1–2 h PO; 20 min IM

Peak: 1 h PO; 4–8 h IM

Half-life: 1.5–2 h

Duration: 1–1.5 days PO or IM

ADVERSE EFFECTS

When used at low doses for replacement therapy, or by the topical or intranasal routes, adverse effects of hydrocortisone are rare. However, signs of Cushing's syndrome can develop with high doses or with prolonged use. If taken for longer than 2 weeks, hydrocortisone should be discontinued gradually. Hydrocortisone possesses some mineralocorticoid activity, so sodium and fluid retention may be noted. A wide range of CNS effects have been reported, including insomnia, anxiety, headache, vertigo, confusion, and depression. Cardiovascular effects may include hypertension and tachycardia. Long-term therapy may result in peptic ulcer disease.

Contraindications: Hydrocortisone is contraindicated in clients with known infections or who are hypersensitive to the drug. Clients with diabetes, osteoporosis, psychoses, liver disease, or hypothyroidism should be treated with caution.

INTERACTIONS

Drug–Drug: Barbiturates, phenytoin, and rifampin may increase hepatic metabolism, thus decreasing hydrocortisone levels. Estrogens potentiate the effects of hydrocortisone. Use with nonsteroidal anti-inflammatory drugs (NSAIDs) increases the risk of peptic ulcers. Cholestyramine and colestipol decrease hydrocortisone absorption. Diuretics and amphotericin B increase the risk of hypokalemia. Anticholinesterase agents may produce severe weakness. Hydrocortisone may cause a decrease in immune response to vaccines and toxoids.

Lab Tests: May increase serum values for glucose, cholesterol, sodium, uric acid, or calcium. May decrease serum values of potassium and T_3/T_4.

Herbal/Food: Use of hydrocortisone with senna, cascara, or buckthorn may cause potassium deficiency with chronic use.

Treatment of Overdose: There is no specific treatment for overdose.

 See the Companion Website for a Nursing Process Focus specific to this drug.

NURSING PROCESS FOCUS Client Receiving Systemic Glucocorticoid Therapy

Assessment	Potential Nursing Diagnoses
Prior to administration: - Obtain a complete health history including allergies, drug history, and possible drug interactions. - Obtain a complete physical examination, focusing on presenting symptoms. - Determine the reason the medication is being administered. - Obtain serum sodium and potassium levels, hematocrit and hemoglobin levels, and blood glucose level, and blood urea nitrogen (BUN) and creatinine levels.	- Infection, Risk for, related to immunosuppression - Injury, Risk for, related to side effects of drug therapy - Knowledge, Deficient, related to drug therapy - Breast-feeding, Interrupted, related to drug therapy

Planning: Client Goals and Expected Outcomes

The client will:
- Exhibit a decrease in the symptoms for which the drug is being given.
- Exhibit no symptoms of infection.
- Demonstrate an understanding of the drug's action by accurately describing drug side effects and precautions.
- Adhere to drug and laboratory studies regimen.

Implementation

Interventions and (Rationales)	Client Education/Discharge Planning
- Monitor vital signs. (Blood pressure may increase because of increased blood volume and potential vasoconstriction effect.)	- Instruct client to report dizziness, palpitations, or headaches.

NURSING PROCESS FOCUS Client Receiving Systemic Glucocorticoid Therapy *(Continued)*

Implementation

Interventions and (Rationales)	Client Education/Discharge Planning
▪ Monitor for infection. Protect client from potential infections. (Glucocorticoids increase susceptibility to infections by suppressing the immune response.)	Instruct client to: ▪ Avoid people with infection. ▪ Report fever, cough, sore throat, joint pain, increased weakness, and malaise. ▪ Consult with the healthcare provider before receiving any immunizations.
▪ Monitor client's compliance with drug regimen. (Sudden discontinuation of these agents can precipitate an adrenal crisis.)	Instruct client: ▪ Never to suddenly stop taking the medication. ▪ In proper use of self-administering tapering dose pack. ▪ To take oral medications with food.
▪ Monitor for symptoms of Cushing's syndrome, such as moon face, buffalo hump, weight gain, muscle wasting, and increased deposits of fat in the trunk. (Symptoms may indicate excessive use of glucocorticoids.)	Instruct client: ▪ To weigh self daily. ▪ That initial weight gain is expected; provide the client with weight gain parameters that warrant reporting. ▪ That there are multiple side effects to therapy and that changes in health status should be reported.
▪ Monitor blood glucose levels. (Glucocorticoids cause an increase in gluconeogenesis and reduce glucose utilization.)	Instruct client to: ▪ Report symptoms of hyperglycemia such as excessive thirst, copious urination, and insatiable appetite. ▪ Adjust insulin doses based on blood glucose levels as directed by the healthcare provider.
▪ Monitor skin and mucous membranes for lacerations, abrasions, or break in integrity. (Glucocorticoids impair wound healing.)	Instruct client to: ▪ Examine skin daily for cuts and scrapes and to cover any injuries with a sterile bandage. ▪ Watch for symptoms of skin infection such as redness, swelling, and drainage. ▪ Notify the healthcare provider of any nonhealing wound or symptoms of infection.
▪ Monitor GI status for peptic ulcer development. (Glucocorticoids decrease gastric mucus production and predispose client to peptic ulcers.)	▪ Instruct client to report GI side effects, such as heartburn, abdominal pain, or tarry stools.
▪ Monitor serum electrolytes. (Glucocorticoids cause hypernatremia and hypokalemia.)	Instruct client to: ▪ Consume a diet high in protein, calcium, and potassium, but low in fat and concentrated simple carbohydrates. ▪ Keep all laboratory appointments.
▪ Monitor changes in musculoskeletal system. (Glucocorticoids decrease bone density and strength and cause muscle atrophy and weakness.)	Instruct client: ▪ To participate in exercise or physical activity, to help maintain bone and muscle strength. ▪ That drug may cause weakness in bones and muscles. ▪ To avoid strenuous activity that may cause injury.
▪ Monitor emotional stability. (Glucocorticoids may produce mood and behavior changes such as depression or feeling of invulnerability.)	▪ Instruct client that mood changes may be expected and to report mental status changes to the healthcare provider.

Evaluation of Outcome Criteria

Evaluate the effectiveness of drug therapy by confirming that client goals and expected outcomes have been met (see "Planning").

▪ The client states that symptoms have decreased.

▪ The client is free from signs of infection.

▪ The client demonstrates an understanding of the drug's action by accurately describing drug side effects and precautions.

▪ The client verbalizes the importance of adhering to drug and laboratory studies regimen.

∞ *See Table 43.4 for a list of drugs to which these nursing actions apply.*

readily inactivated by placental enzymes, as opposed to dexamethasone and betamethasone, which are more likely to reach the fetus in their active state.

Client Teaching. Client education as it relates to glucocorticoid therapy includes the goals of therapy, the reasons for obtaining baseline data such as vital signs and the existence of underlying cardiac and renal disorders, and possible drug side effects. Include the following points when teaching clients about glucocorticoid therapy:

- Report unusual changes in mood or personality, moon face, and buffalo hump, because these are signs of overdosage (Cushing's syndrome).
- Practice reliable contraception and notify your healthcare provider if pregnancy is planned or suspected.
- Do not breast-feed while taking these medications.
- Report wounds that are unusually slow to heal.
- Keep all scheduled appointments and laboratory visits for testing.
- Report fever, which may indicate an underlying infection.

43.11 Pharmacotherapy of Cushing's Syndrome

Cushing's syndrome occurs when high levels of glucocorticoids are present in the body over a prolonged period. Although hypersecretion of these hormones can be due to pituitary (excess ACTH) or adrenal tumors, the most common cause of Cushing's syndrome is long-term therapy with high doses of systemic glucocorticoid medications. Signs and symptoms include adrenal atrophy, osteoporosis, hypertension, increased risk of infections, delayed wound healing, acne, peptic ulcers, general obesity, and a redistribution of fat around the face (moon face), shoulders, and neck (buffalo hump). Mood and personality changes may occur, and the client may become psychologically dependent on the drug. Some glucocorticoids, including hydrocortisone, also have mineralocorticoid activity and can cause retention of sodium and water. Because of their anti-inflammatory properties, glucocorticoids may mask signs of infection, and a resulting delay in antibiotic therapy may result.

Cushing's syndrome has a high mortality rate, and the therapeutic goal is to identify and treat the cause of the excess glucocorticoid secretion. If the cause is overtreatment with glucocorticoid drugs, a gradual reduction in dose is sufficient to reverse the syndrome. When the cause of this hypersecretion is an adrenal tumor or perhaps an ectopic tumor secreting ACTH, surgical removal is indicated.

Clients with severe disease will receive drug therapy to quickly lower serum glucocorticoid levels. Combination therapy with aminoglutethimide (Cytadren) and metyrapone (Metopirone) is sometimes used. Aminoglutethimide suppresses adrenal function within 3 to 5 days; however, therapy is usually limited to 3 months because of its ineffectiveness over time. The antifungal drug ketoconazole (Nizoral) has

been found to be a safer therapy for long-term use. Most antiadrenal agents inhibit the metabolic conversion of cholesterol to adrenal corticosteroids. They are not curative; their use is temporary until the tumor can be removed or otherwise treated with radiation or antineoplastics.

NURSING CONSIDERATIONS

The role of the nurse in antiadrenal therapy for Cushing's Syndrome involves careful monitoring of a client's condition and providing education as it relates to the prescribed drug treatment. Assess and monitor lab values, including platelet count, bilirubin, and prothrombin, for jaundice, bruising, and bleeding, because antiadrenal therapy may cause leukopenia and thrombocytopenia. Monitor for orthostatic hypotension, because the drug causes decreased aldosterone production. Monitor for dizziness and assist with ambulation. Caution the client to change positions slowly. Ketoconazole (Nizoral) administered at high levels is an effective corticosteroid inhibitor. This medication is metabolized in the liver; therefore, hepatic function must be assessed prior to administration and monitored during therapy. Ketoconazole is contraindicated in those with liver dysfunction and those who abuse alcohol. Obtain a thorough history to assess for alcohol intake or possible HIV infection because these medications are contraindicated in these clients.

Lifespan Considerations. Aminoglutethimide is contraindicated during pregnancy. In animal studies, the drug has been shown to prevent fetal implantation and increase the potential for fetal death. Also in pregnant animals, the drug causes an unusual condition known as *pseudohermaphrodism*, in which an individual has the internal reproductive organs of only one gender but exhibits both male and female external genitalia. Ketoconazole has also been shown to be teratogenic and embryotoxic at high doses in animals.

Client Teaching. Client education as it relates to antiadrenal drugs should include the goals of therapy, the reasons for obtaining baseline data such as vital signs and the existence of underlying hematologic disorders, and possible drug side effects. Include the following points when teaching clients about antiadrenal drugs:

- Immediately report unusual bleeding, change in color of stool or urine, or yellowing of eyes or skin.
- Monitor temperature and report fever.
- Change positions slowly to avoid dizziness.
- Take medication with fruit juice or water to enhance absorption.
- Avoid alcohol use.
- Practice reliable contraception and notify your healthcare provider if pregnancy is planned or suspected.
- Keep all scheduled appointments and laboratory visits for testing.
- Practice relaxation techniques, because increased stress may cause adverse effects of the drug.

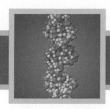

CHAPTER REVIEW

KEY CONCEPTS

The numbered key concepts provide a succinct summary of the important points from the corresponding numbered section within the chapter. If any of these points are not clear, refer to the numbered section within the chapter for review.

43.1 The endocrine system maintains homeostasis by using hormones as chemical messengers that are secreted in response to changes in the internal environment. Negative feedback prevents overresponses by the endocrine system.

43.2 The hypothalamus secretes releasing hormones, which direct the anterior pituitary gland to release specific hormones. The posterior pituitary releases its hormones in response to nerve signals from the hypothalamus.

43.3 Hormones are used in replacement therapy, as antineoplastics, and for their natural therapeutic effects, such as their suppression of body defenses. Hormone blockers are used to inhibit actions of certain hormones.

43.4 Only a few pituitary and hypothalamic hormones, including growth hormone and ACTH, have clinical applications as drugs. Growth hormone and ADH are examples of pituitary hormones used as drugs for replacement therapy.

43.5 The thyroid gland secretes thyroxine (T_4) and triiodothyronine (T_3), which control the basal metabolic rate and affect every cell in the body.

43.6 Hypothyroidism may be treated by administering thyroid hormone agents, especially levothyroxine (T_4).

43.7 Hyperthyroidism is treated by administering agents such as the thioamides that decrease the activity of the thyroid gland or by using radioactive iodide, which kills overactive thyroid cells.

43.8 The adrenal cortex secretes glucocorticoids, gonadocorticoids, and mineralocorticoids. The glucocorticoids mobilize the body for long-term stress and influence carbohydrate, lipid, and protein metabolism in most cells.

43.9 Glucocorticoid release is stimulated by ACTH secreted by the pituitary. ACTH and related agents are rarely used as medications.

43.10 Adrenocortical insufficiency may be acute or chronic. Glucocorticoids are prescribed for adrenocortical insufficiency, allergies, neoplasms and a wide variety of other conditions.

43.11 Antiadrenal drugs may be used to treat severe Cushing's syndrome by inhibiting corticosteroid synthesis. They are not curative, and their use is usually limited to 3 months of therapy.

NCLEX-RN® REVIEW QUESTIONS

1 The nurse recognizes that drugs from which of the following classes cause increased risk for peptic ulcers, decreased wound healing, and increased capillary fragility?

1. Glucocorticoids
2. Antidiuretic hormones
3. Growth hormones
4. Antithyroid hormones

2 When administering hydrocortisone (Cortef, others), the nurse recognizes it may mask which symptoms?

1. Signs and symptoms of infection
2. Signs and symptoms of heart failure
3. Hearing loss
4. Skin infections

3 When hydrocortisone use is discontinued abruptly, the nurse must assess for which side effect?

1. Development of myxedema
2. Circulatory collapse
3. Development of Cushing's syndrome
4. Development of diabetes insipidus

4 A client who is taking levothyroxine (Synthroid) begins to develop weight loss, diarrhea, and stress intolerance. The nurse should be aware that this might be an indication of what hormonal condition?

1. Addison's disease
2. Hyperthyroidism
3. Cushing's syndrome
4. Development of acromegaly

5 What precautions should a client who is receiving radioactive iodine be made aware of? (Select all that apply.)

1. Drink plenty of fluids, especially those high in calcium.
2. Avoid close contact with children or pregnant women for 1 week after administration of the drug.
3. Be aware of symptoms of tachycardia, increased metabolic rate, and anxiety.
4. Wear a mask if around children and pregnant women.
5. Signs and symptoms of hypothyroidism include general weakness, muscle cramps, and dry skin.

CRITICAL THINKING QUESTIONS

1. A 5-year-old girl requires treatment for diabetes insipidus acquired following a case of meningitis. The child has suffered serious complications including blindness and mental retardation. Her diabetes insipidus is being treated with intranasal desmopressin, and the child's mother has been asked to help evaluate the drug's effectiveness using urine volumes and urine specific gravity. Discuss the changes that would indicate that the drug is effective.

2. A 17-year-old adolescent with a history of severe asthma is admitted to the intensive care unit. He is comatose, appears much younger than his listed age, and has short stature. The nurse notes that the asthma has been managed with pred-nisone for 15 days, until 3 days ago. The client's father is extremely anxious and says that he was unable to refill his son's prescription for medicine until he got his paycheck. What is the nurse's role in this situation?

3. A 9-year-old boy has been diagnosed with growth hormone deficiency. His parents have decided to proceed with a prescribed regimen of somatropin (Humatrope). Outline the basic information the parents need to know regarding this regimen, side effects, and evaluation of effectiveness.

See Appendix D for answers and rationales for all activities.

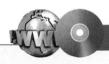

EXPLORE MediaLink

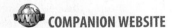
www.prenhall.com/adams

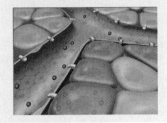

NCLEX-RN® review, case studies, and other interactive resources for this chapter can be found on the companion website at www.prenhall.com/adams. Click on "Chapter 43" to select the activities for this chapter. For animations, more NCLEX-RN® review questions, and an audio glossary, access the accompanying Prentice Hall Nursing MediaLink DVD-ROM in this textbook.

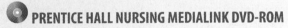

PRENTICE HALL NURSING MEDIALINK DVD-ROM

- **Audio Glossary**
- **NCLEX-RN® Review**

COMPANION WEBSITE

- **NCLEX-RN® Review**
- **Dosage Calculations**
- **Case Study:** Pituitary and hypothalamic hormones
- **Care Plan:** Client with surgically induced hypothyroidism treated with levothyroxine

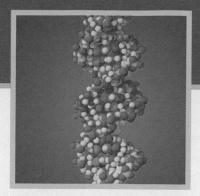

CHAPTER 44

Drugs for Diabetes Mellitus

DRUGS AT A GLANCE

INSULINS
- 🔊 *regular insulin*

ORAL HYPOGLYCEMICS
- 🔊 *glipizide (Glucotrol, Glucotrol XL)*

OBJECTIVES

After reading this chapter, the student should be able to:

1. Describe the endocrine and exocrine functions of the pancreas.
2. Compare and contrast type 1 and type 2 diabetes mellitus.
3. Compare and contrast types of insulin.
4. Describe the signs and symptoms of insulin overdose and underdose.
5. Describe the nurse's role in the pharmacological management of diabetes mellitus.
6. Identify drug classes used to treat type 2 diabetes mellitus.
7. For each of the drug classes listed in Drugs at a Glance, know representative drug examples, and explain the mechanisms of drug action, primary actions, and important adverse effects.
8. Use the Nursing Process to care for clients receiving drug therapy for diabetes mellitus.

MediaLink

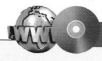

www.prenhall.com/adams

NCLEX-RN® review, case studies, and other interactive resources for this chapter can be found on the companion website at www.prenhall.com/adams. Click on "Chapter 44" to select the activities for this chapter. For animations, more NCLEX-RN® review questions, and an audio glossary, access the accompanying Prentice Hall Nursing MediaLink DVD-ROM in this textbook.

KEY TERMS

diabetic ketoacidosis (DKA) *page 683*

exocrine *page 682*

hyperglycemic effect *page 683*

hyperosmolar nonketotic coma (HNKC)
   page 691

hypoglycemic effect *page 682*

insulin analog *page 684*

insulin resistance *page 689*

islets of Langerhans *page 682*

ketoacids *page 683*

Somogyi phenomenon *page 684*

type 1 diabetes mellitus *page 683*

type 2 diabetes mellitus *page 689*

The pancreas serves unique and vital functions by supplying essential digestive enzymes while also secreting the hormones responsible for glucose homeostasis. From a pharmacological perspective, the most important disorder associated with the pancreas is diabetes mellitus. Millions of people have diabetes, a disease caused by genetic and environmental factors that impair the cellular utilization of glucose. Because glucose is essential to every cell in the body, the effects of diabetes are widespread. Diabetes merits special consideration in pharmacology because the nurse will encounter many clients with this disorder.

44.1 Normal Functions of the Pancreas

Located behind the stomach and between the duodenum and spleen, the pancreas is an organ essential to both the digestive and endocrine systems. It is responsible for the secretion of several enzymes into the duodenum that assist in the chemical digestion of nutrients (Chapter 41 ∞). This is its **exocrine** function. Clusters of cells in the pancreas, called **islets of Langerhans,** are responsible for its endocrine function: the secretion of glucagon and insulin. Alpha cells secrete glucagons, and beta cells secrete insulin (● Figure 44.1). As with other endocrine organs, the pancreas secretes these hormones directly into blood capillaries, where they are available for transport to body tissues. Insulin and glucagon play key roles in maintaining normal glucose levels in the blood.

Insulin secretion is regulated by a number of chemical, hormonal, and neural factors. The most important regulator is the level of glucose in the blood. After a meal, when blood glucose levels rise, the islets of Langerhans secrete insulin, which causes glucose to leave the blood and enter cells. High insulin levels and falling blood glucose levels provide negative feedback to the pancreas to stop secreting insulin.

Insulin affects carbohydrate, lipid, and protein metabolism in most cells of the body. Its most important action is to assist in glucose transport; without insulin, glucose cannot enter cells. A cell may be literally swimming in glucose, but the glucose cannot enter and be used as an energy source by the cell without insulin present. Thus, insulin is said to have a **hypoglycemic effect,** because its presence causes glucose to *leave* the blood and serum glucose to *fall*. The brain is an important exception, because it does not require insulin for glucose transport.

Islet cells in the pancreas also secrete glucagon. Glucagon is an antagonist to insulin with actions opposite those of insulin. When levels of glucose are low, glucagon is secreted. Its primary function is to maintain adequate serum levels of

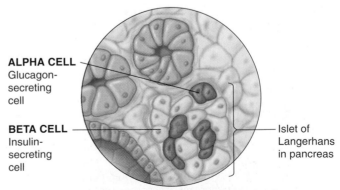

ALPHA CELL
Glucagon-
secreting
cell

BETA CELL
Insulin-
secreting
cell

Islet of
Langerhans
in pancreas

Glucagon—raises blood glucose level
Insulin—lowers blood glucose level

●**Figure 44.1** Glucagon- and insulin-secreting cells in the islets of Langerhans *Source: Pearson Education/PH College.*

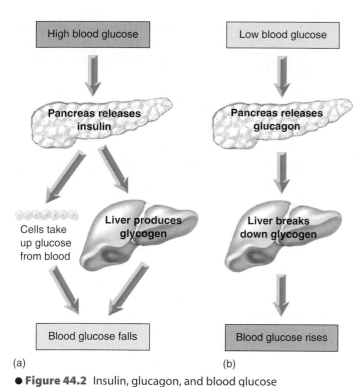

(a) **(b)**

● **Figure 44.2** Insulin, glucagon, and blood glucose

glucose between meals. Thus, glucagon has a **hyperglycemic effect,** because its presence causes blood glucose to *rise.* ● Figure 44.2 illustrates the relationships among blood glucose, insulin, and glucagon.

Blood glucose levels are usually kept within a normal range by insulin and glucagons; however, other hormones and drugs can affect glucose metabolism. *Hyperglycemic* hormones include epinephrine, thyroid hormones, growth hormone, and corticosteroids. Common drugs that can raise blood glucose levels include phenytoin, NSAIDs, and diuretics. Drugs with a *hypoglycemic* effect include alcohol, lithium, angiotensin-converting enzyme (ACE) inhibitors, and beta-adrenergic blockers. It is important that serum glucose be periodically monitored in clients receiving medications that exhibit hypoglycemia or hypoglycemic effects.

DIABETES MELLITUS

Worldwide, approximately 135 million people are thought to have diabetes mellitus (DM); by 2025, this number is expected to have increased to 300 million. The etiology of DM includes a combination of genetic and environmental factors. The recent increase in the frequency of the disease is probably the result of trends toward more sedentary and stressful lifestyles, increasing consumption of highly caloric foods with resultant obesity, and increased longevity.

Diabetes mellitus is a group of metabolic diseases in which there is deficient insulin secretion or decreased sensitivity of insulin receptors on target cells, resulting in hyperglycemia. Diabetes mellitus includes type 1, type 2, gestational diabetes, and other specific types such as those found in Cushing's

syndrome or that are chemically induced. Discussion in this chapter is limited to type 1 and type 2 DM.

44.2 Etiology and Characteristics of Type 1 Diabetes Mellitus

Type 1 diabetes mellitus accounts for 10% of all cases of DM and is one of the most common diseases of childhood. Type 1 DM was previously called *juvenile-onset diabetes,* because it is often diagnosed between the ages of 11 and 13. Because approximately 25% of clients with type 1 DM develop the disease in adulthood, this is not the most accurate name for this disorder. This type of diabetes is also referred to as insulin-dependent diabetes mellitus.

Type 1 DM results from autoimmune destruction of pancreatic beta cells, causing an absolute lack of insulin secretion. The disease is thought to be an interaction of genetic, immunologic, and environmental factors. Because children and siblings of those with DM have a higher risk of acquiring the disorder, there is an obvious genetic component to the disease.

The signs and symptoms of type 1 DM are consistent from client to client, with the most diagnostic sign being sustained hyperglycemia. Following are the typical signs and symptoms.

- Hyperglycemia—fasting blood glucose greater than 126 mg/dl on at least two separate occasions
- Polyuria—excessive urination
- Polyphagia—increased hunger
- Polydipsia—increased thirst
- Glucosuria—high levels of glucose in the urine
- Weight loss
- Fatigue

Untreated DM produces long-term damage to arteries, leading to heart disease, stroke, kidney disease, and blindness. Lack of adequate circulation to the feet may cause gangrene of the toes, requiring amputation. Nerve degeneration is common, with symptoms ranging from tingling in the fingers or toes to complete loss of sensation of a limb. Because glucose is unable to enter cells, lipids are utilized as an energy source and **ketoacids** are produced as waste products. These ketoacids can give the client's breath an acetone-like, fruity odor. More important, high levels of ketoacids lower the pH of the blood, causing **diabetic ketoacidosis (DKA),** and may progress to coma and possible death if untreated.

INSULIN

Insulin first became available as a medication in 1922. Prior to that time, type 1 diabetics were unable to adequately maintain normal blood glucose, experienced many complications, and usually died at a young age. Increased insulin availability and improvements in insulin products, personal blood glucose monitoring devices, and the insulin pump have made it possible for clients to maintain more exact control of their blood glucose levels.

PHARMFACTS

Diabetes Mellitus

- Of the 16 million Americans who have diabetes, 5 million probably are unaware that they have the disease.

- Each day, more than 2,000 people are diagnosed with diabetes.

- Gestational diabetes affects about 4% of all pregnant women in the United States each year—about 135,000 cases.

- Diabetes causes almost 200,000 deaths each year; it is the sixth leading cause of death.

- Diabetes is the leading cause of blindness in adults; each year 12,000 to 24,000 people lose their sight because of diabetes.

- Diabetes is responsible for 50% of nontraumatic lower-limb amputations; 56,000 amputations are performed each year on clients with diabetes.

- Costs for diabetes treatment exceed $100 billion annually—$1 of every $7 of healthcare expenditures.

- Diabetes is the leading cause of end-stage renal disease, accounting for about 40% of new cases.

44.3 Pharmacotherapy With Insulin

Because clients with type 1 DM have a total lack of insulin secretion, the therapeutic goal is to administer insulin as replacement therapy, in normal physiological amounts. Because normal insulin secretion varies greatly in response to daily activities such as eating and exercise, insulin pharmacotherapy must be carefully planned in conjunction with proper meal planning and lifestyle habits. The desired outcome of insulin therapy is to prevent the long-term consequences of the disorder by strictly maintaining blood glucose levels within the normal range.

The fundamental principle to remember about insulin therapy is that the right amount of insulin must be available to cells when glucose is available in the blood. Administering insulin when glucose is *not* available can lead to serious hypoglycemia and coma. This situation occurs when a client administers insulin correctly but skips a meal; the insulin is available to cells, but glucose is not. In another example, the client participates in heavy exercise. The insulin may have been administered on schedule, and food eaten, but the active muscles quickly use up all the glucose in the blood, and the client becomes hypoglycemic. Clients with diabetes who engage in competitive sports need to consume food or sports drinks just prior to or during the activity to maintain their blood sugar at normal levels.

Clients with diabetes who skip or forget their insulin dose face equally serious consequences. Again, remember the fundamental principle of insulin pharmacotherapy: the right amount of insulin must be available to cells when glucose is available in the blood. Without insulin present, glucose from a meal can build up to high levels in the blood, causing hyperglycemia and possible coma. Proper teaching and planning by the nurse is essential to successful outcomes and client compliance with therapy.

Several types of insulin are available, differing in their source, onset, and duration of action. Until the 1980s, the source of all insulin was beef or pork pancreas. Almost all

insulin today, however, is human insulin obtained through recombinant DNA technology because it is more effective, causes fewer allergies, and has a lower incidence of resistance. Pharmacologists have modified human insulin to create certain pharmacokinetic advantages, such as a more rapid onset of action (Humalog) or a more prolonged duration of action (Lantus). These modified forms are called **insulin analogs.**

Doses of insulin are highly individualized for each client to produce precise control of blood glucose levels. Some clients may need two or more injections daily. Two different compatible types of insulin are sometimes mixed, using a standard method, to obtain the desired therapeutic effects. Some of these are marketed in cartridges containing premixed solutions for ease of use. Common insulin preparations are listed in Table 44.1.

The most common route of administration for insulin is subcutaneous, although research is being conducted to discover more convenient routes such as an insulin nasal spray. In 2006, an inhaled form of insulin (Exubera) was approved by the FDA. This insulin is packaged as a dry powder in a device for inhalation through the mouth (● Figure 44.3a). Exubera has a more rapid onset of glucose-lowering activity compared with that of regular human insulin injected subcutaneously. Its duration of action is comparable to that of regular human insulin injected subcutaneously and longer than that of rapid-acting insulin.

Some clients have an insulin pump (● Figure 44.3b). This pump is usually abdominally anchored and is programmed to release small subcutaneous doses of insulin into the abdomen at predetermined intervals, with larger boluses administered manually at mealtime if necessary. Most pumps contain an alarm that sounds to remind clients to take their insulin. Figure 44.3b shows an insulin pump.

The primary adverse effect of insulin therapy is hypoglycemia. Symptoms of hypoglycemia occur when a client with type 1 DM has more insulin in the blood than is needed for the amount of circulating blood glucose. This may occur when the insulin level peaks, during exercise, when the client receives too much insulin owing to a medication error, or if the client skips a meal. Some of the symptoms of hypoglycemia are the same as those of diabetic ketoacidosis. Those that differ and help in determining that a client is hypoglycemic include pale, cool, and moist skin, with blood glucose less than 50 mg/dl and a sudden onset of symptoms. Left untreated, severe hypoglycemia may result in death.

Other adverse effects of insulin include localized allergic reactions at the injection site, generalized urticaria, and swollen lymph glands. Some clients will experience **Somogyi phenomenon,** a rapid decrease in blood glucose, usually during the night, which stimulates the release of hormones that elevate blood glucose (epinephrine, cortisol, and glucagon) resulting in an elevated morning blood glucose level. Additional insulin above the client's normal dose may produce a rapid rebound hypoglycemia.

The hormone glucagon is administered as a replacement therapy for some diabetic clients when they are in a hypoglycemic state and have impaired glucagon secretion.

TABLE 44.1 Insulin Preparations

Drug	Route and Adult Dose (max dose where indicated)	Adverse Effects
INSULIN ANALOGS		
insulin aspart (NovoLog)	Subcutaneous; 0.25–0.7 units/kg/day given 5–10 min before each meal	*Pain and swelling at injection site*
insulin glargine (Lantus)	Type 1 diabetes: subcutaneous; 10 units/day in the evening; if taking NPH insulin bid, give 80% of total daily dose in the evening Type 2 diabetes: subcutaneous; 10 units/day in the evening, and adjust as needed	<u>Anaphylaxis, rash, hypoglycemia (tremors, palpitations, sweating), diabetic ketoacidosis, coma</u>
insulin lispro (Humalog)	Subcutaneous; 5–10 units given 10–15 min with meal	
INSULIN MIXTURES		
NPH 70% Regular 30% (Humulin 70/30, Novolin 70/30)	IM/subcutaneous; individualized doses	
NPH 50% Regular 50%	IM/subcutaneous; individualized doses	
SHORT-ACTING INSULIN (PEAK ACTIVITY BETWEEN 2 AND 4 HOURS)		
Ⓟ insulin, regular (Regular Iletin II, Humulin R, Novolin R)	Subcutaneous; 5–10 units given 15–30 min with meals and in the evening	
INTERMEDIATE-ACTING INSULIN (PEAK ACTIVITY BETWEEN 4 AND 12 HOURS)		
isophane insulin suspension (NPH, NPH Iletin II, Humulin N, Novolin N)	IM/subcutaneous; individualized doses	
insulin zinc suspension (Lente Iletin II, Lente L, Humulin L, Novolin L)	IM/subcutaneous; individualized doses	
LONG-ACTING INSULIN (PEAK ACTIVITY BETWEEN 6 AND 20 HOURS)		
extended insulin zinc suspension (Humulin U, Ultralente)	IM/subcutaneous; individualized doses	
insulin detemir (Levemir)	Subcutaneous; individualized doses	

Italics indicate common adverse effects; <u>underlining</u> indicates serious adverse effects.

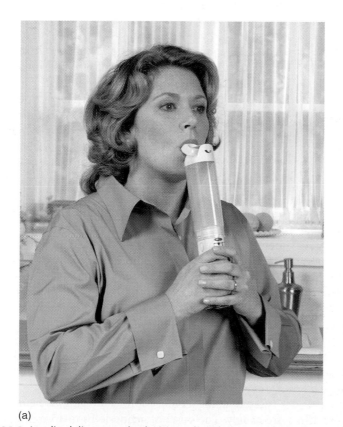

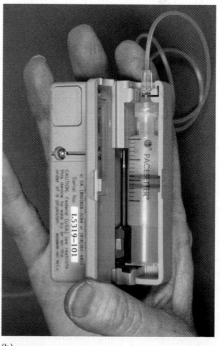

(a)   (b)

● **Figure 44.3** Insulin delivery methods: (a) insulin inhalation device; (b) insulin pump *Source: Pfizer Inc.*

Pr PROTOTYPE DRUG | Regular Insulin *(Humulin R, Novolin R, and others)* | Insulin

ACTIONS AND USES

Regular insulin is prepared from pork pancreas or as human insulin through recombinant DNA technology. It is classified as short-acting insulin, with an onset of 30 to 60 minutes, a peak effect at 2 to 3 hours, and a duration of 5 to 7 hours. Its primary action is to promote the entry of glucose into cells. For the emergency treatment of acute ketoacidosis, it may be given subcutaneously or IV. Regular insulin is also available as Humulin 70/30 (a mixture of 30% regular insulin and 70% isophane insulin) or as Humulin 50/50 (a mixture of 50% of regular and isophane insulin).

ADMINISTRATION ALERTS

- Hypoglycemic reactions may occur quickly if regular insulin is not supported by sufficient food or is given when the client is hypoglycemic.
- Regular insulin is the only type of insulin that may be used for IV injection.
- Rotate injection sites. When the client is hospitalized, use sites not normally used by the client when at home.
- Administer approximately 30 minutes before meals so insulin will be absorbed and available when the client begins to eat.
- Pregnancy category B.

PHARMACOKINETICS

Onset: 30–60 min subcutaneous; 10–30 min IV

Peak: 2–4 h subcutaneous; 30–60 min IV

Half-life: Up to 13 h

Duration: 5–7 h subcutaneous; 30–60 min IV

ADVERSE EFFECTS

The most serious adverse effect of insulin therapy is hypoglycemia. Hypoglycemia may result from taking too much insulin, not properly timing the insulin injection with food intake, or skipping a meal. Dietary carbohydrates must have reached the blood when insulin is injected, otherwise the drug will remove too much glucose, and signs of hypoglycemia—tachycardia, confusion, sweating, and drowsiness—will ensue. If severe hypoglycemia is not quickly treated with glucose, convulsions, coma, and death may follow.

Contraindications: Insulin is contraindicated in clients allergic to the drug or any of its components.

INTERACTIONS

Drug–Drug: The following substances may potentiate hypoglycemic effects: alcohol, salicylates, MAOIs, anabolic steroids, and guanethidine. The following substances may antagonize hypoglycemic effects: corticosteroids, thyroid hormone, and epinephrine. Serum glucose levels may be increased with furosemide or thiazide diuretics. Symptoms of hypoglycemic reaction may be masked with beta-adrenergic blockers.

Lab Tests: May increase urinary vanillylmandelic acid (VMA) and interfere with liver tests and thyroid function tests. May decrease levels of serum potassium, calcium, and magnesium.

Herbal/Food: Garlic, bilberry, and ginseng may potentiate the hypoglycemic effects of insulin.

Treatment of Overdose: Overdose causes hypoglycemia. Mild cases are treated with oral glucose, and severe episodes with parenteral glucagon or intravenous glucose.

 See the Companion Website for a Nursing Process Focus specific to this drug.

Glucagon (1 mg) can be given IV, IM, or subcutaneously to reverse hypoglycemic symptoms in 20 minutes or less, depending on the route.

NURSING CONSIDERATIONS

The role of the nurse in insulin therapy involves careful monitoring of a client's condition and providing education as it relates to the prescribed drug treatment. Be familiar with the onset, peak, and duration of action of the insulin(s) prescribed, as well as any other important aspects of the specific insulin, and convey this information to the client.

Assess the client for signs and symptoms of hypoglycemia as well as the adequacy of glucose monitoring. Hypoglycemia is most likely to occur when insulin reaches its peak effect, during exercise, or during acute illness. Obtain food for the client and determine that the client is ready to eat before administering insulin. Assess the client's level of understanding of the symptoms of insulin reaction, hypoglycemia, and diabetic ketoacidosis. Teach the client to recognize key symptoms, and know what action to take in response to them. Contraindications to insulin include sensitivity to an ingredient in the formulation, and hypoglycemia that would be worsened by administration of insulin. Use with caution in pregnant clients and in those

with severe stress, and infection. Clients with these conditions usually have increased insulin requirements and must be monitored more carefully.

Two of the most frequently prescribed types of insulin are NPH (isophane) and regular insulin. Intermediate or NPH insulin is used to provide a longer acting source of insulin as compared with regular insulin and other types of short-acting insulin. The onset of action for NPH insulin is between 1 and 4 hours, and peak effect occurs in 8 to 12 hours. Its duration is 18 to 24 hours. NPH insulin is normally administered 30 minutes before the first meal of the day, but in some instances a second, smaller dose is taken before the evening meal or at bedtime. Many clients are prescribed insulin that is premixed, such as 70% NPH with 30% regular or rapid acting. If the client is prescribed a premixed insulin solution, it is important that proper instruction be given, especially if the client will be using additional regular or rapid-acting insulin on a sliding scale.

Under some circumstances regular insulin may be given IV, but other types of insulin, including NPH, are to be given only as subcutaneous injections. Intermediate insulin cannot be given IV.

Rapid-acting insulin lispro (Humalog) is being used more frequently. The onset of action is 10 to 15 minutes, which is much faster than the onset of 30 to 60 minutes associated with

NURSING PROCESS FOCUS Clients Receiving Insulin Therapy

Assessment	Potential Nursing Diagnoses
Prior to administration: ■ Obtain a complete health history including allergies, drug history, and possible drug interactions. ■ Assess vital signs. If the client has a fever or elevated pulse, assess further to determine the cause, because infection can alter the amount of insulin required. ■ Assess blood glucose level. ■ Assess appetite and presence of symptoms that indicate the client may not be able to consume or retain the next meal. ■ Assess subcutaneous areas for potential insulin injection sites. ■ Assess knowledge of insulin and ability to self-administer insulin.	■ Injury (hypoglycemia), Risk for, related to adverse effects of drug therapy ■ Knowledge, Deficient, related to need for self-injection ■ Imbalanced Nutrition, Risk for, related to adverse effects of drug therapy ■ Infection, Risk for, related to blood glucose elevations and impaired circulation

Planning: Client Goals and Expected Outcomes

The client will:
■ Immediately report irritability, dizziness, diaphoresis, hunger, behavior changes, and changes in level of consciousness.
■ Demonstrate ability to self-administer insulin.
■ Demonstrate an understanding of lifestyle modifications necessary for successful maintenance of drug therapy.
■ Demonstrate an understanding of the drug's action by accurately describing drug side effects and precautions.

Implementation

Interventions and (Rationales)	Client Education/Discharge Planning
■ Increase frequency of blood glucose monitoring if the client is experiencing fever, nausea, vomiting, or diarrhea. (Illness usually requires adjustments in insulin doses.)	Instruct client: ■ To increase blood glucose monitoring when experiencing fever, nausea, vomiting, or diarrhea.
■ Check urine for ketones if blood glucose is over 300 mg/dl. (Ketones spill into the urine at this glucose level and provide an early sign of diabetic ketoacidosis.)	Instruct client: ■ To check urine for ketones. ■ That ketoacidosis normally develops slowly but is a serious problem that needs to be corrected.
■ Monitor weight on a routine basis. (Changes in weight alter insulin needs.)	■ Instruct client to weigh self on a routine basis at the same time each day, and to report significant changes (plus or minus 10 lb).
■ Monitor vital signs. (Increased pulse and blood pressure are early signs of hypoglycemia. Clients with diabetes may have circulatory problems and impaired kidney function that can increase blood pressure.)	■ Teach client how to take blood pressure and pulse, and to report significant changes.
■ Monitor potassium level. (Insulin causes potassium to move into the cell and may cause hypokalemia.)	■ Instruct client to report the first sign of heart irregularity.
■ Check blood glucose and feed client some form of simple sugar at the first sign of hypoglycemia. (Using a simple sugar will raise blood glucose immediately.)	Advise client: ■ That exercise may increase insulin needs. ■ To check blood glucose before and after exercise and to keep a simple sugar on hand while exercising. ■ Before strenuous exercise, to eat some form of simple sugar or complex carbohydrate to prevent hypoglycemia.

Evaluation of Outcome Criteria

Evaluate the effectiveness of drug therapy by confirming that client goals and expected outcomes have been met (see "Planning"):
■ The client states the need to immediately report irritability, dizziness, diaphoresis, hunger, behavior changes, and changes in LOC.
■ The client demonstrates ability to self-administer insulin.
■ The client verbalizes an understanding of lifestyle modifications necessary for successful maintenance of drug therapy.
■ The client demonstrates an understanding of the drug's action by accurately describing drug side effects and precautions.

∞ *See Table 44.1 for a list of drugs to which these nursing actions apply.*

regular insulin. The peak effect of rapid-acting insulin lispro occurs in 30 to 60 minutes, and its duration of action is 5 hours or less. It is often used with insulin infusion pumps.

Insulin glargine (Lantus) is a newer agent that is a recombinant human insulin analog. It must not be mixed in the syringe with any other insulin and must be administered subcutaneously. Insulin glargine exhibits a constant long-duration hypoglycemic effect with no defined peak effect. It is prescribed once daily, at bedtime.

Long-acting insulin is prescribed for some clients. Protamine zinc (PZI) (Iletin II) has an onset of 4 to 8 hours, a peak effect at 14 to 24 hours, with duration of 36 hours. Extended insulin zinc suspension (Ultralente) has an onset of 4 to 6 hours, a peak of 10 to 30 hours, and duration of 36 hours. A premixed insulin, Novolin Mix (70% N and 30% R) has an onset of 4 to 8 hours, a peak effect of 16 to 18 hours, and duration greater than 36 hours. A new long-acting insulin, insulin detemir (Levemir), was approved in 2005.

When administering insulin, ensure that the units on the syringe match the units on the insulin vial. For example, when U100 insulin is ordered, the vial must be U100 and the syringe must also be calibrated for U100. Although U100 and U50 are the most often used strengths of insulin, U500 is available for clients who have developed insulin resistance and need a much higher dose to manage blood glucose. When U500 insulin is given, a syringe calibrated for U500 is necessary. It is also imperative to understand that not all types of insulin are compatible and may not be mixed together in a single syringe. Clear insulin must be drawn into the syringe first to reduce the possible contamination of a clear insulin by an insulin containing a suspension.

Lifespan Considerations. Gestational diabetes mellitus (GDM) is a condition that is diagnosed during pregnancy and usually is not present after the postpartum period, approximately 6 weeks after delivery. Placental lactogen and destruction of maternal insulin by the placenta contribute to GDM by increasing insulin resistance in the mother. The incidence of GDM has been on the rise since the mid-1990s, and many healthcare providers recommend performing glucose tests at about 24 to 28 weeks' gestation to rule out GDM. Following diagnosis of GDM, changes in dietary and exercise habits are implemented. If these changes are ineffective in controlling blood glucose level, the client will be prescribed a regimen of insulin injections. Educate clients about the potential problems to the fetus and to themselves during the pregnancy, labor, birth, and postpartum if the treatment prescribed by the healthcare provider is not followed. A child born to a mother diagnosed with GDM has a 40% chance of being obese and developing type 2 DM in later life. The mother has an increased potential for developing GDM in future pregnancies. Oral hypoglycemic agents are contraindicated during pregnancy because of their potential teratogenic effects on the fetus.

The geriatric population also presents with specific problems with regard to maintaining a normal blood glucose level. If geriatric clients have been diabetic for most of their life, they may choose to ignore their recommended therapy regimen because they feel it will make little difference at this time in their lifespan. Also, elderly clients frequently display cognitive impairment that distorts their judgment and their desire to maintain their prescribed diet. Monitor these clients closely, because diet is a major factor in the control of blood glucose levels.

Client Teaching. Client education at it relates to insulin therapy should include the goals of therapy, the reasons for obtaining baseline data such as vital signs and the existence of underlying hypoglycemic disorders, and possible drug side effects. Include the following points when teaching clients about insulin therapy:

- Closely monitor blood glucose before each meal and before insulin administration, as directed by the healthcare provider.
- Carry a source of sugar in case of hypoglycemic reactions.
- When in doubt whether symptoms indicate hypoglycemia or hyperglycemia, treat for hypoglycemia. Hypoglycemia progresses rapidly, whereas hyperglycemia progresses slowly.
- Rotate insulin sites to prevent lipodystrophy.
- Do not inject insulin into areas that are raised, swollen, dimpled, or itching.
- Keep insulin vials that are currently in use at room temperature, because at that temperature insulin is less irritating to the skin.
- When not needed, refrigerate insulin to keep it stable.
- Strictly follow the prescribed diet unless otherwise instructed.
- Wear a medic alert bracelet to alert emergency personnel of DM. Notify caregivers, coworkers, and others who may be able to render assistance.
- Use only an insulin syringe calibrated to the same strength as the insulin.
- Use only the type of insulin prescribed by the healthcare provider.

SPECIAL CONSIDERATIONS

Psychosocial and Cultural Impacts on Young Diabetic Clients

For the child or adolescent who has diabetes, there are psychosocial and cultural considerations of compliance with medication and dietary regimens. Even if diagnosed early in life (with learned behaviors regarding the disease parameters), the elementary school years can be difficult for some children with diabetes. Social events such as birthday parties, field trips, and after-school snack time, where sweet treats are the norm, serve as a physical and psychological temptation. During adolescence, when the teen wants to fit in with a peer group, the diabetic regimen can become more difficult. It is during this time that failure to take insulin or to follow dietary guidelines becomes an issue that may negatively affect present and future health. Some teens may have insulin pumps and can more easily take extra insulin to cover foods not usually on their diet. The ability to do this helps teens feel less different from peers, but carried to excess, this practice can also lead to problems. The nurse plays a vital role in educating the client and family and in making referrals to community agencies that may assist in helping the young person keep blood sugar in control while preserving self-esteem.

44.4 Etiology and Characteristics of Type 2 Diabetes Mellitus

There are a number of differences between type 1 and type 2 diabetes mellitus. Because **type 2 diabetes mellitus** first appears in middle-aged adults, it has been referred to as *age-onset diabetes* or *maturity-onset diabetes*. These are inaccurate descriptions of this disorder, however, because increasing numbers of children are being diagnosed with type 2 DM. (See the Lifespan Considerations feature on page 692.) Approximately 90% of all diabetic clients are type 2.

Unlike clients with type 1 DM, those with type 2 DM are capable of secreting insulin, although in deficient amounts. The fundamental problem in type 2 DM, however, is that insulin receptors in the target tissues have become *insensitive* to the hormone. This phenomenon is called **insulin resistance.** Thus, the small amount of insulin secreted does not bind to its cellular receptors in the tissues as efficiently, and less effect is achieved. Clients are often asymptomatic and may have the condition for years before their diagnosis.

Another important difference is that proper diet and exercise can sometimes increase the sensitivity of insulin receptors to the point that drug therapy is unnecessary for type 2 DM. Many clients with type 2 DM are obese, have dyslipidemias, and will need a medically supervised plan to reduce weight gradually and exercise safely. This is an important lifestyle change for such clients; they will need to maintain these healthy lifestyle habits for a lifetime. Clients with poorly managed type 2 DM often suffer from the same complications as clients with type 1 diabetes (e.g., retinopathy, neuropathy, and nephropathy).

ORAL HYPOGLYCEMICS

Type 2 diabetes is usually controlled with oral hypoglycemic agents, which are prescribed after diet and exercise have failed to reduce blood glucose to normal levels. In severe, unresponsive cases, insulin may also be necessary for type 2 diabetics, or it may be required temporarily during times of stress such as illness or loss.

44.5 Pharmacotherapy With Oral Hypoglycemics

All oral hypoglycemics have the common action of lowering blood glucose levels when taken on a regular basis. Many have the potential to cause hypoglycemia; thus, periodic laboratory tests are conducted to monitor blood glucose levels. Oral hypoglycemics are not effective for type 1 DM. The oral hypoglycemics are listed in Table 44.2.

Classification of oral hypoglycemic drugs is based on their chemical structures and mechanisms of action. The five classes of oral hypoglycemic medications used for type 2 diabetes are sulfonylureas, biguanides, thiazolidinediones, alpha-glucosidase inhibitors, and meglitinides. A new drug class, the dipeptidyl peptidase-4 (DPP-4) inhibitors, was approved in 2006. Therapy is usually initiated with a single agent. If therapeutic goals are not achieved with monotherapy, two agents are administered concurrently. Failure to achieve normal blood glucose levels with two oral hypoglycemics usually indicates a need for insulin.

Sulfonylureas The sulfonylureas were the first oral hypoglycemics available, and are divided into first- and second-generation categories. Although drugs from both generations are equally effective at lowering blood glucose, the second-generation drugs exhibit fewer drug–drug interactions. The sulfonylureas act by stimulating the release of insulin from pancreatic islet cells and by increasing the sensitivity of insulin receptors on target cells. The most common adverse effect of sulfonylureas is hypoglycemia, which is usually caused by taking too much medication or not eating enough food. Persistent hypoglycemia from these agents may be prolonged and require administration of dextrose to return glucose to normal levels. Other side effects include weight gain, hypersensitivity reactions, GI distress, and hepatotoxicity. When alcohol is taken with these agents, some clients experience a disulfiram-like reaction, with flushing, palpitations, and nausea.

Biguanides Metformin (Glucophage), the only drug in this class, acts by decreasing the hepatic production of glucose (gluconeogenesis) and reducing insulin resistance. It does not promote insulin release from the pancreas. Most side effects are minor and GI related, such as anorexia, nausea, and diarrhea. Unlike the sulfonylureas, metformin does not cause hypoglycemia or weight gain. Rarely, metformin has been reported to cause lactic acidosis in clients with impaired liver function owing to accumulation of medication in the liver. A new extended-release formulation of metformin (Glumetza) that allows for once-daily dosing was approved in 2005.

Alpha-glucosidase inhibitors The alpha-glucosidase inhibitors such as acarbose (Precose) act by blocking enzymes in the small intestine responsible for breaking down complex carbohydrates into monosaccharides. Because carbohydrates must be in the monosaccharide form to be absorbed, digestion of glucose is delayed. These agents are usually well tolerated and have minimal side effects. The most common side effects are GI related, such as abdominal cramping, diarrhea, and flatulence. Liver function should be monitored, as a small incidence of liver impairment has been reported. Although alpha-glucosidase inhibitors do not produce hypoglycemia when used alone, hypoglycemia may occur when these agents are combined with insulin or a sulfonylurea. Concurrent use of garlic and ginseng may increase the hypoglycemic action of alpha-glucosidase inhibitors.

Thiazolidinediones The thiazolidinediones, or glitazones, reduce blood glucose by decreasing insulin resistance and inhibiting hepatic gluconeogenesis. Optimal lowering of blood glucose may take 3 to 4 months of therapy. The most common adverse effects are fluid retention, headache, and weight gain. Hypoglycemia does not occur with drugs in this class. Liver function should be monitored, because thiazolidinediones may be hepatotoxic; in 2000, troglitazone (Rezulin) was withdrawn from the market because of drug-related deaths due to

TABLE 44.2   Oral Hypoglycemics

Drug	Route and Adult Dose (max dose where indicated)	Adverse Effects
ALPHA-GLUCOSIDASE INHIBITORS		
acarbose (Precose)	PO; 25–100 mg tid (max: 300 mg/day)	*Flatulence, diarrhea, abdominal distension*
miglitol (Glyset)	PO; 25–100 mg tid (max: 300 mg/day)	Hypoglycemia (tremors, palpitations, sweating)
BIGUANIDE		
metformin HCl (Glucophage, Glumetza)	PO; 500 mg 1–3 times/day (max: 3 g/day) Glumetza is an extended-release tablet; 1,000–2,000 mg once/day	*Flatulence, diarrhea, nausea, anorexia, abdominal pain, bitter or metallic taste* Lactic acidosis
MEGLITINIDES		
nateglinide (Starlix)	PO; 60–120 mg tid	*Flu-like symptoms, upper respiratory infection, back pain*
repaglinide (Prandin)	PO; 0.5–4.0 mg bid–qid	Hypoglycemia (tremors, palpitations, sweating)
SULFONYLUREAS, FIRST GENERATION		
acetohexamide (Dimelor, Dymelor)	PO; 250 mg/day (max: 1,500 mg/day)	*Nausea, heartburn, dizziness, headache, drowsiness*
chlorpropamide (Diabinese, Novo-propamide)	PO; 100–250 mg/day (max: 750 mg/day)	Hypoglycemia (tremors, palpitations, sweating), cholestatic jaundice, blood dyscrasias
tolazamide (Tolamide, Tolinase)	PO; 100–500 mg 1–2 times/day (max: 1 g/day)	
tolbutamide (Orinase)	PO; 250–1,500 mg 1–2 times/day (max: 3 g/day)	
SULFONYLUREAS, SECOND GENERATION		
glimepiride (Amaryl)	PO; 1–4 mg/day (max: 8 mg/day)	
glipizide (Glucotrol)	PO; 2.5–20 mg 1–2 times/day (max: 40 mg/day)	
glyburide (DiaBeta, Micronase, Glynase)	PO; 1.25–10 mg 1–2 times/day (max: 20 mg/day)	
THIAZOLIDINEDIONES		
pioglitazone (Actos)	PO; 15–30 mg/day (max: 45 mg/day)	*Upper respiratory infection, myalgia, headache*
rosiglitazone (Avandia)	PO; 2–4 mg 1–2 times/day (max: 8 mg/day)	Hypoglycemia (tremors, palpitations, sweating)
COMBINATION DRUGS AND OTHER AGENTS		
exenatide (Byetta)	Subcutaneous; 5–10 mcg 1–2 times/day	*Nausea, vomiting, diarrhea, nervousness* Hypoglycemia (tremors, palpitations, sweating)
glipizide/metformin (Metaglip)	PO; 2.5/250 mg/day (max: 10 mg glipizide and 2,000 mg metformin/day)	See above for individual drug classes.
glyburide/metformin (Glucovance)	PO; 1.25 mg/250 mg 1–2 times/day (max: 20 mg glyburide and 2,000 mg metformin/day)	
rosiglitazone/glimepride (Avandaryl)	PO; 4 mg/1 mg, 4 mg/2 mg, or 4 mg/4 mg fixed dose rosiglitazone/glimepride daily (max: 8 mg rosiglitazone and 4 mg glimepiride/day)	
pioglitazone/metformin (ACTOplus met)	PO; 15 mg/500 mg or 15 mg/850 mg fixed dose pioglitazone/metformin daily (max: 45 mg pioglitazone and 2,000 mg metformin/day	
rosiglitazone/metformin (Avandamet)	PO; variable dose (max: 8 mg rosiglitazone and 1,000 mg metformin/day)	
sitagliptin (Januvia)	PO; 100 mg once daily	

Italics indicate common adverse effects; underlining indicates serious adverse effects.

hepatic failure. Because of their tendency to promote fluid retention, thiazolidinediones are contraindicated in clients with serious heart failure or pulmonary edema.

Meglitinides   The meglitinides are a newer class of oral hypoglycemics that act by stimulating the release of insulin from pancreatic islet cells in a manner similar to that of the sulfonylureas. Both agents in this class have short durations of action of 2–4 hours. Their efficacy is equal to that of the sulfonylureas, and they are well tolerated. Hypoglycemia is the most common adverse effect.

Newer agents Several new drugs have been approved that act by affecting the incretin–glucose control mechanism. Incretins are hormones secreted by the intestine following a meal, when blood glucose is elevated. Incretins signal the pancreas to increase insulin secretion and the liver to stop producing glucagon. Both of these actions lower blood glucose levels. Diabetic clients are unable to secrete incretins in adequate amounts, thus disrupting an important glucose-control mechanism. Drugs may be used to modify the incretin system in diabetics in two ways: by mimicking the actions of incretins, or by reducing their destruction.

Exenatide (Byetta) is an injectable drug that *mimics* the effects of incretins. Exenatide lower blood glucose by increasing the secretion of insulin, slowing the absorption of glucose, and reducing the action of glucagon. The drug was approved in 2005 as an alternative to metformin in clients who have not achieved adequate glycemic control during metformin or sulfonylurea monotherapy. The drug must be administered subcutaneously, often twice a day, and causes significant nausea, vomiting, and diarrhea in some clients.

In 2006, the FDA approved sitagliptin phosphate (Januvia), the first drug in a class known as the dipeptidyl peptidase-4 (DPP-4) inhibitors. The normal function of the DDP-4 enzyme is to break down incretins. Sitaglipton inhibits DPP-4, thereby reducing the destruction of incretins. Levels of incretin hormones increase, thus decreasing blood glucose levels in clients with type 2 diabetes. Several other DDP-4 inhibitors are in the later stages of clinical trials, and may be approved in the near future, including vildaglipton (Galvus), denaglipton (Redona), aloglipton (Takeda) and saxaglipton.

Pramlintide (Symlin) is a new injectable drug for type 1 and type 2 DM that resembles human amylin, a hormone produced by the pancreas after meals that helps the body regulate blood glucose. Pramlintide slows absorption of glucose and inhibits the action of glucagon. Pramlintide lowers blood glucose levels and promotes weight loss.

Because various oral hypoglycemics work by different mechanisms to lower blood sugar and have different pharmacokinetic properties, combinations of antidiabetic agents have been developed to maximize the therapeutic effects and minimize adverse effects. One popular combination drug is glyburide/metformin (Glucovance), which comes in various strengths such as 1.25/250, 2.5/500, and 5/500.

The American Diabetes Association and the American Association of Clinical Endocrinologists recommend that type 2 diabetics maintain a preprandial blood glucose level below 110 mg/dl. In healthy persons, the beta cells secrete insulin in response to small increases in blood glucose, which is referred to as an *acute insulin response.* This response is diminished at 115 mg/dl, and the higher the glucose level the less likely it is that the beta cells will respond by secreting insulin. Because clients with type 2 diabetes need to secrete some insulin, keeping the blood glucose level below 110 mg/dl before meals optimizes secretion of insulin.

Clients with type 2 DM need to recognize the symptoms of **hyperosmolar nonketotic coma (HNKC),** which is a life-threatening emergency. As with the onset of diabetic

NATURAL THERAPIES

Stevia for Hyperglycemia

Stevia (*Stevia rebaudiana*) is an herb belonging to the sunflower family indigenous to Paraguay that may be helpful to clients with diabetes. Although widely used in Japan and other Asian countries as a sweetener, the FDA has not approved its use for this purpose because there are concerns that substances in the herb may cause mutations. Thus, although not permitted as a food additive, the powdered extract is readily available as a dietary supplement and can be used in place of sugar. Its sweetening power is 300 times that of sugar, but it does not appear to have a negative effect on blood glucose or insulin secretion. In animal experiments, stevia significantly elevated the glucose clearance, an effect that may be beneficial to those with diabetes. Another study done on type 2 diabetic clients showed that stevia reduces postprandial (after eating) blood glucose levels (Gregersen, Jeppesen, et al. 2004). The nurse should strongly encourage all diabetic clients to discuss this supplement and other herbal products with the healthcare provider before taking them.

ketoacidosis in those with type 1 DM, HNKC develops slowly and is caused by insufficient circulating insulin. It is seen most often in older adults. The skin appears flushed, dry, and warm, like in diabetic ketoacidosis. Unlike diabetic ketoacidosis, HNKC does not affect breathing. Blood glucose levels may rise over 600 mg/dl and reach 1,000 to 2,000 mg/dl. HNKC has a higher mortality rate than DKA.

NURSING CONSIDERATIONS

The role of the nurse in oral hypoglycemic therapy involves careful assessment and monitoring of a client's condition and providing education as it relates to the prescribed drug treatment. Assessment of the client with type 2 diabetes includes a physical examination, health history, psychosocial history, and lifestyle history. A comprehensive assessment is needed, because diabetes can affect multiple body systems. Psychosocial factors and lifestyle, as well as knowledge base regarding diabetes, can affect the client's ability to keep his or her blood glucose level within the normal range. The client's lifestyle factors and health history help determine the type of drug prescribed.

Provide clients with information about the importance of keeping blood glucose levels within the normal range. Blood glucose should be monitored daily; urinary ketones should be monitored if blood glucose is over 300 mg/dl. Also monitor intake and output, and review lab studies for liver function abnormalities. Monitor the client for signs and symptoms of illness or infection, because illness can affect the client's medication needs. Use these drugs cautiously in those with impaired renal and hepatic function and those who are malnourished, because these conditions interfere with absorption and metabolism of the oral hypoglycemics. Caution should be used in clients with pituitary or adrenal disorders, because hormones from these sources affect blood glucose levels. Oral hypoglycemics are contraindicated in hypersensitivity, ketoacidosis, or diabetic coma. They are also contraindicated in clients who are pregnant or lactating,

Pr PROTOTYPE DRUG | Glipizide *(Glucotrol, Glucotrol XL)* | Oral Hypoglycemic Agent

ACTIONS AND USES

Glipizide is a second-generation sulfonylurea offering advantages of higher potency, once daily dosing, fewer side effects, and fewer drug–drug interactions than some of the first-generation drugs in this class. Glipizide stimulates the pancreas to secrete more insulin and also increases the sensitivity of insulin receptors at target tissues. Some degree of pancreatic function is required for glipizide to lower blood glucose. Maximum effects are achieved if the drug is taken 30 minutes prior to the first meal of the day. Both immediate-release and extended-release (XL) formulations are available.

ADMINISTRATION ALERTS

- Sustained-release tablets must be swallowed whole and not crushed or chewed.
- Sulfonylureas including glipizide should not be given after the last meal of the day.
- Administer medication as directed by the healthcare provider.
- Pregnancy category C.

PHARMACOKINETICS

Onset: 15–30 min

Peak: 1–2 h

Half-Life: 3–5 h

Duration: Up to 24 h

ADVERSE EFFECTS

Hypoglycemia is less frequent with glipizide than with first-generation sulfonylureas. Elderly clients are prone to hypoglycemia because many have decreased renal and hepatic function, which can cause an increase in the amount of medication circulating in the blood. For this reason, elderly clients are often prescribed a reduced dosage.

Clients should stay out of direct sunlight, because rashes and photosensitivity are possible. Some clients experience mild, GI-related effects such as nausea, vomiting, or loss of appetite.

Contraindications: Contraindications include known hypersensitivity to the drug or diabetic ketoacidosis.

INTERACTIONS

Drug–Drug: Glipizide and other sulfonylureas have the potential to interact with a number of drugs; thus, the client should always consult with a healthcare provider before adding a new medication or herbal supplement. There is a cross-sensitivity of glipizide with sulfonamides and thiazide diuretics. Oral anticoagulants, chloramphenicol, clofibrate, and MAOIs may potentiate the hypoglycemic actions of glipizide. Ingestion of alcohol will result in a disulfiram-like reaction that includes headache, flushing, nausea, and abdominal cramping.

Lab Tests: May increase values of the following: LDH, blood urea nitrogen (BUN), aspartate aminotransferase (AST), alkaline phosphatase, and creatinine.

Herbal/Food: Ginseng, bilberry, and garlic may increase hypoglycemic effects.

Treatment of Overdose: Overdose may cause hypoglycemia, which is usually treated by administering oral glucose. Severe cases may be treated with IV glucose.

 See the Companion Website for a Nursing Process Focus specific to this drug.

---

because safety has not been established, and these drugs may be secreted in breast milk.

Administer oral hypoglycemics as directed by the prescriber. Some oral antidiabetic drugs are given 30 minutes before breakfast so that the drug will have reached the plasma when the client begins to eat. Others such as acarbose (Precose) and miglitol (Glyset) are given with each meal.

Lifespan Considerations. The rapid rise in the incidence of type 2 DM in children is a growing concern for healthcare providers. The disease is reaching epidemic proportions, especially in certain ethnic groups such as African American, Native American, Hispanic, and Asian or Pacific Islander. Children who develop type 2 diabetes are most often overweight and sedentary. Although insulin and metformin are the only two drugs approved by the FDA for treating pediatric type 2 DM, other drugs are sometimes prescribed. Insulin is the most effective agent, although children often respond negatively to daily injections. Metformin has been shown to be safe and effective in children, although drugs from other classes may need to be added to the regimen over time. The guidelines for phar-macotherapy of pediatric type 2 diabetes will likely change rapidly as research determines the best therapies for this age group.

Client Teaching. Client education as it relates to oral hypoglycemic drugs should include the goals of therapy, the reasons for obtaining baseline data such as vital signs and the existence of underlying cardiac and renal disorders, and possible drug side effects. Include the following points when teaching clients about oral hypoglycemics:

- Always carry a source of sugar in case of hypoglycemic reactions.
- Wear a medic alert bracelet to alert emergency personnel of diabetes. Notify caregivers, coworkers, and others who may be able to render assistance.
- Avoid alcohol use.
- Closely monitor blood glucose levels as directed by the healthcare provider.
- Strictly follow the prescribed diet unless otherwise instructed.

Assessment Data	Potential Nursing Diagnoses
Prior to administration: ■ Obtain a complete health history including allergies, drug history, and possible drug interactions. ■ Assess for pain location and level. ■ Assess knowledge of drug and ability to conduct blood glucose testing.	■ Injury (hypoglycemia), Risk for, related to adverse effects of drug therapy ■ Pain (abdominal), related to adverse effects of drug ■ Knowledge, Deficient, related to drug therapy ■ Knowledge, Deficient, related to blood glucose testing

Planning: Client Goals and Expected Outcomes

The client will:
- Describe signs and symptoms that should be reported immediately, including nausea, diarrhea, jaundice, rash, headache, anorexia, abdominal pain, tachycardia, seizures, and confusion.
- Demonstrate an ability to accurately self-monitor blood glucose.
- Demonstrate an understanding of the drug's action by accurately describing drug side effects and precautions.
- Maintain blood glucose within a normal range.

Implementation

Interventions and (Rationales)	Client Education/Discharge Planning
■ Monitor blood glucose at least daily and monitor urinary ketones if blood glucose is greater than 300 mg/dl. (Ketones spill into the urine at high blood glucose levels and provide an early sign of diabetic ketoacidosis.)	■ Teach client how to monitor blood glucose and test urine for ketones, especially when ill.
■ Monitor for signs of lactic acidosis if client is receiving a biguanide. (Mitochondrial oxidation of lactic acid is inhibited, and lactic acidosis may result.)	■ Instruct client to report signs of lactic acidosis such as hyperventilation, muscle pain, fatigue, and increased sleeping.
■ Review lab tests for any abnormalities in liver function. (These drugs are metabolized in the liver and may cause elevations in AST and LDH. Metformin decreases absorption of vitamin B_{12} and folic acid.)	■ Instruct client to report the first sign of yellow skin, pale stools, or dark urine.
■ Obtain accurate history of alcohol use, especially if client is receiving a sulfonylurea or biguanide. (These drugs may cause a disulfiram-like reaction.)	■ Advise client to abstain from alcohol and to avoid liquid OTC medications that may contain alcohol.
■ Monitor for signs and symptoms of illness or infection. (Illness may increase blood glucose levels.)	■ Instruct client to report signs of fatigue, muscle weakness, and nausea and to get adequate rest.
■ Monitor blood glucose frequently especially at the beginning of therapy, in elderly clients, and in those taking a beta-blocker. (Early signs of hypoglycemia may not be apparent.)	Instruct client: ■ To monitor blood glucose before breakfast and dinner and not to skip meals. ■ To monitor signs and symptoms of hypoglycemia and, if present, eat a simple sugar; if symptoms do not improve, call 911. ■ Not to skip meals and to follow a diet specified by the healthcare provider.
■ Monitor weight, weighing at the same time of day each time. (Changes in weight affect the amount of drug needed to control blood glucose.)	■ Instruct client to weigh self each week, at the same time of day, and report any significant loss or gain.
■ Monitor vital signs. (Increased pulse and blood pressure are early signs of hypoglycemia.)	■ Teach client how to take accurate blood pressure, temperature, and pulse.
■ Monitor skin for rashes and itching. (These are signs of an allergic reaction to the drug.)	■ Advise client of the importance of immediately reporting skin rashes and itching that is unaccounted for by dry skin.
■ Monitor activity level. (Dose may require adjustment with change in physical activity.)	Advise client to: ■ Increase activity level to help lower blood glucose. ■ Closely monitor blood glucose when involved in vigorous physical activity.

Evaluation of Outcome Criteria

Evaluate the effectiveness of drug therapy by confirming that client goals and expected outcomes have been met (see "Planning").
- The client accurately describes signs and symptoms that should be reported immediately, including nausea, diarrhea, jaundice, rash, headache, anorexia, abdominal pain, tachycardia, seizures, and confusion.
- The client demonstrates an ability to accurately self-monitor blood glucose.
- The client demonstrates an understanding of the drug's action by accurately describing drug side effects and precautions.
- The client maintains blood glucose within a normal range.

∞ *See Table 44.2 for a list of drugs to which these nursing actions apply.*

- Swallow tablets whole and do not crush sustained-release tablets.
- Take medication 30 minutes before breakfast, or as directed by the healthcare provider.
- Immediately report nervousness, confusion, excessive sweating, rapid pulse, or tremors, because these are signs of overdosage (hypoglycemia).
- Immediately report increased thirst or urine output, decreased appetite, or excessive fatigue, because these are signs of underdosage (hyperglycemia).

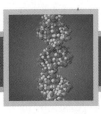

CHAPTER REVIEW

KEY CONCEPTS

The numbered key concepts provide a succinct summary of the important points from the corresponding numbered section within the chapter. If any of these points are not clear, refer to the numbered section within the chapter for review.

44.1 The pancreas is both an endocrine and an exocrine gland. Insulin is released when blood glucose increases, and glucagon when blood glucose decreases.

44.2 Type 1 DM is caused by an absolute lack of insulin secretion due to autoimmune destruction of pancreatic islet cells. If untreated, it results in serious, chronic conditions affecting the cardiovascular and nervous systems.

44.3 Type 1 DM is treated by dietary restrictions, exercise, and insulin therapy. The many types of insulin preparations vary as to their onset of action, time to peak effect, and duration.

44.4 Type 2 DM is caused by a lack of sensitivity of insulin receptors at the target cells and a deficiency in insulin secretion. If untreated, the same chronic conditions result as in type 1 DM.

44.5 Type 2 DM is controlled through lifestyle changes and oral hypoglycemic drugs. More than five classes of drugs are available for the pharmacotherapy of type 2 DM.

NCLEX-RN® REVIEW QUESTIONS

1 A client receives NPH (Isophane) insulin at 0730. Based on an understanding of peak time, the nurse should assess the client for hypoglycemia at what time? Write your answer below.

2 The client is scheduled to receive 5 units of Humalog and 25 units of NPH (Isophane) insulin prior to breakfast. What nursing intervention is most appropriate for this client?

1. Make sure the client's breakfast is ready to eat before administering this insulin.
2. Offer the client a high-carbohydrate snack in 6 hours.
3. Hold the insulin if the blood glucose level is greater than 100 mg/dl.
4. Administer the medications in two separate syringes.

3 The nurse is initiating discharge teaching with the newly diagnosed diabetic. Which of the following statements indicates that the client needs additional teaching?

1. "If I am experiencing hypoglycemia, I should drink 1/2 cup of apple juice."
2. "My insulin needs may increase when I have an infection."
3. "I must draw the NPH insulin first if I am mixing it with regular insulin."
4. "If my blood glucose levels are >300mg/dl, I must check my urine for ketones."

4 What client education should the nurse provide to the diabetic client who is planning an exercise program? (Select all that apply.)

1. Monitor blood glucose levels before and after exercise.
2. Eat a complex carbohydrate prior to strenuous exercise.
3. Exercise may increase insulin needs.
4. Withhold insulin prior to engaging in strenuous exercise.
5. Take extra insulin prior to exercise.

5 During assessment, the client states, "My blood glucose levels range between 80 and 100mg/dl, but my early morning blood glucose levels are 200 mg/dl." This nurse explains that this phenomena is best known as which of the following?

1. Hyperosmolarity
2. Somogyi phenomenon
3. Insulin resistance
4. Diabetic ketoacidosis

CRITICAL THINKING QUESTIONS

1. A 28-year-old woman who is pregnant with her first child is diagnosed with gestational DM. She is concerned about the fact that she might have to take "shots." She tells the nurse at the public health clinic that she doesn't think she can self-administer an injection and asks if there is a pill that will control her blood sugar. She has heard her grandfather talk about his pills to control his "sugar." What should the nurse explain to this client?

2. When reviewing a client's insulin administration record, the nurse notes that the client is routinely rotating injection sites from arm to leg to abdomen. The nurse also notes that the client continues to have fluctuations in his blood glucose levels despite receiving the same amount of insulin. What does the nurse need to explain to this client about site rotation?

3. The client has insulin glargine (Lantus) and regular insulin ordered for every morning. Explain the implications of administering these two types of insulins.

See Appendix D for answers and rationales for all activities.

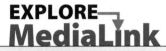

EXPLORE MediaLink

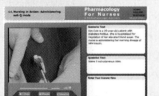

www.prenhall.com/adams

NCLEX-RN® review, case studies, and other interactive resources for this chapter can be found on the companion website at www.prenhall.com/adams. Click on "Chapter 44" to select the activities for this chapter. For animations, more NCLEX-RN® review questions, and an audio glossary, access the accompanying Prentice Hall Nursing MediaLink DVD-ROM in this textbook.

PRENTICE HALL NURSING MEDIALINK DVD-ROM

- **Animation**
  Mechanism in Action: Glipizide (*Glucotrol*)
- **Audio Glossary**
- **NCLEX-RN® Review**
- **Nursing in Action**
  Administering Subcutaneous Medications
  Administering Subcutaneous Medications (Abdomen)

COMPANION WEBSITE

- **NCLEX-RN® Review**
- **Dosage Calculations**
- **Case Study:** Diabetes and insulin
- **Care Plan:** Noncompliant client with type 1 diabetes who is prescribed insulin glargine

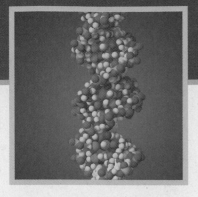

CHAPTER 45

Drugs for Disorders and Conditions of the Female Reproductive System

DRUGS AT A GLANCE

ORAL CONTRACEPTIVES
Estrogen–Progestin Combinations
Monophasic
- ethinyl estradiol with norethindrone (Ortho-Novum 1/35)

Progestin-only Agents
DRUGS FOR EMERGENCY CONTRACEPTION AND PHARMACOLOGIC ABORTION
HORMONE REPLACEMENT THERAPY
Estrogens and Estrogen/Progestin Combinations
- conjugated estrogens (Premarin) and conjugated estrogens with medroxy-progesterone (Prempro)

DRUGS FOR DYSFUNCTIONAL UTERINE BLEEDING
Progestins
- medroxyprogesterone (Provera)

UTERINE STIMULANTS AND RELAXANTS
Oxytocics (Stimulants)
- oxytocin (Pitocin, Syntocinon)

Ergot Alkaloids
Prostaglandins
Tocolytics (Relaxants)
Beta$_2$-adrenergic Agonists
DRUGS FOR FEMALE INFERTILITY AND ENDOMETRIOSIS

OBJECTIVES

After reading this chapter, the student should be able to:

1. Describe the roles of the hypothalamus, pituitary, and ovaries in maintaining female reproductive function.
2. Explain the mechanisms by which estrogens and progestins prevent conception.
3. Explain how drugs may be used to provide emergency contraception and to terminate early pregnancy.
4. Describe the role of drug therapy in the treatment of menopausal and postmenopausal symptoms.
5. Identify the role of the female sex hormones in the treatment of cancer.
6. Discuss the uses of progestins in the therapy of dysfunctional uterine bleeding.
7. Compare and contrast the use of uterine stimulants and relaxants in the treatment of antepartum and postpartum clients.
8. Explain how drug therapy may be used to treat female infertility.
9. Describe the nurse's role in the pharmacological management of disorders and conditions of the female reproductive system.
10. For each of the classes shown in Drugs at a Glance, know representative drugs, and explain the mechanisms of drug action, primary actions, and important adverse effects.
11. Categorize drugs used in the treatment of female reproductive disorders and conditions based on their classification and mechanism of action.
12. Use the Nursing Process to care for clients who are receiving drug therapy for disorders and conditions of the female reproductive system.

MediaLink 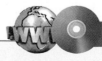 www.prenhall.com/adams

NCLEX-RN® review, case studies, and other interactive resources for this chapter can be found on the companion website at www.prenhall.com/adams. Click on "Chapter 45" to select the activities for this chapter. For animations, more NCLEX-RN® review questions, and an audio glossary, access the accompanying Prentice Hall Nursing MediaLink DVD-ROM in this textbook.

Hormones from the pituitary gland and the gonads provide for the growth and maintenance of the female reproductive organs. Endogenous hormones can be supplemented with natural or synthetic hormones to achieve a variety of therapeutic goals, ranging from replacement therapy, to prevention of pregnancy, to milk production. This chapter examines drugs used to treat disorders and conditions associated with the female reproductive system.

45.1 Hypothalamic and Pituitary Regulation of Female Reproductive Function

Regulation of the female reproductive system is achieved by hormones from the hypothalamus, pituitary gland, and ovary. The hypothalamus secretes **gonadotropin-releasing hormone (GnRH),** which travels a short distance to the pituitary to stimulate the secretion of **follicle-stimulating hormone (FSH)** and **luteinizing hormone (LH).** Both of these pituitary hormones act on the ovary and cause immature ovarian follicles to begin developing. The rising and falling levels of pituitary hormones create two interrelated cycles that occur on a periodic, monthly basis, the ovarian and uterine cycles. The hormonal changes that occur during the ovarian and uterine cycles are illustrated in ● Figure 45.1.

Under the influence of FSH and LH, several ovarian follicles begin the maturation process each month during a woman's reproductive years. On approximately Day 14 of the ovarian cycle, a surge of LH secretion causes one follicle to expel its oocyte, a process called **ovulation.** The ruptured follicle, minus its oocyte, remains in the ovary and is transformed into the hormone-secreting **corpus luteum.** The oocyte, on the other hand, begins its journey through the uterine tube and eventually reaches the uterus. If conception does not occur, the outer lining of the uterus degenerates and is shed to the outside during menstruation.

45.2 Ovarian Control of Female Reproductive Function

As ovarian follicles mature, they secrete the female sex hormones **estrogen** and **progesterone.** Estrogen is actually a generic term for three different hormones: estradiol, estrone, and estriol. Estrogen is responsible for the maturation of the female reproductive organs and for the appearance of secondary

KEY TERMS
corpus luteum   *page 697*
dysfunctional uterine bleeding   *page 708*
endometriosis   *page 715*
estrogen   *page 697*
follicle-stimulating hormone (FSH)   *page 697*
gonadotropin-releasing hormone (GnRH)   *page 697*
hormone replacement therapy (HRT)   *page 705*
infertility   *page 714*
luteinizing hormone (LH)   *page 697*
menopause   *page 705*
ovulation   *page 697*
oxytocics   *page 710*
progesterone   *page 697*
prostaglandin   *page 711*
tocolytic   *page 710*

PHARMFACTS

Female Reproductive Conditions

- There is a wide range of ages at which women reach menopause: 8 of 100 women will stop menstruating before age 40, and 5 of 100 women will continue beyond age 60.

- About half the cases of dysfunctional uterine bleeding are diagnosed in women older than 45; however, 20% of cases occur under in those younger than 20.

- The most common reason why women become pregnant while on oral contraceptives is skipping a dose.

- A nonsmoking woman aged 25 to 29 has a 2 in 100,000 chance of dying from complications due to oral contraceptives. The risk that a woman in this age group will die in an automobile accident is 74 in 100,000.

- Oral contraceptives confer benefits besides contraception. It is estimated that each year they prevent the following:
  51,000 cases of pelvic inflammatory disease
  9,900 hospitalizations for ectopic pregnancy
  27,000 cases of iron-deficiency anemia
  20,000 hospitalizations for certain types of nonmalignant breast disease

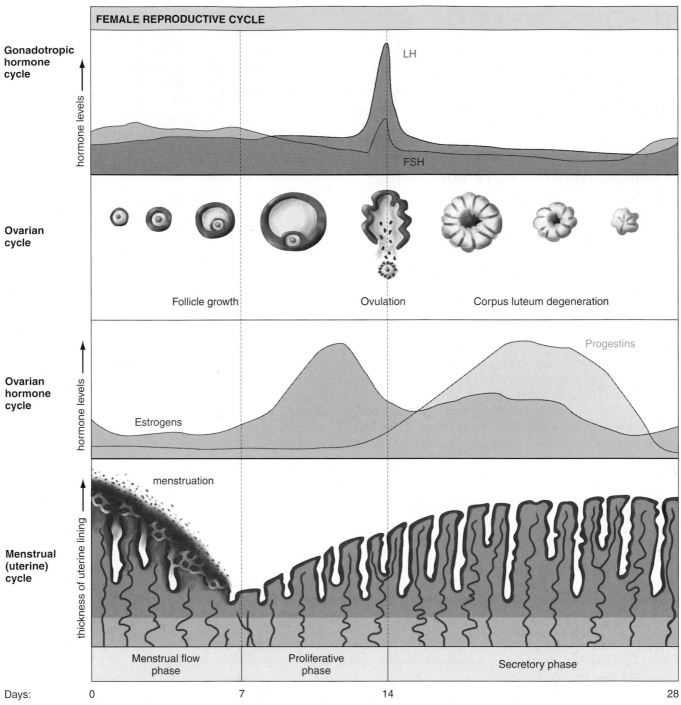

FEMALE REPRODUCTIVE CYCLE

Gonadotropic hormone cycle

hormone levels

LH

FSH

Ovarian cycle

Follicle growth

Ovulation

Corpus luteum degeneration

Ovarian hormone cycle

hormone levels

Progestins

Estrogens

Menstrual (uterine) cycle

thickness of uterine lining

menstruation

Menstrual flow phase

Proliferative phase

Secretory phase

Days: 0   7   14   28

● **Figure 45 .1** Hormonal changes during the ovarian and uterine cycles *Source: Pearson Education/PH College.*

sex characteristics. In addition, estrogen has numerous metabolic effects on nonreproductive tissues, including the brain, kidneys, blood vessels, and skin. For example, estrogen helps maintain low blood cholesterol levels and facilitates calcium uptake by bones to help maintain proper bone density (Chapter 47 ∞). When women enter menopause at about age 50 to 55, the ovaries stop secreting estrogen.

In the last half of the ovarian cycle, the corpus luteum secretes a class of hormones called *progestins,* the most abundant of which is progesterone. In combination with estrogen,

progesterone promotes breast development and regulates the monthly changes of the uterine cycle. Under the influence of estrogen and progesterone, the uterine endometrium becomes vascular and thickens in preparation for receiving a fertilized egg. High progesterone and estrogen levels in the final third of the uterine cycle provide negative feedback to shut off GnRH, FSH, and LH secretion. This negative feedback loop is illustrated in ● Figure 45.2. Without stimulation from FSH and LH, estrogen and progesterone levels fall sharply, the endometrium is shed, and menstrual bleeding begins.

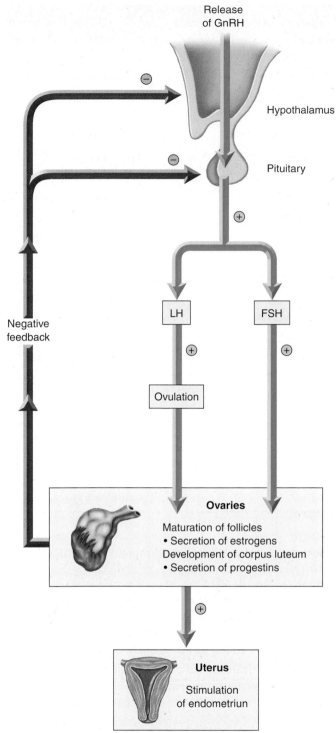

Figure 45.2 Negative feedback control of the female reproductive hormones

CONTRACEPTION

The most widespread pharmacological use of the female sex hormones is to prevent pregnancy.

ORAL CONTRACEPTIVES

Oral contraceptives are drugs used to prevent pregnancy. Commonly referred to as "the pill," most oral contraceptives are a combination of estrogens and progestins. In low doses,

they prevent fertilization by inhibiting ovulation. Selected oral contraceptives are listed in Table 45.1.

45.3 Estrogens and Progestins as Oral Contraceptives

When used appropriately, female sex hormones are nearly 100% effective. Most oral contraceptives contain a combination of estrogen and progestin; a few preparations contain only progestin. The most common estrogen used for contraception is ethinyl estradiol, and the most common progestin is norethindrone.

A large number of oral contraceptive preparations are available, differing in dose and by type of estrogen and progestin. Selection of a specific formulation is individualized to each client, and determined by which drug gives the best contraceptive protection with the fewest side effects. Daily doses of estrogen in oral contraceptives have declined from 150 mcg, 40 years ago, to about 35 mcg in modern formulations. This reduction has resulted in a decrease in estrogen-related adverse effects.

Typically, drug administration of an oral contraceptive begins on Day 5 of the ovarian cycle, and continues for 21 days. During the other 7 days of the month, the client takes a placebo. Although the placebo serves no pharmacological purpose, it does encourage the client to take the pills on a daily basis. Some of these placebos contain iron, which replaces iron lost from menstrual bleeding. If a daily dose is missed, two pills taken the following day usually provide adequate contraception. If more than one day is missed, the client should observe other contraceptive precautions, such as abstinence or using condoms, until the oral contraceptive doses can be resumed at the beginning of the next monthly cycle. ● Figure 45.3 shows a typical monthly oral contraceptive packet with the 28 pills.

Estrogen–progestin oral contraceptives act by providing negative feedback to the pituitary to shut down the secretion of LH and FSH. Without the influence of these pituitary hormones, the ovarian follicle cannot mature, and ovulation is prevented. The estrogen–progestin agents also reduce the likelihood of implantation of the fertilized ovum by making the uterine endometrium less favorable to receive an embryo. In addition to their contraceptive function, these agents are sometimes prescribed to promote timely and regular monthly cycles, and to reduce the incidence of dysmenorrhea.

The three types of estrogen–progestin formulations are monophasic, biphasic, and triphasic. The most common is the monophasic, which delivers a constant amount of estrogen and progestin in every pill. In biphasic agents, the amount of estrogen in each pill remains constant, but the amount of progestin is increased toward the end of the menstrual cycle to better nourish the uterine lining. In triphasic formulations, the amounts of both estrogen and progestin vary in three distinct phases during the 28-day cycle.

The progestin-only oral contraceptives, sometimes called *minipills,* prevent pregnancy primarily by producing thick, viscous mucus at the entrance to the uterus that discourages penetration by sperm. They also tend to inhibit implantation

TABLE 45.1 Selected Oral Contraceptives

Trade Name	Type	Estrogen	Progestin
Alesse	monophasic	ethinyl estradiol; 20 mcg	levonorgestrel; 0.1 mg
Desogen	monophasic	ethinyl estradiol; 30 mcg	desogestrel; 0.15 mg
Loestrin 1.5/30 Fe	monophasic	ethinyl estradiol; 30 mcg	norethindrone; 1.5 mg
Lo/Ovral	monophasic	ethinyl estradiol; 30 mcg	norgestrel; 0.3 mg
Ortho-Cyclen	monophasic	ethinyl estradiol; 35 mcg	norgestimate; 0.25 mg
Yasmin	monophasic	ethinyl estradiol; 30 mcg	drospirenone; 3 mg
Ortho-Novum 10/11	biphasic	ethinyl estradiol; 35 mcg	norethindrone; 0.5 mg (phase 1)
		ethinyl estradiol; 35 mcg	norethindrone; 1.0 mg (phase 2)
Ortho-Novum 7/7/7	triphasic	ethinyl estradiol; 35 mcg	norethindrone; 0.5 mg (phase 1)
		ethinyl estradiol; 35 mcg	norethindrone; 0.75 mg (phase 2)
		ethinyl estradiol; 35 mcg	norethindrone; 1.0 mg (phase 3)
Ortho Tri-Cyclen	triphasic	ethinyl estradiol; 35 mcg	norgestimate; 0.5 mg (phase 1)
		ethinyl estradiol; 35 mcg	norgestimate; 0.75 mg (phase 2)
		ethinyl estradiol; 35 mcg	norgestimate; 1.0 mg (phase 3)
Tri-Levlen	triphasic	ethinyl estradiol; 35 mcg	levonorgestrel; 0.05 mg (phase 1)
		ethinyl estradiol; 40 mcg	levonorgestrel; 0.075 mg (phase 2)
		ethinyl estradiol; 30 mcg	levonorgestrel; 0.125 mg (phase 3)
Triphasil	triphasic	ethinyl estradiol; 30 mcg	norgestrel; 0.05 mg (phase 1)
		ethinyl estradiol; 40 mcg	norgestrel; 0.075 mg (phase 2)
		ethinyl estradiol; 30 mcg	norgestrel; 1.25 mg (phase 3)
Micronor	progestin only	none	norethindrone; 0.35 mg
Nor-Q.D.	progestin only	none	norethindrone; 0.35 mg
Ovrette	progestin only	none	norgestrel; 0.075 mg

MediaLink   The History of Contraception

of a fertilized egg. Minipills are less effective than estrogen–progestin combinations, having a failure rate of 1% to 4%. Their use also results in a higher incidence of menstrual irregularities such as amenorrhea, prolonged menstrual bleeding, or breakthrough spotting. They are generally reserved for clients who are at high risk for side effects from estrogen.

Several long-term formulations of oral contraceptives are available. These extended-duration formulations are equally effective in preventing pregnancy and have the same side-effect profile as oral contraceptives. They offer a major advantage for women who are likely to forget their daily pill, or who prefer a greater ease of use. Examples of alternative formulations are as follows:

- Depo-Provera: Deep IM injection of medroxyprogesterone acetate that provides 3 months of contraceptive protection.
- Lunelle: IM injection of medroxyprogesterone acetate and estradiol cypionate in prefilled syringes that provide 1 month of contraceptive protection.
- Implants: Norplant, which was removed from the U.S. market in 2000, consisted of six small, plastic tubes filled with levonorgestrel implanted subcutaneously under the inner aspect of the upper arm that provided contraception for up to 5 years. Jadelle is a two-rod system of

levonorgestrel that is easier to implant and remove than Norplant and provides 3 years of protection. It has been approved by the FDA but has not yet been marketed. Implanon is a single rod containing the progestin 3-keto-desogestrel that provides 3 years of protection and is being considered by the FDA for approval. Jadelle and Implanon are widely available outside the United States.

- Ortho-Evra: Transdermal patch containing ethinyl estradiol and norelgestromin. The patch is changed every 7 days for the first 3 weeks, followed by no patch during Week 4.
- NuvaRing: A 2-inch-diameter ring containing estrogen and progestin that is inserted into the vagina to provide 3 weeks of contraceptive protection. The ring is removed during Week 4, and a new ring is inserted during the first week of the next menstrual cycle.
- Mirena: Polyethylene cylinder placed in the uterus that releases levonorgestrel. About the size of a quarter and shaped like the letter *T*, Mirena acts locally to prevent conception for 5 years.

Also new in contraceptive therapy is the development of "extended regimen" oral contraceptives. Approved in 2003, Seasonale consists of tablets containing levonorgestrel and ethinyl estradiol that are taken for 84 consecutive days,

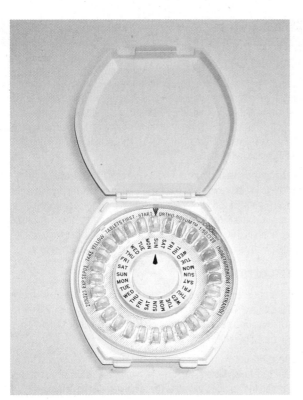

● **Figure 45.3** An oral contraceptive showing the daily doses and the different formulation taken in the last 7 days of the 28-day cycle

followed by 7 inert tablets (without hormones). This allows for continuous contraceptive protection while extending the time between menses; only four periods are experienced per year. Seasonique is similar, but instead of inert tablets for 7 days, the client takes low-dose estrogen tablets. Seasonique, approved in 2006, is claimed by the manufacturer to have a lower incidence of bloating and breakthrough bleeding.

Although oral contraceptives are safe for the large majority of women, there are some potentially serious adverse effects. As with other medications, the higher the dose of estrogen or progesterone, the more likely will be the risk for side effects. With oral contraceptives, however, some side effects are more prominent at *lower* doses. Thus, physicians try to prescribe the oral contraceptive with the lowest dose of hormones that will achieve the therapeutic goal of pregnancy prevention with minimal side effects. Table 45.2 summarizes the adverse effects of the oral contraceptives.

Numerous drug–drug interactions are possible with estrogen and progesterone. Certain anticonvulsants and antibiotics can reduce the effectiveness of oral contraceptives, thus increasing a woman's risk of pregnancy. Because oral contraceptives can reduce the effectiveness of warfarin (Coumadin), insulin, and certain oral hypoglycemic agents, dosage adjustment may be necessary.

The risk of cancer following long-term oral contraceptive use has been extensively studied. Because some studies have shown a small increase in breast cancer incidence, oral contraceptives are contraindicated in clients with known or suspected breast cancer. The incidences of endometrial and ovarian cancers, however, are significantly reduced after long-term oral contraceptive administration. It is likely that the relationship between the long-term use of these drugs and cancer will continue to be a controversial and frequently researched topic.

NURSING CONSIDERATIONS

The role of the nurse in oral contraceptive therapy involves careful monitoring of a client's condition and providing education as it relates to the prescribed drug treatment. Oral contraception is the most effective form of birth control, and many products are available to prevent pregnancy. Oral contraceptives are contraindicated for women with a history of stroke, myocardial infarction (MI), coronary artery disease, thromboembolic disorders, or estrogen-dependent tumors because of increases in estrogen levels and the risk of thrombus formation. Assess for pregnancy before initiating oral contraceptive therapy. Obtain a complete health history including personal or familial history of breast cancer, liver tumors, and hemorrhagic disorders, because these conditions are contraindications to the use of oral

TABLE 45.2	Adverse Effects of Oral Contraceptives (OC)
Adverse Effect	**Prevention**
abnormal menstrual bleeding	Breakthrough bleeding and spotting are common with the low-dose OCs. Client may need a higher dose.
amenorrhea or hypermenorrhea	These side effects are often caused by low amounts of progestins. Dose of progestin may need to be increased.
birth defects	Estrogens are pregnancy category X. Clients should be advised to discontinue OCs if pregnancy is confirmed.
cancer	Women who test positive for the human papillomavirus have a slight increased risk of cervical cancer. These clients should have regular checkups. Because estrogens promote the growth of certain types of breast cancer, clients with a history of this cancer should not take OCs.
hypertension	Risk is increased with age, dose, and length of therapy. Blood pressure should be monitored periodically and antihypertensives prescribed as needed.
increased appetite, weight gain, fatigue, depression, acne, hirsutism	These are common effects often caused by high amounts of progestins. Dose of progestin may need to be lowered.
nausea, edema, breast tenderness	These are common effects often caused by high amounts of estrogen. Dose of estrogen may need to be lowered.
thromboembolic disorders	Risk is increased in clients with certain risk factors. OCs should not be prescribed for clients with a history of thromboembolic disorders, cerebrovascular accidents, or coronary artery disease, or for those who are heavy smokers.

Pr PROTOTYPE DRUG | Ethinyl Estradiol With Norethindrone *(Ortho-Novum 1/35)* | Oral Contraceptive

ACTIONS AND USES

Ortho-Novum is typical of the monophasic oral contraceptives, containing fixed amounts of estrogen (0.035 mg) and progesterone (1 mg) for 21 days, followed by placebo tablets for 7 days. It is nearly 100% effective at preventing conception. Ortho-Novum is also available in biphasic and triphasic preparations. All preparations prevent ovulation by negative feedback control targeted at the hypothalamus and the pituitary gland. When the right combination of estrogen and progestin is present in the bloodstream, the release of FSH and LH is inhibited, thus preventing ovulation. Noncontraceptive benefits of Ortho-Novum include improvement in menstrual cycle regularity and decreased incidence of dysmenorrhea.

ADMINISTRATION ALERTS

- Tablets must be taken exactly as directed.
- If a dose is missed, take as soon as remembered, or take two tablets the next day.
- Pregnancy category X.

PHARMACOKINETICS (PO)

Onset: 1 mo

Peak: 1 mo

Half-life: 6–45 h

Duration: 1 mo

ADVERSE EFFECTS

The most common side effects of Ortho-Novum 1/35 are edema, nausea, abdominal cramps, dysmenorrhea, breast tenderness, fatigue, skin rash, acne, headache, weight gain, midcycle breakthrough bleeding, vaginal candidiasis, photosensitivity, and changes in urinary patterns. Serious cardiovascular side effects are more common in smokers, and include hypertension and thromboembolic disorders.

Contraindications: Oral contraceptives are contraindicated in women with the following conditions: current or past history of thromboembolic disorders, stroke or coronary artery disease; hepatic tumors; known or suspected carcinoma of the breast, endometrium, or other estrogen-dependent tumor; abnormal uterine bleeding; cholestatic jaundice of pregnancy or jaundice with prior oral contraceptive use; known or suspected pregnancy.

INTERACTIONS

Drug–Drug: Rifampin, some antibiotics, barbiturates, anticonvulsants, and antifungals decrease the efficacy of oral contraceptives, increasing the risk of breakthrough bleeding and the possibility of pregnancy. Ortho-Novum may decrease the effects of oral anticoagulants.

Lab Tests: Values of the following may be increased: prothrombin time, certain coagulation factors, thyroid-binding globulin, PBI, T_4, platelet aggregation, and triglycerides. Values of the following may be decreased: antithrombin III, T_3, folate, and vitamin B_{12}.

Herbal/Food: Breakthrough bleeding has been reported with concurrent use of St. John's wort.

Treatment of Overdose: There is specific treatment for overdose.

 See the Companion Website for a Nursing Process Focus specific to this drug.

---

contraceptives. Risks and adverse effects are greater for women who smoke and are older than age 35. Oral contraceptives should be used with caution in clients with hypertension, cardiac or renal disease, liver dysfunction, diabetes, gallbladder disease, and a history of depression.

Monitor blood pressure, because these medications can cause mild to moderate hypertension. Assess vital signs frequently, and monitor for symptoms of thrombophlebitis, such as pain, redness, and tenderness of the calves. Oral contraceptives can mimic certain symptoms of pregnancy, including breast tenderness, nausea, bloating, and chloasma. Reassure the client that these side effects do not indicate pregnancy. Oral contraceptives may increase the risk of certain types of breast cancer; therefore, teach clients how to perform breast self-exams and provide information on routine scheduling of mammograms appropriate for their age bracket.

Client Teaching. Client education as it relates to oral contraceptives should include the goals of therapy, the reasons for assessing baseline data such as vital signs and the existence of underlying cardiovascular disorders, and possible drug side effects. Include the following points when teaching the client about oral contraceptives:

- Take medications as directed by the healthcare provider.
- Follow instructions carefully for missed doses.
- Immediately report calf pain or redness, dyspnea, and chest pain.
- Monitor blood pressure regularly and report elevations.
- Attend a smoking cessation program if appropriate.
- Perform monthly self-examination of breasts.

HOME & COMMUNITY CONSIDERATIONS

Serious Side Effects of Hormone Therapy

Treatment with male and female hormones, although beneficial, also places the client at risk for serious side effects and complications. Emphasize to the client the importance of taking the medications as directed. Recognition of side effects such as calf tenderness, chest pain, dizziness, and abnormal bleeding is essential and must be reported immediately to the healthcare provider. Advise clients who smoke cigarettes to enter a community support group or smoking cessation program, because smoking increases the risk of complications, especially in women older than 35. Inform clients that hormone therapy for emergency contraception or termination of pregnancy may result in excessive vaginal bleeding. This occurrence must be reported to the healthcare provider. Hormone therapy may be used to treat certain malignant tumors in male and in female clients. Side effects include development of characteristics of the opposite gender such as gynecomastia in men, change in libido, and testicular atrophy, and increased facial hair and deepening of the voice in women. These changes may have devastating emotional effects on the client and family. Encourage the client to seek professional help if symptoms of depression or inability to cope occur. Family counseling may also be advised.

NURSING PROCESS FOCUS   Clients Receiving Oral Contraceptive Therapy

Assessment	Potential Nursing Diagnoses
Prior to administration: ■ Obtain a complete health history including cigarette smoking. ■ Obtain a drug history to determine possible drug interactions and allergies. ■ Assess cardiovascular status including hypertension, history of MI, cerebrovascular accident, or thromboembolic disease. ■ Determine whether client is pregnant or lactating.	■ Knowledge, Deficient, related to drug therapy ■ Nausea, related to side effects of drug ■ Noncompliance, related to medication regimen

Planning: Client Goals and Expected Outcomes

The client will:
■ Report effective birth control.
■ Demonstrate an understanding of the drug's action by accurately describing drug side effects and precautions.
■ Take medication exactly as ordered to prevent pregnancy.
■ Immediately report symptoms of thrombophlebitis, difficulty breathing, visual disturbances, or severe headache.

Implementation

Interventions and (Rationales)	Client Education/Discharge Planning
■ Monitor for the development of breast or other estrogen-dependent tumors. (Estrogen may cause tumor growth or proliferation.)	Instruct client to: ■ Immediately report if first-degree relative is diagnosed with any estrogen-dependent tumor. ■ Perform monthly self-examinations of breasts.
■ Monitor for thrombophlebitis or other thromboembolic disease. (Estrogen predisposes to thromboembolic disorders by increasing levels of clotting factors.)	■ Instruct client to immediately report pain in calves, limited movement in legs, dyspnea, sudden severe chest pain, headache, seizures, anxiety, or fear.
■ Monitor for cardiac disorders and hypertension. (These drugs increase blood levels of angiotensin and aldosterone, which increase blood pressure.)	Instruct client to: ■ Immediately report signs of possible cardiac problems such as chest pain, dyspnea, edema, tachycardia, bradycardia, and palpitations. ■ Monitor blood pressure regularly. ■ Report symptoms of hypertension such as headache, flushing, fatigue, dizziness, palpitations, tachycardia, or nosebleeds.
■ Encourage client not to smoke. (Smoking increases risk of thromboembolic disease.)	■ Instruct client to join a smoking cessation program, because the combination of oral contraceptives and smoking greatly increases risk of cardiovascular disease, especially MI, especially if client is older than 35 and smoking 15 or more cigarettes per day.
■ Monitor blood and urine glucose levels. (These drugs increase serum glucose levels.)	Instruct client to: ■ Monitor urine and blood glucose regularly. ■ Contact the healthcare provider if hyperglycemia or hypoglycemia occurs.
■ Monitor client's knowledge level of proper administration. (Incorrect use may lead to pregnancy.)	Instruct client to: ■ Discontinue medication and notify the healthcare provider if significant bleeding occurs at midcycle. ■ Take a missed dose as soon as remembered, or take two tablets the next day. If three consecutive tablets are missed, begin a new compact of tablets, starting 7 days after last tablet was taken. ■ Contact the healthcare provider if two consecutive periods are missed, because pregnancy may have occurred.
■ Encourage compliance with follow-up treatment. (Follow-up is necessary to avoid serious adverse effects.)	Instruct client to: ■ Schedule annual Pap smears. ■ Perform monthly self-breast exams and obtain routine mammograms as recommended by the healthcare provider.

(Continued)

NURSING PROCESS FOCUS Clients Receiving Oral Contraceptive Therapy *(Continued)*

Evaluation of Outcome Criteria

Evaluate the effectiveness of drug therapy by confirming that client goals and expected outcomes have been met (see "Planning").

- The client experiences effective birth control.
- The client demonstrates an understanding of the drug's actions by accurately describing drug side effects and precautions.
- The client demonstrates accurate administration of the drug.
- The client accurately states signs and symptoms to be reported to the healthcare provider.

∞ *See Table 45.1 for a list of drugs to which these nursing actions apply.*

EMERGENCY CONTRACEPTION AND PHARMACOLOGICAL ABORTION

Emergency contraception is the *prevention* of implantation of a fertilized ovum following unprotected intercourse. Pharmacological abortion is the *removal* of an embryo by the use of drugs after implantation has occurred. The treatment goal is to provide effective, immediate prevention or safe termination of pregnancy. Agents used for these purposes are listed in Table 45.3.

45.4 Drugs for Emergency Contraception and Termination of Early Pregnancy

Statistics suggest that more than half the pregnancies in the United States are unplanned. Some of these occur because of the inconsistent use or failure of contraceptive devices; even oral contraceptives have a failure rate of 0.3% to 1%. Emergency contraception following unprotected intercourse offers a means of protecting against unwanted pregnancies. The goal is to prevent implantation of a fertilized ovum.

Emergency contraception can be accomplished by the administration of various doses and combinations of estrogens and progestins. These agents should be administered as soon as possible after unprotected intercourse; if taken more than 72 hours later, they become less effective. By 7 days after intercourse, they are totally ineffective. When used accordingly, these drugs act by preventing ovulation or implantation; they do not induce abortion. Following are the two regimens approved by the FDA.

- Plan B: This regimen involves taking 0.75 mg of levonorgestrel in two doses, 12 hours apart. Recently, the FDA approved Plan B for over-the-counter (OTC) status, making it available to more women. Side effects are rare.

- Preven: A combination of ethinyl estradiol and levonorgestrel, Preven is effective, although nausea and

TABLE 45.3	**Agents for Emergency Contraception and Pharmacological Abortion**	
Drug	**Route and Adult Dose (max dose where indicated)**	**Adverse Effects**
AGENTS FOR EMERGENCY CONTRACEPTION		
ethinyl estradiol and levonorgestrel (Preven)	PO; 1 tablet (0.25 mg levonorgestrel and 0.05 mg ethinyl estradiol) taken within 72 h of unprotected intercourse, followed by two pills 12 h later	*Side effects are rare when only two doses are administered.*
levonorgestrel (Plan B)	PO; 2 tablets within 72 h of unprotected intercourse, followed by 2 tablets 12 h later (0.75 mg in each pill)	
AGENTS FOR PHARMACOLOGICAL ABORTION		
carboprost tromethamine (Hemabate)	IM; initial: 250 mcg (1 ml) repeated at $^1/_2$–3 $^1/_2$-h intervals if indicated by uterine response. Dosage may be increased to 500 mcg (2 ml) if uterine contractility is inadequate after several doses of 250 mcg (1 ml), not to exceed total dose of 12 mg or continuous administration for 1 mo	*Nausea, vomiting, diarrhea, fever* Serious adverse effects are uncommon
dinoprostone (Cervidil, Prepidil, Prostin E₂)	Intravaginal; insert suppository high in vagina, repeat q2–5h until abortion occurs or membranes rupture (max: total dose 240 mg)	*Nausea, vomiting, diarrhea, fever, headache* Uterine spasms, laceration, or hemorrhage
methotrexate with misoprostol	IM; methotrexate (50 mg/m²) followed 5 days later by intravaginal 800 mcg of misoprostol	*Nausea, vomiting, diarrhea, abdominal pain, headache* Uterine hemorrhage
mifepristone (Mifeprex) with misoprostol	PO; Day 1: 600 mg of mifepristone; Day 3 (if abortion has not occurred): 400 mcg of misoprostol	*Nausea, vomiting, diarrhea, abdominal pain, headache* Uterine hemorrhage

Italics indicate common adverse effects; <u>underlining</u> indicates serious adverse effects.

vomiting are common. An antiemetic drug may be indicated to reduce these unpleasant side effects. Preven is administered as two doses, 12 hours apart.

Once the ovum has been fertilized, several pharmacological choices are available for terminating the pregnancy. A single dose of mifepristone (Mifeprex, RU486) followed 36 to 48 hours later by a single dose of misoprostol (Cytotec) is a frequently used regimen. Mifepristone is a synthetic steroid that blocks progesterone receptors in the uterus. If given within 3 days of intercourse, mifepristone alone is almost 100% effective at *preventing* pregnancy. Given up to 9 weeks after conception, mifepristone aborts the implanted embryo. Misoprostol is a prostaglandin that causes uterine contractions, thus increasing the effectiveness of the pharmacological abortion.

Although mifepristone–misoprostol should never be substituted for effective means of contraception such as abstinence or oral contraceptives, these medications do offer women a safer alternative to surgical abortion. The primary adverse effect is cramping that occurs soon after taking misoprostol. The most serious adverse effect is uterine bleeding, which may continue for 1 to 2 weeks after dosing.

A few other agents may be used to induce pharmacological abortion. Methotrexate, an antineoplastic agent, combined with intravaginal misoprostol, usually induces abortion within 24 hours. The prostaglandins carboprost and dinoprostone induce strong uterine contractions that can expel an implanted embryo up to the second trimester.

MENOPAUSE

Menopause is characterized by a progressive decrease in estrogen secretion by the ovaries, resulting in the permanent cessation of menses. Menopause is neither a disease nor a disorder but is a natural consequence of aging that is often accompanied by a number of unpleasant symptoms, some of which respond well to pharmacotherapy.

45.5 Hormone Replacement Therapy

Over the past 20 years, healthcare providers have commonly prescribed **hormone replacement therapy (HRT)** to treat unpleasant symptoms of menopause and to prevent the long-term consequences of estrogen loss listed in Table 45.4. In 2001, more than 66 million prescriptions for Premarin and Prempro were filled, and sales of the two drugs exceeded $2 billion. All this changed, however, in 2002 when the results of a large clinical study, the Women's Health Initiative (WHI) were analyzed.

Data from the WHI research suggest that clients taking combination therapy with estrogen and progestin (Prempro) experienced a small, though significant, increased risk of serious adverse effects such as coronary artery disease, stroke, breast cancer, dementia, and venous thromboembolism. Women taking estrogen alone (Premarin) experienced a slightly increased risk of stroke, but no increased risk of breast cancer or heart disease. The risks were higher in women older than age 60; women aged 50 to 59 actually experienced a slight *decrease* in cardiovascular side effects. The potential adverse effects documented in the WHI study, and others, were significant enough to suggest that the potential benefits of long-term HRT may not outweigh the risks for many women. However, the results of this study remain controversial.

Although there is consensus that HRT does offer relief from the immediate, distressing menopausal symptoms, it is now recommended that women *not* undergo HRT to prevent coronary heart disease. In addition, although HRT appears to prevent osteoporotic bone fractures, women are now encouraged to discuss alternatives with their healthcare provider, as discussed in Chapter 47 ∞. Undoubtedly, research will continue to provide valuable information on the long-term effects of HRT. Until then, the choice of HRT to treat menopausal symptoms remains a highly individualized one, between the client and her healthcare provider.

TABLE 45.4	Potential Consequences of Estrogen Loss Related to Menopause
Stage	**Symptoms/Conditions**
Early Menopause	mood disturbances, depression, irritability
	insomnia
	hot flashes
	irregular menstrual cycles
	headaches
Midmenopause	vaginal atrophy, increased infections, painful intercourse
	skin atrophy
	stress urinary incontinence
	sexual disinterest
Postmenopause	cardiovascular disease
	osteoporosis
	Alzheimer's-like dementia
	colon cancer

If used to treat symptoms of menopause, estrogens are prescribed for the shortest time possible and at the lowest possible dose.

In addition to their use in treating menopausal symptoms, estrogens are used for female hypogonadism, primary ovarian failure, and as replacement therapy following surgical removal of the ovaries, usually combined with a progestin. The purpose of the progestin is to counteract some of the adverse effects of estrogen on the uterus. When used alone, estrogen increases the risk of uterine cancer. Estrogen without progestin is considered appropriate only for clients who have had a hysterectomy.

High doses of estrogens are used to treat prostate and breast cancer. Prostate cancer is usually dependent on androgens for growth; administration of estrogens suppresses androgen secretion. As an antineoplastic hormone, estrogen is rarely used alone. It is one of many agents used in combination for the chemotherapy of cancer, as discussed in Chapter 35 ∞.

NATURAL THERAPIES

Black Cohosh for Menopause

Black cohosh (*Actaea racemosa*) is a perennial that grows in the eastern United States and parts of Canada. Use of the herb has been recorded by Native Americans for more than 100 years. It is used as a hormone balancer in perimenopausal women. Black cohosh has been shown to be effective in the management of menopausal hot flashes (Osmers, et al., 2005). Black cohosh may even help prevent osteoporosis in postmenopausal women. Doses of black cohosh are sometimes standardized by the amount of the chemical 27-deoxyactein, which is an active ingredient. A typical dose of black cohosh ranges from 40 to 80 mg of dried herb per day. (Approximately 1 mg of 27-deoxyactein is present in each 20-mg tablet or in 20 drops of the liquid formulation.)

Although black cohosh was once thought to have phytoestrogenic effects, new research questions its estrogenic effects. So its actual mechanism of action is still unknown. Adverse effects include hypotension, uterine stimulation, and GI complaints such as nausea. Black cohosh can increase the action of antihypertensives, so concurrent use should be avoided.

Pr PROTOTYPE DRUG | Estrogen/Progestin Conjugated Estrogens *(Premarin)* and Conjugated Estrogens with Medroxyprogesterone *(Prempro)* | Hormone Replacement Therapy

ACTIONS AND USES

Premarin contains a mixture of different estrogens. It exerts several positive metabolic effects, including an increase in bone density and a reduction in LDL cholesterol. It may also lower the risk of coronary artery disease and colon cancer in some clients. When used as postmenopausal replacement therapy, estrogen is typically combined with a progestin, as in Prempro. Conjugated estrogens may be administered by the IM or IV route for abnormal uterine bleeding due to hormonal imbalance.

ADMINISTRATION ALERTS

- Use a calibrated dosage applicator for administration of vaginal cream.
- For IM or IV administration of conjugated estrogens, reconstitute by first removing approximately 5 ml of air from the dry-powder vial, then slowly inject the diluent into the vial, aiming it at the side of the vial. Gently agitate to dissolve; do not shake.
- Administer IV push slowly, at a rate of 5 mg/min.
- Both are pregnancy category X.

PHARMACOKINETICS (PO)

Onset: Unknown

Peak: Unknown

Half-life: 4–18

Duration: Unkown

ADVERSE EFFECTS

Adverse effects of Prempro or Premarin include nausea, fluid retention, edema, breast tenderness, abdominal cramps and bloating, acute pancreatitis, appetite changes, acne, mental depression, decreased libido, headache, fatigue, nervousness, and weight gain. Effects are dose dependent. Estrogens, when used alone, have been associated with a higher risk of uterine cancer. Although adding a progestin may exert a protective effect by lowering the risk of uterine cancer, recent studies suggest the progestin may increase the risk of breast cancer following long-term use. The risks of adverse effects increase in clients over age 35.

Contraindications: Conjugated estrogens are contraindicated in pregnant clients and in women with known or suspected carcinoma of the breast or other estrogen-dependent tumor. Caution should be used when treating clients with a history of thromboembolic disease, hepatic impairment, or abnormal uterine bleeding.

INTERACTIONS

Drug–Drug: Drug interactions include a decreased effect of tamoxifen, enhanced corticosteroid effects, decreased effects of anticoagulants, especially warfarin. The effects of estrogen may be decreased if taken with barbiturates or rifampin, and there is a possible increased effect of tricyclic antidepressants if taken with estrogens.

Lab Tests: Values of the following may be increased: prothrombin time, certain coagulation factors, thyroid-binding globulin, PBI, T_4, platelet aggregation, and triglycerides. values of the following may be decreased: antithrombin III, T_3, folate, and vitamin B_{12}.

Herbal/Food: Red clover and black cohosh may interfere with estrogen therapy. Effects of estrogen may be enhanced if combined with ginseng.

Treatment of Overdose: There is no specific treatment for overdose.

 See the Companion Website for a Nursing Process Focus specific to this drug.

NURSING PROCESS FOCUS Clients Receiving Hormone Replacement Therapy

Assessment	Potential Nursing Diagnoses
Prior to administration: ■ Obtain a complete health history including personal or familial history of breast cancer, gallbladder disease, diabetes mellitus, liver or kidney disease. ■ Obtain a drug history to determine possible drug interactions and allergies. ■ Assess cardiovascular status including hypertension, history of MI, cerebrovascular accident, or thromboembolic disease. ■ Determine whether client is pregnant or lactating.	■ Fluid Volume, excess, related to edema secondary to side effect of drug ■ Tissue Perfusion, impaired, related to development of thrombophlebitis, pulmonary or cerebral embolism

Planning: Client Goals and Expected Outcomes

The client will:
■ Report relief from symptoms of menopause.
■ Demonstrate an understanding of the drug's action by accurately describing drug side effects and precautions.
■ Immediately report symptoms of thrombophlebitis, difficulty breathing, visual disturbances, severe headache, and seizure activity.

Implementation

Interventions and (Rationales)	Client Education/Discharge Planning
■ Monitor for thromboembolic disease. (Estrogen increases risk for thromboembolism.)	Instruct client to: ■ Report shortness of breath, feeling of heaviness, chest pain, severe headache, warmth or swelling in affected part, usually the legs or pelvis.
■ Monitor for abnormal uterine bleeding. (If undiagnosed tumor is present, these drugs can increase its size and cause uterine bleeding.)	■ Instruct client to report excessive uterine bleeding or that which occurs between menstruations.
■ Monitor breast health. (Estrogens promote the growth of certain breast cancers.)	■ Instruct client to have regular breast exams, perform monthly breast self-examinations, obtain routine mammograms as recommended by the healthcare and provider.
■ Monitor for vision changes. (These drugs may worsen myopia or astigmatism and cause intolerance of contact lenses.)	Instruct client to: ■ Obtain regular eye exams during HRT. ■ Report changes in vision. ■ Report any difficulty in wearing contact lenses.
■ Encourage client not to smoke. (Smoking increases risk of cardiovascular disease.)	■ Instruct client to avoid smoking and participate in smoking cessation programs, if necessary.
■ Encourage client to avoid caffeine. (Estrogens and caffeine may lead to increased CNS stimulation.)	Instruct client to: ■ Restrict caffeine consumption. ■ Recognize common foods that contain caffeine such as coffee, tea, carbonated beverages, chocolate, and certain OTC medications. ■ Report unusual nervousness, anxiety, or insomnia.
■ Monitor glucose levels. (Estrogens may increase blood glucose levels.)	Instruct client to: ■ Monitor blood and urine glucose frequently if diabetic. ■ Report any consistent changes in blood glucose.
■ Monitor for seizure activity. (Estrogen-induced fluid retention may increase risk of seizures.)	■ Instruct client to be alert for possibility of seizures, even at night, and report any seizure-type symptoms.
■ Monitor client's understanding and proper self-administration. (Improper administration may increase incidence of adverse effects.)	Instruct client to: ■ Administer proper dose and form of medication at proper intervals. ■ Take with food to decrease GI irritation. ■ Take daily dose in the evening to decrease occurrence of side effects. ■ Document any changes in the frequency or pattern of menstrual periods.

(Continued)

NURSING PROCESS FOCUS Clients Receiving Hormone Replacement Therapy *(Continued)*

Evaluation of Outcome Criteria

Evaluate the effectiveness of drug therapy by confirming that client goals and expected outcomes have been met (see "Planning").

- The client verbalizes relief of unpleasant symptoms of menopause.
- The client demonstrates an understanding of the drug's actions by accurately describing drug side effects and precautions.
- The client accurately states signs and symptoms to be reported to the healthcare provider.

∞ *See Table 45.4, under the heading "Estrogens," for a list of drugs to which these nursing actions apply.*

NURSING CONSIDERATIONS

For the use of estrogen-containing products such as oral contraceptives, refer to "Nursing Process Focus: Clients Receiving Oral Contraceptive Therapy" on page 703.

The role of the nurse in HRT involves careful monitoring of a client's condition and providing education as it relates to the prescribed drug treatment. Conjugated estrogens are contraindicated for use in breast cancer (except in clients being treated for metastatic disease) and any suspected estrogen-dependent cancer. These conditions put the client at a higher risk for developing cancer. Assess for pregnancy; conjugated estrogen is contraindicated in pregnancy or for use in women who intend to become pregnant in the immediate future, because it can cause fetal harm. Assess for a history of thromboembolic disease because of potential side effects of the drug. Obtain a complete health history including family history of breast or genital cancer. Cautious use of estrogen therapy must be exercised in a client whose first-degree relative has a history of breast or genital cancer. Estrogen monotherapy places the woman at higher risk for cancer of the female reproductive organs. Obtain a history of CAD, hypertension, cerebrovascular disease, fibrocystic breast disease, breast nodules, or abnormal mammograms.

Because of the risk of thromboembolism, monitor the client closely for signs and symptoms of thrombus or embolus, such as pain in calves, limited movement in legs, dyspnea, sudden severe chest pain, or anxiety. Encourage the client to report signs of depression, decreased libido, headache, fatigue, and weight gain. Because controversy surrounds the long-term use of these drugs as HRT, it is imperative for women to be aware of current research and discuss treatment alternatives with their healthcare provider before beginning pharmacotherapy.

When using these drugs to treat male clients, inform them that secondary female characteristics, such as higher voice, sparse body hair, and increased breast size may develop. Inform the client that impotence may also occur.

Client Teaching. Client education as it relates to HRT should include the goals of therapy, the reasons for obtaining baseline data such as vital signs and the existence of underlying cardiovascular disorders, and possible drug side effects. Include the following points when teaching clients about hormone replacement therapy:

- Immediately report calf tenderness, chest pain, or dyspnea.
- Take with food if GI upset occurs.

- Schedule an annual PAP smear and breast examinations.
- Perform monthly self-examinations of breasts.
- Do not take other prescribed drugs, OTC medications, herbal remedies, or dietary supplements without notifying your healthcare provider.

UTERINE ABNORMALITIES

Dysfunctional uterine bleeding is a condition in which hemorrhage occurs on a noncyclic basis or in abnormal amounts. It is the health problem most frequently reported by women and a common reason for hysterectomy. Progestins are the drugs of choice for treating uterine abnormalities.

45.6 Pharmacotherapy With Progestins

Secreted by the corpus luteum, endogenous progesterone prepares the uterus for implantation of the embryo and pregnancy. If implantation does not occur, levels of progesterone fall dramatically and menses begins. If pregnancy occurs, the ovary continues to secrete progesterone to maintain a healthy endometrium until the placenta develops sufficiently to begin producing the hormone. Whereas the function of estrogen is to cause proliferation of the endometrium, progesterone limits and stabilizes endometrial growth.

SPECIAL CONSIDERATIONS

Estrogen Use and Psychosocial Issues

Because undesirable side effects may occur with estrogen use, the nurse should communicate these prior to implementing drug therapy. The nurse can explore the client's reaction to these potential risks. An assessment of the client's emotional support system should also be made before initiating drug therapy. Hirsutism, loss of hair, or a deepening of the voice can occur in the female client. The male client may develop secondary female characteristics such as a higher voice, lack of body hair, and increased breast size. Impotence may also develop and is typically viewed as a concern by most men.

Clients should be taught that these adverse effects are reversible and may subside with adjustment of dosage or discontinuation of estrogen therapy. This knowledge may allow both male and female clients to remain compliant when adverse effects occur. During therapy, clients may need emotional support to assist in dealing with these body image issues. The nurse can encourage this support, discuss these issues with family members, and refer clients for counseling. For the female client, the nurse can refer to an aesthetician for hair removal or wig fitting. The male client and his sexual partner may need a referral to deal with issues surrounding impotence and its effect on their relationship.

TABLE 45.5	Selected Estrogens and Progestins	
Drug	**Route and Adult Dose (max dose where indicated)**	**Adverse Effects**
ESTROGENS		
estradiol (Estraderm, Estrace)	PO; 1–2 mg/day	*Breakthrough bleeding, spotting, breast tenderness, libido changes*
estradiol cypionate (Dep-Gynogen, Depogen)	IM; 1–5 mg q3–4wk	
estradiol valerate (Delestrogen, Duragen-10, Valergen)	IM; 10–20 mg q4wk	<u>Hypertension, gallbladder disease, thromboembolic disorders, increased cancer risk</u>
estrogen, conjugated (Premarin)	PO; 0.3–1.25 mg/day for 21 days each month	
estropipate (Ogen)	PO; 0.75–6 mg/day for 21 days each month	
ethinyl estradiol (Estinyl, Feminone)	PO; 0.02–0.05 mg/day for 21 days each month	
PROGESTINS		
medroxyprogesterone (Provera, Cycrin)	PO; 5–10 mg/day on Days 1–12 of menstrual cycle Subcutaneous; (Depo-SubQ Provera 104) one injection every 3 months	*Breakthrough bleeding, spotting, breast tenderness, weight gain*
norethindrone (Micronor, Nor-Q.D.)	PO; 0.35 mg/day beginning on Day 1 of menstrual cycle	<u>Amenorrhea, dysmenorrhea, depression thromboembolic disorders</u>
norethindrone acetate (Norlutate)	PO; 5 mg/day for 2 wk, then increase by 2.5 mg/day q2wk (max: 15 mg/day)	
progesterone micronized (Prometrium)	PO; 400 mg at nighttime for 10 days	
ESTROGEN–PROGESTIN COMBINATIONS		
conjugated estrogens, equine/ medroxyprogesterone acetate (Prempro)	PO; 0.625 mg/day continuously or in 25-day cycles	*Breakthrough bleeding, spotting, breast tenderness, weight gain*
estradiol/drospirenone (Angeliq)	PO; 1 tablet daily (fixed-dose 1 mg estradiol/0.5 mg drospirenone)	<u>Amenorrhea, dysmenorrhea, depression, thromboembolic disorders, hypertension</u>
estradiol/norgestimate (Ortho-Prefest)	PO; 1 tablet of 1 mg estradiol for 3 days, followed by 1 tablet of 1 mg estradiol combined with 0.09 mg norgestimate for 3 days. Regimen is repeated continuously without interruption.	
ethinyl estradiol/norethindrone acetate (Femhrt)	PO; 1 tablet daily (2.5 mcg/0.5 mg or 5 mcg/1.0 mg fixed-dose ethinyl estradiol/norethindrone)	

Italics indicate common adverse effects; <u>underlining</u> indicates serious adverse effects.

Dysfunctional uterine bleeding can have a number of causes, including spontaneous abortion, pelvic neoplasms, thyroid disorders, pregnancy, and infection. Types of dysfunctional uterine bleeding include the following conditions:

- Amenorrhea—absence of menstruation
- Oligomenorrhea—infrequent menstruation
- Menorrhagia—prolonged or excessive menstruation
- Breakthrough bleeding—hemorrhage between menstrual periods
- Postmenopausal bleeding—hemorrhage following menopause

Dysfunctional uterine bleeding is often caused by a hormonal imbalance between estrogen and progesterone. Although estrogen increases the thickness of the endometrium, bleeding occurs sporadically unless balanced by an adequate amount of progesterone. Administration of a progestin in a pattern starting 5 days after the onset of menses and continuing for the next 20 days can sometimes reestablish a normal, monthly cyclic pattern. Oral contraceptives may also be prescribed for this disorder.

In cases of heavy bleeding, high doses of conjugated estrogens may be administered for 3 weeks prior to adding medroxyprogesterone for the last 10 days of therapy. Treatment with nonsteroidal anti-inflammatory drugs (NSAIDs) sometimes helps to reduce bleeding and ease painful menstrual flow. If aggressive hormonal therapy fails to stop the heavy bleeding, dilation and curettage (D & C) may be necessary.

Progestins are occasionally prescribed for the treatment of metastatic endometrial carcinoma. In these cases, they are used for palliation, usually in combination with other antineoplastics. Selected progestins and their dosages are listed in Table 45.5.

NURSING CONSIDERATIONS

The role of the nurse in progestin therapy involves careful monitoring of a client's condition and providing education as it relates to the prescribed drug treatment. Obtain baseline data including blood pressure, weight, and pulse. Obtain results of laboratory tests including complete blood count (CBC), liver function, serum glucose, and electrolyte profile. Obtain a thorough health history including a close

Pr PROTOTYPE DRUG | Medroxyprogesterone Acetate *(Provera)* | Progestin

ACTIONS AND USES

Medroxyprogesterone is a synthetic progestin with a prolonged duration of action. As with its natural counterpart, the primary target tissue for medroxyprogesterone is the endometrium of the uterus. It inhibits the effect of estrogen on the uterus, thus restoring normal hormonal balance. Applications include dysfunctional uterine bleeding, secondary amenorrhea, and contraception. Medroxyprogesterone may also be given IM for the palliation of metastatic uterine or renal carcinoma.

ADMINISTRATION ALERTS

- Give PO with meals to avoid gastric distress.
- Observe IM sites for abscess: presence of lump and discoloration of tissue.
- Pregnancy category X.

PHARMACOKINETICS (PO)

Onset: Unknown

Peak: 2–4 h

Half-life: 30 days

Duration: Unknown

ADVERSE EFFECTS

The most common side effects are breakthrough bleeding and breast tenderness. Weight gain, depression, hypertension, nausea, vomiting, dysmenorrhea, and vaginal candidiasis may also occur. The most serious side effect is an increased risk for thromboembolic disease.

Contraindications: Medroxyprogesterone is contraindicated during pregnancy and in women with known or suspected carcinoma of the breast. Caution should be used when treating clients with a history of thromboembolic disease, hepatic impairment, or undiagnosed vaginal bleeding.

INTERACTIONS

Drug–Drug: Serum levels of medroxyprogesterone are decreased by aminoglutethimide, barbiturates, primidone, rifampin, rifabutin, and topiramate.

Lab Tests: May increase values for alkaline phosphatase, glucose tolerance test (GTT), and HDL.

Herbal/Food: St. John's wort may decrease the effectiveness of medroxyprogesterone and cause abnormal menstrual bleeding.

Treatment of Overdose: There is no specific treatment for overdose.

 See the Companion Website for a Nursing Process Focus specific to this drug.

---

family history of breast or genital malignancies, thromboembolic disorders, impaired liver function, and undiagnosed vaginal bleeding. Assess the client for pregnancy or lactation. Clients with allergies to peanuts should avoid the use of Prometrium, because the oral capsules contain peanut oil. Encourage the client to report a history of depression, anemia, diabetes, asthma, seizure disorders, cardiac or kidney disorders, migraine headaches, previous ectopic pregnancies, sexually transmitted infections, unresolved abnormal Pap smears, or previous pelvic surgeries.

Monitor the client for side effects of progestins. Susceptible clients may experience acute intermittent porphyria as a reaction to progesterone. Assess for severe, colicky abdominal pain, vomiting, abdominal distention, diarrhea, and constipation. Common side effects of progesterone include breakthrough bleeding, nausea, abdominal cramps, dizziness, edema, and weight gain. Monitor for amenorrhea; sudden, severe headache; and signs of pulmonary embolism such as sudden severe chest pain and dyspnea; and report such symptoms to the healthcare provider immediately. Progesterone can cause photosensitivity and phototoxicity; monitor for pruritus, sensitivity to light, acne, rash, and alopecia. Phototoxic reactions cause serious sunburn within 5 to 18 hours after sun exposure.

Client Teaching. Client education as it relates to progestins should include goals of therapy, the reasons for obtaining baseline data such as vital signs and the existence of underlying cardiovascular disorders, and possible drug side effects. Include the following points when teaching clients about progestin therapy:

- Monitor blood pressure and vital signs regularly.

- Report severe chest pain, severe headache, or changes in the amount or timing of menstrual flow.
- Avoid prolonged exposure to sunlight; use sunscreen or wear protective clothing when outside.

LABOR AND BREAST-FEEDING

Several agents are used to manage uterine contractions and to stimulate lactation.

OXYTOCICS AND TOCOLYTICS

Oxytocics are agents that *stimulate* uterine contractions to promote the induction of labor. **Tocolytics,** are used to *inhibit* uterine contractions during premature labor. These agents are listed in Table 45.6.

45.7 Pharmacological Management of Uterine Contractions

The most widely used oxytocic is the natural hormone *oxytocin,* which is secreted by the posterior portion of the pituitary gland. The target organs for oxytocin are the uterus and the breast. As the growing fetus distends the uterus, oxytocin is secreted in increasingly larger amounts. The rising blood levels of oxytocin provide a steadily increasing stimulus to the uterus to contract, thus promoting labor and the delivery of the baby and the placenta. As pregnancy progresses, the number of oxytocin receptors in the uterus increases, making it even more sensitive to the effects of the hormone.

TABLE 45.6 Uterine Stimulants and Relaxants

Drug	Route and Adult Dose (max dose where indicated)	Adverse Effects
STIMULANTS (OXYTOCICS)		
oxytocin (Pitocin, Syntocinon)	IV (antepartum); 1 milliunit/min starting dose to a maximum of 20 milliunits/min IV (postpartum); 10 units infused at a rate of 20–40 milliunits/min Nasal; 1 spray or drop 2–3 min before breast-feeding	*Nausea, vomiting, maternal dysrhythmias* Fetal bradycardia, uterine rupture, fetal intracranial hemorrhage, water intoxication, fetal brain hemorrhage
STIMULANTS (OXYTOCICS): Ergot Alkaloids		
ergonovine maleate (Ergotrate)	PO; 1 tablet (0.2 mg) tid–qid after childbirth for a maximum of 1 wk IM/IV; 0.2 mg q2–4h (max: 5 doses)	*Nausea, vomiting, uterine cramping* Shock, severe hypertension, dysrhythmias
methylergonovine maleate (Methergine)	PO; 0.2–0.4 mg bid–qid IM/IV; 0.2–0.4 mg q2–4h (max: 5 doses)	
STIMULANTS (OXYTOCICS): Prostaglandins		
carboprost tromethamine (Hemabate)	IM; initial; 250 mcg (1 ml) repeated at 1 1/2–3 1/2-h intervals if indicated by uterine response	*Nausea, vomiting, diarrhea, headache, chills, uterine cramping*
dinoprostone (Cervidil, Prepidil, Prostin E₂)	Intravaginal; 10 mg	Uterine lacerations or perforation due to intense contractions
misoprostol (Cytotec)	PO; 400 mcg as a single dose	
RELAXANTS (TOCOLYTICS): Beta₂-adrenergic Agonists		
ritodrine hydrochloride (Yutopar)	IV; 50–100 mcg/min starting dose, increased by 50 mcg/min q10min	*Nervousness, tremor, drowsiness*
terbutaline sulfate (Brethine)	PO; 2.5 mg 84–6h	Bronchoconstriction, dysrhythmias, altered maternal and fetal heart rate
RELAXANTS (TOCOLYTICS): Other		
magnesium sulfate (see page 652 for the Prototype Drug box ∞)	IV; 1–4 g in 5% dextrose by slow infusion	*Flushing, sweating, muscle weakness* Complete heart block, circulatory collapse, respiratory paralysis
nifedipine (Procardia) (see page 314 for the Prototype Drug box ∞)	PO; 10 mg as a single dose	*Adverse effects are rare with a single dose.*

Italics indicate common adverse effects; underlining indicates serious adverse effects.

Parenteral oxytocin (Pitocin) may be given to initiate and promote labor contractions. Doses in an IV infusion are increased gradually, every 15 to 60 minutes, until a normal labor pattern is established. After delivery, an IV infusion of oxytocin may be given to control postpartum uterine bleeding by temporarily impeding blood flow to this organ.

In postpartum women, oxytocin is released in response to suckling, which causes milk to be *ejected* (let down) from the mammary glands. Oxytocin does not increase the *volume* of milk production. This function is provided by the pituitary hormone *prolactin,* which increases the synthesis of milk. The actions of oxytocin during breast-feeding are illustrated in Figure 45.4. When given for milk letdown, oxytocin (Pitocin) is given intranasally several minutes before breast-feeding or pumping is anticipated.

Several prostaglandins are also used as uterine stimulants. Unlike most hormones, which travel through the blood to affect distant tissues, **prostaglandins** are local hormones that act directly at the site where they are secreted. Although the body makes dozens of different prostaglandins, only a few have clinical utility. Dinoprostone (Cervidil),

prostaglandin E₂, is used to initiate labor, to prepare the cervix for labor, or to expel a fetus that has died. Mifepristone (Mifeprex, RU486), a synthetic analog of prostaglandin E₁, is used for emergency contraception and for pharmacological abortion, as described in Section 45.4. Carboprost (Hemabate), is a salt of prostaglandin F₂ alpha that can induce pharmacological abortion and may be used to control postpartum bleeding.

Some women enter labor before the baby has reached a normal stage of development. Premature birth is a leading cause of infant death. Tocolytics are uterine relaxants prescribed to inhibit the uterine contractions experienced during premature labor. Suppressing labor allows additional time for the fetus to develop and may permit the pregnancy to reach normal term. Typically, the mother is given a monitor with a sensor that records uterine contractions, and this information is used to determine the doses and timing of tocolytic medications.

Two beta₂-adrenergic agonists are used as tocolytics. Ritodrine (Yutopar) may be given by the oral or IV route to suppress labor contractions. It is more effective when

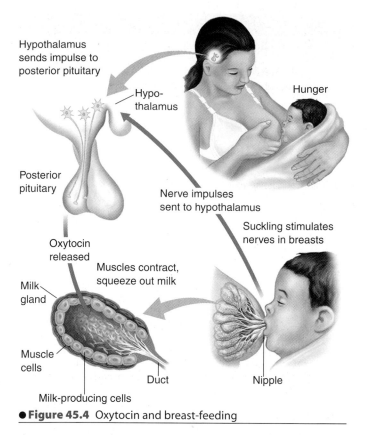

Hypothalamus sends impulse to posterior pituitary

Hypo-thalamus

Hunger

Posterior pituitary

Nerve impulses sent to hypothalamus

Oxytocin released

Suckling stimulates nerves in breasts

Muscles contract, squeeze out milk

Milk gland

Muscle cells

Duct

Nipple

Milk-producing cells

● **Figure 45.4** Oxytocin and breast-feeding

administered before labor intensifies, and normally results in only a 1- to 2-day prolongation of pregnancy. Terbutaline is another beta$_2$-agonist that may be used for uterine relaxation, though it is not approved for this purpose in the United States. The benefits of tocolytics must be carefully weighed against their potential adverse effects, which include tachycardia in both the mother and the fetus.

NURSING CONSIDERATIONS

The role of the nurse in uterine stimulant therapy involves careful monitoring of both the mother's and child's conditions and providing education as it relates to the prescribed drug treatment. Evaluate the client for fetal presentation, especially for the presence of cephalopelvic disproportion.

For oxytocin to be administered safely, the fetus must be viable, and vaginal delivery must be possible. Assess the progression of labor. Assess the client for a history of invasive cervical cancer, active herpes genitalis, or cord prolapse. Obtain a complete health history including gynecological and obstetrics history. Oxytocin is contraindicated in clients with a history of previous uterine or cervical surgery including cesarean section. This drug is not used if the client is a grand multipara, is older than

---

Pr PROTOTYPE DRUG | Oxytocin *(Pitocin, Syntocinon)* | Oxytocic

ACTIONS AND USES

Oxytocin is a natural hormone secreted by the posterior pituitary that is a drug of choice for inducing labor. Oxytocin is given by several different routes depending on its intended action. Given antepartum by IV infusion, oxytocin induces labor by increasing the frequency and force of uterine contractions. It is timed to the final stage of pregnancy, after the cervix has dilated, membranes have ruptured, and presentation of the fetus has occurred. Oxytocin may also be administered postpartum to reduce hemorrhage after expulsion of the placenta, and to aid in returning normal muscular tone to the uterus. A second route of administration is intranasally to promote the ejection of milk from the mammary glands. Milk letdown occurs within minutes after spray or drops are applied to the nostril during breast-feeding.

ADMINISTRATION ALERTS

- Dilute 10 units oxytocin in 1,000 ml IV fluid prior to administration. For postpartum administration, may add up to 40 units in 1,000 ml IV fluid.
- Incidence of allergic reactions is higher when given IM or by IV injection, rather than IV infusion.
- Pregnancy category X.

PHARMACOKINETICS

Onset: 1–3 min nasal; immediate IV

Peak: Unknown

Half-life: 3–5 min

Duration: 20 min nasal; 1 h IV

ADVERSE EFFECTS

When oxytocin is given IV, vital signs of the fetus and mother are monitored continuously to avoid complications in the fetus, such as dysrhythmias or intracranial hemorrhage. Serious complications in the mother may include uterine rupture, seizures, or coma. Risk of uterine rupture increases in women who have delivered five or more children. Though experience has shown the use of oxytocin to be quite safe, labor should be induced by this drug only when there are demonstrated risks to the mother or fetus in continuing the pregnancy.

Contraindications: Antepartum use is contraindicated in the following: significant cephalopelvic disproportion; unfavorable fetal positions that are undeliverable without conversion before delivery; obstetrical emergencies in which the benefit-to-risk ratio for the fetus or mother favors surgical intervention; fetal distress when delivery is not imminent; when adequate uterine activity fails to achieve satisfactory progress; when the uterus is already hyperactive or hypertonic; when vaginal delivery is contraindicated, such as invasive cervical carcinoma, active genital herpes, total placenta previa, vasa previa, and cord presentation or prolapse of the cord.

INTERACTIONS

Drug–Drug: Vasoconstrictors used concurrently with oxytocin may cause severe hypertension.

Lab Tests: Unknown.

Herbal/Food: Ephedra (mahuang) used with oxytocin may lead to hypertension.

Treatment of Overdose: Overdose causes strong uterine contractions, which may lead to uterine lacerations or rupture. Immediate discontinuation of the drug is necessary, along with symptomatic treatment.

NURSING PROCESS FOCUS Clients Receiving Oxytocin	
Assessment	**Potential Nursing Diagnoses**
Prior to administration: ■ Obtain a complete health history including past and present gynecologic and obstetric history. ■ Obtain a drug history to determine possible drug interactions and allergies.	■ Fluid Volume, Excess, related to water intoxication due to antidiuretic hormone effects of drug ■ Injury, Risk to Fetus, related to strong uterine contractions

Planning: Client Goals and Expected Outcomes
The client will: ■ Report an increase in force and frequency of uterine contractions and/or letdown of milk for breast-feeding. ■ Demonstrate an understanding of the drug's action by accurately describing drug side effects and precautions. ■ Immediately report listlessness, headache, confusion, anuria, hypotension, nausea, vomiting, or weight gain.

Implementation	
Interventions and (Rationales)	**Client Education/Discharge Planning**
■ Monitor fetal heart rate. (An increase in force and frequency of uterine contractions may cause fetal distress.)	■ Instruct client about the purpose and importance of fetal monitoring.
■ Monitor maternal status including blood pressure, pulse, and frequency, duration, and intensity of contractions. (Frequent assessment identifies potential complications early.)	■ Instruct client about the importance of monitoring maternal status and the progression of labor.
■ Monitor fluid balance. (Prolonged IV infusion may cause water intoxication.)	■ Instruct client to report drowsiness, listlessness, headache, confusion, anuria, or weight gain.
■ Monitor for postpartum/postabortion hemorrhage. (Oxytocin can be used to control postpartum bleeding.)	Instruct client: ■ About the importance of being monitored frequently after delivery or after abortion. ■ To report severe vaginal bleeding or increase in lochia.
■ Monitor lactation status. (Oxytocin causes milk ejection within minutes after administration.)	Instruct client: ■ That oxytocin does not increase milk production. ■ To monitor for decreased breast pain, redness, or hardness if taking oxytocin to decrease breast engorgement.

Evaluation of Outcome Criteria
Evaluate the effectiveness of drug therapy by confirming that client goals and expected outcomes have been met (see "Planning"). ■ The client reports an increase in force and frequency of contractions and/or letdown of milk for breast-feeding. ■ The client demonstrates an understanding of the drug's actions by accurately describing drug side effects and actions. ■ The client accurately states signs and symptoms to be reported to the healthcare provider.

35 years of age, or has a history of uterine sepsis or traumatic birth. Previous sensitivity or allergic reaction to an ergot derivative contraindicates the use of oxytocin. Dinoprostone use is contraindicated in clients with active cardiac, pulmonary, renal, or hepatic disease. These medications must be used cautiously with vasoconstrictive drugs.

Frequently assess the client in labor, because oxytocin increases the frequency and force of uterine contractions. Discontinue the infusion if fetal distress is detected, to prevent fetal anoxia. Hypertensive crisis may occur if local or regional anesthesia is used in combination with oxytocin.

Uterine hyperstimulation is characterized by contractions that are less than 2 minutes apart, have a force greater than 50 mm Hg, or last longer than 90 seconds. Discontinue oxytocin immediately if hyperstimulation occurs. Monitor fluid balance, because prolonged IV infusion of oxytocin

may cause water intoxication. Assess for symptoms of water intoxication and report immediately. Symptoms include drowsiness, listlessness, headache, confusion, anuria, and weight gain. Assess for side effects of oxytocin, including anxiety, maternal dyspnea, hypotension or hypertension, nausea, vomiting, neonatal jaundice, and maternal or fetal dysrhythmias.

Client Teaching. Client education as it relates to oxytocic drugs should include the goals of therapy; the reasons for obtaining baseline data such as vital signs and the existence of underlying cardiovascular, pulmonary, or renal disorders; and possible drug side effects. Include the following points when teaching clients about oxytocics:

• Be aware that a healthcare provider will continuously monitor for complications of oxytocin therapy and assess fetal status.

• Immediately report headache, increased vaginal bleeding, and prolonged uterine contractions.

FEMALE INFERTILITY

Infertility is defined as the inability to become pregnant after at least 1 year of frequent unprotected intercourse. Infertility is a common disorder, with as many as 25% of couples experiencing difficulty in conceiving children at some point during their reproductive lifetimes. It is estimated that females contribute to approximately 60% of the infertility disorders. Agents used to treat infertility are listed in Table 45.7.

45.8 Pharmacotherapy of Female Fertility

Causes of female infertility are varied, and include lack of ovulation, pelvic infection, and physical obstruction of the uterine tubes. Extensive testing is often necessary to determine the exact cause of the infertility. For women whose infertility has been determined to have an endocrine etiology, pharmacotherapy may be of value. Endocrine disruption of reproductive function can occur at the level of the hypothalamus, pituitary, or ovary, and pharmacotherapy is targeted to the specific cause of the dysfunction.

Lack of regular ovulation is a cause of infertility that can be successfully treated with drug therapy. Clomiphene (Clomid, Serophene) is a drug of choice for female infertility that acts as an antiestrogen. Clomiphene stimulates the release of LH, resulting in the maturation of more ovarian follicles than would normally occur. The rise in LH level is sufficient to induce ovulation in about 90% of treated women. The pregnancy rate of clients taking clomiphene is high, and twins occur in about 5% of treated clients. Therapy is usually begun with a low dose of 50 mg for 5 days, following menses. If ovulation does not occur, the dose is increased to 100 mg for 5 days and then to 150 mg. If ovulation still is not induced, human chorionic gonadotropin (HCG) is added to the regimen. Made by the placenta during pregnancy, HCG is similar to LH and can mimic the LH surge that normally causes ovulation. The use of clomiphene assumes that the pituitary gland is able to respond by secreting LH, and that the ovaries are responsive to LH. If either of these assumptions is false, other treatment options should be considered.

If the endocrine disruption is at the pituitary level, therapy with human menopausal gonadotropin (HMG) or gonadotropin-releasing hormone (GnRH) may be indicated. These therapies are generally indicated only after clomiphene has failed to induce ovulation. HMG is a combination of FSH and LH extracted from the urine of postmenopausal women, who secrete large amounts of these hormones. Also called menotropin (Pergonal, Humegon), HMG acts on the ovaries to increase follicle maturation, and results in a 25% incidence of multiple pregnancies. Successful therapy with HMG assumes that the ovaries are responsive to LH and FSH. Newer formulations use recombinant DNA technology

TABLE 45.7 Agents for Female Infertility	
Drug	**Mechanism**
bromocriptine mesylate (Parlodel)	reduction of high prolactin levels
clomiphene (Clomid, Serophene)	promotion of follicle maturation and ovulation
danazol (Danocrine)	control of endometriosis
HUMAN FSH (PURIFIED FROM THE URINE OF POSTMENOPAUSAL WOMEN)	
urofollitropin (Fertinex, Metrodin)	promotion of follicle maturation and ovulation
RECOMBINANT FSH	
follitropin alfa (Gonal-F)	promotion of follicle maturation and ovulation
follitropin beta (Follistim)	
GnRH AND GnRH ANALOGS	
cetrorelix acetate (Cetrotide)	promotion of follicle maturation and ovulation or control of endometriosis
leuprolide acetate (Lupron, Lupron Depot)	
nafarelin acetate (Synarel)	
ganirelix acetate (Antagon)	
gonadorelin acetate (Lutrepulse)	
goserelin acetate (Zoladex)	
human chorionic gonadotropin (A.P.L., Chorex, Choron 10, Profasi HP, Pregnyl)	promotion of follicle maturation and ovulation
human menopausal gonadotropin–menotropins (Pergonal, Humegon, Repronex)	promotion of follicle maturation and ovulation

to synthesize gonadotropins containing nearly pure FSH, rather than extracting the FSH–LH mixture from urine.

Given IV, gonadorelin (Factrel) is a synthetic analog of GnRH that is prescribed for women unresponsive to clomiphene. GnRH analogs take over the function of the hypothalamus and attempt to restart normal hormonal rhythms. Other medications used to stimulate ovulation are bromocriptine (Parlodel) and HCG.

Endometriosis, a common cause of infertility, is characterized by the presence of endometrial tissue in nonuterine locations such as the pelvis and ovaries. Being responsive to hormonal stimuli, this abnormal tissue can cause pain,

dysfunctional bleeding, and dysmenorrhea. Leuprolide (Lupron) is a GnRH agonist that induces an initial release of LH and FSH, followed by suppression due to the negative feedback effect on the pituitary. Many women experience relief from the symptoms of endometriosis after 3 to 6 months of leuprolide therapy, and the benefits may extend well beyond the treatment period. Leuprolide is also indicated for the palliative therapy of prostate cancer. As an alternative choice, danazol (Danocrine) is an anabolic steroid that suppresses FSH production, which in turn shuts down both ectopic and normal endometrial activity. While leuprolide is given only by the parenteral route, danazol is given orally.

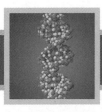

CHAPTER REVIEW

KEY CONCEPTS

The numbered key concepts provide a succinct summary of the important points from the corresponding numbered section within the chapter. If any of these points are not clear, refer to the numbered section within the chapter for review.

45.1 Female reproductive function is controlled by the secretion of GnRH from the hypothalamus, and FSH and LH from the pituitary.

45.2 Estrogens are secreted by ovarian follicles and are responsible for maturation of the sex organs and the secondary sex characteristics of the female. Progestins are secreted by the corpus luteum and prepare the endometrium for implantation.

45.3 Low doses of estrogens and progestins prevent conception by blocking ovulation. Long-term formulations are available that offer greater convenience.

45.4 Drugs for emergency contraception may be administered within 72 hours after unprotected sex to prevent implantation of the fertilized egg. Other agents may be

given to stimulate uterine contractions to expel the implanted embryo.

45.5 Estrogen–progestin combinations are used for hormone replacement therapy during and after menopause; however, their long-term use may have serious adverse effects.

45.6 Progestins are prescribed for dysfunctional uterine bleeding. High doses of progestins are also used as antineoplastics.

45.7 Oxytocics are drugs that stimulate uterine contractions and induce labor. Tocolytics slow uterine contractions to delay labor.

45.8 Medications may be administered to stimulate ovulation, to increase female fertility.

NCLEX-RN® REVIEW QUESTIONS

1 The client is admitted with pain in the calf, shortness of breath, and severe chest pain. A medical history reveals that the client is taking oral contraceptives. Based on this assessment, the client may be experiencing a:

1. Cerebrovascular accident.
2. Hypertensive crisis.
3. Hyperglycemic reaction.
4. Thromboembolism.

2 The nurse includes which of the following discharge instructions to the client receiving HRT?

1. Avoid common foods that contain caffeine.
2. Take medication 30 minutes before meals.
3. Discontinue medication if uterine bleeding begins.
4. Monitor for a sudden increase in LDL cholesterol.

3 The nurse's assessment of the client receiving an IV infusion of oxytocin notes that uterine contractions are 4 minutes apart and 60 seconds in duration. Which of the following nursing interventions is most important based on this assessment?

1. Administer oxygen via facemask.
2. Monitor the client for water intoxication.
3. Position the client on her left side.
4. Discontinue the infusion immediately.

4 The client has made the decision to use Ortho-Novum 1/35 for contraception. The nurse includes which of the following instructions to the client about this medication? (Select all that apply.)

1. Take the first pill of the pack on the fifth day of the menstrual cycle.
2. Placebo must be taken to decrease estrogen-related adverse effects.
3. Possible side effects include intolerance to contact lenses, abdominal cramps, dysmenorrhea, and breast fullness.
4. Barrier contraceptives are needed if a daily dose is missed.
5. Breakthrough bleeding indicates that ovulation has occurred.

5 The client questions the nurses about how she could have become pregnant while she was taking oral contraceptives. Which of the following statements best describes the primary reason why a client would become pregnant while on oral contraceptives?

1. Antibiotics were taken in conjunction with the oral contraceptive.
2. Two or more doses of the oral contraceptive were skipped.
3. The dosage of the estrogen in the oral contraceptive was too low.
4. The oral contraceptive was taken in combination with an anticonvulsant.

CRITICAL THINKING QUESTIONS

1. A 28-year-old woman has a 3-year history of pelvic pain, dyspareunia, and infertility. She has been diagnosed with endometriosis and is prescribed leuprolide (Lupron) once a month per intramuscular injection. Discuss the mechanism of action of leuprolide in managing the client's endometriosis. What information should be included in a teaching plan for a client receiving this drug?

2. A labor and delivery nurse places one fourth of a tablet (crushed) of misoprostol (Cytotec) on the cervix of a client who is being induced because she is 2 weeks past her due date. After several hours, the client begins to have contractions, and the nurse notes late decelerations on the monitor. The nurse flushes the drug out of the client's vagina with saline per hospital protocol. What is the use and action of misoprostol?

3. A nurse is assessing a 32-year-old postpartum client and notes 2+ pitting edema of the ankles and pretibial area. The client denies having "swelling" prior to delivery. The nurse reviews the client's chart and notes that she was induced with oxytocin (Pitocin) over a 23-hour period. What is the relationship between this drug regimen and the client's current presentation? What additional assessments should be made?

See Appendix D for answers and rationales for all activities.

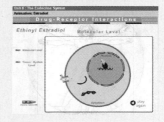

EXPLORE MediaLink

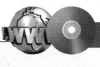

www.prenhall.com/adams

NCLEX-RN® review, case studies, and other interactive resources for this chapter can be found on the companion website at www.prenhall.com/adams. Click on "Chapter 45" to select the activities for this chapter. For animations, more NCLEX-RN® review questions, and an audio glossary, access the accompanying Prentice Hall Nursing MediaLink DVD-ROM in this textbook.

 PRENTICE HALL NURSING MEDIALINK DVD-ROM

- **Animation**
  Mechanism in Action: Ethinyl estradiol with norethindrone (*Ortho-Novum*)
- **Audio Glossary**
- **NCLEX-RN® Review**

 COMPANION WEBSITE

- **NCLEX-RN® Review**
- **Dosage Calculations**
- **Case Study:** Client taking hormone replacement therapy
- **Care Plan:** Client with family history of fibrocystic breast disease and hypertension taking ethinyl estradiol with norethindrone

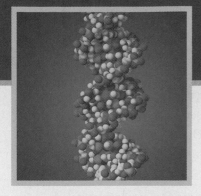

CHAPTER 46

Drugs for Disorders and Conditions of the Male Reproductive System

DRUGS AT A GLANCE

AGENTS FOR MALE HYPOGONADISM
Androgens
  ● *testosterone base (Andro)*
AGENTS FOR MALE INFERTILITY
AGENTS FOR ERECTILE DYSFUNCTION
Phosphodiesterase-5 Inhibitors
  ● *sildenafil (Viagra)*
AGENTS FOR BENIGN PROSTATIC HYPERPLASIA
Alpha₁-adrenergic Blockers
5-alpha-reductase Inhibitors
  ● *finasteride (Proscar)*

OBJECTIVES

After reading this chapter, the student should be able to:

1. Describe the roles of the hypothalamus, pituitary, and testes in maintaining male reproductive function.
2. Explain the role of androgens in the treatment of male hypogonadism.
3. Describe the misuse and dangers associated with the use of anabolic steroids to enhance athletic performance.
4. Discuss the use of androgens as antineoplastic agents.
5. Explain the limited role of drugs in the therapy of male infertility.
6. Describe the pharmacotherapy of erectile dysfunction.
7. Describe the nurse's role in the pharmacological management of disorders and conditions of the male reproductive system.
8. Identify the static and dynamic components of benign prostatic hyperplasia (BPH), and how they lead to client symptoms.
9. For each of the drugs/classes listed in Drugs at a Glance, know representative drugs, and explain the mechanism of drug action, primary actions, and important adverse effects.
10. Categorize drugs used in the treatment of male reproductive disorders and conditions based on their classification and mechanism of action.
11. Use the Nursing Process to care for clients who are receiving drug therapy for disorders and conditions of the male reproductive system.

MediaLink

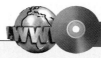

www.prenhall.com/adams

KEY TERMS

anabolic steroids   *page 719*

androgens   *page 718*

azoospermia   *page 721*

benign prostatic hyperplasia (BPH)   *page 725*

corpus cavernosum   *page 723*

follicle-stimulating hormone (FSH)   *page 718*

hypogonadism   *page 718*

impotence   *page 723*

leuteinizing hormone (LH)   *page 718*

libido   *page 719*

oligospermia   *page 721*

testosterone   *page 718*

virilization   *page 719*

As in women, reproductive function in men is regulated by a small number of hormones from the hypothalamus, pituitary, and gonads. Because hormonal secretion in men is relatively constant throughout the adult lifespan, pharmacological treatment of reproductive disorders in men is less complex, and more limited, than in women. This chapter examines drugs used to treat disorders and conditions of the male reproductive system.

46.1 Hypothalamic and Pituitary Regulation of Male Reproductive Function

The same pituitary hormones that control reproductive function in women (Chapter 45 ∞) also affect men. Although the name **follicle-stimulating hormone (FSH)** applies to its target in the female ovary, this same hormone regulates sperm production in men. **Leuteinizing hormone (LH),** more accurately called *interstitial cell–stimulating hormone* (ICSH) in the male reproductive system, regulates the production of testosterone.

Although secreted in small amounts by the adrenal glands in women, **androgens** are considered male sex hormones. The testes secrete **testosterone,** the primary androgen responsible for maturation of the male sex organs and the secondary sex characteristics of men. Unlike the cyclic secretion of estrogen and progesterone in women, testosterone secretion is relatively constant in adult men. If the level of testosterone in the blood rises above normal, negative feedback to the pituitary shuts off the secretion of LH and FSH. The relationship between the hypothalamus, pituitary, and the male reproductive hormones is illustrated in ● Figure 46.1.

Like estrogen, testosterone has metabolic effects in tissues outside the reproductive system. Of particular note is its ability to build muscle mass, which contributes to differences in muscle strength and body composition between men and women.

MALE HYPOGONADISM

ANDROGENS

Androgens include testosterone and related hormones that control many aspects of male reproductive function. Therapeutically they are used to treat hypogonadism and certain cancers. These agents are in Table 46.1.

46.2 Pharmacotherapy With Androgens

Lack of sufficient testosterone secretion by the testes can result in male **hypogonadism.** Insufficient testosterone secretion may be caused by disorders of either the pituitary or the testes. Deficiency in FSH and LH secretion by the pituitary

PHARMFACTS

Male Reproductive Conditions and Disorders

- Erectile dysfunction affects 10 to 15 million Americans—about one in four men older than 65 years.
- Smoking more than 20 cigarettes a day has been shown to produce a 60% higher risk of erectile dysfunction. Ten or fewer cigarettes daily still increases the risk by 16%.
- In the United States 13 million men are estimated to have hypogonadism.
- BPH affects 50% of men older than 60 years, and 90% of men older than 80.
- BPH is the most common benign neoplasm affecting middle-aged and elderly men.
- Approximately 30% of men are subfertile, and at least 2% of men are totally infertile.

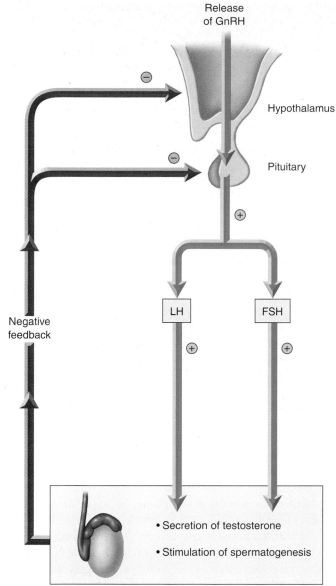

●**Figure 46.1** Hormonal control of the male reproductive hormones

will result in a lack of stimulus to the testes to produce androgens. This condition is known as *secondary* hypogonadism. Lack of FSH and LH secretion may have a number of causes, including Cushing's syndrome, thyroid disorders, estrogen-secreting tumors, and therapy with GnRH agonists such as leuprolide (Lupron). Hypogonadism may be congenital or acquired later in life.

Hypogonadism may also occur in clients with normal pituitary function if the testes are diseased or otherwise unresponsive to FSH-LH. Examples of conditions that may cause testicular failure include mumps, testicular trauma or inflammation, and certain autoimmune disorders. When the condition is caused by a testicular disorder, it is called *primary* hypogonadism.

Symptoms of male hypogonadism include a diminished appearance of the secondary sex characteristics of men: sparse axillary, facial, and pubic hair; increased subcutaneous

fat; and small testicular size. In adult men, lack of testosterone can lead to erectile dysfunction, low sperm counts, and decreased **libido**, or interest in intercourse. Nonspecific complaints may include fatigue, depression, and reduced muscle mass. In young men, lack of sufficient testosterone secretion may lead to delayed puberty.

Pharmacotherapy of hypogonadism includes replacement therapy with testosterone or other androgens. Within days or weeks of initiating therapy, androgens improve libido and correct erectile dysfunction caused by low testosterone levels. Male sex characteristics reappear, a condition called *masculinization* or **virilization.** Depression resolves, and muscle strength rapidly improves. Therapy with androgens is targeted to return serum testosterone to normal levels. Above-normal levels serve no therapeutic purpose and increase the risk of side effects.

Testosterone is available in a number of different formulations. Testosterone cypionate (Depotest, others) and testosterone enanthate (Andro LA) are slowly absorbed after IM injections, which are given every 2 to 4 weeks. Testosterone pellets (Testopel) are implanted subcutaneously, and last 3 to 6 months. Several skin-patch products are available, which release testosterone over a 24-hour period. Testoderm patches are applied to the scrotal area, whereas Testoderm TTS and Androderm patches are applied to the arm, back, or upper buttocks. Two gel systems are available as Testim and Androgel, which are applied to the shoulders, upper arm, or abdomen. The alcohol-based gels dry quickly, and the testosterone is absorbed into the skin in about 30 minutes and released slowly to the blood. A new formulation is a buccal tablet (Striant) that adheres to the gum surface to release the drug over a 12-hour period.

Androgens have important physiological effects outside the reproductive system. Testosterone promotes the synthesis of erythropoietin, which explains why men usually have a slightly higher hematocrit than women. Testosterone has a profound anabolic effect on skeletal muscle, which is the rationale for giving this drug to debilitated clients who have muscle-wasting disease.

Anabolic steroids are testosterone-like compounds with hormonal activity that are taken inappropriately by athletes who hope to build muscle mass and strength, thereby obtaining a competitive edge. When taken in large doses for prolonged periods, anabolic steroids can produce significant adverse effects, some of which may persist for months after discontinuation of the drugs. These agents tend to raise cholesterol levels and may cause low sperm counts and impotence in men. In female athletes, menstrual irregularities are likely, with an obvious increase in masculine appearance. Oral androgens are hepatotoxic, and permanent liver damage may result with prolonged use. Behavioral changes include aggression and psychological dependence. The use of anabolic steroids to improve athletic performance is illegal and strongly discouraged by healthcare providers and athletic associations. Most androgens are classified as Schedule III drugs because of their abuse potential.

TABLE 46.1 Selected Androgens		
Drug	**Route and Adult Dose (max dose where indicated)**	**Adverse Effects**
danazol (Danocrine)	PO; 200–400 mg bid for 3–6 mo	*Acne, gynecomastia, hirsutism and male sex characteristics (in women), sodium and water retention, hypercholesterolemia*
fluoxymesterone (Halotestin)	PO; 2.5–20 mg/day for replacement therapy	
methyltestosterone (Android, Testred)	PO; 10–50 mg/day	
nandrolone phenpropionate (Durabolin, Hybolin)	IM; 50–100 mg/wk	Anaphylaxis, testicular atrophy and oligospermia at high doses
testolactone (Teslac)	PO; 250 mg qid	
℞ testosterone (Andro 100, Histerone, Testoderm)	PO; 10–25 mg q 2–3 days	
testosterone cypionate (Depotest, Andro-Cyp, Depo-Testosterone)	IM; 50–400 mg q 2–4 wk	
testosterone enanthate (Andro L.A., Delatest, Delatestryl)	IM; 50–400 mg q 2–4 wk	

Italics indicate common adverse effects; underlining indicates serious adverse effects.

High doses of androgens are occasionally used as a palliative measure to treat certain types of breast cancer, in combination with other antineoplastics. Because the growth of most prostate carcinomas is testosterone dependent, androgens should not be prescribed for older men unless the possibility of prostate cancer has been ruled out. Clients with prostate carcinoma are sometimes given a GnRH agonist such as leuprolide (Lupron) to reduce circulating testosterone levels.

NURSING CONSIDERATIONS

The role of the nurse in androgen therapy for hypogonadism involves careful monitoring of a client's condition and providing education as it relates to the prescribed drug treatment. Obtain a history that includes questions regarding the possibility of impaired sexual functioning and diminished libido. Conduct a physical assessment for evidence of decreased hormone production, such as decreased or absent body hair, small testes, or delayed signs of puberty. This assessment should also include the client's

SPECIAL CONSIDERATIONS

Androgen Abuse by Athletes

A serious problem with androgens is their abuse by athletes. The drugs have been used and abused to increase weight, muscle mass, and muscle strength. What began as a movement by weightlifters to enhance muscle mass in the early 1960s has progressed into use by athletes in most competitive sports and in all age groups. Teen use has been increasing, and not just among athletes; some report taking the drugs simply to look better. Use of these drugs is further encouraged by the absence of immediate adverse effects; rather, the serious effects of anabolic steroids are long term but not readily observable.

Anabolic steroids may be taken orally or IM. The oral forms are absorbed rapidly; they are sometimes preferred because they are excreted quickly and thus are less likely to be detected in drug screening. The IM injections may be water or oil based, with the oil forms having a prolonged duration and being more detectable. Most U.S. professional sports prohibit the use of androgens for these purposes, and any athlete proved to use them is banned from participation.

emotional status, because depression and mood swings may be symptoms of decreased hormone secretion. Monitor lab results, especially liver enzymes, if the client has a history of anabolic steroid use. Also monitor serum cholesterol, especially in clients with a history of myocardial infarction or angina, as the drug can increase this lab value. Contraindications to androgen therapy include prostatic or male breast cancer, renal disease, cardiac and liver dysfunction, hypercalcemia, benign prostatic hyperplasia (BPH), and hypertension. Androgens must be used cautiously in prepubertal men, older adults, and in men with acute intermittent porphyria.

Monitor for side effects of clients taking androgens, including skin reactions such as pruritus or blistering with topical formulations. Some adverse reactions found to occur in women as a result of androgen use include deepening of the voice, facial hair growth, enlarged clitoris, and irregular menses.

Client Teaching. Client education as it relates to androgen therapy should include the goals of therapy, the reasons for obtaining baseline data such as vital signs and the existence of underlying cardiac or renal disorders, and possible drug side effects. Include the following points when teaching clients about androgen therapy:

• Keep all scheduled laboratory visits for periodic serum cholesterol, serum electrolyte, and liver functions tests.

• Check weight twice a week and report significant increases.

• Report any soreness at injection sites.

• Immediately report prolonged or painful erection (priapism).

• If diabetic, be alert for signs and symptoms of hypoglycemia (shaking, sweating, hunger, anxiety, and dizziness).

• Notify the healthcare provider immediately if pregnancy is planned or suspected.

• Be aware of proper technique in using medication (transdermal patch, oral medication, gel, or injection).

Pr PROTOTYPE DRUG | Testosterone Base *(Andro, others)* | Androgen

ACTIONS AND USES

The primary therapeutic use of testosterone is the treatment of hypogonadism in males by promoting virilization, including enlargement of the sexual organs, growth of facial hair, and a deepening of the voice. In adult males, testosterone administration will increase libido and restore masculine characteristics that may be deficient. Testosterone base acts by stimulating RNA synthesis and protein metabolism. High doses may suppress spermatogenesis. Testosterone base is administered by the IM route, although other salts are available for the transdermal and buccal routes.

ADMINISTRATION ALERTS

- If using a patch, place on hair-free, dry skin of the abdomen, back, thigh, upper arm, or as directed.
- Alternate patch site daily, rotating sites every 7 days.
- Give IM injection into gluteal muscles.
- Pregnancy Category X.

PHARMACOKINETICS

Onset: Unknown

Peak: Unknown

Half-life: Unknown

Duration: 1–3 days

ADVERSE EFFECTS

An obvious side effect of testosterone therapy is virilization, which is usually only of concern when the drug is taken by female clients. Increased libido may also occur. Salt and water are often retained, causing edema, and a diuretic may be indicated. Liver damage is rare, although it is a potentially serious adverse effect with some of the orally administered androgens. Acne and skin irritation is common during therapy.

Contraindications: Testosterone is contraindicated in men with known or suspected breast or prostatic carcinomas and in women who are or may become pregnant (category X). The drug should be used with caution in clients with preexisting renal or hepatic disease.

INTERACTIONS

Drug–Drug: When taken concurrently with oral anticoagulants, testosterone may potentiate hypoprothrombinemia.

Lab Tests: Values of the following may be decreased: T4, thyroxine-binding globulin, serum calcium, and clotting factors II, V, VII, and X. Creatinine may be increased, and cholesterol may be either increased or decreased.

Herbal/Food: Insulin requirements may decrease, and the risk of hepatotoxicity may increase when used with echinacea.

Treatment of Overdose: There is no specific treatment for overdose.

 See the Companion Website for a Nursing Process Focus specific to this drug.

MALE INFERTILITY

It is estimated that 30% to 40% of infertility among couples is caused by difficulties with the male reproductive system. Male infertility may have psychological etiology, which must be ruled out before pharmacotherapy is considered.

46.3 Pharmacotherapy of Male Infertility

Like female infertility, male infertility may have a number of complex causes. **Oligospermia,** the presence of less than 20 million sperm/ml of ejaculate is considered abnormal. **Azoospermia,** the complete absence of sperm in an ejaculate, may indicate an obstruction of the vas deferens or ejaculatory duct that can be corrected surgically. Infections such as mumps, chronic tuberculosis, and sexually transmitted diseases can contribute to infertility. The possibility of erectile dysfunction must be considered and treated, as discussed in Section 46.4. Infertility may occur with or without signs of hypogonadism.

The goal of endocrine pharmacotherapy of male infertility is to increase sperm production. Therapy often begins with IM injections of human chorionic gonadotropin (hCG), three times per week over 1 year. Although hCG is secreted by the placenta, its effects in men are identical to those of LH: increased testosterone secretion and spermatogenesis. Sperm counts are conducted periodically to assess therapeutic progress. If hCG is unsuccessful, therapy with menotropins

(Pergonal) may be attempted. Menotropin consists of a mixture of purified FSH and LH. For infertile clients exhibiting signs of hypogonadism, testosterone therapy also may be indicated.

Other pharmacological approaches to treating male infertility have been attempted. Antiestrogens such as tamoxifen (Nolvadex) and clomiphene (Clomid) have been used to block the negative feedback of estrogen (from the adrenal glands) to the pituitary and hypothalamus, thus increasing the levels of FSH and LH. Testolactone (Teslac), an aromatase inhibitor, has been administered to block the metabolic conversion of testosterone to estrogen. Various nutritional supplements, such as zinc to improve sperm production, L-arginine to improve sperm motility, and vitamins C and E as antioxidants to reduce reactive intermediates, have been tested. Unfortunately these and other therapies have not conclusively been shown to have any positive effect on male infertility.

Drug therapy of male infertility is not as successful as fertility pharmacotherapy in women, because only about 5% of infertile males have an endocrine etiology for their disorder. Many years of therapy may be required. Because of the expense of pharmacotherapy and the large number of injections needed, other means of conception may be explored, such as in vitro fertilization or intrauterine insemination.

ERECTILE DYSFUNCTION

Erectile dysfunction, or **impotence,** is a common disorder in men. The defining characteristic of this condition is the consistent inability to either obtain an erection or

NURSING PROCESS FOCUS Clients Receiving Androgen Therapy

Assessment	Potential Nursing Diagnoses
Prior to administration: • Obtain a complete health history including male breast or prostatic cancer; BPH; cardiac, kidney, or liver disease; diabetes; or hypercalcemia. • Obtain lab results including renal function tests, blood urea nitrogen (BUN), creatinine, and PSA. • Obtain a drug history to determine possible drug interactions and allergies.	• Body Image, Disturbed, related to effects of decreased or increased hormone function • Sexual Dysfunction, related to effects of drug therapy or decreased hormone function • Sleep Pattern, Disturbed, related to effects of drug therapy • Knowledge, Deficient, related to disease process and drug therapy

Planning: Client Goals and Expected Outcomes

The client will:
• Demonstrate improvement of the underlying condition for which testosterone was ordered.
• Demonstrate an ability to correctly self-administer the prescribed drug.
• Demonstrate an understanding of the drug's action by accurately describing drug side effects and precautions.

Implementation

Interventions and (Rationales)	Client Education/Discharge Planning
• Monitor serum cholesterol levels. (Elevated cholesterol levels secondary to testosterone administration may increase client's risk of cardiovascular disease.)	Instruct client to: • Have cholesterol levels measured periodically during therapy. • Modify factors that may lower risk of hypercholesterolemia: decrease fat in diet, increase exercise, decrease consumption of red meat.
• Monitor calcium levels. (Testosterone can cause hypercalcemia.)	Instruct client to: • Have calcium levels checked during therapy. • Recognize and report symptoms of increased serum calcium, including deep bone and flank pain, anorexia, nausea/vomiting, thirst, constipation, lethargy, and psychoses.
• Monitor bone growth in children and adolescents. (Premature epiphyseal closing may occur, leading to growth retardation.)	• Instruct the pediatric caregiver to have bone-age determinations performed on the child every 6 months.
• Monitor input, output, and client weight. (Testosterone can cause retention of salt and water, leading to edema.)	• Instruct client to check weight twice weekly and report increases, particularly if accompanied by dependent edema.
• Monitor blood glucose, especially in clients with diabetes. (Testosterone therapy may affect glucose tolerance.)	Instruct client to: • Monitor blood glucose daily and report significant changes. • Recognize that adjustments may need to be made in hypoglycemic medications and diet.
• Monitor proper self-administration. (Proper self-administration is key to safety and effectiveness.)	Instruct client to: • Mark calendar so medication can be taken/given at appropriate intervals. • Apply transdermal patch to dry, clean scrotal skin that has been dry shaved, and not to use chemical depilatories. • Notify female partner of transdermal patch use; there is a chance of absorbing testosterone, resulting in mild virilization. • Avoid showering or swimming for at least 1 hour after gel application.

Evaluation of Outcome Criteria

Evaluate the effectiveness of drug therapy by confirming that client goals and expected outcomes have been met (see "Planning").
• The client demonstrates improvement in the condition for which the drug was ordered.
• The client demonstrates safe self-administration of the drug.
• The client demonstrates an understanding of the drug's action by accurately describing drug side effects and precautions.

∞ *See Table 46.1 for a list of drugs to which these nursing actions apply.*

to sustain an erection long enough to achieve successful intercourse.

46.4 Pharmacotherapy of Erectile Dysfunction

The incidence of erectile dysfunction increases with age, although it may occur in a male adult of any age. Certain diseases, most notably atherosclerosis, diabetes, stroke, and hypertension, are associated with a higher incidence of the condition. Psychogenic causes may include depression, fatigue, guilt, or fear of sexual failure. In some men, a number of common drugs cause impotence as a side effect, including thiazide diuretics, phenothiazines, selective serotonin reuptake inhibitors (SSRIs), tricyclic antidepressants (TCAs), propranolol (Inderal), and diazepam (Valium). Low testosterone secretion can cause an inability to develop an erection, owing to the loss of libido.

Penile erection has both neuromuscular and vascular components. Autonomic nerves dilate arterioles leading to the major erectile tissues of the penis, called the **corpora cavernosa.** The corpora have vascular spaces that fill with blood to cause rigidity. In addition, constriction of veins draining blood from the corpora allows the penis to remain rigid long enough for successful penetration. After ejaculation, the veins dilate, blood leaves the corpora, and the penis quickly loses its rigidity. Organic causes of erectile dysfunction may include damage to the nerves or blood vessels involved in the erection reflex.

The marketing of sildenafil (Viagra), an inhibitor of the enzyme phosphodiesterase-5, has revolutionized the medical therapy of erectile dysfunction. When sildenafil was approved as the first pharmacological treatment for erectile dysfunction in 1998, it set a record for pharmaceutical sales for any new drug in U.S. history. Prior to the discovery of sildenafil, rigid or inflatable penile prostheses were implanted into the corpora. As an alternative to prostheses, drugs such as alprostadil (Caverject) or the combination of papaverine plus phentolamine were injected directly into the corpora cavernosa just prior to intercourse. Penile injections cause pain and reduce the spontaneity associated with pleasurable intercourse. These alternative therapies are rare today, though they may be used for clients in whom phosphodiesterase-5 inhibitors are contraindicated.

Sildenafil does not cause an erection; it merely *enhances* the erection caused by physical contact or other sexual stimuli. In addition, sildenafil is not as effective in promoting erections in men who do not have erectile dysfunction. Despite considerable research interest, no effects of sildenafil have been shown on female sexual function, and this drug is not approved for use by women.

Two other phosphodiesterase-5 inhibitors have been approved by the FDA. Vardenafil (Levitra), acts by the same mechanism as sildenafil but has a faster onset and slightly longer duration of action. Tadalafil (Cialis) acts within 30 minutes and has a prolonged duration lasting from 24 to 36 hours. Drugs for erectile dysfunction are listed in Table 46.2.

The three phosphodiesterase-5 inhibitors are equally effective at promoting erections in 60% to 80% of male clients, and side effects are similar. The most common side effects are nasal congestion, headache, facial flushing, and dizziness. These drugs produce a 5- to 10-mm fall in blood pressure, but this drop is usually not clinically important. In clients who are taking nitrates or multiple antihypertensive medications, however, this blood pressure change may produce symptoms of hypotension. Phosphodiesterase-5 inhibitors are contraindicated in clients taking nitrates. Tadalafil produces less blood pressure decrease than the other drugs in this class.

NURSING CONSIDERATIONS

The role of the nurse in pharmacotherapy in erectile dysfunction therapy involves careful monitoring of a client's condition and providing education as it relates to the prescribed drug treatment. Obtain a complete physical examination including history of impaired sexual function, cardiovascular disease, and presence of emotional disturbances. Also obtain and monitor results of lab tests related to liver function.

A number of diagnostic tests may be ordered to confirm the diagnosis of erectile dysfunction. Blood is drawn to check for possible metabolic or hormonal causes of erectile dysfunction. Laboratory tests may include testosterone, prolactin, and thyroxin levels. If hormones are the cause of the dysfunction, treatment will be aimed at correcting the abnormality. A nocturnal penile tumescence and rigidity (NPTR) test may be ordered. This test monitors

TABLE 46.2 Agents for Erectile Dysfunction		
Drug	**Route and Adult Dose (max dose where indicated)**	**Adverse Effects**
sildenafil (Viagra)	PO; 50 mg approximately 30–60 min before intercourse (max: 100 mg once/day)	*Nasal congestion, headache, facial flushing, dizziness and blurred vision (sildenafil)*
tadalafil (Cialis)	PO; 10 mg approximately 30 min before intercourse (max: 20 mg once/day)	Hypotension when taken with nitrates, priapism
vardenafil (Levitra)	PO; 10 mg approximately 1 h before intercourse (max: 20 mg once/day)	

Italics indicate common adverse effects; underlining indicates serious adverse effects.

Pr PROTOTYPE DRUG | Sildenafil *(Viagra)* | Erectile Dysfunction Agent

ACTIONS AND USES

Sildenafil acts by relaxing smooth muscle in the corpus cavernosum, thus allowing increased blood flow into the penis. The increased blood flow results in a firmer and longer lasting erection in about 70% of men taking the drug. The onset of action is relatively rapid, less than 1 hour, and its effects last up to 4 hours. Sildenafil blocks the enzyme phosphodiesterase-5.

ADMINISTRATION ALERTS

- Avoid administration of sildenafil with meals, especially high-fat meals, because absorption is decreased.
- Avoid grapefruit juice when administering sildenafil.

PHARMACOKINETICS

Onset: 20–60 min

Peak: 30–120 min

Half-life: 4 h

Duration: Unknown

ADVERSE EFFECTS

The most serious adverse effect, hypotension, occurs in clients concurrently taking organic nitrates for angina. Common side effects include headache, dizziness, flushing, rash, nasal congestion, diarrhea, dyspepsia, UTI, chest pain, or indigestion. Sildenafil can produce blurred vision or changes in color perception in 10% of the clients. Priapism, a sustained erection lasting longer than 6 hours has been reported with sildenafil use and may lead to permanent damage to penile tissues.

Contraindications: Sildenafil is contraindicated in clients taking nitrates and in those with hypersensitivity to the drug.

INTERACTIONS

Drug–Drug: Cimetidine, erythromycin, and ketoconazole will increase serum levels of sildenafil and necessitate lower drug doses. Use with nitrates will result in hypotension. Protease inhibitors (ritonavir, amprenavir, others) will cause increased sildenafil levels, which may lead to toxicity. Rifampin may decrease sildenafil levels, leading to decreased effectiveness.

Lab Tests: Unknown.

Herbal/Food: Unknown.

Treatment of Overdose: There is no specific treatment for overdose.

 See the Companion Website for a Nursing Process Focus specific treatment for overdose.

---

the number of erections during sleep and is used to differentiate between psychological and physiological causes of erectile dysfunction. If the cause is found to be psychological, treatment will usually consist of a combination of psychological and pharmacological therapy. A blood flow test is also used to determine whether there is sufficient arterial and venous flow to the penis. Clients who have diminished or abnormal blood flow may find that the pharmacological agents to treat erectile dysfunction are not effective. These clients may have more success with penile implants.

Sildenafil, vardenafil, and tadalafil are contraindicated with the use of organic nitrates such as nitroglycerin, because they potentiate the hypotensive effect of nitrates. Nitrates are also found in recreational drugs, including amyl nitrate or nitrite, commonly called "poppers." Coadministration of vardenafil or tadalafil with alpha-adrenergic blockers can also lead to profound hypotension. These agents are contraindicated in clients with severe cardiovascular disease and in the presence of anatomical deformities of the penis.

Use in clients with hepatic dysfunction is cautioned, because the drugs are metabolized in the liver, and drug accumulation may lead to toxicity. Clients with cirrhosis or severe decreased liver function should start with lower doses. Clients with leukemia, sickle-cell anemia, multiple myeloma, ulcer, and retinitis pigmentosa should also use sildenafil cautiously.

Monitor for side effects including vision changes such as blurred vision, the inability to differentiate between green and blue, perception of a blue tinge to objects, or photophobia. Also observe safety precautions until it is known whether sensory-perceptual alterations occur, so falls and other accidents can be avoided. Monitor the client for presence of headache, dizziness, flushing, rash, nasal congestion, diarrhea, dyspepsia, UTI, chest pain, or indigestion.

Client Teaching. Client education as it relates to erectile dysfunction agents should include the goals of therapy; the reasons for obtaining baseline data such as vital signs and tests for cardiac and renal disorders, and the existence of underlying disorders such as angina; and possible drug side effects. Include the following points when teaching clients about erectile dysfunction agents:

- Keep all laboratory visits to monitor liver function.
- Do not take more than one dose in a 24-hour period.
- Have vital signs, including blood pressure, checked routinely.
- Take 30–60 minutes prior to sexual activity.
- If taking nitrates or alpha blockers, do not use erectile dysfunction agents.
- Do not share medication.
- Immediately report chest pain.
- Immediately report erection that lasts longer than 4 hours or is painful.

BENIGN PROSTATIC HYPERPLASIA

Benign prostatic hyperplasia (BPH) is the most common benign neoplasm in men. It is characterized by enlargement of the prostate gland that decreases the outflow of urine by obstructing the urethra, causing difficult urination. BPH is not considered to be a precursor to prostate carcinoma.

Symptoms of BPH include increased urinary frequency (usually with small amounts of urine), increased urgency to urinate, postvoid leakage, excessive nighttime urination (nocturia), decreased force of the urine stream, and a sensation that the bladder did not empty completely. The urinary outlet obstruction can lead to serious complications such as urinary infections or renal failure. In advanced cases, a surgical procedure called transurethral resection is needed to restore the patency of the urethra. BPH is illustrated in ● Figure 46.2.

ANTIPROSTATIC AGENTS

Only a few drugs are available for the pharmacotherapy of BPH. Early in the course of the disease, drug therapy may relieve some symptoms. These agents are listed in Table 46.3.

46.5 Pharmacotherapy of Benign Prostatic Hyperplasia

The pathogenessis of BPH involves two components: static and dynamic. The *static factors* relate to anatomical enlargement of the prostate gland. The gland can double or triple its size with aging. This enlargement may cause a physical block of urine outflow at the neck of the bladder. The *dynamic factors* are due to excessive numbers of alpha$_1$-adrenergic receptors located in smooth-muscle cells in the neck of the urinary bladder and in the prostate gland. When activated, the alpha$_1$-adrenergic receptors compress the urethra and provide resistance to urine outflow from the bladder. The two mechanisms of disease, static and dynamic, have led to two different classes of drugs (Table 46.3) used to treat symptoms of BPH. The mechanisms of action of these drugs are shown in Pharmacotherapy Illustrated 46.1.

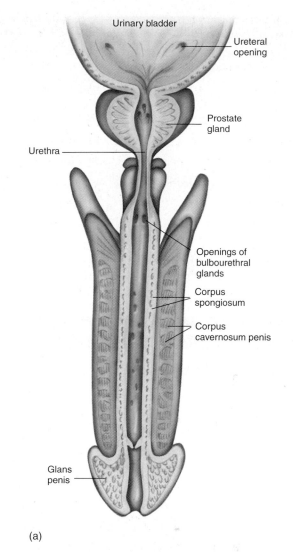

(a)

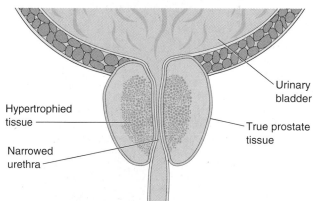

(b)

● **Figure 46.2** Benign prostatic hyperplasia: (a) normal prostate with penis; (b) benign prostatic hyperplasia
Source: Rice, Jane, Medical Terminology with Human Anatomy, 5th ed., © 2005, p. 538. Reprinted by permission of Pearson Education, Inc., Upper Saddle River, NJ.

Certain commonly used medications have been found to worsen symptoms of BPH. Alpha-adrenergic agents, which include decongestants such as pseudoephedrine and

TABLE 46.3 Agents for Benign Prostatic Hyperplasia

Drug	Route and Adult Dose (max dose where indicated)	Adverse Effects
ALPHA ADRENERGIC BLOCKERS		
doxazosin (Cardura) (see page 322 for the Protoype Drug box ∞)	PO; 1–8 mg/day	*Orthostatic hypotension, headache, dizziness*
prazosin (Minipress)	PO; 1 mg qid or bid	<u>First-dose phenomenon (severe hypotension and syncope), tachycardia</u>
tamsulosin (Flomax)	PO; 0.4 mg 30 min after a meal (max: 0.8 mg/day)	
terazosin (Hytrin)	PO; start with 1 mg at bedtime, then 1–5 mg/day (max: 20 mg/day)	
5-ALPHA-REDUCTASE INHIBITORS		
dutasteride (Avodart)	PO; 0.5 mg/day	*Sexual dysfunction, decreased libido, decreased ejaculate volume*
Ⓟ finasteride (Proscar)	PO; 5 mg/day	<u>No serious adverse effects</u>

Italics indicate common adverse effects; <u>underlining</u> indicates serious adverse effects.

PHARMACOTHERAPY ILLUSTRATED

46.1 Mechanisms of Action of Antiprostatic Drugs

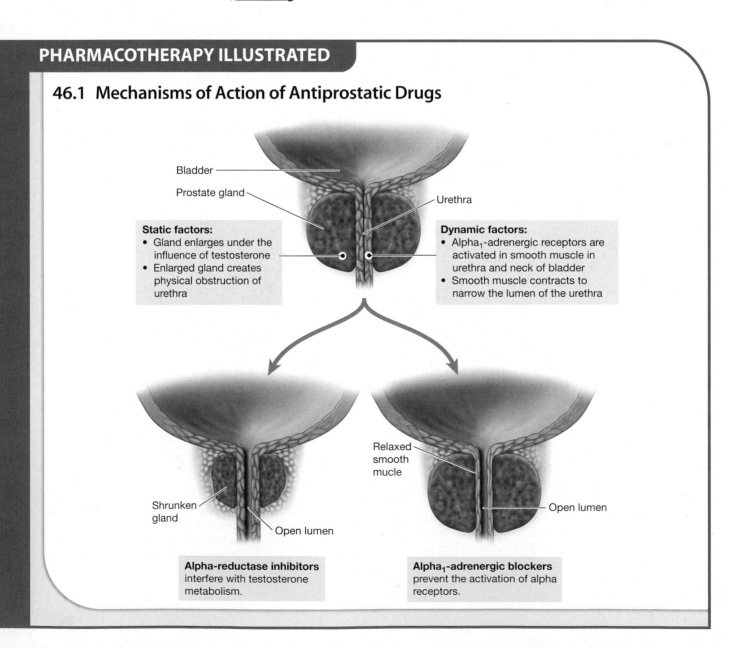

Bladder

Prostate gland

Urethra

Static factors:
- Gland enlarges under the influence of testosterone
- Enlarged gland creates physical obstruction of urethra

Dynamic factors:
- Alpha₁-adrenergic receptors are activated in smooth muscle in urethra and neck of bladder
- Smooth muscle contracts to narrow the lumen of the urethra

Shrunken gland

Open lumen

Relaxed smooth mucle

Open lumen

Alpha-reductase inhibitors interfere with testosterone metabolism.

Alpha₁-adrenergic blockers prevent the activation of alpha receptors.

phenylephrine, may activate alpha$_1$-adrenergic receptors in the bladder neck, causing restriction of urine flow. Drugs with anticholinergic side effects such as antihistamines, TCAs, or phenothiazines may also worsen symptoms. Testosterone and other anabolic steroids may increase prostate enlargement, worsening physical obstruction of the urethra. Drugs that worsen symptoms of BPH should be avoided in elderly men.

Clients who are asymptomatic or who present with mild symptoms generally do not receive pharmacotherapy. Not all BPH is progressive, and many clients never experience moderate or advanced symptoms. Client education such as avoiding caffeine or alcohol intake, eliminating drugs that worsen BPH, and restricting fluids close to bedtime may be sufficient to achieve symptomatic improvement. The client is reevaluated at 6- to 12-month intervals to assess for worsening symptoms.

When symptoms of BPH worsen, pharmacotherapy is indicated. Alpha$_1$-adrenergic blockers are often drugs of choice for treating moderate symptoms of BPH. The selective alpha$_1$-blockers relax smooth muscle in the prostate gland, bladder neck, and urethra, thus easing the urinary obstruction. Doxazosin (Cardura) and terazosin (Hytrin) are of particular value to clients who have both hypertension and BPH; these two disorders occur concurrently in about 25% of men older than 60. In 2005, an extended-release formulation of doxazosin (Cardura XL) was approved for clients with BPH. A third alpha$_1$-blocker,

tamsulosin (Flomax), has no effect on blood pressure, and its only indication is BPH. Drugs in this class improve urine flow and reduce other bothersome symptoms of BPH within 1 to 2 weeks after administration. Primary adverse effects include headache, fatigue, and dizziness. Doxazosin and terazosin are not associated with an increased risk of sexual dysfunction, but ejaculatory dysfunction has been reported with tamsulosin. Reflex tachycardia due to stimulation of baroreceptors is common with alpha-blockers. Additional information on the alpha-blockers and a prototype feature for doxazosin are presented in Chapter 23 ∞.

Some clients are unable to tolerate the cardiovascular side effects of the alpha$_1$-adrenergic blockers. For these clients, the 5-alpha-reductase inhibitors offer an alternative. These agents block an enzyme in the testosterone metabolic pathway, thus eliminating the hormonal signal for prostate growth. The most commonly prescribed drug in this class is finasteride (Proscar), which is featured as a prototype for BPH. These agents may take several months to shrink the size of the prostate; thus, they are not appropriate for severe disease. The 5-alpha-reductase inhibitors produce few side effects, although they can cause sexual dysfunction in some clients.

Antiprostatic drugs have limited efficacy and have value only in treating mild-to-moderate disease, as an alternative to surgery. Because pharmacotherapy alleviates the symptoms but does not cure the disease, these medications must

---

Pr PROTOTYPE DRUG | Finasteride (Proscar) | 5-alpha-reductase Inhibitor

ACTIONS AND USES

Finasteride acts by inhibiting 5-alpha-reductase, the enzyme responsible for converting testosterone to one of its metabolites, 5-alpha-dihydrotestosterone. This active metabolite causes proliferation of prostate cells and promotes enlargement of the gland. Because it inhibits the metabolism of testosterone, finasteride is sometimes called an *antiandrogen*. Finasteride promotes shrinkage of enlarged prostates and subsequently helps restore urinary function. It is most effective in clients with larger prostates. This drug is also marketed as Propecia, which is prescribed to promote hair regrowth in clients with male-pattern baldness. Doses of finasteride are five times higher when prescribed for BPH than when prescribed for baldness.

ADMINISTRATION ALERTS

- Tablets may be crushed for oral administration.
- The pregnant nurse or pharmacist should avoid handling crushed medication, as it may be absorbed through the skin and cause harm to a male fetus.

PHARMACOKINETICS

Onset: 3–6 min

Peak: 1–2 h

Half-life: 5–7 h

Duration: 5–7 days

ADVERSE EFFECTS

Finasteride causes various types of sexual dysfunction in up to 16% of clients, including impotence, diminished libido, and ejaculatory dysfunction.

Contraindications: The only contraindication is hypersensitivity to the drug.

INTERACTIONS

Drug–Drug: Use with anticholinergics may decrease the effects of finasteride.

Lab Tests: Values for DHT and prostate-specific antigen may be decreased. Testosterone levels may be increased.

Herbal/Food: Saw palmetto may potentiate the effects of finasteride.

Treatment of Overdose: There is no specific treatment for overdose.

be taken for the remainder of the client's life, or until surgery is indicated.

NURSING CONSIDERATIONS

The role of the nurse in drug therapy with antiprostatic agents for BPH involves careful monitoring of a client's condition and providing education as it relates to the prescribed drug treatment. Obtain a complete physical examination including history of cardiovascular disease and sexual dysfunction. The exam should include assessing changes in urinary elimination such as urine retention, nocturia, dribbling, difficulty starting urinary stream, frequency, and urgency. If alpha$_1$-adrenergic blockers are prescribed, assess vital signs, especially blood pressure and heart rate. The client may experience hypotension (first-dose phenomenon) with the initial doses, and orthostatic hypotension may persist throughout treatment. Syncope can occur. Monitor the client for evidence of orthostatic hypotension, dizziness, and GI disturbances. Elderly clients are especially prone to the hypotensive and hypothermic effects related to vasodilation caused by these drugs. Alpha-blockers should be used cautiously in clients with asthma or heart failure, because they cause bradycardia and bronchoconstriction.

Use cautiously in clients with decreased hepatic function, because the drugs are metabolized in the liver. Clients with obstructive uropathy should use finasteride cautiously. Monitor the emotional status of clients taking alpha-blockers, because depression is a common side effect. Inform the client that it may take 6 to 12 months of treatment before the maximum benefit from the drug is achieved. Improvement will last only as long as the medication is continued.

Monitor for side effects, including impotence, decreased volume of ejaculate, or decreased libido. Tell the client to report these occurrences to the healthcare provider.

Client Teaching. Client education as it relates to antiprostatic agents should include the goals of therapy; the reasons for obtaining baseline data such as vital signs, tests for cardiac and renal disorders, and the existence of underlying disorders such as asthma; and possible drug side effects. Include the following points when teaching clients about antiprostatic agents:

- Keep all scheduled laboratory visits to evaluate prostate-specific antigen (PSA) levels.
- Immediately report increased difficulty with urination, impotence, decreased libido, or decreased volume of ejaculate.
- Take medication at bedtime, and take the first dose immediately before getting into bed.
- Change positions slowly to prevent dizziness.
- Be aware that women of childbearing age (especially those who are pregnant or breast-feeding) should not touch this medication.
- Do not take any prescribed drugs, OTC medications, herbal remedies, or dietary supplements without notifying the healthcare provider.

NATURAL THERAPIES

Saw Palmetto

Saw palmetto (*Serona repens*) is a bushy palm that grows in the coastal regions of the southern United States. The portion used in supplements is the berries of the plant. More than 2 million men use saw palmetto in the hopes that it will treat BPH. Like finasteride, saw palmetto is thought to help stop a cascade of prostate-damaging enzymes that may create BPH. It also occupies binding sites on the prostate that are typically occupied by dihydrotestosterone (DHT), an enzyme that may trigger BPH. Although several clinical studies have suggested that saw palmetto is as effective as finasteride in treating mild to moderate BPH and produces fewer side effects, new research indicates that it has no benefit in treating BPH (Bent, Kane, et al., 2006).

Saw palmetto may cause damage to the liver and pancreas, so it is vital that the nurse obtain a thorough health and supplement use history, and advise the client of its potential adverse effects.

NURSING PROCESS FOCUS Clients Receiving Finasteride (Proscar)

Assessment	Potential Nursing Diagnoses
Prior to administration: ■ Obtain a complete health history including liver disease and altered urinary functioning. ■ Obtain a drug history to determine possible drug interactions and allergies. ■ Determine whether client has a female partner who is pregnant, is planning to become pregnant, or is breast-feeding.	■ Noncompliance, related to side effects of drug ■ Knowledge, Deficient, related to drug therapy ■ Sexual Dysfunction, related to adverse reaction to drug therapy

Planning: Client Goals and Expected Outcomes

The client will:
- Experience a decreased size of enlarged prostate gland.
- Demonstrate less frequency and urgency and greater force of urine stream.
- Demonstrate an understanding of the drug's action by accurately describing drug side effects and precautions.

NURSING PROCESS FOCUS Clients Receiving Finasteride (Proscar) *(Continued)*

Implementation

Interventions and (Rationales)	Client Education/Discharge Planning
▪ Monitor urinary function. (Finasteride may interfere with PSA test results.)	Instruct client to: ▪ Schedule a prostate and PSA test periodically during therapy. ▪ Recognize and report symptoms of BPH: urinary retention, hesitancy, difficulty starting stream, decreased diameter of stream, nocturia, dribbling, frequency. ▪ Avoid all fluids in the evening, especially caffeine-containing fluids and alcohol, to avoid nocturia. ▪ Drink adequate fluids early in the day to decrease chances of kidney stones and urinary tract infection (UTI).
▪ Monitor female partner for pregnancy. (Finasteride is teratogenic to the male fetus.)	Instruct female sexual partner to: ▪ Avoid semen of man using finasteride. ▪ Avoid touching crushed tablets of finasteride to prevent transdermal absorption and the transfer of medication through placenta to fetus. Instruct client and female sexual partner to: ▪ Use a reliable barrier contraceptive during therapy.
▪ Monitor client's commitment to the medication regimen. (Maximum therapeutic effects may take several months.)	Instruct client to: ▪ Continue medication even if there is no decrease in symptoms for 6 to 12 months, or no increase in hair growth for 3 months. ▪ Recognize that lifelong therapy may be necessary to control symptoms of BPH.
▪ Monitor for adverse reactions. (Adverse reactions may require review of medication by the healthcare provider.)	▪ Instruct client to report impotence, decreased volume of ejaculate, or decreased libido.

Evaluation of Outcome Criteria

Evaluate the effectiveness of drug therapy by confirming that client goals and expected outcomes have been met (see "Planning").
▪ The client exhibits a decreased size of enlarged prostate gland.
▪ The client reports less frequency and urgency, and greater force of urine stream.
▪ The client demonstrates an understanding of the drug's action by accurately describing drug side effects and precautions.

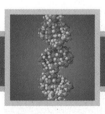

CHAPTER REVIEW

KEY CONCEPTS

The numbered key concepts provide a succinct summary of the important points from the corresponding numbered section within the chapter. If any of these points are not clear, refer to the numbered section within the chapter for review.

46.1 FSH and LH from the pituitary regulate the secretion of testosterone, the primary hormone contributing to the growth, health, and maintenance of the male reproductive system.

46.2 Androgens are used to treat hypogonadism in males, and breast cancer in females. Anabolic steroids are frequently abused by athletes, and can result in serious adverse effects with long-term use.

46.3 Male infertility is difficult to treat pharmacologically; medications include HCG, menotropins, testolactone, and antiestrogens.

46.4 Erectile dysfunction is a common disorder that may be successfully treated with sildenafil (Viagra), an inhibitor of the enzyme phosphodiesterase-5.

46.5 In its early stages, benign prostatic hyperplasia may be treated successfully with drug therapy, including finasteride (Proscar) and alpha₁-adrenergic blockers.

NCLEX-RN® REVIEW QUESTIONS

1 Which of the following nursing assessments would be appropriate for the client receiving testosterone? (Select all that apply.)

1. Monitor for a decrease in hematocrit (Hct).
2. Assess for signs of fluid retention.
3. Assess for increased muscle mass and strength.
4. Check for blood dyscrasias.
5. Assess for muscle wasting.

2 Which of the following nursing assessment findings may be evident in a client who has undergone testosterone therapy?

1. Virilization
2. Electrolyte imbalances
3. Hepatomegaly
4. Precocious puberty

3 The nurse assesses for which of the following medications that may predispose the client to erectile dysfunction?

1. Insulin
2. Nonsteroidal anti-inflammatory drugs (NSAIDs)
3. Phenothiazines
4. Oral hypoglycemics

4 Which of the following questions should the nurse ask prior to the administration of sildenafil (Viagra)?

1. "Are you currently taking medications for angina?"
2. "Do you have a history of diabetes?"
3. "Have you ever had an allergic reaction to dairy products?"
4. "Have you ever been treated for migraine headaches?"

5 The client with a history of BPH is complaining of feeling like he "cannot empty his bladder." The nurse anticipates that the healthcare provider will order what?

1. Tadalafil
2. Sildenafil
3. Testosterone
4. Finasteride (Proscar)

CRITICAL THINKING QUESTIONS

1. A 78-year-old widower has come to see his healthcare provider. The nurse practitioner interviews the client about his past medical history and current health concerns. The client states that he is planning to marry "a very nice lady," but is concerned about his sexual performance. He asks about a prescription for sildenafil (Viagra). What additional assessment data does the nurse need to collect given this client's age?

2. A 16-year-old adolescent goes out for the football team. He is immediately impressed with the size of several junior and senior linemen. One older student offers to "hook him up" with a source for androstenedione (Andro). From a developmental perspective, explain why this young man may be susceptible to anabolic steroid abuse. Can anabolic steroid abuse affect his stature?

3. A 68-year-old man has been diagnosed with BPH. As the nurse prepares to educate him about his prescription for finasteride (Proscar), he says that he has been hearing about the benefits of saw palmetto, an herbal preparation. Discuss the mechanism of action of finasteride and compare it with that of saw palmetto.

See Appendix D for answers and rationales for all activities.

EXPLORE MediaLink

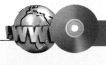 www.prenhall.com/adams

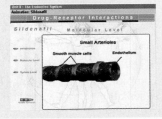

NCLEX-RN® review, case studies, and other interactive resources for this chapter can be found on the companion website at www.prenhall.com/adams. Click on "Chapter 46" to select the activities for this chapter. For animations, more NCLEX-RN® review questions, and an audio glossary, access the accompanying Prentice Hall Nursing MediaLink DVD-ROM in this textbook.

PRENTICE HALL NURSING MEDIALINK DVD-ROM

- **Animation**
  Mechanism in Action: Sildenafil (*Viagra*)
- **Audio Glossary**
- **NCLEX-RN® Review**

 COMPANION WEBSITE

- **NCLEX-RN® Review**
- **Dosage Calculations**
- **Case Study:** Client taking male hormones
- **Care Plan:** Client with erectile dysfunction taking sildenafil

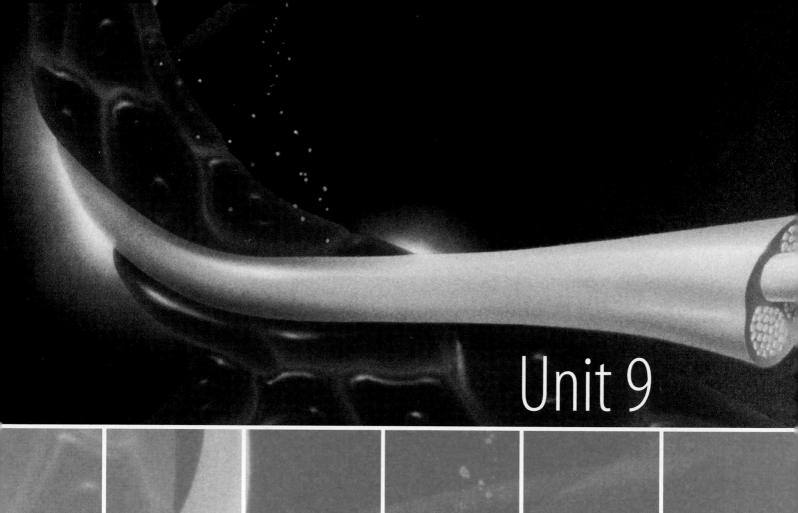

Unit 9

The Integumentary System and Eyes/Ears

CHAPTER 47   Drugs for Bone and Joint Disorders

CHAPTER 48   Drugs for Skin Disorders

CHAPTER 49   Drugs for Eye and Ear Disorders

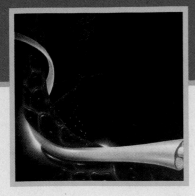

Drugs for Bone and Joint Disorders

DRUGS AT A GLANCE

DRUGS FOR CALCIUM-RELATED DISORDERS
Calcium Supplements
- *calcium gluconate (Kalcinate)*

Vitamin D Therapy
- *calcitriol (Calcijex, Rocaltrol)*

Bisphosphonates
- *etidronate disodium (Didronel)*

Selective Estrogen Receptor Modulators
- *raloxifene (Evista)*

Calcitonin
HORMONE-REPLACEMENT THERAPY
DRUGS FOR JOINT DISORDERS
DISEASE-MODIFYING ANTIRHEUMATIC DRUGS
- *hydroxychloroquine sulfate (Plaquenil Sulfate)*

URIC ACID INHIBITORS
- *colchicine*

OBJECTIVES

After reading this chapter, the student should be able to:

1. Identify major disorders, signs, and symptoms associated with an imbalance of calcium, vitamin D, parathyroid hormone, and calcitonin.
2. Discuss drug treatments for hypocalcemia, osteomalacia, and rickets.
3. Describe the nurse's role in the pharmacological management of disorders caused by calcium and vitamin D deficiency.
4. Identify important disorders characterized by weak, fragile bones and abnormal joints.
5. Explain nonpharmacological therapies used to treat bone and joint disorders.
6. Describe the nurse's role in the pharmacological management of disorders related to bones and joints.
7. For each of the drug classes listed in Drugs at a Glance, know representative drugs, and explain their mechanisms of action, primary actions, and/or important adverse effects.
8. Use the Nursing Process to care for clients receiving drug therapy for bone and joint disorders.

MediaLink

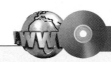

www.prenhall.com/adams

NCLEX-RN® review, case studies, and other interactive resources for this chapter can be found on the companion website at www.prenhall.com/adams. Click on "Chapter 47" to select the activities for this chapter. For animations, more NCLEX-RN® review questions, and an audio glossary, access the accompanying Prentice Hall Nursing MediaLink DVD-ROM in this textbook.

The skeletal system and joints are at the core of body movement. Disorders associated with bones and joints may affect a client's ability to fulfill daily activities and lead to immobility. In addition, the skeletal system serves as the primary repository for calcium, one of the body's most important minerals.

This chapter focuses on the pharmacotherapy of important skeletal and joint disorders such as osteomalacia, osteoporosis, arthritis, and gout. The importance of calcium balance and the action of vitamin D are stressed as they relate to the proper structure and function of bones.

47.1 Normal Calcium Physiology and Vitamin D

One of the most important minerals in the body responsible for bone formation is calcium. This major mineral constitutes about 2% of our body weight. Levels of calcium in the blood are controlled by two endocrine glands: the parathyroid glands, which secrete parathyroid hormone (PTH), and the thyroid gland, which secretes calcitonin, as shown in ● Figure 47.1.

PTH stimulates bone cells called *osteoclasts*. These cells accelerate the process of **bone resorption,** demineralization that breaks down bone into its mineral components. Once bone is broken down (resorbed), calcium becomes available to be transported and used elsewhere in the body. The opposite of this process is **bone deposition,** which is bone building. This process, which removes calcium from the blood to be placed in bone, is stimulated by the hormone calcitonin.

PTH and calcitonin control calcium homeostasis in the body by influencing three major targets: the bones, kidneys, and gastrointestinal (GI) tract. The GI tract is influenced mainly by parathyroid hormone and involves vitamin D. Vitamin D and calcium metabolism are intimately related: calcium disorders are often associated with vitamin D disorders.

Vitamin D is unique among vitamins because the body is able to synthesize it from precursor molecules. In the skin, **cholecalciferol,** the *inactive* form of vitamin D, is synthesized from cholesterol. Exposure of the skin to sunlight or ultraviolet light increases the level of cholecalciferol in the blood. Cholecalciferol can also be obtained from dietary products such as milk or other foods fortified with vitamin D. ● Figure 47.2 illustrates the metabolism of vitamin D.

Following its absorption or formation, cholecalciferol is converted to an intermediate vitamin form called **calcifediol.** Enzymes in the kidneys metabolize calcifediol to **calcitriol,** the *active* form of vitamin D. Parathyroid hormone stimulates the formation of calcitriol at the level of the kidneys. Clients with extensive kidney disease are unable to adequately synthesize calcitriol and thus frequently experience calcium and vitamin D abnormalities.

The primary function of calcitriol is to increase calcium absorption from the GI tract. Dietary calcium is absorbed more efficiently in the presence of active vitamin D and parathyroid hormone, resulting in higher serum levels of calcium, which is then transported to bone, muscle, and other tissues.

The importance of proper calcium balance in the body cannot be overstated. Calcium ion influences the excitability of all neurons. When calcium concentrations are too high (hypercalcemia), sodium permeability decreases across cell membranes. This is a dangerous state, because nerve conduction depends on the proper influx of sodium into cells. When calcium levels in the bloodstream are too low (hypocalcemia), cell membranes become hyperexcitable. If this situation becomes severe, convulsions or muscle spasms may result. Calcium is also important for the normal functioning of other body processes such as blood coagulation and muscle contraction. It is, indeed, a critical mineral for life.

KEY TERMS

acute gouty arthritis *page 746*

autoantibodies *page 746*

bisphosphonates *page 740*

bone deposition *page 733*

bone resorption *page 733*

calcifediol *page 733*

calcitonin *page 733*

calcitriol *page 733*

cholecalciferol *page 733*

disease-modifying antirheumatic drug (DMARD) *page 746*

gout *page 746*

hyperuricemia *page 746*

osteoarthritis (OA) *page 745*

osteomalacia *page 738*

osteoporosis *page 739*

Paget's disease *page 744*

rheumatoid arthritis (RA) *page 745*

selective estrogen receptor modulators (SERMs) *page 743*

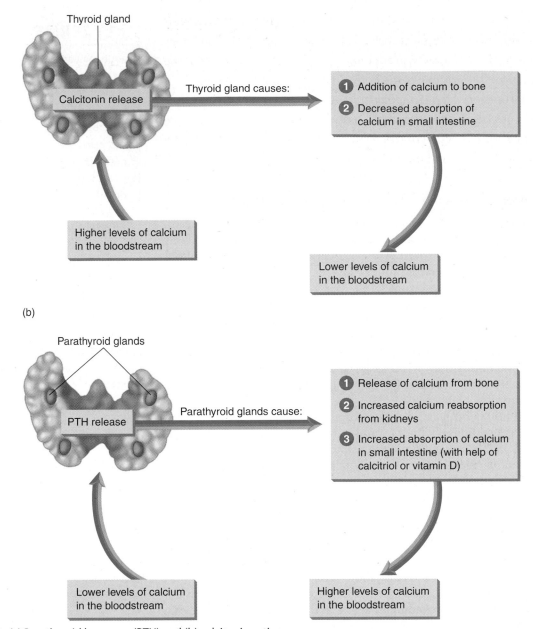

● **Figure 47.1** (a) Parathyroid hormone (PTH) and (b) calcitonin action

CALCIUM-RELATED DISORDERS

Diseases and conditions of calcium and vitamin D metabolism include hypocalcemia, osteomalacia, osteoporosis, and Paget's disease. Therapies for calcium disorders include calcium supplements, vitamin D supplements, bisphosphonates, and several miscellaneous agents.

47.2 Pharmacotherapy of Hypocalcemia

Hypocalcemia is not a disease but a sign of underlying pathology; therefore, diagnosis of the cause of hypocalcemia is essential. One common etiology is hyposecretion of PTH, as occurs when the thyroid and parathyroid glands are diseased or surgically removed. Digestive-related

malabsorption disorders and vitamin D deficiencies also result in hypocalcemia.

Signs and symptoms of hypocalcemia are those of nerve and muscle excitability. Muscle twitching, tremor, or cramping may be evident. Numbness and tingling of the extremities may occur, and convulsions are possible. Confusion and abnormal behavior may be observed.

Unless the hypocalcemia is life threatening, adjustments in diet should be attempted prior to initiating therapy with calcium supplements. Increasing the consumption of calcium-rich foods, especially dairy products, fortified orange juice, cereals, and green leafy vegetables is often sufficient to restore calcium balance.

If a change in diet is not practical or has not proved adequate, effective and inexpensive calcium supplements are readily available over the counter (OTC), in a variety of formulations. Calcium supplements often contain vitamin D.

Sources of Vitamin D

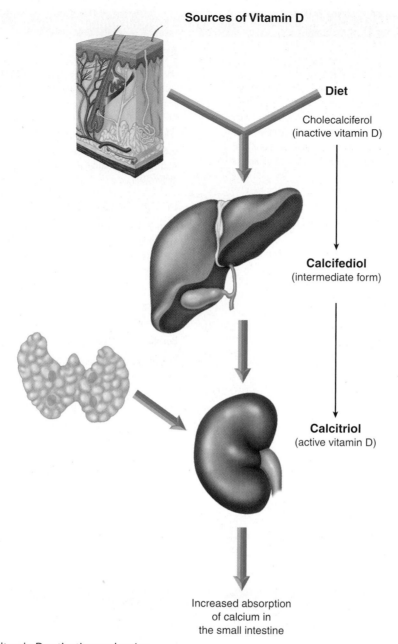

Diet

Cholecalciferol
(inactive vitamin D)

Calcifediol
(intermediate form)

Calcitriol
(active vitamin D)

Increased absorption
of calcium in
the small intestine

● **Figure 47.2** Pathway for vitamin D activation and action

Severe cases of hypocalcemia require IV administration of calcium salts.

Calcium has two major forms: complexed and elemental. Most calcium supplements are in the form of complexed calcium. These products are often compared on the basis of their ability to release elemental calcium into the bloodstream. The greater the ability of complexed calcium to release elemental calcium, the more potent is the supplement. Table 47.1 lists calcium supplements.

NURSING CONSIDERATIONS

The role of the nurse in calcium supplement therapy involves careful monitoring of a client's condition and providing education as it relates to the prescribed drug treatment. Assess for signs and symptoms of calcium imbalance. For

hypercalcemia, assess for drowsiness, lethargy, weakness, headache, anorexia, nausea, vomiting, thirst, and increased urination. Signs and symptoms to assess for hypocalcemia are facial twitching, muscle spasms, paresthesias, and seizures. Obtain baseline and periodic vital signs, serum calcium levels, and ECG to determine the effectiveness of the medication.

Obtain a thorough history to determine pregnancy or lactation, past medical history, and current medications including dietary supplements. A history of fracture should be investigated. Clients with osteoporosis sometimes experience fractures following minimal trauma, which may be the first indication of osteopenic problems. Calcium supplements are contraindicated in clients with a history of renal calculi, digoxin toxicity, dysrhythmias, or hypercalcemia.

Pr PROTOTYPE DRUG | Calcium Gluconate *(Kalcinate)* | Calcium Supplement

ACTIONS AND USES

Calcium gluconate and other calcium compounds are used to correct hypocalcemia, and for osteoporosis and Paget's disease. The objective of calcium therapy is to return serum levels of calcium to normal. People at high risk for developing these conditions include postmenopausal women, those with little physical activity over a prolonged period, and clients taking certain medications such as corticosteroids, immunosuppressive drugs, and some antiseizure medications. Calcium gluconate is available in tablets or as a 10% solution for IV injection.

ADMINISTRATION ALERTS

- Give oral calcium supplements with meals or within 1 hour following meals.
- Administer IV slowly to avoid hypotension, dysrhythmias, and cardiac arrest.
- Pregnancy category B.

PHARMACOKINETICS

Onset: Unknown

Peak: Unknown

Half-life: Unknown

Duration: Unknown

ADVERSE EFFECTS

The most common adverse effect of calcium gluconate is hypercalcemia, caused by taking too much of this supplement. Symptoms include drowsiness, lethargy, weakness, headache, anorexia, nausea and vomiting, increased urination, and thirst. IV administration of calcium may cause hypotension, bradycardia, dysrhythmias, and cardiac arrest.

Contraindications: Calcium salts are contraindicated in clients with ventricular fibrillation, metastatic bone cancer, renal calculi, or hypercalcemia.

INTERACTIONS

Drug–Drug: Concurrent use with digoxin increases the risk of dysrhythmias. Magnesium may compete for GI absorption. Calcium decreases the absorption of tetracyclines. May antagonize the effects of calcium channel blockers.

Lab Tests: May increase values for blood pH and serum calcium. May decrease serum phosphate and potassium levels, and serum and urinary magnesium.

Herbal/Food: Unknown.

Treatment of Overdose: Measures may be taken to treat cardiac abnormalities caused by the resulting hypercalcemia.

 See the Companion Website for a Nursing Process Focus specific to this drug.

Clients who are taking glucocorticoids for exacerbations of COPD or other conditions are more likely to develop a more brittle bone matrix. Other lifestyle patterns predispose individuals to develop a risk for brittle bone matrix (osteopenia and/or osteoporosis). Refer to Section 47.4 for risk factors for osteoporosis.

Lifespan Considerations. The normal bone matrix is formed by a cyclic process in which there is a balance between bone formation and resorption. Aging causes the bone matrix to gradually become more brittle. Although this occurs in both genders, the process is accelerated in women. Decreased estrogen levels in postmenopausal

TABLE 47.1	Calcium Supplements and Vitamin D Therapy	
Drug	**Route and Adult Dose (max dose where indicated)**	**Adverse Effects**
CALCIUM SUPPLEMENTS (ALL DOSES ARE IN TERMS OF ELEMENTAL CALCIUM.)		
calcium carbonate (BioCal, Calcite-500, others)	PO; 1–2 g bid–tid	*Constipation nausea, vomiting*
calcium chloride	IV; 0.5–1 g by slow infusion (1 ml/min) at 1–3 day intervals	Serious adverse effects are observed only with IV administration. Hypercalcemia (drowsiness, lethargy, headache, anorexia, nausea and vomiting, increased urination, and thirst), dysrhythmias, and cardiac arrest
calcium citrate (Citracal)	PO; 1–2 g bid–tid	
Pr calcium gluceptate	IV; 1.1–4.4 g/day; IM; 0.5–1.1 g/day	
calcium gluconate (Kalcinate)	PO; 1–2 g bid–tid	
calcium lactate	PO; 325 mg–1.3 g tid with meals	
calcium phosphate tribasic (Posture)	PO; 1–2 g bid–tid	
VITAMIN D SUPPLEMENTS		
Pr calcifediol (Calderol)	PO; 50–100 mcg/day or every other day	*Side effects are not observed at normal doses.*
calcitriol (Calcijex, Rocaltrol)	PO; 0.25 mcg/day	Overdose produces signs of hypercalcemia, bone pain, lethargy, anorexia, nausea and vomiting, increased urination, hallucinations and dysrhythmias.
ergocalciferol (Deltalin, Calciferol)	PO/IM; 25–125 mcg/day for 6–12 wk	

Italics indicate common adverse effects; <u>underlining</u> indicates serious adverse effects.

NURSING PROCESS FOCUS Clients Receiving Calcium Supplements

Assessment	Potential Nursing Diagnoses
Prior to administration: ■ Obtain a complete health history including allergies, drug history, signs of hypercalcemia or hypocalcemia, and possible drug interactions. ■ Obtain a baseline ECG. ■ Obtain baseline vital signs, especially apical pulse for rate and rhythm, and blood pressure. ■ Obtain lab work, includoing complete blood count (CBC) and electrolytes, especially calcium.	■ Injury, Risk for, related to loss of bone mass and side effects of drug ■ Knowledge, Deficient, related to drug therapy ■ Knowledge, Deficient, related to signs and symptoms to report to healthcare provider ■ Knowledge, Deficient, related to rationale for baseline data and subsequent laboratory data collection for optimal drug regimen

Planning: Client Goals and Expected Outcomes

The client will:
■ Have normal serum calcium levels (8.5–11.5 mg/dl).
■ Demonstrate an understanding of the drug's action by accurately describing drug side effects and precautions.
■ Immediately report side effects and adverse reactions.

Implementation

Interventions and (Rationales)	Client Education/Discharge Planning
■ Monitor electrolytes throughout therapy. (Calcium and phosphorus levels tend to vary inversely: low magnesium levels coexist with low calcium levels.)	■ Teach client importance of routine lab studies, so deviations from normal can be corrected immediately.
■ Monitor for signs and symptoms of hypercalcemia. (Overtreatment may lead to excessive serum calcium levels.)	■ Instruct client to report signs or symptoms of hypercalcemia: drowsiness, lethargy, weakness, headache, anorexia, nausea and vomiting, increased urination, and thirst.
■ Initiate seizure precautions for clients at risk for hypocalcemia. (Low calcium levels may cause seizures.)	■ Instruct client to recognize signs of hypocalcemia, such as facial twitching, muscle spasms, seizures, and paresthesias.
■ Monitor for musculoskeletal difficulties. (Calcium supplements are used to treat osteoporosis, rickets, and osteomalacia.)	Instruct client to: ■ Take special precautions to prevent fractures. ■ Report episodes of sudden pain, joints out of alignment, or inability of client to assume normal positioning.
■ Monitor intake and output. Use cautiously in client with renal insufficiency. (Calcium is excreted by the kidneys.)	■ Instruct client to report any difficulty in urination and to measure intake and output.
■ Monitor cardiac functioning. (Possible side effects may include short QT wave, heart block, hypotension, dysrhythmia, or cardiac arrest with IV administration.)	■ Inform client to recognize and report palpitations, light-headedness, dizziness, or shortness of breath.
■ Monitor injection site during intravenous administration for infiltration. (Extravasation may lead to necrosis.)	■ Instruct client to report pain at IV site.
■ Monitor diet. (Consuming calcium-rich foods may increase effect of drug. Consuming foods rich in zinc may decrease calcium absorption.)	■ Advise client to consume calcium-rich foods and avoid zinc-rich foods.

Evaluation of Outcome Criteria

Evaluate the effectiveness of drug therapy by confirming that client goals and expected outcomes have been met (see "Planning").
■ The client's calcium levels are normal.
■ The client demonstrates an understanding of the drug by accurately describing drug side effects and precautions.
■ The client accurately states signs and symptoms to be reported to the healthcare provider.

∞ *See Table 47.1 for a list of drugs for which these nursing actions apply.*

women cause an increase in osteoclasts, which causes increased resorption of bone. Thus, the bone mass and bone density are decreased, and bones become fragile. Decreased bone mass in men is typically related to decreased levels of testosterone.

Client Teaching.   Client education as it relates to calcium supplements or medications should include the goals of therapy, the reasons for obtaining baseline data such as vital signs and the existence of underlying cardiac and hepatic disorders, and possible drug side effects. Include the following points when teaching clients about calcium supplements or medications:

- Report drowsiness, fatigue, lethargy, headache, loss of appetite, nausea, vomiting, increased urination, thirst, facial twitching, weakness of an extremity, muscle spasms, or seizures.

- Immediately report nausea, vomiting, constipation, or difficulty urinating.

- Take precautions to prevent falls: make sure there are no loose rugs, keep hallways lighted, and use assistive devices such as canes or walkers.

- Exercise daily for optimal bone health and to prevent future complications.

- Consume calcium-rich foods such as salmon, milk, dairy products, dark green vegetables, and soybeans.

- Avoid or limit excessive intake of zinc-rich foods, which decrease the absorption of calcium. Zinc-enriched foods include nuts, legumes, seeds, sprouts, and tofu.

- Avoid or limit alcohol, caffeine, and carbonated beverages, because they affect the absorption of calcium.

- Avoid calcium antacids, because they may increase serum calcium to a harmful level.

47.3 Pharmacotherapy of Osteomalacia

Osteomalacia, referred to as *rickets* in children, is a disorder characterized by softening of bones without alteration of basic bone structure. The cause of osteomalacia and rickets is a lack of adequate vitamin D and calcium, usually as a result of kidney failure or malabsorption of calcium from the GI tract. Signs and symptoms include hypocalcemia, muscle weakness, muscle spasms, and diffuse bone pain, especially in the hip area. Clients may also experience pain in the arms, legs, and spine. Classic signs of rickets in children include bowlegs and a pigeon breast. Children may also develop a slight fever and become restless at night.

Tests performed to verify osteomalacia include bone biopsy, bone radiographs, computed tomography (CT) scan of the vertebral column, and determination of serum calcium, phosphate, and vitamin D levels. Many of these tests are routine for bone disorders and are performed as needed to determine the extent of bone health.

In extreme cases, surgical correction of disfigured limbs may be required. Drug therapy for children and adults consists of calcium supplements and vitamin D. Drugs used for these conditions are summarized in Table 47.1.

Inactive, intermediate, and active forms of vitamin D are available as medications. Clients' vitamin D needs vary depending on how much sunlight they receive. After age 70, the average recommended intake of vitamin D increases from 400 units/day to 600 units/day. In severe cases of malabsorption disorders, clients may receive 50,000 to 100,000 units/day. Because vitamin D is needed to absorb calcium from the GI tract, many supplements combine vitamin D and calcium into a single tablet.

Vitamin D is a fat-soluble vitamin that is stored by the body; therefore, it is possible to consume too much of this vitamin or to show signs of overdose from prescription medications. Excess vitamin D will cause calcium to leave bones and enter the blood. Signs and symptoms of hypercalcemia, such as anorexia, vomiting, excessive thirst, fatigue, and confusion may become evident. Kidney stones may occur, and bones may fracture easily.

NURSING CONSIDERATIONS

The role of the nurse in vitamin D therapy involves careful monitoring of a client's condition and providing education as it relates to the prescribed drug treatment. Obtain a thorough history to assess liver function, intake of fat-soluble vitamins, and current medications. Liver impairment and an accumulation of fat-soluble vitamins may cause toxicity. Assess sclera, skin pigment, bowel movements, and lab results for evidence of liver dysfunction. High levels of vitamin D may cause renal impairment. Obtain liver function tests and urinalysis to establish baseline data, and regularly monitor these values during the course of treatment.

Assess for adverse effects of vitamin D therapy, such as hypercalcemia, headache, weakness, dry mouth, thirst, increased urination, and muscular or bone pain. Monitor calcium, magnesium, and phosphate levels along with urinary calcium and phosphate levels during vitamin D therapy.

Lifespan Considerations.   Recent research has documented a global resurgence of rickets, a childhood disease caused by a deficiency of vitamin D. The promotion of breast-feeding over vitamin D–fortified formulas is thought to be responsible for part of the problem, particularly in mothers who are vitamin D deficient. In addition, the increased use of sunscreens to prevent skin cancer prevents the formation of adequate vitamin D. The replacement of vitamin D–fortified milk with carbonated beverages by children and teens also contributes to the possibility of rickets. Nurses need to emphasize the importance of including extra dietary vitamin D in children and pregnant women.

HOME & COMMUNITY CONSIDERATIONS

Accommodating Those With Bone and Joint Disorders

The American elderly population has increased and will continue to increase over the next decade. As a community, it is important that we accommodate those with bone and joint disorders. Such accommodations as handicapped and wheelchair-accessible sidewalks, bathrooms, and doorways are an issue a community must face now or in the near future, because this population will require assistance with mobility.

Pr PROTOTYPE DRUG | Calcitriol *(Calcijex, Rocaltrol)* | Vitamin D Therapy

ACTIONS AND USES

Calcitriol is the active form of vitamin D. It promotes the intestinal absorption of calcium and elevates serum levels of calcium. This medication is used in cases in which clients have impaired kidney function or have hypoparathyroidism. Calcitriol reduces bone resorption and is useful in treating rickets. The effectiveness of calcitriol depends on an adequate amount of calcium; therefore, it is usually prescribed in combination with calcium supplements. It is available as oral tablets and solutions, and by the IV route.

ADMINISTRATION ALERTS

- Protect capsules from light and heat.
- Pregnancy category C.

PHARMACOKINETICS (PO)

Onset: 2–6 h
Peak: 10–12 h
Half-life: 3–6 h
Duration: 3–5 days

ADVERSE EFFECTS

Side effects include hypercalcemia, headache, weakness, dry mouth, thirst, increased urination, and muscle or bone pain.

Contraindications: This drug should not be given to clients with hypercalcemia or with evidence of vitamin D toxicity.

INTERACTIONS

Drug–Drug: Thiazide diuretics may enhance effects of vitamin D, causing hypercalcemia. Too much vitamin D may cause dysrhythmias in clients receiving digoxin. Magnesium antacids or supplements should not be given concurrently owing to increased risk of hypermagnesemia.

Lab Tests: May increase serum cholesterol, phosphate, magnesium or calcium values; may decrease values for alkaline phosphatase.

Herbal/Food: Ingestion of large amounts of calcium-rich foods may cause hypercalcemia.

Treatment of Overdose: Measures may be taken to treat the resulting hypercalcemia.

 See the Companion Website for a Nursing Process Focus specific to this drug.

MediaLink Mechanism in Action: Calcitriol

Client Teaching. Client education as it relates to vitamin D supplements should include the goals of therapy, the reasons for obtaining baseline data such as vital signs and the existence of underlying cardiac and hepatic disorders, and possible drug side effects. Include the following points when teaching clients about vitamin D therapy:

- Consume dietary sources of vitamin D such as fortified milk, eggs, and fish.
- Take vitamin D as directed, because too much may cause toxic levels.
- Take vitamin D with meals to assist with absorption.
- Immediately report signs of excess vitamin D, such as fatigue, weakness, nausea, vomiting, and changes in the color and/or amount of urine.
- Report yellowing of the skin or whites of the eyes, pale bowel movements, and darkened urine.
- Spend at least 20 minutes/day in sunlight to provide enough vitamin D to prevent disease.
- Avoid alcohol and other hepatotoxic drugs while taking vitamin D.
- Report any changes to your current medications or dietary supplements to the healthcare provider.

47.4 Pharmacotherapy of Osteoporosis

Osteoporosis is the most common metabolic bone disease, responsible for as many as 1.5 million fractures annually. This disorder is usually asymptomatic until the bones become brittle enough to fracture or for a vertebrae to collapse. In some cases, a lack of dietary calcium and vitamin D contributes to bone deterioration. In other cases, osteoporosis is due to disrupted bone homeostasis. Simply stated, bone resorption outpaces bone deposition, and clients develop weak bones. The following are risk factors for osteoporosis:

- Postmenopause
- High alcohol or caffeine consumption
- Anorexia nervosa
- Tobacco use
- Physical inactivity
- Testosterone deficiency, particularly in elderly men
- Lack of adequate vitamin D or calcium in the diet
- Drugs such as corticosteroids, some anticonvulsants, and immunosuppressants that lower calcium levels in the bloodstream

The most common risk factor associated with the development of osteoporosis is the onset of menopause. When women reach menopause, estrogen secretion declines, and bones become weak and fragile. One theory to explain this occurrence is that normal levels of estrogen may limit the life span of osteoclasts, the bone cells that resorb bone. When estrogen levels decrease, osteoclast activity is no longer controlled, and bone demineralization is accelerated, resulting in loss of bone density. In women with osteoporosis, fractures often occur in the hips, wrists, forearms, or spine. The metabolism of calcium in osteoporosis is illustrated in ● Figure 47.3.

Many drug therapies are available for osteoporosis. These include calcium and vitamin D therapy, estrogen replacement

MediaLink National Osteoporosis Foundation

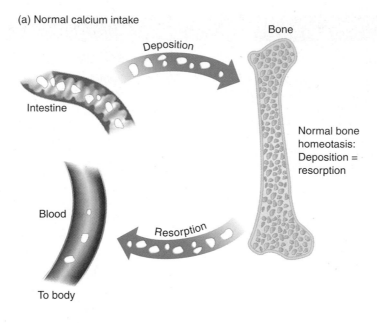

(a) Normal calcium intake

Deposition

Bone

Intestine

Blood

Resorption

To body

Normal bone homeotasis: Deposition = resorption

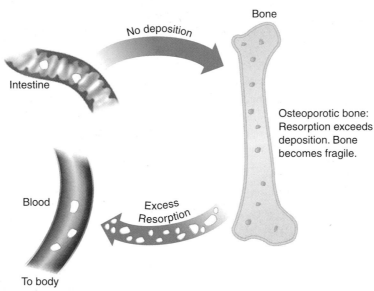

(b) Low calcium intake

No deposition

Bone

Intestine

Blood

Excess Resorption

To body

Osteoporotic bone: Resorption exceeds deposition. Bone becomes fragile.

● **Figure 47.3** Calcium metabolism in osteoporosis

therapy (ERT), estrogen receptor modulators, statins, slow-release sodium fluoride, bisphosphonates, and calcitonin. Teriparatide (Forteo) is a new drug for osteoporosis that is a structural analog of PTH, produced through recombinant DNA technology. Many of these drug classes are also used for other bone disorders or conditions unrelated to the skeletal system. Selected drugs for osteoporosis are listed in Table 47.2.

BISPHOSPHONATES

The most common drug class for treating osteoporosis is the **bisphosphonates.** These drugs are structural analogs of pyrophosphate, a natural substance that inhibits bone resorption. Bisphosphonates inhibit bone resorption by suppressing osteoclast activity, thus increasing bone density and reducing the incidence of fractures by about 50%. Examples include etidronate (Didronel), alendronate (Fosamax), tiludronate (Skelid), and pamidronate (Aredia), which is available as an injectable drug. Adverse effects include GI problems such as nausea, vomiting, abdominal

PHARMFACTS

Osteoporosis

- Osteoporosis is the most prevalent bone disorder in America.
- On a yearly basis, 28 million clients are either diagnosed with osteoporosis or considered to be at extreme risk for this disorder.
- Women are four times more likely to develop osteoporosis than men. Many women with osteoporosis are of postmenopausal age.
- After the age of 50, one of every two women and one of every eight men are likely to develop a fracture related to osteoporosis.

MediaLink Osteoporosis and Related Bone Diseases National Resource Center

TABLE 47.2   Selected Drugs for Osteoporosis

Drug	Route and Adult Dose (max dose where indicated)	Adverse Effects
HORMONAL AGENTS		
calcitonin—human (Cibacalcin)	Paget's disease: subcutaneous; human, 0.5 mg/day; subcutaneous/IM; salmon, 100 international units/day	*Nausea, inflammation at infection site, and flushing of face*
calcitonin—salmon (Calciman, Miacalcin)	Hypercalcemia: subcutaneous/IM; salmon, 4 international units/kg bid Osteoporosis: intranasal; 1 spray/day (200 international units)	<u>Anaphylaxis</u>
raloxifene hydrochloride (Evista)	PO; 60 mg/day	*Hot flashes, sinusitis, flulike symptoms, nausea* <u>Breast pain, vaginal bleeding, pneumonia, and chest pain</u>
teriparatide (Forteo)	Subcutaneous; 20 mcg/day	*Dizziness, depression, insomnia, vertigo, rhinitis, increased cough, leg cramps, nausea, and arthralgia* <u>Syncope, angina</u>
BISPHOSPHONATES		
alendronate sodium (Fosamax)	Osteoporosis treatment: PO; 10 mg/day Osteoporosis prevention: PO; 5 mg/day Paget's disease: PO; 40 mg/day for 6 mo	*Nausea, dyspepsia, diarrhea, bone pain, back pain*
etidronate disodium (Didronel)	PO; 5–10 mg/kg/day for 6 mo or 11–20 mg/kg/day for 3 mo	<u>Bone fractures, nephrotoxicity, hypocalcemia, hypophosphatemia, gastric ulcer, dysrhythmias (pamidronate)</u>
ibandronate (Boniva)	PO; 2.5 mg/day or one 150-mg tablet per mo, taken on the same date each mo	
pamidronate disodium (Aredia)	IV; 15–90 mg in 1,000 ml normal saline or D5W over 4–24 h	
risedronate sodium (Actonel)	PO; 30 mg/day at least 30 min before the first drink or meal of the day for 2 mo	
tiludronate disodium (Skelid)	PO; 400 mg/day taken with 6–8 oz of water 2 h before or after food for 3 mo	

Italics indicate common adverse effects; <u>underlining</u> indicates serious adverse effects.

Pr **PROTOTYPE DRUG** | Etidronate Disodium *(Didronel)* | Bisphosphonate

ACTIONS AND USES

Etidronate is a bisphosphonate that strengthens bones by slowing bone resorption. Effects appear 1 to 3 months after therapy starts and may continue for months after therapy is discontinued. This drug lowers serum alkaline phosphatase, the enzyme associated with bone turnover, without major adverse effects. Etidronate is also used for Paget's disease and to treat hypercalcemia due to malignancy. Both oral and IV forms available.

ADMINISTRATION ALERTS

- Take drug on an empty stomach 2 hours before a meal.
- Pregnancy category B (PO); C (parenteral).

PHARMACOKINETICS

Onset: 4 wk (PO); 24h (IV)

Peak: Unknown

Half-life: 6 h

Duration: Up to 1 y (PO); 10–12 days (IV)

ADVERSE EFFECTS

Side effects of etidronate are diarrhea, nausea, vomiting, GI irritation, and a metallic or altered taste perception. Pathological fractures may occur if the drug is taken longer than 3 months or in cases of chronic overdose. Rarely, high IV doses can cause nephrotoxicity.

Contraindications: Contraindications include clients with osteomalacia or who have hypersensitivity to the drug.

INTERACTIONS

Drug–Drug: Calcium, iron, antacids containing aluminum or magnesium, and certain mineral supplements interfere with the absorption of etidronate and have the potential to decrease its effectiveness.

Lab Tests: Unknown.

Herbal/Food: Food, especially milk and dairy products, interfere with absorption of the drug.

Treatment of Overdose: Hypocalcemia is an expected effect, and may be treated with oral or IV calcium compounds.

 See the Companion Website for a Nursing Process Focus specific to this drug.

NURSING PROCESS FOCUS Clients Receiving Bisphosphonates

Assessment	Potential Nursing Diagnoses
Prior to administration: ■ Obtain a complete health history including allergies, drug history, and possible drug interactions. ■ Assess for presence or history of pathological fractures, hypocalcemia, and hypercalcemia. ■ Assess nutritional status. ■ Obtain lab work to include CBC, pH, electrolytes and renal function studies [blood urea nitrogen (BUN), creatinine, uric acid], serum calcium, phosphorus, and magnesium levels.	■ Knowledge, Deficient, related to drug therapy ■ Fluid Volume, Imbalanced, Risk for, related to adverse reation to drug ■ Nausea, related to side effects of drug ■ Pain, Acute, Bone, related to adverse drug reaction ■ Therapeutic regimen management, Ineffective, related to the fact that therapeutic response may take 1–3 months

Planning: Client Goals and Expected Outcomes

Client will:
- Demonstrate decreased progression of osteoporosis or Paget's disease and is free of pathologic fractures.
- Demonstrate decreased risk for pathological fractures.
- Demonstrate an understanding of the drug's action by accurately describing drug side effects and precautions.
- Demonstrate an understanding of dietary needs and modifications.
- Maintain adequate fluid volume.

Implementation

Interventions and (Rationales)	Client Education/Discharge Planning
■ Monitor for pathological fractures and bone pain. (Drug may cause defective mineralization of newly formed bone.)	■ Instruct client to report any sudden bone or joint pain, inability to correctly position self, or swelling or inflammation over bone or joint.
■ Monitor for GI side effects. (There may be problems with absorption if client has persistent nausea or diarrhea.)	■ Advise client to immediately report new-onset nausea or diarrhea.
■ Monitor calcium lab values: Serum calcium levels should be 9–10 mg/dl. (Through inhibition of bone resorption, drug causes blood levels of calcium to fall.)	Advise client to: ■ Keep lab appointments for baseline and periodic testing. ■ Report symptoms of hypocalcemia (muscle spasms, facial grimacing, convulsions, irritability, depression, and psychoses). ■ Report symptoms of hypercalcemia (increased bone pain, anorexia, nausea/vomiting, constipation, thirst, lethargy, fatigue, confusion, and depression).
■ Monitor kidney function, especially creatinine level. (Etidronate cannot be used in clients whose creatinine level is greater than 5 mg/dl.)	■ Instruct client to report any urinary changes, such as decreased urine production or increased urination.
■ Monitor BUN, vitamin D, urinalysis, and serum phosphate and magnesium levels. (Bisphosphonates may cause renal dysfunction. Monitor for toxic vitamin D levels, and assess for decreased serum phosphate and magnesium levels.)	■ Instruct client to report any weakness, persistent headaches, dry mouth, thirst, increased urination, and muscle or bone pain.
■ Monitor dietary habits. (Diet must have adequate amounts of vitamin D, calcium, and phosphate.)	■ Instruct client to include dietary sources of vitamin D, calcium, and phosphate, including dairy products and green leafy vegetables.
■ Monitor compliance with recommended regimen. (Client may discontinue drug because of perceived lack of response.)	Advise client: ■ That therapy should continue for 6 months maximum, but full therapeutic response may take 1–3 months. ■ That effects continue several months after the drug is discontinued. ■ To avoid vitamins, mineral supplements, antacids, and high-calcium products within 2 hours of taking bisphosphonates.

Evaluation of Outcome Criteria

Evaluate the effectiveness of drug therapy by confirming that client goals and expected outcomes have been met (see "Planning").
- The client demonstrates decreased progression of osteoporosis or Paget's disease and is free of pathologic fractures.
- The client is free of pathological fractures.
- The client demonstrates an understanding of the drug's action by accurately describing drug side effects and precautions.
- The client verbalizes an understanding of dietary requirements and modifications.
- The client maintains adequate fluid intake.

∞ *See Table 47.2, under "Bisphosphonates," for a list of drugs to which these nursing actions apply.*

pain, and esophageal irritation. Because these drugs are poorly absorbed, they should be taken on an empty stomach, as tolerated by the client. Recent studies suggest that once-weekly dosing with bisphosphonates may give the same bone density benefits as daily dosing because of the extended duration of drug action.

NURSING CONSIDERATIONS

The role of the nurse in bisphosphonate drug therapy involves careful monitoring of a client's condition and providing education as it relates to the prescribed drug treatment. Obtain a thorough history to determine risk factors, past medical history (especially a history of fractures), GI conditions, and current medications and dietary supplements. Clients with preexisting vitamin D deficiency or hypocalcemia should be placed on supplements, and these conditions should be corrected prior to initiating bisphosphonate therapy. A complete physical examination should include complete blood count (CBC), pH, chemistry panel, renal and liver function studies, vital signs, and bone density studies such as a dual x-ray absorptiometry (DXA scan) to establish baseline data. Several months of bisphosphonate therapy are required to obtain desired effects.

Lifespan Considerations. Intravenous bisphosphonate therapy has been used in the treatment of osteogenesis imperfecta and hypercalcaemia in children with some success. However, the safety, effectiveness, and dosages of bisphosphonates in children have not been established, so they should be used with caution. Studies in animals show fetal and maternal abnormalities in bones and calcium metabolism; therefore, bisphosphonates should not be used in pregnant or lactating women.

Client Teaching. Client education as it relates to bisphosphonates should include the goals of therapy, the reasons for obtaining baseline data such as vital signs and the existence of underlying cardiac and hepatic disorders, and possible drug side effects. Include the following points when teaching clients about bisphosphonates:

- Immediately report seizures, muscle spasms, facial twitching, and paralysis of extremities.
- Report difficulty urinating, decreased urination, darkened urine, nausea, vomiting, diarrhea, or bone pain.
- Take medication on an empty stomach at least 30 minutes prior to eating, and sit upright during this time to ensure proper absorption of the medication.
- Eat calcium-rich foods such as dairy products, dark green vegetables, canned fish with bones such as salmon, and soybeans.
- Report pain, warmth, or inflammation over joints, or decreased activity.
- Participate in light exercise as often as possible.
- Keep all medications away from children and store as recommended by the manufacturer.

SELECTIVE ESTROGEN RECEPTOR MODULATORS

Selective estrogen receptor modulators (SERMs), a relatively new class of drugs that bind to estrogen receptors, are used in the prevention and treatment of osteoporosis. SERMs may be estrogen agonists or antagonists, depending on the specific drug and the tissue involved. For example, raloxifene (Evista) blocks estrogen receptors in the uterus and breast only; thus, it has no estrogen-like proliferative effects on these tissues that might promote cancer. Raloxifene does, however, decrease bone resorption, thus increasing bone density and reducing the likelihood of fractures. It is most effective at preventing vertebral fractures. Another SERM, tamoxifen, is used to treat breast cancer (see Chapter 37 ∞).

CALCITONIN

Calcitonin is a hormone secreted by the thyroid gland when serum calcium is elevated. As a drug, it is approved for the treatment of osteoporosis in women who are more than 5 years postmenopause. It is available by nasal spray or subcutaneous injection. Calcitonin increases bone density and reduces the risk of vertebral fractures. Side effects are generally minor; the nasal formulation may irritate the nasal mucosa, and allergies are possible. Because parenteral forms cause nausea and vomiting, they are rarely used. In addition to treating osteoporosis, calcitonin is indicated for Paget's disease and hypercalcemia. For osteoporosis, calcitonin is less effective than other therapies and is considered a second-line treatment.

HORMONE REPLACEMENT THERAPY

Until recently, hormone replacement therapy (HRT) with estrogen was one of the most common treatments for osteoporosis in postmenopausal women. HRT is very effective at reducing fractures due to osteoporosis. Unfortunately, because of increased risks of uterine cancer, thromboembolic disease, breast cancer, and other chronic disorders, the

SPECIAL CONSIDERATIONS

The Impact of Ethnicity and Lifestyle on Osteoporosis

Women of Caucasian and Asian American descent have a higher incidence of osteoporosis than those of African American descent, although postmenopausal women are at the highest risk in all ethnic groups. It is important to remember that men also can develop this disease.

Even though medications are available to halt bone deterioration, prevention by establishing and maintaining a healthy lifestyle is the key to conquering osteoporosis. During childhood and adolescence, the focus should be on building bone mass. Children should be encouraged to eat foods high in calcium and vitamin D, exercise regularly, and avoid smoking and excessive use of alcohol. During adulthood, the focus should be on maintaining bone mass and continuing healthy dietary and exercise habits. Vitamin supplements may be taken on the advice of the healthcare provider. Postmenopausal women should focus on preventing bone loss. In addition to maintaining a healthy lifestyle, clients should have bone density tests and should discuss the possibility of taking medication to prevent or treat osteoporosis with their healthcare provider.

Pr PROTOTYPE DRUG | Raloxifene *(Evista)* | Selective Estrogen Receptor Modulator

ACTIONS AND USES

Raloxifene is a selective estrogen receptor modulator (SERM). It decreases bone resorption and increases bone mass and density by acting through the estrogen receptor. Raloxifene is primarily used for the prevention of osteoporosis in postmenopausal women. This drug also reduces serum total cholesterol and LDL (low-density lipoprotein) without lowering HDL (high-density lipoprotein) or triglycerides.

ADMINISTRATION ALERTS

- Take drug exactly as prescribed.
- Give with or without food.
- Pregnancy category X.

PHARMACOKINETICS

Onset: Unknown

Peak: Unknown

Half-life: 27–33 h

Duration: Unknown

ADVERSE EFFECTS

Side effects are hot flashes, migraine headache, flulike symptoms, endometrial disorder, breast pain, and vaginal bleeding. Raloxifene may cause fetal harm when administered to a pregnant woman.

Contraindications: This drug is contraindicated during lactation and pregnancy, and in women who may become pregnant. Clients with a history of venous thromboembolism and those hypersensitive to raloxifene should not take this drug.

INTERACTIONS

Drug–Drug: Concurrent use with warfarin may decrease prothrombin time. Decreased raloxifene absorption will result from concurrent use with ampicillin or cholestyramine. Use of raloxifene with other highly protein-bound drugs (ibuprofen, indomethacin, diazepam, etc.) may interfere with binding sites. Clients should not take cholesterol-lowering drugs or estrogen replacement therapy concurrently with this medication.

Lab Tests: Increases values of apolipoprotein A_1, corticosteroid-binding globulin, and thyroxine-binding globulin. May decrease values of cholesterol, fibrinogen, apolipoprotein B, and lipoprotein (a), calcium, phosphate, total protein, and albumin.

Herbal/Food: Unknown.

Treatment of Overdose: There is no specific treatment for overdose.

 See the Companion Website for a Nursing Process Focus specific to this drug.

---

use of HRT in treating osteoporosis is no longer recommended. Additional information on HRT and the effects of estrogen may be found in Chapter 45 ∞.

47.5 Pharmacotherapy of Paget's Disease

Paget's disease, or *osteitis deformans,* is a chronic, progressive condition characterized by enlarged and abnormal bones. With this disorder, the processes of bone resorption and bone formation occur simultaneously, at a high rate. Excessive bone turnover causes the new bone to be weak and brittle; deformity and fractures may result. The client may be asymptomatic, or have only vague, nonspecific complaints for many years. Symptoms include pain of the hips and femurs, joint inflammation, headaches, facial pain, and hearing loss if bones around the ear cavity are affected. Nerves along the spinal column may be pinched because of compression between the vertebrae.

Medical treatments for osteoporosis are similar to those for Paget's disease. The cause of Paget's disease, however, is quite different. The enzyme alkaline phosphatase (ALP) is elevated in the blood because of the extensive bone turnover: the disease is usually confirmed by early detection of this enzyme in the blood. Calcium is also liberated because of its close association with phosphate. If diag-

nosed early enough, symptoms can be treated successfully. If the diagnosis is made late in the progress of the disease, permanent skeletal abnormalities may develop, and other disorders may appear, including arthritis, kidney stones, and heart disease.

Bisphosphonates are drugs of choice for the pharmacotherapy of Paget's disease. Therapy is usually cyclic, with bisphosphonates administered until serum ALP levels return to normal, followed by several months without the drugs. When the serum ALP level becomes elevated, therapy is begun again. The pharmacological goals are to slow the rate of bone reabsorption and encourage the deposition of strong bone. Calcitonin nasal spray is used as an option for clients who cannot tolerate bisphosphonates.

AVOIDING MEDICATION ERRORS

The evening nurse on duty administers medications at 10:15 P.M. When a nurse enters Ms. Brown's room, Ms. Brown is already in bed and falling asleep. The nurse gently shakes her and says, "I have your 10 P.M. medications, Ms. Brown." Although the client awakens, she is not fully awake. The nurse hands her the medication and a glass of water. Ms. Brown takes the medication and quickly returns to sleeping. In leaving, the nurse notices the room number and realizes that medication was just given to Ms. Crown, who is in a room down the hall from Ms. Brown. What should the nurse have done differently?

See Appendix D for the suggested answer.

Surgery may be indicated in cases of severe bone deformity, degenerative arthritis, or fracture. Clients with Paget's disease should maintain adequate dietary sources of calcium and vitamin D (or supplements) on a daily basis.

JOINT DISORDERS

Joint conditions such as osteoarthritis, rheumatoid arthritis, and gout are frequent indications for pharmacotherapy. Because joint pain is common to all three disorders, analgesics and anti-inflammatory drugs are important components of pharmacotherapy. A few additional drugs are specific to the particular joint pathology.

47.6 Pharmacotherapy of Osteoarthritis and Rheumatoid Arthritis

Arthritis is a general term meaning inflammation of a joint. There are several types of arthritis, each having somewhat different characteristics based on the etiology. Gouty arthritis is presented in Section 47.7.

Nonpharmacological therapies to alleviate the pain of arthritis are common. The use of nonimpact and passive range-of-motion (ROM) exercises to maintain flexibility along with rest is encouraged. Splinting may help keep joints positioned correctly and relieve pain. Other therapies commonly used to relieve pain and discomfort include thermal therapies, meditation, visualization, distraction techniques, and massage therapy. Knowledge of proper body mechanics and posture may offer some benefit. Surgical procedures such as joint replacement and reconstructive surgery may become necessary when other methods are ineffective.

Osteoarthritis

Osteoarthritis (OA), the most common type of arthritis, is due to excessive wear and tear of articular cartilage of the weight-bearing joints; the knee, spine, and hip are particu-

larly affected. Symptoms include localized pain and stiffness, joint and bone enlargement, and limitations in movement. OA is not accompanied by the degree of inflammation associated with other forms of arthritis. Many consider this condition to be a normal part of the aging process. A client with OA is shown in ● Figure 47.4.

The goals of pharmacotherapy for OA include reduction of pain and inflammation. Topical medications (capsaicin cream and balms), nonsteroidal anti-inflammatory drugs (NSAIDs, including aspirin), acetaminophen, COX-2 inhibitors, and tramadol (Ultram) are of value for treatment of OA pain. In acute cases, intra-articular glucocorticoids may be used on a temporary basis. Note that all these therapies are symptomatic; no drugs have been found that significantly modify the course of OA. The student should review Chapters 18 ∞ and 33 ∞ for a complete discussion of drugs for pain and inflammation.

A new type of drug therapy for clients with moderate OA who do not respond adequately to analgesics includes sodium hyaluronate (Hyalgan), a chemical normally found in high amounts within synovial fluid. Administered by injection directly into the knee joint, this drug replaces or supplements the body's natural hyaluronic acid that deteriorated because of the inflammation of osteoarthritis. Treatment consists of one injection per week for three to five injections. By coating the articulating cartilage surface, Hyalgan helps provide a barrier that prevents friction and further inflammation of the joint. Information given to the client prior to administration should include side effects such as pain and/or swelling at the injection site and the avoidance of any strenuous activities for approximately 48 hours after injection.

Rheumatoid Arthritis

Rheumatoid arthritis (RA) occurs at an earlier age than osteoarthritis and has an autoimmune etiology. It is characterized by disfigurement and inflammation of

---

PHARMFACTS

Arthritis

- Between 20 and 40 million people in the United States are affected by osteoarthritis.
- After age 40, more than 90% of the population have symptoms of osteoarthritis in major weight-bearing joints. After 70 years of age, almost all clients have symptoms of osteoarthritis.
- Of the world's population, 1% have rheumatoid arthritis, which most often affects clients between 30 and 50 years of age. Women are three to five times more likely to develop rheumatoid arthritis than men.
- Between 1% and 3% of the U.S. population are affected by gout. Most of the clients are men between the ages of 30 and 60. Most women are affected after menopause.

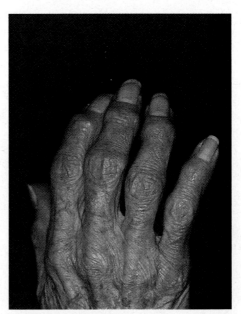

● **Figure 47.4** Client with osteoarthritis

multiple joints. In RA, **autoantibodies** called *rheumatoid factors* activate complement and draw leukocytes into the area, where they attack normal cells. This results in persistent injury and the formation of inflammatory fluid within the joints. Joint capsules, tendons, ligaments, and skeletal muscles may also be affected. Unlike OA, which causes local pain in affected joints, RA may produce systemic manifestations that include infections, pulmonary disease, pericarditis, abnormal numbers of blood cells, and symptoms of metabolic dysfunction such as fatigue, anorexia, and weakness. A client with RA is shown in ● Figure 47.5.

Pharmacotherapy for the symptomatic relief of RA includes the same classes of analgesics and anti-inflammatory drugs used for osteoarthritis. Because of their potent anti-inflammatory action, glucocorticoids may be used for RA flare-ups but are not used for long-term therapy because of their adverse effects.

Unlike with OA, the progression of RA can be modified with some drugs. These **disease-modifying antirheumatic drugs (DMARDs)** belong to several drug classes and have been found to reduce mortality due to RA. Most physicians begin therapy with a DMARD within the first few months after the onset of RA symptoms. Therapy often begins with hydroxychloroquine (Plaquenil), methotrexate (Rheumatrex), or sulfasalazine (Azulfidine), because these drugs have the most research-based evidence for reducing mortality. Gold salts, D-penicillamine (Cuprimine), azathioprine (Imuran), cyclosporine (Neoral), and cyclophosphamide (Cytoxan) have been used in the past but are more toxic than many other DMARDs. Biological agents such as etanercept (Enbrel), infliximab (Remicade), adalimumab (Humira), and anakinra (Kineret) are newer therapies that block steps in the inflammatory response. The biological agents appear to be effective and relatively nontoxic, although they are more expensive than first-line therapies.

DMARDs are administered after pain and anti-inflammatory medications have failed to achieve the desired treatment outcomes. Maximum therapeutic effects may take

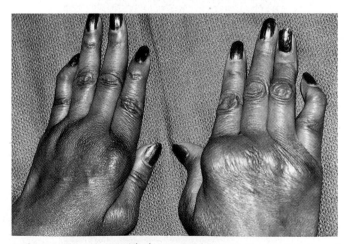

● **Figure 47.5** Client with rheumatoid arthritis *Source: Courtesy of Dr. Jason L. Smith.*

Glucosamine and Chondroitin for Osteoarthritis

Glucosamine is a natural substance that is an important building block of cartilage. With aging, glucosamine is lost with the natural thinning of cartilage. As cartilage wears down, joints lose their normal cushioning ability, resulting in the pain and inflammation of osteoarthritis. Glucosamine sulfate is available as an OTC dietary supplement. Some studies have shown it to be more effective than a placebo in reducing mild arthritis and joint pain. It is purported to promote cartilage repair in the joints. A typical dose is 500 to 10,000 mg/day.

Chondroitin is another dietary supplement purported to promote cartilage repair. It is a natural substance that forms part of the matrix between cartilage cells. Chondroitin is safe and almost free of side effects. A typical dose is 400 to 1,500 mg/day for 1–2 months. Chondroitin is usually combined with glucosamine in specific arthritis formulas. New research shows that glucosamine and chondroitin may be effective only for moderate to severe osteoarthritis pain (Clegg et al., 2006).

several months to achieve. Because many of these drugs can be toxic, clients must be closely monitored. These agents and their side effects are listed in Table 47.3.

47.7 Pharmacotherapy of Gout

Gout is a form of acute arthritis caused by an accumulation of uric acid (urate) crystals. These crystals are the result of increased metabolism of nucleic acids or the reduced excretion of uric acid by the kidneys. Uric acid is the final breakdown product of DNA and RNA metabolism. An important metabolic step in the pharmacotherapy of this disease is the conversion of hypoxanthine to uric acid by the enzyme xanthine oxidase.

In clients with gout, uric acid accumulates and **hyperuricemia,** an elevated blood level of uric acid, occurs. Clients with mild hyperuricemia may be asymptomatic. Once the level of uric acid rises to saturation levels in body fluids, urate crystals form and symptoms appear, usually with a sudden onset.

Gout may be classified as primary or secondary. Primary gout, caused by genetic errors in uric acid metabolism, is most commonly observed in Pacific Islanders. Secondary gout is caused by diseases or drugs that increase the metabolic turnover of nucleic acids, or that interfere with uric acid excretion. Examples of drugs that may cause gout include thiazide diuretics, aspirin, cyclosporine, and alcohol, when ingested on a chronic basis. Conditions that can cause secondary gout include diabetic ketoacidosis, kidney failure, and diseases associated with a rapid cell turnover such as leukemia, hemolytic anemia, and polycythemia.

Acute gouty arthritis occurs when needle-shaped uric acid crystals accumulate in joints, resulting in red, swollen, and inflamed tissue. Attacks have a sudden onset, often occur at night, and may be triggered by diet, injury, or other stresses. Gouty arthritis most often occurs in the big toes, heels, ankles, wrists, fingers, knees, or elbows. Of clients with gout, 90% are men.

TABLE 47.3   Selected Disease-modifying Antirheumatic Drugs

Drug	Route and Adult Dose (max dose where indicated)	Adverse Effects
GOLD AGENTS		
auranofin (Ridaura)	PO; 3–6 mg 1–2 times/day; may increase up to 3 mg tid after 6 mo	*Diarrhea, rash, abdominal cramping, nausea, stomatitis*
aurothioglucose (Gold thioglucose, Solganal)	IM; 10 mg on Week 1; 25 mg on Week 2; then 50 mg/wk to a cumulative dose of 1 g	
gold sodium thiomalate (Myochrysine)	IM; 10 mg on Week 1; 25 mg on Week 2; then 25–50 mg/wk to a cumulative dose of 1 g	<u>Blood dyscrasias, cholestatic jaundice, renal failure, exfoliative dermatitis, anaphylaxis</u>
OTHER ANTIRHEUMATIC AGENTS*		
anakinra (Kineret)	Subcutaneous; 100 mg/day	*Local reactions at injection site (pain, erythema, myalgia), headache* <u>Infections</u>
hydroxychloroquine sulfate (Plaquenil Sulfate)	PO; 400–600 mg/day	*Anorexia, nausea, vomiting, headache, and personality changes* <u>Retinopathy, agranulocytosis, aplastic anemia, seizures</u>
leflunomide (Arava)	PO; Loading dose: 100 mg/day for 3 days Maintenance dose: 10–20 mg/day	*Diarrhea, nausea, rash, alopecia, respiratory infection* <u>Stevens–Johnson syndrome, leucopenia, thrombocytopenia</u>
methotrexate (Folex, Mexate, Rheumatrex) (see page 562 for the Prototype Drug box ∞)	PO; 2.5–5 mg q12h for 3 doses each week	*Headache, glossitis, gingivitis, mild leukopenia, nausea* <u>Ulcerative stomatitis, myelosuppression, aplastic anemia, hepatic cirrhosis, nephrotoxicity, sudden death, pulmonary fibrosis</u>
penicillamine (Cuprimine, Depen)	PO; 125–250 mg/day (max: 1–1.5 g/day)	*Nausea, vomiting, reduced taste perception, metallic taste, proteinuria, pruritus, rashes* <u>Agranulocytosis, hemolytic anemia, aplastic anemia</u>
sulfasalazine (Azulfidine)	PO; 250–500 mg/day (max: 8 g/day)	*Headache, anorexia, nausea, and vomiting* <u>Anaphylaxis, Stevens–Johnson syndrome, agranulocytosis, leukopenia</u>

*Doses for immunosuppressants and biological agents are found in Chapter 32 ∞ .
Italics indicate common adverse effects; <u>underlining</u> indicates serious adverse effects.

The goals of gout pharmacotherapy are twofold: termination of acute attacks and prevention of future attacks. NSAIDs are the drugs of choice for treating the pain and inflammation of acute attacks. Indomethacin (Indocin) is a NSAID that has been widely used for acute gout, although the COX-2 inhibitors are also prescribed.

Uric acid inhibitors such as colchicine, probenecid (Benemid), sulfinpyrazone (Anturane), and allopurinol (Lopurin) are also used for acute gout. Uric acid inhibitors block the accumulation of uric acid in the blood or uric acid crystals within the joints. When uric acid accumulation is blocked, symptoms associated with gout diminish. About 80% of the clients using uric acid inhibitors experience GI complaints such as abdominal cramping, nausea, vomiting, and/or diarrhea. Glucocorticoids are useful for the short-term therapy of acute gout, particularly when the symptoms are in a single joint, and the medication is delivered intra-articularly. These agents are summarized in Table 47.4.

Prophylaxis of gout includes dietary management, avoidance of drugs that worsen the condition, and treatment with antigout medications. Clients should avoid high-purine foods such as meat, legumes, alcoholic beverages, mushrooms, and oatmeal, because nucleic acids will be formed when they are metabolized. Prophylactic therapy includes drugs that lower serum uric acid. Probenecid and

Pr PROTOTYPE DRUG | Hydroxychloroquine Sulfate *(Plaquenil)* | Disease-modifying Antirheumatic Drug

ACTIONS AND USES

Hydroxychloroquine is prescribed for rheumatoid arthritis and lupus erythematosus in clients who have not responded well to other anti-inflammatory drugs. This agent relieves the severe inflammation characteristic of these disorders, although its mechanism of action is not known. For full effectiveness, hydroxychloroquine is most often prescribed with salicylates and glucocorticoids. This drug is also used for prophylaxis and treatment of malaria (Chapter 35 ∞).

ADMINISTRATION ALERTS

- Take at the same time every day.
- Administer with milk to decrease GI upset.
- Store drug in safe place, as it is very toxic to children.
- Pregnancy category C.

PHARMACOKINETICS

Onset: Unknown
Peak: 1–2 h
Half-life: 70–120 h
Duration: Unknown

ADVERSE EFFECTS

Side effects include anorexia, GI disturbances, loss of hair, headache, and mood and mental changes. Possible ocular effects include blurred vision, photophobia, diminished ability to read, and blacked-out areas in the visual field. With high doses or prolonged therapy, these retinal changes may be irreversible in some clients.

Contraindications: Clients hypersensitive to the drug or who exhibit retinal or visual field changes associated with quinoline drugs should not receive hydroxychloroquine.

INTERACTIONS

Drug–Drug: Antacids containing aluminum or magnesium may prevent absorption of hydroxychloroquine. Hydroxychloroquine may increase the risk of liver toxicity when administered with hepatotoxic drugs; alcohol use should be eliminated during therapy. This drug also may lead to increased digoxin levels, and may interfere with the client's response to rabies vaccine.

Lab Tests: Unknown.

Herbal/Food: Unknown.

Treatment of Overdose: Overdose may be life threatening, especially in children. Therapy with anticonvulsants, vasopressors, and antidysrhythmics may be necessary.

 See the Companion Website for a Nursing Process Focus specific to this drug.

sulfinpyrazone are uricosuric drugs that increase the excretion of uric acid by blocking its reabsorption in the kidney. Allopurinol blocks xanthine oxidase, thus inhibiting the formation of uric acid. Prophylactic therapy is used for clients who suffer frequent and acute gout attacks. Drugs for gout are listed in Table 47.4.

NURSING CONSIDERATIONS

The role of the nurse in drug therapy with antigout medications involves careful monitoring of a client's condition and providing education as it relates to the prescribed drug treatment. Obtain a thorough health history including current

TABLE 47.4 Uric Acid–inhibiting Drugs for Gout and Gouty Arthritis

Drug	Route and Adult Dose (max dose where indicated)	Adverse Effects
allopurinol (Lopurin, Zyloprim)	PO (primary); 100 mg/day; may increase by 100 mg/wk (max: 800 mg/day) PO (secondary); 200–800 mg/day for 2–3 days or longer	*Drowsiness, skin rash, diarrhea* Severe skin reactions, bone marrow depression, hepatotoxicity, renal failure
colchicine	PO; 0.5–1.2 mg, followed by 0.5–0.6 mg q1–2h until pain is relieved (max: 4 mg/attack)	*Nausea, vomiting, diarrhea, and GI upset* Bone marrow depression, aplastic anemia, leucopenia, thrombocytopenia and agranulocytosis, severe diarrhea, nephrotoxicity
probenecid (Benemid, Probalan)	PO; 250 mg bid for 1 wk, then 500 mg bid (max: 3 g/day)	*Nausea, vomiting, headache, anorexia, flushed face* Anaphylaxis, severe skin reactions, hepatotoxicity
sulfinpyrazone (Anturane)	PO; 100–200 mg bid for 1 wk, then increase to 200–400 mg bid	*GI distress, rash* Blood dyscrasias, nephrolithiasis

Italics indicate common adverse effects; underlining indicates serious adverse effects.

Pr PROTOTYPE DRUG | Colchicine | Uric Acid Inhibitor

ACTIONS AND USES

Colchicine is a natural product obtained from the autumn crocus, which is grown in gardens and found in meadows throughout the United States and Canada. The drug reduces inflammation associated with acute gouty arthritis by inhibiting the synthesis of microtubules, subcellular structures responsible for helping white blood cells infiltrate an area. Although colchicine has no analgesic properties, clients experience pain relief owing to the reduction in inflammation. It may be taken to prevent or treat acute gout, often in combination with other uric acid-inhibiting agents.

ADMINISTRATION ALERTS

- Take on an empty stomach, when symptoms first appear.
- Pregnancy category C. Parenteral doses must not be given to pregnant women.

PHARMACOKINETICS

Onset: Unknown

Peak: 0.5–2 h

Half-life: 20 min

Duration: Unknown

ADVERSE EFFECTS

Side effects such as nausea, vomiting, diarrhea, and GI upset are more likely to occur at the beginning of therapy. The drug may cause bone marrow toxicity, and aplastic anemia, leucopenia, thrombocytopenia, or agranulocytosis may occur. Colchicine may also directly interfere with the absorption of vitamin B_{12}.

Contraindications: This drug is contraindicated in clients with a known hypersensitivity to colchicine, and in those with serious GI, renal, hepatic, or cardiac impairment. Clients with blood dyscrasias should not receive colchicine.

INTERACTIONS

Drug–Drug: Concurrent use with NSAIDs may increase the risk of GI symptoms. Colchicine may exhibit additive bone marrow toxicity with cyclosporine, phenylbutazone, and other drugs that adversely affect bone marrow. Erythromycin may increase serum colchicine levels. Loop diuretics may decrease colchicine effects. Alcohol or products that contain alcohol may cause skin rashes and result in additive liver damage. Colchicine may increase sensitivity to CNS depressants.

Lab Tests: May interefere with urinary steroid determinations; may give false positive values for urinary erythrocytes and Hgb.

Herbal/Food: Unknown.

Treatment of Overdose: Overdoses (including accidental ingestion of autumn crocus) may cause severe GI distress, shock, paralysis, delirium, respiratory failure, and death.

NURSING PROCESS FOCUS   Clients Receiving Colchicine

Assessment	Potential Nursing Diagnoses
Prior to administration: - Obtain a complete health history including allergies, drug history, and possible drug interactions. - Obtain baseline vital signs. - Obtain lab work to include complete blood count (CBC), platelets, uric acid levels, renal and liver function tests, and urinalysis.	- Activity Intolerance, related to joint pain - Body Image, Disturbed, related to joint swelling - Knowledge, Deficient, related to effects and side effects of drug therapy

Planning: Client Goals and Expected Outcomes

The client will:
- Report a decrease in pain and an increase in function in affected joints.
- Demonstrate an understanding of the drug's action by accurately describing drug side effects and precautions.
- Immediately report side effects and adverse reactions.

Implementation

Interventions and (Rationales)	Client Education/Discharge Planning
- Monitor lab results throughout therapy and perform a Coombs' test for hemolytic anemia. (Agranulocytosis, aplastic anemia, and thrombocytopenia may occur.)	- Teach client importance of routine lab studies, so that deviations from normal can be corrected immediately.
- Monitor for signs of toxicity. (This will evaluate therapeutic drug regimen and prevent complications.)	- Instruct client to report weakness, abdominal pain, nausea, and/or diarrhea.
- Monitor for signs of renal impairment such as oliguria. Record intake and output. (Monitoring allows prevention of renal complications.)	- Instruct client to report a decrease in urine output and to increase fluid intake to 3–4 L/day.

(Continued)

NURSING PROCESS FOCUS Clients Receiving Colchicine (Continued)

Implementation

Interventions and (Rationales)	Client Education/Discharge Planning
▪ Ensure that medication is administered correctly. (Effectiveness of drug regimen and prevention of complications depends on compliance.)	▪ Inform client to take medication on an empty stomach. Medication should be taken at first sign of gout attack.
▪ Monitor for pain and mobility. (This monitoring assesses effectiveness of medication.)	▪ Teach client to report an increase or decrease in discomfort and swelling.

Evaluation of Outcome Criteria

Evaluate the effectiveness of drug therapy by confirming that client goals and expected outcomes have been met (see "Planning").

▪ The client reports a decrease in pain and an increase in function of affected joints.

▪ The client demonstrates an understanding of the drug's actions by accurately describing drug side effects and precautions.

▪ The client accurately states signs and symptoms to report to the healthcare provider.

medications, vital signs, a complete physical examination, and CBC, platelets, liver and renal function studies, uric acid levels, and urinalysis. These tests should be established as baseline data and performed periodically during the course of treatment to assess the effectiveness of the drug.

Lifespan Considerations. Children have low blood levels of uric acid. Unless there is a rare inherited disorder, gout in children is rare. Children who are obese may be at risk for developing gout in adulthood. Pediatric dosing with antigout medications has not been established. The literature has identified that use of antigout medications in children may suppress growth; thus, drugs should be used cautiously in young clients.

Client Teaching. Client education as it relates to antigout medications should include the goals of therapy, the reasons for obtaining baseline data such as vital signs and the existence of underlying cardiac and hepatic disorders, and

possible drug side effects. Include the following points when teaching clients about antigout medications:

- Take the medications as ordered.
- Report rash, headache, anorexia, lower back pain, painful urination, blood in the urine, and decreased urine output.
- Increase your fluid intake to 3 to 4 L/day.
- Avoid alcohol use.
- Limit foods that cause the urine to become more alkaline, leading to kidney stones: milk, fruits, carbonated drinks, most vegetables, molasses, and baking soda.
- Avoid taking aspirin and large doses of vitamin C, because they enhance kidney stone formation.
- Practice reliable contraception and notify your healthcare provider if pregnancy is planned or suspected.

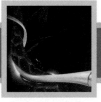

CHAPTER REVIEW

KEY CONCEPTS

The numbered key concepts provide a succinct summary of the important points from the corresponding numbered section within the chapter. If any of points these are not clear, refer to the numbered section within the chapter for review.

47.1 Adequate levels of calcium in the body are necessary to properly transmit nerve impulses, prevent muscle spasms, and provide stability and movement. Adequate levels of vitamin D, parathyroid hormone, and calcitonin are also necessary for these functions.

47.2 Hypocalcemia is a serious condition that requires immediate therapy with calcium supplements, often concurrently with vitamin D.

47.3 Pharmacotherapy of osteomalacia includes calcium and vitamin D supplements.

47.4 Pharmacotherapy of osteoporosis includes bisphosphonates, estrogen modulator drugs, and calcitonin.

47.5 Pharmacotherapy of clients with Paget's disease includes bisphosphonates and calcitonin.

47.6 For osteoarthritis, the main drug therapy is pain medication that includes aspirin, acetaminophen, NSAIDs, COX-2 inhibitors, or stronger analgesics. Drug therapy for rheumatoid arthritis includes analgesics, anti-inflammatory drugs, glucocorticoids, and disease-modifying antirheumatic drugs.

47.7 Gout is characterized by a buildup of uric acid in either the blood or the joint cavities. Drug therapy includes agents that inhibit uric acid buildup or enhance its excretion.

NCLEX-RN® REVIEW QUESTIONS

1 The nurse completing a physical exam on a child diagnosed with osteomalacia would expect to find:

1. Bowlegs and a pigeon breast.
2. Deformities of the fingers and toes.
3. Shortness of breath.
4. The use of crutches for walking.

2 The client's calcium level is reported as 5.6 mg/dl. The nurse should assess the client for:

1. Headache.
2. Anorexia.
3. Muscles spasms.
4. Drowsiness.

3 The client receiving allopurinol (Lopurin) for treatment of gout asks why he should avoid consumption of alcohol. The nurse's response is based on the knowledge that alcohol:

1. Causes liver damage.
2. Interferes with the absorption of antigout medications.
3. Raises uric acid levels.
4. Causes the urine to become more alkaline.

4 The client is admitted with a diagnosis of hypercalcemia. The nurse would assess for which of the following? (Select all that apply.)

1. Cardiac dysrhythmias
2. Fatigue
3. Bone fractures
4. Increased muscle strength
5. Hunger

5 Sodium hyaluronate (Hyalgan) is prescribed for a client with osteoarthritis. The nurse explains this drug will be administered by which method?

1. Intramuscularly
2. Directly into the joint
3. Intravenously
4. Subcutaneously

CRITICAL THINKING QUESTIONS

1. A young woman calls the triage nurse in her healthcare provider's office with questions concerning her mother's medication. The mother, age 76, has been taking alendronate (Fosamax) after a bone-density study revealed a decrease in bone mass. The daughter is worried that her mother may not be taking the drug correctly and asks for information to minimize the potential for drug side effects. What information should the triage nurse incorporate in a teaching plan regarding the oral administration of alendronate?

2. A community health nurse has decided to discuss the benefits of oral calcium supplements with an 82-year-old female client. The client had a stroke 6 years ago and requires help with most activities of daily living. Since her husband's death 18 months ago, she rarely leaves home. She has lost 25 pounds because she "just can't get interested" in her meals. She refuses to drink milk. What considerations must the nurse make before recommending calcium supplementation?

3. A 36-year-old man comes to the emergency department complaining of severe pain in the first joint of his right big toe. The triage nurse inspects the toe and notes that the joint is red, swollen, and extremely tender. Recognizing this as a typical presentation for acute gouty arthritis, what historical data should the nurse obtain relevant to this disease process?

See Appendix D for answers and rationales for all activities.

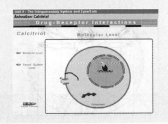

EXPLORE MediaLink

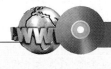

www.prenhall.com/adams

NCLEX-RN® review, case studies, and other interactive resources for this chapter can be found on the companion website at www.prenhall.com/adams. Click on "Chapter 47" to select the activities for this chapter. For animations, more NCLEX-RN® review questions, and an audio glossary, access the accompanying Prentice Hall Nursing MediaLink DVD-ROM in this textbook.

PRENTICE HALL NURSING MEDIALINK DVD-ROM

- **Animation**
  Mechanism in Action: Calcitriol (*Galcijet, Rocatrol*)
- **Audio Glossary**
- **NCLEX-RN® Review**

 COMPANION WEBSITE

- **NCLEX-RN® Review**
- **Dosage Calculations**
- **Case Study:** Drug therapy for arthritis
- **Care Plan:** Client at risk for osteoporosis prescribed raloxifene

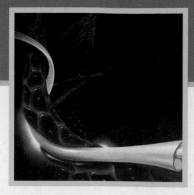

CHAPTER 48

Drugs for Skin Disorders

DRUGS AT A GLANCE

ANTI-INFECTIVES
Antibacterials, Antifungals, and Antivirals
Antiparasitics
Scabicides
 lindane (Kwell)
Pediculicides
DRUGS FOR SUNBURN AND OTHER MINOR BURNS
Local Anesthetics
 benzocaine (Solarcaine, others)
DRUGS FOR ACNE AND ROSACEA
Benzoyl Peroxide
Retinoids
 isotretinoin/13-cis-retinoic acid (Accutane)
Antibiotics
DRUGS FOR DERMATITIS
Topical Glucocorticoids
DRUGS FOR PSORIASIS
Topical Glucocorticoids
Topical Immunomodulators
Systemic Agents

OBJECTIVES

After reading this chapter, the student should be able to:

1. Identify the skin layers and associated structures.
2. Explain the process by which superficial skin cells are replaced.
3. Identify important drug therapies for bacterial, fungal, or viral infections; mite and lice infestations; sunburn; acne vulgaris; rosacea; dermatitis; and psoriasis.
4. Describe the nurse's role in the pharmacological management of skin disorders.
5. For each of the classes listed in Drugs at a Glance, know representative drugs, and explain the mechanisms of drug action, primary actions, and important adverse effects.
6. Use the Nursing Process to care for clients who are receiving drug therapy for skin disorders.

MediaLink

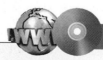

www.prenhall.com/adams

KEY TERMS

acne vulgaris *page 761*

comedone *page 761*

dermatitis *page 765*

eczema *page 765*

erythema *page 754*

excoriation *page 765*

keratolytic *page 761*

nits *page 756*

pediculicides *page 757*

pruritus *page 753*

psoralen *page 768*

retinoid *page 762*

rhinophyma *page 761*

rosacea *page 761*

scabicides *page 757*

seborrhea *page 761*

vitiligo *page 753*

The integumentary system consists of the skin, hair, nails, sweat glands, and oil glands. The largest and most visible of all organs, the skin normally provides an effective barrier between the outside environment and the body's internal organs. At times, however, external conditions become too extreme, or conditions within the body change, resulting in unhealthy skin. When this occurs, pharmacotherapy may be utilized to improve the skin's condition. The purpose of this chapter is to examine the broad scope of skin disorders and the drugs used for skin pharmacotherapy.

48.1 Structure and Function of the Skin

To understand the actions of dermatologic drugs, it is necessary to have a thorough knowledge of skin structure. The skin comprises three primary layers: the epidermis, dermis, and subcutaneous layer. The epidermis is the visible, outermost layer that constitutes only about 5% of the skin depth. The middle layer is the dermis, which accounts for about 95% of the entire skin thickness. The subcutaneous layer lies beneath the dermis. Some textbooks consider the subcutaneous layer as being separate from the skin, and not one of its layers.

Each layer of skin is distinct in form and function and provides the basis for how drugs are injected or topically applied (Chapter 4 ∞). The epidermis has either four or five sublayers depending on its thickness. The five layers from the innermost to outermost are *stratum basale* (also referred to as the *stratum germinativum*), *stratum spinosum*, *stratum granulosum*, *stratum lucidum*, and the strongest layer, the *stratum corneum*. The stratum corneum is referred to as the *horny layer* because of the abundance of the protein keratin, which is also found in the hair, hooves, and horns of many mammals. Keratin forms a barrier that repels bacteria and foreign matter, and most substances cannot penetrate it. The largest amount of keratin is found in those areas subject to mechanical stress, for example, the soles of the feet and the palms of the hands.

The deepest epidermal sublayer, the stratum basale, supplies the epidermis with new cells after older superficial cells have been damaged or lost through normal wear. Over time, these newly created cells migrate from the stratum basale to the outermost layers of the skin. As these cells are pushed to the surface they are flattened and covered with a water-insoluble material, forming a protective seal. On average, it takes a cell about 3 weeks to move from the stratum basale to the body surface. Specialized cells within the deeper layers of the epidermis, called *melanocytes,* secrete the dark pigment *melanin,* which offers a degree of protection from the sun's ultraviolet rays. The number and type of melanocytes determine the overall pigment of the skin. The more melanin, the darker the skin color. In areas where the melanocytes are destroyed, there are milk-white areas of depigmented skin referred to as **vitiligo.**

The second primary layer of skin, the dermis, provides a foundation for the epidermis and accessory structures such as hair and nails. Most receptor nerve endings, oil glands, sweat glands, and blood vessels are found within the dermis.

Beneath the dermis is the subcutaneous layer, or *hypodermis,* consisting mainly of adipose tissue, which cushions, insulates, and provides a source of energy for the body. The amount of subcutaneous tissue varies in an individual, and is determined by nutritional status and heredity.

48.2 Causes of Skin Disorders

Of the many types of skin disorders, some have vague, generalized signs and symptoms, and others have specific and easily identifiable causes. **Pruritus,** or itching, is a general condition associated with dry, scaly skin, or it may be a symptom of mite or lice infestation (Section 48.4). Inflammation, a characteristic

TABLE 48.1	Classification of Skin Disorders
Type	**Examples**
infectious	Bacterial infections: boils, impetigo, infected hair follicles
	Fungal infections: ringworm, athlete's foot, jock itch, nail infection
	Parasitic infections: ticks, mites, lice
	Viral infections: cold sores, fever blisters (herpes simplex), chicken pox, warts, shingles (herpes zoster), measles (rubeola), and German measles (rubella)
inflammatory	Injury and exposure to the sun such as sunburn and other environmental stresses
	Disorders marked by a combination of overactive glands, increased hormone production, and/or infection such as acne, blackheads, whiteheads, rosacea
	Disorders marked by itching, cracking, and discomfort such as eczema (atopic dermatitis), other forms of dermatitis (contact dermatitis, seborrheic dermatitis, stasis dermatitis), and psoriasis
neoplastic	Types of skin cancers: squamous cell carcinoma, basal cell carcinoma, and malignant melanoma. Malignant melanoma is the most dangerous. Benign neoplasms include keratosis and keratoacanthoma.

of burns and other traumatic disorders, occurs when damage to the skin is extensive. Local **erythema** or redness accompanies inflammation and many other skin disorders. Trauma to deeper tissues may cause additional symptoms such as bleeding, bruising, and infections.

Skin disorders are diverse and difficult to classify. These disorders are summarized in Table 48.1. One simple method is to group them into the following general categories.

- *Infectious:* Bacterial, fungal, viral, and parasitic infections of the skin and mucous membranes are relatively common, and are frequent indications for anti-infective pharmacotherapy. A brief overview is presented in Sections 48.3 and 48.4; however, greater detail may be found in the anti-infective chapters of this text (Chapters 34–36 ∞).

- *Inflammatory:* Inflammatory disorders encompass a broad range of pathology that includes acne, burns, eczema, dermatitis, and psoriasis. Pharmacotherapy of inflammatory skin disorders includes many of the agents discussed in Chapter 43 ∞, such as glucocorticoids.

- *Neoplastic:* Neoplastic disease includes malignant melanoma and basal cell carcinoma, which are treated with the therapies described in Chapter 37 ∞ .

Dermatologic signs and symptoms may reflect disease processes occurring elsewhere in the body. Skin abnormalities including color, sizes, types, and character of surface lesions, and skin turgor and moisture may have systemic causes such as liver or renal impairment, cardiovascular insufficiency, metastatic tumors, recent injury, and poor nutritional status. The relationship between the integumentary system and other body systems is depicted in ● Figure 48.1. Common symptoms associated with a range of conditions are listed in Table 48.2.

Although there are many skin disorders, some warrant only localized or short-term pharmacotherapy. Examples include lice infestation, sunburn with minor irritation, and acne. Eczema, dermatitis, and psoriasis are more serious disorders requiring extensive and sometimes prolonged therapy.

SKIN INFECTIONS

The skin is normally populated with microorganisms or flora that include a diverse collection of viruses, fungi, and bacteria. As long as the skin remains healthy and intact, it provides an effective barrier against infection from these organisms. The skin is very dry, and keratin is a poor energy source for microbes. Although perspiration often provides a wet environment, its high salt content discourages microbial growth. Furthermore, the outer layer is continually being sloughed off, and the microorganisms go with it.

48.3 Pharmacotherapy of Bacterial, Fungal, and Viral Skin Infections

Bacterial skin diseases can occur when the skin is punctured or cut, or when the outer layer is abraded through trauma or removed through severe burns. Some bacteria also infect hair follicles. The two most common bacterial infections of the skin are caused by *Staphylococcus* and *Streptococcus,* which are normal skin inhabitants. *S. aureus* is responsible for furuncles, carbuncles, and abscesses of the skin. Both *S. aureus* and *S. pyogenes* can

PHARMFACTS

Skin Disorders

- An estimated 3 million people with new cases of lice infestation are treated each year in the United States.
- Nearly 17 million people in the United States have acne, making it the most common skin disease.
- More than 15 million people in the United States have symptoms of dermatitis.
- Of infants and young children, 10% experience symptoms of dermatitis; roughly 60% of these infants continue to have symptoms into adulthood.
- Psoriasis affects 1% to 2% of the U.S. population. This disorder occurs in all age groups—adults mainly—affecting about the same number of men as women.

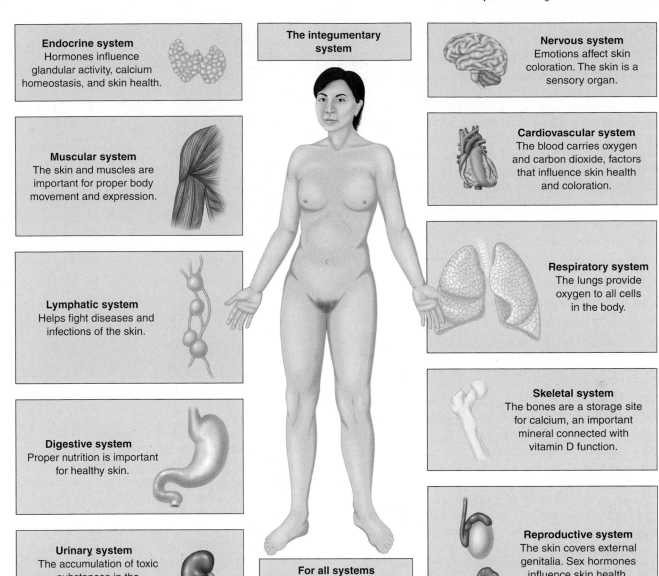

Endocrine system
Hormones influence glandular activity, calcium homeostasis, and skin health.

The integumentary system

Nervous system
Emotions affect skin coloration. The skin is a sensory organ.

Muscular system
The skin and muscles are important for proper body movement and expression.

Cardiovascular system
The blood carries oxygen and carbon dioxide, factors that influence skin health and coloration.

Lymphatic system
Helps fight diseases and infections of the skin.

Respiratory system
The lungs provide oxygen to all cells in the body.

Digestive system
Proper nutrition is important for healthy skin.

Skeletal system
The bones are a storage site for calcium, an important mineral connected with vitamin D function.

Reproductive system
The skin covers external genitalia. Sex hormones influence skin health.

Urinary system
The accumulation of toxic substances in the bloodstream will affect the skin adversely.

For all systems
The skin forms a protective barrier against hazardous conditions.

●**Figure 48.1** Interrelationships of the integumentary system with other body systems

TABLE 48.2	Signs and Symptoms Associated With Changing Health, Age, or a Weakened Immune System
Sign	**Description**
delicate skin, wrinkles, and hair loss	Many degenerative changes occur in the skin; some are found in elderly clients; others are genetically related (fragile epidermis, wrinkles, reduced activity of oil and sweat glands, male pattern baldness, poor blood circulation); hair loss may also be linked to medical procedures, for example, radiation and chemotherapy.
discoloration of the skin	Discoloration is often a sign of an underlying medical disorder (for example, anemia, cyanosis, fever, jaundice, or Addison's disease); some medications have photosensitive properties, making the skin sensitive to the sun and causing erythema.
scales, patches, and itchy areas	Some symptoms may be related to a combination of genetics, stress, and immunity; other symptoms are due to a fast turnover of skin cells; some symptoms develop for unknown reasons.
seborrhea/oily skin and bumps	This condition is usually associated with younger clients; examples include cradle cap in infants and an oily face, chest, arms, and back in teenagers and young adults; pustules, cysts, papules, and nodules represent lesions connected with oily skin.
tumors	Tumors may be genetic or may occur because of exposure to harmful agents or conditions.
warts, skin marks, and moles	Some skin marks are congenital; others are acquired or may be linked to environmental factors.

cause impetigo, a skin disorder commonly occurring in school-age children.

Although many skin bacterial infections are self-limiting, others may be serious enough to require pharmacotherapy. When possible, pharmacotherapy utilizes topical agents applied directly to the infection site. Topical agents offer the advantage of causing fewer side effects, and many are available OTC for self-treatment. If the infection is deep within the skin, affects large regions of the body, or has the potential to become systemic, then oral or parenteral therapy is indicated. Chapter 34 ∞ provides a complete discussion of antibiotic therapy. Some of the more common topical antibiotics include the following:

- Bacitracin ointment (Baciguent)
- Chloramphenicol cream (Chloromycetin)
- Erythromycin ointment (EryDerm, others)
- Gentamicin cream and ointment (Garamycin)
- Mupirocin (Bactroban)
- Neomycin (Myciguent) or neomycin with polymyxin B (Neosporin), cream and ointment
- Tetracycline (Topicycline)

Fungal infections of the skin or nails commonly occur in warm, moist areas of the skin covered by clothing, such as tinea pedis (athlete's foot) and tinea cruris (jock itch). Tinea capitis (ringworm of the scalp) and tinea unguium (nails) are also common. These pathogens are responsive to therapy with topical OTC antifungal agents such as undecylenic acid (Cruex, Desenex, others). More serious fungal infections of the skin and mucous membranes, such as *Candida albicans* infections that occur in immunocompromised clients, require systemic antifungals (Chapter 35 ∞). Clotrimazole (Mycelex, Lotrimin, others) and miconazole (Monistat, others) are common antifungals used for a variety of dermatologic mycoses.

Some viral infections of the skin are considered diseases of childhood. These include varicella (chicken pox), rubeola (measles), and rubella (German measles). Usually, these infections are self-limiting and nonspecific, so treatment is directed at controlling the extent of skin lesions. Viral infections of the skin in adults include herpes zoster (shingles) and herpes simplex (cold sores and genital lesions). Pharmacotherapy of severe or persistent viral skin lesions may include topical or oral antiviral therapy with acyclovir (Zovirax), as discussed in Chapter 36 ∞.

SKIN PARASITES

Common skin parasites include mites and lice. Scabies is an eruption of the skin caused by the female mite, *Sarcoptes scabiei*, which burrows into the skin to lay eggs that hatch after about 5 days. Scabies mites are barely visible without magnification and are smaller than lice. Scabies lesions most commonly occur between the fingers, on the extremities, in axillary and gluteal folds, around the trunk, and in the pubic area, as shown in ● Figure 48.2. The major symptom

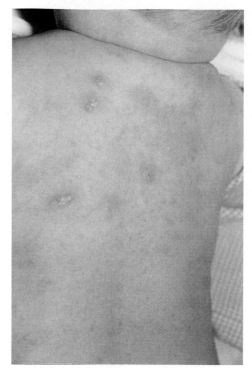

● **Figure 48.2** Scabies *Source: Courtesy of Dr. Jason L. Smith.*

is intense itching; vigorous scratching may lead to secondary infections. Scabies is readily spread through contact with upholstery and shared bed and bath linens.

Lice are larger than mites, measuring from 1 to 4 mm in length. They are readily spread by infected clothing or close personal contact. These parasites require human blood for survival and die within 24 hours without the blood of a human host. Lice (singular: louse) often infest the pubic area or the scalp and lay eggs, referred to as **nits,** which attach to body hairs. Head lice are referred to as *Pediculus capitis* (● Figure 48.3), body lice as *P. corpus*, and pubic lice as *Phthirus pubis.* The pubic louse is referred to as a *crab louse*, because it looks like a tiny crab when viewed under the microscope. Individuals with pubic lice will sometimes say that they have "crabs." Pubic lice may produce sky-blue

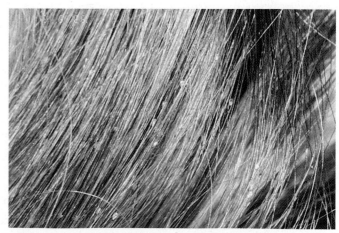

● **Figure 48.3** *Pediculus capitis Source: Courtesy of Dr. Jason L. Smith.*

macules on the inner thighs or lower abdomen. The bite of the louse and the release of saliva into the wound lead to intense itching followed by vigorous scratching. Secondary infections can result from scratching.

48.4 Pharmacotherapy With Scabicides and Pediculicides

Scabicides are drugs that kill mites, and **pediculicides** are drugs that kill lice. Some drugs are effective against both types of parasites. The choice of drug may depend on where the infestation is located, as well as other factors such as age, pregnancy, or breast-feeding.

The current drug of choice for lice is permethrin, a chemical derived from chrysanthemum flowers and formulated as a 1% liquid (Nix). This drug is considered the safest agent, especially for infants and children. Pyrethrin (RID, others) is a related product also obtained from the chrysanthemum plant. Permethrin and pyrethrins, which are also widely used as insecticides on crops and livestock, kill lice and their eggs on contact. These agents are effective in about 90% to 99% of clients, although a repeat application may be needed. Side effects are generally minor and include stinging, itching, or tingling. Malathion (Ovide) is an alternative for resistant organisms.

Permethrin is also a preferred agent for scabies. The 5% cream (Elimite) is applied to the entire skin surface and allowed to remain for 8 to 14 hours before bathing. A single application cures 95% of the clients, although itching may continue for several weeks as the dead mites are removed from the skin. Crotamiton (Eurax) is an alternative scabicide available by prescription as a 10% cream.

The traditional drug of choice for many decades for both mites and lice was lindane (Kwell, Scabene). Lindane was also widely used as an agricultural pesticide in the 1950s and 1960s, causing pollution of waterways and prompting restrictions on its use. Because lindane has the potential to cause serious nervous system toxicity, it is prescribed only after other less toxic drugs have failed to produce a therapeutic response.

All scabicides and pediculicides must be used strictly as directed, because their excessive use can cause serious systemic effects and skin irritation. Drugs for the treatment of lice or mites must not be applied to the mouth, open skin lesions, or eyes, because this will cause severe irritation.

NURSING CONSIDERATIONS

The role of the nurse in scabicide and pediculicide therapy involves careful monitoring of a client's condition and providing education as it relates to the prescribed drug treatment. Before assessing the client, be sure to don gloves. Assess the client's hair and skin for evidence of lice, nits, or scabies. Assess the axilla, neckline, hairline, groin, and beltline areas for evidence of lice, such as visualization of nits, erythema, and pruritus. Look for evidence of scabies—small, pimplelike areas of redness noted in these areas and in webbing between fingers, on wrist, in skin folds, and in genital areas.

Pr PROTOTYPE DRUG | Lindane *(Kwell)* | Scabicide/Pediculocide

ACTIONS AND USES

Lindane is marketed as a cream or lotion for mites, and as a shampoo for head lice. Lindane cream or lotion takes longer to produce its effect; therefore, it is usually left on the body for about 8 to 12 hours before rinsing. Lindane shampoo is applied and left on for at least 5 minutes before rinsing. Clients should be aware that penetration of the skin with mites causes itching, which lasts up to 2 or 3 weeks even after the parasites have been killed. Lindane is absorbed directly into lice, mites, and their eggs, producing seizure and death of the parasites.

Treatment may be reapplied in 24 hours when there is evidence of live lice or in 7 days for continued evidence that live mites are present.

ADMINISTRATION ALERTS

- Do not use on premature infants and children younger than 2 years.
- Do not use on areas of skin that have abrasions, rash, or inflammation.
- Pregnancy category C.

PHARMACOKINETICS

Onset: Rapid

Peak: Unknown

Half-life: 18 h

Duration: 3 h

ADVERSE EFFECTS

Lindane is absorbed across the skin and can cause systemic effects. CNS adverse effects include restlessness, dizziness, tremors, or convulsions (usually after misuse or accidental ingestion), and local irritation. If inhaled, lindane may cause headaches, nausea, vomiting, or irritation of the ears, nose, or throat.

Contraindications: Topical lindane is contraindicated for premature neonates, clients crusted scabies and those with hypersensitivity to the drug. It is also contraindicated for clients with known seizure disorders.

INTERACTIONS

Drug–Drug: No clinically significant interactions have been documented.

Lab Tests: Unknown.

Herbal/Food: Unknown.

Treatment of Overdose: Oral overdose causes CNS excitation and possibly convulsions that can be reversed with diazepam or a barbiturate.

SPECIAL CONSIDERATIONS

Psychosocial and Community Impact of Scabies and Pediculosis

Children and parents, particularly those in relatively affluent areas, may express feeling unclean or that their self-esteem has been lowered when they are diagnosed with scabies or pediculosis. Some clients think that only homeless persons or people of low income get these disorders. Educate the client and family members about the ways in which people contract scabies or pediculosis and the ways in which these infestations may be prevented. Help those affected to maintain their self-esteem and adopt a healthy attitude. Persons with scabies or pediculosis may tend to isolate socially, but this is unnecessary if precautions are taken to not share clothing, combs, or other hygiene supplies or have bodily contact with others.

Scabies or lice can rapidly spread in a school, nursing home, residential treatment center, or hospital and become a community health problem. School nurses must assess the potential for students or clients contacting scabies or lice and take preventive measures. This may include frequent assessments of the hair, scalp, and exposed skin, and elimination of coat and hat racks and opportunities to share or swap clothing and/or towels. School children and their families need education on prevention and treatment. Clients and their families reporting scabies or pediculosis to the nurse should be treated in an accepting, professional, helpful manner.

Obtain a thorough history regarding onset of symptoms and possible exposure to others. Take a history of epilepsy, pregnancy, lactation, allergies, and use of over-the-counter (OTC) or other home remedies to treat the current condition. If the client has lesions, assess the skin for abrasions, rashes, and open areas to determine any sites that might be prone to irritation from the topical medication.

Follow application instructions, and wear gloves when applying medication. Cleanse the lesions and surrounding areas with warm water and soap, and dry thoroughly prior to applying medication. Cleansing of the lesions prior to and between applications of medication reduces the risk of secondary infections. If the medication is applied incorrectly or ingested, the client may experience headaches, nausea, vomiting, dizziness, tremors, restlessness, convulsions, and irritation of the nose, ears, or throat.

Lifespan Considerations. Most medications for the treatment of skin parasites are contraindicated or should be used cautiously in pregnant or lactating women and young children. Assess women of childbearing age for the possibility of pregnancy, and ask if they are breast-feeding. Lindane (Kwell) is contraindicated in premature infants and should not be applied to children younger than 2 years of age because of increased risk of central nervous system (CNS) toxicity. Lindane is used cautiously in children ages 2 to 10 and only after other agents have been unsuccessful in treating the condition. Lower dosages are typically prescribed for children and elderly clients.

Client Teaching. Client teaching regarding scabicides and pediculicides should include the goals of the therapy, the reasons for obtaining baseline data such as vital signs and the existence of underlying disorders, and possible drug side effects. Include the following points when teaching clients about scabicides or pediculicides:

- Follow application instructions exactly.
- After treatment for head lice, remove all nits from the hair shaft with a nit comb or a fine-tooth comb. Remove all nits manually to ensure that the parasite does not recur.
- Notify those who may have been exposed to or have been in close contact with the individual who is infected.
- For a child in day care, notify caregivers so that others may be assessed for possible infestation.
- Keep medication out of reach of children, because it is highly toxic if swallowed or inhaled.
- If breast-feeding, use another source of milk for a minimum of 4 days after using medication.
- If applying medication such as lindane to an infant's skin, do not allow the medication to touch other skin areas.
- To prevent further infestation or recurrence, wash all bedding in hot water and dry in the dryer on maximum heat. If materials are nonwashable, have them dry cleaned.
- Place stuffed animals or other objects that cannot be washed in plastic bags, and ensure that they are sealed completely for 2 weeks.
- Vacuum all carpets and upholstered surfaces, discard the vacuum bag or empty the container, and place in trash outside the household.
- Keep the environmental temperature at 68°F to 72°F and at low humidity to reduce itching and drying of skin.

SUNBURN AND MINOR BURNS

Burns are a unique type of stress that may affect all layers of the skin. Minor, first-degree burns affect only the outer layers of the epidermis, are characterized by redness, and are analogous to sunburn. Sunburn results from overexposure of the skin to ultraviolet light, and is associated with light skin complexions, prolonged exposure to the sun during the more hazardous hours of the day (10 A.M. until 3 P.M.), and lack of protective clothing when outdoors. Chronic sun exposure can result in serious conditions, including eye injury, cataracts, and skin cancer.

48.5 Pharmacotherapy of Sunburn and Minor Skin Irritation

The best treatment for sunburn is prevention. Clients must be reminded of the acute and chronic hazards of exposure to direct sunlight. Liberal application of a lotion or oil having a very high SPF (sun protection factor) that protects against UVA and UVB rays, to areas of skin directly exposed to sunlight is strongly recommended.

In addition to producing local skin damage, sun overexposure releases toxins that may produce systemic effects. The signs and symptoms of sunburn include erythema, intense pain, nausea, vomiting, chills, edema, and headache. These symptoms usually resolve within a matter of hours or days, depending on the severity of the exposure. Once

NURSING PROCESS FOCUS Clients Receiving Lindane (Kwell)	
Assessment	**Potential Nursing Diagnoses**
Prior to administration: • Obtain a complete history including age, allergies, drug history, possible drug interactions, and seizure disorders. • Obtain a social history of close contacts, including household members and sexual partners. • Assess vital signs. • Assess skin for presence of lice and/or mite infestation, skin lesions, raw or inflamed skin, and open areas. • Assess pregnancy and lactation status.	• Knowledge, Deficient, related to no previous experience with lice or mite treatment • Noncompliance, Potential for, related to knowledge deficit and embarrassment • Skin Integrity, Impaired, related to lesions and pruritus

Planning: Client Goals and Expected Outcomes

The client will:
• Be free of lice or mites and experience no reinfestation of self or other family members.
• Verbalize an understanding of how lice and mites are spread, proper administration of lindane, necessary household hygiene, and the need to notify household members, sexual partners, and other close contacts, such as classmates, of infestation.
• Exhibit skin that is intact and free of secondary infection and irritation.
• Demonstrate an understanding of the drug's action by accurately describing drug side effects and precautions.

Implementation

Interventions and (Rationales)	Client Teaching/Discharge Planning
• Monitor for presence of lice or mites. (This determines the effectiveness of drug therapy.)	Instruct client and caregiver to: • Examine for nits on hair shafts; lice on skin or clothes, inner thigh areas, seams of clothes that come in contact with axilla, neckline, or beltline. • Examine for mites between the fingers, on the extremities, in axillary and gluteal folds, around the trunk, and in the pubic area.
• Apply lindane properly. (Proper application is critical to eliminating infestation.)	Instruct client and caregiver: • To wear gloves during application. • To remove all skin lotions, creams, and oil-based hair products completely by scrubbing the whole body well with soap and water, and drying the skin prior to application. • To apply lindane to clean and dry affected body area as directed, using no more than 2 oz per application. • To avoid contact with the product on an infant's skin. • That eyelashes can be treated with the application of petroleum jelly twice a day for 8 days followed by combing to remove nits. • To comb affected hair with a fine-tooth comb, following lindane application, making sure to remove all nits. • To treat all household members and sexual contacts immediately. • To recheck affected hair or skin daily for 1 week after treatment.
• Inform client and caregivers about proper care of clothing and equipment. (Contaminated articles will cause reinfestation.)	Instruct client and caregiver to: • Wash all bedding and clothing in hot water, and to dry-clean all nonwashable items that came in close contact with client. • Clean combs and brushes with lindane shampoo and rinse thoroughly.

Evaluation of Outcome Criteria

Evaluate the effectiveness of drug therapy by confirming that client goals and expected outcomes have been met (see "Planning").
• Client and significant others are free of lice or mites and reinfestation.
• Client verbalizes an understanding of how lice and mites are spread, proper administration of lindane, and necessary household hygiene, and has notified household members, sexual partners, and other close contacts, such as classmates, of infestation.
• The client's skin is intact and free of secondary infection and irritation.
• The client demonstrates an understanding of the drug's action by accurately stating drug side effects and precautions.

Pr PROTOTYPE DRUG | Benzocaine *(Solarcaine, others)* | Topical Anesthetic

ACTIONS AND USES

Benzocaine is an ester-type local anesthetic that provides temporary relief for pain and discomfort in cases of sunburn, pruritus, minor wounds, and insect bites. Its pharmacological action is caused by local anesthesia of skin receptor nerve endings. Preparations are also available to treat specific areas such as the ear, mouth, and throat, and rectal and genital areas.

ADMINISTRATION ALERTS

- Do not use benzocaine to treat clients with open lesions or traumatized mucosal lesions.
- Clients should use preparations only in areas of the body for which the medication is intended.
- Pregnancy category C.

PHARMACOKINETICS

Onset: Immediate

Peak: 1 min

Half-life: Unknown

Duration: 15–30 min

ADVERSE EFFECTS

Benzocaine has a low toxicity; anaphylaxis is rare, though possible. There are some reports of methemoglobinemia in infants. If prescribed in a spray form, avoid inhalation. Inhalation of benzocaine may cause methemoglobinemia.

Contraindications: This drug is contraindicated in clients with hypersensitivity to "caine" anesthetics or to sunscreens containing PABA.

INTERACTIONS

Drug–Drug: Benzocaine may interfere with the activity of some antibacterial sulfonamides.

Lab Tests: Unknown.

Herbal/Food: Unknown.

Treatment of Overdose: Overdose by the topical route is unlikely.

 See the Companion Website for a Nursing Process Focus specific to this drug.

---

sunburn has occurred, medications can only alleviate the symptoms; they do not speed recovery time.

Treatment for sunburn consists of addressing symptoms with soothing lotions, rest, prevention of dehydration, and topical anesthetic agents, if needed. Treatment is usually done on an outpatient basis. Topical anesthetics for minor burns include benzocaine (Solarcaine), dibucaine (Nupercainal), lidocaine (Xylocaine), and tetracaine HCl (Pontocaine). Aloe vera is a popular natural therapy for minor skin irritations and burns. These same agents may also provide relief from minor pain due to insect bites and pruritus. In more severe cases, oral analgesics such as aspirin or ibuprofen may be indicated.

NURSING CONSIDERATIONS

The role of the nurse in drug therapy for sunburn and minor skin irritation involves careful monitoring of a client's condition and providing education as it relates to the prescribed drug treatment. Assess the sunburn, including location, portion of body surface area, edema, erythema, and blistering. For severe cases, especially those sunburns that affect a large portion of the body surface area, assess for fever, chills, weakness, and shock. Obtain a thorough history including sunburn and tanning history, the amount of time the client usually spends in the sun, how easily the client burns, and what type of sun protection is used. If the client uses a sunscreen, obtain the SPF rating. As part of the history, obtain allergies to any medications and use of OTC products or home remedies to treat the sunburn. If topical anesthetics or ointments are ordered, assess the skin for secondary infections, in which these medications are contraindicated. Topical benzocaine (Solarcaine) may cause a

hypersensitivity reaction. For clients using the medication for the first time, a trial application on a small area of skin should be conducted to assess for an allergic reaction. If no adverse effects occur within 30 to 60 minutes, the medication may be applied to the entire area of sunburn.

Lifespan Considerations.   Education regarding sunburn prevention in clients of all ages is important. Infants and young children are vulnerable to sun exposure and should always be protected with a sunscreen with an SPF of 15 or higher.

Client Teaching.   Client education as it relates to sunburn and minor skin irritation should include the goals of therapy, the reasons for obtaining baseline data such as vital signs and the existence of underlying disorders, and possible drug side effects. Include the following points when teaching clients about sunburn and minor skin irritations:

- Avoid applying medication to open or infected areas of skin.
- Drink plenty of water to avoid dehydration.
- Report severe, persistent pain.
- Avoid sun exposure while receiving treatment.
- Prevent sunburn in the future by wearing protective clothing such as long-sleeved shirts and large-brim hats, and by using sunscreen with an SPF of 15 or greater.
- Follow the directions regarding use and reapplication of sunscreen after swimming or sweating.
- Refrigerate topical lotions so they will provide a soothing, cooling effect when applied.
- Avoid the use of benzocaine on infants and young children.

ACNE AND ROSACEA

Acne vulgaris is a common condition, affecting 80% of adolescents. Although acne occurs most often in teenagers, it is not unusual to find clients with acne who are older than 30 years, a condition referred to as *mature acne* or *acne tardive*. Acne vulgaris is more common in men but tends to persist longer in women.

Factors associated with acne vulgaris include **seborrhea,** the overproduction of sebum by oil glands, and abnormal formation of keratin that blocks oil glands. The bacterium *Propionibacterium acnes* grows within oil gland openings and changes sebum to an acidic and irritating substance. As a result, small inflamed bumps appear on the surface of the skin. Other factors associated with acne include androgens, which stimulate the sebaceous glands to produce more sebum. This is clearly evident in teenage boys and in clients who are administered testosterone.

Acne lesions include open and closed comedones. Blackheads, or open **comedones,** occur when sebum has plugged the oil gland, causing it to become black because of the presence of melanin granules. Whiteheads, or closed comedones, develop just beneath the surface of the skin and appear white rather than black.

Rosacea is another skin disorder with lesions affecting mainly the face. Unlike acne, which most commonly affects teenagers, rosacea is a progressive disorder with an onset between 30 and 50 years of age. Rosacea is characterized by small papules or inflammatory bumps without pus that swell, thicken, and become painful, as shown in ● Figure 48.4. The face takes on a reddened or flushed appearance, particularly around the nose and cheek area. With time, the redness becomes more permanent, and lesions resembling acne appear.

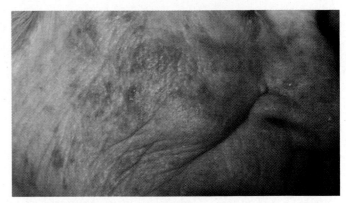

● **Figure 48.4** Rosacea *Source: Courtesy of Dr. Jason L. Smith.*

The soft tissues of the nose may thicken, giving the nose a reddened, bullous, irregular swelling called **rhinophyma.**

Rosacea is exacerbated by factors such as sunlight, stress, increased temperature, and agents that dilate facial blood vessels including alcohol, spicy foods, skin care products, and warm beverages. It affects more women than men, although men more often develop rhinophyma.

48.6 Pharmacotherapy of Acne and Acne-related Disorders

Medications used for acne and related disorders are available OTC and by prescription. Because of their increased toxicity, prescription agents are reserved for more severe, persistent cases. These drugs are listed in Table 48.3.

Benzoyl peroxide (Benzalin, Fostex, others) is the most common topical OTC medication for acne. Benzoyl peroxide has a **keratolytic** effect, which helps dry out and shed the

TABLE 48.3 Drugs for Acne and Acne-related Disorders	
Drug	**Remarks**
OTC AGENT	
benzoyl peroxide (Benzacin, Benzamyclin, others)	Sometimes combined with tetracycline, erythromycin, or clindamycin in severe cases, to fight bacterial infection
PRESCRIPTION AGENTS (TOPICAL)	
adapalene (Differin)	Retinoid-like compound used to treat acne formation
azelaic acid (Azelex, Finacea, others)	For mild to moderate inflammatory acne
sulfacetamide sodium (Cetamide, Klaron, others)	For sensitive skin; sometimes combined with sulfur to promote peeling, as in the condition rosacea; also used for conjunctivitis
tretinoin (Retin-A, others)	To prevent clogging of pore follicles; also used for the treatment of acute promyelocytic leukemia and wrinkles
PRESCRIPTION AGENTS (ORAL)	
ethinyl estradiol (Estinyl)	Oral contraceptives are sometimes used for acne; example: ethinyl estradiol plus norgestimate (Ortho Tri-Cyclen-28).
doxycycline (Doryx, Vibramycin)	Antibiotic; refer to Chapter 34 ∞.
isotretinoin (Accutane)	For acne with cysts or acne formed in small, rounded masses; pregnancy category X
tetracycline hydrochloride (Achromycin, Panmycin, Sumycin) (see page 495 for the Prototype Drug box ∞)	Antibiotic; refer to Chapter 34 ∞.

outer layer of epidermis. In addition, this drug suppresses sebum production and exhibits rapid bacteriostatic action against *P. acnes.* Benzoyl peroxide is available as a topical lotion, cream, or gel in various percent concentrations. The drug is very safe, with local redness, irritation, and drying being the most common side effects. Other keratolytic agents used for severe acne include resorcinol, salicylic acid, and sulfur.

Retinoids are a class of drug closely related to vitamin A that are used in the treatment of inflammatory skin conditions, dermatologic malignancies, and acne. The topical formulations are often drugs of choice for clients with mild to moderate acne. Tretinoin (Retin-A) is an older drug with an irritant action that decreases comedone formation and increases extrusion of comedones from the skin. Tretinoin also has the ability to improve photodamaged skin and is for wrinkle removal. Other retinoids include isotretinoin (Accutane), an oral vitamin A metabolite medication that aids in reducing the size of sebaceous glands, thereby decreasing oil production and the occurrence of clogged pores. Therapy with retinoids may require 8 to 12 weeks to achieve maximum

effectiveness. Common reactions to retinoids include burning, stinging, and sensitivity to sunlight. Adapalene (Differin) is a third-generation retinoid that causes less imitation than the older agents. Additional retinoid-like agents and related compounds used to treat acne are listed in Table 48.3.

Antibiotics are sometimes used in combination with acne medications to lessen the severe redness and inflammation associated with the disorder. Doxycycline (Vibramycin, others) and tetracycline (Achromycin) have been the traditional antibiotics used in acne therapy. Topical erythromycin is an alternative for clients with microorganisms resistant to tetracyclines.

Oral contraceptives containing ethinyl estradiol and norgestimate are also used to help clear the skin of acne. The agents are reserved for women who are unable to take oral antibiotics or when antibiotic therapy has proved ineffective. For the actions and contraindications of oral contraceptives, see Chapter 45 ∞.

Pharmacotherapy for rosacea includes a number of drugs given for acne vulgaris, including isotretinoin (Accutane), topical azelaic acid 20% cream (Finacea, Finevin), sulfacetamide

---

Pr PROTOTYPE DRUG | Isotretinoin *(Accutane)* | Antiacne Agent/Retinoid

ACTIONS AND USES

The principal action of isotretinoin is regulation of skin growth and turnover. As cells from the stratum germinativum grow toward the surface, skin cells are lost from the stratum pore openings, and their replacement is slowed. Isotretinoin also decreases oil production by reducing the size and number of oil glands. Symptoms take 4 to 8 weeks to improve, and maximum therapeutic benefit may take 5 to 6 months. Because of potentially serious adverse effects, this drug is most often reserved for cystic acne or severe keratinization disorders.

ADMINISTRATION ALERTS

- Do not use in clients with a history of severe depression or suicidal ideation.
- Take with meals to minimize GI distress.
- Pregnancy category X.

PHARMACOKINETICS

Onset: Unknown

Peak: 3.2 h

Half-life: 10–20 h

Duration: Unknown

ADVERSE EFFECTS

Isotretinoin is a toxic metabolite of retinol or vitamin A. Common adverse effects are conjunctivitis, dry mouth, inflammation of the lips, dry nose, increased serum concentrations of triglycerides (by 50% to 70%), bone and joint pain, and photosensitivity. Liver function, serum glucose, and serum triglyceride tests should be obtained when taking isotretinoin.

Contraindications: This drug causes birth defects and is contraindicated during lactation, pregnancy, or suspected pregnancy. Pregnancy testing is advised before starting therapy in female clients of childbearing age. Isotretinoin is also contraindicated in clients who have leucopenia or neutropenia or who are hypersensitive to the drug.

INTERACTIONS

Drug–Drug: Use with vitamin A supplements increases the toxicity of isotretinoin. Tetracycline or minocycline use may increase risk of pseudotumor cerebri. concurrent use of hypoglycemic agents may lead to loss of glycemic control as well as increased risk for cardiovascular disease, secondary to elevated triglyceride levels. Isotretinoin decreases blood levels of carbamazepine, possibly leading to increased seizure activity. Isotretinoin is suspected of decreasing the effectiveness of certain contraceptives; therefore, it is critical that female clients of childbearing potential use two forms of effective contraception simultaneously.

Lab Tests: The following values may be increased: plasma triglycerides, cholesterol, alkaline phosphatase (ALP), aspartate aminotransferase (AST), alanine aminotransferase (ALT), lactate dehydrogenase (LDH), fasting blood glucose, creatine phosphokinase (CPK), and serum uric acid. The following values may be decreased: serum HDL, white blood cells, and platelets.

Herbal/Food: The oral absorption of isotretinoin is increased if taken with a high-fat meal. St. John's wort should not be taken with isotretinoin because concurrent use may cause depression. In addition, pregnancies have been reported by users of certain contraceptives who also used St. John's wort.

Treatment of Overdose: Symptoms of overdose are nonspecific and resolve with symptomatic treatment.

NURSING PROCESS FOCUS Clients Receiving Isotretinoin (Accutane)

Assessment	Potential Nursing Diagnosesm
Prior to administration: ▪ Obtain a complete health history including allergies, drug history, and possible drug interactions. ▪ Obtain pregnancy and lactation status. ▪ Assess for history of psychiatric disorders. ▪ Assess vital signs to obtain baseline information.	▪ Body Image, Disturbed, related to presence of acne and possible worsening of symptoms after initiation of treatment ▪ Decisional Conflict, related to desire for pregnancy, and necessity of preventing pregnancy during therapy with isotretinoin ▪ Noncompliance, related to length of treatment time or failure to use effective contraception ▪ Skin Integrity, Impaired, related to inflammation, redness, and scaling secondary to treatment

Planning: Client Goals and Expected Outcomes

The client will:
▪ Experience decreased acne, without side effects or adverse reactions.
▪ Demonstrate acceptance of body image.
▪ Demonstrate an understanding of the drug's action by accurately describing drug side effects and precautions.
▪ Use contraceptive measures to prevent pregnancy while taking medication.
▪ Comply with treatment regimen by keeping all scheduled appointments and laboratory visits for testing.

Implementation

Interventions and (Rationales)	Client Education/Discharge Planning
▪ Monitor lab studies during treatment, including blood glucose. (Monitoring of lab values is important in determining complications or serious side effects.)	▪ Instruct client to keep laboratory appointments prior to therapy and periodically during therapy, and if diabetic, to perform home blood glucose monitoring.
▪ Discuss potential adverse reactions to drug therapy. (Understanding of drug effects is important for compliance.)	Instruct client: ▪ To use two forms of reliable birth control for 1 month before beginning treatment, during treatment, and for 1 month following completion of treatment. ▪ Not to donate blood during treatment and for a minimum of 4 weeks after completion of treatment; isotretinoin in donated blood could cause fetal damage if given to a pregnant woman. ▪ To talk with pediatrician about alternative methods of feeding, if breast-feeding. ▪ To avoid use of vitamin A products.
▪ Monitor for cardiovascular problems. (Use isotretinoin with caution in clients with heart block, especially if client is also taking a beta-blocker.)	▪ Discuss with client importance of complete disclosure regarding medical history and medications.
▪ Monitor emotional health. (Client may become depressed secondary to acne itself, length of treatment, possibility of worsening symptoms at beginning of treatment, changed body image, or drug itself.)	Instruct client: ▪ To report signs of depression immediately and discontinue isotretinoin. ▪ To report any feelings of suicide.
▪ Monitor CBC, blood lipid levels, glucose levels, liver function tests, eye exam, GI status, and urinalysis. (Monitoring of lab values is important in assessing for complications or serious side effects.)	▪ Teach client importance of a complete workup prior to starting isotretinoin therapy and periodically during course of treatment.
▪ Monitor for vision changes. (Corneal opacities and/or cataracts may develop as result of isotretinoin use. Dryness of eyes during treatment is common. Night vision may be diminished during treatment.)	Instruct client: ▪ To report any decreased vision and discontinue use of isotretinoin. ▪ To avoid driving at night if possible. ▪ That use of artificial tears may relieve dry eyes. ▪ That use of contact lenses may need to be discontinued during therapy.
▪ Monitor alcohol use. (Alcohol use with isotretinoin leads to increased triglyceride levels.)	Advise client to: ▪ Eliminate or greatly reduce alcohol use, including alcohol-containing preparations such as mouthwashes or OTC medications, especially products containing acetaminophen. ▪ Read labels for alcohol content.

(Continued)

NURSING PROCESS FOCUS Clients Receiving Isotretinoin (Accutane) *(Continued)*

Implementation

Interventions and (Rationales)	Client Education/Discharge Planning
▪ Monitor skin problems. (This will determine the effectiveness of drug therapy.)	Advise client: ▪ That acne may worsen during beginning of treatment. ▪ To monitor skin for improvement in 4 to 8 weeks; if no improvement is noted, client should contact primary healthcare provider.
▪ Monitor for side effects. (Side effects may point to potential complications and noncompliance with drug regimen.)	▪ Instruct client to be aware of and to report headache (especially if accompanied by nausea and vomiting), fatigue, depression, lethargy, severe diarrhea, rectal bleeding, abdominal pain, visual changes, dry mouth, hematuria, proteinuria, and liver dysfunction (jaundice, pruritus, dark urine).

Evaluation of Outcome Criteria

Evaluate the effectiveness of drug therapy by confirming that client goals and expected outcomes have been met (see "Planning").

▪ The client reports decreased acne, without side effects or adverse reactions.

▪ The client verbalizes acceptance of body image.

▪ The client demonstrates an understanding of the drug's action by accurately drug side effects and precautions.

▪ The client uses contraceptive measures to prevent pregnancy while taking medication.

▪ The client keeps all scheduled appointments and laboratory visits for testing.

---

preparations, and systemic antibiotics. Metronidazole 0.75% to 1% topical preparation (MetroGel, MetroCream), an antibacterial and antiprotozoal preparation is often the drug of choice for rosacea. Crotamiton (Eurax) 10% cream or lotion may also be prescribed if hair follicle mites are present. In addition to medications, some clients receive vascular or carbon dioxide laser surgery for rhinophyma.

NURSING CONSIDERATIONS

The role of the nurse in drug therapy for acne-related disorders includes careful monitoring of a client's condition and providing education as it relates to the prescribed drug treatment. Have the client undress so you can examine the extent of acne. Wear gloves when assessing the skin. Assess the anterior and posterior thorax, because many acne lesions may be found in these areas. Obtain a thorough history including onset of acne, treatments used and their effects, and whether the client is pregnant. Ask about allergies, past medical history, and current medications.

Isotretinoin (Accutane) is contraindicated in individuals with a history of depression and suicidal ideation and during pregnancy. Individuals who are prescribed isotretinoin should sign a consent regarding the understanding of suicidal risks prior to treatment. Obtain a pregnancy test in all female clients of childbearing years. Isotretinoin is also contraindicated for individuals taking carbamazepine for seizures because the drug may decrease the serum levels of carbamazepine, resulting in increased seizure activity. Use of isotretinoin with hypoglycemic agents may lead to a loss of glycemic control and cardiovascular risks, because isotretinoin raises serum triglyceride levels.

Lifespan Considerations. Some acne medications are contraindicated during pregnancy because they may have teratogenic effects to the fetus. Therefore, verification of pregnancy in those individuals who are sexually active is critical in treatment. If assessing a teenager, rapport must be established, because many are embarrassed or have altered body image or low self-esteem issues related to their acne. Establishing rapport prior to assessing and taking a health history allows the client to become comfortable with answering questions.

Client Teaching. Client education as it relates to drugs used to treat acne should include the goals of therapy, the reasons for obtaining baseline data such as vital signs and the existence of underlying psychiatric disorders, and possible drug side effects. Include the following points when teaching clients about drugs to treat acne:

- Report use of any OTC medications or herbal supplements to treat acne.
- Take medications exactly as prescribed and for the designated length of time.
- Practice reliable contraception and notify your healthcare provider if pregnancy is planned or suspected.
- If breast-feeding, select a different method of feeding your baby while on medications to control acne. If you have stopped taking the acne medications, contact your healthcare provider to determine when breast-feeding may resume.
- Immediately report unusual bleeding, bruising, yellow coloration of the skin or eyes, pale stools, and darkened urine.
- If taking isotretinoin, do not donate blood for 30 days after discontinuing the medication.
- If taking isotretinoin and wearing contacts, unusual dryness of the eyes may be experienced while on this medication.
- Keep a food diary to determine foods that may make acne worse, and avoid those foods.

Burdock Root for Acne and Eczema

Burdock root, *Arctium lappa*, comes from a thick, flowering plant sometimes found on the roadsides of Great Britain and North America. It contains several active substances such as bitter glycosides and flavonoids, and it has a range of potential actions in the body: anti-infective, diuretic, mild laxative, and skin detoxifier. Burdock root is sometimes described as an attacker of skin disorders from within because it fights bacterial infections, reduces inflammation, and treats some stages of eczema, particularly the dry and scaling phases. Some claim that it is also effective against boils and sores.

Burdock root is considered safe, having few side effects or drug interactions. It contains 50% inulin, a fiber widely distributed in vegetables and fruits, and is consumed as a regular part of the daily diet in many Asian countries. In many cases, burdock root is combined with other natural products for a better range of effectiveness. Such products include sarsaparilla (*Smilax officinalis*), yellow dock (*Rumex crispus*), licorice root (*Glycyrrhiza glabra*), echinacea (*Echinacea purpurea*), and dandelion (*Taraxacum officinale*).

- Avoid products that will dry or irritate the skin such as cologne, perfumes, and other alcohol-based products.

- Report severe skin irritation or inflammation that develops while taking these medications, and discontinue use.

DERMATITIS

Dermatitis is an inflammatory skin disorder characterized by local redness, pain, and pruritus. Intense scratching may lead to **excoriation,** scratches that break the skin surface and fill with blood or serous fluid to form crusty scales. Dermatitis may be acute or chronic.

Atopic dermatitis, or **eczema,** is a chronic, inflammatory skin disorder with a genetic predisposition. Clients presenting with eczema often have a family history of asthma and hay fever as well as allergies to a variety of irritants such as cosmetics, lotions, soaps, pollens, food, pet dander, and dust. About 75% of clients with atopic dermatitis have had an initial onset before 1 year of age. In those babies predisposed to eczema, breast-feeding seems to offer protection, as it is rare for a breast-fed child to develop eczema before the introduction of other foods. In infants and small children, lesions usually begin on the face and scalp, and then progress to other parts of the body. A frequent and prominent symptom in infants is the appearance of red cheeks.

Contact dermatitis can be caused by a hypersensitivity response, resulting from exposure to specific natural or synthetic allergens such as plants, chemicals, latex, drugs, metals, or foreign proteins. Accompanying the allergic reaction may be various degrees of cracking, bleeding, or small blisters.

Skin Disorders and Self-esteem

The individual who has skin disorders must adhere to the medical regimen to achieve the desired result. An individual's appearance is very important to self-esteem; therefore, skin lesions may cause embarrassment and the potential for limited social contact. Educate clients about the complexity of the skin disorder, the importance of compliance with the medical regimen and lifestyle changes, which are crucial to success in managing the disorder.

Seborrheic dermatitis is sometimes seen in newborns and in teenagers after puberty, and is characterized by yellowish, oily and crusted patches of skin that appear in areas of the face, scalp, chest, back, or pubic area. Bacterial infection or dandruff may accompany these symptoms.

Stasis dermatitis, a condition found primarily in the lower extremities, results from poor venous circulation. Redness and scaling may be observed in areas where venous circulation is impaired or where deep venous blood clots have formed.

48.7 Pharmacotherapy of Dermatitis

Pharmacotherapy of dermatitis is symptomatic and involves lotions and ointments to control itching and skin flaking. Antihistamines may be used to control inflammation and reduce itching, and analgesics or topical anesthetics may be prescribed for pain relief. Atopic dermatitis can be controlled, but not cured, by medications. Part of the management plan must include the identification and elimination of allergic triggers that cause flare-ups.

Topical glucocorticoids are the most effective treatment for controlling the inflammation and itching of dermatitis. Creams, lotions, solutions, gels, and pads containing glucocorticoids are specially formulated to penetrate deep into the skin layers. These dermatologic agents are classified by potency, as listed in Table 48.4. The high-potency agents are

TABLE 48.4	Topical Glucocorticoids for Dermatitis and Related Symptoms
Generic Name	**Trade Names**
HIGHEST LEVEL OF POTENCY	
betamethasone	Benisone, Diprosone, Valisone
clobetasol	Dermovate, Temovate
diflorasone	Florone, Maxiflor, Psorcon
MIDDLE LEVEL OF POTENCY	
amcinonide	Cyclocort
desoximetasone	Topicort, Topicort LP
fluocinonide	Lidex, Lidex-E, others
halcinonide	Halog
mometasone	Elocon
triamcinolone	Aristocort, Kenalog, others
LOWER LEVEL OF POTENCY	
clocortolone	Cloderm
fluocinolone	Fluolar, Synalar, others
flurandrenolide	Cordran, Cordran SP
fluticasone	Flonase
hydrocortisone	Hytone, Locoid, Westcort, others
LOWEST LEVEL OF POTENCY	
alclometasone	Aclovate
desonide	DesOwen, Tridesilon
dexamethasone	Decaderm, Decadron, others

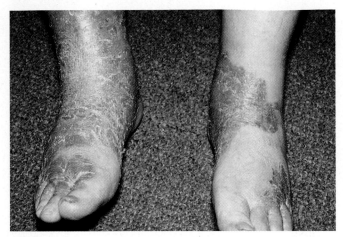

● **Figure 48.5** Psoriasis *Source: Courtesy of Dr. Jason L. Smith.*

used to treat acute flare-ups and are limited to 2 to 3 weeks of therapy. The moderate-potency formulations are for more prolonged therapy of chronic dermatitis. The low-potency glucocorticoids are prescribed for children.

Long-term glucocorticoid use may lead to irritation, redness, hypopigmentation, and thinning of the skin. High-potency formulations are not advised for the head or neck regions because of potential adverse effects. If absorption occurs, topical glucocorticoids may produce undesirable systemic effects including adrenal insufficiency, mood changes, serum imbalances, and loss of bone mass, as discussed in Chapter 43 ∞. To avoid serious adverse effects, careful attention must be given to the amount of glucocorticoid applied, the frequency of application, and how long it has been used.

Several alternatives to the glucocorticoids are available. Clients with persistent atopic dermatitis that does not respond to glucocorticoids may benefit from oral immunosuppressive agents, such as cyclosporine. This drug is generally used for the short-term treatment of severe disease. The topical calcineurin inhibitors pimecrolimus 1% (Elidel) and tacrolimus 0.03%, 0.1% (Protopic) are available for clients older than 2 years of age. These medications may be used over all skin surfaces (including face and neck) because they have fewer side effects than the topical glucocorticoids. Side effects include burning and stinging on broken skin. Although these drugs are not approved for long-term therapy, research has supported their safety over several years of use.

PSORIASIS

Psoriasis is a chronic, noninfectious, inflammatory disorder characterized by red, raised patches of skin covered with flaky, thick, silver scales called *plaques,* as shown in ● Figure 48.5. These plaques shed the scales, which are sometimes grayish. The reason for the appearance of plaques is an extremely fast skin turnover rate, with skin cells reaching the surface in 4 to 7 days instead of the usual 14 days. Plaques are ultimately shed from the surface, while the underlying skin becomes inflamed and irritated. Lesion size varies, and the shape tends to be round. Lesions are usually discovered on the scalp, elbows, knees, and extensor surfaces of the arms and legs, sacrum, and occasionally around the nails. The various forms of psoriasis are described in Table 48.5.

The etiology of psoriasis is incompletely understood. About 50% of the cases have a genetic basis, with a close family member also having the disorder. One theory of causation is that psoriasis is an autoimmune condition, because overactive immune cells release cytokines that increase the production of skin cells. There is also a strong environmental component to the disease: factors such as stress, smoking, alcohol, climate changes, and infections can trigger flare-ups. In addition, certain drugs act as triggers, including angiotensin-converting enzyme (ACE) inhibitors, beta-adrenergic blockers, tetracyclines, and nonsteroidal anti-inflammatory drugs (NSAIDs).

48.8 Pharmacotherapy of Psoriasis

Psoriasis is cosmetically disfiguring, and clients may experience anxiety, embarrassment, or depression, causing them to avoid social interactions. The pharmacological

TABLE 48.5 Types of Psoriasis			
Form of Psoriasis	**Description**	**Most Common Location of Lesions**	**Comments**
guttate (droplike) or eruptive psoriasis	lesions smaller than those of psoriasis vulgaris	upper trunk and extremities	more common in early-onset psoriasis; can appear and resolve spontaneously a few weeks following a streptococcal respiratory infection
psoriatic arthritis	resembles rheumatoid arthritis	fingers and toes at distal interphalangeal joints; can affect skin and nails	about 20% of clients with psoriasis also have arthritis.
psoriasis vulgaris	lesions are papules that form into erythematous plaques with thick, silver or gray plaques that bleed when removed; plaques in dark-skinned individuals often appear purple	skin over scalp, elbows, and knees; lesions possible anywhere on the body	most common form; requires long-term specialized management
psoriatic erythroderma or exfoliative dermatitis	generalized scaling; erythema without lesions	all body surfaces	least common form
pustular psoriasis	eruption of pustules; presence of fever	trunk and extremities; can appear on palms, soles, and nail beds	average age of onset is 50 years

goal of psoriasis pharmacotherapy is to reduce erythema, plaques, and scales to improve the cosmetic appearance of the client, leading to more normal lifestyle activities. The condition is lifelong, and there is no pharmacological cure.

A number of prescription and OTC drugs are available for the treatment of psoriasis, including both topical and systemic agents, as listed in Table 48.6. Combination therapy with two or more agents is common, and drugs are often rotated to achieve the maximum therapeutic response.

TABLE 48.6	Drugs for Psoriasis and Related Disorders	
Drug	**Route and Adult Dose (max dose where indicated)**	**Adverse Effects**
TOPICAL MEDICATIONS*		
calcipotriene (Dovonex)	Topical: Apply thin layer to lesions 1–2 times/day	*Burning, stinging, folliculitis, itching* No serious adverse effects
tacrolimus (Protopic)	Topical: Apply thin layer to affected area bid Oral: Start with 0.05 mg/kg/day; increase to 0.1 mg/kg/day at Week 3 and to 0.15 mg/kg/day at Week 6	The following may occur if the drug is administered PO or IV: *Oliguria, nausea, constipation, diarrhea, headache, abdominal pain, insomnia, peripheral edema, fever* Infections, hypertension, nephrotoxicity, neurotoxicity (tremors, paresthesia, psychosis), hyperkalemia, anemia, hyperglycemia
tazarotene (Tazorac)	Acne: Apply thin film to clean dry area daily Plaque psoriasis: Apply thin film daily in the evening	*Pruritus, burning, stinging, skin irritation, transient worsening of psoriasis* No serious adverse effects
SYSTEMIC MEDICATIONS		
acitretin (Soriatane)	PO; 10–50 mg/day with the main meal	*Dry mouth* Increased triglycerides and cholesterol, paresthesias, rigors, arthralgia
cyclosporine (Sandimmune, Neoral) (see page 466 for the Prototype Drug box ∞)	PO; 1.25 mg/kg bid (max: 4 mg/kg/day)	*Hirsutism, tremor, vomiting* Hypertension, MI, nephrotoxicity, hyperkalemia
etanercept (Enbrel)	Subcutaneous: 25 mg twice/wk or 0.08 mg/kg or 50 mg once/wk	*Local reactions at injection site (pain, erythema, myalgia), abdominal pain, vomiting, headache* Infections, pancytopenia, MI, heart failure
etretinate (Tegison)	PO: 0.75–1 mg/kg/day (max: 1.5 mg/kg/day)	*Fever, headache, fatigue, double vision, nosebleeds, appetite change, sore tongue, nausea, photosensitivity, arthralgia* Pseudotumor cerebri, cardiac thrombotic obstructive events, increased triglycerides and cholesterol, hepatotoxicity, malignant neoplasms
hydroxyurea (Hydrea)	PO: 80 mg/kg q3days or 20–30 mg/kg/day	*Headache, dizziness, fever, chills, nausea, vomiting* Bone marrow depression, convulsions, nephrotoxicity
methotrexate (Mexate, Folex) (see page 562 for the Prototype Drug box ∞)	PO; 2.5–5 mg bid for 3 doses each week (max: 25–30 mg/wk)	*Headache, glossitis, gingivitis, mild leukopenia, nausea* Ulcerative stomatitis, myelosuppression, aplastic anemia, hepatic cirrhosis, nephrotoxicity, sudden death, pulmonary fibrosis

*See Table 48.4 for topical glucocorticoids for psoriasis.
Italics indicate common adverse effects; underlining indicates serious adverse effects.

TOPICAL THERAPIES

Topical glucocorticoids are a primary treatment for psoriasis. Examples include betamethasone (Diprosone) ointment, lotion, or cream and hydrocortisone acetate (Cortaid, Caldecort, others) cream or ointment. Topical glucocorticoids reduce the inflammation associated with fast skin turnover. As in the treatment of dermatitis, high-potency agents are used for acute flare-ups for 2 to 3 weeks. Moderate-and low-potency glucocorticoids are used for chronic therapy.

Topical immunomodulators (TIMS) are another class of agents that suppress the immune system. One example is the calcineurin inhibitor tacrolimus (Protopic) ointment. Other agents applied topically are retinoid-like compounds such as calcipotriene (Dovonex), a synthetic vitamin D ointment, cream, or scalp solution; and tazarotene (Tazorac), a vitamin A derivative gel or cream. These drugs provide the same benefits as topical glucocorticoids but exhibit a lower incidence of adverse effects. Calcipotriene may produce hypercalcemia if applied over large areas of the body or used in higher doses than recommended. This drug is usually not used on an extended basis.

Other skin therapy techniques may be used with or without additional psoriasis medications. These include various forms of tar treatment (coal tar) and anthralin, which are applied to the skin's surface. Tar and anthralin inhibit DNA synthesis and arrest abnormal cell growth. These are considered second-line therapies.

SYSTEMIC THERAPIES

The most often prescribed systemic drug for severe psoriasis is methotrexate. Methotrexate (Folex) is used in the treatment of a variety of disorders, including carcinomas and rheumatoid arthritis, in addition to being used for the treatment of psoriasis. Methotrexate is discussed as a prototype drug on page in Chapter 37 ∞. Other systemic drugs for psoriasis include acitretin (Soriatane) and etretinate (Tegison). These drugs are taken orally to inhibit excessive skin cell growth.

Additionally, drugs used for different disorders, but which provide relief of severe psoriatic symptoms, include hydroxyurea (Hydrea) and cyclosporine (Sandimmune, Neoral). Hydroxyurea is a drug used for sickle-cell anemia. Cyclosporine is an immunosuppressive agent that was presented as a prototype drug on page in Chapter 32 ∞. Etanercept (Enbrel) and infliximab (Remicade), which are biological therapies approved for other autoimmune conditions, have been found to improve symptoms of psoriasis. Etanercept and infliximab are classified as tumor necrosis factor (TNF) blockers.

NONPHARMACOLOGICAL THERAPIES

Phototherapy with UVB and UVA light is used in cases of severe psoriasis. UVB therapy is less hazardous than UVA therapy. The wavelength of UVB is similar to sunlight, and it reduces lesions covering a large area of body that normally resist topical treatments. With close supervision, this type of phototherapy can be administered at home. Keratolytic pastes are often applied between treatments. The second type of phototherapy is referred to as PUVA therapy because **psoralens** are often administered in conjunction with phototherapy. Psoralens are oral or topical agents that when exposed to UV light produce a photosensitive reaction. This reaction reduces the number of lesions, but unpleasant side effects such as headache, nausea, and skin sensitivity still occur, limiting the effectiveness of this therapy. Immunosuppressant drugs such as cyclosporine are not used in conjunction with PUVA therapy, because they increase the risk of skin cancer.

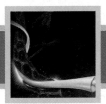

CHAPTER REVIEW

KEY CONCEPTS

The numbered key concepts provide a succinct summary of the important points from the corresponding numbered section within the chapter. If any of these points are not clear, refer to the numbered section within the chapter for review.

48.1 Three layers of skin, epidermis, dermis, and subcutaneous layer, provide effective barrier defenses for the body.

48.2 Skin disorders that may benefit from pharmacotherapy are acne, sunburns, infections, dermatitis, and psoriasis.

48.3 When the skin integrity is compromised, bacteria, viruses, and fungi can gain entrance and cause infections. Anti-infective therapy may be indicated.

48.4 Scabicides and pediculicides are used to treat parasitic mite and lice infestations, respectively. Permethrin is an agent of choice for these infections.

48.5 The pharmacotherapy of sunburn includes the symptomatic relief of pain using soothing lotions, topical anesthetics, and analgesics.

48.6 The pharmacotherapy of acne includes treatment with benzoyl peroxide, retinoids, and antibiotics. Therapies for rosacea include retinoids and metronidazole.

48.7 The most effective treatment for dermatitis is topical glucocorticoids, which are classified by their potency.

48.8 Both topical and systemic drugs, including glucocorticoids, immunomodulators, and methotrexate, are used to treat psoriasis.

NCLEX-RN® REVIEW QUESTIONS

1 The client is treated for head lice with lindane (Kwell). Following treatment, the nurse reinforces instructions to:

1. Remain isolated for 48 hours.
2. Inspect the hair shaft, checking for nits daily for 1 week following treatment.
3. Shampoo with Kwell three times per day.
4. Wash linens with cold water and bleach.

2 Careful attention to directions for application of lindane (Kwell) is emphasized by the nurse. Signs of overapplication include (select all that apply):

1. Nausea and vomiting.
2. Headache.
3. Eye irritation.
4. Diaphoresis.
5. Restlessness.

3 The nurse evaluates the client's understanding of the procedure for application of lindane (Kwell). Which of the following statements requires intervention by the nurse?

1. "The cream should be left on for 8 to 12 hours before rinsing."
2. "I will leave the shampoo on 5 minutes before rinsing."
3. "I will leave the lotion on about 30 minutes before rinsing."
4. "The lotion takes longer to work."

4 The teaching plan for a 24-year-old female receiving isotretinoin (Accutane) for treatment of acne must include:

1. Avoiding the use of oral contraceptives while taking this drug.
2. Avoiding pregnancy while taking this drug.
3. Avoiding using makeup until the treatment is completed.
4. Washing the face with cool water only.

5 Methotrexate (Amethopterin) is prescribed for a client with psoriasis vulgaris. During the physical examination, the nurse expects to find the lesions on the client's:

1. Scalp, elbows, and knees.
2. Upper trunk and extremities.
3. Fingers and toes at distal interphalangeal joints.
4. Palms of hands, soles of feet.

CRITICAL THINKING QUESTIONS

1. A senior nursing student is participating in well-baby screenings at a public health clinic. While examining a 4-month-old infant, the student notes an extensive, confluent diaper rash. The baby's mother is upset and asks the student nurse about the use of OTC corticosteroid ointment and wonders how she should apply the cream. How should the student nurse respond?

2. A 14-year-old girl has been placed on oral doxycycline (Doxy-Caps) for acne vulgaris because she has not responded to topical antibiotic therapy. After 3 weeks of therapy, the client returns to the dermatologist's office complaining about episodes of nausea and epigastric pain. The nurse learns that the client is "so busy with school activities" that she often forgets a morning dose and "doubles up" on the drug before bedtime. Devise a teaching plan relevant to drug therapy that takes into consideration the major side effects of this drug and the cognitive abilities of this client.

3. A 37-year-old woman is referred to a dermatologist for increasing redness and painful "acne" lesions. The client is frustrated with her attempts to camouflage her "teenage face" with makeup. She relates to the nurse that she had acne as a teen but had no further problem until the last 11 months. After consultation, the dermatologist suggests a 3-month trial of isotretinoin (Accutane). What are the specific reproductive considerations for this client? What information should this client be provided in relation to reproductive concerns?

See Appendix D for answers and rationales for all activities.

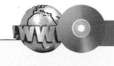

EXPLORE MediaLink

www.prenhall.com/adams

NCLEX-RN® review, case studies, and other interactive resources for this chapter can be found on the companion website at www.prenhall.com/adams. Click on "Chapter 48" to select the activities for this chapter. For animations, more NCLEX-RN® review questions, and an audio glossary, access the accompanying Prentice Hall Nursing MediaLink DVD-ROM in this textbook.

 PRENTICE HALL NURSING MEDIALINK DVD-ROM

- **Audio Glossary**
- **NCLEX-RN® Review**

COMPANION WEBSITE

- **NCLEX-RN® Review**
- **Dosage Calculations**
- **Case Study:** Acne and rosacea
- **Care Plan:** Client with head lice

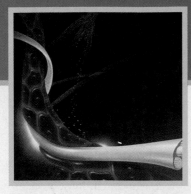
Drugs for Eye and Ear Disorders

DRUGS AT A GLANCE

DRUGS FOR GLAUCOMA
Prostaglandins
 ☞ *latanoprost (Xalatan)*
Beta-adrenergic Blockers
 ☞ *timolol (Timoptic, Timoptic XE)*
Alpha$_2$-adrenergic Agonists
Carbonic Anhydrase Inhibitors
Cholinergic Agonists (miotics)
Nonselective Sympathomimetics
Osmotic Diuretics
DRUGS FOR OPHTHALMIC EXAMINATIONS AND MINOR EYE CONDITIONS
Anticholinergics
Sympathomimetics
Lubricants
DRUGS FOR EAR CONDITIONS
Antibiotics
Cerumen Softeners

OBJECTIVES

After reading this chapter, the student should be able to:

1. Describe eye anatomy relevant to glaucoma development.
2. Identify the major risk factors associated with glaucoma.
3. Compare and contrast the two principal types of glaucoma and explain their reasons for development.
4. Explain the two major mechanisms by which drugs reduce intraocular pressure.
5. Describe the nurse's role in the pharmacological management of eye and ear disorders.
6. Identify examples of drugs for treating glaucoma and explain their basic actions and adverse effects.
7. Identify examples of drugs that dilate or constrict pupils, relax ciliary muscles, constrict ocular blood vessels, or moisten eye membranes.
8. Identify examples of drugs for treating ear conditions.
9. Use the Nursing Process to care for clients who are receiving drug therapy for eye and ear disorders.

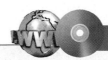

MediaLink

www.prenhall.com/adams

NCLEX-RN® review, case studies, and other interactive resources for this chapter can be found on the companion website at www.prenhall.com/adams. Click on "Chapter 49" to select the activities for this chapter. For animations, more NCLEX-RN® review questions, and an audio glossary, access the accompanying Prentice Hall Nursing MediaLink DVD-ROM in this textbook.

KEY TERMS

aqueous humor *page 771*

closed-angle glaucoma *page 772*

cycloplegic drugs *page 778*

external otitis *page 779*

glaucoma *page 772*

mastoiditis *page 779*

miosis *page 775*

mydriatic drugs *page 778*

open-angle glaucoma *page 772*

otitis media *page 779*

tonometry *page 772*

The eye is vulnerable to a variety of conditions, many of which can be prevented, controlled, or reversed with proper treatment. A simple scratch can cause the client almost unbearable discomfort as well as concern about the effect the damage may have on vision. Other eye disorders may be more bearable, but extremely dangerous—including glaucoma, one of the leading causes of preventable blindness in the world. The first part of this chapter covers various drugs used for the treatment of glaucoma. Drugs used routinely by ophthalmic healthcare providers are also discussed. The remaining part of the chapter presents drugs used for treatment of common ear disorders, including infections, inflammation, and the buildup of ear wax.

49.1 Anatomy of the Eye

A firm knowledge of basic ocular anatomy, shown in ● Figures 49.1 and 49.2, is required to understand eye disorders and their pharmacotherapy. A fluid called **aqueous humor** is found in the anterior cavity of the eye, which has two divisions. The *anterior* chamber extends from the cornea to the anterior iris; the *posterior* chamber lies between the posterior iris and the lens. The aqueous humor originates in the posterior chamber from a muscular structure called the *ciliary body*.

Aqueous humor helps retain the shape of the eye and circulates to bring nutrients to the area and remove wastes. From its origin in the ciliary body, aqueous humor flows from the posterior chamber through the pupil and into the anterior

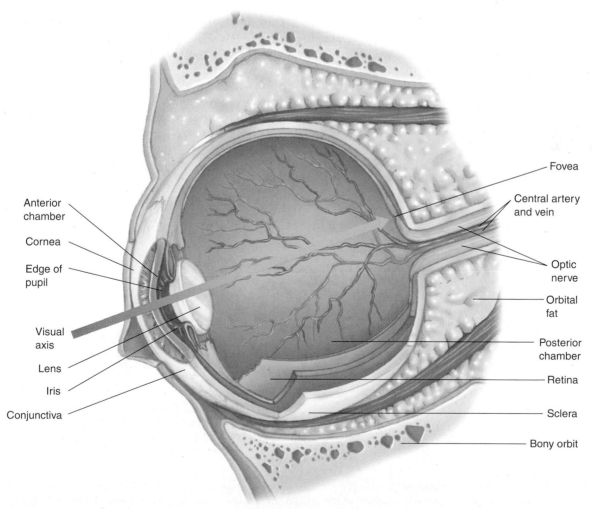

● **Figure 49.1** Internal structures of the eye *Source: Pearson Education/PH College.*

chamber. Within the anterior chamber and around the periphery is a network of spongy connective tissue, or *trabecular meshwork,* that contains an opening called the *canal of Schlemm.* The aqueous humor drains into the *canal of Schlemm* and out of the anterior chamber into the venous system, thus completing its circulation. Under normal circumstances, the rate of aqueous humor production is equal to its outflow, maintaining intraocular pressure (IOP) within a normal range. Interference with either the production or outflow of aqueous humor, however, can lead to an increase in IOP.

GLAUCOMA

Glaucoma occurs when the IOP becomes high enough to cause optic nerve damage, leading to visual field loss, possibly advancing to blindness. Although the median IOP in the population is 15 to 16 mm Hg, this pressure varies greatly with age, daily activities, and even time of day. As a rule, IOPs consistently above 21 mm Hg are considered abnormal. Many clients, however, tolerate IOPs in the mid to high 20s without damage to the optic nerve. IOPs above 30 mm Hg require treatment because they are associated with permanent vision changes. Some clients of Asian descent may experience glaucoma at "normal" IOP values, below 21 mm Hg.

Glaucoma often exists as a *primary* condition without an identifiable cause and is most frequently found in persons older than 60 years. In some cases, glaucoma is associated with genetic factors; it can be congenital in infants and children. Glaucoma can also be *secondary* to eye trauma, infection, diabetes, inflammation, hemorrhage, tumor, or cataracts. Some medications may contribute to the development or progression of glaucoma, including the long-term use of topical glucocorticoids, some antihypertensives, antihistamines, and antidepressants. Other major risk factors associated with glaucoma include high blood pressure, migraine headaches, refractive disorders with high degrees of nearsightedness or farsightedness, and normal aging. Glaucoma is the leading cause of *preventable* blindness.

49.2 Types of Glaucoma

Diagnosis of glaucoma can be difficult, because clients typically do not experience symptoms, and therefore may not seek medical intervention. Glaucoma may occur so gradually that clients do not notice a problem until late in the disease process.

Tonometry is a primary ophthalmic technique that tests for glaucoma by measuring IOP. Clients with unusually thick or thin corneas may have false negatives or false positives during tonometry. Clients who have had Lasik surgery, which removes corneal tissue to correct myopia, may appear to have normal IOPs yet have glaucoma. Other routine refractory and visual field tests are also used to uncover signs of glaucoma.

As shown in Figure 49.2, the two principal types of glaucoma are **closed-angle glaucoma** and **open-angle glaucoma**. Both disorders result from the same problem: a buildup of aqueous humor in the anterior cavity. This buildup is caused either by *excessive production* of aqueous humor or by a *blockage of its outflow*. In either case, IOP increases, leading to progressive damage to the optic nerve. As degeneration of the optic nerve occurs, the client will first notice a loss of visual field, then a loss of central visual acuity, and lastly total blindness. Major differences between closed-angle glaucoma and open-angle glaucoma include how quickly the IOP develops and whether there is narrowing of the anterior chamber angle between the iris and cornea.

Closed-angle glaucoma, also called *acute-* or *narrow-angle* glaucoma accounts for only 5% of all primary glaucoma. The incidence is higher in older adults and in persons of Asian descent. It is typically caused by the normal thickening of the lens and may develop continually over several years. This type of glaucoma is usually unilateral and may

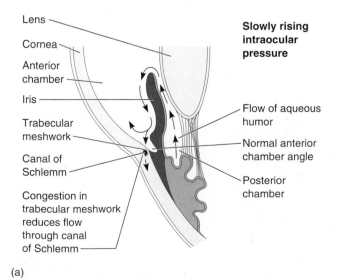

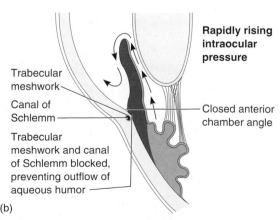

● **Figure 49.2** Forms of primary adult glaucoma: (a) in chronic open-angle glaucoma, the anterior chamber angle remains open, but drainage of aqueous humor through the canal of Schlemm is impaired; (b) in acute closed-angle glaucoma, the angle of the iris and anterior chamber narrows, obstructing the outflow of aqueous humor

be caused by stress, impact injury, or medications. Pressure inside the anterior chamber increases suddenly because the iris is being pushed over the area where the aqueous humor normally drains. The displacement of the iris is due in part to the dilation of the pupil or accommodation of the lens, causing the angle between the posterior cornea and the anterior iris to narrow or close. Signs and symptoms, caused by acute obstruction of the outflow of aqueous humor from the eye, include dull to severe eye pain, headaches, bloodshot eyes, foggy vision with halos around bright lights, and a bulging iris. Ocular pain may be so severe that it causes vomiting. Once the outflow is totally closed, closed-angle glaucoma constitutes an emergency. Laser or conventional surgery is indicated for this condition. Options include iridectomy, laser trabeculoplasty, trabeculectomy, and drainage implants.

Open-angle glaucoma is the most common type, accounting for more than 90% of the cases. It is usually bilateral, with intraocular pressure developing over years. Many clients are asymptomatic. It is called "open-angle" because the iris does not cover the trabecular meshwork; it remains open. Most clients with open-angle glaucoma are treated with medications.

49.3 General Principles of Glaucoma Pharmacotherapy

Some physicians initiate glaucoma pharmacotherapy in all clients with an IOP greater than 21 mm Hg. Because of the expense of pharmacotherapy and the potential for adverse drug effects, other physicians will instead carefully monitor the client through regular follow-up exams and wait until the IOP rises to 28 to 30 mm Hg before initiating drug therapy. If signs of optic nerve damage or visual field changes are evident, the client is treated regardless of the IOP.

Once pharmacotherapy is initiated, reevaluation is performed after 2 to 4 months to check for therapeutic effectiveness. Some of the antiglaucoma drugs take 6 to 8 weeks to reach peak effect. If the therapeutic goals are not achieved with a single agent, it is common to add a second drug from a different class to the regimen to produce an additive decrease in IOP. Some of the agents may continue to have effects on the eye for 2 to 4 weeks after discontinuing the drug.

Drugs for glaucoma work by one of two mechanisms: increasing the outflow of aqueous humor at the canal of Schlemm or decreasing the formation of aqueous humor at the ciliary body. Many agents for glaucoma act by affecting the autonomic nervous system (Chapter 13 ∞).

49.4 Antiglaucoma Drugs

There are many drugs available to treat glaucoma. Although topical drugs are most commonly prescribed, oral medications are also available for severe cases. Agents for glaucoma, listed in Table 49.1, include the following classes:

- Prostaglandins
- Beta-adrenergic blockers
- Alpha$_2$-adrenergic agonists
  Carbonic anhydrase inhibitors
- Cholinergic agonists
  Nonselective sympathomimetics
- Osmotic diuretics

PROSTAGLANDINS

Prostaglandin analogs are a newer therapy for glaucoma, and one of the most effective drug classes. They are often drugs of choice for glaucoma because they have long durations of action and produce fewer adverse effects than the beta-adrenergic blockers.

Prostaglandin analogs decrease IOP by increasing the outflow of aqueous humor. Latanoprost (Xalatan), available as a 0.005% eye drop solution, is one of the most commonly used prostaglandin analogs and is a prototype drug in this chapter. Several new ocular prostaglandins have recently been approved, including bimatoprost (Lumigan), travaprost (Travatan), and unoprostone (Rescula). An occasional side effect of these medications is heightened pigmentation, which turns a blue iris to a more brown color. Many clients experience thicker and longer eyelashes. These drugs cause local irritation, stinging of the eyes, and redness during the first month of therapy. Because of these effects, prostaglandins are normally administered just before bedtime.

BETA-ADRENERGIC BLOCKERS

Before the discovery of the prostaglandin analogs, beta-adrenergic blockers were drugs of choice for open-angle glaucoma. These drugs act by decreasing the production of aqueous humor by the ciliary body, thus lowering IOP. Ophthalmic solutions applied to the affected eye include betaxolol (Betoptic), carteolol (Ocupress), levobunolol (Betagan), metipranolol (OptiPranolol), and timolol (Timoptic, Timoptic XE). They generally produce fewer ocular adverse effects than cholinergic agonists or sympathomimetics. In most clients, the topical administration of beta-blockers does not result in significant systemic absorption. Should absorption occur, however, systemic side effects may include bronchoconstriction, dysrhythmias, and hypotension. Because of the potential for systemic side

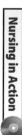

Nursing in Action

Administering Eye Drops

TABLE 49.1 Selected Drugs for Glaucoma

Drug	Route and Adult Dose (max dose where indicated)	Adverse Effects
PROSTAGLANDINS		
bimatoprost (Lumigan)	1 drop 0.03% solution daily in the evening	*Increased length and thickness of eyelashes, darkening of iris, sensation of foreign body in the eye*
latanoprost (Xalatan)	1 drop 0.005% solution daily in the evening	
travoprost (Travatan)	1 drop 0.004% solution daily in the evening	Serious adverse effects that may occur with systemic absorption: respiratory infection/flu, angina, muscle or joint pain
unoprostone isopropyl (Rescula)	1 drop 0.15% solution bid	
BETA-ADRENERGIC BLOCKERS		
betaxolol (Betoptic)	1 drop 0.5% solution bid	*Local burning and stinging, blurred vision, headache*
carteolol (Ocupress)	1 drop 1% solution bid	
levobunolol (Betagan)	1–2 drops 0.25%–0.5% solution 1–2 times/day	Serious adverse effects that may occur with systemic absorption: angina, anxiety, bronchoconstriction, hypertension, dysrhythmias
metipranolol (OptiPranolol)	1 drop 0.3% solution bid	
timolol (Betimol, Timoptic, and others)	1–2 drops of 0.25%–0.5% solution 1–2 times/day Gel (salve): apply daily	
ALPHA₂-ADRENERGIC AGONISTS		
apraclonidine (Iopidine)	1 drop 0.5% solution bid	*Local itching and burning, blurred vision, dry mouth*
brimonidine tartrate (Alphagan)	1 drop 0.2% solution tid	
		Allergic conjunctivitis, conjunctival hyperemia, hypertension
CARBONIC ANHYDRASE INHIBITORS		
acetazolamide (Diamox)	PO; 250 mg 1–4 times/day	*For topical agents: Blurred vision, bitter taste, dry eye, blepharitis, local itching, sensation of foreign body in the eye, headache*
brinzolamide (Azopt)	1 drop 1% solution tid	
methazolamide (Neptazane)	PO; 50–100 mg bid–tid	
		For oral agents: diuresis, electrolyte imbalances, blood dyscrasias, flaccid paralysis, hepatic impairment
CHOLINERGIC AGONISTS		
carbachol (Isopto Carbachol, Miostat)	1–2 drops 0.75%–3% solution in lower conjunctival sac q4h–tid	*Induced myopia, reduced visual acuity in low light, eye redness, headache*
demecarium bromide (Humorsol)	1–2 drops 0.125%–0.25% solution 2 times/wk	
echothiophate iodide (Phosphaline Iodide)	1 drop 0.03%–0.25% solution 1–2 times/day	Serious adverse effects that may occur with systemic absorption: salivation, tachycardia, hypertension, bronchospasm, sweating, nausea, and vomiting
physostigmine sulfate (Eserine sulfate)	1 drop 0.25%–0.5% solution 1–4 times/day	
pilocarpine hydrochloride (Adsorbocarpine, Isopto Carpine, and others).	Acute glaucoma: 1 drop 1%–2% solution q5–10min for 3–6 doses Chronic glaucoma: 1 drop 0.5%–4% solution q4–12h	
NONSELECTIVE SYMPATHOMIMETICS		
dipivefrin HCl (Propine)	1 drop 0.1% solution bid	*Local burning and stinging, blurred vision, headache, photosensitivity*
epinephryl borate (Epinal, Eppy/N)	1–2 drops 0.25%–2% solution 1–2 times/day	
		Tachycardia, hypertension
OSMOTIC DIURETICS		
glycerin anhydrous (Ophthalgan)	PO; 1–1.8 g/kg 1–1.5 h before ocular surgery; may repeat q5h	*Orthostatic hypotension, facial flushing, headache, palpitations, anxiety, nausea*
isosorbide (Ismotic)	PO; 1–3 g/kg 1–2 times/day	
mannitol (Osmitrol)	IV; 1.5–2 mg/kg as a 15%–25% solution over 30–60 min	Severe headache, electrolyte imbalances, edema

Italics indicate common adverse effects; underlining indicates serious adverse effects.

MediaLink Mechanism in Action: Pilocarpine

Pr **PROTOTYPE DRUG** | Latanoprost *(Xalatan)* | Prostaglandin/Antiglaucoma Agent

ACTIONS AND USES

Latanoprost is a prostaglandin analog believed to reduce IOP by increasing the outflow of aqueous humor. The recommended dose is one drop in the affected eye(s) in the evening. It is metabolized to its active form in the cornea, reaching its peak effect in about 12 hours. It is used to treat open-angle glaucoma.

ADMINISTRATION ALERTS

- Remove contact lens before instilling eye drops. Do not reinsert contact for 15 minutes.
- Avoid touching the eye or eyelashes with any part of the eyedropper to avoid cross-contamination.
- Wait 5 minutes before/after instillation of a different eye prescription to administer eye drop(s).
- Pregnancy category C.

PHARMACOKINETICS

Onset: 3–4 h

Peak: 8–12 h

Half-life: 17 min

Duration: Unknown

ADVERSE EFFECTS

Adverse effects include ocular symptoms such as conjunctival edema, tearing, dryness, burning, pain, irritation, itching, sensation of foreign body in eye, photophobia, and/or visual disturbances. The eyelashes on the treated eye may grow thicker, and/or darker. Changes may occur in pigmentation of the iris of the treated eye and in the periocular skin.

Contraindications: The only contraindication is hypersensitivity to the drug.

INTERACTIONS

Drug–Drug: Latanoprost interacts with the preservative thimerosal: If used concurrently with other eye drops containing thimerosal, precipitation may occur.

Lab Tests: Unknown.

Herbal/Food: Unknown.

Treatment of Overdose: Overdose with ophthalmic solution is unlikely.

 See the Companion Website for a Nursing Process Focus specific to this drug.

effects, these drugs should be used with caution in clients with asthma or heart failure.

ALPHA₂-ADRENERGIC AGONISTS

Alpha₂-adrenergic agonists decrease the production of aqueous humor. Apraclonidine (Iopidine) is infrequently used for short-term therapy during eye surgery. Brimonidine (Alphagan) is more commonly prescribed, either as monotherapy or as an adjunct in combination with other antiglaucoma agents. These drugs produce few cardiovascular or pulmonary side effects. The most significant side effects are headache, drowsiness, dry mucosal membranes, blurred vision, and irritated eyelids.

CARBONIC ANHYDRASE INHIBITORS

Carbonic anhydrase inhibitors may be administered topically or systemically to reduce IOP in clients with open-angle glaucoma. They act by decreasing the production of aqueous humor.

Drugs in this class are divided into topical or oral formulations. Dorzolamide (Trusopt) is a frequently used topical antiglaucoma agent, either as monotherapy or in combination with other agents. Dorzolamide and other topical carbonic anhydrase inhibitors are well tolerated and produce few significant adverse effects. Oral formulations such as acetazolamide (Diamox) are very effective at lowering IOP, but are rarely used because they produce more systemic side effects than drugs from other classes. Clients must be cautioned when taking these medications because they contain sulfur and may cause an allergic reaction. Because the oral formulations are diuretics and can reduce IOP quickly, serum electrolytes should be monitored during treatment.

CHOLINERGIC AGONISTS (MIOTICS)

Drugs that activate cholinergic receptors in the eye produce **miosis**, constriction of the pupil, and contraction of the ciliary muscle. These actions physically stretch the trabecular meshwork to allow greater outflow of aqueous humor and a lowering of IOP. Pilocarpine (Adsorbocarpine, Isopto Carpine), the most commonly prescribed antiglaucoma agent in this class, acts directly on cholinergic receptors. Because of their greater toxicity, these drugs are normally used only in clients with open-angle glaucoma who do not respond to other agents. Adverse effects include headache, induced myopia, and decreased vision in low light. The cholinergic agonists are applied topically to the eye. Other actions of the cholinergic agonists are presented in Chapter 13 ∞.

NONSELECTIVE SYMPATHOMIMETICS

Sympathomimetics activate the sympathetic nervous system. Dipivefrin (Propine) and epinephryl borate (Epinal, others) are nonselective sympathomimetics administered topically for open-angle glaucoma. Epinephrine produces mydriasis (pupil dilation) and increases the outflow of aqueous humor, resulting in a slightly lower IOP. Dipivefrin is converted to epinephrine in the eye. If epinephrine reaches the systemic circulation, it increases blood pressure and heart rate. Because of the potential for systemic adverse effects, these agents are second-choice drugs for glaucoma.

Pr PROTOTYPE DRUG | Timolol *(Betimol, Timoptic, Timoptic XE)* | Beta-adrenergic Blocker/Antiglaucoma Agent

ACTIONS AND USES

Timolol is a nonselective beta-adrenergic blocker available in several ophthalmic formulations. Betimol and Timoptic are 0.25% or 0.5% ophthalmic solutions taken twice daily. Timoptic XE and Istalol are long-acting solutions that allow for once daily dosing. Timolol lowers IOP in chronic open-angle glaucoma by reducing the formation of aqueous humor. The drug has no significant effects on visual acuity, pupil size, or accommodation. Treatment may require 2 to 4 weeks for maximum therapeutic effect. As an oral medication, timolol is prescribed to treat mild hypertension, stable angina, prophylaxis of myocardial infarction and migraines.

ADMINISTRATION ALERTS

- Proper administration lessens the danger that the drug will be absorbed systemically, which can mask symptoms of hypoglycemia.
- Pregnancy category C.

PHARMACOKINETICS

Onset: 30 min

Peak: 1–2 h

Half-life: Unknown

Duration: 24 h

ADVERSE EFFECTS

The most common side effects are local burning and stinging on instillation. Vision may become temporarily blurred. In most clients there is not enough absorption to cause systemic adverse effects as long as timolol is applied correctly. If absorption occurs, hypotension or dysrhythmias are possible.

Contraindications: Timolol is contraindicated in clients with asthma, severe chronic obstructive pulmonary disease, sinus bradycardia, second- or third-degree atrioventricular block, heart failure; cardiogenic shock, or hypersensitivity to the drug.

INTERACTIONS

Drug–Drug: Drug interactions may result if significant systemic absorption occurs. Timolol should be used with caution in clients taking other beta-blockers owing to additive cardiac effects. Concurrent use with anticholinergics, nitrates, reserpine, methyldopa, and/or verapamil could lead to hypotension and bradycardia. Epinephrine use could lead to hypertension followed by severe bradycardia.

Lab Tests: Unknown.

Herbal/Food: Unknown.

Treatment of Overdose: Overdose with ophthalmic solution is unlikely, but could result in systemic symptoms such as reduced heart rate and bronchospasm.

 See the Companion Website for a Nursing Process Focus specific to this drug.

OSMOTIC DIURETICS

Osmotic diuretics are occasionally used preoperatively before ocular surgery or during acute closed-angle glaucoma attacks. Examples include glycerin anhydrous (Ophthalgan), isosorbide (Ismotic), and mannitol (Osmitrol). Because they have the ability to quickly reduce plasma volume (Chapter 30 ∞), these drugs are effective in reducing the formation of aqueous humor. Side effects include headache, tremors, dizziness, dry mouth, fluid and electrolyte imbalances, and thrombophlebitis or venous clot formation near the site of IV administration.

NURSING CONSIDERATIONS

The role of the nurse in drug therapy for glaucoma involves careful monitoring of a client's condition and providing education as it relates to the prescribed drug treatment. The initial assessment of a client with glaucoma includes a general health history to determine past and current medical problems and medication regimen. Determine if the client has a history of second- or third-degree heart block, bradycardia, heart failure, or chronic obstructive pulmonary disease (COPD). Antiglaucoma agents that affect the autonomic nervous system may be contraindicated for clients with these conditions because of possible drug absorption into the systemic circulation.

Several preparations used for glaucoma have a potential risk of cardiorespiratory side effects that may occur if the medication is systemically absorbed. Prior to starting drug therapy, establish a baseline blood pressure and pulse. When a beta-blocker is used, teach the client how to check pulse and blood pressure before medication administration. Review the parameters of the pulse and blood pressure with the client and family members to establish guidelines for notifying the healthcare provider. Because the safety of ophthalmic preparations such as beta-blockers during pregnancy or lactation has not been established, obtain information concerning the possibility of pregnancy or breast-feeding.

A key factor in preventing further ocular pathology is client compliance with the medication regimen. Determine any factors that could decrease compliance such as insufficient financial resources, lack of knowledge of the disease, lack of dexterity or skill in inserting eye drops, or difficulty in remembering the dosing schedule. Fear and anxiety about potential blindness and disability may also be evident in the client diagnosed with glaucoma. It is crucial that the client be allowed to verbalize feelings; provide emotional support to the client and family. An explanation of how the disease can be controlled may facilitate compliance as well as alleviate the client's anxiety.

Client Teaching. Client education as it relates to drugs to treat glaucoma should include the goals of therapy, the reasons for obtaining baseline data such as vital signs

NURSING PROCESS FOCUS Clients Receiving Ophthalmic Solutions for Glaucoma

Assessment	Potential Nursing Diagnoses
Prior to drug administration: ■ Obtain a complete health history including allergies, drug history, and possible drug interactions. ■ Obtain a complete physical examination focusing on visual acuity and visual field assessments. ■ Assess for the presence or history of ocular pain.	■ Injury, Risk for, related to visual acuity deficits ■ Self-care, Deficient, related to impaired vision ■ Pain, related to disease process

Planning: Client Goals and Expected Outcomes

The client will:
■ Exhibit no progression of visual impairment.
■ Demonstrate an understanding of the disease process.
■ Demonstrate an understanding of the drug's action by accurately describing drug side effects and precautions.
■ Safely function within own environment without injury.
■ Report absence of pain.

Implementation

Interventions and (Rationales)	Client Education/Discharge Planning
■ Monitor visual acuity, blurred vision, pupillary reactions, extraocular movements, and ocular pain. (Reporting these signs and symptoms is very important to reducing the chances for serious drug-related interactions.)	■ Instruct client to report changes in vision, and headache.
■ Monitor the client for specific contraindications for the prescribed drug. (Ophthalmic solutions may be contraindicated in many physiological conditions.)	■ Instruct client to inform the healthcare provider of all health-related problems and prescribed medications.
■ Remove contact lenses before administering ophthalmic solutions. (When contacts are in place, drug is not administered into the eye; therefore, there is no therapeutic effect.)	■ Instruct client to remove contact lenses prior to administering eye drops and wait 15 minutes before reinserting them.
■ Administer ophthalmic solutions using proper technique. (Improper administration may lead to infection and/or injury to the eye.)	Instruct client to: ■ Wash hands prior to administering eye drops. ■ Avoid touching the tip of the container to the eye, which may contaminate the solution. ■ Administer the eye drop in the conjunctival sac. ■ Apply pressure over the lacrimal sac for 1 minute. ■ Wait 5 minutes before administering other ophthalmic solutions. ■ Schedule glaucoma medications around daily routines such as waking, mealtimes, and bedtime to lessen the chance of missed doses.
■ Monitor for ocular reaction to the drug such as conjunctivitis and lid reactions. (Reactions may result in further damage to the eye.)	■ Instruct client to report itching, drainage, ocular pain, or other ocular abnormalities.
■ Assess IOP readings. (These are used to determine effectiveness of drug therapy.)	■ Instruct client that IOP readings will be taken prior to beginning treatment and periodically during treatment.
■ Monitor color of iris and periorbital tissue of treated eye. (Evaluation of eye color assists in determining the effectiveness of the drug therapy and potential adverse reactions.)	Instruct client that: ■ More brown color may appear in a lighter-colored iris and in the periorbital tissue of the treated eye only. ■ Any pigmentation changes develop over months to years. ■ The eyes may become more bloodshot during the first month of therapy.
■ Monitor for systemic absorption of ophthalmic preparations by taking pulse, blood pressure and heart rate. (Ophthalmic drugs for glaucoma can cause serious cardiovascular and respiratory complications if the drug is systemically absorbed.)	■ Instruct client to immediately report palpitations, chest pain, shortness of breath, or irregularities in pulse.

(Continued)

NURSING PROCESS FOCUS Clients Receiving Ophthalmic Solutions for Glaucoma (Continued)	
Implementation	
Interventions and (Rationales)	**Client Education/Discharge Planning**
▪ Monitor and adjust environmental lighting to aid in client's comfort. (People who have glaucoma are sensitive to excessive light, especially extreme sunlight.)	Instruct client to: ▪ Adjust environmental lighting as needed to enhance vision or reduce ocular pain. ▪ Wear darkened glasses as needed.
▪ Encourage compliance with treatment regimen. (Noncompliance with the drug therapy may result in the total loss of vision.)	Instruct client: ▪ To adhere to the medication schedule for eye drop administration. ▪ About the importance of regular follow-up care with the ophthalmologist or optometrist.

Evaluation of Outcome Criteria

Evaluate the effectiveness of drug therapy by confirming that client goals and expected outcomes have been met (see "Planning").
▪ The client exhibits no progression of visual impairment.
▪ The client verbalizes an understanding of the disease process.
▪ The client demonstrates an understanding of the drug's action by accurately describing drug side effects and precautions.
▪ The client safely functions within own environment without injury.
▪ The client is free of pain.

∞ See Table 49.1 for a list of drugs to which these nursing actions apply.

and underlying cardiac and respiratory disorders, and possible drug side effects. Frequently, the person with glaucoma is elderly, so a caregiver will administer the eye drops or gels. Review the proper method for administering eye medications given in Chapter 4 ∞. Include the following points when teaching clients about ophthalmic solutions:

- Remove obstacles in the home that may cause falls and accidents secondary to impaired vision.

- Remove contact lenses before instilling drops, and wait at least 15 minutes before reinserting them to allow the medication sufficient contact with the eye.

- Remain still after instilling eye drops until blurred vision diminishes.

- Immediately report eye irritation, conjunctival edema, burning, stinging, redness, blurred vision, pain, irritation, itching, sensation of foreign body in the eye, photophobia, or visual disturbances.

- Report adverse reactions to the medication as well as any possibility of pregnancy.

49.5 Pharmacotherapy for Eye Exams and Minor Eye Conditions

Various drugs are used to enhance diagnostic eye examinations. **Mydriatic drugs** dilate the pupil to allow better assessment of retinal structures. **Cycloplegic drugs** not only dilate the pupil but also paralyze the ciliary muscle and prevent the lens from moving during assessment. Agents used for eye examinations include anticholinergics such as atropine (Isopto Atropine) and tropicamide (Mydriacyl), and sympathomimetics such as phenylephrine (Mydfrin).

Mydriatics cause intense photophobia and pain in response to bright light. Mydriatics can worsen glaucoma by impairing aqueous humor outflow and thereby increasing IOP. In addition, strong concentrations of anticholinergics have the potential to affect the central nervous system and cause confusion, unsteadiness, or drowsiness. Cycloplegics cause severe blurred vision and loss of near vision. Scopolamine, an

HOME & COMMUNITY CONSIDERATIONS

Ophthalmic Drugs in the Home Setting

In modern American culture, older adults may live alone or with other elderly family or friends. These people often need to use ophthalmic drugs at home. Assess the ability of the aging individual to safely administer ophthalmic drugs in the home setting. Return demonstration by the client may be critical for the nurse to assess the older adult's dexterity and skill in self-administering eye medications. If needed, seek reasonable alternatives, such as help from a neighbor, family member, or caregiver.

Teaching is critical for positive outcomes in this population. The older adult needs to understand that touching or rubbing the eye can result in infection or damage to the eye. Because vision may already be compromised, the older adult may experience blurred vision that should clear in a reasonable time after using ophthalmic drugs. Caution elderly clients about trying to drive or even ambulate until this unclear vision improves. Additionally, with eye problems, diminished vision puts the older adult at increased risk for falls. Assess the home and make suggestions to improve safety. Care should be taken to label eye medicines to indicate which is for the left eye and which is for the right eye. Scheduling medications around a routine, such as meals, also may help the older adult remember to take the ophthalmic medications as prescribed, increasing necessary compliance for healing.

Pediatric clients are also treated at home for eye disorders. Caregivers in the home are responsible for administrating and ensuring the client's compliance with the drug therapy. The same administration instructions apply to both geriatric and pediatric populations. Caution against touching and rubbing the eyes. In the case of infants, toddlers, and very young children, it may be necessary to use elbow splints and guards to prevent them from being able to reach their eyes.

TABLE 49.2   Drugs for Mydriasis, Cycloplegia, and Lubrication of the Eye

Drug	Route and Adult Dose (max dose where indicated)	Adverse Effects
MYDRIATICS: SYMPATHOMIMETICS		
hydroxyamphetamine (Paredrine)	1 drop 1% solution before eye exam	*Eye pain, photosensitivity, eye irritation, headache*
phenylephrine HCl (Mydfrin, Neo-Synephrine) (see page 138 for the Prototype Drug box ∞)	1 drop 2.5% or 10% solution before eye exam	<u>Hypertension, tremor, dysrhythmias</u>
CYCLOPLEGICS: ANTICHOLINERGICS		
atropine sulfate (Isopto Atropine, others) (see page 148 for the Prototype Drug box ∞)	1 drop 0.5% solution each day	*Eye irritation and redness, dry mouth, local burning or stinging, headache, blurred vision, photosensitivity*
cyclopentolate (Cyclogyl, Pentolair)	1 drop 0.5%–2% solution 40–50 min before eye exam	
homatropine (Isopto Homatropine, others)	1–2 drops 2% or 5% solution before eye exam	<u>Somnolence, tachycardia, convulsions, mental changes</u>
scopolamine hydrobromide (Isopto Hyoscine)	1–2 drops 0.25% solution 1 h before eye exam	
tropicamide (Mydriacyl, Tropicacyl)	1–2 drops 0.5%–1% solution before eye exam	
LUBRICANTS		
lanolin alcohol (Lacri-lube)	Apply a thin film to the inside of the eyelid	*Temporary burning or stinging, eye itching or redness, headache*
methylcellulose (Methulose, Visculose, others)	1–2 drops PRN	
naphazoline HCl (Albalon, Allerest, ClearEyes, others)	1–3 drops 0.1% solution q3–4h PRN	<u>No serious adverse effects</u>
oxymetazoline HCl (OcuClear, Visine LR)	1–2 drops 0.025% solution qid	
polyvinyl alcohol (Liquifilm, others)	1–2 drops PRN	
tetrahydrozoline HCl (Collyrium, Murine Plus, Visine, others)	1–2 drops 0.05% solution bid–tid	

Italics indicate common adverse effects; <u>underlining</u> indicates serious adverse effects.

anticholinergic often used to prevent motion sickness, can cause blurred vision due to cycloplegia, as well as angle-closure glaucoma attacks.

Drugs for minor irritation and dryness come from a broad range of classes. Some agents lubricate only the eye's surface, whereas others are designed to penetrate and affect a specific area of the eye. Vasoconstrictors are commonly used to treat minor eye irritation. Common vasoconstrictors include phenylephrine (Neo-Synephrine), naphazoline (ClearEyes), and tetrahydrozoline (Murine-Plus, Visine). Side effects of the vasoconstrictors are usually minor and include blurred vision, tearing, headache, and rebound vasodilation with redness. Examples of cycloplegic, mydriatic, and lubricant drugs are listed in Table 49.2. A new drug, pemirolast (Alamast), was recently approved for the therapy of allergic conjunctivitis, which can cause intense itching, redness, and tearing.

NATURAL THERAPIES

Bilberry for Eye Health

Bilberry (*Vaccinium myrtillus*), a plant whose leaves and fruit are used medicinally, is found in central and northern Europe, Asia, and North America. It has been shown in clinical studies to increase conjunctival capillary resistance in clients with diabetic retinopathy, thereby providing protection against hemorrhage of the retina. One compound in bilberry, anthocyanoside, has a collagen-stabilizing effect. Increased synthesis of connective tissue (including collagen) is one of the contributing factors that may lead to blindness caused by diabetic retinopathy. Bilberry has also been used to reduce eye inflammation and improve night vision. Bilberry may be taken as a tea to treat nonspecific diarrhea and topically to treat inflammation of the mucous membranes of the mouth and throat.

EAR CONDITIONS

The ear has two major sensory functions: hearing and maintenance of equilibrium and balance. As shown in Figure 49.3, three structural areas, the outer ear, middle ear, and inner ear, carry out these functions.

Otitis, inflammation of the ear, most often occurs in the outer and middle ear compartments. **External otitis**, commonly called *swimmer's ear*, is inflammation of the outer ear that is most often associated with water exposure. **Otitis media**, inflammation of the middle ear, is most often associated with upper respiratory infections, allergies, or auditory tube irritation. Of all ear infections, the most difficult ones to treat are inner ear infections. **Mastoiditis**, or inflammation of the mastoid sinus, can be a serious problem because if left untreated, it can result in hearing loss.

OTIC PREPARATIONS

The basic treatment for ear infection is topical antibiotics in the form of ear drops.

49.6 Pharmacotherapy With Otic Preparations

Chloramphenicol (Chloromycetin, Pentamycetin) and ciprofloxacin (Cipro otic) are commonly used topical otic antibiotics. Systemic antibiotics may be needed in cases when outer ear infections are extensive or in clients with middle- or inner-ear infections.

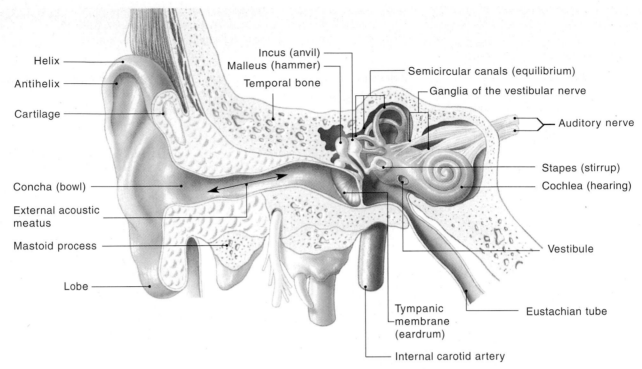

● Figure 49.3 Structures of the external ear, middle ear, and inner ear *Source: Pearson Education/PH College.*

In cases of otitis media, drugs for pain, edema, and itching may also be necessary. Glucocorticoids are often combined with antibiotics or other drugs when inflammation is present. Examples of these drugs are listed in Table 49.3.

Mastoiditis is frequently the result of chronic or recurring bacterial otitis media. The infection moves into the bone and surrounding structures of the middle ear. Antibiotics are usually given for a trial period. If the antibiotics are not effective and symptoms persist, surgery such as mastoidectomy or meatoplasty may be indicated.

Cerumen (ear wax) softeners are also used for proper ear health. When cerumen accumulates, it narrows the ear canal and may interfere with hearing. This procedure usually involves instillation of an earwax softener and then a gentle lavage of the wax-impacted ear with tepid water using an asepto syringe to gently insert the water. An instrument called an *ear loop* may be used to help remove earwax, but should be used only by healthcare providers who are skilled in using it.

NURSING CONSIDERATIONS

The role of the nurse in drug therapy with otic preparations involves careful monitoring of a client's condition and providing education as it relates to the prescribed drug treatment. Before any of the otic preparations are administered, assess the client's baseline hearing and auditory status, symptoms, and any current medical conditions.

Obtain information regarding hypersensitivity to hydrocortisone, neomycin sulfate, or polymyxin B. The use of these medications is contraindicated in the presence of a

TABLE 49.3 Otic Preparations		
Drug	**Route and Adult Dose (max dose where indicated)**	**Adverse Effects**
acetic acid and hydrocortisone (VoSoL HC) aluminum sulfate and calcium acetate (Domeboro)	3–5 drops q4h–qid for 24 h, then 5 drops tid–qid 2 drops 2% solution tid–qid	*Ear irritation, local stinging or burning, dizziness* <u>Allergic reactions (antibiotics)</u>
benzocaine and antipyrine (Auralgan)	Fill ear canal with solution tid for 2–3 days	
carbamide peroxide (Debrox)	1–5 drops 6.5% solution bid for 4 days	
ciprofloxacin hydrochloride and hydrocortisone (Cipro)	3 drops of the suspension instilled into ear bid for 7 days	
polymyxin B, neomycin and hydrocortisone (Cortisporin)	4 drops in ear tid–qid	
triethanolamine polypeptide oleate 10% condensate (Cerumenex)	Fill ear canal with solution; wait 10–20 min	

Italics indicate common adverse effects; <u>underlining</u> indicates serious adverse effects.

perforated eardrum. Chloramphenicol ear drops are contraindicated in hypersensitivity and eardrum perforation. Side effects include burning, redness, rash, swelling, and other signs of topical irritation.

When instilling otic preparations, cleanse the ear thoroughly and remove the cerumen through irrigation. Otic drugs should be warmed to body temperature (but not higher) before instillation. Administer wax emulsifiers according to the manufacturer's guidelines or the healthcare provider's orders.

Lifespan Considerations. Geriatric and pediatric clients frequently experience ear infections (especially otitis media in children). Proper instruction in instillation is needed: with adults and children older than 3 years, the pinna should be held up and back during instillation. With children younger than 3 years of age, the pinna should be gently pulled down and back during instillation. When cerumen accumulates, it narrows the ear canal, and may interfere with hearing. This is especially common in older clients and may be part of the changes associated with aging. Healthcare providers working with elderly clients should be trained to take appropriate measures when removing impacted cerumen. Advise clients not to perform ear wax removal, especially in children, because of the potential for damage to the eardrum. Ear drops are capable of

being absorbed to the systemic circulation and passed on to the fetus or infant in pregnant and lactating women.

Client Teaching. Client education as it relates to otic preparations should include the goals of therapy, the reasons for obtaining baseline data such as hearing/auditory tests and the existence of underlying disorders, and possible drug side effects. Include the following points when teaching clients about otic preparations:

- Lie down while instilling chloramphenicol drops because dizziness may occur.
- Administer ear drops at body temperature by running warm water over the bottle.
- In adults and children older than 3 years, hold the pinna up and back during instillation.
- In children younger than 3 years, gently pull the pinna down and back during instillation.
- Do not touch dropper to the ear.
- Massage the area around the ear gently after instillation to promote thorough administration to the ear canal.
- Lie on the side opposite the affected ear for 5 minutes after instillation.

Nursing in Action Administering Ear Drops

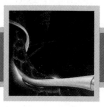

CHAPTER REVIEW

KEY CONCEPTS

The numbered key concepts provide a succinct summary of the important points from the corresponding numbered section within the chapter. If any of these points are not clear, refer to the numbered section within the chapter for review.

49.1 Knowledge of basic eye anatomy is fundamental to understanding eye disorders and pharmacotherapy.

49.2 Glaucoma develops because the flow of aqueous humor in the anterior eye cavity becomes disrupted, leading to increased intraocular pressure. The two principal types of glaucoma are closed-angle glaucoma and open-angle glaucoma. Therapy of acute glaucoma may require laser surgery to correct the underlying pathology.

49.3 The goal of glaucoma pharmacotherapy is to prevent damage to the optic nerve by lowering IOP. Combination therapy may be necessary to achieve this goal.

49.4 Drugs used for glaucoma decrease IOP by increasing the outflow of aqueous humor or by decreasing the formation of aqueous humor. Drug classes include prostaglandins, beta-adrenergic blockers, alpha$_2$-adrenergic agonists, carbonic anhydrase inhibitors, nonselective sympathomimetics, cholinergic agonists, and osmotic diuretics

49.5 Drugs routinely used for eye examinations include mydriatics, which dilate the pupil, and cycloplegics, which cause both dilation and paralysis of the ciliary muscle.

49.6 Otic preparations treat infections, inflammation, and earwax buildup.

NCLEX-RN® REVIEW QUESTIONS

1 A client with a history of glaucoma complains of severe pain in the eye, severe headache, and blurred vision. The appropriate nursing action is to:

1. Document the occurrence; this symptom is expected.
2. Medicate the client with a narcotic analgesic.
3. Notify the physician immediately.
4. Place the client in a quiet darkened environment.

2 The client should be aware of potential side effects of prostaglandins used in the treatment of glaucoma. The nurse should include which of the following in the teaching plan?

1. Hypertension
2. Loss of lashes
3. Dilation of pupils
4. Brown pigmentation of treated eye

3 Beta-adrenergic agents may be used to treat glaucoma. The nurse should teach the clients and family to:

1. Monitor urine output.
2. Monitor blood glucose.
3. Monitor pulse and blood pressure.
4. Monitor respiratory rate.

4 The nurse emphasizes to the client with glaucoma the importance of notifying the physician performing an eye examination of a glaucoma diagnosis because of potential adverse reactions to which drugs?

1. Antibiotic drops
2. Cycloplegic drops
3. Anti-inflammatory drops
4. Anticholinergic mydriatic drops

5 The client is prescribed timolol (Timoptic) for treatment of glaucoma. The nurse assesses for which of the following medical disorders during the history and physical, which may be a contraindication to the use of this drug? (Select all that apply.)

1. Heart block
2. Congestive heart failure
3. Liver disease
4. COPD
5. Renal disease

CRITICAL THINKING QUESTIONS

1. A 3-year-old girl is playing nurse with her dolls. She picks up her mother's flexible metal necklace and places the tips of the necklace in her ears for her "stethoscope." A few hours later, she cries to her mother that her "ears hurt." The child's mother takes her to see the healthcare provider at an after-hours clinic. An examination reveals abrasions in the outer ear canal and some dried blood. The healthcare provider prescribes corticosporin otic drops. What does the nurse need to teach the mother about instillation of this medication?

2. A 64-year-old man has been diagnosed with primary open-angle glaucoma. He has COPD following a 40-year history of smoking. Is he a candidate for treatment with timolol (Timoptic)? Why or why not? Is there a preferred agent?

3. To determine a client's ability to administer glaucoma medications, the nurse asks the 82-year-old woman to instill her own medications prior to discharge. The nurse notes that the client is happy to cooperate and watches as the client quickly drops her head back, opens her eyes, and drops the medication directly onto her cornea. The client blinks several times, smiles at the nurse, and says, "There, it is no problem at all!" What correction should the nurse make in the client's technique?

See Appendix D for answers and rationales for all activities.

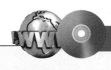

EXPLORE MediaLink

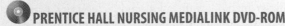

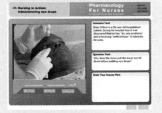

NCLEX-RN® review, case studies, and other interactive resources for this chapter can be found on the companion website at www.prenhall.com/adams. Click on "Chapter 49" to select the activities for this chapter. For animations, more NCLEX-RN® review questions, and an audio glossary, access the accompanying Prentice Hall Nursing MediaLink DVD-ROM in this textbook.

PRENTICE HALL NURSING MEDIALINK DVD-ROM

- **Animation**
  Mechanism in Action: Pilocarpine (*Adsorbocarpine*)
- **Audio Glossary**
- **NCLEX-RN® Review**
- **Nursing in Action**
  Administering eye drops
  Administering ear drops

 COMPANION WEBSITE

- **NCLEX-RN® Review**
- **Dosage Calculations**
- **Case Study:** Client with glaucoma
- **Care Plan:** Client with open-angle glaucoma treated with timolol

GLOSSARY

A-delta fibers nerves that transmit sensations of sharp pain

Absence seizure seizure with a loss or reduction of normal activity, including staring and transient loss of responsiveness

Absorption the process of moving a drug across body membranes

Acetylcholine primary neurotransmitter of the parasympathetic nervous system; also present at somatic neuromuscular junctions and at sympathetic preganglionic nerves

Acetylcholinesterase (AchE) enzyme that degrades acetylcholine within the synaptic cleft, enhancing effects of the neurotransmitter

Acidosis condition of having too much acid in the blood; plasma pH below 7.35

Acne vulgaris condition characterized by small inflamed bumps that appear on the surface of the skin

Acquired immunodeficiency syndrome (AIDS) infection caused by the human immunodeficiency virus (HIV)

Acquired resistance the capacity of a microbe to no longer be affected by a drug following anti-infective pharmacotherapy

Action potential electrical changes in the membrane of a muscle or nerve cell due to changes in membrane permeability

Activated partial thromboplastin time (PTT) blood test used to determine how long it takes clots to form to regulate heparin dosage

Active immunity resistance resulting from a previous exposure to an antigen

Acute gouty arthritis condition in which uric acid crystals accumulate in the joints of the big toes, ankles, wrists, fingers, knees, or elbows, resulting in red, swollen, or inflamed tissue

Acute radiation syndrome life-threatening symptoms resulting from acute exposure to ionizing radiation, including nausea, vomiting, severe leukopenia, thrombocytopenia, anemia, and alopecia

Addiction the continued use of a substance despite its negative health and social consequences

Addison's disease hyposecretion of glucocorticoids and aldosterone by the adrenal cortex

Adenohypophysis anterior portion of the pituitary gland

Adjuvant chemotherapy technique in which antineoplastics are administered *after* surgery or radiation to effect a cure

Adolescence period from 13 to 16 years of age

Adrenergic relating to nerves that release norepinephrine or epinephrine

Adrenergic antagonist drug that blocks the actions of the sympathetic nervous system

Adrenocorticotropic hormone (ACTH) hormone secreted by the anterior pituitary that stimulates the release of glucocorticoids by the adrenal cortex

Aerobic pertaining to an oxygen environment

Aerosol suspension of minute liquid droplets or fine solid particles in a gas

Affinity chemical attraction that impels certain molecules to unite with others to form complexes

Afterload pressure that must be overcome for the ventricles to eject blood from the heart

Agonist drug that is capable of binding with receptors to induce a cellular response

Akathisia inability to remain still; constantly moving

Aldosterone hormone secreted by the adrenal cortex that increases sodium reabsorption in the distal tubule of the kidney

Alkalosis condition of having too many basic substances in the blood; plasma pH above 7.45

Alkylation process by which certain chemicals attach to DNA and change its structure and function

Allergic reaction acquired hyperresponse of body defenses to a foreign substance (allergen)

Alopecia hair loss

Alpha-receptor type of subreceptor found in the sympathetic nervous system

Alzheimer's disease most common dementia, characterized by loss of memory, delusions, hallucinations, confusion, and loss of judgment

Amenorrhea lack of normal menstrual periods

Amide type of chemical linkage found in some local anesthetics involving carbon, nitrogen, and oxygen (–NH–CO–)

Amyloid plaques abnormal protein fragments related to neuronal damage; a sign of Alzheimer's disease observed during autopsy

Anabolic steroids compounds resembling testosterone with hormonal activity commonly abused by athletes

Anaerobic pertaining to an environment without oxygen

Analgesic drug used to reduce or eliminate pain

Anaphylactic shock type of shock caused by an acute allergic reaction

Anaphylaxis acute allergic response to an antigen that results in severe hypotension and may lead to life-threatening shock if untreated

Anastomoses natural communication networks among the coronary arteries

Androgens steroid sex hormones that promote the appearance of masculine characteristics

Anemia lack of adequate numbers of red blood cells, or decreased oxygen-carrying capacity of the blood

Angina pectoris acute chest pain on physical or emotional exertion due to inadequate oxygen supply to the myocardium

Angiotensin II chemical released in response to falling blood pressure that causes vasoconstriction and release of aldosterone

Angiotensin-converting enzyme (ACE) enzyme responsible for converting angiotensin I to angiotensin II

Anions negatively charged ions

Anorexia loss of appetite

Anorexiant drug used to suppress appetite

Antacid drug that neutralizes stomach acid

Antagonist drug that blocks the response of another drug

Antepartum prior to the onset of labor

Anthrax microorganism that can cause severe disease and high mortality in humans

Antibiotic substance produced by a microorganism that inhibits or kills other microorganisms

Antibody protein produced by the body in response to an antigen; used interchangeably with the term *immunoglobulin*

Anticholinergic drug that blocks the actions of the parasympathetic nervous system

Anticoagulant agent that inhibits the formation of blood clots

Antidepressant drug that alters levels of two important neurotransmitters in the brain, norepinephrine and serotonin, to reduce depression and anxiety

Antiemetic drug that prevents vomiting

Antiflatulent agent that reduces gas bubbles in the stomach and intestines, thereby decreasing bloating and discomfort

Anti-infective general term for any medication that is effective against pathogens

Antipyretic drug that lowers body temperature

Antiretroviral drug that is effective against retroviruses

Antithrombin III protein that prevents abnormal clotting by inhibiting thrombin

Antitussive drug used to suppress cough

Anxiety state of apprehension and autonomic nervous system activation resulting from exposure to a nonspecific or unknown cause

Anxiolytics drugs that relieve anxiety

Apoprotein protein component of a lipoprotein

Apothecary system of measurement older system of measurement that uses drams; rarely used

Aqueous humor fluid that fills the anterior and posterior chambers of the eye

Aromatase inhibitor hormone inhibitor that blocks the enzyme aromatase, which normally converts adrenal androgen to estradiol

ASAP order (as soon as possible) order that should be available for administration to the patient within 30 minutes of the written order

Assessment appraisal of a patient's condition that involves gathering and interpreting data

Asthma chronic inflammatory disease of the lungs characterized by airway obstruction

Astringent effect drops or spray used to shrink swollen mucous membranes, or to loosen secretions and facilitate drainage

Atherosclerosis condition characterized by a buildup of fatty plaque and loss of elasticity of the walls of the arteries

Atonic seizure very-short-lasting seizure during which the patient may stumble and fall for no apparent reason

Atrioventricular (AV) node cardiac tissue that receives electrical impulses from the sinoatrial node and conveys them to the ventricles

Atrioventricular bundle cardiac tissue that receives electrical impulses from the AV node and sends them to the bundle branches; also known as the *bundle of His*

Attention-deficit disorder (ADD) inability to focus attention on a task for a sufficient length of time

Attention-deficit hyperactivity disorder (ADHD) disorder typically diagnosed in childhood and adolescence characterized by hyperactivity as well as attention, organization, and behavior control issues

Aura sensory cue such as bright lights, smells, or tastes that precedes a migraine

Autoantibodies proteins called *rheumatoid factors* released by B lymphocytes that tear down the body's own tissue

Automaticity ability of certain myocardial cells to spontaneously generate an action potential

Autonomic nervous system portion of the peripheral nervous system that governs involuntary actions of the smooth muscle, cardiac muscle, and glands

Azole term for the major class of drugs used to treat mycoses

Azoospermia complete absence of sperm in an ejaculate

Bacteriocidal substance that kills bacteria

Bacteriostatic substance that inhibits the growth of bacteria

Balanced anesthesia use of multiple medications to rapidly induce unconsciousness, cause muscle relaxation, and maintain deep anesthesia

Baroreceptors nerves located in the walls of the atria, aortic arch, vena cava, and carotid sinus that sense changes in blood pressure

Basal metabolic rate resting rate of metabolism in the body

Baseline data patient information that is gathered before pharmacotherapy is implemented

B cell lymphocyte responsible for humoral immunity

Beneficence ethical principle of doing good

Benign not life threatening or fatal

Benign prostatic hypertrophy/hyperplasia (BPH) nonmalignant enlargement of the prostate gland

Benzodiazepines major class of drugs used to treat anxiety disorders

Beriberi deficiency of thiamine

Beta-lactam ring chemical structure found in most penicillins and some cephalosporins

Beta-lactamase (penicillinase) enzyme present in certain bacteria that is able to inactivate many penicillins and some cephalosporins

Beta-receptor type of subreceptor found in the sympathetic nervous system

Bile acid resin drug that binds bile acids, thus lowering cholesterol

Bioavailability ability of a drug to reach the bloodstream and its target tissues

Biologics substances that produce biologic responses within the body; they are synthesized by cells of the human body, animal cells, or microorganisms

Bioterrorism intentional use of infectious biological agents, chemical substances, or radiation to cause widespread harm or illness

Bipolar disorder syndrome characterized by extreme and opposite moods, such as euphoria and depression

Bisphosphonates class of drugs that block bone resorption by inhibiting osteoclast activity

Blood–brain barrier anatomical structure that prevents certain substances from gaining access to the brain

Bone deposition opposite of bone resorption; the process of depositing mineral components into bone

Bone resorption process of bone demineralization or the breaking down of bone into mineral components

Botanical plant extract used to treat or prevent illness

Bradykinesia difficulty initiating movement and controlling fine muscle movements

Bradykinin chemical released by cells during inflammation that produces pain and side effects similar to those of histamine

Breakthrough bleeding hemorrhage at abnormal times during the menstrual cycle

Broad-spectrum antibiotic anti-infective that is effective against many different gram-positive and gram-negative organisms

Bronchospasm rapid constriction of the airways

Buccal route administration of a tablet or capsule by placing it in the oral cavity between the gum and the cheek

Buffer chemical that helps maintain normal body pH by neutralizing strong acids or bases

Bundle branch electrical conduction pathway in the heart leading from the AV bundle and through the wall between the ventricles

C fibers nerves that transmit dull, poorly localized pain

Calcifediol substance formed in the first step of vitamin D formation

Calcineurin intracellular messenger molecule to which immunosuppressants bind

Calcitonin hormone secreted by the thyroid gland that increases the deposition of calcium in bone

Calcitriol substance transformed in the kidneys during the second step of the conversion of vitamin D to its active form

Calcium channel blocker drug that blocks the flow of calcium ions into myocardial cells

Calcium ion channel pathway in a plasma membrane through which calcium ions enter and leave

Camptothecins class of antineoplastics that inhibit the enzyme topoisomerase

Cancer/carcinoma malignant disease characterized by rapidly growing, invasive cells that spread to other regions of the body and eventually kill the host

Capsid protein coat that surrounds a virus

Carbonic anhydrase enzyme that forms carbonic acid by combining carbon dioxide and water

Cardiac decompensation condition during heart failure in which the heart can no longer handle the workload, and symptoms such as dyspnea on exertion, fatigue, pulmonary congestion, and peripheral edema appear

Cardiac output amount of blood pumped by a ventricle in 1 minute

Cardiac remodeling change in the size, shape, and structure of the myocardial cells (myocytes) that occurs over time in heart failure

Cardiogenic shock type of shock caused by a diseased heart that cannot maintain circulation to the tissues

Cardioversion/defibrillation conversion of fibrillation to a normal heart rhythm

Carotene class of yellow-red pigments that are precursors to vitamin A

Catecholamines class of agents secreted in response to stress that include epinephrine, norepinephrine, and dopamine

Cathartic substance that causes complete evacuation of the bowel

Cations positively charged ions

CD4 receptor protein that accepts HIV and allows entry of the virus into the T4 lymphocyte

Central nervous system (CNS) division of the nervous system consisting of the brain and spinal cord

Chemical name strict chemical nomenclature used for naming drugs established by the International Union of Pure and Applied Chemistry (IUPAC)

Chemoreceptors nerves located in the aortic arch and carotid sinus that sense changes in oxygen content, pH, or carbon dioxide levels in the blood

Chemotherapy drug treatment of cancer

Chief cells cells located in the mucosa of the stomach that secrete pepsinogen, an inactive form of the enzyme pepsin that chemically breaks down proteins

Cholecalciferol vitamin D_3 formed in the skin by exposure to ultraviolet light

Cholinergic relating to nerves that release acetylcholine

Chronic bronchitis recurrent disease of the lungs characterized by excess mucus production, inflammation, and coughing

Chronic obstructive pulmonary disease (COPD) generic term used to describe several pulmonary conditions characterized by cough, mucus production, and impaired gas exchange

Chyme semifluid, partly digested food that is passed from the stomach to the duodenum

Clinical investigation second stage of drug testing that involves clinical phase trials

Clinical phase trials testing of a new drug in selected patients

Clonic spasm multiple, rapidly repeated muscular contractions

Closed-angle glaucoma acute glaucoma that is caused by decreased outflow of aqueous humor from the anterior chamber

Clotting factors substances contributing to the process of blood hemostasis

Coagulation process of blood clotting

Coagulation cascade complex series of steps by which blood flow stops

Colloid type of IV fluid consisting of large organic molecules that are unable to cross membranes

Colony-stimulating factors hormones that regulate the growth and maturation of specific WBC populations

Combination drug drug product with more than one active generic ingredient

Comedone type of acne lesion that develops just beneath the surface of the skin (whitehead) or as a result of a plugged oil gland (blackhead)

Complement a series of proteins involved in the nonspecific defense of the body that promote antigen destruction

Complementary and alternative medicine (CAM) treatments that consider the health of the whole person and promote disease prevention

Complementary and alternative therapies treatments considered outside the realm of conventional Western medicine

Compliance taking a medication in the manner prescribed by the healthcare provider, or, in the case of OTC drugs, following the instructions on the label

Conjugates side chains that, during metabolism, make drugs more water soluble and more easily excreted by the kidney

Constipation infrequent passage of abnormally hard and dry stools

Contractility the strength with which the myocardial fibers contract

Controlled substance in the United States, a drug whose use is restricted by the Comprehensive Drug Abuse Prevention and Control Act; in Canada, a drug subject to guidelines outlined in the Canadian Narcotic Control Act

Convulsion uncontrolled muscle contraction or spasm that occurs in the face, torso, arms, or legs

Coronary arterial bypass graft (CABG) surgical procedure performed to restore blood flow to the myocardium by using a section of the saphenous vein or internal mammary artery to go around the obstructed coronary artery

Coronary arteries vessels that bring oxygen and nutrients to the myocardium

Corpus cavernosum tissue in the penis that fills with blood during an erection

Corpus luteum ruptured follicle that remains in the ovary after ovulation and secretes progestins

Corpus striatum area of the brain responsible for unconscious muscle movement; a point of contact for neurons projecting from the substantia nigra

Crohn's disease chronic inflammatory bowel disease affecting the ileum and sometimes the colon

Cross-tolerance situation in which tolerance to one drug makes the patient tolerant to another drug

Crystalloid type of IV fluid resembling blood plasma minus proteins that is capable of crossing membranes

Culture set of beliefs, values, religious rituals, and customs shared by a group of people

Culture and sensitivity test laboratory exam used to identify bacteria and to determine which antibiotic is most effective

Cushing's syndrome condition of having an excessive concentration of corticosteroids in the blood; caused by excessive secretion by the adrenal glands or by overdosage with corticosteroid medication

Cyclooxygenase (COX-1 and COX-2) key enzyme in the prostaglandin metabolic pathway that is blocked by aspirin and other NSAIDs

Cycloplegic drugs drugs that relax or temporarily paralyze ciliary muscles and cause blurred vision

Cytokines chemicals produced by white blood cells, such as interleukins, leukotrienes, interferon, and tumor necrosis factor, that guide the immune response

Cytotoxic T cell lymphocyte responsible for cell-mediated immunity that kills target cells directly or by secreting cytokines

Defecation evacuation of the colon; bowel movement

Delusions false ideas and beliefs not founded in reality

Dementia degenerative disorder characterized by progressive memory loss, confusion, and the inability to think or communicate effectively

Dependence strong physiological or psychological need for a substance

Depolarization reversal of the plasma membrane charge such that the inside is made less negative

Depression disorder characterized by depressed mood, lack of energy, sleep disturbances, abnormal eating patterns, and feelings of despair, guilt, and misery

Dermatitis inflammatory condition of the skin characterized by itching and scaling

Dermatophytic relating to a superficial fungal infection

Designer drug substance produced in a laboratory and intended to mimic the effects of another psychoactive controlled substance

Diabetes insipidus disorder marked by excessive urination due to lack of secretion of antidiuretic hormone

Diabetes mellitus, type 1 metabolic disease characterized by hyperglycemia caused by a lack of secretion of insulin by the pancreas

Diabetes mellitus, type 2 chronic metabolic disease caused by insufficient secretion of insulin by the pancreas, and a lack of sensitivity of insulin receptors

Diabetic ketoacidosis a type of metabolic acidosis due to an excess of ketone bodies, most often occurring when diabetes mellitus is uncontrolled

Diarrhea abnormal frequency and liquidity of bowel movements

Diastolic pressure blood pressure during the relaxation phase of heart activity

Dietary fiber ingested substance that is neither digested nor absorbed that contributes to the fecal mass

Dietary supplement nondrug substance regulated by the DSHEA

Dietary Supplement Health and Education Act of 1994 (DSHEA) primary law in the United States regulating herb and dietary supplements

Digitalization procedure in which the dose of cardiac glycoside is gradually increased until tissues become saturated with the drug, and the symptoms of heart failure diminish

Disease-modifying antirheumatic drugs (DMARD) drugs from several classes that modify the progression of rheumatoid arthritis; include hydroxychloroquine (Plaquenil), methotrexate (Rheumatrex), and sulfasalazine (Azulfidine)

Distribution the process of transporting drugs through the body

Diuretic substance that increases urine output

Dopamine type-D_2 receptor receptor for dopamine in the basal nuclei of the brain that is associated with schizophrenia and antipsychotic drugs

Drug general term for any substance capable of producing biological responses in the body

Drug–protein complex drug that has bound reversibly to a plasma protein, particularly albumin, that makes the drug unavailable for distribution to body tissues

Dry powder inhaler (DPI) device used to convert a solid drug to a fine powder for the purpose of inhalation

Dysentery severe diarrhea that may include bleeding

Dysfunctional uterine bleeding hemorrhage that occurs at abnormal times or in excessive quantity during the menstrual cycle

Dyslipidemia abnormal (excess or deficient) level of lipoproteins in the blood

Dysrhythmia abnormality in cardiac rhythm

Dystonia severe muscle spasms, particularly of the back, neck, tongue, and face; characterized by abnormal tension starting in one area of the body and progressing to other areas

Eclampsia pregnancy-induced hypertensive disorder

Ectopic focus, pacemaker cardiac tissue outside the normal cardiac conduction pathway that generates action potentials

Eczema also called *atopic dermatitis*; a skin disorder with unexplained symptoms of inflammation, itching, and scaling

Efficacy the ability of a drug to produce a desired response

Electrocardiogram (ECG) device that records the electrical activity of the heart

Electroconvulsive therapy (ECT) treatment used for serious and life-threatening mood disorders in patients who are unresponsive to pharmacotherapy

Electroencephalogram (EEG) diagnostic test that records brainwaves through electrodes attached to the scalp

Electrolytes charged substances in the blood such as sodium, potassium, calcium, chloride, and phosphate

Embolus blood clot carried in the bloodstream

Emesis vomiting

Emetic drug used to induce vomiting

Emetic potential usually applied to antineoplastic agents; degree to which an agent is likely to trigger the vomiting center in the medulla, resulting in nausea and vomiting

Emphysema terminal lung disease characterized by permanent dilation of the alveoli

Endogenous opioids chemicals produced naturally within the body that decrease or eliminate pain; they closely resemble the actions of morphine

Endometriosis presence of endometrial tissue in nonuterine locations such as the pelvis and ovaries; a common cause of infertility

Endothelium inner lining of a blood vessel

Enteral nutrition nutrients supplied orally or by feeding tube

Enteral route administration of drugs orally, and through nasogastric or gastrostomy tubes

Enteric coated referring to tablets that have a hard, waxy coating designed to dissolve in the alkaline environment of the small intestine

Enterohepatic recirculation recycling of drugs and other substances by the circulation of bile through the intestine and liver

Enzyme induction process in which a drug changes the function of the hepatic microsomal enzymes and increases metabolic activity in the liver

Epilepsy disorder of the CNS characterized by seizures and/or convulsions

Ergocalciferol activated form of vitamin D

Ergosterol lipid substance in fungal cell membranes

Erythema redness associated with skin irritation

Erythrocytic stage phase in malaria during which infected red blood cells rupture, releasing merozoites and causing fever and chills

Erythropoietin hormone secreted by the kidney that regulates the process of red blood cell formation, or erythropoiesis

Ester type of chemical linkage found in some local anesthetics involving carbon and oxygen (–CO–O–)

Estrogen class of steroid sex hormones secreted by the ovary

Ethnic referring to people having a common history and similar genetic heritage

Evaluation, systematic objective assessment of the effectiveness and impact of interventions

Excoriation scratch that breaks the skin surface and fills with blood or serous fluid to form a crusty scale

Excretion the process of removing substances from the body

Expectorant drug used to increase bronchial secretions

External otitis commonly called *swimmer's ear*, an inflammation of the outer ear

Extracellular fluid (ECF) compartment body fluid lying outside cells, which includes plasma and interstitial fluid

Extrapyramidal side effects symptoms of acute dystonia, akathisia, parkinsonism, and tardive dyskinesia often caused by antipsychotic drugs

Febrile seizure tonic–clonic motor activity lasting 1 to 2 minutes with rapid return of consciousness that occurs in conjunction with elevated body temperature

Ferritin one of two protein complexes that maintain iron stores inside cells (hemosiderin is the other)

Fetal–placental barrier special anatomical structure that inhibits entry of many chemicals and drugs to the fetus

Fibrillation type of dysrhythmia in which the chambers beat in a highly disorganized manner

Fibrin an insoluble protein formed from fibrinogen by the action of thrombin in the blood clotting process

Fibrinogen blood protein that is converted to fibrin by the action of thrombin in the blood coagulation process

Fibrinolysis removal of a blood clot

Fight-or-flight response characteristic set of signs and symptoms produced when the sympathetic nervous system is activated

Filtrate fluid in the nephron that is filtered at Bowman's capsule

First-pass effect mechanism whereby drugs are absorbed across the intestinal wall and enter into the hepatic portal circulation

Five rights of drug administration principles that offer simple and practical guidance for nurses to use during drug preparation, delivery, and administration

Folic acid/folate B vitamin that is a coenzyme in protein and nucleic acid metabolism

Follicle-stimulating hormone (FSH) hormone secreted by the anterior pituitary gland that regulates sperm or egg production

Follicular cells cells in the thyroid gland that secrete thyroid hormone

Food and Drug Administration (FDA) U.S. agency responsible for the evaluation and approval of new drugs

Formulary list of drugs and drug recipes commonly used by pharmacists

Frank–Starling law the greater the degree of stretch on the myocardial fibers, the greater will be the force by which they contract

Frequency response curve graphical representation that illustrates interpatient variability in responses to drugs

Fungi kingdom of organisms that includes mushrooms, yeasts, and molds

Gamma-aminobutyric acid (GABA) neurotransmitter in the CNS

Ganglion collection of neuron cell bodies located outside the CNS

Gastroesophageal reflux disease (GERD) regurgitation of stomach contents into the esophagus

General anesthesia medical procedure that produces unconsciousness and loss of sensation throughout the entire body

Generalized anxiety disorder (GAD) difficult-to-control, excessive anxiety that lasts 6 months or more, focuses on a variety of life events, and interferes with normal day-to-day functions

Generalized seizures seizures that travel throughout the entire brain

Generic name nonproprietary name of a drug assigned by the government

Genetic polymorphism changes in enzyme structure and function due to mutation of the encoding gene

Glucocorticoid class of hormones secreted by the adrenal cortex that help the body respond to stress

Glycoprotein IIb/IIIa enzyme that binds fibrinogen and von Willebrand's factor to begin platelet aggregation and blood coagulation

Goal any object or objective that the patient or nurse seeks to attain or achieve

Gonadotropin-releasing hormone hormone secreted by the hypothalamus that stimulates the secretion of follicle-stimulating hormone (FSH) and luteinizing hormone (LH)

Gout metabolic disorder characterized by the accumulation of uric acid in the bloodstream or joint cavities

Graded dose response relationship between and measurement of the patient's response obtained at different doses of a drug

Gram-negative bacteria that do not retain a purple stain because they have an outer envelope

Gram-positive bacteria that stain purple because they have no outer envelope

Graves' disease syndrome caused by hypersecretion of thyroid hormone

Growth fraction the ratio of the number of replicating cells to resting cells in a tumor

H^+, K^+-ATPase enzyme responsible for pumping acid onto the mucosal surface of the stomach

H_1-receptor site located on smooth-muscle cells in the bronchial tree and blood vessels that is stimulated by histamine to produce bronchodilation and vasodilation

H_2-receptor site located on cells of the digestive system that is stimulated by histamine to produce gastric acid

H_2-receptor antagonist drug that inhibits the effects of histamine at its receptors in the GI tract

Hallucination seeing, hearing, or feeling something that is not real

Heart failure (HF) disease in which the heart muscle cannot contract with sufficient force to meet the body's metabolic needs

Helicobacter pylori bacterium associated with a large percentage of peptic ulcer disease

Helminth type of flat, round, or segmented worm

Helper T cell lymphocyte that coordinates both the humoral and cell-mediated immune responses and that is the target of the human immunodeficiency virus

Hematopoiesis process of erythrocyte production that begins with primitive stem cells that reside in bone marrow

Hemophilia hereditary lack of a specific blood clotting factor

Hemosiderin one of two protein complexes that maintain iron stores inside cells (ferritin is the other)

Hemostasis the slowing or stopping of blood flow

Hemostatic drug used to inhibit the normal removal of fibrin, used to speed clot formation, and keep the clot in place for a longer period

Hepatic microsomal enzyme system as it relates to pharmacotherapy, liver enzymes that inactivate drugs and accelerate their excretion; sometimes called the P-450 system

Hepatitis viral infection of the liver

Herb plant with a soft stem that is used for healing or as a seasoning

High-density lipoprotein (HDL) lipid-carrying particle in the blood that contains high amounts of protein and lower amounts of cholesterol; considered to be "good" cholesterol

Highly active antiretroviral therapy (HAART) drug therapy for HIV infection that includes high doses of multiple medications given concurrently

Hippocampus region of the brain responsible for learning and memory; a part of the limbic system

Histamine chemical released by mast cells in response to an antigen that causes dilation of blood vessels, bronchoconstriction, tissue swelling, and itching

HIV-AIDS acronym for human immunodeficiency virus–acquired immune deficiency syndrome; characterized by profound immunosuppression that leads to opportunistic infections and malignancies not commonly found in patients with functioning immune defenses

HMG-CoA reductase primary enzyme in the biochemical pathway for the synthesis of cholesterol

Holistic viewing a person as an integrated biological, psychosocial, cultural, communicating whole, existing and functioning within the communal environment

Hormone chemical secreted by endocrine glands that acts as a chemical messenger to affect homeostasis

Hormone replacement therapy (HRT) drug therapy, consisting of estrogen and progestin combinations; used to treat symptoms associated with menopause

Host flora normal microorganisms found in or on a patient

Household system of measurement older system of measurement that uses teaspoons, tablespoons, and cups

Humoral immunity branch of the immune system that produces antibodies

Hydrolysis breakdown of a substance into simpler compounds by the addition or taking up of water

Hypercholesterolemia high levels of cholesterol in the blood

Hyperemia increase in blood supply to a part or tissue space causing swelling, redness, and pain

Hyperglycemia high glucose level in the blood

Hyperlipidemia excess amount of lipids in the blood

Hypernatremia high sodium level in the blood

Hyperosmolar nonketotic coma life-threatening metabolic condition that occurs in people with type 2 diabetes

Hypertension high blood pressure

Hyperuricemia elevated blood level of uric acid, which causes gout

Hypervitaminosis excess intake of vitamins

Hypnotic drug that causes sleep

Hypoglycemia low glucose level in the blood

Hypogonadism below-normal secretion of the steroid sex hormones

Hyponatremia low sodium level in the blood

Hypovolemic shock type of shock caused by loss of fluids such as occurs during hemorrhage, extensive burns, or severe vomiting or diarrhea

Idiosyncratic response unpredictable and unexplained drug reaction

Ileum third portion of the small intestine extending from the jejunum to the ileocecal valve

Illusion distorted perception of actual sensory stimuli

Immune response specific reaction of the body to foreign agents involving B and/or T lymphocytes

Immunosuppressant any drug, chemical, or physical agent that lowers the immune defense mechanisms of the body

Impotence inability to obtain or sustain an erection; also called *erectile dysfunction*

Infant child younger than 1 year

Infertility inability to become pregnant after at least 1 year of frequent, unprotected intercourse

Inflammation nonspecific body defense that occurs in response to an injury or antigen

Influenza common viral infection; often called flu

Inotropic agent drug or chemical that changes the force of contraction of the heart

Inotropic effect change in the strength or contractility of the heart

Insomnia inability to fall asleep or stay asleep

Insulin analog modified human insulin with pharmacokinetic advantages, such as more rapid onset of action or prolonged duration of action

Insulin resistance occurs in type 2 diabetes mellitus; although insulin is secreted, insulin receptors in target tissues become *insensitive* to insulin, binding of insulin to these receptors decreases, less effect is achieved

Interferon type of cytokine secreted by T cells in response to antigens to protect uninfected cells

Interleukin class of cytokines synthesized by lymphocytes, monocytes, macrophages, and certain other cells that enhance the capabilities of the immune system

Intermittent claudication condition caused by insufficient blood flow to skeletal muscles in the lower limbs, resulting in ischemia of skeletal muscles and severe pain on walking, especially in calf muscles

Intervention action that produces an effect or that is intended to alter the course of a disease or condition

Intracellular fluid (ICF) compartment body fluid that is inside cells; accounts for about two thirds of the total body water

Intracellular parasite infectious microbe that lives inside host cells

Intradermal (ID) medication administered into the dermis layer of the skin

Intramuscular (IM) delivery of medication into specific muscles

Intravenous (IV) administration of medications and fluids directly into the bloodstream

Intrinsic factor chemical substance secreted by the parietal cells in the stomach that is essential for the absorption of vitamin B_{12}

Ionizing radiation radiation that is highly penetrating and can cause serious biological effects

Irritable bowel syndrome inflammatory disease of the small or large intestine, characterized by intense abdominal cramping and diarrhea

Islets of Langerhans cell clusters in the pancreas responsible for the secretion of insulin and glucagon

Jejunum middle portion of the small intestine between the duodenum and the ileum

Kaposi's sarcoma vascular cancer that first appears on the skin and then invades internal organs; frequently occurs in AIDS patients

Kappa receptor type of opioid receptor

Keratolytic action that promotes shedding of old skin

Ketoacid acidic waste product of lipid metabolism that lowers the pH of the blood

Latent phase period of HIV infection during which there are no symptoms

Laxative drug that promotes defecation

Lecithin phospholipid that is an important component of cell membranes

Leukemia cancer of the blood characterized by overproduction of white blood cells

Leukotriene chemical mediator of inflammation stored and released by mast cells; effects are similar to those of histamine

Libido interest in sexual activity

Limbic system area in the brain responsible for emotion, learning, memory, motivation, and mood

Lipodystrophy atrophy increase or decrease of subcutaneous fat at an insulin injection site, resulting in an indenture or a raised area

Lipoprotein substance carrying lipids in the bloodstream that is composed of proteins bound to fat

Liposome small sac of lipids designed to carry drugs inside it

Loading dose comparatively large dose given at the beginning of treatment to rapidly obtain the therapeutic effect of a drug

Local anesthesia loss of sensation to a limited part of the body without loss of consciousness

Long-term insomnia inability to sleep for more than a few nights, often caused by depression, manic disorders, and chronic pain

Low-density lipoprotein (LDL) lipid-carrying particle that contains relatively low amounts of protein and high amounts of cholesterol; considered to be "bad" cholesterol

Low-molecular-weight heparins (LMWHs) drugs closely resembling heparin that inhibit blood clotting

Lutinizing hormone (LH) secreted by the pituitary gland, triggers ovulation in the female and stimulates sperm production in the male

Lymphoma cancer of lymphatic tissue

Macromineral (major mineral) inorganic compound needed by the body in amounts of 100 mg or more daily

Maintenance dose dose that keeps the plasma drug concentration continuously in the therapeutic range

Malaria tropical disease characterized by severe fever and chills caused by the protozoan *Plasmodium*

Malignant life threatening or fatal

Mania condition characterized by an expressive, impulsive, excitable, and overreactive nature

Mast cell connective tissue cell located in tissue spaces that releases histamine following injury

Mastoiditis inflammation of the mastoid sinus

Mechanism of action the way in which a drug exerts its effects

Median effective dose (ED$_{50}$) dose required to produce a specific therapeutic response in 50% of a group of patients

Median lethal dose (LD$_{50}$) often determined in preclinical trials, the dose of drug that will be lethal in 50% of a group of animals

Median toxicity dose (TD$_{50}$) dose that will produce a given toxicity in 50% of a group of patients

Medication drug after it has been administered

Medication administration record (MAR) documentation of all pharmacotherapies received by the patient

Medication error any preventable event that may cause or lead to inappropriate medication use or patient harm while the medication is in the control of the healthcare provider, patient, or consumer

Medication error index categorization of medication errors according to the extent of the harm an error can cause

Menopause period of time during which females stop secreting estrogen and menstrual cycles cease

Menorrhagia prolonged or excessive menstruation

Metabolism total of all biochemical reactions in the body

Metastasis travel of cancer cells from their original site to a distant tissue

Metered dose inhaler (MDI) device used to deliver a precise amount of drug to the respiratory system

Methadone maintenance treatment of opioid dependence by using methadone

Methylxanthine chemical derivative of caffeine

Metric system of measurement most common system of drug measurement that uses grams and liters

Micromineral (trace mineral) inorganic compound needed by the body in amounts of 20 mg or less daily

Middle-age adulthood person from 40 to 65 years of age

Migraine severe headache preceded by auras that may include nausea and vomiting

Minimum effective concentration amount of drug required to produce a therapeutic effect

Miosis constriction of the pupil

Monoamine oxidase (MAO) enzyme that destroys norepinephrine in the nerve terminal

Monoamine oxidase inhibitor (MAOIs) drug inhibiting monoamine oxidase, an enzyme that terminates the actions of neurotransmitters such as dopamine, norepinephrine, epinephrine, and serotonin

Mood disorder change in behavior such as clinical depression, emotional swings, or manic depression

Mood stabilizer drug that levels mood that is used to treat bipolar disorder and mania

Mu receptor type of opioid receptor

Mucolytic drug used to loosen thick mucus

Mucosa layer inner lining of the alimentary canal that provides a surface area for the various acids, bases, and enzymes to break down food

Mucositis inflammation of the epithelial lining of the digestive tract

Muscarinic type of cholinergic receptor found in smooth muscle, cardiac muscle, and glands

Muscle spasm involuntary contraction of a muscle or group of muscles, which become tightened, develop a fixed pattern of resistance, and result in a diminished level of functioning

Mutation permanent, inheritable change to DNA

Myasthenia gravis motor disorder caused by a destruction of nicotinic receptors on skeletal muscles and characterized by profound muscular fatigue

Mycoses diseases caused by fungi

Mydriatic drug agent that causes pupil dilation

Myocardial infarction blood clot blocking a portion of a coronary artery that causes necrosis of cardiac muscle

Myocardial ischemia lack of blood supply to the myocardium due to a constriction or obstruction of a blood vessel

Myoclonic seizure seizure characterized by brief, sudden contractions of a group of muscles

Myxedema condition caused by insufficient secretion of thyroid hormone

Narcotic natural or synthetic drug related to morphine; may be used as a broader legal term referring to hallucinogens, CNS stimulants, marijuana, and other illegal drugs

Narrow-spectrum antibiotic anti-infective that is effective against only one or a small number of organisms

Nausea uncomfortable wavelike sensation that precedes vomiting

NDA review third stage of new drug evaluation by the FDA

Nebulizer device used to convert liquid drugs into a fine mist for the purpose of inhalation

Negative feedback in homeostasis, the shutting off of first hormone in a pathway by the last hormone or product in the pathway

Negative symptoms in schizophrenia, symptoms that subtract from normal behavior, including a lack of interest, motivation, responsiveness, or pleasure in daily activities

Neoplasm abnormal swelling or mass; same as *tumor*

Nephron structural and functional unit of the kidney

Nerve agent chemical used in warfare or by bioterrorists that can affect the central nervous system and cause death

Neurofibrillary tangles bundles of nerve fibers found in the brain of patients with Alzheimer's disease on autopsy

Neurogenic shock type of shock resulting from brain or spinal cord injury

Neurohypophysis posterior portion of the pituitary gland

Neurolepanalgesia type of general anesthesia that combines fentanyl with droperidol to produce a state in which patients are conscious though insensitive to pain and unconnected with surroundings

Neuroleptic malignant syndrome potentially fatal condition caused by certain antipsychotic medications characterized by an extremely high body temperature, drowsiness, changing blood pressure, irregular heartbeat, and muscle rigidity

Neuromuscular blocker drug used to cause total muscle relaxation

Neuropathic pain caused by injury to nerves and typically described as burning, shooting, or numb pain

Nicotinic type of cholinergic receptor found in ganglia of both the sympathetic and parasympathetic nervous systems

Nit egg of the louse parasite

Nociceptor receptor connected with nerves that receive and transmit pain signals to the spinal cord and brain

Nonmaleficence ethical obligation to not harm the patient

Nonspecific body defense defense such as inflammation that protects the body from invasion by general hazards

Nonspecific cellular response drug action that is independent of cellular receptors and is not associated with other mechanisms, such as changing the permeability of cellular membranes, depressing membrane excitability, or altering the activity of cellular pumps

Norepinephrine (NE) primary neurotransmitter in the sympathetic nervous system

Nosocomial infection infection acquired in a healthcare setting such as a hospital, physician's office, or nursing home

Nurse Practice Act legislation designed to protect the public by defining the legal scope of practice of nurses

Nursing diagnosis clinically based judgment about the patient and his or her response to health and illness

Nursing process five-part decision-making system that includes assessment, nursing diagnosis, planning, implementation, and evaluation

Objective data information gathered through physical assessment, laboratory tests, and other diagnostic sources

Obsessive-compulsive disorder recurrent, intrusive thoughts or repetitive behaviors that interfere with normal activities or relationships

Older adulthood person older than age 65

Oligomenorrhea infrequent menstruation

Oligospermia presence of less than 20 million sperm in an ejaculate

Oncogene gene responsible for the conversion of normal cells into cancer cells

Open-angle glaucoma chronic, simple glaucoma caused by hindered outflow of aqueous humor from the anterior chamber

Opiate substance closely related to morphine extracted from the poppy plant

Opioid substance obtained from the unripe seeds of the poppy plant; natural or synthetic morphinelike substance

Orthostatic hypotension fall in blood pressure that occurs when changing position from recumbent to upright

Osmolality number of dissolved particles, or solutes, in 1 kg (1 L) of water

Osmosis process by which water moves from areas of low solute concentration (low osmolality) to areas of high solute concentration (high osmolality)

Osteoarthritis disorder characterized by degeneration of joints; particularly the fingers, spine, hips, and knees

Osteomalacia rickets in children; caused by vitamin D deficiency, characterized by softening of the bones without alteration of basic bone structure

Osteoporosis condition in which bones lose mass and become brittle and susceptible to fracture

Otitis media inflammation of the middle ear

Ototoxicity having an adverse effect on the organs of hearing

Outcome objective measures of goals

Ovulation release of an egg by the ovary

Oxytocin hormone secreted by the posterior pituitary gland that stimulates uterine contractions and milk ejection

Paget's disease disorder of bone formation and resorption characterized by weak, enlarged, and deformed bones

Palliation form of cancer chemotherapy intended to alleviate symptoms rather than cure the disease

Panic disorder anxiety disorder characterized by intense feelings of immediate apprehension, fearfulness, terror, or impending doom, accompanied by increased autonomic nervous system activity

Parafollicular cells cells in the thyroid gland that secrete calcitonin

Paranoia having an extreme suspicion and delusion that one is being followed and that others are trying to inflict harm

Parasympathetic nervous system portion of the autonomic nervous system that is active during periods of rest and that results in the rest or relaxation response

Parasympathomimetic drug that mimics the actions of the parasympathetic nervous system

Parenteral route dispensation of medications via a needle into the skin layers

Parietal cell cell in the stomach mucosa that secretes hydrochloric acid

Parkinson's disease degenerative disorder of the nervous system caused by a deficiency of the brain neurotransmitter dopamine that results in disturbances of muscle movement

Parkinsonism having tremor, muscle rigidity, stooped posture, and a shuffling gait

Partial (focal) seizure seizure that starts on one side of the brain and travels a short distance before stopping

Partial agonist medication that produces a weaker, or less efficacious, response than an agonist

Passive immunity immune defense that lasts 2 to 3 weeks; obtained by administering antibodies

Pathogen organism that is capable of causing disease

Pathogenicity ability of an organism to cause disease in humans

Pediculicides medications that kill lice

Pegylation process that attaches polyethylene glycol (PEG) to an interferon to extend its pharmacological activity

Pellagra deficiency of niacin

Peptic ulcer erosion of the mucosa in the alimentary canal, most commonly in the stomach and duodenum

Percutaneous transluminal coronary angioplasty (PTCA) procedure by which a balloon-shaped catheter is used to compress fatty plaque against an arterial wall for the purpose of restoring normal blood flow

Perfusion blood flow through a tissue or organ

Peripheral nervous system division of the nervous system containing all nervous tissue outside the CNS, including the autonomic nervous system

Peripheral resistance amount of friction encountered by blood as it travels through the vessels

Peristalsis involuntary wavelike contraction of smooth muscle lining the alimentary canal

Pernicious (megaloblastic) anemia type of anemia usually caused by lack of secretion of intrinsic factor

pH measure of the acidity or alkalinity of a solution

Pharmacodynamics study of how the body responds to drugs

Pharmacogenetics area of pharmacology that examines the role of genetics in drug response

Pharmacokinetics study of how drugs are handled by the body

Pharmacological classification method for organizing drugs on the basis of their mechanism of action

Pharmacology the study of medicines; the discipline pertaining to how drugs improve or maintain health

Pharmacopoeia medical reference indicating standards of drug purity, strength, and directions for synthesis

Pharmacotherapy treatment or prevention of disease by means of drugs

Phobia fearful feeling attached to situations or objects such as snakes, spiders, crowds, or heights

Phosphodiesterase enzyme in muscle cells that cleaves phosphodiester bonds; its inhibition increases myocardial contractility

Phospholipid type of lipid that contains two fatty acids, a phosphate group, and a chemical backbone of glycerol

Photosensitivity condition in which the skin is highly sensitive to sunlight

Physical dependence condition of experiencing unpleasant withdrawal symptoms when a substance is discontinued

Planning linkage of strategies or interventions to established goals and outcomes

Plaque fatty material that builds up in the lining of blood vessels and may lead to hypertension, stroke, myocardial infarction, or angina

Plasma cell cell derived from B lymphocytes that produces antibodies

Plasma half-life ($t_{1/2}$) the length of time required for the plasma concentration of a drug to decrease by half after administration

Plasmid small piece of circular DNA found in some bacteria that is able to transfer resistance from one bacterium to another

Plasmin enzyme formed from plasminogen that dissolves blood clots

Plasminogen protein that prevents fibrin clot formation; precuror of plasmin

Polarized condition in which the inside of a cell is more negatively charged than the outside of the cell

Polyene antifungal class containing amphotericin B and nystatin

Polypharmacy the taking of multiple drugs concurrently

Positive symptoms in schizophrenia, symptoms that add to normal behavior, including hallucinations, delusions, and a disorganized thought or speech pattern

Postmarketing surveillance evaluation of a new drug after it has been approved and used in large numbers of patients

Postpartum occurring after childbirth

Postsynaptic neuron in a synapse, the nerve that has receptors for the neurotransmitter

Post-traumatic stress disorder type of anxiety that develops in response to reexperiencing a previous life event that was psychologically traumatic

Potassium ion channel pathway in a plasma membrane through which potassium ions enter and leave

Potency the strength of a drug at a specified concentration or dose

Preclinical investigation procedure implemented after a drug has been licensed for public use, designed to provide information on use and on occurrence of side effects

Preload degree of stretch of the cardiac muscle fibers just before they contract

Prenatal preceding birth

Preschool child child from 3 to 5 years of age

Presynaptic neuron nerve that releases the neurotransmitter into the synaptic cleft when stimulated by an action potential

PRN order (Latin: *pro re nata*) medication is administered as required by the patient's condition

Prodrug drug that becomes more active after it is metabolized

Progesterone hormone secreted by the corpus luteum and placenta responsible for building up the uterine lining in the second half of the menstrual cycle and during pregnancy

Prolactin hormone secreted by the anterior pituitary gland that stimulates milk production in the mammary glands

Prostaglandins class of local hormones that promote local inflammation and pain when released by cells in the body

Protease viral enzyme that is responsible for the final assembly of the HIV virions

Prothrombin blood protein that is converted to thrombin in blood coagulation

Prothrombin activator enzyme in the coagulation cascade that converts prothrombin to thrombin; also called *prothrombinase*

Prothrombin time blood test used to determine the time needed for plasma to clot for the regulation of warfarin dosage

Proton pump inhibitor drug that inhibits the enzyme H^+, K^+-ATPase

Prototype drug well-understood model drug with which other drugs in a pharmacological class may be compared

Protozoan single-celled animal

Provitamin inactive chemical that is converted to a vitamin in the body

Pruritus itching associated with dry, scaly skin

Psoralen drug used along with phototherapy for the treatment of psoriasis and other severe skin disorders

Psychedelic substance that alters perception and reality

Psychological dependence intense craving for a drug that drives people to continue drug abuse

Psychology science that deals with normal and abnormal mental processes and their impact on behavior

Purine building block of DNA and RNA, either adenine or guanine

Purkinje fibers electrical conduction pathway leading from the bundle branches to all portions of the ventricles

Pyrimidine building block of DNA and RNA, either thymine or cytosine in DNA, and cytosine and uracil in RNA

Rapid eye movement (REM) sleep stage of sleep characterized by quick, scanning movements of the eyes

Reabsorption movement of filtered substances from the kidney tubule back into the blood

Reasonable and prudent action defines the standard of care as the actions that a reasonable and prudent nurse with equivalent preparation would do under similar circumstances

Rebound insomnia increased sleeplessness that occurs when long-term antianxiety or hypnotic medication is discontinued

Receptor the structural component of a cell to which a drug binds in a dose-related manner, to produce a response

Recommended Dietary Allowance (RDA) amount of vitamin or mineral needed each day to avoid a deficiency in a healthy adult

Red-man syndrome rash on the upper body caused by certain anti-infectives

Reflex tachycardia temporary increase in heart rate that occurs when blood pressure falls

Refractory period time during which the myocardial cells rest and are not able to contract

Releasing hormone hormone secreted by the hypothalamus that affects secretions in the pituitary gland

Renin–angiotensin system series of enzymatic steps by which the body raises blood pressure

Respiration exchange of oxygen and carbon dioxide in the lungs; also, the process of deriving energy from metabolic reactions

Rest-and-digest response signs and symptoms produced when the parasympathetic nervous system is activated

Reticular activating system (RAS) responsible for sleeping and wakefulness and performs an alerting function for the cerebral cortex; includes the reticular formation, hypothalamus, and part of the thalamus

Reticular formation portion of the brain affecting awareness and wakefulness

Retinoid compound resembling vitamin A used in the treatment of severe acne and psoriasis

Reverse cholesterol transport the process by which cholesterol is transported away from body tissues to the liver

Reverse transcriptase viral enzyme that converts RNA to DNA

Reye's syndrome potentially fatal complication of infection associated with aspirin use in children

Rhabdomyolisis breakdown of muscle fibers usually due to muscle trauma or ischemia

Rheumatoid arthritis systemic autoimmune disorder characterized by inflammation of multiple joints

Rhinophyma reddened, bullous, irregular swelling of the nose

Risk management system of reducing medication errors by modifying policies and procedures within the institution

Rosacea chronic skin disorder characterized by clusters of papules on the face

Routine order order not written as STAT, ASAP, NOW, or PRN

Salicylism poisoning due to aspirin and aspirin-like drugs

Sarcoma cancer of connective tissue such as bone, muscle, or cartilage

Scabicide drug that kills scabies mites

Scabies skin disorder that results when the female mite burrows into the skin and lays eggs

Scheduled drug in the United States, a term describing a drug placed into one of five categories based on its potential for misuse or abuse

Schizoaffective disorder psychosis with symptoms of both schizophrenia and mood disorders

Schizophrenia psychosis characterized by abnormal thoughts and thought processes, withdrawal from other people and the outside environment, and apparent preoccupation with one's own mental state

School-age child child from 6 to 12 years of age

Scurvy deficiency of vitamin C

Seborrhea skin condition characterized by overactivity of oil glands

Second messenger cascade of biochemical events that initiates a drug's action by either stimulating or inhibiting a normal activity of the cell

Secretion in the kidney, movement of substances from the blood into the tubule after filtration has occurred

Sedative substance that depresses the CNS to cause drowsiness or sleep

Sedative–hypnotic drug with the ability to produce a calming effect at lower doses and to induce sleep at higher doses

Seizure symptom of epilepsy characterized by abnormal neuronal discharges within the brain

Selective estrogen receptor modulator (SERM) drug that produces an action similar to estrogen in body tissues; used for the treatment of osteoporosis in postmenopausal women

Selective serotonin reuptake inhibitor (SSRI) drug that selectively inhibits the reuptake of serotonin into nerve terminals; used mostly for depression

Septic shock type of shock caused by severe infection in the bloodstream

Serotonin syndrome set of signs and symptoms associated with overmedication with antidepressants that includes altered mental status, fever, sweating, and lack of muscular coordination

Shock condition in which there is inadequate blood flow to meet the body's metabolic needs

Short-term or behavioral insomnia inability to sleep that is often attributed to stress caused by a hectic lifestyle or the inability to resolve day-to-day conflicts within the home or workplace

Single order medication that is to be given only once, and at a specific time, such as a preoperative order

Sinoatrial (SA) node pacemaker of the heart located in the wall of the right atrium that controls the basic heart rate

Sinus rhythm number of beats per minute normally generated by the SA node

Situational anxiety anxiety experienced by people faced with a stressful environment

Sleep debt lack of sleep

Social anxiety fear of crowds

Sociology study of human behavior within the context of groups and societies

Sodium ion channel pathway in a plasma membrane through which sodium ions enter and leave

Somatic nervous system nerve division that provides voluntary control over skeletal muscle

Somatostatin synonym for growth hormone inhibiting factor from the hypothalamus

Somatotropin another name for growth hormone

Somogyi phenomenon rapid decrease in blood glucose level that stimulates the release of hormones (epinephrine, cortisol, glucagon) resulting in an elevated morning blood glucose

Spasticity inability of opposing muscle groups to move in a coordinated manner

Specialty supplement nonherbal dietary product used to enhance a wide variety of body functions

Spirituality the capacity to love, to convey compassion and empathy, to give and forgive, to enjoy life, and to find peace of mind and fulfillment in living

Stable angina type of angina that occurs in a predictable pattern, usually relieved by rest

Standards of care the skills and learning commonly possessed by members of a profession

Standing order order written in advance of a situation that is to be carried out under specific circumstances

STAT order any medication that is needed immediately and is to be given only once

Status epilepticus condition characterized by repeated seizures or one prolonged seizure attack that continues for at least 30 minutes

Stem cell cell that resides in the bone marrow and is capable of maturing into any type of blood cell

Steroid type of lipid consisting of four rings that is a structural component of certain hormones and drugs

Sterol nucleus ring structure common to all steroids

Strategic National Stockpile (SNS) program designed to ensure the immediate deployment of essential medical materials to a community in the event of a large-scale chemical or biological attack

Stroke volume amount of blood pumped out by a ventricle in a single beat

Subcutaneous medication delivered beneath the skin

Subjective data information gathered regarding what a patient states or perceives

Sublingual route administration of medication by placing it under the tongue and allowing it to dissolve slowly

Substance abuse self-administration of a drug that does not conform to the medical or social norms within the patient's given culture or society

Substance P neurotransmitter within the spinal cord involved in the neural transmission of pain

Substantia nigra location in the brain where dopamine is synthesized that is responsible for regulation of unconscious muscle movement

Superficial mycosis fungal disease of the hair, skin, nails, and mucous membranes

Superinfection new infection caused by an organism different from the one causing the initial infection; usually a side effect of anti-infective therapy

Surgical anesthesia stage 3 of anesthesia, in which most major surgery occurs

Sustained release tablets or capsules designed to dissolve slowly over an extended time

Sympathetic nervous system portion of the autonomic system that is active during periods of stress and results in the fight-or-flight response

Sympathomimetic drug that stimulates or mimics the sympathetic nervous system

Synapse junction between two neurons consisting of a presynaptic nerve, a synaptic cleft, and a postsynaptic nerve

Synaptic transmission process by which a neurotransmitter reaches receptors to regenerate the action potential

Systemic mycosis fungal disease affecting internal organs

Systolic pressure blood pressure during the contraction phase of heart activity

Tardive dyskinesia unusual tongue and face movements such as lip smacking and wormlike motions of the tongue that occur during pharmacotherapy with certain antipsychotics

Taxanes alkaloids isolated from the bark of the Pacific yew and used for antineoplastic activity; current drugs include paclitaxel (Taxol) and docetaxel (Taxotere), but more than 19 others are being investigated

T cell type of lymphocyte that is essential for the cell-mediated immune response

Tension headache common type of head pain caused by stress and relieved by nonnarcotic analgesics

Teratogen drug or other agent that causes developmental birth defects

Testosterone primary androgen responsible for maturation of male sex organs and secondary sex characteristics of men; secreted by testes

Tetrahydrocannabinol (THC) the active chemical in marijuana

Therapeutic classification method for organizing drugs on the basis of their clinical usefulness

Therapeutic index the ratio of a drug's LD_{50} to its ED_{50}

Therapeutic range the dosage range or serum concentration that achieves the desired drug effects

Therapeutics the branch of medicine concerned with the treatment of disease and suffering

Three checks of drug administration in conjunction with the five rights, these ascertain patient safety and drug effectiveness

Thrombin enzyme that causes clotting by catalyzing the conversion of fibrinogen to fibrin

Thrombocytopenia reduction in the number of circulating platelets

Thromboembolic disorder condition in which the patient develops blood clots

Thrombolytic drug used to dissolve existing blood clots

Thrombopoietin hormone produced by the kidneys that controls megakaryocyte activity

Thrombus blood clot obstructing a vessel

Thyrotoxic crisis acute form of hyperthyroidism that is a medical emergency; also called *thyroid storm*

Tissue plasminogen activator (tPA) natural enzyme and a drug that dissolves blood clots

Titer measurement of the amount of a substance in the blood

Tocolytic drug used to inhibit uterine contractions

Tocopherol generic name for vitamin E

Toddlerhood term applied to children from 1 to 3 years of age

Tolerance process of adapting to a drug over a period of time and subsequently requiring higher doses to achieve the same effect

Tonic spasm single, prolonged muscular contraction

Tonic–clonic seizure seizure characterized by intense jerking motions and loss of consciousness

Tonicity the ability of a solution to cause a change in water movement across a membrane owing to osmotic forces

Tonometry technique for measuring intraocular tension and pressure

Topoisomerase enzyme that assists in the repair of DNA damage

Total parenteral nutrition (TPN) nutrition provided through a peripheral or central vein

Toxic concentration level of drug that will result in serious adverse effects

Toxin chemical produced by a microorganism that is able to cause injury to its host

Toxoid substance that has been chemically modified to remove its harmful nature but is still able to elicit an immune response in the body

Trade name proprietary name of a drug assigned by the manufacturer; also called the brand name or product name

Tranquilizer older term sometimes used to describe a drug that produces a calm or tranquil feeling

Transferrin protein complex that transports iron to sites in the body where it is needed

Transplant rejection recognition by the immune system of a transplanted tissue as foreign and subsequent attack on the tissue

Tricyclic antidepressant (TCA) class of drugs used in the pharmacotherapy of depression

Triglyceride type of lipid that contains three fatty acids and a chemical backbone of glycerol

Tubercle cavity-like lesion in the lung characteristic of infection by *Mycobacterium tuberculosis*

Tumor abnormal swelling or mass

Tyramine form of the amino acid tyrosine that is found in foods such as cheese, beer, wine, and yeast products

Ulcerative colitis inflammatory bowel disease of the colon

Undernutrition lack of adequate nutrition to meet the metabolic demands of the body

Unstable angina severe angina that occurs frequently and that is not relieved by rest

Urinalysis diagnostic test that examines urine for the presence of blood cells, proteins, pH, specific gravity, ketones, glucose, and microorganisms

Vaccination immunization inoculation with a vaccine or toxoid to prevent disease

Vaccine biological material that confers protection against infection; preparation of microorganism particles that is injected into a patient to stimulate the immune system, with the intention of preventing disease

Vasomotor center area of the medulla that controls baseline blood pressure

Vasospastic or Prinzmetal's angina type of angina in which the decreased myocardial blood flow is caused by *spasms* of the coronary arteries

Vendor Managed Inventory (VMI) supplies and pharmaceuticals that are shipped after a chemical or biological threat has been identified

Ventilation process by which air is moved into and out of the lungs

Very-low-density lipoprotein (VLDL) lipid-carrying particle that is converted to LDL in the liver

Vesicant agent that can cause serious tissue injury if it escapes from an artery or vein during an infusion or injection (extravasation); many antineoplastics are vesicants

Vestibular apparatus portion of the inner ear responsible for the sense of position

Vinca alkaloid chemical obtained from the periwinkle plant that has antineoplastic activity

Virilization appearance of masculine secondary sex characteristics

Virion particle of a virus capable of causing an infection

Virulence the severity of disease that a pathogen is able to cause

Virus nonliving particle containing nucleic acid that is able to cause disease

Vitamin organic compound required by the body in small amounts

Vitiligo milk-white areas of depigmented skin

Vomiting center area in the medulla that controls the vomiting reflex

Von Willebrand's disease decrease in quantity or quality of von Willebrand factor (vWF), which acts as a carrier of factor VIII and has a role in platelet aggregation

Withdrawal physical signs of discomfort associated with the discontinuation of an abused substance

Withdrawal syndrome symptoms that result when a patient discontinues taking a substance on which he or she was dependent

Yeast type of fungus that is unicellular and divides by budding

Young adulthood term applied to persons from 18 to 40 years of age

Zollinger–Ellison syndrome disorder of excess acid secretion in the stomach resulting in peptic ulcer disease

APPENDIX A
Canadian Drugs and Their U.S. Equivalents

U.S. Drug Name	Canadian Drug Name
acebutolol hydrochloride (Sectral)	Monitan
acetaminophen (Tylenol)	Abenal, Atasol, Campain, others
acetazolamide (Diamox)	Acetazolam, Apo-Acetazolamide
acetohexamide (Dymelor)	Dimelor
albuterol (Proventil, Salbutamol)	Gen-Salbutamol, Novosalmol
allopurinol (Lopurin, Zyloprim)	Alloprin A, Apo-allopurinol-A
altretamine, hexamethylmelamine (Hexalen)	Hexastat
aminophylline (Truphylline)	Paladron, Corophyllin
amitriptyline hydrochloride (Elavil)	Apo-Amitripyline, Levate, Novotriptyn
amoxicillin (Amoxil, Trimox, Wymox)	Apo-Amoxi
ampicillin (Polycillin, Omnipen)	Novo-Ampicillin, Penbritin
asparaginase (Elspar)	Kidrolase A
aspirin (ASA, others)	Novasen, Astrin, Entrophen, others
atenolol (Tenormin)	Apo-Atenolol
atropine sulfate (Isopto Atropine, others)	Atropair
bacampicillin hydrochloride (Spectrobid)	Penglobes
benztropine mesylate (Cogentin)	Apo-Benztropine, Bensylate, PMS Benztropine
betamethasone (Celestone, Betacort, others)	Betnelan, Betaderm, others
bretylium tosylate (Bretylol)	Bretylate
brompheniramine maleate (Codimal-A, Dimetapp)	Dimetane
calcium carbonate (BioCal, Calcite-500, others)	Apo-Cal, Calsan, Caltrate
carbamazepine (Tegretol)	Apo-Carbamazepine, Mazepine
carbenicillin indanyl (Geocillin, Geopen)	Geopen Oral
cephalexin (Keflex)	Ceporex, Novolexin
cetirizine (Zyrtec)	Reactine
chloral hydrate (Noctec)	Novochlorhydrate
chloramphenicol (Chlorofair, Chloromycetin, Chloroptic, Fenicol)	Novochlorocap, Pentamycetin
chlordiazepoxide hydrochloride (Librium)	Medilium, Novopoxide, Solium
chlorthalidone (Hygroton)	Novothalidone, Uridon
chlorpropamide (Chloronase, Diabinese, Glucamide)	Apo-Chlorpropamide, Novopropamide
chlorpheniramine maleate (Chlor-Trimeton, others)	Chlor-Tripolon, Novopheniram
chlorpromazine hydrochloride (Thorazine)	Largactil, Novochlorpromazine
cimetidine (Tagamet)	Apo-Cimetidine, Novocimetine, Peptol
cisplatin (Platinol)	Abiplatin
clindamycin hydrochloride (Cleocin)	Dalacin C
clonazepam (Klonopin)	Rivotril
clonidine hydrochloride (Catapres)	Dixaril
clorazepate dipotassium (Tranxene)	Novoclopate
clotrimazole (Gyne-Lotrimin, Mycelex, Femizole)	Canesten, Clotrimaderm, Myclo-Gyne
cloxacillin (Tegopen)	Apo-Cloxi, Novocloxin
codeine	Paveral
colchicine	Novocolchicine
colestipol (Colestid)	Cholestabyl
cyclizine hydrochloride (Marezine)	Marzine
cyclophosphamide (Cytoxan, Neosar)	Procytox
cyproheptadine hydrochloride (Periactin)	Vimicon
danazol (Danocrine)	Cyclomen

U.S. Drug Name	**Canadian Drug Name**
dexamethasone (Decadron, Dexasone, Hexadrol, Maxidex)	Deronil, Oradexon
dextroamphetamine sulfate (Dexedrine)	Oxydess II
diazepam (Valium)	Apo-Diazepam, Diazemuls, E-Pam
diethylstilbestrol (DES, Stilbestrol)	Honval
diltiazem (Cardizem, Dilacor, Tiamate, Tiazac)	Apo-Dilitaz
dimenhydrinate (Dramamine)	Apo-Dimenhydrinate, Gravol
diphenhydramine hydrochloride (Benadryl, others)	Allerdryl
dipyridamole (Persantine)	Apo-Dipyridamole
disopyramide phosphate (Norpace, Napamide)	Rythmodan
docusate (Surfak, Dialose, Colace)	Regulax
dopamine hydrochloride (Dopastat, Intropin)	Revimine
doxepin hydrochloride (Sinequan)	Triadapin
doxycycline hyclate (Doryx, Doxy, Monodox, Vibramycin)	Apo-Doxy, Doxycin
econazole nitrate (Spectazole)	Ecostatin
epinephrine (Adrenalin, Bronkaid, Primatene)	SusPhrine
ergocalciferol (Deltalin, Calciferol)	Ostoforte, Radiostol
ergotamine tartrate (Ergostat)	Gynergen
erythromycin (E-mycin, Erythrocin)	Novorythro, Erythromid, Apo-Erythro-S
estradiol valerate (Delestrogen, Duragen-10, Valergen)	Femogex
flucytosine (Ancobon)	Ancotil
fluoxymesterone (Halotestin)	Ora Testryl
flurazepam (Dalmane)	Apo-Flurazepam, Novoflupam
furosemide (Lasix)	Furomide
gentamicin sulfate (Garamycin, G-mycin, Jenamicin)	Cydomycin
glyburide (DiaBeta, Micronase, Glynase)	Euglucon
griseofulvin (Fulvicin)	Grisovin-FP
haloperidol (Haldol)	Peridol
heparin sodium (Hep-lock)	Calcilean, Hepalean
hydralazine hydrochloride (Apresoline)	Novo-Hylazin
hydrochlorothiazide (HydroDIURIL, HCTZ)	Apo-Hydro, Urozide
hydrocodone bitartrate (Hycodan)	Robidone
hydrocortisone (Cetacort, Cortaid, Solu-Cortef)	Rectocort, Cortiment
hydroxyzine (Atarax, Vistaril)	Apo-Hydroxyzine
ibuprofen (Advil, Motrin, others)	Amersol
imipramine hydrochloride (Tofranil)	Impril, Novopramine
indapamide (Lozol)	Lozide
isoniazid (INH, Laniazid, Nydrazid, Teebaconin)	Isotamine, PMS Isoniazid
isosorbide dinitrate (Isordil, Sorbitrate, Dilatrate-SR)	Coronex, Novosorbide
ketoprofen (Actron, Orudis, Oruvail)	Rhodis
lidocaine hydrochloride (Xylocaine)	Xylocard
lithium carbonate (Eskalith)	Carbolith, Duralith, Lithizine
lorazepam (Ativan)	Apo-Lorazepam
loxapine succinate (Loxitane)	Loxapac
meclizine (Antivert, Bonine)	Bonamine
methyldopa (Aldomet)	Apo-Methyldopa
methyltestosterone (Android, Testred)	Metandren
metoclopramide (Reglan)	Emex, Maxeran
metoprolol tartrate (Toprol, Lopressor)	Betaloc, Norometoprol, Apo-Metoprolol
morphine sulfate (Astramorph PF, Duramorph, others)	Epimorph, Statex
naproxen (Naprosyn, Anaprox)	Apo-Naproxen, Naxen, Novonaprox
nifedipine (Procardia, Adalat)	Apo-Nifed, Novo-Nifedin
nitrofurantoin (Furadantin, Furalan, Furanite, Macrobid, Macrodantin)	Apo-Nitrofurantoin, Nephronex, Novofuran

U.S. Drug Name	**Canadian Drug Name**
norethindrone acetate	Aygestin, Norlutate
nystatin (Mycostatin, Nilstat, Nystex)	Nadostine, Nyaderm
omeprazole (Prilosec)	Losec
oxazepam (Serax)	Ox-Pam, Zapex
oxymetazoline hydrochloride (Afrin 12 Hour, Neo-Synephrine 12 Hour, others)	Nafrine
penicillin G sodium/potassium (Pentids)	Megacillin
penicillin V (Pen-Vee K, Veetids, Betapen-VK)	Apo-Pen-VK, Nadopen-V
pentamidine isoethionate (Pentam 300, Nebupent)	Pentacarinat
pentobarbital sodium (Nembutal)	Novopentobarb
phenylephrine hydrochloride (Mydfrin, Neo-Synephrine)	AK-Dilate Dionephrine
pilocarpine hydrochloride (Adsorbocarpine, Isopto Carpine, others)	Pilocarpine, Miocarpine
prednisolone (Delta-Cortef, Key-Pred, Prelone, others)	Diopred, Inflamase, Pediapred
prednisone (Deltasone, Meticorten)	Apo-Prednisone, Winpred
primidone (Mysoline)	Apo-Primidone
probenecid (Benemid, Probalan)	Benuryl
procarbazine hydrochloride (Matulane)	Natulan
prochlorperazine (Compazine)	Prorazin, Stemetil
procyclidine hydrochloride (Kemadrin)	Procyclid
promethazine (Pentazine, Phenazine, Phenergan, others)	Histantil
propoxyphene hydrochloride (Darvon); propoxyphene napsylate (Darvon-N)	Novopropoxyn
propranolol hydrochloride (Inderal)	Apo-Propranolol, Detensol, Novopranol
propylthiouracil (PTU)	Propyl-Thyracil
protriptyline hydrochloride (Vivactil)	Triptil
psyllium hydrophilic mucilloid (Metamucil, Naturcil)	Karasil
pyrazinamide (PZA)	Tebrazid
quinidine sulfate (Quinidex)	Apo-Quinidine, Novoquinidin
quinine sulfate (Quinamm)	Novoquinine
ranitidine (Zantac)	Apo-Ranitidine
rifampin (Rifadin, Rimactane)	Rofact
scopolamine (Hyoscine, Transderm-Scop)	Transderm-V
secobarbital (Seconal)	Novosecobarb
spironolactone (Aldactone)	Novospiroton
sulfasalazine (Azulfidine)	PMS Sulfasalazine, others
sulfinpyrazone (Anturan)	Antazone, Anturane, others
tamoxifen citrate (Nolvadex)	Nolvadex-D, Tamofen
testosterone (Andro 100, Histerone, Testoderm)	Malogen
testosterone enanthate (Testone LA, Delatest, Delatestryl)	Malogex
tetracycline hydrochloride (Achromycin, Panmycin, Sumycin)	Novotetra
theophylline (Theo-Dur)	Pulmopylline, Somophyllin-12
thioguanine (TG)	Lanvis
thioridazine hydrochloride (Mellaril)	Novoridazine
tolbutamide (Orinase)	Mobenol, Novobutamide
trifluoperazine hydrochloride (Stelazine)	Novoflurazine, Solazine, Terfluzine
trihexyphenidyl hydrochloride (Artane)	Aparkane, Apo-Trihex, Novohexidyl
tripelennamine hydrochloride (PBZ-SR, Pelamine)	Pyribenzamine
Tums	Apo-Cal
valproic acid (Depakene)	Epival
verapamil hydrochloride (Calan, Isoptin, Verelan)	Novo-Veramil, Nu-Verap
vinblastine sulfate (Velban)	Velbe
warfarin sodium (Coumadin)	Warfilone

Rank	Market Name	Generic Name
1.	Hydrocodone w/APAP	hydrocodone w/APAP
2.	Lipitor	atorvastatin
3.	Amoxicillin	amoxicillin
4.	Lisinopril	lisinopril
5.	Hydrochlorothiazide	hydrochlorothiazide
6.	Atenolol	atenolol
7.	Zithromax	azithromycin
8.	Lasix	furosemide
9.	Alprazolam	alprazolam
10.	Toprol XL	metoprolol
11.	Albuterol Aerosol	albuterol
12.	Norvasc	amlodipine
13.	Synthroid	levothyroxine
14.	Metformin	metformin
15.	Zoloft	sertraline
16.	Lexapro	escitalopram
17.	Ibuprofen	ibuprofen
18.	Cephalexin	cephalexin
19.	Ambien	zolpidem
20.	Prednisone	prednisone
21.	Nexium	esomeprazole magnesium
22.	Triamterene/HCTZ	triamterene/HCTZ
23.	Propoxyphene N/APAP	propoxyphene N/APAP
24.	Zocor	simvastatin
25.	Singulair	montelukast
26.	Prevacid	lansoprazole
27.	Metoprolol tartrate	metoprolol
28.	Prozac	fluoxetine
29.	Lorazepam	lorazepam
30.	Plavix	clopidogrel
31.	Oxycodone w/APAP	oxycodone/APAP
32.	Advair Diskus	salmeterol/fluticasone
33.	Fosamax	alendronate
34.	Effexor XR	venlafaxine
35.	Warfarin	warfarin
36.	Paxil	paroxetine
37.	Clonazepam	clonazepam
38.	Zyrtec	cetirizine
39.	Protonix	pantoprazole
40.	Potassium Chloride	potassium chloride
41.	Acetaminophen/Codeine	acetaminophen/codeine
42.	Trimethoprim/Sulfamethoxazole	TMZ-SMZ
43.	Neurontin	gabapentin
44.	Premarin	conjugated estrogens
45.	Flonase	fluticasone propionate
46.	Desyrel	trazodone

Rank	Market Name	Generic Name
47.	Cyclobenzaprine	cyclobenzaprine
48.	Elavil	amitriptyline
49.	Levaquin	levofloxacin
50.	Tramadol	tramadol
51.	Cipro	ciprofloxacin
52.	Lotrel	amlodipine/benazepril
53.	Ranitidine hydrochloride	ranitidine
54.	Allegra	fexofenadine
55.	Levoxyl	levothyroxine
56.	Diovan	valsartan
57.	Enalapril	enalapril
58.	Valium	diazepam
59.	Anaprox/Naprosyn	naproxen
60.	Diflucan	fluconazole
61.	Zestoretic	lisinopril/HCTZ
62.	Klor-Con	potassium chloride
63.	Altace	ramipril
64.	Wellbutrin XL	bupropion
65.	Celebrex	celecoxib
66.	Viagra	sildenafil citrate
67.	Vibra-Tabs	doxycycline hyclate
68.	Zetia	ezetimibe
69.	Avandia	rosiglitazone maleate
70.	Mevacor	lovastatin
71.	Diovan HCT	valsartan HCT
72.	Soma	carisoprodol
73.	Yasmin 28	drospirenone and ethinyl estradiol
74.	Allopurinol	allopurinol
75.	Clonidine	clonidine
76.	Methylprednisolone	methylprednisolone
77.	Actos	pioglitazone hydrochloride
78.	Pravachol	pravastatin
79.	Actonel	risedronate
80.	Ortho Evra	norelgestromin/ethinyl estradiol
81.	Celexa	citalopram
82.	Verapamil SR	verapamil
83.	Isosorbide	isosorbide
84.	Penicillin VK	penicillin
85.	Micronase	glyburide
86.	Adderall XR	amphetamine
87.	Nasonex	mometasone furoate monohydrate
88.	Folic Acid	folic acid
89.	Seroquel	quetiapine fumarate
90.	Cozaar	losartan potassium
91.	Tricor	fenofibrate

Rank	Market Name	Generic Name	Rank	Market Name	Generic Name
92.	Coreg	carvedilol	139.	Cymbalta	duloxetine hydrochloride
93.	Concerta	methylphenidate HCl	140.	Nitrofurantoin	nitrofurantoin
94.	Vytorin	ezetimibe	141.	Promethazine/Codeine	promethazine/codeine
95.	Lantus	insulin glargine rDNA origin injection	142.	Benicar	olmesartan medoxomil
			143.	Remeron	mirtazapine
96.	Phenergan	promethazine	144.	Bisoprolol/HCTZ	bisoprolol/HCTZ
97.	Mobic	meloxicam	145.	Clarinex	desloratadine
98.	Flomax	tamsulosin hydrochloride	146.	Oxycodone	oxycodone
99.	Crestor	rosuvastatin calcium	147.	Minocycline	minocycline
100.	Glucotrol XL	glipizide extended release	148.	Imitrex	sumatriptan
			149.	Relafen	nabumetone
101.	Ortho Tri-Cyclen Lo	norgestimate/ethinyl estradiol	150.	Zyprexa	olanzapine
			151.	Lamictal	lamotrigine
102.	Restoril	temazepam	152.	Zyrtec Syrup	cetirizine HCl
103.	Prilosec	omeprazole	153.	Glycolax	polyethylene glycol
104.	Omnicef	cefdinivir	154.	Zovirax	acyclovir
105.	Albuterol Nebulizer Solution	albuterol sulfate	155.	Inderal	propranolol
106.	Risperdal	risperidone	156.	Nasacort AQ	triamcinolone acetonide
107.	Aciphex	rabeprazole sodium	157.	Aricept	donepezil hydrochloride
108.	Digitek	digoxin	158.	Fioricet	butalbital/acetaminophen/ caffeine
109.	Aldactone	spironolactone			
110.	Valtrex	valacyclovir hydrochloride	159.	Niaspan	niacin
111.	Xalatan	latanoprost	160.	Zithromax	azithromycin
112.	Fortamet	metformin	161.	Depakote	divalproex sodium
113.	Hyzaar	losartan potassium/ hydrochlorothiazide	162.	Buspar	buspirone
			163.	Tri-Sprintec	norgestimate/ethinyl estradiol
114.	Accupril	quinapril			
115.	Clindamycin	clindamycin	164.	Methotrexate	methotrexate
116.	Metronidazole	metronidazole	165.	OxyContin	oxycodone HCl
117.	Triamcinolone	triamcinolone	166.	Rhinocort Aqua	budesonide
118.	Topamax	topiramate	167.	Benicar HCT	olmesartan medoxomil- hydrochlorothiazide
119.	Combivent	ipratropium bromide and albuterol sulfate			
			168.	Hytrin	terazosin
120.	Lotensin	benazepril	169.	Skelaxin	metaxalone
121.	Gemfibrozil	gemfibrozil	170.	Lotrisone	clotrimazole/betamethasone
122.	Avapro	irbesartan	171.	Cialis	tadalafil
123.	Amaryl	glimepiride	172.	Avalide	irbesartan/ hydrochlorothiazide
124.	Trinessa	norgestimate/ethinyl estradiol			
			173.	Fexofenadine	fexofenadine
125.	Estradiol	estradiol	174.	Ortho Tri-Cyclen	norgestimate/ethinyl estradiol
126.	Hydroxyzine	hydroxyzine			
127.	Metoclopramide	metoclopramide	175.	Wellbutrin SR	bupropion SR
128.	Allegra-D 12 Hour	fexofenadine and pseudoephedrine	176.	Benzonatate	benzonatate
			177.	Patanol	olopatadine hydrochloride
129.	Cardura	doxazosin mesylate	178.	Quinine	quinine
130.	Coumadin	warfarin	179.	Cartia XT	diltiazem hydrochloride
131.	Glipizide	glipizide	180.	Humalog	insulin lispro, rDNA origin
132.	Voltaren	diclofenac	181.	Paxil CR	paroxetine hydrochloride
133.	Evista	raloxifene hydrochloride	182.	Aviane	levonorgestrel and ethinyl estradiol
134.	Tiazac	diltiazem hydrochloride			
135.	Detrol LA	tolterodine tartrate	183.	Lanoxin	digoxin
136.	Meclizine	meclizine	184.	Amphetamine Mixed Salts	amphetamine
137.	Glucovance	glyburide/metformin	185.	Famotidine	famotidine
138.	Strattera	atomoxetine HCl	186.	Digoxin	digoxin

Rank	Market Name	Generic Name	Rank	Market Name	Generic Name
187.	Levothroid	levothyroxine	194.	Etodolac	etodolac
188.	Nifedipine ER	nifedipine	195.	Tenoretic	atenolol/chlorthalidone
189.	Nortriptyline	nortriptyline	196.	Phentermine	phentermine
190.	Tussionex	hydrocodone polistirex and chlorpheniramine polistirex	197.	Ultracet	tramadol/acetaminophen
			198.	Zanaflex	tizanidine
191.	NitroQuick	nitroglycerin	199.	Zyrtec-D	cetirizine hydrochloride and pseudoephedrine
192.	Phenytoin	phenytoin			
193.	Endocet	budesonide	200.	Depakote ER	divalproex

Source: Data from PharmaTrends 2005, *NDCHealth, Inc.* www.rxlist.com

General References

Audesirk, T., Audesirk, G., & Beyers, B. E. (2005). *Biology: Life on earth* (7th ed.). Upper Saddle River, NJ: Prentice Hall.

Beers, M. H., & Berkow, R. (Eds.). (2006). *Merck manual: Diagnosis and therapy* (18th ed.). Whitehouse Station, NJ: Merck & Co.

Holland, N., & Adams, M. (2007). *Core concepts in pharmacology* (2nd ed.). Upper Saddle River, NJ: Prentice Hall.

Krogh, D. (2005). *Biology: A guide to the natural world* (3rd ed.). Upper Saddle River, NJ: Prentice Hall.

LeMone, P., & Burke, K. M. (2004). *Medical-surgical nursing: Critical thinking in client care* (3rd ed.). Upper Saddle River, NJ: Prentice Hall.

Martini, F. H. (2004). *Fundamentals of human anatomy and physiology* (6th ed.). San Francisco: Benjamin Cummings.

Medical Economics (Ed.). (2004). *Physician's desk reference for herbal medicines* (3rd ed.). Montvale, NJ: Author.

Medical Economics (Ed.). (2001). *Physician's desk reference for nutritional supplements.* Montvale, NJ: Author.

Medical Economics (Ed.). (2006). *Physician's desk reference* (60th ed.). Montvale, NJ: Author.

Mulvihill, M. L., Zelman, P., Holdaway, P., Tompary, E., & Turchany, J. (2006). *Human diseases: A systemic approach* (6th ed.). Upper Saddle River, NJ: Prentice Hall.

Rice, J. (2005). *Medical terminology with human anatomy* (5th ed.). Upper Saddle River, NJ: Prentice Hall.

Silverthorn, D. U. (2006). *Human physiology: An integrated approach* (4th ed.). San Francisco: Benjamin Cummings.

Wilson, B. A., Shannon, M. T., Shields, K. L., & Strang, C. L. (2004). *Nurse's drug guide 2007.* Upper Saddle River, NJ: Prentice Hall.

Chapter 1

Carrico, J. M. (2000). Human Genome Project and pharmacogenomics: Implications for pharmacy. *Journal of the American Pharmaceutical Association, 40*(1), 115–116.

Newton, G. D., Pray, W. S., & Popovich, N. G. (2001). New OTC drugs and devices 2000: A selective review. *Journal of the American Pharmaceutical Association, 41*(2), 273–282.

Ng, R. (2004). *Drugs: From discovery to approval.* Hoboken, NJ: Wiley.

Oates, J. A. (2006). The science of drug therapy. In L. L. Brunton, J. S. Lazo, & K. L. Parker (Eds.), *Goodman & Gilman's The pharmacological basis of therapeutics* (11th ed., pp. 117–136). New York: McGraw-Hill.

Olsen, D. P. (2000). The patient's responsibility for optimum healthcare. *Disease Management & Health Outcomes, 7*(2), 57–65.

Chapter 2

Bond, C. A., Raehl, C. L., & Franke, T. (2001). Medication errors in United States hospitals. *Pharmacotherapy, 21*(9), 1023–1036.

Brass, E. P. (2001). Drug therapy: Changing the status of drugs from prescription to over-the-counter availability. *New England Journal of Medicine, 345,* 810–816.

Brown, S. D., & Landry, F. J. (2001). Recognizing, reporting, and reducing adverse drug reactions. *Southern Medical Journal, 94*(4), 370–373.

Force, M. V., Deering, L., Hubbe, J., Andersen, M., Hagemann, B., Cooper-Hahn, M., et al. (2006). Effective strategies to increase reporting of medication errors in hospitals. *Journal of Nursing Administration, 36*(1) 34–41.

Gaither, C. A., Kirking, D. M., Ascione, F. J., & Welage, L. S. (2001). Consumers' views on generic medications. *Journal of the American Pharmaceutical Association, 41*(5), 729–736.

Phillips, K. A., Veenstra, D. L., Oren, E., Lee, J. K., & Sardee, W. (2001). Potential role of pharmacogenomics in reducing adverse drug reactions: A systematic review. *Journal of the American Medical Association, 286,* 2270–2279.

Chapter 3

Barbera, J., Macintyre, A., Gostin, L., Inglesby, T., O'Toole, T., Diatele, C., et al. (2000). Large-scale quarantine following biological terrorism in the United States: Scientific examination, logistic and legal limits, and possible consequences. *Journal of the American Medical Association, 286*(21), 2711–2717.

Bartlett, J. G., Sifton, D. W., & Kelly, G. L. (Eds.). (2002). *PDR guide to biological and chemical warfare response.* Montvale, NJ: Medical Economics.

Blendon, R. J., Des Roches, C. M., Benson, J. M., Herrmann, M. J., Taylor-Clark, K., & Weldon, K. J. (2003). The public and the smallpox threat. *New England Journal of Medicine, 348*(5), 426–432.

Bozeman, W. P., Dilbero, D., & Schauben, J. L. (2002). Biologic and chemical weapons of mass destruction. *Emergency Medical Clinics of North America, 20*(4), xii, 975–993.

Cangemi, C. W. (2002). Occupational response to terrorism. *American Association of Occupational Health Nurses Journal, 50*(4), 190–196.

Chyba, C. F. (2001). Biological security in a changed world. *Science, 293*(5539), 2349.

Crupi, R. S., Asnis, D. S., Lee, C. C., Santucci, T., Marino, M. J., & Flanz, B. J. (2003). Meeting the challenge of bioterrorism: Lessons learned from West Nile virus and anthrax. *American Journal of Emergency Medicine, 21*(1), 77–79.

Donnellan, C. (2002). New law funds nursing's role in bioterrorism response: The ANA establishes the National Nurses Response Team. *American Journal of Nursing, 102*(8), 23.

Fidler, D. P. (2001). The malevolent use of microbes and the rule of law: Legal challenges presented by bioterrorism. *Clinical Infectious Diseases, 33*(5), 686–689.

Henderson, D. A., Inglesby, T. V., & O'Toole, T. (2002). *Bioterrorism: Guidelines for medical and public health management.* Chicago, IL: American Medical Association.

Hughes, J. M. (2001). Emerging infectious diseases: A CDC perspective. *Emerging Infectious Diseases, 7*(3, Suppl.), 494–496.

Khan, A. S., Swerdlow, D. L., & Juranek, D. D. (2001). Precautions against biological and chemical terrorism directed at food and water supplies. *Public Health Reports, 116*(1), 3–14.

Kimmel, S. R., Mahoney, M. C., & Zimmerman, R. K. (2003). Vaccines and bioterrorism: Smallpox and anthrax. *Journal of Family Practice, 52*(1), S56–S61.

McLaughlin, S. (2001). Thinking about the unthinkable. Where to start planning for terrorism incidents. *Health Facilities Management, 14*(7), 26–30, 32.

Morse, A. (2002). Bioterrorism preparedness for local health departments. *Journal of Community Health Nursing, 19*(4), 203–211.

Mortimer, P. P. (2003). Can postexposure vaccination against smallpox succeed? *Clinical Infectious Diseases, 36*(5), 622–629.

O'Connell, K. P., Menuey, B. C., & Foster, D. (2002). Issues in preparedness for biologic terrorism: A perspective for critical care nursing. *American Association of Critical-Care Nurses Clinical Issues, 13*(3), 452–469.

O'Toole, T. (2001). Emerging illness and bioterrorism: Implications for public health. *Journal of Urban Health, 78*(2), 396–402.

Rose, M. A., & Larrimore, K. L. (2002). Knowledge and awareness concerning chemical and biological terrorism: Continuing education implications. *Journal of Continuing Education in Nursing, 33*(6), 253–258.

Salazar, M. K., & Kelman, B. (2002). Planning for biological disasters. Occupational health nurses as "first responders." *American Association of Occupational Health Nurses Journal, 50*(4), 174–181.

Spencer, R. C., & Lightfoot, N. F. (2001). Preparedness and response to bioterrorism. *Journal of Infection, 43*(2), 104–110.

Stephenson, J. (2003). Smallpox vaccine program launched amid concerns raised by expert panel, unions. *Journal of the American Medical Association, 289*(6), 685–686.

Stillsmoking, K. (2002). Bioterrorism:—Are you ready for the silent killer? *Association of PeriOperative Registered Nurses Journal, 76*(3), 434, 437–442, 444–446.

Tasota, F. J., Henker, R. A., & Hoffman, L. A. (2002). Anthrax as a biological weapon: An old disease that poses a new threat. *Critical Care Nurse, 22*(5), 21–32, 34.

Chapter 4

Armitage, G., & Knapman, H. (2003). Adverse events in drug administration: A literature review. *Journal of Nursing Management, 11*(2), 130–140.

Berman, A. J., Snyder, S., Kozier, B., & Erb, G. (2008). *Kozier & Erb's Fundamentals of Nursing Concepts, Process, and Practice,* 8th ed. Upper Saddle River, NJ: Prentice Hall.

Billups, S. J., Malone, D. C., & Carter, B. L. (2000). The relationship between drug therapy noncompliance and patient characteristics, health-related quality of life, and health care costs. *Pharmacotherapy, 20*(8), 941–949.

Blais, K. K., Hayes, J., Kozier, B., & Erb, G. (2002). *Professional nursing practice: Concepts and perspectives* (4th ed.). Upper Saddle River, NJ: Prentice Hall.

Deedwania, P. C. (2002). The changing face of hypertension: Is systolic blood pressure the final answer? *Archives of Internal Medicine, 162*(5), 506–508.

Hallgren, J., Tengvall-Linder, M., Persson, M., Wahlgren, C. F. (2003). Stevens-Johnson syndrome associated with ciprofloxacin: A review of adverse cutaneous events reported in Sweden as associated with this drug. *Journal of the American Academy of Dermatology, 49* (5 Suppl), S267–S269.

Koo, M. M., Krass, I., & Aslani, P. (2003). Factors influencing consumer use of written drug information. *Annals of Pharmacotherapy, 37*(2), 259–267.

Kozma, C. M. (2002). Why aren't we doing more to enhance medication compliance? *Managed Care Interface, 15*(1), 59–60.

Lesaffre, E., & de Klerk, E. (2000). Estimating the power of compliance-improving methods. *Controlled Clinical Trials, 21*(6), 540–551.

Madlon, K., Diane, J., & Mosch, F. S. (2000). Liquid medication dosing errors. *Journal of Family Practice, 49*(1), 741–744.

Olsen, J. L., Giangrasso, A. P., & Shrimpton, D. M. (2004). *Medical dosage calculations* (8th ed.). Upper Saddle River, NJ: Prentice Hall.

Seal. R. (2000). How to promote drug compliance in the elderly. *Community Nurse, 6*(1), 41–42.

Smith, D. I. (2001). Taking control of your medicines. Newsletter 1(1). *Consumer Health Information Corporation.* Retrieved from www.consumer-health.com

Smith, S., Duell, D., & Martin, B. (2000). *Clinical nursing skills: Basic to advanced skills* (5th ed.). Upper Saddle River, NJ: Prentice Hall Health.

Urquhart, J. (2000). Erratic patient compliance with prescribed drug regimens: Target for drug delivery systems. *Clinical Pharmacology and Therapeutics, 67*(4), 331–334.

Wooten, J. (2001). Toxic epidermal necrolysis. *Nursing 2001 64*(10), 35–38.

Chapter 5

Bateman, D. N. (2001). Introduction to pharmacokinetics and pharmacodynamics. *Journal of Toxicology: Clinical Toxicology, 39*(3), 207.

Bhattaram, V. B., Graefe, U., Kohlert, C., Veit, M., & Derendorf, H. (2002). Pharmacokinetics and bioavailability of herbal medicinal products. *Phytomedicine, 9,* 1–33.

Brunton, L. L., Lazo, J. S., & Parker, K. L. (Eds.). (2006). *Goodman & Gilman's The pharmacological basis of therapeutics* (11th ed.). New York: McGraw-Hill.

Buxton, I. L. O. (2006). Pharmacokinetics and pharmacodynamics: The dynamics of drug absorption, distribution, action, and elimination. In L. L. Brunton, J. S. Lazo, K. L. Parker (Eds.), *Goodman & Gilman's The pharmacological basis of therapeutics* (11th ed., pp. 1–40). New York: McGraw-Hill.

Doucet, J., Jego, D., Noel, D., Geffroy, C. E., Capet, C., Coquard, A., et al. (2002). Preventable and nonpreventable risk factors for adverse drug events related to hospital admission in the elderly. *Clinical Drug Investigation, 22*(6), 385–392.

Kanneh, K. (2002a). Paediatric pharmacological principles: An update part 2, Pharmacokinetics: Absorption and distribution. *Paediatric Nursing, 14*(9), 39–44.

Kanneh, K. (2002b). Paediatric pharmacological principles: An update part 3, Pharmacokinetics: Metabolism and excretion. *Paediatric Nursing, 14*(10), 39–43.

Levy, R. H., Thummel, K. E., Trager, W. F., Hansten, P. D., & Eichelbaum, M. (Eds.). (2000). *Metabolic drug interactions.* Philadelphia: Lippincott, Williams & Wilkins.

Rollins, D. E. (2000). Clinical pharmacokinetics. In A. R. Gennaro (Ed.), *Remington: The science and practice of pharmacy* (pp. 1145–1155). Philadelphia: Lippincott, Williams & Wilkins.

Scott, G. N., & Elmer, G. W. (2002). Update on natural product–drug interactions. *American Journal of Health-System Pharmacy, 59*(4), 339–347.

Suggs, D. M. (2000). Pharmacokinetics in children: History, considerations, and applications. *Journal of the American Academy of Nurse Practitioners, 12*(6), 236–240.

White, R. J., & Park, G. (2001). Safe drug prescribing in the critically ill. In G. Park & M. Shelly (Eds.), *Pharmacology of the critically ill.* London: BMI Books.

Chapter 6

Berg, M. J. (2002, August 31–September 5). *Does sex matter?* Paper presented at the Congress of the 62nd International Pharmaceutical Federation. Nice, France. Title also appears in *Medscape Pharmacists, 3*(2).

Bottles, K. (2001). A revolution in genetics: Changing medicine, changing lives. *Physician Executive, 27,* 58–63.

Buxton, I. L. O. (2006). Pharmacokinetics and pharmacodynamics: The dynamics of drug absorption, distribution, action, and elimination. In L. L. Brunton, J. S. Lazo, & K. L. Parker (Eds.), *Goodman & Gilman's The pharmacological basis of therapeutics* (11th ed., pp. 1–40). New York: McGraw-Hill.

du Souich, P. (2001). In human therapy, is the drug–drug interaction or the adverse drug reaction the issue? *Canadian Journal of Clinical Pharmacology, 8,* 153–161.

Ginsburg, G. S., & McCarthy, J. J. (2001). Personalized medicine: Revolutionizing drug discovery and patient care. *Trends in Biotechnology, 19,* 491–496.

Hughes, R. (2001). *A manual of pharmacodynamics.* New Delhi, India: B. Jain.

Kramer, T. (2003). Side effects and therapeutic effects. *Medscape General Medicine, 5*(1).

Kuo, G. M. (2003). Pharmacodynamic basis of herbal medicine. *Annals of Pharmacotherapy, 37*(2), 308.

Ma, M. K., Woo, M. A., & McLeod, H. L. (2002). Genetic basis of drug metabolism. *American Journal of Health-System Pharmacy, 59*(21), 2061–2069.

Nightingale, C. H., Murakawa, T., & Ambrose, P. G. (Eds.). (2002). *Antimicrobial pharmacodynamics in theory and clinical practice.* New York: Marcel Dekker.

Oates, J. A. (2006). The science of drug therapy. In L. L. Brunton, J. S. Lazo, & K. L. Parker (Eds.), *Goodman & Gilman's The pharmacological basis of therapeutics* (11th ed., pp. 117–136). New York: McGraw-Hill.

Relling, M. V., & Dervieux, T. (2001). Pharmacogenetics and cancer therapy. *Nature Reviews Cancer, 1,* 99–108.

Roses, A. D. (2001). Pharmacogenetics. *Human Molecular Genetics, 10,* 2261–2267.

Ross, J. S., & Ginsburg, G. S. (2003). The integration of molecular diagnostics with therapeutics. *American Journal of Clinical Pathology, 119*(1), 26–36.

Steimer, W., & Potter, J. M. (2001). Pharmacogenetic screening and therapeutic drugs. *Clinica Chimica Acta, 315,* 137–155.

Wortman, M. (2001). Medicine gets personal. *Technology Review,* (January/February), 72–78.

Chapter 7

Berman, A. J., Snyder, S., Kozier, B., & Erb, G. (2008). *Kozier & Erb's Fundamentals of Nursing Concepts, Process, and Practice,* 8th ed. Upper Saddle River, NJ: Prentice Hall.

Carpenito, L. J. (2000). *Nursing diagnosis: Application to nursing practice* (8th ed.). Philadelphia: J.B. Lippincott.

D'Amica, D., & Barbarito, C. (2007). Health and physical assessment in nursing. Upper Saddle River, NJ: Prentice Hall.

Gardner, P. (2003). *Nursing process in action.* New York: Thompson Delmar Learning.

Hogan, M. A., Bowles, D., & White, J. E. (2003). *Nursing fundamentals: Reviews & rationales.* Upper Saddle River, NJ: Prentice Hall.

Jahraus, D., Sokolosky, S., Thurston, N., & Guo, D. (2002). Evaluation of an education program for patients with breast cancer receiving radiation therapy. *Cancer Nursing, 24*(4), 266–275.

North American Nursing Diagnosis Association. (2003). *Nursing diagnoses: Definitions and classification 2003–2004.* Philadelphia: Author.

Smith, S. F., Duell, D. J., & Martin, B. C. (2004). *Clinical nursing skills* (6th ed.). Upper Saddle River, NJ: Prentice Hall.

Chapter 8

American Academy of Pediatrics, Committee on Drugs. (2001). The transfer of drugs and other chemicals into human breast milk. *Pediatrics, 3,* 776–782.

Auerbach, K. G. (2000). Breastfeeding and maternal medication use. *Journal of Obstetric, Gynecologic, and Neonatal Nursing, 28*(5), 554–563.

Ball, J. W., & Bindler, R. C. (2003). *Pediatric nursing: Caring for children.* Upper Saddle River, NJ: Prentice Hall.

Beers, M. H., & Berkow, R. (Eds.). (2000). *The Merck manual of geriatrics* (3rd ed.). Whitehouse Station, NJ: Merck & Company, Inc.

Bressler, R., & Katz, M. (2003). *Geriatric pharmacology* (2nd ed.). New York: McGraw-Hill Professional.

Briggs, G. G. (2002). Drug effects on the fetus and breast-fed infant. *Clinical Obstetrics and Gynecology, 45*(1), 6–21, 170–171.

Buehler, B., Delimont, D., van Waes, M., & Finnell, R. (1990). Prenatal prediction of risk of the fetal hydantoin syndrome. *New England Journal of Medicine, 22*(322), 1567–1572.

Dellasega, C., Klinefelter, J. M., & Halas, C. J. (2000). Psychoactive medications and the elderly patient. *Clinician Reviews, 10*(6), 53–74.

Hale, T. W. (2004) Maternal medications during breastfeeding. *Clinical Obstetrics and Gynecology 47*(3): 696–711.

Heinrich, J. (2001). Pediatric drug research: Substantial increase in studies of drugs for children but some challenges remain. Testimony before the Committee on Health, Education, Labor and Pensions, U.S. Senate, Washington, DC.

Leipzig, R. M. (Ed.). (2003). *Drug prescribing for older adults: An evidence-based approach.* Philadelphia: American College of Physicians.

Little, B., & Gilstrap, L. (Eds.). (1998). Introduction to drugs in pregnancy. In *Drugs and pregnancy* (2nd ed., p. 523). New York: Chapman & Hall.

Nice, F. J., Snyder, J. L., & Kotansky, B. C. (2000). Breastfeeding and over-the-counter medications. *Journal of Human Lactation, 16*(4), 319–331.

O'Mahony, D., & Martin, U. (1999). *Practical therapeutics for the older patient.* Indianapolis: Wiley.

Rosenbaum, M., & Irwin, K. (1998). Pregnancy, drugs, and harm reduction. In *Drug addiction research and the health of women* (pp. 309–318). Rockville, MD: United States Department of Health and Human Services, National Institutes of Health.

Spencer, J. P., Gonzalez, L. S., III, & Barnhart, D. J. (2001). Medications in the breast-feeding mother. *American Family Physician, 64,* 19–126.

Chapter 9

Bates, D. W., Clapp, M., Federico, F., Goldmann, D., Kaushal, R., Landrigan, C., et al. (2001). Medication errors and adverse drug events in pediatric inpatients. *Journal of the American Medical Association, 285*(16), 2114–2120.

Berman, A. J., Snyder, S., Kozier, B., & Erb, G. (2008). *Kozier & Erb's Fundamentals of Nursing Concepts, Process and Practice,* 8th ed. Upper Saddle River, NJ: Prentice Hall.

Burns, J. P., Mitchell, C., Griffith, J. L., & Truog, R. D. (2001). End-of-life care in the pediatric intensive care: Attitudes and practices of pediatric critical care physicians and nurses. *Critical Care Medicine, 29*(3), 658–664.

Cohen, M. R. (2000). Preventing medication errors related to prescribing. In M. R. Cohen (Ed.), *Medication errors. Causes, preventions, and risk management.* Sudbury, MA: Jones and Bartlett.

Committee on Drugs and Committee on Hospital Care. (2003). Prevention of medication errors in the pediatric inpatient setting. *Pediatrics, 112,* 431–436.

Federal Drug Administration. (2001, October 1). Med error reports to FDA show a mixed bag. Drug Topics. Retrieved from www.drugtopics.com

Goldman, E. (2006, May 1). PDA-based drug dose calculator slashes NICU med errors. *Family Practice News,* p. 55.

Guido, G. W. (2001). *Legal and ethical issues in nursing* (3rd ed.). Upper Saddle River, NJ: Prentice Hall.

Institute for Safe Medical Practices. (2000). Discussion paper on adverse event and error reporting in healthcare. January 24, 2000.

Joanna Briggs Institute. (2006). Strategies to reduce medication errors with reference to older adults. *Nursing Standard, 20,* 53–57.

Kane-Gill, S., & Weber, R. J. (2006). Principles and practices of medication safety in the ICU. *Critical Care Clinics, 22,* 273–290.

Koczmara, C., Jelincic, V., & Perri, D. (2006). Communication of medication orders by telephone—"writing it right." *Dynamics, 17,* 20–24.

Lazarou, J., Pomeranz, B. H., & Corey, P. N. (1998). Incidence of adverse drug reactions in hospitalized patients. A meta-analysis of prospective studies. *Journal of American Medical Association, 279*(15), 1200–1205.

Meadows, M. (2003) Strategies to reduce medication errors. How the FDA is working to improve medication safety and what you can do help. *FDA Consumer 37*(3): 20–27.

Mitchell, A. (2001). Challenges in pediatric pharmacotherapy: Minimizing medication errors. *Medscape Pharmacists, 2*(1), 1–8.

National Coordinating Council for Medication Error and Reporting (NCC MERP). *Recommendations to enhance accuracy in prescription writing.* Adopted Sept. 4, 1996. Revised June 2, 2005. Retrieved July 18, 2006, from http://www.nccmerp.org/council/council1996-09-04.html

O'Dell K. (2006). Allergy documentation: Strategies for patient safety. *Oklahoma Nurse, 51,* 16.

Page, K., & McKinney, A. A. (2006). Addressing medication errors: The role of undergraduate nurse education. *Nurse Education Today,* July 11 (epub).

Phillips, J., Beam, S., Brinker, A., Holquist, C., Honig, P., Lee, L. Y., et al. (2001). Retrospective analysis of mortalities associated with medication errors. *American Journal of Health-System Pharmacy, 58,* 1835–1841.

Santell J. P., & Cousins, D. (2004). Preventing medication errors that occur in the home. *U.S. Pharmacist 29*(9): 64–68.

Shuttleworth A. (2006). How to keep up to date with practice. *Nursing Times, 102,* 54–55.

USP. (2003). Pediatric population can benefit from USP recommendations. *Quality Review, 7.*

Chapter 10

Andrus, M. R., & Roth, M. T. (2002). Health literacy: A review. *Pharmacotherapy, 22*(3), 282–302.

Bushy, A. (1999). Social and cultural factors affecting health care and nursing practice. In J. Lancaster, *Nursing issues in leading and managing change* (pp. 267–292). St. Louis: Mosby.

Chen, J. (2002, October 20–23). *The role of ethnicity in medication use.* Paper presented at the American College of Clinical Pharmacy 2002 Annual Meeting, Albuquerque, NM.

Chin, J. L. (2000). Viewpoint: Culturally competent health care. *Public Health Reports, 115*(1), 25–33.

Crow, K., & Matheson, L. (2000). Informed consent and truth-telling: Cultural directions for healthcare providers. *Journal of Nursing Administration, 30*(3), 148–152.

Davidhizar, R. (2002). Strategies for providing culturally appropriate pharmaceutical care to the Hispanic patient. *Hospital Pharmacy, 37*(5), 505–510.

Gallagher, R. M. (2002). *The pain–depression conundrum: Bridging the body and mind.* Medscape clinical update based on session presented at the 21st Annual Scientific Meeting of the American Pain Society. Retrieved from http://www.medscape.com/viewprogram/2030

Humma, L. M., & Terra, S. G. (2002). Pharmacogenetics and cardiovascular disease: Impact on drug response and applications to disease management. *American Journal of Health-System Pharmacy, 59*(13), 1241–1252.

Kudzma, E. C. (2001). Cultural competence: Cardiovascular medications. *Progress in Cardiovascular Nursing, 16*(4), 152–160, 169.

Leininger, M. M. (Ed.). (2001). *Culture care diversity and universality: A theory of nursing.* Sudbury, MA: Jones & Bartlett.

Martin, L., Miracle, A. W., & Bonder, B. R. (2001). *Culture in clinical care.* Thorofare, NJ: Slack.

Nichols-English, G., & Poirier, S. (2000). Optimizing adherence to pharmaceutical care plans. *Journal of the American Pharmaceutical Association, 40*(4), 475–485.

Richardson, L. G. (2003). Psychosocial issues in patients with congestive heart failure. *Progressive Cardiovascular Nursing, 18*(1), 19–27.

Sleath, B., & Wallace, J. (2002). Providing pharmaceutical care to Spanish-speaking patients. *Journal of the American Pharmaceutical Association, 42,* 799–801.

Spector, R. E. (2004). *Cultural diversity in health and illness* (6th ed.). Upper Saddle River, NJ: Prentice Hall.

Wick, J. Y. (1996). Culture, ethnicity, and medications. *Journal of the American Pharmaceutical Association, 9,* 557–564.

Chapter 11

Blumenthal, M. (Ed.). (2000). *Herbal medicine: Expanded commission E monographs.* Austin, TX: American Botanical Council.

Ebadi, M. (2002). *Pharmacodynamic basis of herbal medicine.* Boca Raton, FL: CRC Press.

Fontaine, K. L. (2005). *Complementary and alternative therapies for nursing practice.* Upper Saddle River, NJ: Prentice Hall.

Foster, S., & Hobbs, C. (2002). *A field guide to Western medicinal plants and herbs.* Boston and New York: Houghton Mifflin.

Goldman, P. (2001). Herbal medicines today and the roots of modern pharmacology. *Annals of Internal Medicine, 135*(8), 594–597.

Hardy, M. L. (2000). Herbs of special interest to women. *Journal of the American Pharmaceutical Association, 40*(2), 234–242.

Marcus, D. M., & Snodgrass, W. R. (2005). Do no harm: Avoidance of herbal medicines during pregnancy. *Obstetrics & Gynecology, 105,* 1119–1122.

Medical Economics Staff (Ed.). (2000). *Physician's desk reference for herbal medicines* (2nd ed.). Montvale, NJ: Medical Economics.

The review of natural products: 2005 (4th ed.). Missouri: Facts and Comparisons®, Publisher.

Scott, G. N., & Elmer, G. W. (2002). Update on natural product–drug interactions. *American Journal of Health-System Pharmacy, 59*(4), 339–347.

Sierpina, V. S., Wollschlaeger, B., & Blumenthal, M. (2003). Ginkgo biloba. *American Family Physician, 68*(5), 923–926.

White House Commission on Complementary and Alternative Medicine Policy. (2000, March) Final report. Retrieved from http://govinfo.library.unt.edu/whccamp/

Chapter 12

Barangan, C. J., & Alderman, E. M. (2002). Management of substance abuse. *Pediatrics in Review, 23*(4), 123–131.

Chychula, N. M., & Sciamanna, C. (2002). Help substance abusers attain and sustain abstinence. *Nurse Practitioner, 27*(11), 30–47.

Fraschini, F., Demartini, G., & Esposti, D. (2002). Pharmacology of silymarin. *Clinical Drug Investigation, 22*(1), 51–65.

Freese, T. E., Miotto, K., & Reback, C. J. (2002). The effects and consequences of selected club drugs. *Journal of Substance Abuse Treatment, 23*(2), 151–156.

Gable, R. (2006). The toxicity of recreational drugs. *American Scientist, 94*(3), 206.

Hardie, T. L. (2002). The genetics of substance abuse. *American Association of Critical Care Nursing Clinical Issues, 13*(4), 511–522.

Haseltine, E. (2001). The unsatisfied mind: Are reward centers in your brain wired for substance abuse? *Discover, 22*(11), 88.

Jason, L. A., Davis, M. I., Ferrari, J. R., & Bishop, P. D. (2001). A review of research and implications for substance abuse recovery and community research. *Journal of Drug Education, 31*(1), 1–28.

Kandel, D. B. (2003). Does marijuana use cause the use of other drugs? *Journal of the American Medical Association, 289*(4), 482–483.

Manoguerra, A. S. (2001). Methamphetamine abuse. *Journal of Toxicology: Clinical Toxicology, 38*(2), 187.

Naegle, M. A., & D'Avanzo, C. E. (2001). *Addictions and substance abuse: Strategies for advanced practice nursing.* Upper Saddle River, NJ: Prentice Hall.

Sindelar, J. L., & Fiellin, D. A. (2001). Innovations in treatment for drug abuse: Solutions to a public health problem. *Annual Review of Public Health, 22,* 249.

Song, Z., Deaciuc, I., Song, M., Lee, D. Y., Liu, Y., Ji, X., et al. (2006). Silymarin protects against acute ethanol-induced hepatotoxicity in mice. *Alcoholism, Clinical and Experimental Research, 30*(3), 407–413.

Tuttle, J., Melnyk, B. M., & Loveland-Cherry, C. (2002). Adolescent drug and alcohol use. Strategies for assessment, intervention, and prevention. *Nursing Clinics of North America, 37*(3), ix, 443–460.

Wasilow-Mueller, S., & Erickson, C. K. (2001). Drug abuse and dependency: Understanding gender differences in etiology and management. *Journal of the American Pharmaceutical Association, 41*(1), 78–90.

Chapter 13

Bouchard, R., Weber, A. R., & Geiger, J. D. (2002). Informed decision-making on sympathomimetic use in sports and health. *Clinical Journal of Sports Medicine, 12*(4), 209–224.

Chapple, C. R., Yamanishi, T., & Chess-Williams, R. (2002). Muscarinic receptor subtypes and management of the overactive bladder. *Urology, 60* (5 Suppl. 1), 82–88; discussion 88–89.

Cilliers, L., & Retief, F. P. (2003). *Poisons, poisoning, and the drug trade in ancient Rome.* Retrieved from www.sun.ac.za

Defilippi, J., & Crismon, M. L. (2003). Drug interactions with cholinesterase inhibitors. *Drugs and Aging, 20*(6), 437–444.

Herbison, P., Hay-Smith, J., Ellis, G., & Moore, K. (2003). Effectiveness of anticholinergic drugs compared with placebo in the treatment of overactive bladder: Systematic review. *British Medical Journal, 326,* 841–844.

Kolpuru, S. (2003). Doctor corner: Approach to a case of Down syndrome. *Pediatric OnCall™.* Retrieved from www.pediatriconcall.com

Lemstra, A. W., Eikelenboom, P., & van Gool, W. A. (2003). The cholinergic deficiency syndrome and its therapeutic implications. *Gerontology, 49*(1), 55–60.

McCrory, D. C., & Brown, C. D. (2002). Anticholinergic bronchodilators versus beta$_2$-sympathomimetic agents for acute exacerbations of chronic obstructive pulmonary disease. *Cochrane Database of Systematic Reviews, 2003*(1), CD003900.

Medical Economics (Ed.). (2000). *PDR for herbal medicines.* Montvale, NJ: Author.

Miller, C. A. (2002). Anticholinergics: The good and the bad. *Geriatric Nursing, 23*(5), 286–287.

MSN Health. (2003). *Drugs & herbs: Phenylephrine ophthalmic.* Retrieved from www.content.health.msn.com

National Parkinson Foundation. (2004). *What you should know about acetylcholine, anticholinergic drugs, the autonomic nervous system, and Botox.* Retrieved from www.parkinson.org

National Toxicology Program, National Institutes of Health. (2001). *NTP chemical repository: Phenylephrine.* Retrieved from www.ntp-server.hiehs.nih.gov

Rodrigo, G. J., & Rodrigo, C. (2002). The role of anticholinergics in acute asthma treatment: An evidence-based evaluation. *Chest, 121*(6), 1977–1987.

Roe, C. M., Anderson, M. J., & Spivack, B. (2002). Use of anticholinergic medications by older adults with dementia. *Journal of the American Geriatrics Society, 50,* 836–842.

ThinkQuest On-line Library. (2003). *Poisonous plants and animals. Atropa belladonna, deadly nightshade.* Retrieved from www.library.thinkquest.org

Wang, H. E. (2002). Street drug toxicity resulting from opiates combined with anticholinergics. *Prehospital Emergency Care, 6*(3), 351–354.

Westfall, T. C., & Westfall, D. P. (2005) Neurotransmission: The autonomic and somatic motor nervous systems. In L. L. Brunton, J. S. Lazo, & K. L. Parker (Eds.), *Goodman & Gilman's The pharmacological basis of therapeutics* (11th ed., pp. 137–182). New York: McGraw-Hill.

Chapter 14

Andai-Otlong, D. (2006). Patient education guide: Anxiety disorders. *Nursing 2006, 36*(3), 48–49.

Baldessarini, R. J. (2005). Drug therapy of depression and anxiety disorders. In L. L. Brunton, J. S. Lazo, & K. L. Parker (Eds.), *Goodman & Gilman's The pharmacological basis of therapeutics* (11th ed., pp. 429–460). New York: McGraw-Hill.

Charney, D. S., Mihic, J., & Harris, A. (2006). Hypnotics and sedatives. In L. L. Brunton, J. S. Lazo, & K. L. Parker (Eds.), *Goodman & Gilman's The pharmacological basis of therapeutics* (11th ed., pp. 401–428). New York: McGraw-Hill.

Ernst, E. (2006). Herbal remedies for anxiety—a systematic review of controlled clinical trials. *Phytomedicine 13*(3): 205–208.

Gorman, J. N. (2001). Generalized anxiety disorder. *Clinical Cornerstone, 3*(3), 37–46.

Health A to Z. (2003). *Benzodiazepines.* Retrieved from www.healthatoz.com

Kennedy, D. O., Little, W., Haskell, C. F., Schoey, A. B. (2006). Anxiolytic effects of a combination of *Melissa officinalis* and *Valerian officinalis* during laboratory induced stress. *Phytotherapy Research 20*(2): 96–102.

Lippmann, S., Mazour, I., & Shahab, H. (2001). Insomnia: Therapeutic approach. *Southern Medical Journal, 94*(9), 866–873.

Medical Economics (Ed.). (2001). *PDR for nutritional supplements.* Montvale, NJ: Author.

National Institute for Drug Abuse (NIDA). (2006). *Prescription medications*. Retrieved from www.nida.nih.gov/drugpages/prescription.html

Smock, T. K. (2001). *Physiological psychology: A neuroscience approach*. Upper Saddle River, NJ: Prentice Hall.

The Nurse Practitioner: The American Journal of Primary Health Care (2005). *Medication update; FDA: Antidepressants a risk for kids*. Retrieved from www.tnpj.com

United States Drug Enforcement Agency (DEA). (2003). *Benzodiazepines*. Retrieved from www.usdoj.gov/dea

United States Drug Enforcement Agency (DEA). (2003). *Depressants*. Retrieved from www.usdoj.gov/dea

Vitiello, M. V. (2000). Effective treatment of sleep disturbances in older adults. *Clinical Corner, 2*(5), 16–27.

Chapter 15

Burstein, A. H., Horton, R. L., Dunn, T., Alfaro, R. H., Piscitelli, S. C., & Theodore, W. (2000). Lack of effect of St. John's wort on carbamazepine pharmacokinetics in healthy volunteers. *Clinical Pharmacology and Therapeutics, 68*, 6.

Johnson, K. (2002). Epilepsy and pregnancy. *Medscape Ob/Gyn & Women's Health, 7*(2).

Murphy, P. A., & Blaylock, R. L. (2001). *Treating epilepsy naturally: A guide to alternative and adjunct therapies*. New York: McGraw-Hill Contemporary Books.

Pack, A. M., & Morrell, M. J. (2003). Treatment of women with epilepsy. *Seminars in Neurology, 22*(3), 289–298.

Patel, P., & Mageda, M. (2002, April). *Vitamin K deficiency*. E-Medicine: Instant access to the minds of medicine. Retrieved from www.emedicine.com

Snelson, C., & Dieckman, B. (2000, June). Recognizing and managing purple glove syndrome. *Critical Care Nurse, 20*(3), 54–61.

Tierney, L. M., McPhee, S. J., & Papadakis, M. A. (Eds.). (2002). The nervous system. In M. J. Minoff (Ed.), *Current medical diagnosis and treatment* (ch. 24). New York: Lange Medical Books/McGraw-Hill Medical.

Trimble, M., & Schmitz, B. (Eds.). (2002). *The neuropsychiatry of epilepsy*. New York: Cambridge University Press.

United States National Library, National Institutes of Health. (2003). *Neural tube defects*. Retrieved from www.nlm.nih.gov/medlineplus

University of Illinois at Chicago, College of Pharmacy Drug Information Center. (2003). *Is there an interaction between phenytoin and enteral feedings?* Retrieved from www.uic.edu

Wyllie, E. (2001). *The treatment of epilepsy: Principles and practice* (3rd ed.). Philadelphia: Lippincott, Williams & Wilkins.

Chapter 16

American Academy of Pediatrics. (2000). Diagnosis and evaluation of the child with attention deficit–hyperactivity disorder. *Pediatrics, 105*(5), 1158–1170.

Aschenbrenner, D. S. (2005). Drug watch. *American Journal of Nursing, 105*(11), 87–89.

Baldessarini, R. J. (2006). Drug therapy of depression and anxiety disorders. In L. L. Brunton, J. S. Lazo, & K. L. Parker (Eds.), *Goodman & Gilman's The pharmacological basis of therapeutics* (11th ed., pp. 429–460). New York: McGraw-Hill.

Bodkin J. A., & Amsterdam, J. D. (2002). Transdermal selegiline in major depression: A double-blind, placebo-controlled study in outpatients. *Journal of Psychiatry, 159*(11), 1869–1875.

Desai, H. D., & Jann, M. W. (2000). Major depression in women: A review of the literature. *Journal of the American Pharmaceutical Association 40*(4), 525–537.

Eli Lilly & Company. (2003). *Strattera: Safety information for health care professionals*. Indianapolis, IN: Author. Retrieved from www.strattera.com.

Fugh-Berman, A. (2000). Herb-drug interactions. *Lancet, 355*(9198), 134–138.

Gastpar, M., Singer, A., Zeller, K. (2006) Comparative efficacy and safety of a once-daily dosage of hypericum extract STW3-VI and citalopram in patients with moderate depression: A double-blind, randomised, multicentre, placebo-controlled study. *Pharmacopsychiatry 39*(2): 66–75.

Janicak, P. (2002). *TMS vs. ECT in depressed patients*. (Research report). Chicago: University of Illinois.

Lin, K. M. (1982). Cultural aspects in mental health for Asian Americans. In A. Gaw (Ed.), *Cross cultural psychiatry* (pp. 69–73). Boston: John Wright.

Medical Economics (Ed.). (2000). *PDR for herbal medicines*. Montvale, NJ: Author.

Moses, S. (2003). *Family practice notebook: Imipramine*. Lino Lakes: MN: Family Practice Notebook, LLC. Retrieved from www.fpnotebook.com

National Association of State Boards of Education. (2003). The use and abuse of Ritalin. *Policy Update, 7*(18).

Spector, R. E. (2000). *Cultural diversity in health and illness*. Upper Saddle River, NJ: Prentice Hall.

The Nurse Practitioner: The American Journal of Primary Health Care (2004). *Medication update: Antidepressant treats neuropathy in diabetes*. Retrieved from www.tnpj.com

Chapter 17

Bailey, K. (2003). Aripiprazole: The newest antipsychotic agent for the treatment of schizophrenia. *Psychosocial Nursing and Mental Health Services, 41*(2), 14–18.

Baldessarini, R. J., & Tarazi, F. I. (2006). Pharmacotherapy of psychosis and mania. In L. L. Brunton, J. S. Lazo, & K. L. Parker (Eds.), *Goodman & Gilman's The pharmacological basis of therapeutics* (11th ed., pp. 461–500). New York: McGraw-Hill.

Barclay, L. (2002, July 1). Quetiapine well-tolerated, effective in refractory schizophrenia. *Medscape Medical News*. Retrieved from www.medscape.com

Barthel, R. (2002, October 27). Early interventions in psychosis. *Medscape Medical News*. Retrieved from www.medscape.com

Brown University Child and Adolescent Psychopharmacology Update. (2002, July 19). *Drugs in the pipeline: New drugs and indications for children and adolescents*. Retrieved from www.medscape.com

Brown University Geriatric Psychopharmacology Update. (2002, December 9). *Treating bipolar disorder in older adults: Gaps in knowledge remain*. Retrieved from www.medscape.com

Burns, M. J. (2001). The pharmacology and toxicology of atypical antipsychotic agents. *Journal of Toxicology: Clinical Toxicology, 39*(1), 1.

Cada, D., Levien, T., & Baker, D. (2003). Aripiprazole. *Hospital Pharmacy, 38*(3), 247–254.

Kneisl, C. R., Wilson, H. S., & Trigoboff, E. (2004). *Contemporary psychiatric–mental health nursing*. Upper Saddle River, NJ: Prentice Hall.

Medical Economics (Ed.). (2000). *PDR for herbal medicines*. Montvale, NJ: Author.

Medscape Medical News. (2003, February 13). *Dispensing errors reported for serzone and seroquel*. Retrieved from www.medscape.com

Vitiello, B. (2001). Psychopharmacology for young children: Clinical needs and research opportunities. *Pediatrics, 108*(4), 983.

Wahlbeck, K., Cheine, M., & Essali, M. A. (2002, April 1). Clozapine versus typical neuroleptic medication for schizophrenia. *Cochrane Review Abstracts*. Retrieved from www.medscape.com

Chapter 18

Barkin, R. L., & Barkin, D. (2001). Pharmacologic management of acute and chronic pain: Focus on drug interactions and patient-specific pharmacotherapeutic selection. *Southern Medical Journal, 94*(8), 756–812.

Bayer ASA side effects and ASA drug interactions. (2003). Retrieved from www.rxlist.com/cgi/generic/asa_ad.htm

Bell, J., Kimber, J., Mattick, R., Ali, R., Lintzers, N., Monhert, B., et al. (2003). *Interim clinical guidelines: Use of naltrexone in relapse prevention for opioid dependence* (abbreviated version). Washington, DC: Office of Disease Prevention and Health Promotion, United States Department of Health and Human Services. Retrieved from www.health.gov

Broadbent, C. (2000). The pharmacology of acute pain. Part 3. *Nursing Times, 96*(26), 39.

Clinical aspects of G6PD deficiency, (2003). Retrieved from www.rialto.com

Diamond, M. (2003). *Emergency treatment of headache*. Chicago: Internal Medicine Department, Columbus Hospital. Retrieved from www.usdoctor.com

Evans, R. W., & Taylor, F. R. (2006). "Natural" or alternative medications for migraine prevention. *Headache: The Journal of Head and Face Pain 46*(6): 1012–1018.

Glajchen, M. (2001). Chronic pain. Treatment barriers and strategies for clinical practice. *Journal of the American Board of Family Practice, 14*(3), 178–183.

Guay, D. R. P. (2001). Adjunctive agents in the management of chronic pain. *Pharmacotherapy, 21*(9), 1070–1081.

Gunsteuin, H., & Akil, H. (2006). Opioid analgesics. In L. L. Brunton, J. S. Lazo, & K. L. Parker (Eds.), *Goodman & Gilman's The pharmacological basis of therapeutics* (11th ed., pp. 569–620). New York: McGraw-Hill.

Khouzam, H. R. (2000). Chronic pain and its management in primary care. *Southern Medical Journal, 93*(10), 946–952.

Moses, S. (Ed.). (2002). Subarachnoid hemorrhage. *Family Practice Notebook*. Retrieved from www.fpnotebook.com/NEU33.htm

National Reye's Syndrome Foundation, Inc. (2000). *Aspirin or salicylate-containing medications*. Retrieved from www.reyessyndrome.org/aspirin.htm

Office of Disease Prevention and Health Promotion, United States Department of Health and Human Services. (2003). *Section 11: Gastrointestinal system*. Retrieved from www.health.gov

Tepper, S. J., & Rapoport, A. M. (1999). The triptans: A summary. *CNS Drugs, 12*(5), 403–417.

Tfelt-Hansen, P., DeVries, P., & Sexena, P. R. (2000). Triptans in migraine: A comparative review of pharmacology, pharmacokinetics, and efficacy. *Drugs, 60*(6), 1259–1287.

Chapter 19

Catterall, W. A., & Mackie, K. (2006). Local anesthetics. In L. L. Brunton, J. S. Lazo, & K. L. Parker (Eds.), *Goodman & Gilman's The pharmacological basis of therapeutics* (11th ed., pp. 367–384). New York: McGraw-Hill.

Colbert, B. J., & Mason, B. J. (2006). *Integrated cardiopulmonary pharmacology*. Upper Saddle River, NJ: Prentice Hall.

Evers, A., & Crowder, C. M. (2006). General anesthetics. In L. L. Brunton, J. S. Lazo, & K. L. Parker (Eds.), *Goodman & Gilman's The pharmacological basis of therapeutics* (11th ed., pp. 337–366). New York: McGraw-Hill.

KidsHealth for Parents. (2003). *Your child's anesthesia*. The Nemours Foundation. Retrieved from http://www.kidshealth.org

Nagelhout, J. J., Nagelhout, K., & Zaglaniczny, V. H. (2001). *Handbook of nurse anesthesia* (2nd ed.). Philadelphia: W. B. Saunders.

National Institutes of Health. (2003). *General anesthesia*. Retrieved from http://www.search.nlm.nih.gov/medlineplus

Chapter 20

About Alzheimer's. Retrieved from www.alzfdn.org

Alzheimer's disease; Unraveling the mystery: The search for new treatments. (2003, April 11). Retrieved from www.alzheimers.org

Birks, J., Grimley-Evans, J., & Van Dongen, M. (2003). Ginkgo biloba for cognitive impairment and dementia. *Medscape*. Retrieved from www.medscape.com

Borek, C. (2006). Garlic reduces dementia and heart-disease risk. *Journal of Nutrition, 136*(3 Suppl); 810S–812S.

Capozza, K. (2003, April 2). Drug slows progression of Alzheimer's. *Medline Plus*. Retrieved from www.nlm.nih.gov/medlineplus

Cummings, J. L. (2000). Treatment of Alzheimer's disease. *Clinical Corner, 3*(4), 27–39.

Dooley, M., & Lamb, H. M. (2000). Donepezil: A review of its use in Alzheimer's disease. *Drugs and Aging, 16*(3), 199–226.

Gruetzner, H. (2001). *Alzheimer's: A caregiver's guide and sourcebook* (3rd ed.). Indianapolis: Wiley.

Hristove, A. H., & Koller, W. C. (2000). Early Parkinson's disease: What is the best approach in treatment? *Drugs and Aging, 17*(3), 165–181.

Kahle, P., & Haass, C. (Eds.). (2003). *Molecular mechanisms in Parkinson's disease*. Georgetown, TX: Landes Bioscience/Eurekah.com

Lambert, D., & Waters, C. H. (2000). Comparative tolerability of the new generation antiparkinson agents. *Drugs and Aging, 16*(1), 55–65.

Richter, R. (Ed.). (2003). *Alzheimer's disease: The physician's guide to practical management*. Totowa, NJ: Human Press.

Sierpina, V. S., Wollschlaeger, B., & Blumenthal M. Ginkgo biloba. *American Family Physician 68*(5): 923–926.

Standaert, D. G., & Young, A. B. (2006). Treatment of central nervous system degenerative disorders. In L. L. Brunton, J. S. Lazo, & K. L. Parker (Eds.), *Goodman & Gilman's The pharmacological basis of therapeutics* (11th ed., pp. 527–546). New York: McGraw-Hill.

Chapter 21

American Society for Aesthetic Plastic Surgery. (2003). *Your image*. Retrieved from http://surgery.org/EFFECTIVE_METHODS.HTML

Dystonia Medical Research Foundation. (2003a). *Botulism toxin injections*. Retrieved from http://www.dystonia-foundation.org/treatment/botox.asp

Dystonia Medical Research Foundation. (2003b). *Complementary therapy*. Retrieved from http://www.dystonia-foundation.org/treatment/comp.asp

Dystonia Medical Research Foundation. (2003c). *Dystonia defined*. Retrieved from http://www.dystonia-foundation.org/defined/

National Institutes of Health. (2003). *Spasticity*. Retrieved from http://www.nlm.nih.gov/medlineplus/ency/article/003297.htm

National Institutes of Health, National Institute of Neurological Disorders and Stroke. (2003). *NINDS spasticity information page*. Retrieved from http://nindsupdate.ninds.nih.gov/health_and_medical/disorders/spasticity_doc.htm

Nelson, A. J., Ragan, B. G., Bell, G. W., Ichiyama, R. M., Iwamoto, G. A. (2004). Capsaic in-based analgesic balm decreases pressor responses evoked by muscle afferents. *Medicine & Science in Sports & Exercise, 36*(3): 444–450.

Chapter 22

American Association of Clinical Endocrinologists. (2002). Medical guidelines for clinical practice for the diagnosis and treatment of dyslipidemia and prevention of atherogenesis [Amended version]. *Endocrine Practice, 6*(2), March/April 2000.

Ballantyne, C. M., O'Keefe, J. H., Jr., & Gotto, A. M., Jr. (2005). *Dyslipidemia essentials*. Royal Oak, MI: Physician's Press.

Illingworth, D. R. (2000). Management of hypercholesterolemia. *Medical Clinics of North America, 84*(1), 23–42.

Kreisberg, R. A. (2000). Art and science of statin use. *Clinical Review*, (Spring), 47–51.

Levy, H. B., & Kohlhaas, H. K. (2006). Considerations for supplementing with coenzyme Q10 during statin therapy. *Annals of Pharmacotherapy, 40*(2), 290–294.

Littarru, G. P., & Tiano, L. (2005). Clinical aspects of coenzyme Q10: An update. *Current Opinion in Clinical Nutrition and Metabolic Care, 8*(6), 641–646.

Mahley, R. W., & Bersot, T. P. (2006). Drug therapy for hypercholesterolemia and dyslipidemia. In L. L. Brunton, J. S. Lazo, & K. L. Parker (Eds.), *Goodman & Gilman's The pharmacological basis of therapeutics* (11th ed., pp. 933–964). New York: McGraw-Hill.

Maltin, L. (2002, April 9). *Statin drugs may fight Alzheimer's, too.* Retrieved from my.webmd.com/content/ article/16/1626_50907

McLoughlin, C. (2004). Statins. *Professional Nurse, 19*(11), 51–52.

Nichols, N. (2004). Clinical practice guidelines for the management of dyslipidemia. *Canadian Journal of Cardiovascular Nursing, 14*(2), 7–10.

Nutrition and Metabolism Advisory Committee. (2001). *Plant sterols and stanols: A position statement*. Melbourne, Australia: Heart Foundation.

Robinson, A. W., Sloan, H. L., & Arnold, G. (2001). Use of niacin in the prevention and management of hyperlipidemia. *Progress in Cardiovascular Nursing, 16*(1), 14–20.

U. S. Food and Drug Administration Center for Food Safety and Applied Nutrition, Office of Nutritional Products, Labeling, and Dietary Supplements. (2001, February). *New dietary ingredients in dietary supplements* (updated September 10, 2001). Washington, DC: Author.

Xydakis, A. M., & Ballantyne, C. M. (2004). Management of metabolic syndrome: Statins. *Endocrinology and Metabolism Clinics of North America, 33*(3), 509–523.

Young, K. L., Allen, J. K., & Kelly, K. M. (2001). HDL cholesterol: Striving for healthier levels. *Clinical Review, 11*(5), 50–61.

Chapter 23

Biujsee, B., Feskens, E. J., Kok, F. J., & Kromhout, D. (2006). Cocoa intake, blood pressure, and cardiovascular mortality. *Archives of Internal Medicine, 166*, 411–417.

Chang, W. T., Shao, Z. H., Vanden Hoek, T. L., McEntee, E., Mehendale, S. R., Li, J., et al. (2006). Cardioprotective effects of grape seed proanthocyanidins, baicalin, and wogonin. *American Journal of Chinese Medicine, 34*(2), 363–365.

Chaudhry, S. I., Krumholz, H. M., & Foody, J. M. (2004). Systolic hypertension in older persons. *Journal of the American Medical Association, 292*(9), 1074–1080.

Colbert, B. J., & Mason, B. J. (2001). *Integrated cardiopulmonary pharmacology*. Upper Saddle River, NJ: Prentice Hall.

Ding, E. L., Hutfless, S. M., Ding, X., & Girotra, S. (2006). Chocolate and prevention of cardiovascular disease: A systematic review. *Nutrition and Metabolism, 3*, 2.

Grassi, D., Lippi, C., Necozione, S., Desideri, G., & Ferri, C. (2005). Short-term administration of dark chocolate is followed by a significant increase in insulin sensitivity and a decrease in blood pressure in healthy persons. *American Journal of Clinical Nutrition, 81*(3), 611–614.

Hajjar, I. M., Grim, C. E., George, V., & Kotchen, T. A. (2001). Impact of diet on blood pressure and age-related changes in blood pressure in the U.S. population: Analysis of NHANES III. *Archives of Internal Medicine, 161*, 589.

Hoffman, B. B. (2006). Therapy of hypertension. In L. L. Brunton, J. S. Lazo, & K. L. Parker. (Eds.), *Goodman & Gilman's The pharmacological basis of therapeutics* (11th ed., pp. 845–868). New York: McGraw-Hill.

Klag, M. J., Wang, N. Y., Meoni, L. A., Brancati, F. L., Cooper, L. A., Liang, K. Y., et al. (2002). Coffee: Intake and risk of hypertension. The Johns Hopkins Precursors Study. *Archives of Internal Medicine, 162*, 657–662.

National High Blood Pressure Education Program. National Heart, Lung & Blood Institute. (2003). *JNC-7 Express: The Seventh Report of the Joint National Committee on Prevention, Detection, Evaluation, and Treatment of High Blood Pressure*. Bethesda, MD: Author.

National High Blood Pressure Education Program Working Group on High Blood Pressure in Children and Adolescents. (2004). The fourth report on the diagnosis, evaluation, and treatment of high blood pressure in children and adolescents. *Pediatrics, 114*(Suppl. 2), 555–576.

National Institutes of Health. (2003). NHLBI issues new high blood pressure clinical practice guidelines. *NIH NEWS*. Retrieved June 14, 2005, from http://www.nhlbi.nih.gov

Oates, J. A., & Brown, N. J. (2006). Antihypertensive agents and the drug therapy of hypertension. In L. L. Brunton, J. S. Lazo, & K. L. Parker (Eds.), *Goodman & Gilman's The pharmacological basis of therapeutics* (11th ed., pp. 871–900). New York: McGraw-Hill.

Poudre Valley Health System. (2003). *Herbal medicines and dietary supplements: Information for people with heart disease*. Retrieved from www.pvhs.org

Simpson, C. (2003). *Autonomic nervous system agents: Adrenergics and adrenergic blocking agents*. Retrieved from www.cotc.tech.oh.us

Thadhani, R., Camargo, C. A., Jr., Stampfer, M. J., Curhan, G. C., Willett, W. C., & Rimm, E. B. (2002). Prospective study of moderate alcohol consumption and risk of hypertension in young women. *Archives of Internal Medicine, 162*, 569–574.

Woods, A. D. (2001). Improving the odds against hypertension. *Nursing 2001, 31*(8), 36–42.

Vlachopoulos, C., Aznaouridis, K., Alexopoulos, N., Economou, E., Andreadou, I., & Stefanadis, C. (2005). Effect of dark chocolate on arterial function in healthy individuals. *American Journal of Hypertension, 18*(6): 785–971.

Chapter 24

Albrant, D. H. (2001). Drug treatment protocol: Management of chronic systolic heart failure. *Journal of the American Pharmaceutical Association, 41*(5), 672–681.

Chang, W. T., Dao, J., & Shao, Z. H. (2005). Hawthorn: Potential roles in cardiovascular disease. *American Journal of Chinese Medicine, 33*(1), 1–10.

Gomberg-Maitland, M., Baran, D. A., & Fuster, V. (2001). Treatment of congestive heart failure: Guidelines for the primary care health care provider and the heart failure specialist. *Archives of Internal Medicine, 161,* 342–352.

Jamali, A. H., Tang, A. H. W., Khot, U. N., & Fowler, M. B. (2001). The role of angiotensin receptor blockers in the management of chronic heart failure. *Archives of Internal Medicine, 161,* 667–672.

Kennedy, E. B., & Ignatavicius, D. D. (2006). Interventions for clients with cardiac problems. In D. D. Ignatavicius & L. H. Workman, (Eds.), *Medical–surgical nursing critical thinking for collaborative care* (5th ed, pp. 749–776). St. Louis, MO: Elsevier Saunders.

Opie, L. H., & Gersh, B. J. (Eds.). (2001). *Drugs for the heart* (5th ed.). Philadelphia: W. B. Saunders.

Paul, S. (2002). Balancing diuretic therapy in heart failure: Loop diuretics, thiazides, and antagonists. *Congestive Heart Failure, 8*(6), 307–312.

Pittler, M. H., Schmidt, K., & Ernst, E. (2003). Hawthorn extract for treating chronic heart failure: Meta-analysis of randomized trials. *American Journal of Medicine, 114*(8), 665–674.

Richardson, L. G. (2003). Psychosocial issues in patients with congestive heart failure. *Progress in Cardiovascular Nursing, 18*(1), 19–27.

Rocco, T. P., & Fang, J. C. (2006). Pharmacotherapy of congestive heart failure. In L. L. Brunton, J. S. Lazo, & K. L. Parker (Eds.), *Goodman & Gilman's The pharmacological basis of therapeutics* (11th ed., pp. 869–898). New York: McGraw-Hill.

Sperelakis, N., Kurachi, Y., Terzic, A., & Cohen, M. (Eds.). (2001). *Heart physiology and pathophysiology* (4th ed.). San Diego: Academic Press.

Steering Committee and Membership of the Advisory Council to Improve Outcomes Nationwide in Heart Failure. (1999). Consensus recommendations for the management of chronic heart failure. *American Journal of Cardiology, 83*(2A), 1A–38A.

Tankanow, R., Tamer, H. R., Streetman, D. S., Smith, S. G., Welton, J. L., Annesley, T., et al. (2003). Interaction study between digoxin and a preparation of hawthorn (*Crataegus oxyacantha*). *Journal of Clinical Pharmacology, 43*(6), 637–642.

Van Bakel, A. B., & Chidsey, G. (2000). Management of advanced heart failure. *Clinical Corner, 3*(2), 25–35.

Vasant, B. P., & Moliterno, D. J. (2000). Glycoprotein IIb/IIIa antagonist and fibrinolytic agents: New therapeutic regimen for acute myocardial infarction. *Journal of Invasive Cardiology, 12*(B), 8B–15B.

Chapter 25

Ambrose, J., & Dangas, G. (2000). Unstable angina: Current concepts of pathogenesis and treatment. *Archives of Internal Medicine, 160,* 25–37.

Awtry, E. H., & Loscalzo, J. (2000). Aspirin. *Circulation, 101*(10), 1206–1218.

Danchin, N., & Durand, E. (2003). Acute myocardial infarction. *Clinical Evidence, 10,* 37–63.

Freestone, B., Lip, G. Y. H., Scott, P. A., & Pancioli, A. M. (2003). Stroke prevention. *Clinical Evidence, 11,* 257–283.

Kreisberg, R. A. (2000). Overview of coronary heart disease and selected risk factors. *Clinical Review,* (Spring), 4–9.

Kurth, T., Glynn, R. J., Walker, A. M., Chan, K. A., Buring, J. E., Hennekens, C. H., et al. (2003). Inhibition of clinical benefits of aspirin on first myocardial infarction by nonsteroidal antiinflammatory drugs. *Circulation, 108*(10), 1191–1195.

Levine, G. N., Ali, M. N., & Schafer, A. I. (2001). Antithrombotic therapy in patients with acute coronary syndromes. *Archives of Internal Medicine, 161,* 937–948.

Michel, T. (2006). Treatment of myocardial ischemia. In L. L. Brunton, J. S. Lazo, & K. L. Parker (Eds.), *Goodman & Gilman's The pharmacological basis of therapeutics* (11th ed., pp. 823–844). New York: McGraw-Hill.

Parchure, N., & Brecker, S. J. (2002). Management of acute coronary syndromes. *Current Opinions in Critical Care, 8*(3), 230–235.

Priglinger, U., & Huber, K. (2000). Thrombolytic therapy in acute myocardial infarction. *Drugs and Aging, 16*(4), 301–312.

Staniforth, A. D. (2001). Contemporary management of chronic stable angina. *Drugs and Aging, 18*(2), 109–121.

Tong, G. M., & Rude, R. K. (2005). Magnesium deficiency in critical illness. *Journal of Intensive Care Medicine, 20*(1), 3–17.

Ueshima, K. (2005). Magnesium and ischemic heart disease: A review of epidemiological, experimental, and clinical evidences. *Magnesium Research, 18*(4), 275–284.

Chapter 26

Beattie, W. S., & Elliot, R. F. (2005). Magnesium supplementation reduces the risk of arrhythmia after cardiac surgery. *Evidence-based Cardiovascular Medicine, 9*(1), 82–5.

Berry, C., Rankin, A. C., & Brady, A. (2004). Bradycardia and tachycardia occurring in older people: An introduction. *British Journal of Cardiology, 11*(1), 61–64.

Dayer, M., & Hardman, S. (2002). Special problems with antiarrhythmic drugs in the elderly: Safety, tolerability, and efficacy. *American Journal of Geriatric Cardiology, 11*(6), 370–375.

Ellison, K. E., Stevenson, W. G., Sweeney, M. O., Epstein, L. M., & Maisel, W. H. (2003). Management of arrhythmias in heart failure. *Congestive Heart Failure, 9*(2), 91–99.

Haugh, K. H. (2002). Antidysrhythmic agents at the turn of the twenty-first century: A current review. *Critical Care Nursing Clinics of North America, 14*(1), 53–69.

Huikuri, H. V., Castellanos, A., & Myerburg, R. J. (2001). Medical progress: Sudden death due to cardiac arrhythmias. *New England Journal of Medicine, 345,* 1473–1482.

Kern, L. S. (2004). Postoperative atrial fibrillation: New directions in prevention and treatment. *Journal of Cardiovascular Nursing, 19*(2), 103–115.

Piotrowski, A. A., & Kalus, J. S. (2004). Magnesium for the treatment and prevention of atrial tachyarrhythmias. *Pharmacotherapy, 24*(7), 879–895.

Podrid, P. J., & Kowey, P. R. (Eds.). (2001). *Cardiac arrhythmia: Mechanisms, diagnosis, and management* (2nd ed.). Philadelphia: Lippincott, Williams, & Wilkins.

Roden, D. M. (2006). Antiarrhythmic drugs. In L. L. Brunton, J. S. Lazo, & K. L. Parker (Eds.), *Goodman & Gilman's The pharmacological basis of therapeutics* (11th ed., pp. 899–932). New York: McGraw-Hill.

Somberg, J. C., Cao, W., Cvetanovic, I., Ranade, V. V., & Molnar, J. (2005). The effect of magnesium sulfate on action potential duration and cardiac arrhythmias. *American Journal of Therapeutics, 12*(3), 218–222.

Tong, G. M., & Rude, R. K. (2005). Magnesium deficiency in critical illness. *Journal of Intensive Care Medicine, 20*(1), 3–17.

Ueshima, K. (2005). Magnesium and ischemic heart disease: A review of epidemiological, experimental, and clinical evidences. *Magnesium Research, 18*(4), 275–284.

Chapter 27

Allison, G. L., Lowe, G. M., & Rahman, K. (2006). Aged garlic extract and its constituents inhibit platelet aggregation through multiple mechanisms. *Journal of Nutrition, 136*(Suppl. 3), 782S–788S.

Alligood, K. A., & Iltz, J. L. (2001). Update on antithrombotic use and mechanism of action. *Progress in Cardiovascular Nursing, 16*(2), 81–85.

Coumadin: Prescription drug reference. (2003). Retrieved from www.healthsquare.com

Hiatt, W. R. (2001). Drug therapy: Medical treatment of peripheral arterial disease and claudication. *New England Journal of Medicine, 344,* 1608–1621.

Rahman, K., & Lowe, G. M. (2006). Garlic and cardiovascular disease: A critical review. *Journal of Nutrition, 136*(3), 736S–740S.

Chapter 28

Bailey, L. B., Rampersaud, G. C., & Kauwell, G. P. (2003). Folic acid supplements and fortification affect the risk for neural tube defects, vascular disease, and cancer: Evolving science. *Journal of Nutrition, 133*(6), 1961S–1968S.

Dharmarajan, T. S., Adiga, G. U., & Norkus, E. P. (2003). Vitamin B_{12} deficiency. Recognizing subtle symptoms in older adults. *Geritrics, 58*(3), 30–34, 37–38.

Eden, A. N. (2003). Preventing iron deficiency in toddlers: A major public health problem. *Contemporary Pediatrics, 20*(2), 57–67.

Edroso, R. (2003). Understanding HIV fatigue: What's dragging you down? *WebMDHealth.* Retrieved from http://my.webmd.com

Kaushansky, K., & Kipps, T. J. (2006). Hematopoietic agents: Growth factors, minerals, & vitamins. In L. L. Brunton, J. S. Lazo, & K. L. Parker (Eds.), *Goodman & Gilman's The pharmacological basis of therapeutics* (11th ed., pp. 1433–1466). New York: McGraw-Hill.

Oh, R., & Brown, D. L. (2003). Vitamin B_{12} deficiency. *American Family Health Care Provider, 67*(5), 979–986.

Rampersaud, G. C., Kauwell, G. P., & Bailey, L. B. (2003). Folate: A key to optimizing health and reducing disease risk in the elderly. *Journal of the American College of Nutrition, 22*(1), 1–8.

Somer, E. (2003). Ironing out anemia. *WebMDHealth.* Retrieved from http://my.webmd.com

Chapter 29

Baumgartner, J. D., & Calandra, T. (1999). Treatment of sepsis: Past and future avenues. *Drugs, 57*(2), 127–132.

Dellinger, R. P. (2003). Cardiovascular management of septic shock. *Critical Care Medicine, 31*(3), 946–955.

Hasdai, D., Berger, P. B., Battler, A., & Holmes, D. R. (2002). *Cardiogenic shock: Diagnosis and treatment.* Totowa, NJ: Humana Press.

Kolecki, P., & Menckhoff, C. R. (2001, December 11). Hypovolemic shock. *eMedicine Journal, 2*(12).

Menon, V., & Fincke, R. (2003). Cardiogenic shock: A summary of the randomized SHOCK trial. *Congestive Heart Failure, 9*(1), 35–39.

Moser-Wade, D. M., Bartley, M. K., & Chiari-Allwein, H. L. (2000). Shock: Do you know how to respond? *Nursing 2000, 30*(10), 34–40.

Von Rosenstiel, N., von Rosenstiel, I., & Adam, D. (2001). Management of sepsis and septic shock in infants and children. *Paediatric Drugs, 3*(1), 9–27.

Chapter 30

Costello-Boerrigter, L. C., Boerrigter, G., & Burnett, J. C. (2003). Revisiting salt and water retention: New diuretics, aquaretics, and natriuretics. *Medical Clinics of North America, 87*(2), 475–491.

Howell, A. B., Reed, J. D., Krueger, C. G., Winterbottom, R., Cunningham, D. G., & Leahy, M. (2005). A-type cranberry proanthocyanidins and uropathogenic bacterial anti-adhesion activity. *Phytochemistry, 66*(18), 2281–2291.

Jackson, E. K. (2006). Diuretics. In L. L. Brunton, J. S. Lazo, & K. L. Parker (Eds.), *Goodman & Gilman's The pharmacological basis of therapeutics* (11th ed., pp. 737–770). New York: McGraw-Hill.

Jepson, R. G., Mihaljevic, L., & Craig, J. (2006). Cranberries for preventing urinary tract infections. *Cochrane Database of Systemic Reviews 2004*(1), CD001321.

Reiss, B., & Evans, M. (1996). *Pharmacological aspects of nursing care* (5th ed.) Albany, New York: Delmar Publishing.

Skidmore-Roth, L. (2005). *2005 Mosby's Nursing Drug Reference.* St. Louis, MO: Elsevier Mosby.

Williams, B., & Baer, C. (1998). *Essentials of clinical pharmacology in nursing* (3rd ed.). Springhouse, PA: Springhouse Corp.

Chapter 31

Chio, P. T. L., Gordon, Y., Quinonez, L. G., et al. (1999). Crystalloids vs. colloids in fluid resuscitation: A systemic review. *Critical Care Medicine, 27*(1), 200–203.

Rose, B. D. (2000). *Clinical physiology of acid-base and electrolyte disorders* (5th ed.). New York: McGraw-Hill.

Wilmore, D. (2000). Nutrition and metabolic support in the 21st century. *Journal of Parenteral & Enteral Nutrition 4*(1), 1–4.

Chapter 32

Agnew, L. L., Guffogg, S. P., Matthias, A., Lehmann, R. P., Bone, K. M., & Watson, K. (2005). Echinacea intake induces an immune response through altered expression of leucocyte hsp70, increased white cell counts, and improved erythrocyte antioxidant defences. *Journal of Clinical Pharmacy and Therapeutics, 30*(4), 363–369.

Capriotti, T. (2001). Monoclonal antibodies: Drugs that combine pharmacology and biotechnology. *MedSurg Nursing, 10*(2), 89.

Centers for Disease Control and Prevention (2003). *Fact sheet: Racial and ethnic disparities in health care.* Retrieved from http://www.cdc.gov/od/oc/media/pressrel/fs020514b/htm

Centers for Disease Control and Prevention. (2003). *National Vaccine Program Office: Immunization laws.* Retrieved from http://www.cdc.gov/od/nvpo/law.htm

Children's Defense Fund. (2003). *Every child deserves a healthy start.* Retrieved from www.childrensdefense.org

Fitzgerald, K. A., O'Neill, L. A., & Gearing, A. J. (Eds.). (2001). *The cytokine factsbook* (2nd ed.). Burlington, MA: Elsevier Science & Technology Books.

Goel, V., Lovlin, R., Chang, C., Slama, J. V., Barton, R., Gahler, R., et al. A proprietary extract from the echinacea plant (*Echinacea purpurea*) enhances systemic immune response during a common cold. *Phytotherapy Research, 19*(8), 689–694.

Karam, U. S., & Reddy, K. R. (2003). Pegylated interferons. *Clinical Liver Disease, 7*(1), 139–148.

Krensky, A. M., Strom, T. B., & Bluestone, J. A. (2006). Immunomodulators: Immunosuppressive agents, tolerogens, and immunostimulants. In L. L. Brunton, J. S. Lazo, & K. L. Parker (Eds.),

Goodman & Gilman's The pharmacological basis of therapeutics (11th ed., pp. 1463–1484). New York: McGraw-Hill.

Neuzil, K. M. (2003). *Adult immunizations: A review of current recommendations.* Retrieved from www.medscape.com

Santamaria, P. (2003). *Cytokines and autoimmune disease.* New York: Kluwer Academic/Plenum.

Schoop, R., Klein, P., Suter, A., Johnston, S. L. (2006). Echinacea in the prevention of induced rhinovirus colds: A meta-analysis. *Clinical Therapeutics, 28*(2), 174–183.

Sharma, M., Arnason, J. T., Burt, A., & Hudson, J. B. (2006). Echinacea extracts modulate the pattern of chemokine and cytokine secretion in rhinovirus-infected and uninfected epithelial cells. *Phytotherapy Research, 20*(2), 147–152.

Sur, D. K., Wallis, D. H., & O'Connell, T. X. (2003). Vaccinations in pregnancy. *American Family Physician, 68,* E299–E309.

Thomson, A. W., & Lotze, M. T. (2003). *The cytokine handbook* (4th ed., vols. 1–2). Burlington, MA: Elsevier Science & Technology Books.

Chapter 33

Baigent, C., & Patrono, C. (2003). Selective cyclooxygenase-2 inhibitors, aspirin, and cardiovascular disease: A reappraisal. *Arthritis and Rheumatism, 48*(1), 12–20.

Fitzgerald, G. A., & Patrono, C. (2001). Drug therapy: The coxibs, selective inhibitors of cyclooxygenase-2. *New England Journal of Medicine, 345,* 433–442.

Galley, H. F. (2002). *Critical care focus: Vol. 10. Inflammation and immunity.* London: BMJ Books.

Jackson, L. M., & Hawkey, C. J. (2000). COX-2 selective nonsteroidal anti-inflammatory drugs: Do they really offer any advantages? *Drugs, 59*(6), 1207–1216.

Oh, R. (2005). Practical applications of fish oil (omega-3 fatty acids) in primary care. *Journal of the American Board of Family Practice, 18*(1), 28–36.

Sklar, G. E. (2002). Hemolysis as a potential complication of acetaminophen overdose in a patient with glucose-6-phosphate dehydrogenase deficiency. *Pharmacotherapy, 22*(5), 656–658.

Chapter 34

Barclay, L. (2003). Linezolid treats resistant gram-positive infections in children. *Pediatric Infectious Diseases Journal, 23,* 677–685.

Chambers, H. F. (2006). General considerations of antimicrobial therapy. In L. L. Brunton, J. S. Lazo, & K. L. Parker (Eds.), *Goodman & Gilman's The pharmacological basis of therapeutics* (11th ed., pp. 1095–1110). New York: McGraw-Hill.

Diekema, D., & Jones, R. (2001). Oxazolidinones: A review. *Drugs, 59*(1), 7–16.

Gilbert, D. N., Moellering, R. C., & Sande, M. A. (2001). *The Sanford guide to antimicrobial therapy 2001* (31st ed.). Hyde Park, VT: Antimicrobial Therapy, Inc.

Moran, G. J., & Mount, J. (2003). Update on emerging infections: News from the Centers for Disease Control and Prevention. *Annals of Emergency Medicine, 41*(1), 148–151.

Petri, W. A. (2006). Sulfonamides, trimethoprim-sulfamethoxazole, quinolones, and agents for urinary tract infections. In L. L. Brunton, J. S. Lazo, & K. L. Parker (Eds.), *Goodman & Gilman's The pharmacological basis of therapeutics* (11th ed., pp. 1111–1126). New York: McGraw-Hill.

Petri, W. A. (2006). Penicillins, cephalosporins, and other beta-lactam antibiotics. In L. L. Brunton, J. S. Lazo, & K. L. Parker (Eds.), *Goodman & Gilman's The pharmacological basis of therapeutics* (11th ed., pp. 1127–1154). New York: McGraw-Hill.

Petri, W. A. (2006). Chemotherapy of tuberculosis, *Mycobacterium avium* complex disease, and leprosy. In L. L. Brunton, J. S. Lazo, & K. L. Parker (Eds.), *Goodman & Gilman's The pharmacological basis of therapeutics* (11th ed., pp. 1203–1224). New York: McGraw-Hill.

Sheff, B. (2001). Taking aim at antibiotic-resistant bacteria. *Nursing 2001, 31*(11), 62–68.

Small, P. M., & Fujiwara, P. I. (2001). Medical progress: Management of tuberculosis in the United States. *New England Journal of Medicine, 345,* 189–200.

Spector, R. E. (2000). *Cultural diversity in health and illness.* Upper Saddle River, NJ: Prentice Hall.

Wooten, J., & Sakind, A. (2003). Superbugs: Unmasking the threat. *RN, 66*(3), 37–43.

Chapter 35

Bennet, J. E. (2006). Antifungal agents. In L. L. Brunton, J. S. Lazo, & K. L. Parker (Eds.), *Goodman & Gilman's The pharmacological basis of therapeutics* (11th ed., pp. 1225–1242). New York: McGraw-Hill.

Centers for Disease Control and Prevention. (1993). Recommendations of the International Task Force of Disease Eradication. *MMWR. Morbidity and Mortality Weekly Report, 42*(RR16), 1–25.

Dickson, R., Awasthi, S., Demellweek, C., & Williamson, P. (2003). Anthelmintic drugs for treating worms in children: Effects on growth and cognitive performance. *Cochrane Database of Systematic Reviews, 2005*(2), CD000371. Retrieved from http://www.medscape.com

Furness, B. W., Beach, M. J., & Roberts, J. M. (2000). Giardiasis surveillance United States, 1922–1997. *Morbidity Mortality Weekly Report CDC Surveillance Summary, 49*(SS-7), 1–16.

Kontoyiannis, D. P., Mantadakis, E., & Samonis, G. (2003). Systemic mycoses in the immunocompromised host: An update in antifungal therapy. *Journal of Hospital Infection, 53*(4), 243–258.

Martin, K. W., Ernst, E. (2004). Herbal medicines for treatment of fungal infections: A systematic review of controlled clinical trials. *Mycoses, 47*(3–4), 87–92.

Pray, W. S. (2001). Treatment of vaginal fungal infections. *U.S. Pharmacist, 26*(9).

Satchell, A. C., Saurajen, A., Bell, C., Barnetson, R. S. (2002). Treatment of dandruff with 5% tea tree oil shampoo. *Journal of the American Academy of Dermatology, 47*(6), 852–855.

Shapiro, T. A., & Goldberg, D. E. (2006). Chemotherapy of protozoal infections: Malaria. In L. L. Brunton, J. S. Lazo, & K. L. Parker (Eds.), *Goodman & Gilman's The pharmacological basis of therapeutics* (11th ed., pp. 869–898). New York: McGraw–Hill.

Steile, R. W. (2002). Focus on infection, prevention, detection, and treatment. *Medscape Medical News.* Retrieved from http://www.medscape.com

Re, V. L., & Gluckman, S. J. (2003). Prevention of malaria in travelers. *American Family Physician, 68,* 509–514, 515–516.

Wilson, C. (2005). Recurrent vulvovaginitis candidiasis: An overview of traditional and alternative therapies. *Advance for Nurse Practitioners, 13*(5), 24–29.

Chapter 36

Almuente, V. (2002). Herbal therapy in patients with HIV. *Medscape Pharmacists, 3*(2), 1–4.

Duggan, J., Peterson, W. S., Schutz, M., Khuder, S., & Chakraborty, J. (2001). Use of complementary and alternative therapies in HIV-infected patients. *AIDS Patient Care and STDS, 15,* 159–167.

Goldschmidt, R. H., & Dong, B. J. (2001). Treatment of AIDS and HIV-related conditions. *Journal of the American Board of Family Practice, 14*(4), 283–309.

HIV Panel on Clinical Practices for Treatment of HIV Infection. (2000). *Guidelines for the use of antiretroviral agents in HIV-infected adults and adolescents.* Washington DC: U.S. Department of Health and Human Services. Retrieved from http://www.hivatis.org/guidelines/adult/Feb0501/

Idemyor, V. (2003). Twenty years since human immunodeficiency virus discovery: Considerations for the next decade. *Pharmacotherapy, 23,* 384–387.

Kirkbride, H. A., & Watson, J. (2003). Review of the use of neuraminidase inhibitors for prophylaxis of influenza. *Communicable Disease and Public Health, 6*(2), 123–127.

Kuritzkes, D. R., Boyle, B. A., Gallant, J. E., Squires, K. E., & Zolopa, A. (2003). Current management challenges in HIV: Antiretroviral resistance. *AIDS Reader, 13*(3), 133–135, 138–142.

Lesho, E. P., & Gey, D. C. (2003). Managing issues related to antiretroviral therapy. *American Family Physician, 68,* 675–686, 689–690.

Mills, E., Montori, V., Perri, D., Phillips, E., & Koren, G. (2005). Natural health product–HIV drug interactions: A systematic review. *International Journal of STDs and AIDS, 16*(3), 181–186.

Ofotokun, I., & Pomeroy, C. (2003). Sex differences in adverse reactions to antiretroviral drugs. *Topics in HIV Medicine, 11*(2), 55–59.

Sandhu, R. S., Prescilla, R. P., Simonelli, T. M., & Edwards, D. J. (2003). Influence of goldenseal root on the pharmacokinetics of indinavir. *Journal of Clinical Pharmacology, 43*(11), 1283–1288.

Walker, B. D. (2002). Immune reconstitution and immunotherapy in HIV infection. *Medscape Clinical Update.* Retrieved from http://www.medscape.com/viewprogram/2435

Chapter 37

Birner, A. (2003). Safe administration of oral chemotherapy. *Clinical Journal of Oncology Nursing, 2,* 158–162.

Breed, C. D. (2003). Diagnosis, treatment, and nursing care of patients with chronic leukemia. *Seminars in Oncology Nursing, 19*(2), 109–117.

Buzdar, A. U. (2000). Tamoxifen's clinical applications: Old and new. *Archives of Family Medicine, 9,* 906–912.

Dalton, R. R., & Kallab, A. M. (2001). Chemoprevention of breast cancer. *Southern Medical Journal, 94*(1), 7–15.

Hood, L. E. (2003). Chemotherapy in the elderly: Supportive measures for chemotherapy-induced myelotoxicity. *Clinical Journal of Oncology Nursing, 7*(2), 185–190.

Lee, S. O., Yeon Chun, J., Nadiminty, N., Trump, D. L., Ip, C., Dong, Y., et al. (2006). Monomethylated selenium inhibits growth of LNCaP human prostate cancer xenograft accompanied by a decrease in the expression of androgen receptor and prostate-specific antigen (PSA). *The Prostate, 66*(10), 1070–1075.

Moran, P. (2000). Cellular effects of cancer chemotherapy administration. *Journal of Infusion Nursing, 23*(1), 44.

Peters, U., Chatterjee, N., Church, T. R., Mayo, C., Sturup, S. Foster, C. B., et al. (2006). High serum selenium and reduced risk of advanced colorectal adenoma in a colorectal cancer early detection program. *Cancer Epidemiology, Biomarkers, and Prevention, 15*(2), 315–320.

Reid, M. E., Duffield-Lillico, A. J., Sunga, A., Fakih, M., Alberts, D. S., & Marshall, J. R. (2006). Selenium supplementation and colorectal adenomas: An analysis of the nutritional prevention of cancer trial. *International Journal of Cancer, 118*(7), 1777–1781.

Rieger, P. (2001). *Biotherapy: A comprehensive overview* (2nd ed.). Sudbury, MA: Jones and Bartlett.

Rugo, H. (2001, October 15). *How to succeed with breast cancer adjuvant therapy.* Retrieved from http://healthology.com

Smith, B., Waltzman, R., & Rugo, H. (2002, December 10). *Living longer with cancer: Preserving quality of life.* Retrieved from http://healthology.com

U.S. Preventive Services Task Force. (2003). Chemoprevention of breast cancer: Recommendations and rationale. *American Family Physician, 67*(6), 1309–1314.

Wood, L. (2001). Innovative antineoplastic agents. *Journal of Infusion Nursing, 24*(1), 48–55.

Chapter 38

Berger, W. E. (2003). Overview of allergic rhinitis. *Annals of Allergy, Asthma, and Immunology, 90*(6, Suppl. 3), 7–12.

Braunstahl, G., & Hellings, P. W. (2003). Allergic rhinitis and asthma: The link further unraveled. *Current Opinion in Pulmonary Medicine, 9*(1), 46–51.

Nathan, R. A. (2003). Pharmacotherapy for allergic rhinitis: A critical review of leukotriene receptor antagonists compared with other treatments. *Annals of Allergy, Asthma, and Immunology, 90*(2), 182–190.

Raeburn, D., & Giembycz, M. A. (Eds.). (2001). *Rhinitis: Immunopathology and pharmacotherapy.* Boston: Birkhauser.

Rogers, D. F. (2003). Airway hypersecretion in allergic rhinitis and asthma: New pharmacotherapy. *Current Allergy and Asthma Reports, 3*(3), 238–248.

Rosenwasser, L. J. (2002). Treatment of allergic rhinitis. *American Journal of Medicine, 16*(113, Suppl. 9A), 17S–24S.

Chapter 39

Altman, E. E. (2004). Update on COPD. Today's strategies improve quality of life. *Advance for Nurse Practitioners, 12*(3), 49–54.

Celli, B. (2003). *Pharmacotherapy in chronic obstructive pulmonary disease.* New York: Marcel Dekker.

Colbert, B. J., & Mason, B. J. (2001). *Integrated cardiopulmonary pharmacology.* Upper Saddle River, NJ: Prentice Hall.

Fink, J. (2000). Metered dose inhalers, dry powder inhalers, and transitions. *Respiratory Care, 45,* 623–635.

Luggen, A. S. (2004). Pharmacology tips: Medications that complicate asthma control in older people. *Geriatric Nursing, 25*(3), 184.

Matsuyama, W., Mitsuyama, H., Watanabe, M., Oonakahara, K., Higashimoto, I., Osame, M., et al. (2005). Effects of omega-3 polyunsaturated fatty acids on inflammatory markers in COPD. *Chest, 128*(6), 3817–3827.

Rogers, D. F. (2003). Airway hypersecretion in allergic rhinitis and asthma: New pharmacotherapy. *Current Allergy Asthma Reports, 3*(3), 238–248.

Roy, S. R. (2003). Asthma. *Southern Medical Journal, 96*(11), 1061–1067.

Stevens, N. (2003). Inhaler devices for asthma and COPD: Choice and technique. *Professional Nurse, 18*(11), 641–645.

Undem, B. J. (2006). Pharmacotherapy of asthma. In L. L. Brunton, J. S. Lazo, and K. L. Parker (Eds.), *Goodman & Gilman's The pharmacological basis of therapeutics* (11th ed., pp. 717–735). New York: McGraw-Hill.

Vega, C. (2005). Budesonide/formoterol may be effective for maintenance and acute relief of asthma. *American Journal of Respiratory Critical Care Medicine, 171,* 129–136.

Weir, P. (2004). Quick asthma assessment: A stepwise approach to treatment. *Advance for Nurse Practitioners, 12*(1), 53–56.

Wheeler, L. (2003, Mar-April). The last word: Asthma management in schools. *FDA Consumer, 37*(2).

Chapter 40

Chaiyakunapruk, N., Nathisuwan S., Leeprakobboon K., & Leelasettagool C. (2006). The efficacy of ginger for the prevention of postoperative nausea and vomiting: A meta-analysis. *American Journal of Obstetrics and Gynecology, 194,* 95–99.

Hoogerwerf, W. A., & Pasricha, P. J. (2006). Pharmacotherapy of gastric acidity, peptic ulcers, and gastroesophageal reflux disease. In L. L. Brunton, J. S. Lazo, and K. L. Parker (Eds.), *Goodman & Gilman's The pharmacological basis of therapeutics* (11th ed., pp. 967–982). New York: McGraw-Hill.

Huggins, R. M., Scates, A. C., & Latour, J. K. (2003). Intravenous proton-pump inhibitors versus H$_2$-antagonists for treatment of GI bleeding. *Annals of Pharmacotherapy, 37*(3), 433–437.

Meurer, L. N., & Bower, D. J. (2002). Management of *Helicobacter pylori* infection. *American Family Physician, 65,* 1327–1336, 1339.

Patel, A. S., Pohl, J. F., & Easley, D. J. (2003). What's new: Proton pump inhibitors and pediatrics. *Pediatrics in Review, 24*(1), 12–15.

Petersen, A. M. (2003). *Helicobacter pylori:* An invading microorganism? A review. *FEMS Immunology and Medical Microbiology, 36*(3), 117–126.

Sharma, P., & Vakil, N. (2003). Review article: *Helicobacter pylori* and reflux disease. A*limentary Pharmacology and Therapeutics, 17*(3), 297–305.

Stanghellini, V. (2003). Management of gastroesophageal reflux disease. *Drugs Today, 39*(Suppl A), 15–20.

Vanderhoff, B. T., & Tahboub, R. M. (2002). Proton pump inhibitors: An update. *American Family Physician, 66,* 273–280.

Chapter 41

Cole, L. (2002). Unraveling the mystery of acute pancreatitis. *Dimensions of Critical Care Nursing, 21,* 86–91.

Feagan, B. G., Dieckgraefe, B. K., & Hanauer, S. B. (2006). *Advances in the treatment of Crohn's disease: From research to clinical practice.* Retrieved May 25, 2006, from http://www.medscape.com/viewprogram/5211.

Glazer, G. (2001). Long-term pharmacotherapy of obesity: A review of efficacy and safety. *Archives of Internal Medicine, 161,* 1814–1824.

Guglietta, A. (2003). *Pharmacotherapy of gastrointestinal inflammation.* Basel, Switzerland: Birkhauser Verlag.

Knutson, D., Greenberg, G., & Cronau, H. (2003). Management of Crohn's disease: A practical approach. *American Family Physician, 68,* 707–714, 717–718.

Mitchell, R. M. S., Byrne, M. F., & Baillie, J. (2003). Pancreatitis. *Lancet, 361,* 1447–1456.

Pasricha, P. J. (2006). Treatment of disorders of bowel motility and water flux; antiemetics; agents used in biliary and pancreatic disease. In L. L. Brunton, J. S. Lazo, and K. L. Parker (Eds.), *Goodman & Gilman's The pharmacological basis of therapeutics* (11th ed., pp. 983–1008). New York: McGraw-Hill.

Pray, W. S., and Pray, J. J. (2005). Diarrhea: Sweeping changes in the OTC market. *U.S. Pharmacist, 30*(1).

Sellin, J. H., and Pasricha, P. J. (2006). Pharmacotherapy of inflammatory bowel disease. In L. L. Brunton, J. S. Lazo, and K. L. Parker (Eds.), *Goodman & Gilman's The pharmacological basis of therapeutics* (11th ed., pp. 1009–1020). New York: McGraw-Hill.

Spanier, J. A., Howden, C. W., & Jones, M. P. (2003). A systematic review of alternative therapies in the irritable bowel syndrome. *Archives of Internal Medicine, 163*(3), 265–274.

Teitelbaum, J. (2005). Probiotics and the treatment of infectious diarrhea. *Pediatric Infectious Disease Journal, 24*(3), 267–268.

Wald, A. (2003). Is chronic use of stimulant laxatives harmful to the colon? *Journal of Clinical Gastroenterology, 36*(5), 386–389.

Weigle, D. S. (2003). Pharmacological therapy of obesity: Past, present, and future. *Journal of Clinical Endocrinology and Metabolism, 88*(6), 2462–2469.

Chapter 42

Bailey, L. B., Rampersaud, G. C., & Kauwell, G. P. (2003). Folic acid supplements and fortification affect the risk for neural tube defects, vascular disease, and cancer: Evolving science. *Journal of Nutrition 133*(6), 1961S–1968S.

Bhagavan, N. V. (2002). *Medical biochemistry.* Burlington, MA: Harcourt/Academic Press.

Dharmarajan, T. S., Adiga, G. U., & Norkus, E. P. (2003). Vitamin B$_{12}$ deficiency. Recognizing subtle symptoms in older adults. *Geriatrics, 58*(3), 30–34, 37–38.

Douglas, R. M., Hemilä, H., Chalker, E., & Treacy, B. Vitamin C for preventing and treating the common cold. *Cochrane Database of Systematic Reviews, 2004*(4), CD000980.

Eden, A. N. (2003). Preventing iron deficiency in toddlers: A major public health problem. *Contemporary Pediatrics, 20*(2), 57–67.

Edroso, R. (2003). Understanding HIV fatigue: What's dragging you down? *WebMDHealth.* Retrieved from http://my.webmd.com

Joque, L., & Jatoi, A (2005). Total parenteral nutrition in cancer patients: Why and when? *Nutrition in Clinical Care, 8*(2), 89–92.

Kaushansky, K., & Kipps, T. J. (2006). Hematopoietic agents: Growth factors, minerals, and vitamins. In L. L. Brunton, J. S. Lazo, and K. L. Parker (Eds.), *Goodman & Gilman's The pharmacological basis of therapeutics* (11th ed., pp. 1433–1466). New York: McGraw-Hill.

Levine, M., Rumsey, S. C., Daruwala, R., Park, J. B., & Wang, Y. (1999). Criteria and recommendations for vitamin C intake. *Journal of the American Medical Association, 281,* 1415–1423.

McDermott, J. H. (2000). Antioxidant nutrients: Current dietary recommendations and research update. *Journal of the American Pharmaceutical Association, 40*(6), 785–799.

Morin, K. (2005). Infant nutrition: Water-soluble vitamins. *American Journal of Maternal/Child Nursing, 30*(4), 271.

Oh, R. C., & Brown, D. L. (2003). Vitamin B12 deficiency. *American Family Physician, 67,* 979–986, 993–994.

Padayatty, S. J., Katz, A., Wang, Y., Eck, P., Kwon, O., Lee, J. H., et al. (2003). Vitamin C as an antioxidant: Evaluation of its role in disease prevention. *Journal of the American College of Nutrition, 22*(1), 18–35.

Padula, C. A., Kenny, A. Planchon, C., & Lamoureux, C. (2004). *American Journal of Nursing, 104*(7), 62–69.

Perrotta, S., Nobili, B., Rossi, F., Di Pinto, D., Cucciolla, V., Borriello, A., et al. (2003). Riboflavin (vitamin B$_2$) and health. *American Journal of Clinical Nutrition, 77*(6), 1352–1360.

Ragione, F. (2003). Vitamin A and infancy. Biochemical, functional, and clinical aspects. *Vitamins and Hormones, 66,* 457–591.

Rampersaud, G. C., Kauwell, G. P., & Bailey, L. B. (2003). Folate: A key to optimizing health and reducing disease risk in the elderly. *Journal of the American College of Nutrition, 22*(1), 1–8.

Risser, N., & Murphy, M. (2004). Literature review: Enteral nutrition. *Nurse Practitioner: American Journal of Primary Health Care, 29*(3), 49–59.

Somer, E. (2003). Ironing out anemia. *WebMDHealth.* Retrieved from http://my.webmd.com

Chapter 43

Demester, N. (2001). Diseases of the thyroid: A broad spectrum. *Clinical Review, 11*(7), 58–64.

Farwell, A. P., & Braverman, L. E. (2006). Thyroid and antithyroid drugs. In L. L. Brunton, J. S. Lazo, and K. L. Parker (Eds.), *Goodman & Gilman's The pharmacological basis of therapeutics* (11th ed., pp. 1511–1540). New York: McGraw-Hill.

Griffiths, H., & Jordan, S. (2002). Corticosteroids: Implications for nursing practice. *Nursing Standard, 17*(12), 43–53.

Holcomb, S. S. (2002). Thyroid diseases: A primer for the critical care nurse. *Dimensions of Critical Care Nursing, 21*(4), 127–133.

Margioris, A. N., & Chrousos, G. P. (Eds). (2001). *Adrenal disorders.* Totowa, NJ: Humana Press.

Parker, K. L., & Schimmer, B. P. (2006). Pituitary hormones and their hypothalamic releasing factors. In L. L. Brunton, J. S. Lazo, and K. L. Parker (Eds.), *Goodman & Gilman's The pharmacological basis of therapeutics* (11th ed., pp. 1489–1510). New York: McGraw-Hill.

Schori-Ahmed, D. (2003). Defenses gone awry: Thyroid disease. *RN, 66*(6), 38–43.

Winqvist, O., Rorsman, F., & Kämpe, O. (2000). Autoimmune adrenal insufficiency: Recognition and management. *BioDrugs, 13*(2), 107–114.

Chapter 44

American Diabetes Association. (2001). Standards of care. *Diabetes Care, 24*(Suppl. 1), 33–43.

Bates, N. (2002). Overdose of insulin and other diabetic medication. *Emergency Nurse, 10*(7), 22–26.

Bohannon, N. J. V. (2002). Treating dual defects in diabetes: Insulin resistance and insulin secretion. *American Journal of Health-System Pharmacists 59*(Suppl. 9), S9–S13.

Chen, S. W. (2002). Insulin glargine: Basal insulin of choice? *American Journal of Health-System Pharmacists, 59*, 609.

Cole, L. (2002). Unraveling the mystery of acute pancreatitis. *Dimensions of Critical Care Nursing, 21*, 86–91.

Davis, S. N. (2006). Insulin, oral hypoglycemic agents, and the pharmacology of the endocrine pancreas. In L. L. Brunton, J. S. Lazo, and K. L. Parker (Eds.), *Goodman & Gilman's The pharmacological basis of therapeutics* (11th ed., pp. 1613–1646). New York: McGraw-Hill.

Gottlieb, S. W. (2003). Just the facts: The importance of diabetic research. *Diabetes Forcast, 56*, 39–42.

Gregersen, S., Jeppesen, P. B., Holst, J. J., & Hermansen, K. (2004). Antihyperglycemic effects of stevioside in type 2 diabetic subjects. *Metabolism, 53*(1), 73–76.

Harrigan, R. A., Nathan, M. S., & Beattie, P. (2001). Oral agents for the treatment of type 2 diabetes mellitus: Pharmacology, toxicity, and treatment. *Annals of Emergency Medicine, 38*(1), 68.

Hovens, M. M., Tamsma, J. T., Beishuizen, E. D., & Huisman, M. V. (2005). Pharmacological strategies to reduce cardiovascular risk in type 2 diabetes mellitus: An update. *Drugs, 65*(4), 433–445.

Hjelm, K., Mufunda, E., Nambozi, G., & Kemp, J. (2003). Preparing nurses to face the pandemic of diabetes mellitus: A literature review. *Journal of Advanced Nursing, 41*, 424–435.

Mantis, A. K., et al. (2001). Continuous subcutaneous insulin infusion therapy for children and adolescents: An option for routine diabetes care. *Pediatrics, 107*, 351–357.

McKnight-Menci, H., Sababu, S., & Kelly, S. D. (2005). The care of children and adolescents with type 2 diabetes. *Journal of Pediatric Nursing, 20*(2), 96–106.

Mokdad, A. H., Bowman, B. A., & Ford, E. S. (2001). The continuing epidemics of obesity and diabetes in the United States. *Journal of the American Medical Association, 286*, 1195–1200.

Chapter 45

Conley, C. (2003). *Hormonal therapy for breast cancer: Current issues,* http://healthology.com

Frackiewicz, E. J., & Shiovitz, T. M. (2001). Evaluation and management of premenstrual syndrome and premenstrual dysphoric disorder. *Journal of the American Pharmaceutical Association, 41*(3), 437–447.

Leeman, L., Fontaine, P., King, V., Klein, M. C., & Ratcliffe, S. (2003). The nature and management of labor pain: Part II. Pharmacologic pain relief. *American Family Physician, 68*, 1115–1120, 1121–1122.

Loose, D. S., & Stancel, G. M. (2006). Estrogens. In L. L. Brunton, J. S. Lazo, and K. L. Parker (Eds.), *Goodman & Gilman's The pharmacological basis of therapeutics* (11th ed., pp. 1541–1572). New York: McGraw-Hill.

Ludwig, M., Westergaard, L. G., Diedrich, K., & Andersen, C. Y. (2003). Developments in drugs for ovarian stimulation. *Best Practice and Research. Clinical Obstetrics and Gynecology, 17*(2), 231–247.

Nelson, A. (2000). Contraceptive update Y2K: Need for contraception and new contraceptive options. *Clinical Corner, 3*(1), 48–62.

Olds, S. B., London, M. L., Ladewig, P. A., & Davidson, M. R. (2004). *Maternal–newborn nursing and women's health care* (7th ed.). Upper Saddle River, NJ: Prentice Hall Health.

Osmers R., Friede M., Liske E., Schnitker, J., Freudenstein, J., & Henneicke-von Zepelin, H. H. (2005). Efficacy and safety of isopropanolic black cohosh extract for climacteric symptoms. *Obstetrics and Gynecology, 105*(5 pt 1), 1074–1083.

Shepherd, J. E. (2001). Effects of estrogen on cognition, mood, and degenerative brain diseases. *Journal of the American Pharmaceutical Association, 41*(2), 221–228.

Understanding the WHI study: Assessing the results. (2003). Retrieved from http://www.premarin.com/pdf/Risk.Tearsheet.pdf

Chapter 46

Bent, S., Kane, C., Shinohara, K., Neuhaus, J., Hudes, E. S., Goldberg, H., et al. (2006). Saw palmetto for benign prostatic hyperplasia. *New England Journal of Medicine, 354*(6), 557–566.

Bullock, T. L., & Andriole, G. L. (2006). Emerging drug therapies for benign prostatic hyperplasia. *Expert Opinion on Emergency Drugs, 11*(1), 111–123.

Carrier, S. (2003). Pharmacology of phosphodiesterase 5 inhibitors. *Canadian Journal of Urology, 10*(Suppl. 1), 12–16.

Gordon, A. E., & Shaughnessy, A. F. (2003). Saw palmetto for prostate disorders. *American Family Physician, 67*(6), 1281–1283.

Kassabian, V. S. (2003). Sexual function in patients treated for benign prostatic hyperplasia. *Lancet, 361*(9351), 60–62.

Khastgir, J., Arya, M., Shergill, I. S., Kalsi, J. S., Minhas, S., & Mundy, A. R. (2002). Current concepts in the pharmacotherapy of benign prostatic hyperplasia. *Expert Opinion on Pharmacotherapy, 3*(12), 1727–1737.

Mcleod, D. G. (2003). Hormonal therapy: Historical perspective to future directions. *Urology, 61*(2, Suppl. 1), 3–7.

Padma-Nathan, H., Saenz de Tejada, I., Rosen, R. C., & Goldstein, I. (Eds.). (2001). *Pharmacotherapy for erectile dysfunction.* London: Taylor & Francis.

Steiner, B. S. (2002). Hypogonadism in men. A review of diagnosis and treatment. *Advance for Nurse Practioners, 10*(4), 22–27, 29.

Snyder, P. J. (2006). Androgens. In L. L. Brunton, J. S. Lazo, and K. L. Parker (Eds.), *Goodman & Gilman's The pharmacological basis of therapeutics* (11th ed., pp. 1573–1586). New York: McGraw-Hill.

Susman, E. (2003). ACC: *Investigative anti-impotence drug appears with antihypertensive medications*. Retrieved from http://www.docguide.com/news/content.nsf/PatientResAllCateg/Erectile%20Dysfunction?OpenDocument#News

Thiyagarajan, M. (2002). Alpha-adrenoceptor antagonists in the treatment of benign prostate hyperplasia. *Pharmacology, 65*(3), 119–128.

Chapter 47

Burke, A., Smyth, E. M., & Fitzgerald, G. A. (2006). Analgesic–antipyretic agents; pharmacotherapy of gout. In L. L. Brunton, J. S. Lazo, and K. L. Parker (Eds.). *Goodman & Gilman's The pharmacological basis of therapeutics* (11th ed., pp. 671–716). New York: McGraw-Hill.

Burke, S. (2001). Boning up on osteoporosis. *Nursing 2001, 31*(10), 36–42.

Cashman, J. N. (2000). Current pharmacotherapeutic strategies in rheumatic diseases and other pain states. *Clinical Drug Investigation, 19*(Suppl. 2), 9–20.

Clegg, D. O., Reda, D. J., Harris, C. L., Klein, M. A., O'Dell, J. R., Hooper, M. M., et al. (2006). Glucosamine, chondroitin sulfate, and the two in combination for painful knee osteoarthritis. *New England Journal of Medicine, 354*(8), 795–808.

Curry, L. C., & Hogstel, M. O. (2002). Osteoporosis. *American Journal of Nursing, 102,* 26–32.

Friedman, P. A. (2006). Agents affecting mineral ion homeostasis and bone turnover. In L. L. Brunton, J. S. Lazo, and K. L. Parker (Eds.), *Goodman & Gilman's The pharmacological basis of therapeutics* (11th ed., pp. 1647–1677). New York: McGraw-Hill.

Love, C. (2003). Dietary needs for bone health and the prevention of osteoporosis. *British Journal of Nursing, 12*(1), 12–21.

Olsen, N. J., & Stein, C. M. (2004). New drugs for rheumatoid arthritis. *New England Journal of Medicine, 350*(21), 2167–2179.

Prestwood, K. M. (2000). Prevention and treatment of osteoporosis. *Clinical Corner, 2*(6), 34–44.

Sanofi-synthelabs. (2003). *Hyalgan–sodium hyaluronate solutions*. Retrieved from http://www.sanofi-synthelabous.com

Secrist, J. (2003). Osteoporosis. Part IV. Rapid review of drug therapies (A to Z) for preventing male osteoporosis/fractures. *Urology Nursing, 23*(2), 168–174.

Watts, N. B. (2003). Bisphosphonate treatment of osteoporosis. *Clinical Geriatric Medicine,19*(2), 395–414.

Chapter 48

Bayliffe, A. I., Brigandi, R. A., Wilkins, H. J., & Levick, M. P. (2004). Emerging therapeutic targets in psoriasis. *Current Opinions in Pharmacology, 4*(3), 306–310.

Feldman, S. (2000). Advances in psoriasis treatment. *Dermatology Online 6*(1), 4.

Fox, L. P., Merk, H. F., & Bickers, D. R. (2006). Dermatological pharmacology. In L. L. Brunton, J. S. Lazo, and K. L. Parker (Eds.), *Goodman & Gilman's The pharmacological basis of therapeutics* (11th ed., pp. 1679–1706). New York: McGraw-Hill.

Lebwohl, M. (2003). Psoriasis. *Lancet, 361,* 1197–1206.

Leung, D. Y., & Boguniewicz, M. (2003). Advances in allergic skin diseases. *Journal of Allergy and Clinical Immunology, 111*(Suppl. 3), S805–S812.

Lindow, K. B., & Warren, C. (2001). Understanding rosacea: A guide to facilitating care. *American Journal of Nursing, 101,* 44–51.

Murphy, K. D., Lee, J. O., & Herndon, D. N. (2003). Current pharmacotherapy for the treatment of severe burns. *Expert Opinion on Pharmacotherapy, 4*(3), 369–384.

Oprica, C., Emtestam, L., & Nord, C. E. (2001). Overview of treatments for acne. *Dermatology Nursing, 14,* 242–246.

Roos, T. C., & Merk, H. F. (2000). Important drug interactions in dermatology. *Drugs, 59*(2), 181–192.

Smith, G. (2003). Cutaneous expression of cytochrome P-450 CYP25: Individuality in regulation by therapeutic agents for psoriasis and other skin diseases. *Lancet, 361,* 1336–1344.

Smolinski, K. N., & Yan, A. C. (2004). Acne update: 2004. *Current Opinion in Pediatrics, 16*(4), 385–391.

Chapter 49

APhA Drug Treatment Protocols. (2000). Management of pediatric acute otitis media: Introduction by D. H. Albrant. *Journal of the American Pharmaceutical Association, 40*(5), 599–608.

Beers, S. L., & Abramo, T. J. (2004). Otitis externa review. *Pediatric Emergency Care, 20*(4), 250–256.

Henderer, J. D., & Rapuano, C. J. (2006). Ocular pharmacology. In L. L. Brunton, J. S. Lazo, and K. L. Parker (Eds.), *Goodman & Gilman's The pharmacological basis of therapeutics* (11th ed., pp. 1707–1737). New York: McGraw-Hill.

Hoyng, P. F. J., & van Beek, L. M. (2000). Pharmacological therapy for glaucoma: A review. *Drugs, 59*(3), 411–434.

Leibovitz, E., & Dagan, R. (2001a). Otitis media therapy and drug resistance: Part 1. Management principles. *Infections in Medicine, 18*(4), 212–216.

Leibovitz, E., & Dagan, R. (2001b). Pediatric infection: Otitis media therapy and drug resistance: Part 2. Current concepts and new directions. *Infections in Medicine, 18*(5), 263–270.

Pray, S. (2001). Swimmer's ear: An ear canal infection. *U.S. Pharmacist, 26*(8).

Schwartz, K. A., & Budenz, D. B. (2004). Current management of glaucoma. *Current Opinion in Ophthalmology, 15*(2), 119–126.

Tripathi, R. C., Tripathi, B. J., & Haggerty, C. (2003). Drug-induced glaucomas: Mechanism and management. *Drug Safety, 26*(11), 749–767.

APPENDIX D Answers

CHAPTER 1
Answers to Critical Thinking Questions

1 The client may choose OTC medications rather than more effective prescription medications for a variety of reasons. OTC medications do not require the client to see a physician to write a prescription for the drug. By not seeing a physician, the client saves time and money. OTC medications are obtained much more easily than prescription drugs. Clients often think they can effectively treat themselves and that OTC medications do not have as many side effects as prescription medications.

2 The FDA is the agency responsible for determining whether prescription and OTC drugs may be used for therapy. By reviewing the availability of safe, effective drugs, the FDA is responsible for keeping unsafe and ineffective drugs off the market. Another of the agency's goals is to improve the health of Americans and ensure that drug information is clear and easily understandable. Over the years, the scope of the FDA has been broadened to include information on biologics, which include serums, vaccines, and blood products. The FDA also has the authority to recommend civil penalties if the guidelines are not followed and to remove dietary supplements that cause a significant risk to the public.

3 The FDA takes part in the postmarketing surveillence stage of the drug approval process. In this phase, the drug is monitored for harmful effects in the larger population. The FDA holds public meetings to receive feedback from clients and organizations regarding the safety and effectiveness of new drug therapies.

CHAPTER 2
Answers to Critical Thinking Questions

1 The therapeutic classification is a method of organizing drugs based on their therapeutic usefulness in treating particular diseases. The pharmacological classification refers to how an agent works at the molecular, tissue, and body system levels. A beta-adrenergic blocker is pharmacological; an oral contraceptive is therapeutic; a laxative is therapeutic; a folic acid antagonist is pharmacological; an antianginal agent is therapeutic.

2 Prototype drugs have predictable actions and adverse effects within the same drug class. All other drugs within this pharmacological class are compared with the prototype drugs.

3 Generic advantages include cost savings to the client and the fact that only one name is assigned for the drug; therefore, the name is less complicated and easier to remember. However, because generic drug formularies may be different, the inert ingredients may be somewhat different and, consequently, may affect the ability of the drug to reach the target cells and produce an effect.

4 Schedules refer to the potential for abuse. These schedules help the nurse identify the potential for abuse and require the nurse to maintain complete records for all quantities. The higher the abuse potential, the more restrictions are placed on the prescriber and the filling of refills.

CHAPTER 3
Answers to NCLEX-RN® Review Questions

1 Answers: 3, 5
Rationale: Anthrax affects the respiratory system. Fever, persistent cough, and dyspnea are all initial symptoms of inhaled anthrax.

Cognitive Level: Analysis. *Nursing Process:* Assessment. *Client Need:* Physiological Integrity.

2 Answer: 2
Rationale: The potassium iodine protects only the thyroid gland from I-131. No other body organs are protected by this medication. *Cognitive Level:* Analysis. *Nursing Process:* Implementation. *Client Need:* Physiological Integrity.

3 Answer: 1
Rationale: Overstimulation of the neurotransmitter acetylcholine causes convulsions and loss of consciousness within seconds. *Cognitive Level:* Analysis. *Nursing Process:* Assessment. *Client Need:* Physiological Integrity.

4 Answer: 3
Rationale: The antibiotic ciprofloxacin (Cipro) has been used for both prophylaxis and treatment of anthrax. *Cognitive Level:* Analysis. *Nursing Process:* Planning. *Client Need:* Physiological Integrity.

5 Answer: 2
Rationale: The CDC has categorized biological threats based on their potential impact on public health. The goal of biological terrorism is to cause widespread casualties. *Cognitive Level:* Analysis. *Nursing Process:* Assessment. *Client Need:* Safe, Effective Care Environment.

Answers to Critical Thinking Questions

1 Mass vaccination of the general public for anthrax and smallpox should be avoided at this time because there is ongoing controversy regarding the safety and effectiveness of these vaccines.

2 Clients who survive nuclear and radiation exposure are at risk for developing cancers over time. Symptoms of exposure are difficult to treat pharmacologically. KI tablets, if taken prior to or immediately after radiation exposure, can prevent up to 100% of radioactive iodine from entering the thyroid gland and damaging the thyroid tissues.

3 Nurses must be prepared to respond within their community to any type of emergency. Nurses are often found working in various community agencies and in the emergency departments of communities that may be affected.

CHAPTER 4
Answers to NCLEX-RN® Review Questions

1 Answer: 1
Rationale: The primary responsibility of the nurse is to ensure client safety when administering prescribed medications. Client compliance includes much more than watching the client take medications. Accurate physician orders are a part of ensuring safe medication administration. *Cognitive Level:* Comprehension. *Nursing Process:* Implementation. *Client Need:* Health Promotion and Maintenance.

2 Answer: 4
Rationale: When a client demonstrates or verbalizes what has been taught, the nurse is using the evaluation portion of the nursing process. *Cognitive Level:* Comprehension. *Nursing Process:* Assessment. *Client Need:* Health Promotion and Maintenance.

3 Answer: 3

Rationale: This question asks for the highest priority; therefore, all the answers are correct, but one should stand out as the first action the nurse should take. Think about client safety. In this example, the drug has been newly prescribed; therefore, notifying the physician of the client's reaction takes priority so that new medication orders can be received to address the allergic reaction and to discontinue the present order. **Cognitive Level:** Analysis. **Nursing Process:** Implementation. **Client Need:** Physiological Integrity.

4 Answer : 2

Rationale: *STAT* means immediately. *ASAP* orders should be administered within 30 minutes. **Cognitive Level:** Application. **Nursing Process:** Implementation. **Client Need:** Physiological Integrity.

5 Answers: 2 and 3

Rationale: Enteric-coated tablets are designed to dissolve in the alkaline environment of the small intestine. Sustained-release medications dissolve very slowly over an extended period for a longer duration. Liquid forms or finely crushed tablets are the preferred forms. **Cognitive Level:** Application. **Nursing Process:** Implementation. **Client Need:** Physiological Integrity.

Answers to Critical Thinking Questions

1 Although the nurse is responsible for safe medication administration, errors continue because many disciplines are responsible for safe and accurate drug administration. Many steps are involved in the safe administration of medications, and there are multiple points where errors can occur.

2 To help ensure drug compliance, the nurse and client should formulate an individualized plan of care using the nursing process. Including the client in this process enables the client to participate fully, which encourages compliance with the treatment plan.

3 The IV route has the fastest onset because medications are administered directly into the bloodstream. IV medications also bypass the digestive system and the first-pass effect. When administering parental medications (IV, intradermal, subcutaneous, and IM routes), the nurse must ensure that aseptic techniques are strictly used.

4 The metric system is much more accurate than the household or apothecary system. Using the metric system helps ensure that the safest, most accurate doses are prepared and administered.

CHAPTER 5
Answers to NCLEX-RN® Review Questions

1 Answer: 1

Rationale: The blood–brain barrier may cause difficulty in treating tumors. Most antitumor medications do not cross the blood–brain barrier. **Cognitive Level:** Analysis. **Nursing Process:** Assessment. **Client Need:** Physiological Integrity.

2 Answer: 1

Rationale: The liver is the primary site of drug metabolism. Clients with severe liver damage, such as that caused by cirrhosis, will require reductions in drug dosage because of the decreased metabolic activity. **Cognitive Level:** Analysis. **Nursing Process:** Implementation. **Client Need:** Physiological Integrity.

3 Answer: 4

Rationale: Some oral drugs are rendered inactive by hepatic metabolic reactions, during the process known as the first-pass effect. An alternative route may need to be assessed. **Cognitive Level:**

Application. **Nursing Process:** Implementation. **Client Need:** Physiological Integrity.

4 Answer: 3

Rationale: The kidneys are the primary site of excretion. Renal failure increases the duration of the drug's action because of decreased excretion. The client must be assessed for drug toxicity. **Cognitive Level:** Analysis. **Nursing Process:** Assessment. **Client Need:** Physiological Integrity.

5 Answers: 1, 2, 3

Rationale: Glandular activity is an elimination mechanism in which water-soluble drugs are excreted into saliva, sweat, and breast milk. Secretion of drugs in the bile is known as *biliary excretion*. **Cognitive Level:** Application. **Nursing Process:** Implementation. **Client Need:** Physiological Integrity.

Answers to Critical Thinking Questions

1 For most medications, the greatest barrier is crossing the many membranes that separate the drug from its target cells. A drug taken by mouth must cross the plasma membranes of the mucosal cells of the gastrointestinal tract and the capillary endothelial cells to enter the bloodstream. To leave the bloodstream, it must again cross capillary cells, travel through interstitial fluid, and enter target cells by passing through their plasma membranes. Depending on the mechanism of action, the drug may also need to enter cellular organelles, such as the nucleus, which are surrounded by additional membranes. While seeking their target cells and attempting to pass through the various membranes, drugs are subjected to numerous physiological substances such as stomach acids and digestive enzymes.

2 The plasma half-life is the time required for the concentration of the medication in the plasma to decrease to half its initial value after administration. This value is important to nurses because the longer the half-life, the longer it takes the medication to be excreted. The medication will then produce a longer effect in the body. The half-life determines how often a medication will be administered. Renal and hepatic diseases will prolong the half-life of drugs, increasing the potential for toxicity.

3 The degree of ionization of a drug affects its absorption. The pH of the local environment directly influences drug absorption through its ability to ionize the drug. The relationship between pH and drug excretion can be used in critical situations to either increase or decrease excretion of the drug.

4 Many oral drugs are rendered inactive by hepatic metabolic reactions. Alternative routes of delivery that bypass the first-pass effect (sublingual, rectal, or parenteral routes) may need to be considered for these drugs.

CHAPTER 6
Answers to NCLEX-RN® Review Questions

1 Answer: 2

Rationale: Unpredictable and unexplained drug reactions are labeled *idiosyncratic*. **Cognitive Level:** Analysis. **Nursing Process:** Implementation. **Client Need:** Physiological Integrity.

2 Answer: 1

Rationale: An antagonist occupies a receptor site and prevents endogenous chemicals from acting. An agonist produces the same type of response as the endogenous substance. A partial agonist is a medication that produces a weaker response than an agonist. **Cognitive Level:** Application. **Nursing Process:** Implementation. **Client Need:** Physiological Integrity.

3 Answer: 2

Rationale: The most important property is efficacy. *Efficacy* is the magnitude of the maximal response that can be produced from a drug. *Cognitive Level:* Application. *Nursing Process:* Implementation. *Client Need:* Physiological Integrity.

4 Answer: 1

Rationale: The term *efficacious* refers to the response that can be produced from a particular drug. *Cognitive Level:* Application. *Nursing Process:* Implementation. *Client Need:* Physiological Integrity.

5 Answers: 2, 4

Rationale: Narcotic analgesics have a greater efficacy than aspirin and ibuprofen in providing pain relief. *Cognitive Level:* Application. *Nursing Process:* Implementaion. *Client Need:* Physiological Integrity.

Answers to Critical Thinking Questions

1 The other 50% of the clients experienced no effect from the dose.

2 An agonist binds to the receptor and produces the same or a greater response than the endogenous chemical. An antagonist occupies a receptor site and prevents the endogenous substance from acting. Antagonists compete with agonists for binding sites. An antihistamine would most likely be an antagonist.

CHAPTER 7
Answers to NCLEX-RN® Review Questions

1 Answer: 3

Rationale: NANDA classifies a nursing diagnosis as a clinical judgment about individual, family, or community responses to actual or potential health/life processes. Per NANDA, nursing diagnoses provide the basis for the selection of nursing interventions to achieve outcomes for which the nurse is accountable. *Cognitive Level:* Analysis. *Nursing Process:* Assessment. *Client Need:* Health Promotion and Maintenance.

2 Answer: 3

Rationale: Clients must be able to swallow without difficulty to take pills, capsules, and enteric-coated tablets. Clients should be able to sit up to swallow medication. Enteral drugs are not added to IV fluid. *Cognitive Level:* Analysis. *Nursing Process:* Assessment. *Client Need:* Physiological Integrity.

3 Answers: 1, 3

Rationale: Noncompliance assumes that the client has been properly educated about medications and has made a deliberate decision not to take them. The client also needs further education regarding self-injection of insulin, injection sites, and how to prevent complications. *Cognitive Level:* Analysis. *Nursing Process:* Diagnosis. *Client Need:* Safe, Effective Care Environment.

4 Answer: 4

Rationale: Once pharmacotherapy is initiated, ongoing assessment is conducted to determine the presence of therapeutic effects or adverse effects. *Cognitive Level:* Analysis. *Nursing Process:* Assessment. *Client Need:* Physiological Integrity.

5 Answer: 4

Rationale: The purpose of evaluation in the nursing process is to determine whether the goals and outcomes have been adequately met by the client. *Cognitive Level:* Application. *Nursing Process:* Assessment. *Client Need:* Health Promotion and Maintenance.

Answers to Critical Thinking Questions

1 The nurse would need to determine that the client's poor eating habits are related to a nontherapeutic environment. The nurse should determine whether indicators of noncompliance exist, such as unused medications, missed medical appointments, and other signs of progression of the disease process. The nurse should also determine whether the financial cost of therapy is affecting compliance. He or she should also evaluate the type and quality of diabetic education that the client and her mother received. The nurse should use open-ended questions to encourage the client's mother to verbalize her concerns about her daughter's diagnosis and well-being. He or she should determine whether the client's mother has unrealistic expectations about her daughter's ability to manage her disease process (i.e., diet, medications, exercise). The nurse should also speak with the client regarding her understanding of the disease and its management. The nurse should also treat the client and her mother with respect in a nonjudgmental manner.

2 Depending on the system of nursing diagnosis being used, the instructor could modify this question. The question assumes that the student has a basic understanding of the pathophysiology of diabetes and the use of subcutaneous insulin pumps. Typical nursing diagnoses would include the following:

- Ineffective Coping, Risk for, related to complex self-care regimen
- Therapeutic Regimen Management, Ineffective, Risk for, related to insufficient knowledge of condition and medication regimen
- Nutrition, Imbalanced: Less Than Body Requirements, related to intake less than energy expenditure
- Infection, Risk for, related to site for organism invasion

3 The client's bill of rights states that a client is entitled to information about drug therapy including name of drug, purpose, action, and potential side effects. The nurse is the professional who is responsible for client–family education. Failing to teach can affect the client's ability to safely self-administer medications and may affect compliance with pharmacological therapy. The nurse should routinely integrate teaching as a critical part of drug administration, allow the client time to ask questions, and evaluate the client's level of understanding.

CHAPTER 8
Answers to NCLEX-RN® Review Questions

1 Answer: 3

Rationale: Isotretinoin (Accutane) is FDA pregnancy category X and is contraindicated during pregnancy. It should not be used at all during pregnancy. *Cognitive Level:* Application. *Nursing Process:* Implementation. *Client Need:* Physiological Integrity.

2 Answer: 4

Rationale: Administration immediately after breast-feeding allows as much time as possible for the medication to be excreted from the mother's body prior to the next feeding. The other options do not provide enough time for the medication to be excreted. *Cognitive Level:* Analysis. *Nursing Process:* Implementation. *Client Need:* Physiological Integrity.

3 Answer: 3

Rationale: Medications should be stored in child-resistant containers and out of reach of children. Clients with arthritic hands may request special easy-to-open medication containers to make self-administration easier. These two situations may be in conflict if elders and children are present in the same home. Toddlers are at risk for poisoning. *Cognitive Level:* Analysis. *Nursing Process:* Evaluation. *Client Needs:* Physiological Integrity.

4 Answer: 4

Rationale: Toddlers may resist taking medications. Short explanations followed by immediate (kind but firm) drug administration are best.

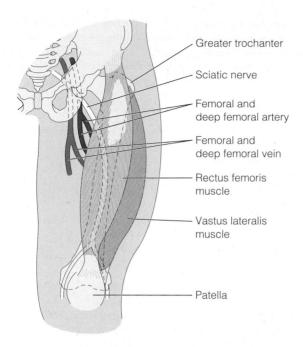

Greater trochanter

Sciatic nerve

Femoral and
deep femoral artery

Femoral and
deep femoral vein

Rectus femoris
muscle

Vastus lateralis
muscle

Patella

Children should not be told that medicine is candy for safety reasons. A toddler is not able to make a decision regarding medication administration. When medication is mixed with liquids or other food products, a small amount should be used; 8 oz is too much liquid to use for mixing. *Cognitive Level:* Analysis. *Nursing Process:* Implementation. *Client Need:* Physiological Integrity.

5 Answer: vastus lateralis
Rationale: The middle third of the vastus lateralis muscle is the preferred site for intramuscular injection in the newborn. The middle third of the rectus femoris is an alternate site, but its proximity to major vessels and the sciatic nerve requires caution in using this site for injection. *Cognitive Level:* Comprehension. *Nursing Process:* Implementation. *Client Need:* Physiological Integrity.

Answers to Critical Thinking Questions

1 Pyelonephritis is frequently associated with preterm labor in pregnancy. Before initiating antibiotic therapy, the nurse should first determine the client's gestational age. The potential for a drug to be teratogenic is highest during the first trimester. The nurse should also look up the pregnancy classification of the antibiotic. Selected agents, such as tetracyclines, should not be used during pregnancy. The nurse should address any concerns regarding the drug category with the prescriber.

2 Prior to considering a sedative agent, the nurse should assess the client for other physical causes of confusion. For example, in the frail elderly, alterations in electrolytes, drug side effects, and rapid environmental changes can contribute to confusion. Attempts at reorientation should be made. The nurse should determine how diazepam (Valium) is distributed and metabolized. Valium is a fat-soluble drug; thus, because elderly clients have increased total body fat, the drug has a much longer half-life. In addition, numerous drugs decrease the metabolism of diazepam and may contribute to an increased half-life and enhanced CNS depression. If sedation is deemed necessary, other drugs should be considered.

3 This question requires the student to go back to Chapter 4 to review techniques of drug administration for infants. The nurse should consult with the pharmacist regarding the need to repeat the dose. Many oral elixirs are absorbed, to some degree, in the mucous membranes of the oral cavity. Therefore, the nurse may not need to repeat the dose. The nurse should consider using an oral syringe to accurately measure and administer medications to infants. The syringe tip

should be placed in the side of the mouth, not forced over the tongue. Conditions affecting the GI tract, such as gastroenteritis, can affect drug absorption because of their effect on peristalsis.

CHAPTER 9
Answers to NCLEX-RN® Review Questions

1 Answer 4
Rationale: Nurse practice acts encompass all aspects of nursing, including the definition of professional nursing, medication administration, and definition of standards of care. *Cognitive Level:* Analysis. *Nursing Process:* Implementation. *Client Need:* Safe, Effective Care Environment.

2 Answer: 3
Rationale: The nurse is responsible for documenting medication errors and completing an incident report for review by the facility's quality assurance personnel. *Cognitive Level:* Analysis. *Nursing Process:* Implementation. *Client Need:* Safe, Effective Care Environment.

3 Answer: 1
Rationale: Prior to administering medications, the nurse should assess renal and liver function and impairments of other body systems that may affect pharmacotherapy. This is especially important when administering medications to elderly and severely debilitated clients. *Cognitive Level:* Analysis. *Nursing Process:* Assessment. *Client Need:* Physiological Integrity.

4 Answer: 4
Rationale: The Food and Drug Administration (FDA) and the National Coordinating Council for Medication Error Reporting and Prevention (NCC MERP) encourage nurses and other healthcare professionals to report medication errors. This aids in examining interdisciplinary causes of medication errors and developing methods to prevent them, thereby promoting medication safety. *Cognitive Level:* Analysis. *Nursing Process:* Implementation. *Client Need:* Safe, Effective Care Environment.

5 Answers: 1, 3, 4, 5
Rationale: When the nurse administers a medication to the wrong client, the nurse must immediately assess the client, including vital signs, and notify the physician. The medication should be documented on the MAR, and a facility incident report must be completed. The nurse should not document that a medication error occurred in the client's record, but should note that the medication was administered, include initial and ongoing assessment findings, indicate that the physician was notified, and document any new orders that were obtained. The nurse should then complete the facility incident report identifying the facts of the error. *Cognitive Level:* Analysis. *Nursing Process:* Implementation. *Client Need:* Safe, Effective Care Environment.

Answers to Critical Thinking Questions

1 The nurse should be well organized in preparing for drug administration. The MAR must be assessed at the beginning of the shift, and the nurse should develop a system that will serve as a reminder of when drugs are due to be administered. In most institutions, regularly scheduled drugs may be administered 30 minutes before and 30 minutes after the assigned time. If administered within this time frame, the drugs are considered to have been given "on time." Institutional policies vary and should be consulted.

2 This order as written does not contain an indication for "right dose." Tylenol 3 is a combination drug of acetaminophen and codeine, given orally. The typical mistake is to assume that the healthcare provider meant for the client to have 1 tablet by mouth. The nurse should not make this assumption because of the risk of an unintended drug error. Prior to administering the dose, the nurse should consult with the healthcare provider to clarify the intent of the order.

3 There are numerous persons potentially "at fault" in this scenario. The nurse is ultimately responsible for the dosage error because a quick check of a drug handbook and a simple dosage calculation might have revealed that the dosage was too high. The prescriber was also responsible for writing the wrong dosage; however, the nurse should have notified the healthcare provider to have the dosage corrected. The pharmacist was also responsible for not checking to see that the dosage was correct for the age and weight of the client. There are numerous possibilities for error. Nurses must work within an institution's medical error reporting system to ensure that such errors are identified and that mechanisms to prevent subsequent errors can be implemented.

CHAPTER 10
Answers to NCLEX-RN® Review Questions

1 Answer: 2
Rationale: Many cultural groups believe in using herbs and other alternative therapies either along with or in place of traditional medicines. The nurse should interpret how these herbal and alternative therapies will affect the desired pharmacotherapeutic outcomes. *Cognitive Level:* Assessment. *Nursing Process:* Application. *Client Need:* Physiological Integrity.

2 Answer: 3
Rationale: Up to 48% of English-speaking clients do not have the basic ability to read, understand, and act on health information. This rate is even higher among non-English-speaking individuals and older clients. The nurse must be aware of the client's literacy level and take appropriate action to ensure that information is understood. *Cognitive Level:* Assessment. *Nursing Process:* Analysis. *Client Need:* Health Promotion and Maintenance.

3 Answer: 2
Rationale: Women seek health care earlier than men. Men and women are both affected by Alzheimer's disease; however, women are one and a half to three times more likely to develop the disease. *Cognitive Level:* Analysis. *Nursing Process:* Diagnosis. *Client Need:* Health Promotion and Maintenance.

4 Answer: 2
Rationale: When clients have strong spiritual or religious beliefs, these may greatly influence their perceptions of illness and their preferred modes of treatment. Ill health and spiritual issues can have an impact on wellness, nursing care, and pharmacotherapy. *Cognitive Level:* Analysis. *Nursing Process:* Assessment. *Client Need:* Psychosocial Integrity.

5 Answers: 1, 2, 4
Rationale: When taken with CNS depressants, St. John's wort may potentiate sedation. When taken with cyclosporine, St. John's wort may decrease cyclosporine levels. St. John's wort in combination with MAOIs may cause a hypertensive crisis. St. John's wort has little to no effect on blood glucose levels. *Cognitive Level:* Analysis. *Nursing Process:* Diagnosis. *Client Need:* Physiological Integrity.

Answers to Critical Thinking Questions

1 The primary concern for this client would be the potential for drug–food interactions. Warfarin (Coumadin) achieves its anticoagulant effect by interfering with the synthesis of vitamin K–dependent clotting factors. The anticoagulant effect of Coumadin can be decreased by a diet high in vitamin K. Fresh greens and tomatoes from the garden are excellent sources of vitamin K. The nurse must include questions related to the dietary intake of these foods. It is common for rural people to "eat out of their gardens" during the growing season. The nurse must also determine whether other medications have been added to the client's regimen that could interfere with the action of Coumadin.

2 As women age, they experience a 10% decrease in total body water. In general, body weight also decreases in this aging population. The nurse should carefully assess the client's current weight and compare it with the previously documented weight. In addition, because this client's body weight has decreased, she may also have decreased serum protein. The dose of furosemide is dependent on the degree of protein binding; therefore, less serum protein could make the drug more pharmacologically active. The client may need to have the dosage adjusted.

3 This textbook includes a reference to community health statistics in the United States. Many of the statistics relate to healthcare concerns among rural citizens. These statistics, and the student's own perceptions, can lead to a general discussion about the impact of culture and ethnicity on health care. The primary point of any discussion is to emphasize the limited access to care that the culture of poverty creates. This client is more affected by poverty and a transient living style than by either culture or ethnicity in the matter of managing his own health care.

CHAPTER 11
Answers to NCLEX-RN® Review Questions

1 Answer: 4
Rationale: Some herbal products contain ingredients that may serve as agonists or antagonists to prescription drugs. Herbal supplements should not be taken without discussing their use with the healthcare provider. Herbal supplements are considered less potent than prescription medications, but when similar drugs are taken together, there is the potential for adverse reactions. *Cognitive Level:* Analysis. *Nursing Process:* Implementation. *Client Need:* Physiological Integrity.

2 Answer: 1
Rationale: Natural products contain many active ingredients, many of which have not been tested or identified. Clients with known allergies to food products or medicines should seek medical advice before using herbal supplements. Dietary supplements must state that the product is not intended to diagnose, treat, cure, or prevent any disease. *Cognitive Level:* Analysis. *Nursing Process:* Implementation. *Client Need:* Physiological Integrity.

3 Answer: 2
Rationale: Saw palmetto is used to relieve urinary problems related to prostate enlargement. Cranberry juice (or the berries) is used to prevent urinary tract infections. Soy, evening primrose, and black cohosh are used for menopausal symptoms. *Cognitive Level:* Analysis. *Nursing Process:* Implementation. *Client Need:* Physiological Integrity.

4 Answer: 4
Rationale: Feverfew may interact with aspirin, heparin, NSAIDs, and warfarin to cause increased bleeding. *Cognitive Level:* Analysis. *Nursing Process:* Assessment. *Client Need:* Physiological Integrity.

5 Answers: 1, 2, 3, 5
Rationale: Serotonin syndrome is a rare but potentially life-threatening medical condition that may occur when clients are taking two or more drugs, one of which is a selective serotonergic medication. Symptoms include agitation, dizziness, sweating, and headache. Clients should discontinue use of the medication and seek medical

care immediately. *Cognitive Level:* Analysis. *Nursing Process:* Assessment. *Client Need:* Physiological Integrity.

Answers to Critical Thinking Questions

1 Tamoxifen is a selective estrogen receptor modulator (SERM) that acts by preventing estrogen from binding to the estrogen receptor in breast cells. Therefore, breast cell proliferation is inhibited. Many women assume that because they are taking a SERM, that estrogen replacement is indicated. In fact, tamoxifen's effect in tissues other than the breast is similar to that of estrogen. Tamoxifen does not cause menopause and does not prevent pregnancy. If the client takes a "natural" soy product, it may interfere with the desired action of tamoxifen. Her concern should be acknowledged, but she should be warned not to consume any herbal product without first consulting her healthcare provider.

2 Both garlic and ginseng have a potential drug interaction with the anticoagulant warfarin (Coumadin). It is known that ginseng is capable of inhibiting platelet activity. When taken in combination with an anticoagulant, these herbal products are capable of producing increased bleeding potential.

3 St. John's wort interacts with multiple drugs. It is important that the client stop taking St. John's wort at least 3 weeks prior to the surgery, because it can potentiate sedation when combined with CNS depressants and opiate analgesics. St. John's wort can also decrease the effects of anticoagulants.

CHAPTER 12
Answers to NCLEX-RN® Review Questions

1 Answer: 2
Rationale: Some clients and healthcare professionals believe that therapeutic use of scheduled drugs creates large numbers of addicted clients. Prescription drugs rarely cause addiction when used according to accepted medical protocols. The risk of addiction for prescription medications is primarily a function of the dose and the length of therapy. *Cognitive Level:* Application. *Nursing Process:* Implementation. *Client Need:* Physiological Integrity.

2 Answer: 2
Rationale: Tolerance is a biological condition that occurs when the body adapts to a substance after repeated administration. Over time, higher doses of the drug are required to produce the same initial effect. *Cognitive Level:* Application. *Nursing Process:* Assessment. *Client Need:* Physiological Integrity.

3 Answer: 4
Rationale: Use of marijuana slows motor activity, decreases coordination, and causes disconnected thoughts, feelings of paranoia, and euphoria. It increases thirst and craving for food, especially chocolate and other candies. Heroin produces a brief, intense rush of euphoria sought by addicts. Individuals experience a range of CNS effects from extreme pleasure to slowed body activities and profound sedation. Signs include constricted pupils, an increase in the pain threshold, and respiratory depression. Crack cocaine produces feelings of intense euphoria, a decrease in hunger, analgesia, illusions of physical strength, and increased sensory perception. Larger doses magnify these effects and also cause rapid heartbeat, sweating, dilation of the pupils, and an elevated body temperature. Large doses of barbiturates drugs suppress the respiratory centers in the brain. The user may stop breathing or lapse into a coma. *Cognitive Level:* Analysis. *Nursing Process:* Assessment. *Client Need:* Physiological Integrity.

4 Answer: 3
Rationale: Clients experiencing alcohol withdrawal typically experience tremors, fatigue, anxiety, abdominal cramping, hallucinations, confusion, seizures, and delirium. *Cognitive Level:* Analysis. *Nursing Process:* Assessment. *Client Need:* Physiological Integrity.

5 Answers: 1, 2, 4
Rationale: Symptoms of nicotine withdrawal include irritability, anxiety, restlessness, headaches, increased appetite, insomnia, inability to concentrate, and a decrease in heart rate and blood pressure. *Cognitive Level:* Application. *Nursing Process:* Implementation. *Client Need:* Physiological Integrity.

Answers to Critical Thinking Questions

1 The National Institute on Drug Abuse offers a link titled Info-Facts, which provides a great deal of information about MDMA (www.drugabuse.gov/infofacts/ecstasy.html). This drug is a neurotoxic agent. When taken in high doses it can produce malignant hyperthermia, which can lead to muscle damage and renal and cardiovascular system failure. Physical symptoms of MDMA use include muscle tension, nausea, rapid eye movement, faintness, chills, sweating, increased heart rate and blood pressure, and involuntary teeth clenching.

2 The NIDA InfoFacts sheet on steroids (www.drugabuse/steroids.html.gov) points out that aggression is a common psychiatric side effect of anabolic steroid abuse. Research indicates that users may experience paranoid jealousy, extreme irritability, delusions, and impaired judgment. Other symptoms are extreme mood changes and maniclike symptoms, even when the user reports feeling "good."

3 The principal danger associated with prolonged use of barbiturates is tolerance and physical addiction. Barbiturates generally lose their effectiveness as hypnotics within 2 weeks of continued use. This client is demonstrating signs of developing tolerance. He needs to discontinue the drug gradually to decrease the risk of complications associated with sudden withdrawal. These symptoms include severe anxiety, tremors, marked excitement, delirium, and rebound rapid eye movement (REM) sleep. Today, nonbarbiturates are usually prescribed as first-line hypnotics.

CHAPTER 13
Answers to NCLEX-RN® Review Questions

1 Answer: 1
Rationale: Adrenergic agonists stimulate the sympathetic nervous system and produce symptoms of the fight-or-flight response. Nausea, vomiting, nervousness, bronchial dilation, and hypertension are potential adverse reactions related to the use of adrenergic agonists. Hypotension is a potential adverse reaction related to the use of adrenergic antagonists. *Cognitive Level:* Assessment. *Nursing Process:* Application. *Client Need:* Physiological Integrity.

2 Answers: 1, 2, 4
Rationale: Anticholinergics are used in the treatment of peptic ulcer disease, irritable bowel syndrome, and bradycardia because they suppress the effects of acetylcholine and stimulate the sympathetic nervous system. Anticholinergics may cause decreased sexual function because the parasympathetic impulses are blocked. Urine retention is a potential side effect of anticholinergics. *Cognitive Level:* Analysis. *Nursing Process:* Diagnosis. *Client Need:* Physiological Integrity.

3 Answer: 1
Rationale: Potential adverse reactions associated with the use of adrenergic antagonists include tachycardia, edema, and heart failure. Bronchodilation is associated with the use of adrenergic agonists. *Cognitive Level:* Analysis. *Nursing Process:* Assessment. *Client Need:* Physiological Integrity.

4 Answer: 3

Rationale: The nurse should monitor elderly clients for episodes of dizziness caused by CNS stimulation from the parasympathomimetic. Diaphoresis and dizziness are potential side effects related to the use of bethanechol. Bethanechol is used to treat nonobstructive urinary retention. *Cognitive Level:* Application. *Nursing Process:* Implementation. *Client Need:* Physiological Integrity.

5 Answer: 2

Rationale: Anticholinergic medications slow intestinal motility; therefore, constipation is a potential side effect. Heartburn and hypothermia are not associated with the use of benztropine. *Cognitive Level:* Application. *Nursing Process:* Assessment. *Client Need:* Physiological Integrity.

Answers to Critical Thinking Questions

1 Terbutaline (Brethine) is a sympathomimetic that was originally prescribed for the treatment of asthma. Terbutaline promotes bronchodilation and therefore reduces bronchospasm by inducing smooth-muscle relaxation. Today, terbutaline has found widespread use as a tocolytic because it also produces smooth-muscle relaxation in the uterus. Because terbutaline is a sympathomimetic, the nurse should prepare the client for potential adverse reactions such as nervousness, tremor, and tachycardia. The nurse should also teach the client to take the medication exactly as directed and on schedule, and instruct on the signs and symptoms of preterm labor in case they occur again.

2 Bethanechol is a direct-acting cholinergic agent that works by stimulating the parasympathetic nervous system. The desired effect, in this case, is an increase in smooth-muscle tone in the bladder. Any side effects would be related to an overstimulation of the parasympathetic nervous system. Following are suggested nursing diagnoses.

- Injury, Risk for, related to side effects of cholinergic agents (hypotension, bradycardia, and syncope)
- Comfort, Alteration in, related to abdominal cramping, nausea, and vomiting
- Individual Therapeutic Management, Ineffective, Risk for, related to side effects and precautions of using cholinergic agents

3 Benztropine (Cogentin) is an anticholinergic. Blocking the parasympathetic nerves allows the sympathetic nervous system to dominate. The drug is given as an adjunct in Parkinson's disease to reduce muscular tremor and rigidity. Anticholinergics affect many body systems and produce a wide variety of side effects. The nurse should monitor for decreased heart rate, dilated pupils, decreased peristalsis, and decreased salivation in addition to decreased muscular tremor and rigidity. Many of the side effects of anticholinergics are dose dependent. Adverse effects include typical signs of sympathetic nervous system stimulation.

CHAPTER 14
Answers to NCLEX-RN® Review Questions

1 Answer: 3

Rationale: CNS side effects for lorazepam (Ativan) include amnesia, weakness, disorientation, ataxia, blurred vision, diplopia, nausea, and vomiting. *Cognitive Level:* Analysis. *Nursing Process:* Assessment. *Client Need:* Physiological Integrity.

2 Answer: 4

Rationale: The nurse should recognize that this medication is ordered for insomnia. Therefore, the client should be experiencing relief from insomnia and reporting feeling rested when awakening. *Cognitive Level:* Analysis. *Nursing Process:* Evaluation. *Client Need:* Physiological Integrity.

3 Answers: 1, 2, 4

Rationale: Stevens–Johnson syndrome is a potentially fatal medication reaction that may occur within 1 to 4 days of therapy and is characterized by fever, chills, malaise, blisterlike lesions, and skin sloughing of 10% of the body. *Cognitive Level:* Analysis. *Nursing Process:* Assessment. *Client Need:* Physiological Integrity.

4 Answer: 3

Rationale: Benzodiazepines should not be stopped abruptly. The physician should decide when and how to discontinue the medication. *Cognitive Level:* Analysis. *Nursing Process:* Evaluation. *Client Need:* Physiological Integrity.

5 Answer: 2

Rationale: The statement by the client needs to show clearly that the expected benefit of the medication therapy has been experienced by the client. *Cognitive Level:* Analysis. *Nursing Process:* Evaluation. *Client Need:* Physiological Integrity.

Answers to Critical Thinking Questions

1 Pain is emphasized as being the fifth vital sign. The assessment and appropriate management of pain is a nursing function. A nurse might be tempted to give this client a sleeping medication alone, fearing the side effects that might occur if given in combination with an opioid narcotic. Secobarbital is a short-acting barbiturate. Barbiturates are not effective analgesics and generally do not produce significant hypnosis in clients with severe pain. The barbiturate may intensify the client's reaction to painful stimuli. Administering a barbiturate with a potent analgesic appears to reduce analgesic requirements by about 50%. The nurse may need to consult with the healthcare provider regarding lowering the dose of narcotic.

2 The student may immediately recognize lorazepam (Ativan) as an antianxiety agent. The assumption might be that the purpose of the drug in this case is to control anxiety related to the client's diagnosis and treatment. After consulting the handbook, the student will discover that lorazepam also has an off-label use as an antiemetic.

3 The student should consider conducting a thorough assessment of the client's sleep patterns. In addition, the student should consider nonpharmacological interventions. In older adults, the total amount of sleep does not change; however, the quality of sleep deteriorates. Time spent in REM sleep and stages 3 and 4 NREM sleep shortens. Older adults awaken more often during the night. This sleep disturbance can be compounded by the presence of a chronic illness. The alteration in sleep patterns may also be due to changes in the CNS that affect the regulation of sleep. After a thorough assessment, the nurse should discuss age-related issues, health concerns, and environmental factors that may be affecting the quality of sleep.

CHAPTER 15
Answers to NCLEX-RN® Review Questions

1 Answer: 3

Rationale: Seizures may be caused by inflammation, head injuries, or low blood sugar levels. Rapid-growing, space-occupying lesions in the brain, which increase intracranial pressure, may cause seizures, but not tumors, within the muscles. *Cognitive Level:* Analysis. *Nursing Process:* Evaluation. *Client Need:* Physiological Integrity.

2 Answer: 3

Rationale: The influx of sodium into a neuron enhances neuronal activity. The delay of an influx suppresses neurotransmitter frequency. *Cognitive Level:* Analysis. *Nursing Process:* Assessment. *Client Need:* Physiological Integrity.

3 Answer: 2

Rationale: GABA drugs mimic GABA by stimulating the influx of chloride ions into the neuron, leading to the suppression of neuron firing. *Cognitive Level:* Analysis. *Nursing Process:* Assessment. *Client Need:* Physiological Integrity.

4 Answer: 3

Rationale: Valproic acid may produce an idiosyncratic response in children, including restlessness and psychomotor agitation. *Cognitive Level:* Analysis. *Nursing Process:* Assessment. *Client Need:* Physiological Integrity.

5 Answer: 3

Rationale: Carbamazepine affects vitamin K metabolism and may lead to blood dyscrasias and bleeding. *Cognitive Level:* Application. *Nursing Process:* Implementation. *Client Need:* Physiological Integrity.

6 Answers: 1, 2, 4

Rationale: The phenytoin-like drugs are used to treat partial seizures. Diazepam (Valium) is a benzodiazepine that is used to treat tonic–clonic seizures and status epilepticus. *Cognitive Level:* Analysis. *Nursing Process:* Implementation. *Client Need:* Physiological Integrity.

Answers to Critical Thinking Questions

1 Carbamazepine (Tegretol) is the second most widely prescribed antiepileptic drug in the United States. Common side effects are drowsiness, dizziness, nausea, ataxia, and blurred vision. Serious and sometimes fatal blood dyscrasias secondary to bone marrow suppression have occurred with carbamazepine. The client's hematocrit suggests anemia, and the petechiae and bruising suggest thrombocytopenia. The nurse practitioner should evaluate the client for complaints of fever and sore throat that would suggest leukopenia. This client needs immediate evaluation by the healthcare provider responsible for monitoring the seizure disorder.

2 This question requires that the student consult a laboratory reference manual. The therapeutic drug level of phenytoin (Dilantin) is 5 to 20 mg/dl. Clients may become drug toxic and demonstrate signs of CNS depression. Exaggerated effects of Dilantin can be seen if the drug has been combined with alcohol or other agents. Dilantin also demonstrates dose-dependent metabolism. When hepatic enzymes necessary for metabolism are saturated, any increase in drug concentration results in a disproportionate increase in plasma concentration level.

3 Long-term phenytoin therapy can produce an androgenic stimulus. Reported skin manifestations include acne, hirsutism, and an increase in subcutaneous facial tissue—changes that have been characterized as "Dilantin facies." These changes, coupled with the risk for gingival hypertrophy, may be difficult for the adolescent to cope with. In addition, the adolescent with a seizure disorder may be prohibited from operating a motor vehicle at the very age when driving becomes key to achieving young-adult status. The thoughtful nurse will consider the range of possible support groups for this client once she is discharged and will encourage the client to discuss her concerns about the drug regimen with her healthcare provider.

CHAPTER 16
Answers to NCLEX-RN® Review Questions

1 Answer: 1

Rationale: The therapeutic dose range of lithium is 0.6 to 1.5 mEq/L. A reading of 0.95 mEq/L is within normal limits. *Cognitive Level:*

Analysis. *Nursing Process:* Implementation. *Client Need:* Physiological Integrity.

2 Answer: 3

Rationale: Methylphenidate (Ritalin) is a Schedule II drug with potential to cause drug dependence when used over an extended period. The drug holiday is to decrease the risk of dependence and to evaluate behavior. *Cognitive Level:* Application. *Nursing Process:* Implementation. *Client Need:* Physiological Integrity.

3 Answers: 1, 2, 5

Rationale: Diarrhea, ataxia, hypotension, edema, slurred speech, and muscle weakness are signs of lithium toxicity. Dehydration can lead to lithium toxicity. *Cognitive Level:* Analysis. *Nursing Process:* Assessment. *Client Need:* Physiological Integrity.

4 Answer: 2

Rationale: Taking St. John's wort with an MAOI could result in hypertensive crisis; clients should always consult with their healthcare provider before taking any medications or OTC drugs/herbal remedies. *Cognitive Level:* Application. *Nursing Process:* Implementation. *Client Need:* Physiological Integrity.

5 Answer: 3

Rationale: Nardil is an MAOI. This class of drugs has many drug and food interactions that may cause a hypertensive crisis. *Cognitive Level:* Analysis. *Nursing Process:* Planning. *Client Need:* Physiological Integrity.

Answers to Critical Thinking Questions

1 Methylphenidate (Ritalin) therapy is usually administered twice a day, with one dose before breakfast and one dose before lunch. A child in school would be required to visit a school nurse to receive a dose of Ritalin before lunch. Amphetamine (Adderall) requires once-a-day dosing and may be better accepted by the child and his or her family because treatment can be privately managed at home. Although many children cope effectively with treatment for ADHD, a 12-year-old girl might be concerned about being "singled out" for therapy. She is old enough to realize her problems in performance. The self-esteem of children in this age group is tied to success in school, a characteristic of Erikson's developmental stage of industry versus inferiority. Children who have difficulty in school perceive themselves as being inferior to peers. Helping the child with ADHD pharmacologically may require the healthcare provider to be sensitive to social factors such as dosage regimens.

2 The nurse should teach the client that it might take 2 to 4 weeks before she begins to notice therapeutic benefit. The nurse should help the client identify a support person or network to help assist as she works through her grief. The nurse also needs to instruct the client that both caffeine and nicotine are CNS stimulants and decrease the effectiveness of the medication.

3 The use of any drug during pregnancy must be carefully evaluated. Sertraline (Zoloft) is a pregnancy category B drug, which means that studies indicate no risk to animal fetuses, although safety in humans has not been established. The prescriber must weigh risks and benefits of any medication during pregnancy. The nurse should recognize this client's risk for ineffective coping, as evidenced by her history of depression, and help the client identify support groups in the community. She may be functioning in some degree of isolation from family or other parenting women, which is typical of women who suffer postpartum depression. Identifying community resources for the client is one intervention designed to provide more holistic care.

Answer to Avoiding Medication Errors

1 Unless there is a physician's order, it is never permissible to leave medications at the bedside of a client. It is possible that the client will deliberately discard them, save them for a later overdose, or forget to take them. It is also possible that the medications could be inadvertently removed with the food tray or taken by another client. Always supervise all medication administration and be certain that the drug is swallowed. Never leave medications unattended in a client's room. If there are concerns that the client may not have swallowed the medications, ask the client to open his or her mouth. The risk that a depressed client will take an intentional overdose increases as the medication begins to work and gives the client more energy to carry out a suicide plan.

CHAPTER 17
Answers to NCLEX-RN® Review Questions

1 Answer: 4
Rationale: Symptoms of psychosis are likely to return and manifest as agitation, distrust, and frustration. *Cognitive Level:* Analysis. *Nursing Process:* Implementation. *Client Need:* Physiological Integrity.

2 Answer: 2
Rationale: Acute dystonias occur early in the course of therapy. These are severe muscle spasms, particularly of the back, neck, tongue, and face. *Cognitive Level:* Analysis. *Nursing Process:* Planning. *Client Need:* Physiological Integrity.

3 Answer: 1
Rationale: Concurrent therapy with anticholinergic Parkinson's medications reduces EPS. *Cognitive Level:* Analysis. *Nursing Process:* Implementation. *Client Need:* Physiological Integrity.

4 Answers: 1, 2, 4
Rationale: Aluminum- and magnesium-based antacids decrease absorption of haloperidol (Haldol). Haldol also has a high incidence of EPS. Haldol must be taken as ordered for therapeutic results to occur. It is contraindicated in Parkinson's disease, seizure disorders, alcoholism, and severe mental depression. The sustained-release forms must not be opened or crushed. *Cognitive Level:* Analysis. *Nursing Process:* Implementation. *Client Need:* Physiological Integrity.

5 Answer: 3
Rationale: Fluphenazine (Prolixin) is a phenothiazine drug. Use is contraindicated in clients with CNS depression, bone marrow depression, and alcohol withdrawal. *Cognitive Level:* Analysis. *Nursing Process:* Assessment. *Client Need:* Physiological Integrity.

Answers to Critical Thinking Questions

1 The client is exhibiting signs of EPS. Initially, the nurse would assess the client to ensure he had sustained no recent neck injury or trauma, but if the neck spasms started spontaneously, the nurse would then assess for the possibility of EPS. The client probably needs to be on a medication such as benztropine (Cogentin) to decrease the EPS effects. The client should be taught to recognize the symptoms of EPS and to seek medical evaluation when the symptoms occur.

2 The client is elderly; thus, safety is a priority when administering this medication. Postural hypotension and dizziness are common; therefore, the client needs to move and change position slowly. Constipation is also a concern for a client on this medication, especially elderly clients.

3 The nurse should initially assess whether the client has been taking the medication as ordered or has altered the dose in any way. It is not uncommon for a young person to "cheek" the medication or attempt to cut back on the dose because of the lack of desire to take the medication on a continual basis—especially when the client begins to

feel better. It is important that the client understand the necessity of being on this medication for a lifetime, and that the dose is not to be adjusted without consulting a healthcare provider.

CHAPTER 18
Answers to NCLEX-RN® Review Questions

1 Answer: 2
Rationale: When used concurrently with medication, nonpharmacological techniques may allow for lower doses and possibly fewer drug-related adverse effects. Relaxation techniques and imagery may also be used in the acute care setting. *Cognitive Level:* Analysis. *Nursing Process:* Implementation. *Client Need:* Physiological Integrity.

2 Answer: 3
Rationale: Some opioid agonists, such as morphine, activate both mu and kappa receptors. *Cognitive Level:* Analysis. *Nursing Process:* Implementation. *Client Need:* Physiological Integrity.

3 Answer: 3
Rationale: Vicodin is a combination drug of hydrocodone and acetaminophen. Acetaminophen can be hepatotoxic, and this client has hepatitis B, a chronic liver disorder. *Cognitive Level:* Application. *Nursing Process:* Implementation. *Client Need:* Physiological Integrity.

4 Answers: 4, 5
Rationale: Opioids activate mu and kappa receptors that may cause profound respiratory depression. The client's respiratory rate should remain above 12 breaths per minute. Although the client may also become drowsy, he or she should not become unresponsive after administration of morphine sulfate. *Cognitive Level:* Analysis. *Nursing Process:* Implementation. *Client Need:* Physiological Integrity.

5 Answer: 2
Rationale: Opioids suppress intestinal contractility, increase anal sphincter tone, and inhibit fluids into the intestines, which can lead to constipation. *Cognitive Level:* Application. *Nursing Process:* Implementation. *Client Need:* Physiological Integrity.

Answers to Critical Thinking Questions

1 The nurse should initially manage the client's airway, breathing, and circulation (ABCs) by opening the airway and providing oxygen support, and then stop the PCA pump. Although the nurse's first reaction may be to go directly to the PCA to stop the medication, it is important initially to manage the client's airway before stopping the PCA because it is unknown how long the client has been hypoxic. The nurse then needs to administer IV naloxone (Narcan), which is a narcotic antagonist. After these initial steps have been completed and the client is stabilized, the nurse must inform the healthcare provider of this adverse effect of the morphine.

2 Sumatriptan (Imitrex) is not recommended for clients with CAD, diabetes, or hypertension because of the drug's vasoconstrictive properties. The nurse should refer the client to the healthcare provider for review of medications and possible adverse reactions related to sumatriptan.

3 The client should be taught not to take any medication, including OTC medications, without the approval of the healthcare provider. This client is taking an anticoagulant, and aspirin increases bleeding time. The client needs to be taught how to recognize the signs and symptoms of bleeding related to the anticoagulant therapy. The client should review with the healthcare provider all her medications. Possibly, her anti-inflammatory medication can be changed from aspirin to another drug for treatment of arthritis.

CHAPTER 19
Answers to NCLEX-RN® Review Questions

1 Answer: 1

Rationale: The throat is anesthetized during a gastroscopy. Monitor the client for return of the gag reflex before the patient drinks or eats. Ensuring an airway is the priority when caring for these clients. Abdominal pain, ability to stand, and ability to urinate are not priorities. *Cognitive Level:* Application. *Nursing Process:* Assessment. *Client Need:* Physiological Integrity.

2 Answer: 4

Rationale: Solutions of lidocaine containing preservatives or epinephrine are intended for local anesthesia only and must never be given IV for dysrhythmias. *Cognitive Level:* Analysis. *Nursing Process:* Implementation. *Client Need:* Physiological Integrity.

3 Answer: 3

Rationale: The first step of the nursing process is assessment. Assessment of prior knowledge provides the basis for the development of a teaching plan. The other options take place after a thorough assessment. *Cognitive Level:* Application. *Nursing Process:* Assessment. *Client Need:* Physiological Integrity.

4 Answer: 3

Rationale: Nitrous oxide suppresses the pain mechanisms within the CNS, thereby causing analgesia. It does not produce complete loss of consciousness or profound relaxation of skeletal muscles. Nitrous oxide does not induce stage 3 analgesia or cause a loss of consciousness. *Cognitive Level:* Analysis. *Nursing Process:* Implementation. *Client Need:* Physiological Integrity.

5 Answers: 1, 4

Rationale: Succinylcholine (Anectine) can cause complete paralysis of the diaphragm and intercostal muscles. Bradycardia and respiratory depression are expected. Mechanical ventilation should be available. *Cognitive Level:* Analysis. *Nursing Process:* Assessment. *Client Need:* Physiological Integrity.

Answers to Critical Thinking Questions

1 The nurse should question the healthcare provider regarding this order. Lidocaine is an appropriate choice for a local anesthesia but not if it includes epinephrine. Epinephrine has alpha-adrenergic properties, is a potent vasoconstrictor, and may cause cardiac dysrhythmias in this elderly client. Epinephrine is traditionally not used in the areas of "fingers, nose, penis, and toes," because these areas may suffer adverse effects from the vasoconstrictive properties of the drug.

2 The nurse understands that this drug is a depolarizing medication and therefore has the potential to increase potassium release. The nurse is aware that this client is on digoxin (Lanoxin) and has renal failure, and therefore is not a good candidate for this drug because of the potential hyperkalemia that may result in life-threatening cardiac dysrhythmias.

3 The priority postoperative drug is St. John's wort because it may prolong the effects of anesthesia and opioids in the client's system, causing depression of the CNS and respiratory system. The client should also be monitored for postoperative bleeding related to the use of ibuprofen. The digoxin concentration should be at a therapeutic level prior to surgery to decrease possible adverse effects of the cardiovascular system postoperatively.

CHAPTER 20
Answers to NCLEX-RN® Review Questions

1 Answer: 2

Rationale: Extrapyramidal symptoms may be life threatening without intervention. The client should be immediately transported to the emergency department. Diphenhydramine must be given parenterally for effective treatment. The drug dosage should not be increased, because symptoms may become worse. *Cognitive Level:* Analysis. *Nursing Process:* Implementation. *Client Need:* Physiological Integrity.

2 Answer: 2

Rationale: Pharmacotherapy does not cure or stop the disease process but does improve the client's ability to perform normal activities such as eating, bathing, and walking. Depending on the drug therapy, EPS may be an adverse effect. *Cognitive Level:* Analysis. *Nursing Process:* Implementation. *Client Need:* Physiological Integrity.

3 Answer: 4

Rationale: A decrease in kidney and liver function may slow the metabolism and excretion of the drug, leading to overdose and toxicity. Levodopa does not cause the urine to turn orange. It is not reasonable for a client to monitor his or her blood pressure every 2 hours during the first 2 weeks of therapy. *Cognitive Level:* Analysis. *Nursing Process:* Implementation. *Client Need:* Physiological Integrity.

4 Answer: 1

Rationale: The cause is unknown; however, structural damage consisting of amyloid plaques and neurofibrillary tangles has been found within the brain at autopsy. Alzheimer's disease has not been associated with intracranial bleeding, loss of circulation to the brain, or loss of dopamine receptors. *Cognitive Level:* Application. *Nursing Process:* Implementation. *Client Need:* Physiological Integrity.

5 Answers: 1, 3

Rationale: Symptoms of overdose include severe nausea and vomiting, sweating, salivation, hypotension, bradycardia, convulsions, and increased muscle weakness, including respiratory muscles. Tachycardia, hypertension, emotional withdrawal, tachypnea, and increased muscle strength are not associated with overdose of these drugs. *Cognitive Level:* Analysis. *Nursing Process:* Assessment. *Client Need:* Physiological Integrity.

Answers to Critical Thinking Questions

1 The client should reassess with a healthcare provider the need for regular Mylanta. This drug contains magnesium, which may cause increased absorption and toxicity. The client needs teaching on decreasing foods that contain vitamin B_6 (for example, bananas, wheat germ, and green vegetables) because vitamin B_6 may also cause an increase in the absorption of the medication. Teaching should include information about a potential loss of glycemic control (because this patient is diabetic) and safety issues related to postural hypotension.

2 A client on benztropine (Cogentin) has a decreased ability to tolerate heat. Arizona in July is hot, so the patient should be taught to avoid hot climates, if at all possible, or to increase rest periods, avoid exertion, and observe for signs of heat intolerance. When symptoms occur, the client must immediately get out of the heat and rest.

3 The nurse should refer the client and his wife to a healthcare provider regarding the appropriateness of this medication (this is not a nursing function). The couple should be educated regarding safety issues such as postural hypotension and bradycardia that may occur with this medication. Anorexia is also a potential problem; this client has diabetes and thus may have glycemic issues.

CHAPTER 21
Answers to NCLEX-RN® Review Questions

1 Answers: 1, 2, 5

Rationale: Adverse reactions to cyclobenzaprine include drowsiness, dizziness, dry mouth, rash, and tachycardia. Because medication can cause drowsiness and dizziness, ensuring client safety must be a priority. Usually, clients experiencing back pain have orders for limited ambulation until muscle spasms have subsided. *Cognitive Level:* Analysis. *Nursing Process:* Implementation. *Client Need:* Physiological Integrity.

2 Answer: 4

Rationale: An adverse effect of botulinum is pain. The drug is injected directly into the muscle. Pain associated with injections is usually blocked by a local anesthetic. Treatment with botulinum helps improve muscle strength, but therapeutic effects are usually delayed by a few days. *Cognitive Level:* Analysis. *Nursing Process:* Implementation. *Client Need:* Physiological Integrity.

3 Answer: 1

Rationale: Elevated serum liver enzymes should be reported to the physician. Cyclobenzaprine may cause serious liver damage. The medication should be held until the healthcare provider has been notified. *Cognitive Level:* Analysis. *Nursing Process:* Implementation. *Client Need:* Physiological Integrity.

4 Answer: 3

Rationale: Verapamil is a calcium channel blocker. Administer the medication, but remember that the client is at increased risk of ventricular fibrillation and cardiovascular collapse when taking this drug with dantrolene sodium. Therefore, monitor cardiovascular status closely. Neurological and renal function monitoring are not the priority assessment. *Cognitive Level:* Analysis. *Nursing Process:* Implementation. *Client Need:* Physiological Integrity.

5 Answer: 4

Rationale: Clients should be instructed to report side effects such as muscle weakness, drowsiness, dry mouth, dizziness, nausea, diarrhea, tachycardia, erratic blood pressure, photosensitivity, and urine retention. Until effects are known, the client should not drive. It may take a few hours for the drug to become effective. *Cognitive Level:* Analysis. *Nursing Process:* Evaluation. *Client Need:* Physiological Integrity.

Answers to Critical Thinking Questions

1 The nurse would anticipate a decrease in the client's spasticity after 1 week of therapy. If there has been no improvement in 45 days, the medication regimen is usually discontinued. In this case, the nurse should evaluate the client's muscle firmness, pain experience, range of motion, and ability to maintain posture and alignment when in a wheelchair. When spasticity is used to maintain posture, dantrolene should not be used. In this case, the client's spasticity involved only the lower extremities.

2 Leg and foot cramps have anecdotally been associated with tamoxifen, an antiestrogenic drug. Tamoxifen, which has been shown to reduce the recurrence of some breast cancers, has been demonstrated to preserve bone density. Tamoxifen has several side effects that affect lifestyle, including the potential for weight gain and leg cramps. The nurse should assess the following factors before responding to this client's concerns:

- What is the client's activity level? Muscle cramps are associated with muscle fatigue.
- Does she take exogenous calcium?
- Can she tolerate dietary sources of calcium?

Interventions for leg cramps include the following:
- Stretching exercises before sleep
- Daily calcium and magnesium supplements
- Increasing dietary calcium intake
- Drinking a glass of tonic water (containing quinine) at bedtime

This client needs to relate her concerns to the oncologist. A healthcare provider may consider starting the client on quinine 200 to 300 mg at bedtime. This is an off-label use and requires careful client evaluation.

3 Cyclobenzaprine (Flexeril) has been demonstrated to produce significant anticholinergic activity. Students should recall that anticholinergics block the action of the neurotransmitter acetylcholine at the muscarinic receptors in the parasympathetic nervous system. This allows the activities of the sympathetic nervous system to dominate. In this case, the result has been a decrease in oral secretions and relaxation of the smooth muscle of the GI tract. Decreased peristalsis and motility can result in constipation. The anticholinergic effect is also responsible for urine retention because of increased constriction of the internal sphincter.

CHAPTER 22
Answers to NCLEX-RN® Review Questions

1 Answer: 2

Rationale: Diarrhea, not constipation, is a potential side effect of HMG-CoA reductase inhibitors. Bile acid resins are not absorbed from the small intestine and may cause constipation and hemorrhoids. Hypokalemia may occur with use of bile acid resins. *Cognitive Level:* Analysis *Nursing Process:* Assessment. *Client Need:* Physiological Integrity.

2 Answer: 3

Rationale: Nicotinic acid is used to decrease VLDL levels, and because LDL is synthesised from VLDL, there is a resultant reduction in LDL cholesterol levels. *Cognitive Level:* Analysis. *Nursing Process:* Evaluation. *Client Need:* Physiological Integrity.

3 Answers: 1, 2, 4, 5

Rationale: Side effects of nicotinic acid include nausea, diarrhea, excess gas, flushing, and hot flashes. Constipation is associated with bile acid resins. *Cognitive Level:* Application. *Nursing Process:* Assessment. *Client Need:* Physiological Integrity.

4 Answer: 3

Rationale: The nurse teaches the client with a diagnosis of hyperlipidemia about lipids in the body. The nurse informs the client that the major storage form of fat in the body is triglycerides. *Cognitive Level:* Analysis. *Nursing Process:* Implementation. *Client Need:* Health Promotion and Maintenance.

5 Answer: 3

Rationale: Optimal LDL levels should be less than 100 mg/dl. HDL levels less than 40 mg/dl are considered low. *Cognitive Level:* Analysis. *Nursing Process:* Assessment. *Client Need:* Physiological Integrity.

Answers to Critical Thinking Questions

1 Photosensitivity is a major problem with atorvastatin (Lipitor), so the client must take precautions such as using sunscreen, wearing sunglasses and protective clothing, and staying out of the direct sun as much as possible. This will probably be a lifestyle change for this client, and education with reinforcement is necessary.

2 This medication has the possibility of causing esophageal irritation, so taking the proper fluids or food with this medication is important. Pulpy fruit such as applesauce could be used for dual purposes with this drug, because the applesauce works for the esophageal irritation, and it also may help prevent the constipation caused by the drug.

3 The nurse should advise this client to seek medical advice before self-medicating—especially because this client has diabetes, and many drugs affect hyperglycemic medications and blood glucose levels. Niacin can cause hyperglycemia in this client, so serum glucose levels should be evaluated. The flushing and hot flashes are normal side effects of this medication.

Answer to Avoiding Medication Errors

The nurse should have administered Questran at least 4 hours before or 2 hours after digoxin and tetracycline because there is decreased absorption if they are administered together.

CHAPTER 23
Answers to NCLEX-RN® Review Questions

1 Answer: 2
Rationale: Lasix was prescribed as an adjunct treatment for hypertension. Blood pressure within normal limits indicates that treatment has been effective. Absence of edema, weight loss, and frequency of voiding is related to fluid status. **Cognitive Level:** Analysis. **Nursing Process:** Evaluation. **Client Need:** Physiological Integrity.

2 Answer: 1
Rationale: HCTZ is a thiazide diuretic. It acts on the kidney tubules to decrease the reabsorption of sodium. When reabsorption is blocked, more sodium is sent into the urine. The most common side effect of HCTZ is electrolyte sodium and potassium depletion. The client's potassium level is decreased at 2.8 mEq/ml. Administering HCTZ could further deplete the client's potassium level. **Cognitive Level:** Analysis. **Nursing Process:** Diagnosis. **Client Need:** Physiological Integrity.

3 Answer: 2
Rationale: The advantage of using two drugs is that lower doses of each may be used, resulting in fewer side effects and better client compliance. **Cognitive Level:** Application. **Nursing Process:** Planning. **Client Need:** Physiological Integrity.

4 Answer: 3
Rationale: ACE inhibitors block the effects of angiotensin II, decreasing blood pressure through two mechanisms: lowering peripheral resistance and decreasing blood volume. **Cognitive Level:** Application. **Nursing Process:** Assessment. **Client Need:** Physiological Integrity.

5 Answers: 2, 3, 4, 5
Side effects of ACE inhibitors include persistent cough and postural hypotension. Hyperkalemia may occur and can be a major concern for those with diabetes or renal impairment and in clients taking potassium-sparing diuretics. Though rare, the most serious adverse effect of ACE inhibitors is the development of angioedema. **Cognitive Level:** Analysis. **Nursing Process:** Assessment. **Client Need:** Physiological Integrity.

Answers to Critical Thinking Questions

1 Traditionally, if the client has a systolic blood pressure of less than 110 mm Hg, the dose should be held unless verified with the healthcare provider that the dose should be given. The client is on a low-sodium, low-protein diet, which may contribute to hypotension. Because the client has mild renal failure, the excretion of the drug may be prolonged and also contribute to the hypotensive effects. If the healthcare provider wants the client to receive the benazepril (Lotensin), then the BP should be rechecked at 30 minutes and 60 minutes after the medication is given. The client should be cautioned about postural hypotension.

2 Atenolol (Tenormin) is a beta₁-adrenergic blocker that works directly on the heart. The nurse and the client need to be aware that the client's heart rate will rarely go above 80 beats per minute because of the action of the medication. Tachycardia is one of the adrenergic signs of hypoglycemia that would not be evident with this client. Both the nurse and client need to be aware of the more subtle signs of hypoglycemia (or any other condition that may be

recognized by tachycardia) that would not be evident with a client on beta-blocking medications.

3 The nurse must be careful that the client's blood pressure is not lowered too dramatically, or hypotension may occur. This is an example of a case in which 120/80 mm Hg is not necessarily an ideal blood pressure reading. Typically, the blood pressure is not lowered below 160 mm Hg systolic. The client is reevaluated and then (often many hours later) the blood pressure is brought down further. This drip is light sensitive and must remain covered with foil during infusion. Once prepared, the drip is stable for only 24 hours. Nitroprusside is a cyanide by-product; therefore, any client on this drug must be monitored for cyanide toxicity.

CHAPTER 24
Answers to NCLEX-RN® Review Questions

1 Answer: 3
Rationale: Digoxin helps increase the contractility of the heart. The heart rate will increase with the use of digoxin. **Cognitive Level:** Analysis. **Nursing Process:** Evaluation. **Client Need:** Physiological Integrity.

2 Answer: 2
Rationale: Normal serum potassium level is 3.5 to 5.0 mEq/L. Hypokalemia may predispose the client to digitalis toxicity. **Cognitive Level:** Analysis. **Nursing Process:** Implementation. **Client Need:** Physiological Integrity.

3 Answer: 3
Rationale: ACE inhibitors can cause severe hypotension with initial doses. The nurse should monitor the client closely for several hours. **Cognitive Level:** Analysis. **Nursing Process:** Implementation. **Client Need:** Physiological Integrity.

4 Answer: 2
Rationale: Potassium levels should be closely monitored. Encouraging the eating of foods rich in potassium could help maintain potassium levels. **Cognitive Level:** Application. **Nursing Process:** Planning. **Client Need:** Physiological Integrity.

5 Answers: 1, 3, 4, 5
Rationale: Side effects of this medication may include cough, headache, dizziness, change in sensation of taste, vomiting and diarrhea, and hypotension. Hyperkalemia may occur, especially when the drug is taken concurrently with potassium-sparing diuretics. **Cognitive Level:** Analysis. **Nursing Process:** Assessment. **Client Need:** Physiological Integrity.

Answers to Critical Thinking Questions

1 The nurse should first note improved signs of perfusion if this medication is effective. The nurse would evaluate the patient's skin signs, blood pressure, heart rate, and urine output. If the medication is effective, all these will be within normal limits, or at least improved from the client's baseline. The ECG may show improvement with a normal sinus rhythm once the digoxin (Lanoxin) has reached therapeutic level.

2 The nurse understands that there is a cross-sensitivity between sulfa and furosemide (Lasix) and therefore would inform the healthcare provider of the client's allergy status so a different diuretic might be utilized. Morphine is an appropriate medication for this client, not only for its analgesic and sedative effects but also for the increased venous capacitance that it causes.

3 This diabetic client needs to be educated about the importance of regular glucose checks, because this medication may cause the blood sugar to vary sporadically. Typically, hypoglycemia is more of a problem, so the client needs to be especially aware of the symptoms and treatment of hypoglycemia. Safety should be emphasized, especially regarding postural hypotension.

CHAPTER 25
Answers to NCLEX-RN® Review Questions

1 Answer: 2

Rationale: At the initial onset of chest pain, sublingual nitroglycerin is administered to assist in the diagnosis, and three doses may be taken 5 minutes apart. Pain that persists 5 to 10 minutes after the initial dose may indicate an MI, and the client should seek medical assistance. *Cognitive Level:* Application. *Nursing Process:* Implementation. *Client Need:* Physiological Integrity.

2 Answer: 4

Rationale: Antianginal drugs act by decreasing myocardial oxygen demand. This is accomplished by decreasing heart rate, preload, contractility, and afterload. *Cognitive Level:* Application. *Nursing Process:* Implementation. *Client Need:* Physiological Integrity.

3 Answer: 1

Rationale: Beta-blockers decrease the workload of the heart by slowing heart rate and reducing contractility. Calcium channel blockers decrease peripheral resistance. Nitrates relax arterial and venous smooth muscles. *Cognitive Level:* Application. *Nursing Process:* Assessment. *Client Need:* Physiological Integrity.

4 Answer: 4

Rationale: Clients are often instructed to remove the transdermal patch for 6 to 12 hours each day or withhold the nighttime dose of the oral medications to delay the development of tolerance. Because the oxygen demands of the heart during sleep are diminished, the client with stable angina experiences few anginal episodes during this drug-free interval. *Cognitive Level:* Application. *Nursing Process:* Implementation. *Client Need:* Physiological Integrity.

5 Answers: 4, 2, 1, 3, 5

Rationale: Prior to administering nitrates for chest pain, the nurse must first assess location, quality, and intensity of pain. Nitrates should not be administered if the client is hypotensive or if the heart rate is below 60 beats per minute. Once nitrates are administered, blood pressure must be monitored, because hypotension may occur. Documentation of interventions and outcomes is essential to the client's health history. *Cognitive Level:* Application. *Nursing Process:* Implementation. *Client Need:* Physiological Integrity.

Answers to Critical Thinking Questions

1 The nurse needs to verify blood pressure. A major adverse effect of nitroglycerin is hypotension. If the systolic blood pressure remains below 100 mm Hg, the nurse needs to notify the healthcare provider of the client's chest pain and blood pressure.

2 Beta-blockers slow the heart rate to a desired 50 to 65 beats per minute (bpm). Many clients suffer from postural hypotension if the heart rate drops below 60 bpm; therefore, the nurse needs to educate the client about the necessity of changing positions slowly. The nurse must be aware that a cardinal sign of decreasing cardiac output is tachycardia—a heart rate greater than 100 bpm for the client not on beta-blockers. If the client is on beta-blocking medication, the heart rate may not go above 80 to 85 bpm and is considered tachycardia for this type of client.

3 Diltiazem (Cardizem) has been given to lower the heart rate and to decrease the myocardial oxygen consumption for this client with chest pain. The nurse must monitor closely for hypotension, because this medication lowers the heart rate but also lowers the blood pressure, and this client already has a borderline low blood pressure of 100/60 mm Hg. The client should be on a cardiac monitor with frequent monitoring of blood pressure.

CHAPTER 26
Answers to NCLEX-RN® Review Questions

1 Answer: 3

Rationale: There is increased incidence of hypoglycemia with type 1 diabetes mellitus, because propranolol may inhibit glycogenolysis. *Cognitive Level:* Application. *Nursing Process:* Assessment. *Client Need:* Physiological Integrity.

2 Answer: 1

Rationale: Studies have shown that because of a lack of specific drug-metabolizing enzyme, Asians metabolize propranolol more quickly than Caucasians; thus, the drug has a significantly greater effect on heart rate for Asians. *Cognitive Level:* Analysis. *Nursing Process:* Assessment. *Client Need:* Physiological Integrity.

3 Answer: 2

Rationale: Sodium channel blockers are the largest group of antidysrhythmics and act by slowing the rate of impulse conduction across the heart. *Cognitive Level:* Analysis. *Nursing Process:* Assessment. *Client Need:* Physiological Integrity.

4 Answers: 1, 3, 4

Rationale: Because antidysrhythmics can slow the heart rate, the client may experience hypotension, dizziness, or weakness. *Cognitive Level:* Analysis. *Nursing Process:* Assessment. *Client Need:* Physiological Integrity.

5 Answer: 3

Rationale: Calcium influx into the cells signals release of stored calcium. Intracellular calcium is responsible for the contraction of cardiac muscles. *Cognitive Level:* Analysis. *Nursing Process:* Assessment. *Client Need:* Physiological Integrity.

Answers to Critical Thinking Questions

1 Propranolol (Inderal) is a nonselective beta-adrenergic blocker, which means it acts on both the intended system (heart) and the lungs. This may cause the client to have untoward lung problems such as shortness of breath; therefore, this client should not be taking propranolol.

2 The client should be monitored closely for hypotension, especially in the first few weeks of treatment, and should be taught about postural hypotension. Pulmonary toxicity is a major complication of this drug, so the client should be monitored for cough or shortness of breath. Because both digoxin (Lanoxin) and amiodarone (Cordarone) slow the heart rate, the client must be monitored closely for bradycardia. Safety and pulmonary symptoms are priorities of care for this client. Amiodarone often increases the effects of digoxin and warfarin (Coumadin) and thus must be closely monitored.

3 Bradycardia is a potential problem for a client taking verapamil (Isoptin) and digoxin. The client may exhibit signs of decreased cardiac output, such as pale skin, chest pain, dyspnea, hypotension, and altered level of consciousness. The client needs to be taught how to recognize the signs of decreasing cardiac output as well as how to assess heart rate.

Answer to Avoiding Medication Errors

Don't administer the medication. Research the correct dosage and administration. The correct dose of lidocaine is 1–1.5 mg/kg IV every 3 to 5 minutes up to a maximum dose of 3 mg/kg. It should be given over a 2-minute period, and you should obtain an apical heart rate. The instructions regarding the continuous infusion are unclear. Lidocaine is generally administered 1–4 mg/minute after a bolus dose. Never proceed with drug administration until you are confident of the correct parameters for the particular medication.

CHAPTER 27
Answers to NCLEX-RN® Review Questions

1 Answer: 4

Rationale: Prothrombinase converts prothrombin to thrombin. Thrombin then converts fibrinogen to long strands of fibrin, which provide a framework for the clot. Thrombin and fibrin are formed only after the injury occurs. Fibrin strands form an insoluble web over the injured area to stop blood loss. *Cognitive Level:* Analysis. *Nursing Process:* Implementation. *Client Need:* Physiological Integrity.

2 Answer: 2

Rationale: Anticoagulants do not change the viscosity of the blood. Instead, anticoagulants exert a negative charge on the surface of the platelets, so that clumping or aggregation of cells is inhibited. *Cognitive Level:* Analysis. *Nursing Process:* Implementation. *Client Need:* Physiological Integrity.

3 Answers: 1, 2, 3

Rationale: Enoxaparin is a low-molecular-weight heparin (LMWH). This class of drugs has fewer side effects, including being less likely to cause thrombocytopenia. Clients and family can be taught to give subcutaneous injections at home. Teaching should include not taking any other medications without first consulting the healthcare provider and recognizing the signs and symptoms of bleeding. *Cognitive Level:* Analysis. *Nursing Process:* Implementation. *Client Need:* Physiological Integrity.

4 Answer: 2

Rationale: PT is the lab test for monitoring the effectiveness of warfarin (Coumadin) therapy. During therapeutic anticoagulation, PT should increase to one to two times the client's baseline level. PT is also reported as an international normalized ratio (INR). INR values of 2 to 3.5 are considered therapeutic. *Cognitive Level:* Analysis. *Nursing Process:* Assessment. *Client Need:* Physiological Integrity.

5 Answer: 2

Rationale: Changes in peripheral pulses, paresthesias, positive Homans' sign, and prominence of superficial veins indicate that clotting is occurring in peripheral arterial or venous vasculature. *Cognitive Level:* Analysis. *Nursing Process:* Assessment. *Client Need:* Physiological Integrity.

Answers to Critical Thinking Questions

1 The nurse should question the healthcare provider about this order. No client who appears to be having a CVA (brain attack) should have heparin until a CT scan of the brain has been done. Approximately 20% of CVAs are hemorrhagic; these types of CVAs must be ruled out before an anticoagulant is given.

2 The major adverse effect of a fibrinolytic drug is bleeding. All tubes (nasogastric, Foley, or endotracheal) must be inserted, blood needs to be drawn, and IVs need to be inserted before the medication is given, or the drugs may potentiate bleeding in this client.

3 Whether the nurse gives this drug or is teaching the client to self-administer the medication, proper placement of the needle in the abdomen is vital. The injection must be given at least 1 to 2 inches away from the umbilicus. Major blood vessels run close to the umbilicus, and if the LMWH is given near one of these vessels, there is an increased chance of bleeding into the abdomen or formation of a large (and often initially occult) hematoma in the abdomen.

Answer to Avoiding Medication Errors

Most prescribers recommend that mothers not breast-feed while taking warfarin (Coumadin). Heparin is considered safe for breast-feeding mothers. Warfarin is pregnancy category X. Heparin is not excreted into the breast milk.

CHAPTER 28
Answers to NCLEX-RN® Review Questions

1 Answer: 1 tablet

Rationale: 1 gram = 1000 mg. 1000 mg divided by 3 is 333 mg. One tablet will be administered. *Cognitive Level:* Application. *Nursing Process:* Implementation. *Client Need:* Physiological Integrity.

2 Answer: 3

Rationale: Secreted by the kidney, erythropoietin travels to the bone marrow, where it interacts with receptors on hematopoietic stem cells with the message to increase erythrocyte production. The primary signal for the increased secretion of erythropoietin is a reduction in oxygen reaching the kidney. *Cognitive Level:* Analysis. *Nursing Process:* Assessment. *Client Need:* Physiological Integrity.

3 Answer: 2

Rationale: This medication does not cure the primary disease condition; however, it helps reduce the anemia that dramatically affects the client's ability to function. The hematocrit and hemoglobin levels will provide reference for evaluating the drug's effectiveness. *Cognitive Level:* Analysis. *Nursing Process:* Evaluation. *Client Need:* Physiological Integrity.

4 Answer: 1

Rationale: This drug increases the risk of thromboembolic disease. The client should be monitored for early signs of CVA or MI. *Cognitive Level:* Analysis. *Nursing Process:* Assessment. *Client Need:* Safe, Effective Care.

5 Answer: 2

Rationale: Intrinsic factor is required for vitamin B_{12} to be absorbed from the intestine. The most profound consequence of vitamin B_{12} deficiency is pernicious anemia or megaloblastic anemia. *Cognitive Level:* Analysis. *Nursing Process:* Assessment. *Client Need:* Physiological Integrity.

Answers to Critical Thinking Questions

1 Clients with chronic renal failure often have decreased secretion of endogenous erythropoietin and therefore require a medication such as epoetin alfa (Epogen) to stimulate RBC production and reduce the potential of becoming anemic (or to decrease the effects of anemia). Teaching points should include the importance of monitoring blood pressure for hypertension. Side effects such as nausea, vomiting, constipation, redness/pain at the injection site, confusion, numbness, chest pain, and difficulty breathing should be reported to the healthcare provider. The client should also be instructed to maintain a healthy diet and follow any dietary restrictions necessary because of renal failure.

2 Clients who are receiving filgrastim (Neupogen) should have their vital signs assessed every 4 hours (especially pulse and temperature) to monitor for signs of infection related to a low WBC count. Other nursing interventions include assessing for signs and symptoms of myocardial infarction, dysrhythmias, and hepatic dysfunction during treatment.

3 Clients taking this drug need to be educated about the GI distress that may occur while on iron supplements. This medication may be taken with food to reduce the potential for GI upset. Constipation is a common complaint of clients on this medication, so preventive measures need to be taken. The client needs to ensure that this medication has a child-resistant cap and is safely secured, because overdose of iron supplements is a common toxicology emergency for children.

CHAPTER 29
Answers to NCLEX-RN® Review Questions

1 Answer: 1
Rationale: Lactated Ringer's is a crystalloid solution that contains electrolytes in a concentration similar to that of plasma. It leaves the blood and enters the cells, replacing fluids and promoting urinary output. *Cognitive Level:* Application. *Nursing Process:* Evaluation. *Client Need:* Physiological Integrity.

2 Answers: 1, 2
Rationale: With increased cardiac output, renal function should improve, and there should be an increase in urine output. BUN and creatinine levels should be normal. Blood pressure should increase. *Cognitive Level:* Analysis. *Nursing Process:* Evaluation. *Client Need:* Physiological Integrity.

3 Answer: 2
Rationale: Dobutamine is beneficial when shock is caused by heart failure. The drug increases contractility and has the potential to cause dysrhythmias. *Cognitive Level:* Analysis. *Nursing Process:* Assessment. *Client Need:* Physiological Integrity.

4 Answer: 3
Rationale: Anaphylactic reactions may occur with the use of plasma protein fraction (Plasmanate). Symptoms include periorbital edema, urticaria, wheezing, and respiratory difficulties. *Cognitive Level:* Analysis. *Nursing Process:* Assessment. *Client Need:* Physiological Integrity.

5 Answer: 1
Rationale: Albumin is a colloid solution. Colloids pull fluid into the vascular space. Circulatory overload may occur. The nurse should assess the client for symptoms of heart failure. *Cognitive Level:* Analysis. *Nursing Process:* Assessment. *Client Need:* Physiological Integrity.

Answers to Critical Thinking Questions

1 A major action of this vasopressor medication is the positive inotropic effect it has on a damaged myocardium that is having difficulty maintaining a good cardiac output (and, therefore, blood pressure). Nursing assessments include constant monitoring of blood pressure, heart rate and rhythm, fluid volume status, and urine output. The drip must be slowly tapered to a point at which the blood pressure is well maintained, normally a systolic blood pressure of greater than 100 mm Hg. The nurse must never consider a blood pressure reading as okay and shut off the vasopressor drip—the client may immediately become acutely hypotensive.

2 This isotonic solution is appropriate for this client. Based on history and assessment, the client is demonstrating signs of being hypovolemic (heart rate of 122 bpm) and requires a solution that will meet the intracellular need. The client must be monitored for hypernatremia and hyperchloremia if more than 3 L of normal saline is given. As the client responds to the fluid, the nurse will note a corresponding decrease in the heart rate.

3 This is not an appropriate IV solution for a client with a head injury. Once this IV solution is infused into the client, it is considered to be a hypotonic solution that moves fluids into the cells. A client with an increased ICP cannot tolerate an increase of fluid at the cellular level because this may cause the brain to herniate and lead to death.

CHAPTER 30
Answers to NCLEX-RN® Review Questions

1 Answer: 1
Rationale: Because the kidneys excrete most drugs, clients with renal failure will need a significantly lower dosage of medications that may damage the kidneys, to avoid fatal consequences. *Cognitive Level:* Analysis. *Nursing Process:* Implementation. *Client Need:* Physiological Integrity.

2 Answer: 1
Rationale: Potassium is a serious side effect of loop diuretics, and this is a serious concern for clients being treated with digoxin (Lanoxin). *Cognitive Level:* Analysis. *Nursing Process:* Evaluation. *Client Need:* Physiological Integrity.

3 Answer: 3
Rationale: Rapid excretion of large amounts of fluid predisposes the client to potassium deficits and is manifested by hypotension, dizziness, cardiac dysrhythmias, and fainting. Polydipsia is not associated with hypokalemia, but with diabetes. Hypertension is an indication for the use of diuretics. Diarrhea can be associated with hyperkalemia. *Cognitive Level:* Analysis. *Nursing Process:* Assessment. *Client Need:* Physiological Integrity.

4 Answer: 2
Mannitol increases osmolarity of glomerular filtrate, which raises osmotic pressure in renal tubules and decreases absorption of water and electrolytes. Although mannitol increases urine output, it does not draw excess fluid from tissue spaces and should be used with caution in clients with CHF. Acetazolamide (Diamox) is used to decrease intraocular fluid pressure clients with open-angle glaucoma. Bumetanide (Bumex) and ethacrynic acid (Edecrin) are loop diuretics. *Cognitive Level:* Analysis. *Nursing Process:* Assessment. *Client Need:* Physiological Integrity.

5 Answers: 2, 4
Rationale: Type 2 diabetes is the most common cause of chronic renal failure; hypertension is the second leading cause. *Cognitive Level:* Application. *Nursing Process:* Assessment. *Client Need:* Physiological Integrity.

Answers to Critical Thinking Questions

1 Losartan (Cozaar) is an angiotensin II receptor antagonist commonly prescribed for hypertension. Because some clients do not respond adequately to monotherapy, a drug that offers combined therapy, Hyzaar, is added. Hyzaar combines losartan with hydrochlorothiazide, a diuretic. This combination decreases blood pressure initially by reducing blood volume and arterial resistance. Over time, the diuretic is effective in maintaining the desired change in sodium balance with a resultant decrease in the sensitivity of vessels to norepinephrine. Angiotensin II–receptor antagonists appear to prevent the hypokalemia associated with thiazide therapy.

2 The nurse should carefully monitor fluid status. Because the primary concern is cardiopulmonary, the nurse should assess and document lung sounds, vital signs, and urine output. Depending on the client's condition, a Foley catheter may be inserted to permit the measurement of hourly outputs. Daily weights should be obtained. Edema should be evaluated and documented, as well as status of mucous membranes and skin turgor. Because furosemide (Lasix) is a loop diuretic, the nurse would anticipate a rapid and profound diuresis. Therefore, the nurse should also observe for signs of dehydration and potassium depletion over the course of therapy.

3 Cerebral edema occurs as a result of the body's response to an initial head trauma. In this case, the client sustained a skull fracture and underwent the trauma of required surgery. The nurse should explain to the mother that mannitol (Osmitrol) helps reduce swelling or cerebral edema at the site of her son's injury. The nurse might explain that the drug helps "pull" water from the site of injury and carry it to the kidneys, where it is eliminated. The client's mother should understand that the goal of decreasing swelling is to promote tissue recovery.

Nurses must be sensitive to the fact that family members may have severe emotional reactions to a client's injury and need help to focus on short-term goals for recovery when the long-term prognosis is not known. For additional information on the action or administration of mannitol, students should consult a drug handbook.

CHAPTER 31
Answers to NCLEX-RN® Review Questions

1 Answer: 2
Rationale: Thirst is the most important regulator of fluid intake. *Cognitive Level:* Analysis. *Nursing Process:* Assessment. *Client Need:* Physiological Integrity.

2 Answer: 2
Rationale: Dextran 40, a plasma volume expander, causes fluid to move rapidly from the tissues to vascular spaces, which places the client at risk for fluid overload. *Cognitive Level:* Analysis. *Nursing Process:* Implementation. *Client Need:* Physiological Integrity.

3 Answers: 1, 4
Rationale: Hypernatremia is defined as serum sodium levels higher than 148 mEq/L. A slight increase in sodium can be managed by diet. The healthcare provider should be notified of any elevated lab values. *Cognitive Level:* Analysis. *Nursing Process:* Implementation. *Client Need:* Physiological Integrity.

4 Answer: 4
Rationale: Hyperkalemia, a serum potassium level greater than 5 mEq/L, predisposes the client to cardiac and muscle irregularities such as cramping in the calves, paresthesia of the toes, and palpitations. *Cognitive Level:* Analysis. *Nursing Process:* Diagnosis. *Client Need:* Physiological Integrity.

5 Answer: 3
Rationale: Sodium bicarbonate acts by directly raising the pH of body fluids. It is the drug of choice for restoring plasma pH to normal limits. *Cognitive Level:* Analysis. *Nursing Process:* Implementation. *Client Need:* Physiological Integrity.

Answers to Critical Thinking Questions

1 Aggressive treatment with loop diuretics is a common cause of hypokalemia. As in this example, hypokalemia can produce a myriad of sequelae including dysrhythmias. KCl is indicated for clients with low potassium levels and is preferred over other potassium salts because chloride is simultaneously replaced. The nurse administering KCl must keep in mind several critical concerns to safeguard the client. The primary concern is the risk of potassium intoxication. High plasma concentrations of potassium may cause death through cardiac depression, arrhythmias, or arrest. The signs and symptoms of potassium overdose include mental confusion, weakness, listlessness, hypotension, and ECG abnormalities. In a client with heart disease, cardiac monitoring may be indicated during potassium infusion. Students should consult their drug handbooks and look up the maximum rates for infusing KCl in adults and children.

To prevent potassium intoxication, the nurse should carefully regulate the infusion of IV fluids. Most institutions require that any solution containing KCl be administered using an infusion pump. Prior to beginning and throughout the infusion, the nurse should assess the client's renal function (BUN and creatinine levels). A client with diminished renal function is more likely to develop hyperkalemia.

2 The student should recognize from an intravascular standpoint that this client is dehydrated despite her appearance. The client's elevated hematocrit and hemoglobin are indications of her degree of "dehydration." Most pregnant women present with dilution anemia. This client does not. The midwife recognizes the need to increase the intravascular fluid compartment to promote renal and uterine perfusion.

3 Excessive renal fluid loss due to diuretic therapy, such as with furosemide (Lasix), can contribute to fluid volume deficits in clients taking these medications. Because pharmacotherapy with thiazide or loop diuretics such as furosemide is the most common cause of potassium loss, clients taking these diuretics are usually instructed to take oral potassium supplements to prevent hypokalemia.

Answer to Avoiding Medication Errors

1 Student nurses are held to the same standard as nurses holding a license. Like the student nurse, the nursing instructor and the primary nurse are responsible if they checked the medication dosage prior to administration and did not question the order. The physician is responsible because the order was incorrect, but the errors should have been identified prior to reaching the client. The nurse manager retains accountability for the unit.

CHAPTER 32
Answers to NCLEX-RN® Review Questions

1 Answer: 4
Rationale: Due to immune system suppression by the medication, infections are common. *Cognitive Level:* Application. *Nursing Process:* Diagnosis. *Client Need:* Physiological Integrity.

2 Answer: 4
Rationale: Grapefruit juice increases cyclosporine levels 50% to 200%, resulting in drug toxicity. Hand washing is important to prevent infection. Renal toxicity and hypertension are adverse effects of cyclosporine therapy. *Cognitive Level:* Analysis. *Nursing Process:* Assessment. *Client Need:* Physiological Integrity.

3 Answer: 2
Rationale: Seventy-five percent of clients on cyclosporine experience decreased renal output because of physiological changes in the kidneys, such as microcalcification and interstitial fibrosis. The serum creatinine test is a good indicator of renal function. *Cognitive Level:* Analysis. *Nursing Process:* Assessment. *Client Need:* Physiological Integrity.

4 Answers: 1, 2, 4, 5
Rationale: Pregnancy, renal or liver disease, and metastatic cancer are contraindications to the use of immunostimulant drugs. Infection, immunodeficiency disease, and cancer are indications for use of these drugs. *Cognitive Level:* Analysis. *Nursing Process:* Assessment. *Client Need:* Physiological Integrity.

5 Answer: 1
Rationale: Active immunity occurs when the client has received the vaccine. Passive immunity is achieved by directly administering antibodies to a client. A titer is a measurement of the amount of antibody produced after a vaccine. *Cognitive Level:* Application. *Nursing Process:* Assessment. *Client Need:* Physiological Integrity.

Answers to Critical Thinking Questions

1 Sirolimus (Rapamune) is an immunosuppressant. The nurse should assess for any signs and symptoms of bleeding or jaundice and infection. The nurse should question the client regarding activities that may cause bleeding. The nurse should also assess for signs and symptoms of liver impairment. The nurse should notify the healthcare provider of the laboratory findings and educate the client to report any bleeding to the healthcare provider. The client should also report signs and symptoms of infection.

2 The client needs the protection of this passive form of immunity after an exposure to such an illness. The gamma globulin will act as a protective mechanism for 3 weeks while the client is in the window of opportunity for developing hepatitis A. This drug does not stimulate the client's immune system but will help protect the client from developing the disease. The nurse should inform the client that the shot is far less debilitating than the disease.

3 Cyclosporine is a toxic medication with many serious adverse effects. The nurse must understand that this drug cannot be given with grapefruit juice; clients who take this medication need their kidney function assessed regularly (not because of the kidney transplant but because cyclosporine reduces urine output). The nurse also must assess whether this client is taking steroids, which are often given concurrently with cyclosporine, as the serum glucose will need to be monitored regularly.

Answer to Avoiding Medication Errors

Methotrexate is given for rheumatoid arthritis in smaller doses than when used in cancer chemotherapy. It is thought to block metabolism of folic acid. For rheumatoid arthritis, clients take 10 to 12 mg once a week. It may modify the disease manifestations, or it may just improve symptoms and quality of life.

CHAPTER 33
Answers to NCLEX-RN® Review Questions

1 Answer: 3
Rationale: Acetaminophen has analgesic and antipyretic properties, but no anti-inflammatory actions. *Cognitive Level:* Analysis. *Nursing Process:* Implementation. *Client Need:* Physiological Integrity.

2 Answer: 3
Rationale: High doses of asprin can produce side effects of tinnitus, dizziness, headache, and sweating. *Cognitive Level:* Analysis. *Nursing Process:* Implementation. *Client Need:* Physiological Integrity.

3 Answer: 4
Rationale: Side effects that need to be reported immediately include difficulty breathing; heartburn; chest, abdomen, or joint or bone pain; nosebleed; blood in sputum when coughing, vomitus, urine, or stools; fever; chills or signs of infection; increased thirst or urination; fruity breath odor; falls; or mood swings. *Cognitive Level:* Analysis. *Nursing Process:* Implementation. *Nursing Process:* Physiological Integrity.

4 Answer: 4
Rationale: Monitor for development of Cushing's syndrome (adrenocortical excess) with signs and symptoms of bruising and a characteristic pattern of fat deposits in the cheeks (moon face), shoulders (buffalo hump), and abdomen. *Cognitive Level:* Analysis. *Nursing Process:* Diagnosis. *Client Need:* Physiological Integrity.

5 Answers: 1, 2, 3
Rationale: Prolonged, high fever can break down body tissues, reduce mental acuity, and lead to delirium or coma and death. *Cognitive Level:* Analysis. *Nursing Process:* Assessment. *Client Need:* Physiological Integrity.

Answers to Critical Thinking Questions

1 This client has many potential problems related to the use of prednisone over a sustained period. The primary current concern is the hyperglycemia—an adverse effect of the prednisone that can become serious when the client is diabetic. Blood pressure must be monitored for potential hypertension, which is related to sodium retention and, therefore, increased water retention caused by the prednisone. The client is also at high risk for infection while on prednisone because of suppression of the immune system, also related to the diabetes.

2 The nurse should give the client celecoxib (Celebrex) for the elbow inflammation and pain. This medication should provide adequate relief of the symptoms for this client. Ensure that the client is not allergic to sulfa prior to giving this medication. The client should not take acetaminophen (Tylenol) because of related potential liver compromise secondary to alcohol abuse. The client should not take ibuprofen (Motrin) because of the potential for gastric bleeding. The client's stomach is already at risk because of alcohol abuse, and the chance for bleeding is elevated because of potential liver problems secondary to alcohol abuse.

3 The nurse should educate the mother that aspirin and aspirin-containing products should not be given to children younger than age 18. These drugs have been implicated in the development of Reye's syndrome. Acetaminophen is the antipyretic of choice for treating most fevers. The nurse should also further question the mother regarding the length and severity of symptoms.

CHAPTER 34
Answers to NCLEX-RN® Review Questions

1 Answer: 1
Rationale: A superinfection is a side effect of antibiotic therapy. The antibiotic destroys the body's normal flora, resulting in another infection. The other options do not describe a superinfection. *Cognitive Level:* Application. *Nursing Process:* Implementation. *Client Need:* Physiological Integrity.

2 Answer: 2
Rationale: Many people will discontinue medication after improvement is noted. All antibiotic regimens must be completed to prevent recurrence of infection. Some penicillins (amoxicillin) should be taken with meals, whereas all others should be taken 1 hour before or 2 hours after meals. Penicillins should be used with caution during breast-feeding. *Cognitive Level:* Analysis. *Nursing Process:* Implementation. *Client Need:* Physiological Integrity.

3 Answer: 4
Rationale: This drug has the ability to cause permanent mottling and discoloration of teeth, and therefore is not good for children younger than 8 years of age. Tetracyclines have one of the broadest spectrums of the antibiotics and are contraindicated in pregnancy. *Cognitive Level:* Analysis. *Nursing Process:* Implementation. *Client Need:* Physiological Integrity.

4 Answer: 4
Rationale: This anti-infective is noted for its toxic effects on kidneys and vestibular apparatus. Clients should be monitored for ototoxicity and nephrotoxicity during and after therapy. Aminoglycosides do not cause discoloration of the teeth. Fluid intake should be increased with aminoglycosides. Aminoglycosides are poorly absorbed from the GI tract and are administered parentally for systemic bacterial infections. *Cognitive Level:* Analysis. *Nursing Process:* Implementation. *Client Need:* Physiological Integrity.

5 Answers: 1, 2, 3
Rationale: For the medication to reach the microorganism, it is critical that the medicine be taken for 6 to 12 months, and possibly as long as 24 months. Antitubercular drugs are also used for prevention and treatment. Multiple drug therapy is necessary because the Mycobacteria grow slowly, and resistance is common. Using multiple drugs in different combinations during the long treatment period lowers the potential for resistance and increases the chances for successful therapy. *Cognitive Level:* Analysis. *Nursing Process:* Implementation. *Client Need:* Physiological Integrity.

Answers to Critical Thinking Questions

1 This client should not be on tetracycline (Achromycin) while pregnant because tetracycline is a category D drug that has teratogenic effects on the fetus. Counseling should be provided for alternative sources of care for her acne as well as for use of drugs when pregnant.

2 No, the nurse should not give the erythromycin. This client has a history of hepatitis B, and this medication is metabolized by the liver. An alternative type of antibiotic should be utilized.

3 This medication is typically reserved for more serious infections because of its higher potential for toxicity. Renal function is a priority assessment for this client. The nurse should monitor urine output, urine protein, and serum BUN and creatinine on a regular basis. A secondary priority is hearing assessment, because ototoxicity is common for clients on gentamicin.

Answer to Avoiding Medication Errors

The nurse should have questioned the physician regarding Bactrim, which contains sulfamethoxazole. Because the client has an allergy to sulfa drugs, he would be allergic to Bactrim as well. Some individuals experience nausea, a side effect of sulfa drugs. True allergies involve histamine-mediated responses and result in symptoms such as a rash or hives. In severe cases, bronchospasm and cardiovascular compromise are possible. Because the drug is a large tablet, it is permissible to break the tablet in half and provide a large glass of water.

CHAPTER 35
Answers to NCLEX-RN® Questions

1 Answer: 3
Rationale: Systemic antifungal drugs have little or no antibacterial activity. Fluid intake should be increased with this medication because it can affect renal function. The full course of therapy should be completed. All intramuscular sites have the potential to bruise. *Cognitive Level:* Analysis. *Nursing Process:* Implementation. *Client Need:* Physiological Integrity.

2 Answer: 2
Rationale: The client needs to be assessed for preexisting cardiovascular disease, and an ECG should be done. Quinine therapy does not require a consent to be signed, but education is needed. All medication should be continued unless otherwise specified. *Cognitive Level:* Analysis. *Nursing Process:* Implementation. *Client Need:* Physiological Integrity.

3 Answer: 4
Rationale: Chloroquine (Aralen) is the classic antimalarial for treating the acute stage. Proguanil (Paludrine) is the prototype antimalarial for prophylaxis. Rizatriptan (Maxalt) is used in the treatment of migraines. *Cognitive Level:* Analysis. *Nursing Process:* Implementation. *Client Need:* Physiological Integrity.

4 Answers: 1, 2, 3, 4
Rationale: Play habits and hygiene of children can contribute to the transmission and reinfestation of pinworms and roundworms. It is important that all family members understand the importance of hand washing to prevent the transmission of worms. Correct hand washing should be taught, and children should not be allowed to play in sandboxes that are left uncovered. Children should also wear shoes when outside playing to prevent skin invasion. *Cognitive Level:* Analysis. *Nursing Process:* Implementation. *Client Need:* Safe, Effective Care Environment.

5 Answer: 2
Rationale: Clients using antihelminthic therapy should practice reliable contraception because these drugs must be used cautiously in clients who are pregnant or lactating. The complete course of medication should be taken. Family members living in close contact may require antihelminthic therapy also. Itching, fatigue, and abdominal pain are side effects that should be reported to the healthcare provider. *Cognitive Level:* Analysis. *Nursing Process:* Implementation. *Client Need:* Physiological Integrity.

Answers to Critical Thinking Questions

1 As always, the ABCs are a priority for any client and must be considered. The nurse must monitor the client's airway for evidence of bronchospasm or decreased gas exchange, such as coughing, poor color, and decreased oxygen saturation. The nurse must understand that leukopenia is a problem for these clients (related to the amphotericin B and the client's own depressed immune status); therefore, prevention of infection is always a priority. The client's renal status (urine output, serum BUN, and creatinine) also must be closely monitored because approximately 30% of clients on this medication suffer renal damage.

2 This client has vaginal candidiasis, so it must be stressed that her partner be treated concurrently or reinfection may result. Alcohol must be avoided while on this medication to prevent profound vomiting. It is important to stress that alcohol is found not only in alcoholic drinks but also in products such as cough medicine, vanilla, and, at times, even in perfume that is absorbed via the dermis.

3 This drug can have profound adverse effects, and the client must be carefully screened and educated about this drug prior to taking it. The client must have a baseline physical assessment, including an ECG and blood pressure assessment, liver and renal function tests, and a hearing and visual assessment screening. Because the client may suffer permanent organ damage while taking this medication, baseline information is crucial.

CHAPTER 36
Answers to NCLEX-RN® Questions

1 Answer: 2
Rationale: Drug therapy has not produced a cure but has resulted in a number of therapeutic successes. There is no vaccine for HIV. *Cognitive Level:* Application. *Nursing Process:* Implementation. *Client Need:* Physiological Integrity.

2 Answers: 3, 4
Rationale: Two laboratory tests used to guide pharmacotherapy are an absolute CD4 count and an HIV RNA measurement. Clotting factors and a CBC do not provide information for guiding HIV-AIDS therapy. *Cognitive Level:* Analysis. *Nursing Process:* Implementation. *Client Need:* Physiological Integrity.

3 Answer: 1
Rationale: The medicine should be taken on an empty stomach for maximum absorption. *Cognitive Level:* Analysis. *Nursing Process:* Implementation. *Client Need:* Physiological Integrity.

4 Answer: 1
Rationale: Adequate immunity is achieved about 2 weeks after vaccination. Influenza vaccination should occur annually. All high-risk populations should be vaccinated. The influenza vaccination should be administered early in the season. *Cognitive Level:* Analysis. *Nursing Process:* Implementation. *Client Need:* Physiological Integrity.

5 Answer: 2
Rationale: The best treatment for viral hepatitis is prevention through immunization, which is available for HAV and HBV. *Cognitive Level:* Analysis. *Nursing Process:* Implementation. *Client Need:* Physiological Integrity.

Answers to Critical Thinking Questions

1 The best approach to influenza infection is *prevention* through annual vaccination. Those who benefit greatly from vaccinations include residents of long-term care facilities. The drug amantadine (Symmetrel) is used to prevent and treat influenza. The nurse should work with the healthcare provider to obtain an order and make arrangements to administer the medication.

2 This medication may cause bone marrow suppression. This client is already immunocompromised, and the potential for leukopenia is high. The client should be taught to watch for any evidence of infection, monitor temperature, and have regular lab tests. The client also needs instruction about the importance of good hand washing and safeguarding against potential sources of infection.

3 The nurse should inform the healthcare provider that the medication needs to be administered over a minimum of 1 hour, and that the nurse is unable to give the medication as a bolus or IV piggyback for less than 1 hour. The IV site must be monitored closely for potential infiltration while the medication is infusing. If this occurs, the IV must be stopped immediately.

CHAPTER 37
Answers to NCLEX-RN® Review Questions

1 Answer: 2
Rationale: Effectiveness of chemotherapy is increased by use of multiple drugs from different classes that attack cancer cells at different points in the cell cycle. Thus, lower doses of each individual agent can be used to reduce side effects. A third benefit of combination chemotherapy is reduced incidence of drug resistance. *Cognitive Level:* Application. *Nursing Process:* Implementation. *Client Need:* Physiological Integrity.

2 Answer: 3
Rationale: For maximum effect, clients starting therapy with agents with high emetic potential should be given an antiemetic prior to the start of treatment. *Cognitive Level:* Application. *Nursing Process:* Implementation. *Client Need:* Physiological Integrity.

3 Answers: 4, 5
Rationale: Client and family members should avoid receiving live virus vaccinations or becoming exposed to chicken pox. The client could have an exacerbation or a more pronounced episode of chicken pox. The client should also avoid crowds. *Cognitive Level:* Analysis. *Nursing Process:* Implementation. *Client Need:* Physiological Integrity.

4 Answer: 3
Rationale: The nurse should monitor for blood dyscrasias resulting from bone marrow suppression by monitoring the CBC with differential and platelet count. *Cognitive Level:* Analysis. *Nursing Process:* Evaluation. *Client Need:* Physiological Integrity.

5 Answer: 2
Rationale: The most serious side effect of vincristine is nervous system toxicity. Paralytic ileus is likely in young children. *Cognitive Level:* Analysis. *Nursing Process:* Implementation. *Client Need:* Physiological Integrity.

Answers to Critical Thinking Questions

1 The client needs to be taught strategies for coping with the side effects of the chemotherapy regimen. A major focus is nutritional issues. The client should always take antiemetics 1 hour prior to

chemotherapy, eat small frequent meals, drink high-calorie liquids if unable to eat solid food, and increase fluids if diarrhea occurs.

2 The client and family should be taught about the potential for infection related to immunosuppression. The nurse should stress frequent washing of hands, avoiding large crowds, self-assessing temperature accurately at home, and knowing when to call the healthcare provider. Nurses take these basics for granted even though clients often have misconceptions about them.

3 The nurse should remain with the solution and call for someone to bring the chemo spill kit immediately. While waiting for the spill kit, the nurse may cover the contaminated fluid with paper towels (the nurse must not touch the solution without wearing protective equipment). The nurse should clean up the spill and dispose of the waste per hospital protocols. At no time should the chemotherapy spill be left unattended.

CHAPTER 38
Answers to NCLEX-RN® Review Questions

1 Answer: 1
Rationale: Prolonged use of oxymetazoline causes hypersecretion of mucus and worsening nasal congestion, resulting in increased daily use. This medication should not be used for longer than 3 days and should be used only as directed. *Cognitive Level:* Application. *Nursing Process:* Implementation. *Client Need:* Physiological Integrity.

2 Answers: 2, 3
Rationale: The device delivers a metered spray that regulates the dosage and keeps it consistent. Use of intranasal glucocorticoids may require 2 to 4 weeks. Side effects include drying and bleeding of the nasal cavity. Saline nasal sprays may be used to alleviate drying. The medication should be used as prescribed. *Cognitive Level:* Application. *Nursing Process:* Implementation. *Client Need:* Physiological Integrity.

3 Answer: 1
Rationale: First-generation H_1-receptor antagonists are contraindicated in clients with a history of dysrhythmias and heart failure. These medications can cause vasodilation of vessels owing to H_1 stimulation. These medications have no relationship to weight gain or peptic ulcer disease. *Cognitive Level:* Analysis. *Nursing Process:* Assessment. *Client Need:* Physiological Integrity.

4 Answers: 1, 2, 5
Rationale: The device must be primed prior to initial use. The nose should be cleared prior to administration, not afterward, so that medication remains in the nasal cavity. Any excess that drains into the mouth must not be swallowed but should be spit out. *Cognitive Level:* Application. *Nursing Process:* Implementation. *Client Need:* Physiological Integrity.

5 Answer: 1
Rationale: A major side effect of antihistamines relates to their anticholinergic effects. Anticholinergic effects can also cause urinary hesitancy and should not be used in clients with a history of prostatic hypertrophy. *Cognitive Level:* Analysis. *Nursing Process:* Assessment. *Client Need:* Physiological Integrity.

Answers to Critical Thinking Questions

1 The nurse needs to ensure that the client understands the potential side effects related to the anticholinergic effects of this medication. The client (based on age) is at higher risk for urine retention, glaucoma (or other visual changes), and constipation.

2 Although codeine is a more powerful antitussive, it can cause dependence and constipation. Dextromethorphan is a more appropriate choice for this client initially, with codeine syrup as a potential later choice for more severe cough symptoms.

3 Intranasal glucocorticoids, such as Flonase, may take as long as 2 to 4 weeks to work. The medication should not be discontinued prematurely. If a decongestant spray is being used along with the Flonase, the decongestant should always be administered first to clear the nasal passages, which will facilitate adequate application of the glucocorticoid mist.

Answer to Avoid Medication Errors

The nurse should not have massaged the injection site because doing so may contribute to increased bruising and tissue injury. Subcutaneous injections can be given at a 45° to 90° angle, depending on the size of the person.

CHAPTER 39
Answers to NCLEX-RN® Review Questions

1 Answer: 2
Rationale: An aerosol is a suspension of minute liquid droplets or fine solid particles in a gas. Aerosol therapy can give immediate relief for bronchospasm or can loosen thick mucus. The major advantage of aerosol therapy is that it delivers medications to the immediate sites of action, thus reducing systemic side effects. The main disadvantage is that the precise dose received by the client is difficult to measure because it depends on the client's breathing pattern and the correct use of the aerosol device. *Cognitive Level:* Application. *Nursing Process:* Implementation. *Client Need:* Physiological Integrity.

2 Answer: 2
Rationale: Beta-adrenergic agonists (sympathomimetics) act by relaxing bronchial smooth muscle, resulting in bronchodilation that lowers airway resistance and makes breathing easier for the client. Beta-adrenergic agonists do not liquefy or reduce mucus production. *Cognitive Level:* Analysis. *Nursing Process:* Implementation. *Client Need:* Physiological Integrity.

3 Answer: 4
Rationale: Tolerance may develop to the therapeutic effects of the beta-adrenergic agonists; therefore, the client must be instructed to seek medical attention if the drugs become less effective with continued use. Increased heart rate is a side effect of beta-adrenergic agonists. The client should not change the medication dosage without first consulting the prescriber. *Cognitive Level:* Analysis. *Nursing Process:* Implementation. *Client Need:* Physiological Integrity.

4 Answer: 3
Rationale: Anticholinergic bronchodilators should be used cautiously in elderly men with benign prostatic hyperplasia and in clients with glaucoma. An enlarged liver and diarrhea have no relationship to the use of ipratropium. *Cognitive Level:* Analysis. *Nursing Process:* Implementation. *Client Need:* Physiological Integrity.

5 Answers: 3, 4
Rationale: If taken for longer than 10 days, oral glucocorticoids can produce significant adverse effects, including adrenal gland atrophy, peptic ulcers, and hyperglycemia. Long-term oral glucocorticoids can cause osteoporosis. Changes in level of consciousness may be related to oxygenation levels and need to be reported to the healthcare provider. *Cognitive Level:* Analysis. *Nursing Process:* Assessment. *Client Need:* Physiological Integrity.

Answers to Critical Thinking Questions

1 The nurse needs to ensure that the client understands the potential side effects related to anticholinergic effects of this medication. The client (based on age) is at higher risk for urine retention, glaucoma (or other visual changes), and constipation. These are also common problems for clients who are taking this medication.

2 Once the client's condition begins to improve, the nurse should assess the father's understanding of the asthma regimen. The client should receive instruction on the side effects of glucocorticoid therapy. Glucocorticoids can suppress the hypothalamic–pituitary axis. Abruptly discontinuing a glucocorticoid after long-term therapy (greater than 10 days) can produce cardiovascular collapse. The client needs to be instructed on the dosage regimen for prednisone, which may include an incremental decrease in the drug dosage when discontinuing the drug. The client should be monitored for hyperglycemia, peptic ulcer disease, signs and symptoms of GI bleeding, and mood changes.

3 Key client education points of emphasis regarding administering medications via an inhaler include the following:

1. Shake the canister well immediately before each use.
2. Exhale completely to the end of a normal breath.
3. With the inhaler in the upright position, place the mouthpiece just inside the mouth and use the lips to form a tight seal.
4. While pressing down on the inhaler, take a slow, deep breath and hold for approximately 10 seconds.
5. Wait approximately 2 minutes before taking a second inhalation of the drug.
6. Rinse the mouth with water after each use (especially after using steroid inhalers, because the drug may cause fungal infections of the mouth and throat).

CHAPTER 40
Answers to NCLEX-RN® Review Questions

1 Answer: 3
Rationale: Antacids are generally combinations of aluminum hydroxide and magnesium hydroxide. Hypermagnesemia can develop with use of OTC antacids while on renal dialysis because the kidneys are unable to excrete excess magnesium. Hyperkalemia is a complication of renal failure. Hypernatremia can occur with use of antacids. *Cognitive Level:* Analysis. *Nursing Process:* Implementation. *Client Need:* Physiological Integrity.

2 Answer: 1
Rationale: Two or more antibiotics are used to lower the potential for bacterial resistance and increase the effectiveness of therapy. Bacterial infections can recur, requiring future treatment. *Cognitive Level:* Analysis. *Nursing Process:* Implementation. *Client Need:* Physiological Integrity.

3 Answer: 1
Rationale: Ginger may be used to strengthen the upper GI tract. Peppermint may be used to induce a sense of calm but may make esophageal reflux more pronounced. Basil and green tea have no effect on the GI tract. *Cognitive Level:* Analysis. *Nursing Process:* Implementation. *Client Need:* Physiological Integrity.

4 Answer: 3

Rationale: Bismuth compounds may be added to the regimen treatment of *Helicobacter pylori*. These products inhibit bacterial growth and prevent *H. pylori* from adhering to the gastric mucosa. None of the other options is used in the treatment of *H. pylori*. *Cognitive Level:* Analysis. *Nursing Process:* Implementation. *Client Need:* Physiological Integrity.

5 Answers: 1, 2, 3, 5

Rationale: Risk factors associated with peptic ulcer disease include a family history of peptic ulcer disease; blood group O; smoking tobacco; caffeine, aspirin, glucocorticoid, and NSAID use; excessive stress; and *H. pylori*. Type 2 diabetes mellitus has not been associated with peptic ulcer disease. *Cognitive Level:* Analysis. *Nursing Process:* Assessment. *Client Need:* Physiological Integrity.

Answers to Critical Thinking Questions

1 Regular use of aluminum hydroxide (Amphojel) may cause hypercalcemia because calcium and phosphorus have a reciprocal relationship; that is, if the calcium goes up, the phosphorus goes down. A client with low serum phosphorus often exhibits signs of increasing weakness. The treatment is to replace the aluminum hydroxide with a different antacid and take oral phosphorus supplements until serum phosphorus returns to a normal level.

2 The stomach is empty during the sleep cycle, the time when the protective protein peptide TFF2 is most effective at repairing the mucoprotective lining of the stomach. For the TFF2 protein to reach its maximum effectiveness, the person needs a minimum of 6 hours of uninterrupted sleep, which is uncommon in people who sleep during the daytime.

3 This client has a history of PUD; therefore, alcohol and smoking are contraindicated because they will exacerbate the condition. This client is on ranitidine (Zantac), and smoking decreases the effectiveness of the medication. Alcohol is a depressant and can cause increased drowsiness in combination with ranitidine. This client should be advised to stop smoking and drinking alcohol if PUD is to be resolved.

CHAPTER 41
Answers to NCLEX-RN® Review Questions

1 Answer: 1

Rationale: When contents lost from the stomach are strongly acidic, vomiting may change the pH of the blood, resulting in metabolic acidosis. With severe loss, acid–base disturbances can lead to vascular collapse. Clients' respirations may increase with prolonged vomiting. Esophageal tears with prolonged vomiting occur rarely. *Cognitive Level:* Analysis. *Nursing Process:* Assessment. *Client Need:* Physiological Integrity.

2 Answer: 1

Rationale: Dramamine is most effective when taken at least 20 to 60 minutes before intended use. The other options are not within the range of optimal effectiveness. *Cognitive Level:* Application. *Nursing Process:* Implementation. *Client Need:* Physiological Integrity.

3 Answer: 1

Rationale: Stress is one of the major factors in developing IBS. *Helicobacter pylori* is associated with development of peptic ulcers. GERD is associated with esophageal disorders. *Cognitive Level:* Analysis. *Nursing Process:* Assessment. *Client Need:* Physiological Integrity.

4 Answers: 2, 5

Rationale: Prochlorperazine (Compazine) and promethazine hydrochloride (Phenergan) can cause the anticholinergic side effects of dry mouth, constipation, urine retention, and a rapid heart rate. Peppermint induces a calming effect. Loperamide (Imodium, Kaopectate) is an antidiarrheal. *Cognitive Level:* Analysis. *Nursing Process:* Implementation. *Client Need:* Physiological Integrity.

5 Answers: 1, 2, 3, 4

Rationale: Sibutramine (Meridia) is a CNS agent that is contraindicated in clients with a history of hypertension, CAD, and renal and hepatic impairments. The client should be assessed for abdominal pain after medication has been initiated. *Cognitive Level:* Analysis. *Nursing Process:* Assessment. *Client Need:* Physiological Integrity.

Answers to Critical Thinking Questions

1 A priority for the nurse would be to assess the potential for dehydration. The nurse would assess the client for possible hypotension and tachycardia. The cause of this ongoing diarrhea needs to be investigated by the physician.

2 The client needs to be informed that prochlorperazine (Compazine) is administered in its own syringe and must not be mixed with any other drug. The nurse could notify the healthcare provider that the client wants a change of antiemetic to one that can be combined with an analgesic and given in the same syringe.

3 This client needs to take a contact laxative to stimulate the nerve endings and facilitate a bowel movement. A bulk-forming laxative promotes bowel regularity. The liquid stool may be a result of fecal impaction, in which only liquid seeps out. If this client has ongoing bowel irregularity problems, the bulk-forming laxative may be helpful later. The nurse should educate the client to drink plenty of fluids when taking bulk-forming laxatives.

CHAPTER 42
Answers to NCLEX-RN® Review Questions

1 Answer: 1

Rationale: Enlargement of the thyroid gland, known as *goiter*, develops when there is a low iodide intake. Increased metabolic rate and weight loss are related to hyperthyroidism. *Cognitive Level:* Analysis. *Nursing Process:* Assessment. *Client Need:* Physiological Integrity.

2 Answers: 2, 3, 4

Rationale: Circulatory collapse, complete heart block, and respiratory failure are all known to occur in clients receiving magnesium sulfate intravenously. The therapy should be used cautiously in clients with renal impairment. *Cognitive Level:* Analysis. *Nursing Process:* Assessment. *Client Need:* Physiological Integrity.

3 Answer: 3

Rationale: Hypomagnesemia should be assessed. Clients experiencing hypomagnesemia may experience general weakness, dysrhythmias, hypertension, loss of deep tendon reflexes, and respiratory depression. *Cognitive Level:* Analysis. *Nursing Process:* Assessment. *Client Need:* Physiological Integrity.

4 Answer: 4

Rationale: Alcohol is known for its ability to inhibit the absorption of thiamine and folic acid. Alcohol abuse is the most common cause of thiamine deficiency. *Cognitive Level:* Analysis. *Nursing Process:* Implementation. *Client Need:* Physiological Integrity.

5 Answer: 3

Rationale: Vitamin K should be given to the client to improve clotting. Without vitamin K, abnormal prothrombin is produced and blood clotting is affected. *Cognitive Level:* Analysis. *Nursing Process:* Implementation. *Client Need:* Physiological Integrity.

Answers to Critical Thinking Questions

1 The client is experiencing a normal reaction to the niacin but should be instructed to follow up with the healthcare provider for guidance on the appropriate dose of niacin to take.

2 This client should be instructed to see a healthcare provider regarding the appropriate doses of vitamins. Vitamin A can cause increased intracranial pressure, which could be the cause of the headaches. Clients need to be instructed about the appropriate amounts of vitamins and potential adverse effects—especially when taking megadoses of vitamins.

3 This client needs to be assessed for possible renal calculi. The client is taking 500 mg of vitamin C daily to prevent an upper respiratory infection, but vitamin C is contraindicated in clients with a history of renal calculi because the vitamin may exacerbate the problem.

CHAPTER 43
Answers to NCLEX-RN® Review Questions

1 Answer: 1

Rationale: Glucocorticoids can cause increased risk of peptic ulcers, decreased wound healing, and increased capillary fragility. Glucocorticoids place the client at increased risk for infection. The other options do not cause increased risk for peptic ulcers, delayed wound healing, or infection. *Cognitive Level:* Analysis. *Nursing Process:* Implementation. *Client Need:* Physiological Integrity.

2 Answer: 1

Rationale: This drug may mask the signs and symptoms of infection. Hydrocortisone is contraindicated in clients with known infections or hypersensitivity to the drug. Skin infections, heart failure, and hearing loss are not associated with the use of hydrocortisone. *Cognitive Level:* Analysis. *Nursing Process:* Implementation. *Client Need:* Physiological Integrity.

3 Answer: 2

Rationale: Circulatory collapse can occur if hydrocortisone use is discontinued abruptly. The client may experience nausea, vomiting, lethargy, and confusion, progressing to coma and death. Diabetes insipidus is caused by ADH deficiency. Myxedema is related to hypothyroidism. Cushing's syndrome is caused by excess glucocorticoids. *Cognitive Level:* Analysis. *Nursing Process:* Assessment. *Client Need:* Physiological Integrity.

4 Answer: 2

Rationale: The client may have the hormonal condition hyperthyroidism. Symptoms of hyperthyroidism include diarrhea, stress intolerance, and weight loss. The other disease processes are not related to the thyroid gland. *Cognitive Level:* Analysis. *Nursing Process:* Implementation. *Client Need:* Physiological Integrity.

5 Answers: 2, 5

Rationale: Because small doses of radiation will be emitted for up to 1 week, clients should avoid close contact with children or pregnant women after administration of the drug. Radioactive iodine is used to permanently decrease thyroid function. Clients may experience hypothyroidism, including signs and symptoms such as general weakness, muscle cramps, and dry skin. Fluids do not affect radiation

levels. *Cognitive Level:* Application. *Nursing Process:* Implementation. *Client Need:* Physiological Integrity.

Answers to Critical Thinking Questions

1 To answer this question the student should refer to a medical–surgical text or a laboratory manual. A child with diabetes insipidus produces large amounts of pale or colorless urine with a low specific gravity of 1.001 to 1.005. Daily urine volume may be 4 to 10 L or more and result in excessive thirst and rapid dehydration. Desmopressin is a synthetic analog of ADH. It may be administered intranasally and therefore may be better tolerated by a child. With pharmacotherapy, there should be an immediate decrease in urine production and an increase in urine concentration. The child's mother or caregiver should be taught to use a urine dipstick to check specific gravity during the initiation of therapy. A normal specific gravity would range from 1.005 to 1.030 and would indicate that the kidneys are concentrating urine. The caregiver also should be taught to monitor urine volume, color, and odor until a dosing regimen is established.

2 The nurse must be empathetic with the client's father and allow him to express his concerns. He may feel guilty about contributing to his son's current health crisis. Once the client's condition begins to improve, the nurse should assess the father's understanding of the asthma regimen. The father and the client should receive instruction about the side effects of glucocorticoid therapy. Glucocorticoids used for anti-inflammatory purposes can suppress the hypothalamic–pituitary axis. Abruptly discontinuing a glucocorticoid after long-term therapy (more than 10 days) can produce cardiovascular collapse. The father needs to be instructed about the dosage regimen for prednisone, which may include an incremental decrease in the drug dosage when discontinuing the drug. The nurse might also be concerned about the economic needs of this family. Referrals to a resource providing financial support for medication would be appropriate.

3 This question requires the student to use an additional resource such as a drug handbook. In this situation, the parents need to be instructed about the following points:

a. Drug action: The drug stimulates growth of most body tissues, especially epiphyseal plates; it also increases cellular size.

b. Instructions for reconstituting the medication, site selection, and technique for IM or subcutaneous injection.

c. Dosing schedule: Somatropin injections are usually scheduled 48 hours apart.

d. Pain and swelling at the injection site.

e. Importance of regular follow-up with the healthcare provider, including checks on height, weight, and bone age.

Answer to Avoiding Medication Errors

No. The infant's weight of 2000 g is equivalent to 2 kg. Therefore, 25 mg/kg/day would be 50 mg. When given in two equally divided doses, the correct dose is 25 mg.

CHAPTER 44
Answers to NCLEX-RN® Review Questions

1 Answer: 1600

Rationale: The onset of NPH is between 1 and 4 hours, and it peaks between 8 and 12 hours. *Cognitive Level:* Application. *Nursing Process:* Assessment. *Client Need:* Physiological Integrity.

2 Answer: 1
Rationale: Humalog is a rapid-acting insulin that is administered for elevated glucose levels and should be given 0 to 15 minutes before breakfast. Hypoglycemic reactions may occur rapidly if Humalog insulin is not supported by sufficient food intake. The medication can be mixed in one syringe. *Cognitive Level:* Application. *Nursing Process:* Implementation. *Client Need:* Physiological Integrity.

3 Answer: 3
Rationale: Additional teaching is needed. The clear solution (regular insulin) should be drawn into the syringe first followed by the cloudy solution (NPH). The other options demonstrate an understanding of discharge instructions. *Cognitive Level:* Analysis. *Nursing Process:* Evaluation. *Client Need:* Physiological Integrity.

4 Answers: 1, 2, 3, 4
Rationale: The client needs to understand that exercise may increase insulin needs. Blood glucose levels should be monitored prior to starting and after ending exercise, and addressed appropriately. A complex carbohydrate should be consumed prior to strenuous exercise. *Cognitive Level:* Analysis. *Nursing Process:* Implementation. *Client Need:* Physiological Integrity.

5 Answer: 2
Rationale: Somogyi phenomenon occurs when there is a rapid drop in blood glucose levels during the night, which stimulates the release of blood glucose–elevating hormones. The result is an elevated morning glucose level. Insulin resistance occurs when the body is unable to adequately utilize the insulin it produces. Diabetes ketoacidosis occurs when the blood sugar is elevated and the body is producing ketoacids. Hyperosmolarity occurs with elevated blood glucose levels. *Cognitive Level:* Analysis. *Nursing Process:* Implementation. *Client Need:* Physiological Integrity.

Answers to Critical Thinking Questions

1 The nurse should first explain that management of type 1 diabetes is initiated with diet, exercise, and home blood glucose monitoring. Compliance with prescribed regimens may reduce the client's fasting and postprandial blood glucose values to acceptable levels. Mothers with type 1 diabetes must keep their blood glucose level within a very narrow range to prevent the numerous complications that can occur because of elevated blood glucose during pregnancy. These complications can range from fetal deformity to fetal macrosomia and its subsequent sequelae. Some authorities recommend that the fasting blood glucose levels be maintained at or below 100 mg/dl and the postprandial glucose below 120 mg/dl. The nurse should prepare the client for insulin therapy in case diet and exercise fail to maintain control. Oral hypoglycemic agents cross placental membranes and have been implicated as teratogenic agents. Their use is not recommended during pregnancy.

2 Absorption rates of subcutaneous insulin vary among various body areas. It is known that the abdomen has the fastest rate of absorption, followed by the arms, thighs, and buttocks. It is also generally accepted that exercise of a body area can increase the rate of insulin absorption. Rotating from arm, to leg, to abdomen for injections affects glucose control levels because of the variation in absorption rates. For this reason, systematic rotation within one area at a time is recommended. The nurse in this situation should review a correct system of rotation for this client.

3 Insulin glargine (Lantus) is a newer agent that is a recombinant human insulin analog. It must not be mixed in the syringe with any other insulin and must be administered subcutaneously. Insulin glargine appears to have a constant long-duration hypoglycemic effect with no defined peak effect. It is prescribed once daily, at bedtime.

The nurse should question the order for Lantus to be administered every morning.

CHAPTER 45
Answers to NCLEX-RN® Review Questions

1 Answer 4
Rationale: Use of oral contraceptives puts a client at risk for thromboembolism, which is manifested by calf pain, shortness of breath, and chest pain. *Cognitive Level:* Analysis. *Nursing Process:* Assessment. *Client Need:* Physiological Integrity.

2 Answer: 1
Rationale: Caffeine and estrogen may lead to increased CNS stimulation. *Cognitive Level:* Analysis. *Nursing Process:* Implementation. *Client Need:* Physiological Integrity.

3 Answer: 2
Rationale: The assessment of the client is within normal parameters for a client in labor. Antidiuretic hormone can cause water intoxication in clients with prolonged IV infusion of oxytocin. *Cognitive Level:* Analysis. *Nursing Process:* Assessment. *Client Need:* Physiological Integrity.

4 Answers: 1, 2
Rationale: Barrier contraception is needed only when two or more doses are missed. Placebos are usually iron, which has no effect on estrogen-related adverse effects. Side effects include intolerance to contact lenses, abdominal cramps, dysmenorrhea, breast fullness, headache, acne, skin rash, hypertension, and thromboembolic disorders. *Cognitive Level:* Analysis. *Nursing Process:* Implementation. *Client Need:* Physiological Integrity.

5 Answer: 2
Rationale: Although some antibiotics and anticonvulsants can reduce the efficacy of oral contraceptives, the most common cause of pregnancy in clients using oral contraceptives is skipping two or more doses. *Cognitive Level:* Analysis. *Nursing Process:* Implementation. *Client Need:* Physiological Integrity.

Answers to Critical Thinking Questions

1 The student should be able to use this example to help illustrate neuroendocrine control of the female reproductive system. Leuprolide acetate is a synthetic GnRH agonist that acts by stimulating the anterior pituitary to secrete FSH and LH. The pituitary receptors become desensitized, which causes a decrease in FSH and LH secretion. Consequently, estrogen production, which is dependent on ovarian stimulation, is diminished and the patient's menstrual cycle is suppressed. The goal of suppressing the menstrual cycle is to decrease hormonal stimuli to abnormal endometriotic tissue. It is expected that amenorrhea will result and that endometriosis lesions will decrease. A decrease in lesions will likely enhance the patient's fertility or improve her level of comfort during menstruation. The patient will remain on this drug therapy for approximately 6 months. Menstrual periods usually resume 2 months after the completion of therapy.

2 Misoprostol (Cytotec) is a prostaglandin that may be prescribed as an antiulcer agent. The drug also has two off-label uses, which include cervical ripening prior to induction of labor, or termination of pregnancy when used with mifepristone. It is known that prostaglandins have a role in the initiation of labor, as has been demonstrated with the vaginal application of prostaglandin E. Misoprostol is a prostaglandin E analog that has clearly been demonstrated to produce uterine contractions. In this example, the fetus was not tolerating the uterine contractions and the nurse used correct judgment in quickly acting to remove the drug.

3 Oxytocin exerts an antidiuretic effect when administered in doses of 20 milliunits/min or greater. Urine output decreases, and fluid retention increases. Most patients begin a postpartum diuresis and are able to balance fluid volumes relatively quickly. However, the nurse should evaluate the patient for signs of water intoxication, which include drowsiness, listlessness, headache, and oliguria.

CHAPTER 46
Answers to NCLEX-RN® Review Questions

1 Answers: 2, 3
Rationale: A side effect of testosterone therapy is fluid retention. Testosterone is also used to increase muscle mass and strength. The hematocrit usually increases with the use of testosterone, because it promotes the synthesis of erythropoietin. *Cognitive Level:* Analysis. *Nursing Process:* Assessment. *Client Need:* Physiological Integrity.

2 Answer: 1
Rationale: The primary use of testosterone is to treat hypogonadism in men with delayed puberty. Testosterone therapy promotes normal gonadal development and often restores reproductive function. Secondary sex characteristics or virilization also occur. *Cognitive Level:* Analysis. *Nursing Process:* Assessment. *Client Need:* Physiological Integrity.

3 Answer: 3
Rationale: In men, some medications such as phenothiazines, thiazide diuretics, SSRIs, TCAs, propranolol, and diazepam cause impotence because of low testosterone secretion. *Cognitive Level:* Analysis. *Nursing Process:* Assessment. *Client Need:* Physiological Integrity.

4 Answer: 1
Rationale: Life-threatening hypotension is an adverse effect in clients who are taking sildenafil (Viagra) and organic nitrates. *Cognitive Level:* Analysis. *Nursing Process:* Assessment. *Client Needs:* Physiological Integrity.

5 Answer: 4
Rationale: Finasteride promotes shrinking of enlarged prostates and helps restore urinary function. Tadalafil and sildenafil are used in clients experiencing erectile dysfunction. Testosterone is used in the treatment of hypogonadism. *Cognitive Level:* Analysis. *Nursing Process:* Implementation. *Client Need:* Physiological Integrity.

Answers to Critical Thinking Questions

1 This client's age puts him at risk for a variety of health problems. Conditions such as renal or hepatic dyfunction may alter the manner in which the drug is metabolized or excreted. The potential impact on clients with coronary artery disease who are using nitrates has been well documented. Because the client is requesting a prescription for sildenafil (Viagra), the nurse should ensure that the history includes the following data: sexual dysfunction, cardiovascular disease and use of organic nitrates, severe hypotension, and renal or hepatic impairment—which requires a decrease in the prescribed dose. Nurses can be effective in initiating conversations about sexuality. Studies have shown that clients are often forthcoming with concerns about sexual performance when an interviewer is open and professional.

2 According to Erikson's theory of psychosocial development, this young man is in the stage of identity versus isolation. The family has been replaced in its influence largely by the adolescent's peer group. This young man's desire to be accepted as an athlete and a team mem-

ber may produce a willingness to do what it takes to fit in. In addition, the young man may have aspirations of a career in sports and recognize the need to be in optimum physical condition. This client may not realize that the use of testosterone in immature men has not been associated with significant increases in muscle mass. Such an increase has been documented only in mature men. In addition, testosterone can produce premature epiphyseal closure, potentially affecting this young man's adult height.

3 Finasteride (Proscar), an androgen inhibitor, is used to shrink the prostate and relieve symptoms associated with BPH. Finasteride inhibits 5-alpha-reductase, an enzyme that converts testosterone to the potent androgen 5-alpha-dihydrotestosterone (DHT). The prostate gland depends on this androgen for its development, but excessive levels can cause prostate cells to increase in size and divide. A regimen of 6 to 12 months may be necessary to determine client response. Saw palmetto is an herbal preparation derived from a shrublike palm tree that is native to the southeastern United States. This phytomedicine compares pharmacologically with finasteride in that it is an antiandrogen. The mechanism of action is virtually the same in these two agents. Authorities note no significant adverse effects of saw palmetto extract and no known drug–drug interactions. Just as with finasteride, long-term use is required.

CHAPTER 47
Answers to NCLEX-RN® Review Questions

1 Answer: 1
Rationale: Osteomalacia, referred to as *rickets* in children, is a disorder characterized by softening of bones without alteration in basic bone structure. Classic signs of rickets in children include bowlegs and a pigeon breast. Shortness of breath, crutch walking, and finger and toe deformities are not associated with osteomalacia. *Cognitive Level:* Analysis. *Nursing Process:* Assessment. *Client Need:* Physiological Integrity.

2 Answer: 3
Rationale: A normal serum calcium level is 8.5–11.5 mg/dl. Signs of hypocalcemia include seizures, muscle spasms, facial twitching, and paresthesias. Anorexia, headache, and drowsiness may be associated with hypercalcemia. *Cognitive Level:* Analysis. *Nursing Process:* Assessment. *Client Need:* Physiological Integrity.

3 Answer: 3
Rationale: Gout is a metabolic disorder characterized by the accumulation of uric acid in the bloodstream or joint cavities. Alcohol increases uric acid levels. Although long-term alcohol use may affect the liver, it is not related to uric acid. Alcohol does not affect the absorption of antigout medications. Alcohol increases urine acidity. *Cognitive Level:* Analysis. *Nursing Process:* Assessment. *Client Need:* Physiological Integrity.

4 Answers: 1, 2, 3
Rationale: Signs and symptoms of hypercalcemia include anorexia, vomiting, excessive thirst, fatigue, and confusion. Kidney stones may occur, and bones may fracture easily. Cardiac dysrhythmias may occur, because calcium ions influence the excitability of all neurons. Whenever calcium concentrations are too high, sodium permeability decreases across cell membranes. This is a dangerous state, because nerve conduction depends on the proper influx of sodium into cells. *Cognitive Level:* Analysis. *Nursing Process:* Assessment. *Client Need:* Physiological Integrity.

5 Answer: 2
Rationale: Sodium hyaluronate (Hyalgan) is administered by injection directly into the knee joint. This medication replaces or supplements

the body's natural hyaluronic acid that deteriorated because of the inflammation of osteoarthritis. All other routes are incorrect. *Cognitive Level:* Analysis. *Nursing Process:* Implementation. *Client Need:* Physiological Integrity.

Answers to Critical Thinking Questions

1 Alendronate (Fosamax) is poorly absorbed after oral administration and can produce significant GI irritation. It is important that the client be educated regarding several elements of drug administration. To promote absorption, the drug should be taken first thing in the morning with 8 oz of water before food or beverages are ingested or any other medications are taken. It has been shown that certain beverages, such as orange juice and coffee, interfere with drug absorption. By delaying eating for 30 minutes or more, the client is promoting absorption of the drug. Additionally, the client should be taught to sit upright after taking the drug to reduce the risk of esophageal irritation. Alendronate must be used carefully in clients with esophagitis or gastric ulcer. If the client misses a dose, she should be told to skip it and not to double the next dose. Alendronate has a long half-life, and missing an occasional dose will do little to interfere with the therapeutic effect of the drug.

2 Frail elderly clients may be susceptible to hypocalcemia caused by dietary deficiencies of calcium and vitamin D or decreased physical activity and lack of exposure to sunshine. This client has all these risk factors. She is uninterested in eating, has physical limitations, and is not able to get out of the house into the sunshine without assistance. Orally administered calcium requires vitamin D for absorption to take place. Because this client does not consume milk, the most recognizable source of vitamin D, she needs to be encouraged to increase her intake of other dietary sources of this vitamin. Foods rich in vitamin D include canned salmon, cereals, lean meats, beans, and potatoes. To promote the effectiveness of calcium supplementation, the nurse must remember the importance of drug–nutrient interactions.

3 The triage nurse should obtain information about the onset of symptoms, degree of discomfort, and frequency of attacks. A familial history of gout can be predictive, because primary gout is inherited as an X-linked trait. A past medical history of renal calculi may also be predictive of acute gouty arthritis. The nurse should ask the client questions about his diet and fluid intake. An attack of gout can be precipitated by alcohol intake (particularly beer and wine), starvation diets, and insufficient fluid intake. In addition, the nurse should obtain information about prescribed drugs and the use of OTC drugs containing salicylates. Thiazide diuretics and salicylates can precipitate an attack. The nurse should also ask about recent lifestyle events. Stress, illness, trauma, or strenuous exercise can precipitate an attack of gouty arthritis.

Answer to Avoiding Medication Errors

This error occurred because the nurse administered the medication to the wrong client. Clients must be correctly identified by checking the identification band or by another identifying method and not by relying on clients to respond to calling them by name. When there are two clients with similar names, it is particularly important to double-check the room number and identification band. Perhaps Ms. Brown was responding to being awoken. Best practice requires that proper client identification occur prior to any medication administration. The nurse must adhere to the five rights of medication administration:

1. Right patient
2. Right drug
3. Right dose
4. Right route
5. Right time

CHAPTER 48
Answers to NCLEX-RN® Review Questions

1 Answer: 2
Rationale: To ensure the effectiveness of drug therapy, clients should inspect hair shafts after treatment, checking for nits by combing with a fine-toothed comb after the hair is dry. This procedure must be conducted daily for at least 1 week after treatment. The client does not require isolation. Linens should be washed with hot water; bleach is not required. Lindane (Kwell) should be used only after other less toxic medications have failed. *Cognitive Level:* Analysis. *Nursing Process:* Implementation. *Client Need:* Physiological Integrity.

2 Answers: 1, 2, 5
Rationale: The directions for scabicides and pediculicides must be followed carefully. If these doses are overapplied, wrongly applied, or accidentally ingested, the client may experience headaches; nausea or vomiting; irritation of the nose, ears, or throat; dizziness; tremors; restlessness; or convulsions. Eye irritation does not occur with overapplication. *Cognitive Level:* Analysis. *Nursing Process:* Implementation. *Client Need:* Physiological Integrity.

3 Answer: 3
Rationale: Creams or lotions take longer to produce their effect; therefore, they are usually left on the body for about 8 to 12 hours before rinsing. Lindane shampoo is applied and left on for at least 5 minutes before rinsing. *Cognitive Level:* Analysis. *Nursing Process:* Implementation. *Client Need:* Physiological Integrity.

4 Answer: 2
Rationale: Isotretinoin (Accutane) is a vitamin A metabolite that aids in reducing the size of sebaceous glands, thereby decreasing oil production and the occurrence of clogged pores. Isotretinoin is not recommended during pregnancy because of possible harmful effects to the fetus. Oral contraceptives may be used to help clear acne. Makeup may help cover some of the acne, but the face should be washed at least twice a day with warm water and a mild soap. *Cognitive Level:* Analysis. *Nursing Process:* Implementation. *Client Need:* Physiological Integrity.

5 Answer: 1
Rationale: Lesions of psoriasis vulgaris are papules that form into thick erythematosus plaques that are silver or gray and bleed when removed. The lesions are found primarily over the scalp, elbows, and knees and not on other surfaces of the body. *Cognitive Level:* Analysis. *Nursing Process:* Assessment. *Client Need:* Physiological Integrity.

Answers to Critical Thinking Questions

1 To establish a rapport with the baby's mother, the nurse should first respond to the mother's anxiety. She should validate that the baby's condition is cause for concern and commend the mother for seeking medical guidance. The nursing student should recognize that the availability of OTC preparations can be a temptation to a young mother who only wants to see her infant more comfortable and relieved of symptoms.

However, the student nurse must also recognize that topical use of corticosteroid ointments can be potentially harmful, especially for young children. Corticosteroids, when absorbed by the skin in large enough quantities over a long period can result in adrenal suppression and skin atrophy. Children have an increased risk of toxicity from topically applied drugs because of their greater ratio of skin surface area to weight compared with that of adults. The student nurse should ensure that the healthcare provider at the public health clinic sees this patient. Once a drug treatment modality is prescribed, the student nurse should make sure that the baby's mother understands the correct method for drug administration.

2 According to Piaget, this 14-year-old client is capable of formal operations, the highest level of cognitive development. A young person in this age group is able to think logically and make decisions regarding healthcare problems and take control of a treatment regimen. To safely self-medicate, the teenager needs information about the medication, its administration, and side effects. Teenagers need clear instructions and often respond to a caregiver outside the family as a resource for information.

The nurse should recognize that this patient is experiencing GI side effects that are common in doxycycline and all tetracycline treatment. Recent studies have demonstrated cases of esophagitis in teenage patients. To develop an effective teaching plan, the nurse will need to assess the client's dosing regimen and current dietary patterns. A teaching plan would include the following:

- Encouraging oral fluids to maintain hydration even if nausea occurs
- Drinking a full glass of water with the medication to reduce gastric irritation
- Sitting up for 30 minutes after the nighttime dose to reduce gastric irritation and reflux
- Consuming small frequent meals to ensure adequate nutrition
- Taking the drug 1 hour before or 2 hours after meals to promote its absorption and effectiveness. (If nausea persists, however, the patient should be encouraged to take the doxycycline with food.)
- Taking doxycycline with milk products or antacids decreases the absorption of the drug. Therefore, other remedies for GI irritation will need to be discussed with the healthcare provider.

3 This patient's presentation is typical of rosacea. To prevent long-term changes in the skin, therapy should be aggressive despite the fact that this patient is also of childbearing age. Isotretinoin (Accutane) is a pregnancy category X drug and has a picture of a fetus overlaid by the "No" symbol on the package. Reported teratogenic effects include severe CNS abnormalities such as hydrocephalus, microcephalus, cranial nerve deficits, and compromised intelligence scores.

This patient needs to understand that she must use contraception while receiving drug therapy and for up to 6 months after therapy is discontinued. She should not begin therapy unless she first demonstrates a negative pregnancy test. In addition, she should be taught to begin therapy on the second or third day of her normal menstrual cycle. Teenagers who are on isotretinoin should anticipate monthly pregnancy tests.

CHAPTER 49
Answers to NCLEX-RN® Review Questions

1 Answer: 3
Rationale: Closed-angle glaucoma is an acute type of glaucoma that is caused by stress, impact injury, or medications. Pressure inside the anterior chamber increases suddenly because the iris is pushed over the area where the aqueous fluid normally drains. Signs and symptoms include intense headaches, difficulty concentrating, bloodshot eyes, blurred vision, and a bulging iris. Closed-angle glaucoma constitutes an emergency. All other options are inappropriate in this emergency. *Cognitive Level:* Application. *Nursing Process:* Implementation. *Client Need:* Physiological Integrity.

2 Answer: 4
Rationale: Side effects include eye irritation, conjunctival edema, burning, stinging, redness, blurred vision, pain, itching, the sensation of a foreign body in the eye, photophobia, and visual disturbances. The client may experience the phenomenon of increasing amounts of brown pigmentation in the treated eye only and thickening of the eyelashes and hair adjacent to the treated eye. General body symptoms such as flulike symptoms, rash, or headache may occur. Loss of lashes, hypertension, and dilation of the pupils do not occur with the use of prostaglandins. *Cognitive Level:* Analysis. *Nursing Process:* Implementation. *Client Need:* Physiological Integrity.

3 Answer: 3
Rationale: Beta-adrenergic drugs may reduce resting heart rate and blood pressure. The client and family should be taught how to check the pulse and blood pressure before administration and to notify the physician if extremes occur. Beta-adrenergic drugs do not affect urine output, respiratory rate, or glucose levels. *Cognitive Level:* Analysis. *Nursing Process:* Implementation. *Client Need:* Physiological Integrity.

4 Answer: 4
Rationale: Some drugs are specifically designed for examining the eyes of clients. These include cycloplegic drugs to relax ciliary muscles and mydriatic drugs to dilate the pupils. One has to be especially careful with anticholinergic mydriatics, because these drugs can worsen glaucoma by impairing aqueous humor outflow and thereby increasing intraocular pressure. *Cognitive Level:* Analysis. *Nursing Process:* Implementation. *Client Need:* Physiological Integrity.

5 Answers: 1, 2, 4
Rationale: The nurse needs to notify the healthcare provider if the client has second- or third-degree heart block, bradycardia, cardiac failure, CHF, or COPD because Timolol may be contraindicated for clients with these conditions. If the drug is absorbed systemically, it will worsen these conditions. Proper administration lessens the danger that the drug will be absorbed systemically. The renal and hepatic systems are not affected by Timolol. *Cognitive Level:* Analysis. *Nursing Process:* Assessment. *Client Need:* Physiological Integrity.

Answers to Critical Thinking Questions

1 Cortisporin Otic is a combination of neomycin, polymyxin B, and 1% hydrocortisone. The technique for instilling this drug applies to most eardrops. The nurse needs to instruct the mother to position her daughter in a side-lying position with the affected ear facing up. The mother needs to inspect the ear for the presence of drainage or cerumen and, if present, gently remove it with a cotton-tipped applicator. Any unusual odor or drainage could indicate a ruptured tympanic membrane and should be reported to the healthcare provider. Next, the mother should be taught to straighten the child's external ear canal by pulling down and back on the auricle to promote distribution of the medication to deeper external ear structures. After the drops are instilled, the mother can further promote medication distribution by gently pressing on the tragus of the ear. The mother should be taught to keep her daughter in a side-lying position for 3 to 5 minutes after the drops are instilled. If a cotton ball has been prescribed, the cotton ball should be placed in the ear without applying pressure. The cotton ball can be removed in 15 minutes.

2 Timoptic, a beta-adrenergic blocking agent, is contraindicated in individuals with COPD. This agent has been known to produce bronchospasm by blocking the stimulation of beta$_2$-adrenergic receptors. When beta$_2$-receptors are stimulated, relaxation of bronchial smooth muscles is facilitated. Timolol is contraindicated in COPD, an air-trapping disorder, and may be contraindicated in chronic asthma. In both cases, the beta-adrenergic blocking effect of timolol could be potentially life threatening. Betaxolol (Betoptic) is also a beta-adrenergic blocking agent but is considered safer for use in clients with COPD who require treatment for glaucoma.

3 All ophthalmic agents should be administered in the conjunctival sac. The cornea is highly innervated, and direct application of medication to the cornea can result in excessive burning and stinging. The conjunctival sac normally holds one or two drops of solution. The client should be reminded to place pressure on the inner canthus of the eye following administration of the medication to prevent the medication from flowing into the nasolacrimal duct. This maneuver helps prevent systemic absorption of medication and decreases the risk of side effects commonly associated with antiglaucoma agents.

I. CALCULATING DOSAGE USING RATIOS AND PROPORTIONS

A. A *ratio* is used to express a relationship between two or more quantities. Ratios may be written using the following notations.

1:10 means 1 part of drug A to 10 parts of solution/solvent

In drug calculations, ratios are usually expressed as a fraction:

$$\frac{1 \text{ part drug A}}{10 \text{ parts solution}} = \frac{1}{10}$$

A *proportion* shows the relationship between two ratios. It is a simple and effective means for calculating certain types of doses.

$$\frac{\text{Dose on hand}}{\text{Quantity on hand}} = \frac{\text{Desired dose}}{\text{Quantity desired } (X)}$$

Using cross multiplication, we can write the same formula as follows:

$$\text{Quantity desired } (X) = \frac{\text{Desired dose}}{\text{Dose on hand} \times \text{quantity on hand}}$$

Example 1: The healthcare provider orders erythromycin 500 mg. It is supplied in a liquid form containing 250 mg in 5 mL. How much drug should the nurse administer?

To calculate the dosage, use the formula:

$$\frac{\text{Dose on hand (250 mg)}}{\text{Quantity on hand (5 ml)}} = \frac{\text{Desired dose (500 mg)}}{\text{Quantity desired } (X)}$$

Then, cross-multiply:

$$250 \text{ mg} \times X = 5 \text{ ml} \times 500 \text{ mg}$$

Therefore, the dose to be administered is 10 ml.

B. The same proportion method can be used to solve solid dosage calculations.

Example 2: The healthcare provider orders methotrexate 20 mg/day. The methotrexate is available in 2.5-mg tablets. How many tablets should the nurse administer each day?

$$\frac{\text{Dose on hand (2.5 mg)}}{1 \text{ tablet}} = \frac{\text{Desired dose (20 mg)}}{\text{Quantity desired } (X \text{ tablets})}$$

Cross-multiplication gives:

$$2.5 \text{ mg } X = 20 \text{ mg} \times 1 \text{ tablet}$$

Therefore the nurse should administer 8 tablets daily.

II. CALCULATING DOSAGE BY WEIGHT

Doses for pediatric clients are often calculated by using body weight. The nurse must use caution to convert between pounds and kilograms, as necessary (see Table 4.2 in Chapter 4, page 31). Use the formula:

$$\text{Body weight} \times \text{amount/kg} = X \text{ mg of drug}$$

Example 3: The healthcare provider orders 10 mg/kg of methsuximide for a client who weighs 90 kg. How much should be administered?
The client should receive 900 mg of methsuximide.

Example 4: The healthcare provider orders 5 mg/kg/day of amiodarone. The client weighs 110 pounds. How much of the drug should be administered daily?

Step 1: Convert pounds to kilograms.

$$110 \text{ lb} \times 1 \text{ kg/2.2 lb} = 50 \text{ kg}$$

Step 2: Perform the drug calculation.

$$50 \text{ kg (body weight)} \times 5 \text{ mg/kg} = 250 \text{ mg}$$

The client should receive 250 mg of amiodarone per day.

III. CALCULATING DOSAGE BY BODY SURFACE AREA

Many antineoplastic drugs and most pediatric doses are calculated using body surface area (BSA).

The formula for BSA in metric units is:

$$\text{BSA} = \sqrt{\frac{\text{weight (kg)} \times \text{height (cm)}}{3600}}$$

The formula for BSA in household units is

$$\text{BSA} = \sqrt{\frac{\text{weight (lb)} \times \text{height (inches)}}{3131}}$$

Example 5: The healthcare provider orders 10 mg/m^2 of an antibiotic for a child who is 2 feet tall and weighs 30 lb. How many milligrams should be administered?

Step 1: Calculate the BSA of the child.

$$\text{BSA} = \sqrt{\frac{30 \times 24}{3131}}$$

$$\text{BSA} = \sqrt{\frac{720}{3131}}$$

$$\text{BSA} = \sqrt{0.230} = 0.48 \text{ m}^2$$

Step 2: Calculate the drug amount.

$$10 \text{ mg/m}^2 \times 0.48 \text{ m}^2$$

The nurse should administer 4.8 mg of the antibiotic to the child.

IV. CALCULATING IV INFUSION RATES

Intravenous fluids are administered over time in units of ml/min or gtt/min (gtt = drops). The basic equation for IV drug calculations is as follows:

$$\frac{\text{ml of solution} \times \text{gtt/ml}}{\text{h of administration} \times 60 \text{ min/h}} = \frac{\text{gtt}}{\text{min}}$$

Example 6: The healthcare provider orders 1,000 ml of 5% normal saline to infuse over 6 hours. What is the flow rate?

$$\frac{1{,}000 \; \cancel{\text{ml}} \times 10 \text{ gtt/}\cancel{\text{ml}}}{6 \; \cancel{\text{h}} \times 60 \text{ min/}\cancel{\text{h}}} = \frac{28 \text{ gtt}}{\text{min}}$$

Other IV conversion formulas you may use include the following:

mcg/kg/h S ml/h

$$\cancel{\text{kg}} \times \frac{\cancel{\text{mcg/kg}}}{\text{h}} \times \frac{\cancel{\text{mg}}}{1{,}000 \; \cancel{\text{mcg}}} \times \frac{\text{ml}}{\cancel{\text{mg}}} = \frac{\text{ml}}{\text{h}}$$

mcg/m^2/h S ml/h

$$\cancel{\text{m}^2} \times \frac{\cancel{\text{mcg/m}^2}}{\text{h}} \times \frac{\cancel{\text{mg}}}{1{,}000 \; \cancel{\text{mcg}}} \times \frac{\text{ml}}{\cancel{\text{mg}}} = \frac{\text{ml}}{\text{h}}$$

mcg/kg/min S gtt/min

$$\cancel{\text{kg}} \times \frac{\cancel{\text{mcg/kg}}}{\text{min}} \times \frac{\cancel{\text{mg}}}{1{,}000 \; \cancel{\text{mcg}}} \times \frac{\cancel{\text{ml}}}{\cancel{\text{mg}}} \times \frac{10 \text{ gtt}}{\cancel{\text{ml}}} = \frac{\text{gtt}}{\text{min}}$$

INDEX

Page numbers followed by *f* indicate figures and those followed by *t* indicate tables, boxes, or special features. The titles of special features (e.g., Home and Community Considerations, PharmFacts, Special Considerations) are also capitalized.

Prototype drugs appear in **boldface,** drug classifications are in SMALL CAPS, and trade names are capitalized and cross-referenced to their generic name. Diseases, disorders, and conditions are in red type.

A

AAPMC (antibiotic-associated pseudomembranous colitis), 491, 502
abacavir, 537t
abarelix, 568t, 569
abbreviations:
  to avoid, 30t, 92t
  drug administration, 30t
abciximab, 358, 386t
Abel, John Jacob, 3
Abelcet. *See* **amphotericin B**
Abenal. *See* **acetaminophen**
Abilify. *See* aripiprazole
Abiplatin. *See* cisplatin
abortion, pharmacological, drugs for:
  carboprost tromethamine, 704t, 705
  dinoprostone, 704t, 705
  methotrexate with misoprostol, 704t, 705
  mifepristone with misoprostol, 704t, 705
Abreva. *See* docosanol
absence (petit mal) seizure, 172t, 173t, 176, 783
absorption:
  definition, 48, 783
  factors affecting, 48–49, 49f
  mechanisms, 48, 48f
  in older adults, 86
  in pregnancy, 77
acamprosate calcium, 122
acarbose, 689, 690t
Accolate. *See* **zafirlukast**
Accupril. *See* quinapril
Accutane. *See* **isotretinoin**
ACE inhibitors. *See* ANGIOTENSIN-CONVERTING ENZYME (ACE) INHIBITORS
acebutolol, 79t, 140t, 367t, 797
Acel-Imune. *See* diphtheria, tetanus, and pertussis vaccine
Acetadote. *See* acetylcysteine
acetaminophen, 479t
  actions and uses, 479t
  administration alerts, 479t
  adverse effects, 233t, 479t
  Canadian/U.S. trade names, 797
  in cold/allergy combination drugs, 582t
  ethnic/racial considerations, 480t
  interactions, 479t

overdose treatment, 479t
  pharmacokinetics, 479t
  route and adult dose, 233t
acetaminophen/codeine, 800
Acetazolam. *See* acetazolamide
acetazolamide:
  Canadian/U.S. trade names, 797
  for glaucoma, 774t, 775
  for pancreatitis, 638
  for renal failure, 433, 433t
acetic acid and hydrocortisone, 780t
acetohexamide, 690t, 797
acetylation, 104
acetylcholine (Ach):
  definition, 783
  physiology, 134–35, 143
  receptors. *See* cholinergic receptors
acetylcholinesterase (AchE), 136, 269, 783
acetylcholinesterase inhibitors. *See*
  CHOLINERGICS (PARASYMPATHOMIMETICS), INDIRECT ACTING
acetylcysteine, 479t, 589t
acetylsalicylic acid. *See* **aspirin**
acetyltransferase, 104, 104t
Achromycin. *See* **tetracycline**
acid–base balances, 446, 447t. *See also* acidosis; alkalosis
acidophilus, 114t, 629, 629t
acidosis:
  causes, 426t, 447t
  definition, 446, 447f, 783
  natural therapy with seaweeds, 447t
  nursing considerations, 447–48
    client teaching, 449
  pharmacotherapy, 447, 448t
Aciphex. *See* rabeprazole
acitretin, 767t, 768
Aclovate. *See* alclometasone
acne tardive, 761
acne vulgaris:
  characteristics, 761, 783
  natural therapy with burdock root, 765t
  pharmacotherapy
    adapalene, 761t, 762
    azelaic acid, 761t
    benzoyl peroxide, 761–62, 761t
    doxycycline. *See* doxycycline
    erythromycin, 762
    ethinyl estradiol. *See* ethinyl estradiol
    nursing considerations, 764
      client teaching, 764
      lifespan considerations, 764
    sulfacetamide, 761t
    tetracycline. *See* **tetracycline**
    tretinoin, 761t, 762
Acova. *See* argatroban
acquired immune deficiency syndrome (AIDS), 534, 783. *See also* HIV-AIDS

acquired resistance, 487, 487f, 783
acromegaly, 664t, 665
Actaea racemosa. See black cohosh
ACTH. *See* adrenocorticotropic hormone; corticotropin
ACTH-40. *See* repository corticotropin
ACTH-80. *See* repository corticotropin
Acthar. *See* corticotropin
ActHIB. *See* haemophilus type B conjugate vaccine
Actidil. *See* triprolidine
Actifed. *See* triprolidine
Actifed Cold and Allergy caplets, 582t
Actifed Cold and Allergy tablets, 582t
Actinomycin-D. *See* dactinomycin
action potentials, 363, 783
Actiq. *See* fentanyl
Activase. *See* **alteplase**
activated partial thromboplastin time (aPTT), 380, 383, 783
active immunity, 457, 459f, 783
active transport, 47
Actonel. *See* risedronate sodium
ACTOplus met. *See* pioglitazone/metformin
Actos. *See* pioglitazone
Actron. *See* ketoprofen
acute gouty arthritis, 746, 783
acute insulin response, 691
acute pain, 224
acute radiation syndrome, 24, 783
acyclovir, 545t
  actions and uses, 545t
  administration alerts, 545t
  adverse effects, 544t, 545t
  interactions, 545t
  pharmacokinetics, 545t
  prescription ranking, 801
  route and adult dose, 544t
  for viral skin lesions, 756
A-δ (A-delta) fibers, 225, 783
Adalat. *See* **nifedipine**
adalimumab, 465t, 746
Adamsite, 24t
adapalene, 761t, 762
Adapin. *See* doxepin
Adderall. *See* D- and L-amphetamine racemic mixture
addiction, 14, 118, 783. *See also* substance abuse
Addison's disease, 664t, 674, 783
adefovir, 548, 548t
Adenocard. *See* adenosine
adenohypophysis, 662, 783
Adenoscan. *See* adenosine
adenosine, 367t, 374
ADH. *See* antidiuretic hormone
ADHD. *See* attention deficit–hyperactivity disorder

847

adjuvant chemotherapy, 554, 783
adolescence, 84, 783
adolescents. *See* children
ADP RECEPTOR BLOCKERS:
   drugs classified as
      clopidogrel. *See* **clopidogrel**
      ticlopidine, 358, 386, 386*t*
   mechanisms of action, 386
adrenal atrophy, 674
adrenal gland:
   disorders
      Addison's disease, 664*t*, 674, 783
      adrenocortical insufficiency, 674
      Cushing's syndrome. *See* Cushing's
         syndrome
      overview, 664*t*
   function, 673, 674*f*
adrenal medulla, 134
Adrenalin. *See* **epinephrine**
adrenergic, 134, 783
ADRENERGIC AGONISTS (SYMPATHOMIMETICS):
   actions and uses, 136–37, 137*t*
   ALPHA-. *See* ALPHA-ADRENERGIC AGONISTS
   BETA-. *See* BETA-ADRENERGIC AGONISTS
   classification, 136
   mechanisms of action, 136–37, 794
   nursing considerations, 137–138
      client teaching, 138
      lifespan considerations, 138
   nursing process focus, 139–40*t*
ADRENERGIC ANTAGONISTS (SYMPATHOLYTICS):
   ALPHA-. *See* ALPHA-ADRENERGIC
      ANTAGONISTS
   BETA-. *See* BETA-ADRENERGIC ANTAGONISTS
   clinical applications, 138, 140–41, 140*t*
   definition, 783
   nursing considerations, 141
      client teaching, 141
      lifespan considerations, 141
   nursing process focus, 142*t*
ADRENERGIC NEURON BLOCKERS:
   guanadrel, 321*t*
   guanethidine, 191, 321*t*
   reserpine, 321*t*
adrenergic receptors:
   location and responses, 135*t*
   types, 134, 135*f*, 135*t*
adrenocortical insufficiency, 674
adrenocorticotropic hormone (ACTH):
   definition, 783
   preparations, 673–74
   production, 663*t*, 673
Adriamycin. *See* **doxorubicin**
Adrucil. *See* fluorouracil
Adsorbocarpine. *See* pilocarpine
Advair Diskus. *See* salmeterol/fluticasone
Advil. *See* ibuprofen
aerobic, 485, 783
AeroBid. *See* flunisolide
aerosol, 595, 783
affinity, 49, 783
African Americans:
   ACE inhibitor effects, 320*t*

angina incidence, 348*t*
cancer incidence, 553*t*
depression treatment considerations,
   187*t*
G6PD deficiency, 525*t*
glaucoma incidence, 773*t*
heart failure incidence, 330*t*
mental illness treatment, 212*t*
pain management, 225*t*
tobacco use and mortality rates, 126*t*
Afrin. *See* **oxymetazoline; phenylephrine**
Aftate. *See* tolnaftate
afterload, 331, 331*f*, 783
Agenerase. *See* amprenavir
age-onset diabetes. *See* diabetes mellitus,
   type 2
Aggrastat. *See* tirofiban
agonist, 61, 783
AIDS (acquired immune deficiency syndrome), 534, 783. *See also*
   HIV-AIDS
akathisia, 213*t*, 214, 783
AK-Dilate Dionephrine. *See* **phenylephrine**
Akineton. *See* biperiden hydrochloride
Alazide, 309*t*
Albalon. *See* naphazoline HCl
albendazole, 528*t*
Albenza. *See* albendazole
Albuminar. *See* **normal serum albumin**
Albutein. *See* **normal serum albumin**
albuterol:
   actions and uses, 137*t*
   in anaphylaxis, 419
   for asthma, 597, 597*t*
   Canadian/U.S. trade names, 797
   prescription ranking, 800, 801
alclometasone, 765*t*
alcohol:
   dependency characteristics, 120*t*
   effects, 121–22
   fetal effects, 80*t*
   metabolism, 122
   toxicity signs, 120*t*
alcohol abuse:
   adverse health effects, 122
   chronic pancreatitis and, 638, 638*t*
   cultural and environmental
      influences, 101*t*
   vitamin B_1 deficiency and, 644
   withdrawal symptoms, 120*t*, 122
Aldactazide, 309*t*, 428
Aldactone. *See* **spironolactone**
aldesleukin, 461*t*, 462
Aldomet. *See* methyldopa
Aldoril, 309*t*
aldosterone, 317, 431, 673, 783
aldosterone antagonist, 335, 431. *See also*
   spironolactone
aldosterone receptor blocker, 317. *See also*
   eplerenone
alemtuzumab, 570, 571*t*
alendronate, 741*t*, 800
Alesse, 700*t*

Aleve. *See* naproxen sodium
Alfenta. *See* alfentanil hydrochloride
alfentanil hydrochloride, 255*t*, 256*t*
Alimta. *See* pemetrexed
alkaline phosphatase (ALP), 744
alkalosis:
   causes, 447*t*
   definition, 449, 783
   nursing considerations, 449–50
      client teaching, 450
   pharmacotherapy, 448*t*, 449, 449*t*
Alka-Seltzer. *See* **sodium bicarbonate**
Alkeran. *See* melphalan
ALKYLATING AGENTS:
   adverse effects, 558, 559*t*
   drugs classified as
      altretamine, 559*t*, 797
      busulfan, 559*t*
      carboplatin, 559*t*
      cisplatin, 559*t*, 797
      dacarbazine, 559*t*
      nitrogen mustards
         chlorambucil, 559*t*
         cyclophosphamide. *See*
         cyclophosphamide
         estramustine, 559*t*
         ifosfamide, 559*t*
         mechlorethamine, 559*t*
         melphalan, 559*t*
      nitrosoureas
         carmustine, 557, 559*t*
         lomustine, 559*t*
         streptozocin, 559*t*
      oxaliplatin, 559*t*
      procarbazine, 559*t*, 799
      temozolomide, 559*t*
      thiotepa, 559*t*
   mechanisms of action, 555, 555*f*, 557,
      558*f*
   nursing considerations, 558–59
      client teaching, 559–60
   nursing process focus, 572–73*t*
   pharmacotherapy with, 558
alkylation, 557, 558*f*, 783
Allegra. *See* **fexofenadine**
Allegra-D 12 Hour. *See* fexofenadine with
   pseudoephedrine
Allerdryl. *See* **diphenhydramine**
Allerest. *See* naphazoline HCl
allergen, 418, 580
allergic reaction, 29, 783
allergic rhinitis:
   pathophysiology, 580, 580*f*
   pharmacotherapy
      H_1-receptor antagonists. *See* H_1-
         RECEPTOR ANTAGONISTS
      intranasal glucocorticoids. *See*
         INTRANASAL GLUCOCORTICOIDS
      therapeutic approach, 580–81
Allium sativum. *See* garlic
Alloprin A. *See* allopurinol
allopurinol:
   Canadian/U.S. trade names, 797

for gout, 747, 748, 748*t*
prescription ranking, 800
almotriptan, 238*t*
aloe, drug interactions:
amiodarone, 372*t*
atropine, 148*t*
chlorothiazide, 430*t*
prednisone, 477*t*
aloglipton, 691
alopecia, 556, 783
alosetron, 630
Aloxi. *See* palonosetron
ALP (alkaline phosphatase), 744
alpha cells, 682, 682*f*
alpha interferons. *See* INTERFERONS
alpha (α) receptors, 135*t*, 137, 783
ALPHA-ADRENERGIC AGONISTS
(SYMPATHOMIMETICS):
adverse effects, 137, 137*t*, 321*t*
drugs classified as
apraclonidine, 774*t*, 775
brimonidine, 774*t*, 775
clonidine. *See* clonidine
dexmedetomidine HCl, 137*t*, 165*t*
dopamine. *See* **dopamine**
epinephrine. *See* **epinephrine**
guanabenz, 321*t*
metaraminol, 137*t*
methyldopa, 137*t*, 321*t*, 798
norepinephrine. *See* **norepinephrine**
oxymetazoline. *See* **oxymetazoline**
phenylephrine. *See* **phenylephrine**
pseudoephedrine. *See*
pseudoephedrine
intranasal use. *See* DECONGESTANTS
mechanisms of action, 307*f*, 322
for specific conditions
glaucoma, 774*t*, 775
hypertension, 321*t*, 322
nasal congestion. *See* DECONGESTANTS
overview, 137, 137*t*
shock, 414, 414*t*
ALPHA-ADRENERGIC ANTAGONISTS
(SYMPATHOLYTICS):
adverse effects, 321, 321*t*, 726*t*, 727
drugs classified as
carteolol, 321*t*, 773, 774*t*
carvedilol, 140*t*, 333*t*, 801
doxazosin. *See* **doxazosin**
labetalol, 321*t*
phentolamine, 140*t*, 723
prazosin. *See* **prazosin**
tamsulosin, 726*t*, 727, 801
terazosin, 140*t*, 321*t*, 726*t*, 801
mechanisms of action
in benign prostatic hypertrophy, 726*f*
in heart failure, 332*f*
in hypertension, 307*f*
overview, 140*t*
nursing considerations, 322, 728
nursing process focus, 142*t*
for specific conditions
benign prostatic hypertrophy, 726*t*, 727

hypertension, 321–22, 321*t*
overview, 140, 140*t*
Alphagan. *See* brimonidine
ALPHA-GLUCOSIDASE INHIBITORS:
adverse effects, 690*t*
characteristics, 689
drugs classified as
acarbose, 689, 690*t*
miglitol, 690*t*
route and adult doses, 690*t*
5-ALPHA-REDUCTASE INHIBITORS:
adverse effects, 726*t*, 727
drugs classified as
dutasteride, 726*t*
finasteride. *See* **finasteride**
mechanisms of action, 726*f*, 727
nursing considerations, 728
client teaching, 728
alprazolam, 162*t*, 800
alprostadil, 723
Altace. *See* ramipril
alteplase, 388*t*
actions and uses, 388*t*
administration alerts, 388*t*
adverse effects, 388*t*
interactions, 388*t*
overdose treatment, 388*t*
pharmacokinetics, 388*t*
route and adult dose, 388*t*
alternative healthcare systems, 109*t*
alternative therapies. *See* complementary
and alternative therapies
altretamine, 559*t*, 797
aluminum hydroxide, 620*t*
actions and uses, 620*t*
administration alerts, 620*t*
adverse effects, 619*t*, 620*t*
interactions, 620*t*
pharmacokinetics, 620*t*
route and adult dose, 619*t*
aluminum sulfate and calcium
acetate, 780*t*
Alupent. *See* metaproterenol
Alurate. *See* aprobarbital
alveoli, 594
Alzheimer's disease:
caregiving concerns, 268*t*
characteristics, 261*t*, 268–69, 783
incidence, 262*t*
living with, 262*t*
natural therapy with ginkgo biloba and
garlic, 263*t*
pharmacotherapy
acetylcholinesterase inhibitors
adverse effects, 269, 269*t*
donepezil. *See* **donepezil**
galantamine, 269*t*
mechanisms of action, 270*f*
rivastigmine, 269, 269*t*
tacrine, 269, 269*t*
memantine, 269–70
nursing considerations, 271–72
client teaching, 272

therapeutic approach, 269–71
sleep disruptions in, 262*t*
Amanita muscaria, 136
amantadine, 263, 263*t*, 546, 547*t*
Amaryl. *See* glimepiride
ambenonium, 143*t*
Ambenyl Cough Syrup, 590*t*
Ambien. *See* **zolpidem**
AmBisome. *See* **amphotericin B**
amcinonide, 765*t*
amebiasis, 526, 526*t*
amenorrhea, 709, 783
Amerge. *See* naratriptan
Americaine. *See* **benzocaine**
American Pharmaceutical Association
(APhA), 6*f*
Amersol. *See* **ibuprofen**
Amethopterin. *See* **methotrexate**
Amicar. *See* **aminocaproic acid**
Amidate. *See* etomidate
amides, 246, 248*f*, 783. *See also* LOCAL
ANESTHETICS
amikacin, 498*t*, 507*t*
Amikin. *See* amikacin
amiloride, 310*t*, 431*t*
Amin-Aid, 655
amino acids, as dietary supplement, 114*t*
aminocaproic acid, 390*t*
actions and uses, 390*t*
administration alerts, 390*t*
adverse effects, 390*t*
interactions, 390*t*
pharmacokinetics, 390*t*
route and adult dose, 390*t*
aminoglutethimide, 568*t*, 678
AMINOGLYCOSIDES:
adverse effects, 497, 498*t*
drugs classified as
amikacin, 498*t*, 507*t*
gentamicin. *See* **gentamicin**
kanamycin, 498*t*, 507*t*
neomycin, 497, 498*t*
netilmicin, 498*t*
paromomycin, 497, 498*t*, 526*t*
streptomycin, 498*t*, 507*t*
tobramycin, 498*t*
nursing considerations, 497–98
client teaching, 499
pharmacotherapy with, 497
aminophylline, 597*t*, 600, 797
amiodarone, 372*t*
actions and uses, 372*t*
administration alerts, 372*t*
adverse effects, 367*t*, 372, 372*t*
hypothyroidism and, 667
interactions, 113*t*, 372*t*
overdose treatment, 372*t*
pharmacokinetics, 372*t*
route and adult dose, 367*t*
Amitiza. *See* lubiprostone
amitriptyline:
adverse effects, 159*t*, 189*t*, 238*t*
Canadian/U.S. trade names, 797

amitriptyline (*continued*)
  genetic polymorphisms affecting
    metabolism, 104t
  prescription ranking, 800
  for specific conditions
    depression, 189t
    migraine, 238t, 239
    panic disorders, 159t
amlodipine, 313t, 350t, 800
amlodipine/benazepril, 800
ammonium chloride, 449t
  actions and uses, 449t
  administration alerts, 449t
  adverse effects, 449t
  interactions, 449t
  nursing considerations, 449–50
    client teaching, 450
  overdose treatment, 449t
  pharmacokinetics, 449t
amobarbital:
  as general anesthesia adjunct,
    256t
  for sedation and insomnia, 164t
  for seizures, 175t
  for status epilepticus, 174
amoxapine, 189t
amoxicillin:
  adverse effects, 489t
  Canadian/U.S. trade names, 797
  for *H. pylori,* 620
  mechanisms of action, 490
  prescription ranking, 800
  route and adult dose, 489t
amoxicillin–clavulanate, 489t, 490
Amoxil. *See* amoxicillin
amphetamines:
  abuse, 124–25
  adverse effects, 79t, 203, 204t
  dependency characteristics, 120t
  drugs classified as
    D- and L-amphetamine racemic
      mixture, 203, 204t
    dextroamphetamine. *See*
      dextroamphetamine
    methamphetamine, 124–25, 203, 204t
  toxicity signs, 120t
  for weight loss, 635
  withdrawal symptoms, 120t
Amphotec. *See* **amphotericin B**
amphotericin B, 517t
  actions and uses, 517t
  administration alerts, 517t
  adverse effects, 516t, 517t
  interactions, 517t
  nursing process focus, 518t
  pharmacokinetics, 517t
  route and adult dose, 516t
ampicillin, 489t, 490, 797
amprenavir, 537t
amyl nitrite, 350t
amyloid plaques, 267, 270f, 783
amyotrophic lateral sclerosis, 261t
Amytal. *See* amobarbital

anabolic steroids, 113t, 719, 720t, 783
anaerobic, 485, 783
Anafranil. *See* clomipramine
anakinra, 465t, 746, 747t
analgesics:
  definition, 226, 783
  nonopioid
    acetaminophen. *See* **acetaminophen**
    centrally-acting
      clonidine. *See* clonidine
      tramadol, 233t, 800, 802
    nonsteroidal anti-inflammatory drugs.
      See NONSTEROIDAL ANTI-INFLAMMATORY
      DRUGS (NSAIDs)
  opioid. *See* OPIOID (NARCOTIC) ANALGESICS
anaphylactic shock, 410, 410t, 412t, 783
anaphylaxis:
  definition, 29, 418, 783
  drugs causing, 419
  inflammatory mediators in, 473
  pharmacotherapy
    epinephrine. *See* **epinephrine**
    nursing considerations, 420
      client teaching, 420–21
    therapeutic approach, 418–20
  prevention, 420t
  recurrent, 421t
  symptoms, 29, 418, 419f
Anaprox. *See* naproxen sodium
anastomoses, 346, 783
anastrozole, 568t, 569
Ancobon. *See* flucytosine
Ancotil. *See* flucytosine
Andro. *See* **testosterone**
Andro 100. *See* **testosterone**
Andro L.A. *See* testosterone enanthate
Andro-Cyp. *See* testosterone cypionate
Androderm, 719. *See also* **testosterone**
Androgel, 719. *See also* **testosterone**
ANDROGEN ANTAGONISTS:
  adverse effects, 568t
  bicalutamide, 568t, 569
  flutamide, 568t, 569
  nilutamide, 568t, 569
  route and adult doses, 568t
ANDROGENS:
  abuse, 719, 720t
  adverse effects, 568t, 720, 720t
  for cancer chemotherapy, 568t, 569
  drugs classified as
    danazol, 714t, 715, 720t, 797
    fluoxymesterone, 568, 568t, 720t, 798
    methyltestosterone, 720t, 798
    nandrolone phenpropionate, 720t
    testolactone, 568, 568t, 720t, 721
    testosterone. *See* **testosterone**
    testosterone cypionate, 719, 720t
    testosterone enanthate, 719, 720t, 799
  functions, 719, 783
  nonreproductive effects, 719
  nursing considerations, 720
    client teaching, 720
  nursing process focus, 722t

  production, 673
  route and adult dose, 720t
  route and adult doses, 568t
Android. *See* methyltestosterone
Anectine. *See* **succinylcholine**
anemia:
  causes, 401
  classification, 401, 401t
  definition, 401, 783
  pernicious, 402
  pharmacotherapy
    folic acid. *See* **folic acid/folate**
    iron. *See* IRON SALTS
    nursing considerations, 403, 404–6
      client teaching, 403, 406
      lifespan considerations, 406
      nursing process focus, 405t
    vitamin B_{12}. *See* **vitamin B_{12}**
  in renal failure, 426t
Anergan. *See* promethazine
anesthetics:
  general. *See* GENERAL ANESTHETICS
  local. *See* LOCAL ANESTHETICS
Angeliq. *See* estradiol/drospirenone
angina pectoris:
  definition, 346
  ethnic/racial considerations, 348t
  gender considerations, 348t
  incidence, 347t
  nonpharmacological management, 348
  pathophysiology, 346–47
  pharmacotherapy
    beta-adrenergic antagonists. *See*
      BETA-ADRENERGIC ANTAGONISTS
    calcium channel blockers. *See* CALCIUM
      CHANNEL BLOCKERS
    mechanisms of action, 349f
    nursing considerations, 350–51,
      352–53, 354–55
      client teaching, 351, 353, 355
      nursing process focus, 352t
    organic nitrates. *See* ORGANIC NITRATES
    overview, 350t
    therapeutic approach, 348–49
  symptoms, 347
Angiomax. *See* bivalirudin
angiotensin II, 317, 783
ANGIOTENSIN II RECEPTOR BLOCKERS (ARBs):
  adverse effects, 317
  drugs classified as
    candesartan, 316t, 334
    eprosartan, 316t
    irbesartan, 316t, 801
    losartan, 316t, 800
    olmesartan medoxomil, 316t, 801
    telmisartan, 316t
    valsartan, 316t, 334, 800
  mechanisms of action, 307f, 316–17
  for specific conditions
    heart failure, 334
    hypertension, 309t, 317
angiotensin-converting enzyme (ACE),
    317, 783

ANGIOTENSIN-CONVERTING ENZYME (ACE) INHIBITORS:
adverse effects, 33*t*, 316*t*, 317, 320, 333*t*
drugs classified as
benazepril, 316*t*, 801
captopril, 316*t*, 333*t*, 358
enalapril. *See* **enalapril**
fosinopril, 316*t*, 333*t*
lisinopril. *See* **lisinopril**
moexipril, 316*t*
perindopril, 316*t*
quinapril, 333*t*, 801
ramipril, 316*t*, 333*t*, 800
trandolapril, 316*t*
ethnic/racial considerations, 320*t*
mechanisms of action, 307*f*, 316–17, 332*f*, 334
nursing process focus, 318–19*t*
for specific conditions
heart failure
nursing considerations, 334–35
route and adult doses, 333*t*
therapeutic approach, 334
hypertension
nursing considerations, 317–20
nursing process focus, 318–19*t*
route and adult doses, 309*t*
therapeutic approach, 317
myocardial infarction, 358
anidulafungin, 516, 516*t*
anions, 442, 442*t*, 783
anise, 247*t*
anisindione, 382*t*
anistreplase, 388*t*
anorexia, 613, 783
anorexiants:
characteristics, 635, 783
drugs classified as
orlistat, 635
sibutramine. *See* **sibutramine**
nursing considerations, 636–37
client teaching, 636–37
lifespan considerations, 636–37
ANP (atrial natriuretic peptide), 342
Ansaid. *See* flurbiprofen
Antabuse. *See* disulfiram
ANTACIDS:
adverse effects, 619*t*
definition, 619, 783
drugs classified as
aluminum hydroxide. *See* **aluminum hydroxide**
calcium carbonate. *See* calcium carbonate
calcium carbonate with magnesium hydroxide, 619*t*
magaldrate, 619*t*
magnesium hydroxide, 619*t*
magnesium hydroxide and aluminum hydroxide, 619*t*
magnesium hydroxide and aluminum hydroxide with simethicone, 619*t*
sodium bicarbonate. *See* **sodium bicarbonate**

mechanisms of action, 614*f*
nursing considerations, 619–20
client teaching, 619–20
pharmacotherapy with, 619
route and adult doses, 619*t*
Antagon. *See* ganirelix
antagonism, 488
antagonist, 62, 783
Antazone. *See* sulfinpyrazone
antepartum, 783
anterior chamber, 771, 771*f*
ANTERIOR PITUITARY AGENTS:
adverse effects, 664*t*
drugs classified as
corticotropin, 664*t*, 673–74
cosyntropin, 664*t*, 674
somatrem, 664*t*, 665
somatropin, 664*t*, 665
thyrotropin, 664*t*
route and adult doses, 664*t*
anthrax:
characteristics, 784
clinical manifestations, 22*t*
pathophysiology, 21–22
prophylaxis and treatment, 22
vaccine, 22
ANTIANEMIC AGENTS:
definition, 784
drugs classified as
folic acid. *See* **folic acid/folate**
iron. *See* IRON SALTS
vitamin B$_{12}$. *See* **vitamin B$_{12}$**
nursing considerations, 403, 404–6
client teaching, 403, 406
lifespan considerations, 406
nursing process focus, 405*t*
ANTIBACTERIALS:
acquired resistance, 487, 487*f*
adverse effects. *See* specific drugs and drug classes
allergy to, 489
drugs classified as
aminoglycosides. *See* AMINOGLYCOSIDES
antituberculosis drugs. *See* ANTITUBERCULOSIS DRUGS
aztreonam, 503*t*
carbapenems
ertapenem, 503*t*, 506
imipenem-cilastatin, 503*t*, 506
meropenem, 503*t*, 506
cephalosporins. *See* CEPHALOSPORINS
chloramphenicol, 503*t*, 778, 797
clindamycin, 502, 503*t*, 797, 801
cyclic lipopeptides
daptomycin, 503*t*, 506
fluoroquinolones. *See* FLUOROQUINOLONES
fosfomycin, 503*t*
glycylcyclines
tigecycline, 494*t*, 506
ketolides
telithromycin, 504*t*, 506
lincomycin, 503*t*

macrolides. *See* MACROLIDES
methenamine, 503*t*
metronidazole. *See* **metronidazole**
nitrofurantoin, 503*t*, 798, 801
oxazolidinones
linezolid, 503*t*, 505
penicillins. *See* PENICILLINS
streptogramins
quinupristin–dalfopristin, 503*t*, 505
sulfonamides. *See* SULFONAMIDES
tetracyclines. *See* TETRACYCLINES
vancomycin, 504*t*, 506
ethnic/racial considerations, 488*t*
for *H. pylori*, 614*f*, 620
host factors, 488–89
nursing considerations. *See* specific drugs and drug classes
nursing process focus, 504–5*t*
prophylactic, 487
selection, 487–88
antibiotic, 486, 784
antibiotic-associated pseudomembranous colitis (AAPMC), 491, 502
ANTIBIOTICS. *See* ANTIBACTERIALS; ANTI-INFECTIVES
ANTIBODIES, MONOCLONAL. *See* MONOCLONAL ANTIBODIES
antibody, 456, 457*f*, 784
anticancer drugs. *See* ANTINEOPLASTICS
ANTICHOLINERGICS:
adverse effects, 147*t*, 267*t*
definition, 784
drugs classified as
atropine. *See* **atropine**
benztropine. *See* **benztropine**
biperiden hydrochloride, 267*t*
cyclopentolate, 147*t*, 779*t*
dicyclomine, 147*t*, 630, 638
diphenhydramine. *See* **diphenhydramine**
glycopyrrolate, 147*t*
homatropine, 779*t*
ipratropium bromide. *See* **ipratropium bromide**
oxybutynin, 147*t*
procyclidine hydrochloride, 267*t*, 799
propantheline, 147*t*
scopolamine. *See* scopolamine
tiotropium, 597*t*, 599
trihexyphenidyl, 147*t*, 267*t*, 799
tropicamide, 779*t*
mechanisms of action, 147, 264*f*, 267, 784
nursing considerations, 149–50
client teaching, 150
lifespan considerations, 150
nursing process focus, 148–49*t*
for specific conditions
asthma
mechanisms of action, 599
nursing considerations, 599–600
route and adult doses, 597*t*
overview, 146–47
Parkinson's disease

ANTICHOLINERGICS *(continued)*
    mechanisms of action, 264f, 267
    nursing considerations, 267–68
    route and adult doses, 267t
ANTICOAGULANTS:
    adverse effects, 382, 382t
    definition, 381, 784
    drugs classified as
        anisindione, 382t
        direct thrombin inhibitors. *See* DIRECT
            THROMBIN INHIBITORS
        fondaparinux, 382t
        heparin. *See* **heparin**
        low-molecular-weight heparins. *See*
            LOW-MOLECULAR-WEIGHT HEPARINS
        warfarin. *See* **warfarin**
    home care considerations, 380t
    mechanisms of action, 381, 381t
    nursing considerations, 382–84
        client teaching, 384
        lifespan considerations, 383
    nursing process focus, 385t
    pharmacotherapy with, 381–82
    for specific conditions
        myocardial infarction, 358
        thromboembolic disease,
            381–82, 382t
ANTIDEPRESSANTS:
    adverse effects. *See specific drugs and drug*
        classes
    black box warning, 188
    drugs classified as
        atypical antidepressants. *See* ATYPICAL
            ANTIDEPRESSANTS
        monamine oxidase inhibitors. *See*
            MONOAMINE OXIDASE INHIBITORS
        selective serotonin reuptake inhibitors.
            See SELECTIVE SEROTONIN REUPTAKE
            INHIBITORS
        tricyclic antidepressants. *See* TRICYCLIC
            ANTIDEPRESSANTS
    mechanisms of action, 188, 784
    nursing considerations. *See specific drugs*
        and drug classes
    nursing process focus, 197–99t
    for specific conditions
        Alzheimer's disease, 271
        anxiety, 158–59, 160t
        depression, 188, 189t
        panic disorders, 159–60, 159t
ANTIDIARRHEALS:
    acidophilus, 114t, 629, 629t
    adverse effects, 628t
    drugs classified as
        bismuth subsalicylate, 620, 628t
        furazolidone, 628t
        opioid
            camphorated opium tincture, 628t
            difenoxin with atropine, 628t
            diphenoxylate with atropine. *See*
            diphenoxylate with atropine
        loperamide, 628t
    nursing considerations, 629–30

        client teaching, 630
        lifespan considerations, 630
    nursing process focus, 631t
    pharmacotherapy with, 629
    route and adult doses, 628t
antidiuretic hormone (ADH):
    in blood pressure control, 304–5
    in fluid balance, 439
    nursing considerations, 666
        client teaching, 666
        lifespan considerations, 666
    pharmacotherapy with, 665. *See also*
        vasopressin
    production, 663f
ANTIDYSRHYTHMICS:
    adverse effects. *See specific drugs and drug*
        classes
    classification, 365, 366t
    drugs classified as
        adenosine, 367t, 368t, 374
        beta-adrenergic antagonists
            acebutolol, 79t, 140t, 367t, 797
            esmolol, 140t, 367t
            ethnic/racial considerations, 371t
            nursing considerations, 371
            propranolol. *See* **propranolol**
            therapeutic approach, 371
        calcium channel blockers
            diltiazem. *See* **diltiazem**
            nursing considerations, 373–74
            therapeutic approach, 373
            verapamil. *See* **verapamil**
        digoxin. *See* **digoxin**
        potassium channel blockers. *See*
            POTASSIUM CHANNEL BLOCKERS
        sodium channel blockers. *See* SODIUM
            CHANNEL BLOCKERS
    nursing process focus, 370t
ANTIEMETICS:
    adverse effects, 634t
    drugs classified as
        antihistamines and anticholinergics,
          633
            cyclizine hydrochloride, 634t, 797
            dimenhydrinate, 633, 634t, 798
            diphenhydramine. *See* **diphenhy-**
            dramine
            hydroxyzine, 137, 634t, 798, 801
            meclizine, 633, 634t, 798, 801
            scopolamine, 633, 634t
        cannabinoids
            dronabinol, 633, 634t
            nabilone, 633, 634t
        glucocorticoids
            characteristics, 633
            dexamethasone. *See* dexamethasone
            methylprednisolone. *See*
            methylprednisolone
        lorazepam. *See* **lorazepam**
        neurokinin receptor antagonist
            aprepitant, 633, 634t
        phenothiazines
            characteristics, 633

            metoclopramide, 634t, 798, 801
            perphenazine. *See* perphenazine
            prochlorperazine. *See* **prochlorpera-**
            zine
            promethazine. *See* promethazine
        selective serotonin receptor
          inhibitors
            characteristics, 633
            dolasetron, 634t
            granisetron, 634t
            ondansetron, 634t
            palonosetron, 634t
    nursing considerations, 633
        client teaching, 635
    route and adult doses, 634t
antifibrinolytics. *See* HEMOSTATICS
antiflatulent, 619, 784
ANTIFUNGALS:
    azoles
        adverse effects, 519–20, 519t
        drugs classified as
            butoconazole, 519t
            clotrimazole. *See* clotrimazole
            econazole, 519t, 798
            fluconazole. *See* **fluconazole**
            itraconazole, 30t, 518, 519t, 521
            ketoconazole. *See* ketoconazole
            miconazole, 519t, 521, 756
            oxiconazole, 519t
            sertaconazole, 519t
            sulconazole, 519t
            terconazole, 519t
            tioconazole, 519t
            voriconazole, 519t
        mechanisms of action, 517
        nursing considerations, 520
            client teaching, 520
        pharmacotherapy with, 517, 518–20
        route and adult doses, 519t
    mechanisms of action, 515
    superficial
        adverse effects, 520t
        drugs classified as
            butenafine, 520t
            ciclopirox olamine, 520t
            griseofulvin, 520t, 521, 798
            haloprogin, 520t
            naftifine, 520t
            nystatin. *See* **nystatin**
            terbinafine, 520t, 521
            tolnaftate, 520t, 521
            undecylenic acid, 520t, 521, 756
        nursing considerations, 521–22
            client teaching, 521
        nursing process focus, 522–23t
        pharmacotherapy with, 520–21
        route and adult doses, 520t
    systemic
        adverse effects, 516t
        drugs classified as
            amphotericin B. *See* **amphotericin B**
            anidulafungin, 516, 516t
            caspofungin, 516, 516t

flucytosine, 515, 516, 516*t*, 798
micafungin, 516*t*
nursing considerations, 516
client teaching, 517
lifespan considerations, 517
nursing process focus, 518*t*
pharmacotherapy with, 516*t*, 756
route and adult doses, 516*t*
antigen, 418, 455
ANTIGLAUCOMA DRUGS:
adverse effects, 774*t*
drugs classified as
alpha$_2$-adrenergic agonists
apraclonidine, 774*t*, 775
brimonidine, 774*t*, 775
beta-adrenergic antagonists
betaxolol, 773, 774*t*
carteolol, 140*t*, 773, 774*t*
levobunolol, 773, 774*t*
metipranolol, 773, 774*t*
timolol. *See* **timolol**
carbonic anhydrase inhibitors
acetazolamide. *See* acetazolamide
brinzolamide, 774*t*
dorzolamide, 775
methazolamide, 774*t*
miotics (cholinergic agonists)
carbachol, 774*t*
demecarium, 774*t*
physostigmine, 774*t*
pilocarpine, 143*t*, 774*t*, 775
prostaglandins
bimatoprost, 773, 774*t*
latanoprost. *See* **latanoprost**
travoprost, 773, 774*t*
unoprostone, 773, 774*t*
sympathomimetics
dipivefrin, 774*t*, 775
epinephryl borate, 774*t*, 775
nursing considerations, 776
client teaching, 776, 778
nursing process focus, 777–78*t*
route and adult doses, 774*t*
ANTIHELMINTHICS:
adverse effects, 528*t*
drugs classified as
albendazole, 528*t*
diethylcarbamazine, 528*t*
ivermectin, 528*t*
mebendazole. *See* **mebendazole**
praziquantel, 528*t*
pyrantel, 528*t*
nursing considerations, 529–30
client teaching, 530
pharmacotherapy with, 528–29
route and adult doses, 528*t*
ANTIHISTAMINES. *See* H$_1$-RECEPTOR
ANTAGONISTS; H$_2$-RECEPTOR
ANTAGONISTS
ANTIHYPERTENSIVES:
drugs classified as
adrenergic agonists. *See* ALPHA-
ADRENERGIC AGONISTS

adrenergic antagonists. *See*
ALPHA-ADRENERGIC ANTAGONISTS;
BETA-ADRENERGIC ANTAGONISTS
calcium channel blockers. *See* CALCIUM
CHANNEL BLOCKERS
diuretics. *See* DIURETICS
vasodilators. *See* VASODILATORS
mechanisms of action, 307*f*
selection of, 306–8
ANTI-INFECTIVES:
acquired resistance, 487, 487*f*
allergy to, 489
antibacterials. *See* ANTIBACTERIALS
antifungals. *See* ANTIFUNGALS
antihelminthics. *See* ANTIHELMINTHICS
antimalarials. *See* ANTIMALARIALS
antiprotozoals. *See* ANTIPROTOZOALS
antituberculosis drugs. *See*
ANTITUBERCULOSIS DRUGS
definition, 486, 784
for *H. pylori*, 620
host factors, 488–89
mechanisms of action, 486, 486*f*
prophylactic use, 487
selection, 487–88
topical, 756
Antilirium. *See* physostigmine
ANTIMALARIALS:
adverse effects, 523*t*
drugs classified as
atovaquone and proguanil, 523*t*
chloroquine. *See* **chloroquine**
hydroxychloroquine. *See*
hydroxychloroquine
mefloquine, 523*t*
primaquine, 523*t*
pyrimethamine, 523*t*
quinine, 523*t*, 799, 801
nursing considerations, 524–25
client teaching, 525
pharmacotherapy with, 524
route and adult doses, 523*t*
ANTIMETABOLITES:
adverse effects, 561, 561*t*
drugs classified as
folic acid antagonists
methotrexate. *See* **methotrexate**
pemetrexed, 561*t*
purine analogs
cladribine, 561*t*
clofarabine, 561
fludarabine, 561*t*
mercaptopurine, 555*f*, 561*t*
nelarabine, 561*t*
pentostatin, 561*t*
thioguanine, 561*t*, 562*f*, 799
pyrimidine analogs
azacitidine, 561, 561*t*
capecitabine, 561*t*
cytarabine, 555*f*, 561, 561*t*
floxuridine, 561*t*
fluorouracil, 555, 555*f*, 561*t*, 562*f*
gemcitabine, 561*t*

mechanisms of action, 466, 555*f*, 561
nursing considerations, 561, 563
client teaching, 563
nursing process focus, 572–73*t*
pharmacotherapy with, 561
route and adult doses, 561*t*
ANTIMICROBIALS. *See* ANTI-INFECTIVES
ANTIMIGRAINE DRUGS:
adverse effects, 238*t*
drugs classified as
ergot alkaloids. *See* ERGOT ALKALOIDS
triptans
almotriptan, 238*t*
eletriptan, 238*t*
frovatriptan, 238*t*
naratriptan, 238*t*
rizatriptan, 238*t*
sumatriptan. *See* **sumatriptan**
zolmitriptan, 238*t*
nursing considerations, 239–41
client teaching, 241
nursing process focus, 240*t*
route and adult doses, 238*t*
Antiminth. *See* pyrantel
ANTINEOPLASTICS:
administration considerations, 557
adverse effects, 556–57, 557*t*
cell kill and, 555, 556*f*
classification, 557
drugs classified as
alkylating agents, 559*t*. *See also*
ALKYLATING AGENTS
antimetabolites, 561*t*. *See also*
ANTIMETABOLITES
antitumor antibiotics, 564*t*. *See also*
ANTITUMOR ANTIBIOTICS
arsenic trioxide, 571*t*
asparaginase, 555*f*, 571, 571*t*, 797
bexarotene, 571*t*
biologic response modifiers, 570–71, 571*t*
bortezomib, 571*t*
camptothecins. *See* CAMPTOTHECINS
erlotinib, 571*t*
gefitinib, 571*t*
hormone antagonists, 568*t*. *See also*
HORMONE ANTAGONISTS
hormones, 568*t*. *See also* HORMONES
hydroxyurea, 571*t*
imatinib mesylate, 571, 571*t*
levamisole, 571*t*
mitotane, 571, 571*t*
monoclonal antibodies, 571*t*. *See also*
MONOCLONAL ANTIBODIES
pegaspargase, 571*t*
sorafenib, 571*t*
taxanes, 566*t*. *See also* TAXANES
topoisomerase inhibitors, 566*t*. *See also*
TOPOISOMERASE INHIBITORS
vinca alkaloids, 566*t*. *See also* VINCA
ALKALOIDS
zoledronic acid, 571*t*
growth fraction and success of, 554–55
mechanisms of action, 554–55, 555*f*

ANTINEOPLASTICS (*continued*)
nadir, 557
nursing considerations
alkylating agents, 558–60
antimetabolites, 561, 563
antitumor antibiotics, 563, 565
hormones and hormone antagonists,
569–70
natural product extracts, 566–67
nursing process focus, 572–73*t*
in older adults, 570*t*
pharmacotherapy protocols and
strategies, 556
route and adult doses, 557*t*
ANTIPLATELET AGENTS:
adverse effects, 386*t*
drugs classified as
abciximab, 358, 386*t*
aspirin. *See* **aspirin**
cilostazol, 386, 386*t*
clopidogrel. *See* **clopidogrel**
dipyridamole, 386*t*, 798
eptifibatide, 386*t*
pentoxifylline, 386, 386*t*
ticlopidine, 358, 386, 386*t*
tirofiban, 386*t*
mechanisms of action, 381*t*, 384, 386
for myocardial infarction and stroke
prevention, 358
nursing considerations, 386–87
client teaching, 387
lifespan considerations, 387
route and adult doses, 386*t*
ANTIPROTOZOALS:
adverse effects, 526*t*
drugs classified as
antimalarial. *See* ANTIMALARIALS
iodoquinol, 526*t*
metronidazole. *See* **metronidazole**
paromomycin, 497, 498*t*, 526*t*
pentamidine, 526*t*, 799
sodium stibogluconate, 526*t*
tinidazole, 526*t*, 527
trimetrexate, 526*t*
nursing considerations, 527
client teaching, 527
route and adult doses, 526*t*
ANTIPSYCHOTICS:
adverse effects, 213–14,
213*t*, 478
drugs classified as
atypical antipsychotics. *See* ATYPICAL
ANTIPSYCHOTICS
conventional (typical) antipsychotics
nonphenothiazines. *See*
NONPHENOTHIAZINES
phenothiazines. *See* PHENOTHIAZINES
dopamine system stabilizers, 221
mechanisms of action, 211*f*
nursing process focus, 216–17*t*
ANTIPYRETICS:
definition, 784
drugs classified as

acetaminophen. *See* **acetaminophen**
aspirin. *See* **aspirin**
ibuprofen. *See* **ibuprofen**
nursing considerations, 478–79
client teaching, 479–80
lifespan considerations, 479
nursing process focus, 480*t*
therapeutic approach, 478
ANTIRETROVIRALS:
adverse effects, 537*t*
compliance, psychosocial issues, 538*t*
definition, 784
drugs classified as
fusion inhibitor
enfuvirtide, 536, 537*t*
protease inhibitors. *See* PROTEASE
INHIBITORS
reverse transcriptase inhibitors
abacavir, 537*t*
delavirdine, 537*t*
didanosine, 537*t*, 543
efavirenz, 113*t*, 537*t*, 538
emtricitabine, 537*t*
lamivudine, 537*t*, 543, 548
nevirapine. *See* **nevirapine**
stavudine, 537*t*, 543
tenofovir, 536, 537*t*
zalcitabine, 537*t*
zidovudine. *See* **zidovudine**
mechanisms of action, 534
nursing considerations, 539–40
client teaching, 540, 543
nursing process focus, 541–42*t*
pharmacotherapy with, 537–38
for postexposure prophylaxis following
occupational exposure to HIV, 543
for prevention of perinatal HIV
transmission, 543
route and adult doses, 537*t*
ANTISEIZURE DRUGS:
adverse effects, 175*t*, 178*t*
drugs classified as
GABA potentiators
barbiturates, 175*t*. *See also*
BARBITURATES
benzodiazepines, 175*t*. *See also*
BENZODIAZEPINES
gabapentin. *See* gabapentin
mechanisms of action, 173, 174*f*
primidone, 79*t*, 175*t*, 799
tiagabine, 175, 175*t*
topiramate, 175*t*, 200, 801
hydantoins
fosphenytoin, 178*t*
nursing considerations, 178–80
phenytoin. *See* **phenytoin**
phenytoin-like agents
carbamazepine. *See* carbamazepine
felbamate, 178, 178*t*
lamotrigine. *See* lamotrigine
nursing considerations, 178–80
valproic acid. *See* **valproic acid**
zonisamide, 178, 178*t*, 180

succinimides
ethosuximide. *See* **ethosuximide**
mechanisms of action, 180
methsuximide, 180*t*
nursing considerations, 181
phensuximide, 180*t*
herb–drug interactions, 113*t*
nursing process focus, 182–83*t*
route and adult doses, 175*t*, 178*t*
for specific conditions
anxiety, 165*t*
bipolar disorder, 200*t*
ANTISPASMODICS:
adverse effects, 279*t*
characteristics, 278–79
drugs classified as
botulinum toxin type A, 278–79,
279*t*, 281*t*
botulinum toxin type B, 278–79, 279*t*
dantrolene sodium. *See* **dantrolene
sodium**
quinine, 279*t*
home care considerations, 281*t*
mechanisms of action, 278, 278*f*
nursing considerations, 279
client teaching, 281
lifespan considerations, 281
nursing process focus, 280*t*
route and adult doses, 279*t*
antithrombin III, 381, 784
Antithymocyte Globulin. *See* lymphocyte
immune globulin
ANTITHYROID AGENTS:
adverse effects, 668*t*
drugs classified as
methimazole, 668*t*, 670
potassium iodide, 24–25, 653, 668, 672
potassium iodide and iodine, 668*t*
propylthiouracil. *See* **propylthiouracil**
radioactive iodine, 80, 653, 668*t*, 670
nursing considerations, 673
client teaching, 673
lifespan considerations, 672–73
nursing process focus, 671–72*t*
pharmacotherapy with, 670, 672
route and adult doses, 668*t*
ANTITUBERCULOSIS DRUGS:
adverse effects, 507*t*
drugs classified as
first-line agents
ethambutol, 507*t*
isoniazid. *See* **isoniazid**
pyrazinamide, 507*t*, 799
rifampin, 194, 507*t*, 508, 799
rifapentine, 507*t*
Rifater, 507*t*
streptomycin, 507*t*
second-line agents
amikacin, 507*t*
capreomycin, 507*t*
ciprofloxacin. *See* **ciprofloxacin**
cycloserine, 507*t*
ethionamide, 507*t*

kanamycin, 507t
ofloxacin, 507t
nursing considerations, 508–9
client teaching, 509
nursing process focus, 509–10t
pharmacotherapy with, 506–8
route and adult doses, 507t
ANTITUMOR ANTIBIOTICS:
adverse effects, 563, 564t
drugs classified as
bleomycin, 555f, 564t
dactinomycin, 564t
daunorubicin, 564t
daunorubicin liposomal, 564t
doxorubicin. See **doxorubicin**
doxorubicin liposomal, 564t
epirubicin, 564t
idarubicin, 563, 564t
mitomycin, 564t
mitoxantrone, 564t
plicamycin, 563, 564t
valrubicin, 563, 564t
mechanisms of action, 555, 555f
nursing considerations, 563, 565
client teaching, 565
nursing process focus, 572–73t
pharmacotherapy with, 563
route and adult doses, 564t
ANTITUSSIVES:
adverse effects, 589t
definition, 784
drugs classified as
benzonatate, 589, 589t, 801
codeine. See codeine
dextromethorphan. See
dextromethorphan
hydrocodone bitartrate. See
hydrocodone bitartrate
nursing considerations, 590–91
client teaching, 590–91
pharmacotherapy with, 589
route and adult doses, 589t
Antivert. See meclizine
ANTIVIRALS:
for herpesviruses
nursing considerations, 545–46
client teaching, 546
systemic agents
acyclovir. See **acyclovir**
adverse effects, 544t
cidofovir, 544t
famciclovir, 544t
foscarnet, 544t
ganciclovir, 544t
route and adult doses, 544t
valacyclovir, 544t, 801
therapeutic approach, 544–45
topical agents
adverse effects, 544t
docosanol, 544t
idoxuridine, 544t, 545
penciclovir, 544t
route and adult doses, 544t

trifluridine, 544t, 545
vidarabine, 544t, 545
for HIV/AIDS. See ANTIRETROVIRALS
for influenza
adverse effects, 547t
amantadine, 263, 263t, 546, 547t
oseltamivir, 546, 547t
rimantadine, 546, 547t
route and adult doses, 547t
zanamivir, 546, 547t
Anturan. See sulfinpyrazone
Anturane. See sulfinpyrazone
anxiety:
brain regions responsible for,
155–56, 155f
causes, 156t
definition, 154, 784
incidence, 156t
insomnia and, 156–57
model for stress management, 156f
nonpharmacologic management,
156, 156f
performance, 154
pharmacotherapy
antidepressants, 159t, 160t. See also
ANTIDEPRESSANTS
benzodiazepines, 162t. See also
BENZODIAZEPINES
nursing considerations, 161–62
client teaching, 162–63
lifespan considerations, 162
nursing process focus, 166t
therapeutic approach, 156, 158–60
situational, 154
social, 154
anxiolytics, 156, 784
Anzemet. See dolasetron
Aparkane. See trihexyphenidyl
A.P.L. See human chorionic gonadotropin
Apo-Acetazolamide. See acetazolamide
Apo-allopurinol-A. See allopurinol
Apo-Amitriptyline. See amitriptyline
Apo-Amoxi. See amoxicillin
Apo-Atenolol. See **atenolol**
Apo-Benztropine. See **benztropine**
Apo-Cal. See calcium carbonate
Apo-Carbamazepine. See carbamazepine
Apo-Chlorpropamide. See chlorpropamide
Apo-Cimetidine. See cimetidine
Apo-Cloxi. See cloxacillin
Apo-Diazepam. See **diazepam**
Apo-Dilitaz. See **diltiazem**
Apo-Dimenhydrinate. See dimenhydrinate
Apo-Dipyridamole. See dipyridamole
Apo-Doxy. See doxycycline
Apo-Erythro-S. See **erythromycin**
Apo-Flurazepam. See flurazepam
Apo-Hydro. See **hydrochlorothiazide**
Apo-Hydroxyzine. See hydroxyzine
Apo-Lorazepam. See **lorazepam**
Apo-Methyldopa. See methyldopa
Apo-Metoprolol. See **metoprolol**
Apo-Naproxen. See naproxen

Apo-Nifed. See **nifedipine**
Apo-Nitrofurantoin. See nitrofurantoin
Apo-Prednisone. See **prednisone**
Apo-Primidone. See primidone
Apo-Propranolol. See **propranolol**
apoprotein, 289, 784
Apo-Quinidine. See quinidine sulfate
Apo-Ranitidine. See ranitidine HCl
apothecary system of measurement,
31, 31t, 784
Apo-Trihex. See trihexyphenidyl
appetite, 635
appetite suppressants. See anorexiants
apraclonidine, 774t, 775
aprepitant, 633, 634t
Apresazide, 309t, 428
Apresoline. See **hydralazine**
aprobarbital, 164t
aprotinin, 390t
Aptivus. See tipranavir
aPTT (activated partial thromboplastin
time), 380, 383, 783
AquaMEPHYTON. See vitamin K
Aquasol A. See **vitamin A**
Aquasol E. See vitamin E
Aquatab. See benzthiazide
Aquatag. See benzthiazide
Aquatensen. See methyclothiazide
aqueous humor, 771, 784
Aralen. See **chloroquine**
Aramine. See metaraminol
Aranesp. See darbepoetin alfa
Arava. See leflunomide
ARBs. See ANGIOTENSIN II RECEPTOR
BLOCKERS
ardeparin, 382t
Aredia. See pamidronate disodium
argatroban, 382, 382t
Aricept. See **donepezil**
Arimidex. See anastrozole
aripiprazole, 218t, 221
Aristocort. See triamcinolone
Arixtra. See fondaparinux
arnica, 383t, 384t
Aromasin. See exemestane
AROMATASE INHIBITORS:
anastrozole, 568t, 569
exemestane, 568t, 569
letrozole, 568t, 569
mechanisms of action, 569, 784
Arranon. See nelarabine
arrhythmias. See dysrhythmias
arsenic trioxide, 571t
Artane. See trihexyphenidyl
arthritis, 745, 745t. See also gout;
osteoarthritis; rheumatoid arthritis
Arthropan. See choline salicylate
articaine, 248t
ASA. See **aspirin**
Asacol. See mesalazine
ASAP order, 31, 784
Ascaris lumbricoides, 528t
ascorbic acid. See vitamin C

Ascorbicap. *See* vitamin C
Asendin. *See* amoxapine
Asians:
  depression treatment
    considerations, 187*t*
  pain management, 225*t*
  propranolol sensitivity, 371*t*
asparaginase, 555*f*, 571, 571*t*, 797
aspergillosis, 515*t*
Aspergillus fumigatus, 515*t*
aspirin, 235*t*
  actions and uses, 235*t*, 384, 474
  administration alerts, 235*t*
  adverse effects, 233*t*, 235*t*, 386*t*,
    473*t*, 474, 479
  breast-feeding and, 79*t*
  Canadian/U.S. trade names, 797
  interactions, 113*t*, 235*t*
  overdose treatment, 235*t*
  pharmacokinetics, 235*t*
  route and adult dose, 233*t*, 386*t*, 473*t*
  for specific conditions
    cardiovascular event risk
      reduction, 479*t*
    fever, 478–80
    myocardial infarction, 358
assessment:
  definition, 67, 784
  related to drug administration, 68–69, 68*t*
Astelin. *See* azelastine
astemizole, 30*t*
asthma:
  causes/triggers, 596*t*
  characteristics, 784
  incidence, 596*t*
  management in schools, 599*t*
  pathophysiology, 595*f*, 596–97
  pharmacotherapy
    bronchodilators. *See* BRONCHODILATORS
    inhaled glucocorticoids. *See* INHALED
      GLUCOCORTICOIDS
    leukotriene modifiers. *See* LEUKOTRIENE
      MODIFIERS
    mast cell stabilizers. *See* MAST CELL
      STABILIZERS
Astramorph PF. *See* **morphine sulfate**
Astrin. *See* **aspirin**
astringent effect, 37, 784
Atacand. *See* candesartan
Atarax. *See* hydroxyzine
Atasol. *See* **acetaminophen**
atazanavir, 537*t*
atenolol, 353*t*
  actions and uses, 140*t*, 353*t*
  administration alerts, 353*t*
  adverse effects, 79*t*, 165*t*, 238*t*, 353*t*
  Canadian/U.S. trade names, 797
  interactions, 353*t*
  mechanisms of action, 140*t*
  overdose treatment, 353*t*
  prescription ranking, 800, 802
  for specific conditions
    angina and myocardial infarction, 350*t*

anxiety, 165*t*
    hypertension, 321*t*
    migraine, 238*t*
atenolol/chlorthalidone, 802
atherosclerosis, 287, 346, 347*f*, 784
athletes, androgen abuse by, 719, 720*t*
athlete's foot, 515*t*, 520
Ativan. *See* **lorazepam**
Atolone. *See* triamcinolone
atomoxetine, 204, 204*t*, 801
atonic seizure, 172*t*, 784
atopic dermatitis, 765. *See also* dermatitis
atorvastatin, 295*t*
  actions and uses, 295*t*
  administration alerts, 295*t*
  adverse effects, 292*t*, 295*t*
  interactions, 295*t*
  pharmacokinetics, 295*t*
  prescription ranking, 800
  route and adult dose, 292*t*
atovaquone and proguanil, 523*t*
atrial fibrillation, 362, 362*t*, 363*t*
atrial flutter, 363*t*
atrial natriuretic peptide (ANP), 342
atrial tachycardia, 363*t*
atrioventricular (AV) bundle, 364, 784
atrioventricular (AV) node, 363, 784
Atripla, 536
Atromid-S. *See* clofibrate
Atropa belladonna, 146
Atropair. *See* **atropine**
atropine, 148*t*
  actions and uses, 147, 147*t*, 148*t*
  administration alerts, 148*t*
  adverse effects, 148*t*
  Canadian/U.S. trade names, 797
  interactions, 148*t*
  overdose treatment, 148*t*
  pharmacokinetics, 148*t*
  for specific conditions
    as cycloplegic, 779*t*
    as nerve agent antidote, 23
Atrovent. *See* **ipratropium bromide**
attention deficit–hyperactivity disorder
    (ADHD):
  characteristics, 202–3, 202*t*, 784
  pharmacotherapy
    methylphenidate. *See* **methylphenidate**
    nursing considerations, 204
      client teaching, 205
    nursing process focus, 205–6*t*
    therapeutic approach, 125,
      203–4, 204*t*
ATYPICAL ANTIDEPRESSANTS:
  adverse effects, 160, 160*t*, 189*t*
  drugs classified as
    bupropion, 188, 189*t*, 203, 800
    duloxetine, 188, 189*t*, 801
    maprotiline, 188, 189*t*
    mirtazapine, 188, 189*t*, 801
    nefazodone, 188, 189*t*
    trazodone, 160*t*, 188, 189*t*, 800
    venlafaxine, 160*t*, 188, 189*t*, 800

nursing process focus, 197–99*t*
  route and adult doses, 160*t*, 189*t*
  for specific conditions
    ADHD, 203–4
    anxiety, 160*t*
    depression, 188, 189*t*
ATYPICAL ANTIPSYCHOTICS:
  adverse effects, 218, 218*t*
  characteristics, 218
  drugs classified as
    aripiprazole, 218*t*, 221
    clozapine. *See* **clozapine**
    olanzapine, 218*t*, 271, 801
    quetiapine fumarate, 218*t*, 800
    risperidone, 218, 218*t*, 271, 801
    ziprasidone, 218*t*
  mechanisms of action, 218
  nursing considerations, 218–19
    client teaching, 219
    lifespan considerations, 219
  nursing process focus, 220–21*t*
  route and adult doses, 218*t*
Augmentin, 490
aura, 237, 784
Auralgan. *See* benzocaine and antipyrine
auranofin, 747*t*
aurothioglucose, 747*t*
autoantibodies, 746, 784
automaticity, 363, 784
autonomic nervous system:
  divisions, 131–32, 132*f*
  drugs affecting, classification, 136
  functions, 131, 132*f*, 784
  neurotransmitters and receptors, 134–35,
    135*f*, 135*t*
  synapse structure and function,
    132–34, 133*f*
AV (atrioventricular) bundle, 364, 784
AV (atrioventricular) node, 363, 784
Avalide. *See* irbesartan/hydrochlorothiazide
Avandamet. *See* rosiglitazone/metformin
Avandaryl. *See* rosiglitazone/glimepiride
Avandia. *See* rosiglitazone
Avapro. *See* irbesartan
Avastin. *See* bevacizumab
Avelox. *See* moxifloxacin
Aventyl. *See* nortriptyline
Avodart. *See* dutasteride
Avonex. *See* interferon beta-1a
Axert. *See* almotriptan
Axid. *See* nizatidine
Aygestin. *See* norethindrone
azacitidine, 561, 561*t*
Azactam. *See* aztreonam
azatadine, 581*t*
azathioprine, 465*t*, 466, 630, 746
azelaic acid, 761*t*, 762
azelastine, 581*t*, 582
Azelex. *See* azelaic acid
azithromycin, 496, 496*t*, 508, 800, 801
Azmacort. *See* triamcinolone
azole, 784
azole antifungals. *See* ANTIFUNGALS, azoles

azoospermia, 721, 784
Azopt. *See* brinzolamide
AZT. *See* **zidovudine**
aztreonam, 503*t*
Azulfidine. *See* sulfasalazine

B

B cell, 456, 784
bacampicillin, 489*t*, 797
Baciguent. *See* bacitracin ointment
bacilli, 485
Bacillus anthracis, 21. *See also* anthrax
Bacillus Calmette-Guérin (BCG) vaccine,
    461*t*, 462
bacitracin ointment, 756
baclofen, 276, 276*t*
bacteremia, 485*t*
bacteria, 484*t*, 485, 485*t*. *See also specific
    bacteria and diseases*
bacteriocidal, 486, 784
bacteriostatic, 486, 784
Bactocill. *See* oxacillin
Bactrim. *See* **trimethoprim–
    sulfamethoxazole**
Bactroban. *See* mupirocin
baking soda. *See* **sodium bicarbonate**
balanced anesthesia, 249, 784
Banflex. *See* orphenadrine
Baraclude. *See* entecavir
BARBITURATES:
    adverse effects, 164*t*, 175*t*
    dependency characteristics, 120*t*
    dependency risk, 163
    drugs classified as
        intermediate acting
            amobarbital. *See* amobarbital
            aprobarbital, 164*t*
            butabarbital sodium, 164*t*, 256*t*
        long acting
            mephobarbital, 164*t*, 174
            phenobarbital. *See* **phenobarbital**
        short acting
            pentobarbital sodium. *See*
                pentobarbital sodium
            secobarbital. *See* secobarbital
    in general anesthesia
        amobarbital. *See* amobarbital
        butabarbital sodium, 256*t*
        etomidate, 255*t*
        methohexital sodium, 255*t*
        pentobarbital sodium. *See* pentobarbi-
            tal sodium
        propofol, 255*t*
        secobarbital. *See* secobarbital
    genetic polymorphisms affecting
        metabolism, 104*t*
    herb–drug interactions, 113*t*
    for specific conditions
        sedation and insomnia, 163, 164*t*
        seizures
            mechanisms of action, 173–74, 174*f*
            nursing considerations, 174–76
            route and adult doses, 175*t*

toxicity signs, 120*t*
uses, 163
withdrawal symptoms, 120*t*
baroreceptors, 304–5, 784
basal ganglia, 211, 211*f*
basal metabolic rate, 666, 784
baseline data, 67, 784
basiliximab, 465*t*, 466
BayHep B. *See* hepatitis B immunoglobulin
BayRab. *See* rabies immune globulin
BayRho-D. *See* Rho(D) immune globulin
BayTet. *See* tetanus immune globulin
BCG (Bacillus Calmette-Guérin) vaccine,
    461*t*, 462
beclomethasone, 604*t*
    actions and uses, 604*t*
    administration alerts, 604*t*
    adverse effects, 601*t*, 604*t*
    inhaled, 601*t*
    intranasal, 585*t*
    pharmacokinetics, 604*t*
    route and adult dose, 601*t*
Beclovent. *See* **beclomethasone**
Beconase. *See* **beclomethasone**
Beesix. *See* vitamin B$_6$
behavioral (short-term) insomnia, 157, 794
belladonna, 147
Benadryl. *See* **diphenhydramine**
Benadryl Allergy/Cold caplets, 582*t*
benazepril, 316*t*, 801
bendroflumethiazide, 429*t*
beneficence, 90, 784
Benemid. *See* probenecid
Benicar. *See* olmesartan medoxomil
benign, 553*t*, 784
benign prostatic hypertrophy (BPH):
    characteristics, 784
    incidence, 718*t*
    natural therapy with saw palmetto, 728*t*
    pathophysiology, 725, 725*f*, 726*f*
    pharmacotherapy
        alpha-adrenergic antagonists
            adverse effects, 726*t*, 727
            doxazosin. *See* **doxazosin**
            mechanisms of action, 322, 727
            prazosin. *See* **prazosin**
            tamsulosin, 726*t*, 727, 801
            terazosin, 726*t*, 727
        alpha-reductase inhibitors
            adverse effects, 726*t*, 727
            dutasteride, 726*t*
            finasteride. *See* **finasteride**
            mechanisms of action, 726*f*, 727
        nursing considerations, 728
        client teaching, 728
        nursing process focus, 728–29*t*
        therapeutic approach, 727
    symptoms, 725
benign tumor, 553*t*
Benisone. *See* betamethasone
Bensylate. *See* **benztropine**
Bentyl. *See* dicyclomine
Benuryl. *See* procarbazine

Benylin. *See* **dextromethorphan**
Benzacin. *See* benzoyl peroxide
Benzalin. *See* benzoyl peroxide
Benzamyclin. *See* benzoyl peroxide
benzocaine, 760*t*
    administration alerts, 760*t*
    adverse effects, 248*t*, 760*t*
    interactions, 760*t*
    otic preparation, 780*t*
    pharmacokinetics, 760*t*
    uses, 247–48
benzocaine and antipyrine, 780*t*
BENZODIAZEPINES:
    abuse, 121
    adverse effects, 162*t*, 175*t*
    definition, 784
    dependency characteristics, 120*t*
    drugs classified as
        alprazolam, 162*t*, 800
        chlordiazepoxide, 162*t*
        clonazepam. *See* clonazepam
        clorazepate, 162*t*, 175*t*, 797
        diazepam. *See* diazepam
        estazolam, 162*t*
        halazepam, 161, 162*t*
        lorazepam. *See* lorazepam
        midazolam, 30*t*, 161, 255*t*
        oxazepam, 162*t*, 799
        quazepam, 162*t*
        temazepam, 162*t*, 801
        triazolam, 162*t*
    herb–drug interactions, 113*t*
    route and adult doses, 162*t*, 175*t*
    for specific conditions
        Alzheimer's disease, 271
        anxiety and insomnia
            adverse effects, 162*t*
            mechanisms of action, 161
            nursing considerations, 162–63
            nursing process focus, 166*t*
            route and adult doses, 162*t*
        as general anesthesia adjunct, 255*t*
        seizures
            adverse effects, 175*t*
            indications, 176
            mechanisms of action, 176
            nursing considerations, 176–77
            route and adult doses, 175*t*
        as skeletal muscle relaxant, 276, 276*t*
    structure, 160
    toxicity signs, 120*t*
    uses, 161
    withdrawal symptoms, 120*t*
benzonatate, 589, 589*t*, 801
benzoyl peroxide, 761–62, 761*t*
benzthiazide, 310*t*, 429*t*
benztropine, 268*t*
    actions and uses, 264*f*, 268*t*
    administration alerts, 268*t*
    adverse effects, 267*t*, 268*t*
    Canadian/U.S. trade names, 797
    interactions, 268*t*
    overdose treatment, 268*t*

benztropine (*continued*)
  pharmacokinetics, 268*t*
  route and adult dose, 267*t*
  uses, 147, 147*t*
bepridil, 350*t*
beractant, 606*t*
beriberi, 646, 784
beta cells, 682, 682*f*
beta (β) receptors, 135*t*, 137, 784
BETA-ADRENERGIC AGONISTS
        (SYMPATHOMIMETICS):
  adverse effects, 597*t*, 774*t*
  drugs classified as
    albuterol. *See* albuterol
    bitolterol mesylate, 597*t*
    dipivefrin, 774*t*, 775
    dobutamine. *See* dobutamine
    dopamine. *See* **dopamine**
    epinephrine. *See* **epinephrine**
    epinephryl borate, 774*t*, 775
    formoterol, 137*t*, 597, 597*t*
    isoetharine HCl, 597, 597*t*
    isoproterenol. *See* isoproterenol
    levalbuterol, 597, 597*t*
    metaproterenol, 137*t*, 597, 597*t*
    metaraminol, 137*t*
    norepinephrine. *See* **norepinephrine**
    pirbuterol acetate, 597, 597*t*
    pseudoephedrine. *See*
        pseudoephedrine
    ritodrine, 137*t*, 711, 711*t*
    salmeterol. *See* **salmeterol**
    terbutaline. *See* terbutaline
  genetic polymorphisms affecting
        metabolism, 104*t*
  for specific conditions
    asthma. *See* BRONCHODILATORS
    glaucoma, 774*t*, 775
    heart failure, 342
    overview, 137, 137*t*
    shock, 414–15, 414*t*
    as tocolytic, 711–12, 711*t*
BETA-ADRENERGIC ANTAGONISTS
        (SYMPATHOLYTICS):
  adverse effects, 321, 321*t*, 350*t*, 367*t*
  drugs classified as
    acebutolol, 79*t*, 140*t*, 367*t*, 797
    atenolol. *See* **atenolol**
    betaxolol, 773, 774*t*
    bisoprolol, 321*t*, 801
    carteolol, 140*t*, 321*t*, 773, 774*t*
    carvedilol, 140*t*, 333*t*, 801
    esmolol, 140*t*, 367*t*
    levobunolol, 773, 774*t*
    metipranolol, 773, 774*t*
    metoprolol. *See* **metoprolol**
    nadolol, 140*t*
    propranolol. *See* **propranolol**
    sotalol, 140*t*, 367*t*, 371
    timolol. *See* **timolol**
  mechanisms of action
    in angina, 349*f*
    in dysrhythmias, 371

  in heart failure, 332*f*, 336
  in hypertension, 307*f*
  overview, 140–41
nursing process focus, 142*t*, 323–24*t*
  for specific conditions
    angina
      nursing considerations, 352–53
      route and adult doses, 350*t*
      therapeutic approach, 351–52
    anxiety, 165*t*
    dysrhythmias
      ethnic/racial considerations, 371*t*
      nursing considerations, 371
      route and adult doses, 367*t*
      therapeutic approach, 371
    glaucoma, 773, 774*t*
    heart failure
      nursing considerations, 337
      route and adult doses, 333*t*
      therapeutic approach, 336
    hypertension
      nursing considerations, 323–24
      nursing process focus, 323–24*t*
      overview, 140–41
      route and adult doses, 321*t*
      therapeutic approach, 320
    migraine, 238*t*, 239
    myocardial infarction, 350*t*, 358
    overview, 140–41, 140*t*, 320–21
Betacort. *See* betamethasone
Betaderm. *See* betamethasone
Betagen. *See* levobunolol
beta-lactam ring, 490, 784
beta-lactamase, 490, 490*f*, 784
BETA-LACTAMASE INHIBITORS, 490
Betalin 12. *See* **vitamin B$_{12}$**
Betalins. *See* vitamin B$_1$
Betaloc. *See* **metoprolol**
betamethasone:
  for adrenocortical insufficiency, 675*t*
  adverse effects, 476*t*
  Canadian/U.S. trade names, 797
  for dermatitis, 765*t*
  for psoriasis, 768
  for severe inflammation, 476*t*
Betapace. *See* sotalol
Betapen. *See* penicillin V
Betapen-VK. *See* penicillin V
Betaseron. *See* interferon beta-1b
betaxolol, 773, 774*t*
bethanechol, 144*t*
  actions and uses, 143, 143*t*, 144*t*
  administration alerts, 144*t*
  adverse effects, 144*t*
  classification, 143*t*
  as general anesthesia adjunct, 256*t*, 258
  interactions, 144*t*
  overdose treatment, 144*t*
Betimol. *See* **timolol**
Betnelan. *See* betamethasone
Betoptic. *See* betaxolol
bevacizumab, 571, 571*t*
bexarotene, 571*t*

Bextra. *See* valdecoxib
Bexxar. *See* tositumomab
Biamine. *See* vitamin B$_1$
Biaxin. *See* clarithromycin
bicalutamide, 568*t*, 569
Bicillin. *See* penicillin G benzathine
BiCNU. *See* carmustine
BIGUANIDES:
  adverse effects, 690*t*
  characteristics, 689
  metformin, 689, 690*t*, 800, 801
  route and adult dose, 690*t*
bilberry, 110*t*, 686*t*, 779*t*
BILE ACID RESINS:
  adverse effects, 292*t*, 293–94
  drugs classified as
    cholestyramine. *See* **cholestyramine**
    colesevelam, 292*t*, 294
    colestipol, 292*t*, 797
    fenofibrate, 292*t*, 800
  mechanisms of action, 293, 294*f*, 784
  nursing considerations, 294–95
    client teaching, 295
    lifespan considerations, 295
  pharmacotherapy with, 293–94
  route and adult doses, 292*t*
biliary excretion, 52
Biltricide. *See* praziquantel
bimatoprost, 773, 774*t*
bioavailability, 14, 784
BioCal. *See* calcium carbonate
BIOLOGIC RESPONSE MODIFIERS. *See also*
        HEMATOPOIETIC GROWTH FACTORS;
        IMMUNOSTIMULANTS
  for cancer chemotherapy, 570–71, 571*t*
  definition, 461
biological-based therapies, 109*t*. *See also*
        herbal therapies
biologics, 4, 784. *See also* BIOLOGIC RESPONSE
        MODIFIERS
Biologics Control Act, 5, 6*f*
bioterrorism:
  chemical and biologic agents
    anthrax, 21–22, 22*t*
    blister/vesicant agents, 24*t*
    blood agents, 24*t*
    categories, 20*t*
    characteristics, 19–20, 19*t*
    choking/vomiting agents, 24*t*
    ionizing radiation, 23–25
    nerve agents, 24*t*
    poliovirus, 21–22
    smallpox, 22
    toxic chemicals, 23
  definition, 19, 784
biotin. *See* vitamin B complex
biotransformation, 50
biperiden hydrochloride, 267*t*
bipolar disorder:
  characteristics, 196, 199, 784
  pharmacotherapy
    lithium. *See* **lithium**
    nursing considerations, 202

client teaching, 202
  lifespan considerations, 202
  nursing process focus, 201–2t
  therapeutic approach, 200–201
bisacodyl, 626t
bismuth subsalicylate, 620, 628t
BISPHOSPHONATES:
  adverse effects, 740, 741t
  drugs classified as
    alendronate, 741t, 800
    etidronate disodium. *See* **etidronate disodium**
    ibandronate, 741t
    pamidronate disodium, 741t
    risedronate sodium, 741t, 800
    tiludronate disodium, 741t
  mechanisms of action, 740, 784
  nursing considerations, 743
    client teaching, 743
    lifespan considerations, 743
  nursing process focus, 742t
  for Paget's disease, 744
  route and adult doses, 741t
bitolterol mesylate, 597, 597t
bivalirudin, 382, 382t
black cohosh, 110t, 112f, 706t
Blastomyces dermatitidis, 515t
blastomycosis, 515t
Blenoxane. *See* bleomycin
bleomycin, 555f, 564t
blister/vesicant agents, bioterrorism, 24t
Blocadren. *See* **timolol**
blood agents, bioterrorism, 24t
blood clots, 379
blood pressure:
  factors affecting, 303–4, 304f
  physiological regulation, 304–5, 305f
  variation throughout the lifespan, 303t
blood products:
  for shock, 411
  types
    fresh frozen plasma, 413t
    packed red blood cells, 413t
    plasma protein fraction, 413t
    whole blood, 413t
blood volume, 304, 304f
blood–brain barrier, 50, 784
body fluid compartments, 438, 438f
body surface area (BSA), 845
Bonamine. *See* meclizine
bone deposition, 733, 785
bone disorders:
  osteomalacia. *See* osteomalacia
  osteoporosis. *See* osteoporosis
  Paget's disease, 744
bone resorption, 733, 785
Bonine. *See* meclizine
Boniva. *See* ibandronate
boosters, 457
Borrelia burgdorferi, 485t
bortezomib, 571t
botanical, 108, 785. *See also* herbal therapies

botulinum toxin type A, 278–79, 279t, 281t
botulinum toxin type B, 278–79, 279t
Bowman's capsule, 424
BPH. *See* benign prostatic hypertrophy
bradykinesia, 262, 785
bradykinin, 472t, 785
brand-name drugs:
  vs. generics, 14
  marketing and promotional spending, 14t
breakthrough bleeding, 701, 701t, 709, 785
breast-feeding:
  client teaching about drug therapy during, 81–82
  drug therapy considerations, 79–80, 80f
  drugs with adverse effects during, 79t, 80t
  oxytocin function in, 712f
Brethaire. *See* terbutaline
Brethine. *See* terbutaline
Bretylate. *See* bretylium
bretylium, 367t, 371, 797
Bretylol. *See* bretylium
Brevibloc. *See* esmolol
Brevital. *See* methohexital sodium
brimonidine, 774t, 775
brinzolamide, 774t
broad-spectrum antibiotics, 487, 785.
  See also ANTIBACTERIALS
broad-spectrum penicillins, 489t, 490.
  See also PENICILLINS
bromocriptine:
  adverse effects during breast-feeding, 79t
  for female infertility, 714t, 715
  for Parkinson's disease, 263, 263t
brompheniramine, 581t, 582, 797
bronchioles, 594–95, 596f
BRONCHODILATORS:
  drugs classified as
    anticholinergics
      adverse effects, 597t, 599
      ipratropium bromide. *See* **ipratropium bromide**
      pharmacotherapy with, 599
      route and adult doses, 597t
      tiotropium, 597t, 599
    beta-agonists/sympathomimetics
      adverse effects, 597–98, 597t
      albuterol. *See* albuterol
      bitolterol mesylate, 597, 597t
      epinephrine. *See* **epinephrine**
      formoterol, 137t, 597, 597t
      isoetharine, 597, 597t
      isoproterenol. *See* isoproterenol
      levalbuterol, 597, 597t
      metaproterenol, 137t, 597, 597t
      pharmacotherapy with, 596–98
      pirbuterol acetate, 597t
      route and adult doses, 597t
      salmeterol. *See* **salmeterol**
      terbutaline. *See* terbutaline
    methylxanthines

adverse effects, 597t, 600
  aminophylline, 597t, 600, 797
  pharmacotherapy with, 600
  route and adult doses, 597t
  theophylline, 113t, 597t, 600, 799
mechanisms of action, 595
nursing considerations
  anticholinergics, 599–600
  beta-agonists/sympathomimetics, 598
  methylxanthines, 600–601
nursing process focus, 602–3t
bronchospasm, 595, 785
Bronkaid. *See* **epinephrine**
Bronkometer. *See* isoetharine
Bronkosol. *See* isoetharine
BSA (body surface area), 845
buccal route, 33–34, 33t, 34f, 785
buckthorn, drug interactions:
  atropine, 148t
  hydrocortisone, 676t
  phenytoin, 179t
  prednisone, 477t
budesonide, 585t, 601t, 801, 802
buffers, 446, 785
bumetanide:
  adverse effects, 310t, 333t
  for heart failure, 333t
  for hypertension, 310t
  for renal failure, 428, 428t
Bumex. *See* bumetanide
Buminate. *See* **normal serum albumin**
bundle branches, 364, 785
bundle of His, 364
bupivacaine, 248t
Buprenex. *See* buprenorphine hydrochloride
buprenorphine hydrochloride, 226f, 227t, 232
bupropion, 188, 189t, 203, 800
burdock root, 765t
BuSpar. *See* buspirone
buspirone, 165, 165t, 271, 801
busulfan, 559t
butabarbital, 164t, 256t
butalbital/acetaminophen/caffeine, 801
butenafine, 520t
Butisol. *See* butabarbital
butoconazole, 519t
butorphanol tartrate, 226f, 227t
Byetta. *See* exenatide

C

C fibers, 225, 785
Ca^{++}. *See* calcium
CABG (coronary artery bypass graft), 348, 786
CAD (coronary artery disease), 346, 348t
Cafergot. *See* ergotamine with caffeine
caffeine, 104t, 125
Calan. *See* **verapamil**
Calcidrine Syrup, 590t
calcifediol, 733, 735f, 785

Calciferol. *See* ergocalciferol
Calciject. *See* calcium chloride
Calcijex. *See* **calcitriol**
Calcilean. *See* **heparin**
Calciman. *See* calcitonin–salmon
Calcimax. *See* calcium lactate
calcineurin, 466, 785
CALCINEURIN INHIBITORS:
   cyclosporine. *See* **cyclosporine**
   pimecrolimus, 766
   tacrolimus. *See* tacrolimus
calcipotriene, 767t, 768
Calcite-500. *See* calcium carbonate
calcitonin:
   functions, 733, 734f, 785
   for osteoporosis, 741t, 743
   for Paget's disease, 744
calcitonin–human, 741t
calcitonin–salmon, 741t
Calcitrans. *See* calcium chloride;
   calcium gluceptate
calcitriol, 739t. *See also* vitamin D
   actions and uses, 739t
   administration alerts, 739t
   adverse effects, 736t, 739t
   formation, 733, 735f, 785
   interactions, 739t
   overdose treatment, 739t
   pharmacokinetics, 739t
   route and adult dose, 736t
calcium (Ca⁺⁺):
   functions, 651, 733
   imbalances, 442t, 651. *See also*
      hypercalcemia; hypocalcemia
   in myocardial cells, 364
   in osteoporosis, 740f
   pharmacotherapy with. *See* CALCIUM SALTS
   physiology, 733, 734f
calcium acetate, 426t
calcium carbonate:
   as antacid, 619t
   for calcium deficiency disorders, 650t, 736t
   Canadian/U.S. trade names, 797
   for renal failure, 426t
calcium carbonate with magnesium
      hydroxide, 619t
CALCIUM CHANNEL BLOCKERS (CCBs):
   adverse effects, 313t, 350t, 367t
   drugs classified as
      amlodipine, 313t, 350t, 800
      bepridil, 350t
      diltiazem. *See* **diltiazem**
      felodipine, 313t
      isradipine, 313t
      nicardipine, 313t, 324, 350t
      nifedipine. *See* **nifedipine**
      nimodipine, 238t
      nisoldipine, 313t
      verapamil. *See* **verapamil**
   mechanisms of action, 785
      in angina, 349f, 354
      in dysrhythmias, 373
      in hypertension, 307f, 311–14

   nursing process focus, 315–16t
   for specific conditions
      angina
         nursing considerations, 354–55
         route and adult doses, 350t
         therapeutic approach, 353–54
      dysrhythmias
         nursing considerations, 373–74
         route and adult dose, 367t
         therapeutic approach, 372
      hypertension
         nursing considerations, 314–16
         nursing process focus, 315–16t
         route and adult doses, 313t
         therapeutic approach, 311–13
      migraine, 238t
      myocardial infarction, 350t
calcium chloride, 442t, 736t
calcium citrate, 650t, 736t
calcium gluceptate, 650t, 736t
calcium gluconate, 736t
   actions and uses, 736t
   administration alerts, 736t
   adverse effects, 650t, 736t
   interactions, 736t
   overdose treatment, 736t
   pharmacokinetics, 736t
   route and adult dose, 650t, 736t
calcium ion channels, 364, 366f, 785
calcium lactate, 650t
calcium phosphate tribasic, 650t
calcium polycarbophil, 626t
CALCIUM SALTS:
   adverse effects, 650t, 736t
   drugs classified as
      calcium acetate, 426t
      calcium carbonate. *See* calcium
         carbonate
      calcium carbonate with magnesium
         hydroxide, 619t
      calcium chloride, 736t
      calcium citrate, 650t, 736t
      calcium gluceptate, 650t, 736t
      calcium gluconate. *See* **calcium
         gluconate**
      calcium lactate, 650t, 736t
      calcium phosphate tribasic, 650t, 736t
   nursing considerations, 652–53, 735
      client teaching, 653, 737–38
      lifespan considerations, 736–37
   nursing process focus, 737t
   route and adult doses, 650t, 736t
Calderol. *See* calcifediol
calfactant, 606t
Cal-Lac. *See* calcium lactate
Calphron. *See* calcium acetate
Calsan. *See* calcium carbonate
Caltrate. *See* calcium carbonate
CAM (complementary and alternative
      medicine), 108, 785. *See also* com-
      plementary and alternative therapies
Campain. *See* **acetaminophen**
Campath. *See* alemtuzumab

camphorated opium tincture, 628t
Camptothecus acuminata, 565, 566
Campral. *See* acamprosate calcium
CAMPTOTHECINS:
   characteristics, 566, 785
   drugs classified as
      irinotecan, 566, 566t
      topotecan, 555f, 566, 566t
   nursing considerations, 566–67
      client teaching, 567
   pharmacotherapy with, 566
Canada:
   drug approval and regulation process,
      9, 9t
   drug names with U.S. equivalents,
      797–99
   regulations restricting drugs of abuse,
      15–16
   three-schedule system, 16t
Canadian Food and Drugs Act, 9, 15
canal of Schlemm, 772
cancer:
   causes, 553, 553t, 554t
   characteristics, 552, 785
   incidence, 553t
   lifestyle changes for prevention, 553–54
   metastasis, 552, 552f
   natural therapy with selenium for
      prevention, 554t
   pharmacotherapy. *See* ANTINEOPLASTICS
   radiation therapy, 554t
   surgery, 554
Cancidas. *See* caspofungin
candesartan, 316t, 334
Candida albicans, 515t
candidiasis, 515t
Canestan. *See* clotrimazole
cannabinoids. *See also* marijuana
   characteristics, 122
   drugs classified as
      dronabinol, 633, 634t
      nabilone, 633, 634t
Cannabis sativa, 122. *See also* marijuana
capecitabine, 561t
Capoten. *See* captopril
Capozide, 309t
capreomycin, 507t
capsaicin, 745
Capsicum annum. See cayenne
capsid, 533, 785
capsules:
   administration guidelines, 32–33, 33t
   types, 32
captopril, 316t, 333t, 358
Carafate. *See* sucralfate
carbachol, 774t
carbamazepine:
   adverse effects, 178t, 200t
   for bipolar disorder, 200, 200t
   Canadian/U.S. trade names, 797
   interactions, 191
   for seizures, 173t, 178, 178t
carbamide peroxide, 780t

CARBAPENEMS:
    ertapenem, 503*t*, 506
    imipenem-cilastatin, 503*t*, 506
    meropenem, 503*t*, 506
carbenicillin, 489*t*, 490, 797
carbidopa, 113*t*
carbidopa-levodopa, 263*t*
Carbocaine. *See* mepivacaine
Carbolith. *See* **lithium**
carbonic anhydrase, 433, 785
CARBONIC ANHYDRASE INHIBITORS:
    adverse effects, 433*t*
    drugs classified as
        acetazolamide. *See* acetazolamide
        brinzolamide, 774*t*
        dichlorphenamide, 433*t*
        dorzolamide, 775
        methazolamide, 433*t*, 774*t*
    for renal failure, 433
carbonyl iron, 404
carboplatin, 559*t*
carboprost tromethamine, 704*t*, 705,
    711, 711*t*
carcinogens, 553, 554*t*
carcinoma, 552, 553*t*, 785
Cardene. *See* nicardipine
cardiac decompensation, 331, 785
CARDIAC GLYCOSIDES:
    adverse effects, 333*t*
    drugs classified as
        digitoxin, 338
        digoxin. *See* **digoxin**
    for heart failure
        nursing considerations, 339–41
            client teaching, 341
            nursing process focus, 340*t*
            route and adult dose, 333*t*
            therapeutic approach, 338–39
    mechanisms of action, 332*f*
cardiac output, 303, 304*f*, 331
cardiac remodeling, 331, 785
cardiogenic shock, 410, 412*t*, 785
Cardioquin. *See* quinidine polygalacturonate
cardiotonic drugs. *See* INOTROPIC AGENTS
cardioversion, 364, 785
Cardizem. *See* **diltiazem**
Cardura. *See* **doxazosin**
Cardura XL. *See* **doxazosin**
Carimune NF. *See* immune globulin
carisoprodol, 276*t*, 800
carmustine, 557, 559*t*
carotenes, 644, 785
carteolol, 140*t*, 773, 774*t*
Cartia XT. *See* **diltiazem**
Cartrol. *See* carteolol
carvedilol, 140*t*, 333*t*, 801
cascara sagrada bark:
    drug interactions
        atropine, 148*t*
        hydrocortisone, 676*t*
        phenytoin, 179*t*
    standardization, 110*t*
    uses, 110*t*

Casec, 655
Casodex. *See* bicalutamide
caspofungin, 516, 516*t*
castor oil, 626*t*
Cataflam. *See* diclofenac
Catapres. *See* clonidine
catecholamines, 134, 785
cathartic, 626, 785
catheter ablation, 364
cations, 442, 442*t*, 785
Caverject. *See* alprostadil
cayenne, 277*t*
CBER (Center for Biologics Evaluation and
    Research), 6
CCBs. *See* CALCIUM CHANNEL BLOCKERS
CCNU. *See* lomustine
CD4 receptor, 534, 785
CDER (Center for Drug Evaluation and
    Research), 6
Cebid. *See* vitamin C
Ceclor. *See* cefaclor
cecum, 625*f*
Cedax. *See* ceftibuten
CeeNU. *See* lomustine
cefaclor, 492*t*
cefadroxil, 492*t*
Cefadyl. *See* cephapirin
cefazolin, 492*t*
cefdinir, 492*t*, 801
cefditoren pivoxil, 492*t*
cefepime, 492*t*
cefixime, 492*t*
Cefizox. *See* ceftizoxime
cefmetazole, 492*t*
Cefobid. *See* cefoperazone
cefonicid, 492*t*
cefoperazone, 492*t*
Cefotan. *See* cefotetan
cefotaxime, 493*t*
    actions and uses, 493*t*
    administration alerts, 493*t*
    adverse effects, 492*t*, 493*t*
    interactions, 493*t*
    pharmacokinetics, 493*t*
    route and adult dose, 492*t*
cefotetan, 492*t*
cefoxitin, 492*t*
cefpodoxime, 492*t*
cefprozil, 492*t*
ceftazidime, 492*t*
ceftibuten, 492*t*
Ceftin. *See* cefuroxime
ceftizoxime, 492*t*
ceftriaxone, 492*t*
cefuroxime, 492*t*
Cefzil. *See* cefprozil
Celebrex. *See* celecoxib
celecoxib, 233*t*, 473*t*, 800
Celestone. *See* betamethasone
Celexa. *See* citalopram
cell cycle, 555, 555*f*
CellCept. *See* mycophenolate mofetil
cell-mediated immunity, 459–61

cellular receptors, 60–61, 61*f*
Center for Biologics Evaluation and
    Research (CBER), 6
Center for Drug Evaluation and Research
    (CDER), 6
Center for Food Safety and Applied
    Nutrition (CFSAN), 6
central nervous system (CNS):
    definition, 785
    degenerative diseases, 261, 261*t*. *See also*
        Alzheimer's disease; Parkinson's
        disease
    depressants
        alcohol. *See* alcohol
        barbiturates. *See* BARBITURATES
        benzodiazepines. *See* BENZODIAZEPINES
        nonbenzodiazepines. *See* NONBENZOD-
        IAZEPINE, NONBARBITURATE CNS
        DEPRESSANTS
        opioids. *See* opioid(s)
    divisions, 131, 132*f*
    stimulants
        amphetamines. *See* amphetamines
        caffeine, 104*t*, 125
        cocaine. *See* cocaine
        methylphenidate.
            See **methylphenidate**
        pemoline, 203, 204*t*
cephalexin, 492*t*, 797, 800
CEPHALOSPORINS:
    adverse effects, 492*t*, 493
    allergy to, 493
    drugs classified as
        first-generation
            cefadroxil, 492*t*
            cefazolin, 492*t*
            cephalexin, 492*t*, 797, 800
            cephapirin, 492*t*
            cephradine, 492*t*
            characteristics, 493
        fourth-generation
            cefepime, 492*t*
            characteristics, 493
        second-generation
            cefaclor, 492*t*
            cefmetazole, 492*t*
            cefonicid, 492*t*
            cefotetan, 492*t*
            cefoxitin, 492*t*
            cefprozil, 492*t*
            cefuroxime, 492*t*
            characteristics, 493
            loracarbef, 492*t*
        third-generation
            cefdinir, 492*t*, 801
            cefditoren pivoxil, 492*t*
            cefixime, 492*t*
            cefoperazone, 492*t*
            cefotaxime. *See* **cefotaxime**
            cefpodoxime, 492*t*
            ceftazidime, 492*t*
            ceftibuten, 492*t*
            ceftizoxime, 492*t*

CEPHALOSPORINS (*continued*)
    ceftriaxone, 492*t*
    characteristics, 493
  nursing considerations, 493–94
    client teaching, 494
  pharmacotherapy with, 492–93
  route and adult doses, 492*t*
cephapirin, 492*t*
cephradine, 492*t*
Ceporex. *See* cephalexin
cerebral palsy, 275*t*
Cerebyx. *See* fosphenytoin
Certiva. *See* diphtheria, tetanus, and
    pertussis vaccine
Cerubidine. *See* daunorubicin
cerumen softeners, 780
Cerumenex. *See* triethanolamine polypep-
    tide oleate 10% condensate
Cervidil. *See* dinoprostone
Cesamet. *See* nabilone
Cetacort. *See* **hydrocortisone**
Cetamide. *See* sulfacetamide
cetirizine:
  for allergic rhinitis, 581*t*
  Canadian/U.S. trade names, 797
  prescription ranking, 800, 801, 802
cetirizine/pseudoephedrine, 802
cetrorelix, 714*t*
Cetrotide. *See* cetrorelix
cetuximab, 571, 571*t*
cevimeline HCl, 143*t*
CFSAN (Center for Food Safety and Ap-
    plied Nutrition), 6
Chagas' disease, 526*t*
chamomile, 163*t*, 177*t*
chemical name, 13, 785
chemoprophylaxis, 487
chemoreceptor trigger zone (CTZ), 632
chemoreceptors, 304, 785
chemotherapy, 554, 785. *See also* ANTINEO-
    PLASTICS
Cheracol Syrup, 590*t*
chief cells, 612, 785
childbirth, depression after, 186
Childhood Vaccine Act, 6, 6*f*
children:
  anesthesia in, 254
  diabetes in, psychosocial and cultural
    impact, 688*t*
  drug administration challenges, 29*t*, 72, 94*t*
  drug administration guidelines
    adolescents, 84
    preschoolers, 83
    school-age children, 83, 84*f*
    toddlers, 82
  drug research and labeling for, 83*t*
  Giardia infections, 528*t*
  helminthic infections, 527*t*
  HIV infection, 544*t*
  medication error prevention, 95*t*
  ophthalmic drug administration, 778*t*
  pain expression and perception, 231*t*
  seizure etiologies, 171*t*

Chirocaine. *See* levobupivacaine
Chlamydia trachomatis, 485*t*
chloral hydrate, 165*t*, 797
chlorambucil, 559*t*
chloramphenicol, 503*t*, 778, 797
chloramphenicol cream, 756
chlordiazepam, 104*t*
chlordiazepoxide, 162*t*, 797
chloride (Cl⁻):
  functions, 651*t*
  imbalances, 442*t*
  recommended dietary allowance, 651*t*
Chlorofair. *See* chloramphenicol
Chloromag. *See* magnesium chloride
Chloromycetin. *See* chloramphenicol cream
Chloronase. *See* chlorpropamide
chloroprocaine, 248*t*
Chloroptic. *See* chloramphenicol
chloroquine, 525*t*
  actions and uses, 525*t*
  administration alerts, 525*t*
  adverse effects, 523*t*, 525*t*
  interactions, 525*t*
  overdose treatment, 525*t*
  pharmacokinetics, 525*t*
  resistance, 524
  route and adult dose, 523*t*
chlorothiazide, 430*t*
  actions and uses, 430*t*
  adverse effects, 429*t*, 430*t*
  interactions, 430*t*
  overdose treatment, 430*t*
  pharmacokinetics, 430*t*
  route and adult dose, 310*t*, 429*t*
  for specific conditions
    renal failure, 429*t*
chlorphenesin, 276*t*
chlorpheniramine, 581*t*, 582, 797
chlorpromazine, 213*t*
  actions and uses, 213*t*
  administration alerts, 213*t*
  adverse effects, 212*t*, 213–14, 213*t*
  Canadian/U.S. trade names, 797
  interactions, 213*t*
  overdose treatment, 213*t*
  pharmacokinetics, 213*t*
  route and adult dose, 212*t*
chlorpropamide, 690*t*, 797
chlorprothixene, 215*t*
chlorthalidone, 310*t*, 429*t*, 797
Chlor-Trimeton. *See* chlorpheniramine;
    pseudoephedrine
Chlor-Trimeton Allergy/Decongestant
    tablets, 582*t*
Chlor-Tripolon. *See* chlorpheniramine
chlorzoxazone, 276*t*
chocolate, 308*t*
choking/vomiting agents, bioterrorism, 24*t*
cholecalciferol, 733, 735*f*, 785
cholera, 485*t*
Cholestabyl. *See* colestipol
cholesterol:
  biosynthesis and excretion, 291, 293*f*

dietary restriction, 291
functions, 287
high levels. *See* hyperlipidemia
laboratory values, 290, 290*t*
in lipoproteins, 289, 289*f*
types, 289, 289*f*
cholesterol absorption inhibitors.
    See ezetimibe
cholestyramine, 297*t*
  actions and uses, 297*t*
  administration alerts, 297*t*
  adverse effects, 292*t*, 297*t*
  interactions, 297*t*
  pharmacokinetics, 297*t*
  route and adult dose, 292*t*
choline salicylate, 233*t*
cholinergic, 135, 785
cholinergic crisis, 147
cholinergic receptors:
  locations and responses, 135*t*
  types, 135–36, 135*f*, 135*t*
CHOLINERGICS (PARASYMPATHOMIMETICS):
  characteristics, 791
  DIRECT-ACTING
    drugs classified as
      bethanechol. *See* **bethanechol**
      cevimeline HCl, 143*t*
      pilocarpine, 143*t*, 774*t*, 775, 799
    mechanisms of action, 143
    nursing considerations, 144
    nursing process focus, 145*t*
  INDIRECT-ACTING
    adverse effects, 269, 269*t*
    for Alzheimer's disease, 269–71, 269*t*
    drugs classified as
      ambenonium, 143*t*
      donepezil. *See* **donepezil**
      edrophonium, 143*t*
      galantamine hydrobromide,
        143*t*, 269*t*
      neostigmine, 143, 143*t*
      physostigmine, 143, 143*t*, 774*t*
      pyridostigmine, 143, 143*t*
      rivastigmine, 143*t*, 269, 269*t*
      tacrine, 143*t*, 269, 269*t*
    mechanisms of action, 143
    nursing considerations,
      144, 146, 271–72
      client teaching, 146, 272
      lifespan considerations, 146
      nursing process focus, 145*t*
  MIOTICS (ANTIGLAUCOMA DRUGS)
    drugs classified as
      carbachol, 774*t*
      demecarium, 774*t*
      physostigmine, 774*t*
      pilocarpine, 774*t*, 775
    nursing process focus, 145–46*t*
cholinesterase. *See* acetylcholinesterase
cholinesterase inhibitors. *See* CHOLINERGICS,
    INDIRECT-ACTING
chondroitin, 114*t*, 746*t*
Chorex. *See* human chorionic gonadotropin

Choron 10. *See* human chorionic gonadotropin
chromium, 653*t*
chronic bronchitis, 606, 785
chronic obstructive pulmonary disease (COPD):
   characteristics, 605–6, 785
   natural therapy with fish oils, 606*t*
   pharmacotherapy, 605–6
chronic pain, 224
chyme, 624, 785
Cialis. *See* tadalafil
Cibacalcin. *See* calcitonin–human
ciclopirox olamine, 520*t*
cidofovir, 544*t*
ciliary body, 771
cilostazol, 386, 386*t*
cimetidine, 191, 615*t*, 638, 797
Cinobac. *See* cinoxacin
cinoxacin, 499*t*
Cipro. *See* ciprofloxacin
ciprofloxacin, 500*t*
   actions and uses, 500*t*
   administration alerts, 500*t*
   adverse effects, 499*t*, 500*t*
   interactions, 500*t*
   pharmacokinetics, 500*t*
   prescription ranking, 800
   route and adult dose, 499*t*
   for specific conditions
      anthrax prophylaxis and treatment, 22, 499
      ear infections, 778, 780*f*
      tuberculosis, 507*t*
circadian rhythm, 667*t*
cirrhosis, 122, 122*t*
cisplatin, 559*t*, 797
citalopram, 160*t*, 189*t*, 271, 800
Citanest. *See* prilocaine
Citracal. *See* calcium citrate
Citrucel. *See* methylcellulose
CK (creatine kinase), 355*t*
Cl⁻. *See* chloride
cladribine, 561*t*
Claforan. *See* **cefotaxime**
Clarinex. *See* desloratadine
clarithromycin, 496*t*, 508, 620
Claritin. *See* loratadine
clavulanate, 490
ClearEyes. *See* naphazoline HCl
clemastine, 581*t*, 582
Cleocin. *See* clindamycin
clindamycin, 502, 503*t*, 504*t*, 797, 801
clinical investigation, in drug development, 7, 7*f*, 785
clinical phase trials, in drug development, 7, 785
Clinoril. *See* sulindac
Cloar. *See* clofarabine
clobetasol, 765*t*
clocortolone, 765*t*
Cloderm. *See* clocortolone
clofarabine, 561

clofibrate, 292*t*
Clomid. *See* clomiphene
clomiphene, 714, 714*t*, 721
clomipramine, 159*t*, 188
clonazepam:
   adverse effects, 162*t*, 276*t*
   Canadian/U.S. trade names, 797
   as muscle relaxant, 276*t*
   prescription ranking, 800
   for seizures, 175*t*
clonic spasm, 275, 785
clonidine:
   actions and uses, 137*t*
   Canadian/U.S. trade names, 797
   interactions, 191
   prescription ranking, 800
   for specific conditions
      ADHD, 203
      hypertension, 321*t*
      pain management, 233*t*, 234
clopidogrel, 387*t*
   actions and uses, 358, 387*t*
   administration alerts, 387*t*
   adverse effects, 386*t*, 387*t*
   interactions, 387*t*
   overdose treatment, 387*t*
   pharmacokinetics, 387*t*
   prescription ranking, 800
   route and adult dose, 386*t*
clorazepate, 162*t*, 175*t*, 797
closed-angle glaucoma, 772–73, 772*f*, 785
Clostridium botulinum, 278
Clostridium difficile, 491
Clostridium perfringens, 502
Clotrimaderm. *See* clotrimazole
clotrimazole
   actions and uses, 518, 521, 756
   adverse effects, 519*t*
   Canadian/U.S. trade names, 797
   prescription ranking, 801
   route and adult dose, 519*t*
clotting disorders, 378*t*, 380–81
clotting factors, 378, 785
clove oil, 247*t*
cloxacillin, 489*t*, 490, 797
clozapine, 219*t*
   actions and uses, 219*t*
   administration alerts, 219*t*
   adverse effects, 218*t*, 219*t*
   contraindications, 219
   interactions, 219
   overdose treatment, 219*t*
   route and adult dose, 218*t*
Clozaril. *See* **clozapine**
CNS. *See* central nervous system
coagulation, 378, 785
coagulation cascade, 378, 379*f*, 785
cobalt, 653*t*
Cobex. *See* **vitamin B₁₂**
cocaine:
   adverse effects during breast-feeding, 79*t*
   characteristics, 125
   dependency characteristics, 120*t*

effects, 125
fetal effects, 80*t*
as local anesthetic, 247
toxicity signs, 120*t*
withdrawal symptoms, 120*t*
cocci, 485
Coccidioides immitis, 515*t*
coccidioidomycosis, 515*t*
codeine:
   adverse effects, 227*t*, 589*t*
   as antitussive, 589, 589*t*
   Canadian/U.S. trade names, 797
   in combination cold drugs, 480*t*
   genetic polymorphisms affecting metabolism, 104, 104*t*
   mechanisms of action, 226*f*
   for pain management, 227*t*
   route and adult dose, 227*t*, 589*t*
Codiclear DH Syrup, 590*t*
Codimal DH, 590*t*
Codimal-A. *See* brompheniramine
coenzyme Q10, 114*t*, 295, 295*t*
Cogentin. *See* **benztropine**
Cognex. *See* tacrine
cognitive-behavioral therapy, 187
Colace. *See* docusate
colchicine, 749*t*
   actions and uses, 749*t*
   administration alerts, 749*t*
   adverse effects, 748*t*, 749*t*
   Canadian/U.S. trade names, 797
   interactions, 749*t*
   nursing process focus, 749–50*t*
   overdose treatment, 749*t*
   pharmacokinetics, 749*t*
   route and adult dose, 748*t*
colesevelam, 292*t*, 294
Colestid. *See* colestipol
colestipol, 292*t*, 797
colfosceril, 606*t*
COLLOIDS:
   characteristics, 440–41, 785
   nursing considerations, 413–14, 441–42
      client teaching, 414, 442
   for shock, 411, 413*t*
   types
      5% albumin, 440*t*
      dextran 40. *See* **dextran 40**
      dextran 70, 413*t*, 414, 440*t*
      hetastarch, 413*t*, 414, 440*t*
      normal serum albumin. *See* **normal serum albumin**
      plasma protein fraction, 413*t*, 414, 440*t*
Collyrium. *See* tetrahydrozoline
colon, 624, 625*f*
COLONY-STIMULATING FACTORS (CSFs):
   adverse effects, 395*t*
   drugs classified as
      filgrastim. *See* **filgrastim**
      pegfilgrastim, 395*t*, 398
      sargramostim, 395*t*, 398
   mechanisms of action, 398, 785
   nursing considerations, 398–99

COLONY-STIMULATING FACTORS (CSFs) (*continued*)
  client teaching, 399
  nursing process focus, 400*t*
  pharmacotherapy with, 398
  route and adult doses, 395*t*
combination drugs, 13*t*, 14, 785
Combipres, 309*t*
Combivent. *See* ipratropium bromide with albuterol sulfate
comedones, 761, 785
common cold:
  characteristics, 588–89
  natural therapy with vitamin C, 647*t*
  pharmacotherapy
    antihistamines. *See* H₁-RECEPTOR ANTAGONISTS
    antitussives. *See* ANTITUSSIVES
    combination drugs, 590*t*
    decongestants. *See* DECONGESTANTS
    expectorants. *See* EXPECTORANTS
Compazine. *See* **prochlorperazine**
Compleat regular, 655
complement, 472*t*, 785
complementary and alternative medicine (CAM), 108, 785
complementary and alternative therapies:
  attitudes toward, 109*t*
  cultural and ethnic influences, 102
  definition, 4, 786
  herbal. *See* herbal therapies
  for HIV, 548*t*
  types, 109*t*
complex partial seizure, 172*t*
compliance:
  definition, 29, 786
  factors affecting, 29–30
Comprehensive Drug Abuse Prevention and Control Act, 15
Comtan. *See* entacapone
Concerta. *See* **methylphenidate**
conduction pathway, heart, 363
congestive heart failure, 331. *See also* heart failure
conjugated estrogens with medroxyprogesterone, 706*t*
  actions and uses, 706*t*
  administration alerts, 706*t*
  adverse effects, 706*t*, 709*t*
  interactions, 706*t*
  pharmacokinetics, 706*t*
  prescription ranking, 800
  route and adult dose, 709*t*
conjugates, 50, 786
conjugation, 487
constipation:
  definition, 625, 786
  incidence, 624*t*
  pathophysiology, 625
  pharmacotherapy. *See* LAXATIVES
contact dermatitis, 765
CONTRACEPTIVES:
  Depo-Provera, 700

emergency. *See* emergency contraception
implants
  desogestrel, 700
  Implanon, 700
  Jadelle, 700
  levonorgestrel, 700
  Norplant, 700
  Lunelle, 700
  Mirena, 700
  NuvaRing, 700
  oral. *See* ORAL CONTRACEPTIVES
  Ortho-Evra, 700
  patch, 700
contractility, 331, 786
Controlled Drug and Substances Act (Canada), 16
controlled substances, 15, 786
Controlled Substances Act of 1970, 15
convulsions, 170, 786
COPD. *See* chronic obstructive pulmonary disease
copper, 653*t*
Cordarone. *See* **amiodarone**
Cordran. *See* flurandrenolide
Cordran SP. *See* flurandrenolide
Coreg. *See* carvedilol
Corgard. *See* nadolol
coronary arteries, 346, 786
coronary artery bypass graft (CABG), 348, 786
coronary artery disease (CAD), 346, 348*t*
Coronex. *See* **isosorbide dinitrate**
Corophyllin. *See* aminophylline
corpora cavernosa, 723, 786
corpus luteum, 697, 786
corpus striatum, 262, 264*f*, 786
Correctol. *See* phenolphthalein
Cortaid. *See* **hydrocortisone**
Cortef. *See* **hydrocortisone**
corticosteroids. *See* GLUCOCORTICOIDS
corticotropin, 664*t*, 673–74
corticotropin zinc hydroxide, 674
Cortiment. *See* **hydrocortisone**
cortisone, 476*t*, 675*t*
Cortisporin. *See* polymyxin B, neomycin, and hydrocortisone
Cortistan. *See* cortisone
Cortone. *See* cortisone
Cortrophin-Zinc. *See* corticotropin zinc hydroxide
Cortrosyn. *See* cosyntropin
Cosmegen. *See* dactinomycin
cosyntropin, 664*t*, 674
Cotazym. *See* **pancrelipase**
Coumadin. *See* **warfarin**
Covera-HS. *See* **verapamil**
Covert. *See* ibutilide
COX. *See* cyclooxygenase
COX-2 inhibitors. *See* cyclooxygenase-2 (COX-2) inhibitors
Cozaar. *See* losartan
CPK (creatinine phosphatase), 355*t*
crab louse, 756
cranberry, 110*t*, 433*t*

creatine kinase (CK), 355*t*
creatinine phosphatase (CPK), 355*t*
Creon. *See* pancreatin
Crestor. *See* rosuvastatin
Crixivan. *See* indinavir
Crohn's disease, 630, 786
cromolyn, 586, 601*t*, 605
cross-tolerance, 120, 786
crotamiton, 757, 764
Cruex. *See* miconazole
cryptococcosis, 515*t*
Cryptococcus neoformans, 515*t*
cryptosporidiosis, 526*t*
Cryptosporidium, 526*t*
CRYSTALLOIDS:
  characteristics, 440, 786
  mechanisms of action, 440
  nursing considerations, 413–14
    client teaching, 414
  for specific conditions
    fluid replacement, 440, 440*t*
    shock, 411, 413*t*
  types
    5% dextrose in 0.2% saline, 440*t*
    5% dextrose in lactated Ringer's, 440*t*
    5% dextrose in normal saline, 440*t*
    5% dextrose in plasma-lyte 56, 440*t*
    5% dextrose in water (D5W), 413*t*, 440*t*
    hypertonic saline, 413*t*, 440*t*
    hypotonic saline, 440
    lactated Ringer's, 413*t*, 440*t*
    normal saline, 413*t*, 440*t*
    Plasmalyte, 413*t*
    plasma-lyte 56, 440*t*
    plasma-lyte 148, 440*t*
Crystamine. *See* **vitamin B₁₂**
Crysticillin. *See* penicillin G procaine
CSFs. *See* COLONY-STIMULATING FACTORS
CTZ (chemoreceptor trigger zone), 632
Cubicin. *See* daptomycin
culture, 102, 786. *See also* ethnic/racial considerations
culture and sensitivity testing, 488, 786
Cuprimine. *See* penicillamine
Cushing's syndrome:
  definition, 786
  glucocorticoid therapy and, 477
  nursing considerations, 678
    client teaching, 678
    lifespan considerations, 678
  pathophysiology, 678, 786
  pharmacotherapy, 664*t*, 678
  symptoms, 678
cutaneous anthrax, 22*t*
Cyanabin. *See* **vitamin B₁₂**
cyanocobalamin. *See* **vitamin B₁₂**
cyanogen chloride, 24*t*
CYCLIC LIPTOPEPTIDES:
  daptomycin, 503*t*, 506
cyclizine hydrochloride, 634*t*, 797
cyclobenzaprine, 277*t*
  actions and uses, 277*t*

administration alerts, 277t
adverse effects, 276t, 277t
interactions, 277t
overdose treatment, 277t
pharmacokinetics, 277t
prescription ranking, 800
Cyclocort. *See* amcinonide
Cycloflex. *See* **cyclobenzaprine**
Cyclogyl. *See* cyclopentolate
Cyclomen. *See* danazol
cyclooxygenase (COX):
forms, 233, 474, 474t, 786
functions, 233, 234f
in inflammation, 474
cyclooxygenase-2 (COX-2) inhibitors:
actions and uses, 233
adverse effects, 233t
celecoxib, 233t, 473t, 800
route and adult dose, 233t
cyclopentolate, 147t, 779t
cyclophosphamide, 560t
actions and uses, 560t
administration alerts, 560t
adverse effects, 559t, 560t
Canadian/U.S. trade names, 797
interactions, 560t
mechanisms of action, 555, 555f
pharmacokinetics, 560t
route and adult dose, 559t
for specific conditions
cancer, 559t, 560t
immunosuppression, 465t
rheumatoid arthritis, 746
CYCLOPLEGICS:
atropine, 779t
characteristics, 778, 779, 786
cyclopentolate, 779t
homatropine, 779t
scopolamine, 779t
tropicamide, 779t
cycloserine, 507t
cyclosporine, 466t
actions and uses, 466, 466t
administration alerts, 466t
adverse effects, 465t, 466t
interactions, 30t, 113t, 466t
pharmacokinetics, 466t
for specific conditions
dermatitis, 766
immunosuppression, 465t, 466t
psoriasis, 767t, 768
rheumatoid arthritis, 746
Cycrin. *See* **medroxyprogesterone acetate**
Cydomycin. *See* **gentamicin**
Cyklokapron. *See* tranexamic acid
Cylert. *See* pemoline
Cymbalta. *See* duloxetine
cyproheptadine, 581t, 797
Cytadren. *See* aminoglutethimide
cytarabine, 555f, 561, 561t
CytoGam. *See* cytomegalovirus immune globulin
cytokines, 459, 786

cytomegalovirus immune globulin, 458t
Cytomel. *See* liothyronine
Cytosar-U. *See* cytarabine
Cytotec. *See* misoprostol
cytotoxic T cells, 459, 786
Cytovene. *See* ganciclovir
Cytoxan. *See* **cyclophosphamide**

D

D- and L-amphetamine racemic mixture, 203, 204t, 800
D4T. *See* stavudine
D5W. *See* 5% dextrose in water
dacarbazine, 559t
daclizumab, 465t, 466
dactinomycin, 564t
Dalacin C. *See* clindamycin
Dalgan. *See* dezocine
Dalmane. *See* flurazepam
dalteparin, 382t
danaparoid, 382t
danazol, 714t, 715, 720t, 797
Danocrine. *See* danazol
dantrolene sodium, 279t
actions and uses, 278f, 279t
administration alerts, 279t
adverse effects, 279t
interactions, 279t
pharmacokinetics, 279t
daptomycin, 503t, 506
Daranide. *See* dichlorphenamide
Daraprim. *See* pyrimethamine
darbepoetin alfa, 395t, 396
darunavir, 537t, 539
Darvocet-N 50, 228
Darvon. *See* propoxyphene hydrochloride
Darvon-N. *See* propoxyphene napsylate
daunorubicin, 564t
daunorubicin liposomal, 564t
DaunoXome. *See* daunorubicin liposomal
Daypro. *See* oxaprozin
DDAVP. *See* desmopressin
DDC. *See* zalcitabine
DDI. *See* didanosine
debrisoquin hydroxylase, 104, 104t
Debrox. *See* carbamide peroxide
Decaderm. *See* dexamethasone
Decadron. *See* dexamethasone
Declomycin. *See* demeclocycline
decoction, 111t
DECONGESTANTS:
adverse effects, 587t
drugs classified as
ephedrine, 587t
ipratropium bromide. *See* **ipratropium**
naphazoline, 587t, 779, 779t
oxymetazoline. *See* **oxymetazoline**
phenylephrine. *See* **phenylephrine**
pseudoephedrine. *See* pseudo-doephedrine
tetrahydrozoline, 587t, 779, 779t
xylometazoline, 587t
nursing considerations, 588

client teaching, 588
pharmacotherapy with, 587
route and adult doses, 587t
deep vein thrombosis (DVT), 378t, 380
defecation, 626, 786
deferoxamine, 404t
defibrillation, 364, 785
Delatest. *See* testosterone enanthate
Delatestryl. *See* testosterone enanthate
delavirdine, 537t
Delestrogen. *See* estradiol valerate
Delta-Cortef. *See* prednisolone
Deltalin. *See* ergocalciferol
Deltasone. *See* **prednisone**
deltoid site, 41
delusions, 210, 786
Demadex. *See* torsemide
demecarium, 774t
demeclocycline, 494t
dementia, 263t, 268, 786. *See also* Alzheimer's disease
Demerol. *See* meperidine
denaglipton, 691
Denavir. *See* penciclovir
Depade. *See* naltrexone hydrochloride
Depakene. *See* **valproic acid**
Depakote. *See* **valproic acid**
Depakote ER. *See* **valproic acid**
Depen. *See* penicillamine
dependence. *See also* substance abuse
definition, 14, 786
opioid, 120t, 232
Dep-Gynogen. *See* estradiol cypionate
DepoCyt. *See* cytarabine
Depogen. *See* estradiol cypionate
depolarization, 364, 786
Depo-Medrol. *See* methylprednisolone
Depo-Provera, 700. *See also* **medroxyprogesterone acetate**
Depotest. *See* testosterone cypionate
Depo-Testosterone. *See* testosterone cypionate
depression:
assessment, 187
characteristics, 186–87
definition, 186, 786
ethnic/racial considerations in treatment, 187t
incidence, 186, 187t
natural therapy with St. John's wort, 193t
nonpharmacological therapy, 187–88
pharmacotherapy
atypical antidepressants. *See* ATYPICAL ANTIDEPRESSANTS
monamine oxidase inhibitors. *See* MONOAMINE OXIDASE INHIBITORS
nursing process focus, 197–99t
selective serotonin reuptake inhibitors. *See* SELECTIVE SEROTONIN REUPTAKE INHIBITORS
tricyclic antidepressants. *See* TRICYCLIC ANTIDEPRESSANTS

dermatitis:
  characteristics, 765, 786
  pharmacotherapy
    immunosuppressants, 766
    pimecrolimus, 766
    tacrolimus, 766
    topical glucocorticoids,
      765–66, 765t
dermatologic preparations, 34
dermatophytic infections, 515, 786. *See also*
      mycoses
dermis, 753
Dermovate. *See* clobetasol
Deronil. *See* dexamethasone
DES. *See* diethylstilbestrol
Desenex. *See* undecylenic acid
Desferal. *See* deferoxamine
desflurane, 252t
designer drugs, 118, 786
desipramine, 159t, 189t, 204
desirudin, 382, 382t
desloratadine, 581t, 801
desmopressin, 664t, 665–66
Desogen, 700t
desogestrel, 700, 700t
desonide, 765t
DesOwen. *See* desonide
desoximetasone, 765t
Desoxyn. *See* methamphetamine
Desyrel. *See* trazodone
Detensol. *See* **propranolol**
Detrol LA. *See* tolterodine tartrate
development, 76
dexamethasone:
  adverse effects, 476t
  Canadian/U.S. trade names, 798
  for specific conditions
    adrenocortical insufficiency, 675t
    cancer chemotherapy, 568t
    dermatitis, 765t
    nausea and vomiting, 633, 634t
    severe inflammation, 476t
Dexasone. *See* dexamethasone
dexbrompheniramine, 581t, 582
Dexchlor. *See* dexchlorpheniramine
dexchlorpheniramine, 581t
Dexedrine. *See* dextroamphetamine
Dexferrum. *See* iron dextran
dexmedetomidine HCl, 137t, 165t
dextran 40, 441t
  actions and uses, 441t
  administration alerts, 441t
  adverse effects, 441t
  characteristics, 440–41, 440t
  interactions, 441t
  pharmacokinetics, 441t
  for shock, 411, 413t
dextran 70, 413t, 414
dextran 75, 414
dextroamphetamine:
  for attention deficit–hyperactivity
      disorder, 203, 204t
  Canadian/U.S. trade names, 798

uses, 124
  for weight control, 635
dextromethorphan, 590t
  actions and uses, 589, 590t
  administration alerts, 590t
  adverse effects, 589t, 590t
  interactions, 194, 590t
  pharmacokinetics, 590t
  route and adult dose, 589t
5% dextrose in 0.2% saline, 440t
5% dextrose in lactated Ringer's, 440t
5% dextrose in normal saline, 440t
5% dextrose in plasma-lyte 56, 440t
5% dextrose in water (D5W), 413t, 440t
dezocine, 227t
DHEA, 114t
DiaBeta. *See* glyburide
diabetes insipidus, 664t, 665, 786
diabetes mellitus:
  in children, psychosocial and cultural
      impact, 688t
  complications, 684t
  gestational, 688
  herbal therapy, 691t
  impact on community resources, 694t
  incidence, 683, 684t
  pharmacotherapy. *See* INSULINS;
      ORAL HYPOGLYCEMICS
  renal failure in, 424t
  type 1, 683, 786
  type 2, 689, 786
diabetic ketoacidosis (DKA), 683, 786
Diabinese. *See* chlorpropamide
Dialose. *See* docusate
Diamox. *See* acetazolamide
Diapid. *See* lypressin
diarrhea:
  definition, 628, 786
  ethnic/racial considerations, 630t
  natural therapy with acidophilus,
      629, 629t
  pathophysiology, 628
  pharmacotherapy. *See* ANTIDIARRHEALS
diastolic pressure, 302–3, 303t, 786. *See also*
      blood pressure
Diazemuls. *See* **diazepam**
diazepam, 177t
  actions and uses, 177t
  administration alerts, 177t
  adverse effects, 162t, 175t, 177t
  Canadian/U.S. trade names, 798
  genetic polymorphisms affecting
      metabolism, 104t
  interactions, 177t
  overdose treatment, 177t
  pharmacokinetics, 177t
  prescription ranking, 800
  for specific conditions
    anxiety, 162t
    as general anesthesia adjunct, 255t
    seizures, 173t, 175t, 177
    as skeletal muscle relaxant, 276t
diazoxide, 324, 324t, 325

dibucaine, 248t, 760
dichlorphenamide, 433t
diclofenac, 233t, 473t, 801
dicloxacillin, 489t
dicyclomine, 147t, 630, 638
didanosine, 537t, 543
Didronel. *See* **etidronate disodium**
diet, cultural and ethnic influences, 102
dietary fiber, 625, 786
Dietary Supplement Health and Education
      Act, 6, 6f, 111, 786
dietary supplements:
  definition, 111–12, 786
  herbal. *See* herbal therapies
  nonherbal, 114, 114t
  for older adults, 109t
diethylcarbamazine, 528t
diethylstilbestrol, 568t, 569, 798
difenoxin with atropine, 628t
Differin. *See* adapalene
diffusion, 47
diflorasone, 765t
Diflucan. *See* **fluconazole**
diflunisal, 233t, 473t
digestion, 611–12, 624
Digibind. *See* digoxin immune Fab
digitalis glycosides. *See* CARDIAC GLYCOSIDES
Digitalis lanata, 338
Digitalis purpurea, 338
digitalization, 339, 786
digitoxin, 338
digoxin, 339t
  actions and uses, 339t
  administration alerts, 339t
  adverse effects, 333t, 339t, 368t, 417t
  interactions, 113t, 339t, 352
  overdose treatment, 339t
  pharmacokinetics, 339t
  prescription ranking, 801
  for specific conditions
    dysrhythmias, 368t, 374
    heart failure, 333t
    shock, 417, 417t
digoxin immune Fab, 339t, 341
dihydroergotamine mesylate, 238t, 239
Dilacor. *See* **diltiazem**
Dilacor XR. *See* **diltiazem**
Dilantin. *See* **phenytoin**
Dilatrate. *See* **isosorbide dinitrate**
Dilaudid. *See* hydromorphone hydrochloride
diltiazem, 354t
  actions and uses, 354t
  administration alerts, 354t
  adverse effects, 350t, 354t, 367t
  Canadian/U.S. trade names, 798
  interactions, 354t
  overdose treatment, 354t
  pharmacokinetics, 354t
  prescription ranking, 801
  for specific conditions
    angina and myocardial infarction, 350t
    dysrhythmias, 367t
    hypertension, 313t

Dimelor. *See* acetohexamide
dimenhydrinate, 633, 634*t*, 798
Dimetane. *See* brompheniramine
Dimetapp. *See* brompheniramine
Dimetapp Cold and Allergy Elixir, 582*t*
DIN (Drug Identification Number), 9
dinoprostone, 704*t*, 705, 711*t*
Diovan. *See* valsartan
Diovan HCT. *See* valsartan
Dipentum. *See* olsalazine
DIPEPTIDYL PEPTIDASE-4 (DPP-4) INHIBITORS:
    sitagliptin, 690*t*, 691
diphenhydramine, 583*t*
    actions and uses, 583*t*
    administration alerts, 583*t*
    adverse effects, 581*t*, 583*t*
    Canadian/U.S. trade names, 798
    interactions, 583*t*
    pharmacokinetics, 583*t*
    for specific conditions
        allergic rhinitis, 581*t*
        anaphylaxis, 419
        extrapyramidal side effects, 262
        insomnia, 167
        nausea and vomiting, 634*t*
        Parkinson's disease, 267*t*
diphenoxylate with atropine, 629*t*
    actions and uses, 629*t*
    administration alerts, 629*t*
    adverse effects, 628*t*, 629*t*
    interactions, 629*t*
    overdose treatment, 629*t*
    pharmacokinetics, 629*t*
    route and adult dose, 628*t*
diphtheria, tetanus, and pertussis
    vaccine, 460*t*
dipivefrin, 774*t*, 775
Dipred. *See* prednisolone
Diprivan. *See* propofol
Diprosone. *See* betamethasone
dipyridamole, 386*t*, 798
DIRECT THROMBIN INHIBITORS.
    See also ANTICOAGULANTS
    drugs classified as
        argatroban, 382, 382*t*
        bivalirudin, 382, 382*t*
        desirudin, 382, 382*t*
        lepirudin, 382, 382*t*
    mechanisms of action, 382
dirithromycin, 496*t*
Disalcid. *See* salsalate
DISEASE-MODIFYING ANTIRHEUMATIC DRUGS
    (DMARDs):
    adverse effects, 747*t*
    characteristics, 786
    drugs classified as
        anakinra, 465*t*, 746, 747*t*
        auranofin, 747*t*
        aurothioglucose, 747*t*
        gold sodium thiomalate, 747*t*
        hydroxychloroquine sulfate.
            See **hydroxychloroquine sulfate**
        leflunomide, 747*t*

methotrexate. *See* **methotrexate**
    penicillamine, 746, 747*t*
    sulfasalazine. *See* sulfasalazine
    pharmacotherapy with, 746
    route and adult dose, 747*t*
disodium phosphate, 442*t*. *See also*
    phosphorus/phosphate
disopyramide phosphate, 367*t*, 798
distribution:
    definition, 49, 786
    factors affecting, 49–50, 49*f*
    mechanisms, 48*f*, 49
    in older adults, 86
    in pregnancy, 77
disulfiram, 122
Ditropan. *See* oxybutynin
Diucardin. *See* hydroflumethiazide
Diulo. *See* metolazone
Diupres, 309*t*
Diurese. *See* trichlormethiazide
DIURETICS:
    carbonic anhydrase inhibitors. *See*
        CARBONIC ANHYDRASE INHIBITORS
    combination drugs, 428
    definition, 786
    home care considerations, 433*t*
    loop. *See* LOOP DIURETICS
    mechanisms of action, 304, 307*f*, 332*f*,
        427–28, 427*f*
    osmotic. *See* OSMOTIC DIURETICS
    potassium-sparing. *See* POTASSIUM-SPARING
        DIURETICS
    for specific conditions
        heart failure
            nursing considerations, 335–36
            route and adult doses, 333*t*
            therapeutic approach, 335
        hypertension
            nursing considerations, 309–11
            nursing process focus, 312–13*t*
            route and adult doses, 310*t*
            therapeutic approach, 308–10
        renal failure
            nursing considerations, 428–29,
            430–31, 431–32
            nursing process focus, 434–35*t*
            route and adult doses, 428*t*, 429*t*,
            431*t*, 432*t*
    thiazide. *See* THIAZIDE DIURETICS
Diuril. *See* **chlorothiazide**
divalproex sodium. *See* **valproic acid**
Dixaril. *See* clonidine
DKA (diabetic ketoacidosis), 683, 786
DMARDs. *See* DISEASE-MODIFYING
    ANTIRHEUMATIC DRUGS
dobutamine:
    actions and uses, 137*t*
    adverse effects, 417*t*
    mechanisms of action, 417
    for specific conditions
        heart failure, 342
        shock, 417, 417*t*
Dobutrex. *See* dobutamine

docetaxel, 565, 566*t*
docosanol, 544*t*
docusate, 626, 626*t*, 798
dofetilide, 367*t*, 371
dolasetron, 634*t*
Dolobid. *See* diflunisal
Dolophine. *See* methadone
DOM, 124
Domeboro. *See* aluminum sulfate and
    calcium acetate
donepezil, 271*t*
    actions and uses, 143*t*, 147, 270*f*, 271*t*
    administration alerts, 271*t*
    adverse effects, 269*t*, 271*t*
    classification, 143*t*
    interactions, 271*t*
    mechanisms of action, 270*f*
    overdose treatment, 271*t*
    pharmacokinetics, 271*t*
    prescription ranking, 801
    route and adult dose, 269*t*
dopamine, 417*t*
    actions and uses, 137*t*, 417*t*
    administration alerts, 417*t*
    adverse effects, 417*t*
    Canadian/U.S. trade names, 798
    interactions, 417*t*
    overdose treatment, 417*t*
    pharmacokinetics, 417*t*
    for specific conditions
        heart failure, 342
        shock, 417*t*
DOPAMINE SYSTEM STABILIZERS, 221
dopamine type 2 (D$_2$) receptors, 211,
    211*f*, 786
DOPAMINERGICS:
    adverse effects, 263*t*
    drugs classified as
        amantadine, 263, 263*t*, 546, 547*t*
        bromocriptine. *See* bromocriptine
        carbidopa-levodopa, 263*t*
        entacapone, 263, 263*t*
        levodopa. *See* **levodopa**
        pergolide, 263, 263*t*
        pramipexole dihydrochloride,
            263, 263*t*, 264*f*
        ropinirole hydrochloride, 263,
            263*t*, 264*f*
        selegiline hydrochloride, 263, 263*t*
        tolcapone, 263, 263*t*
    for Parkinson's disease
        mechanisms of action, 264*f*
        nursing considerations, 264–65
            client teaching, 265
        nursing process focus, 266–67*t*
        route and adult doses, 263*t*
        therapeutic approach, 262–64
Dopastat. *See* **dopamine**
Doral. *See* quazepam
Doriglute. *See* glutethimide
dornase alfa, 591
dorsogluteal site, 41
Doryx. *See* doxycycline

dorzolamide, 775
dose–response relationship, 59, 59f
Dovonex. *See* calcipotriene
doxazosin, 322t
    actions and uses, 140t, 322t
    administration alerts, 322t
    adverse effects, 321t, 322t
    interactions, 322t
    overdose treatment, 322t
    pharmacokinetics, 322t
    prescription ranking, 801
    for specific conditions
        benign prostatic hypertrophy, 726t, 727
        hypertension, 321t
doxepin, 159t, 189t, 798
Doxil. *See* doxorubicin liposomal
doxorubicin, 564t
    actions and uses, 564t
    administration alerts, 564t
    adverse effects, 564t
    interactions, 564t
    overdose treatment, 564t
    pharmacokinetics, 564t
    route and adult dose, 564t
doxorubicin liposomal, 564t
Doxy. *See* doxycycline
Doxycin. *See* doxycycline
doxycycline:
    for acne, 761t, 762
    adverse effects, 494, 494t
    Canadian/U.S. trade names, 798
    mechanisms of action, 494
    prescription ranking, 800
    route and adult dose, 494t
DPI (dry powder inhaler), 595, 595f, 786
DPT. *See* diphtheria, tetanus, and pertussis vaccine
Dramamine. *See* dimenhydrinate
Drixoral. *See* dexbrompheniramine; pseudoephedrine
Drixoral Allergy and Sinus Extended Release tablets, 582t
dronabinol, 633, 634t
drop attacks. *See* atonic seizure
droperidol, 255, 256t
drospirenone, 700t, 800
drug(s):
    administration. *See* drug administration
    administration errors. *See* medication errors
    Canadian approval process, 9, 9t
    consumer spending on, 5
    costs for older adults, 8
    definition, 4, 786
    development costs, 8
    dosage calculations, 845–46
    FDA approval process
        recent changes, 7–8
        stages, 7–8, 7f
        time length, 7–8, 8t
    interactions
        with grapefruit juice, 30t

over-the-counter, 5
    passage through plasma membranes, 47–48. *See also* pharmacokinetics
    prescription, 4–5
    reactions. *See* drug reactions
    regulations and standards, 5–6, 5f
drug administration. *See also* pharmacotherapy
    abbreviations, 30t
    compliance and, 29–30
    enteral
        buccal, 33–34, 33t, 34f
        disadvantages, 32–33
        drug forms, 33t
        gastrostomy tube, 33t, 34
        guidelines, 33t
        nasogastric tube, 33t, 34
        sublingual, 33, 33t, 34f
        tablets and capsules, 31–32, 33t
    guidelines
        five rights, 29
        overview, 32
        three checks, 29
    inhaled, 595
    lifespan considerations
        breast-feeding. *See* breast-feeding
        children. *See* children
        infants. *See* infants
        older adults. *See* older adults
        pregnancy. *See* pregnancy
        young and middle-aged adults, 84–85
    nurse's responsibilities, 28–29
    Nursing Process in
        assessment, 68–69, 68t
        evaluation, 72–73
        goals and outcomes, 70–71
        interventions, 71–72, 72t
        nursing diagnoses, 69–70, 70t
    orders, 30–31
    parenteral
        guidelines, 40–41t
        intradermal, 38, 39f
        intramuscular, 39, 41, 42f
        intravenous, 42f, 43, 43f
        subcutaneous, 38–39, 41f
    pediatric. *See* children; infants
    time schedules, 30–31
    topical
        guidelines, 36–37t
        nasal, 37, 38f
        ophthalmic, 35–36, 35f
        otic, 36f, 37
        rectal, 37–38
        for systemic vs. local effects, 34–35
        transdermal, 35, 35f
        types, 34
        vaginal, 37, 38f
    transdermal, 35, 35f
Drug Identification Number (DIN), 9
drug interactions:
    absorption and, 49
    with grapefruit juice, 30t
    with herbal therapies, 96t, 113t

drug–protein complexes, 49, 50f, 786
drug reactions:
    anaphylaxis. *See* anaphylaxis
    Steven-Johnson syndrome, 28t
    toxic epidermal necrolysis, 28t
dry powder inhaler (DPI), 595, 595f, 786
DTIC-Dome. *See* dacarbazine
Dulcolax. *See* bisacodyl
duloxetine, 188, 189t, 801
duodenal ulcer, 613
duodenum, 625, 625f
Durabolin. *See* nandrolone phenpropionate
Duragen-10. *See* estradiol valerate
Duragesic. *See* fentanyl
Duralith. *See* **lithium**
Duramorph. *See* **morphine sulfate**
Duranest. *See* etidocaine
Duraquin. *See* quinidine gluconate
Duricef. *See* cefadroxil
dutasteride, 726t
Duvoid. *See* **bethanechol**
Dyazide, 309t, 428
Dyclone. *See* dyclonine
dyclonine, 248t
Dymelor. *See* acetohexamide
Dynabac. *See* dirithromycin
DynaCirc. *See* isradipine
Dynapen. *See* dicloxacillin
Dyrenium. *See* triamterene
dysentery, 526, 786
dysfunctional uterine bleeding:
    causes, 709
    definition, 708, 787
    pharmacotherapy
        estrogens, 709
        nonsteroidal anti-inflammatory drugs, 709
        progestins. *See* PROGESTINS
    types, 709
dyslipidemia, 289, 787. *See also* hyperlipidemia
dysrhythmias:
    classification, 362–63, 363t
    definition, 362, 787
    incidence, 362, 362t
    magnesium for, 374t
    nonpharmacological therapy, 364
    pharmacotherapy. *See* ANTIDYSRHYTHMICS
dystonia, 213t, 214, 275t, 277, 787

E
ear:
    anatomy, 779, 780f
    disorders, 779–80
    pharmacotherapy. *See* otic preparations
Eber's Papyrus, 3
ECG (electrocardiogram), 364, 365f, 787
echinacea:
    drug interactions, 113t
        amiodarone, 372t
        cyclophosphamide, 560t
        methotrexate, 56t
        naloxone hydrochloride, 231t

sumatriptan, 239*t*

testosterone, 721*t*

for immune system enhancement, 462*t*

uses, 110*t*

Echinacea purpurea. See echinacea

ECHINOCANDINS:

anidulafungin, 516, 516*t*

caspofungin, 516, 516*t*

echothiophate iodide, 774*t*

eclampsia, 171, 787

econazole, 519*t*, 798

Ecostatin. *See* econazole

Ecstasy, 124

ECT (electroconvulsive therapy), 187, 787

ectopic foci/pacemakers, 364, 787

eczema, 765, 765*t*, 787. *See also* dermatitis

ED$_{50}$ (median effective dose), 58, 58*f*, 790

Edecrin. *See* ethacrynic acid

edrophonium, 143*t*

EEG. *See* electroencephalogram

efavirenz, 113*t*, 537*t*, 538

Effexor. *See* venlafaxine

Effexor XR. *See* venlafaxine

efficacy, 59–60, 60*f*, 787

Efudex. *See* fluorouracil

Elavil. *See* amitriptyline

Eldepryl. *See* selegiline hydrochloride

elderly clients. *See* older adults

electrocardiogram (ECG), 364, 365*f*, 787

electroconvulsive therapy (ECT), 187, 787

electroencephalogram (EEG):

definition, 787

in diagnosis of sleep and seizure

disorders, 158, 170*f*

normal vs. abnormal, 170*f*

electrolytes:

definition, 442, 787

diuretic effects on, 308

functions, 442

imbalances, 442, 442*t. See also*

specific electrolytes

important in human physiology, 442*t*

renal regulation, 443, 443*f*

eletriptan, 238*t*

Eleutherococcus senticosus. See ginseng

Eligard. *See* leuprolide

Elimite. *See* permethrin

Ellence. *See* epirubicin

Elocon. *See* mometasone

Eloxatin. *See* oxaliplatin

Elspar. *See* asparaginase

embolus, 380, 787

Emcyt. *See* estramustine

Emend. *See* aprepitant

emergency contraception, drugs for:

ethinyl estradiol and levonorgestrel,

704, 704*t*

levonorgestrel, 704, 704*t*

emergency preparedness, nurse's role, 20–21

emesis, 632, 787. *See also* nausea and

vomiting

emetic, 633, 787

emetic (emetogenic) potential, 556, 633, 787

Emex. *See* metoclopramide

Eminase. *See* anistreplase

emphysema, 606, 787

Empirin with Codeine No. 2, 228

emtricitabine, 537*t*

Emtriva. *See* emtricitabine

Emulsoil. *See* castor oil

E-Mycin. *See* **erythromycin**

enalapril, 318*t*

actions and uses, 318*t*

administration alerts, 318*t*

adverse effects, 316*t*, 318*t*, 333*t*

interactions, 318*t*

overdose treatment, 318*t*

pharmacokinetics, 318*t*

prescription ranking, 800

for specific conditions

heart failure, 333*t*

hypertension, 316*t*

enalaprilat, 324

Enbrel. *See* etanercept

endocarditis, 485*t*

Endocet. *See* budesonide

endocrine system, 661–62, 661*f*

endogenous opioids, 225, 225*f*, 787.

See also opioid(s)

endometriosis, 485*t*, 715, 787

endothelium, 304, 787

Enduron. *See* methyclothiazide

enflurane, 252*t*

enfuvirtide, 536, 537*t*

Engerix-B. *See* **hepatitis B vaccine**

enoxacin, 499*t*

enoxaparin, 358, 382*t*, 383

Ensure-Plus, 655

entacapone, 263, 263*t*

Entamoeba histolytica, 526, 526*t*

entecavir, 548, 548*t*

enteral nutrition:

definition, 654, 787

formulas, 654–56

nursing considerations, 655

client teaching, 655

routes, 654

enteral route, 32, 787. *See also*

drug administration, enteral

enteric-coated tablets, 32, 787

Enterobius vermicularis, 528*t*

Enterococcus faecalis, 487

Enterococcus faecium, 487, 505

enterohepatic recirculation, 52, 52*f*, 787

Entrophen. *See* **aspirin**

enzyme induction, 50, 787

E-Pam. *See* **diazepam**

ephedra:

drug interactions

digoxin, 339*t*

oxytocin, 712*t*

removal from market, 636

ephedrine, 587*t*

epidermis, 753

Epidermophyton floccosum, 515*t*

epidural anesthesia, 246*f*, 246*t*

epilepsy, 170, 172*t*, 787.

See also seizures

Epimorph. *See* **morphine sulfate**

Epinal. *See* epinephryl borate

epinephrine, 420*t*

actions and uses, 137*t*, 420*t*, 597*t*

administration alerts, 420*t*

adverse effects, 420*t*, 597*t*

Canadian/U.S. trade names, 798

interactions, 420*t*

nursing considerations, 420–21

overdose treatment, 420*t*

pharmacokinetics, 420*t*

for specific conditions

anaphylaxis, 419

asthma, 597*t*

heart failure, 342

epinephryl borate, 774*t*, 775

EpiPen, 421*t. See also* **epinephrine**

epirubicin, 564*t*

Epival. *See* **valproic acid**

Epivir. *See* lamivudine

Epivir HBV. *See* lamivudine

eplerenone, 317, 431, 431*t*

epoetin alfa, 396*t*

actions and uses, 396*t*

administration alerts, 396*t*

adverse effects, 395*t*, 396*t*

interactions, 396*t*

nursing considerations, 395–97, 398

nursing process focus, 397*t*

overdose treatment, 396*t*

pharmacokinetics, 396*t*

route and adult dose, 395*t*

Epogen. *See* **epoetin alfa**

Eppy/N. *See* epinephryl borate

eprosartan, 316*t*

EPS. *See* extrapyramidal side effects

Epsom salts. *See* **magnesium sulfate**

eptifibatide, 386*t*

Equanil. *See* meprobamate

Eraxis. *See* anidulafungin

Erbitux. *See* cetuximab

Ercaf. *See* ergotamine with caffeine

erectile dysfunction:

causes, 718*t*, 723

definition, 723

incidence, 718*t*

pathophysiology, 723

pharmacotherapy

alprostadil, 723

nursing considerations, 723–24

client teaching, 724, 725*t*

papaverine plus phentolamine, 723

sildenafil. *See* **sildenafil**

tadalafil, 723, 723*t*, 801

vardenafil, 723, 723*t*

Ergamisol. *See* levamisole

ergocalciferol (vitamin D$_2$),

644, 787, 798. *See also* vitamin D

ergonovine maleate, 711*t*

Ergostat. *See* ergotamine

ergosterol, 515, 787

ERGOT ALKALOIDS:
    dihydroergotamine mesylate, 238*t*, 239
    ergotamine, 79*t*, 238*t*, 239, 798
    ergotamine with caffeine, 238*t*
ergotamine, 79*t*, 238*t*, 239, 798
ergotamine with caffeine, 238*t*
Ergotrate. *See* ergonovine maleate
erlotinib, 571*t*
Ertaczo. *See* sertaconazole
ertapenem, 503*t*, 506
eruptive psoriasis, 766*t*
EryDerm. *See* **erythromycin**, ointment
erythema, 754
Erythrocin. *See* **erythromycin**
erythrocyte sedimentation rate (ESR), 355*t*
erythrocyte stage, malaria, 524, 787
Erythromid. *See* **erythromycin**
erythromycin, 497*t*
    for acne, 762
    actions and uses, 497*t*
    administration alerts, 497*t*
    adverse effects, 497*t*
    Canadian/U.S. trade names, 798
    interactions, 30*t*, 497*t*
    ointment, 756
    pharmacokinetics, 497*t*
erythropoietin, 395, 787. *See also* **epoetin
    alfa;** hematopoietic growth factors
Escherichia coli, 484*t*, 485*t*
escitalopram oxalate, 161*t*
    actions and uses, 161*t*
    administration alerts, 161*t*
    adverse effects, 160*t*, 161*t*
    interactions, 161*t*
    overdose treatment, 161*t*
    pharmacokinetics, 161*t*
    prescription ranking, 800
    for specific conditions
        anxiety, 160*t*
        depression, 189*t*
Eserine sulfate. *See* physostigmine
Eskalith. *See* **lithium**
esmolol, 140*t*, 367*t*
esomeprazole, 617, 617*t*, 800
esophageal reflux, 611. *See also* gastro-
    esophageal reflux disease
ESR (erythrocyte sedimentation rate), 355*t*
essential hypertension, 305. *See also*
    hypertension
estazolam, 162*t*
esters, 246, 248*f*, 787. *See also*
    LOCAL ANESTHETICS
Estinyl. *See* ethinyl estradiol
Estrace. *See* estradiol
Estraderm. *See* estradiol
estradiol, 709*t*, 801
estradiol cypionate, 709*t*
estradiol valerate, 709*t*, 798
estradiol/drospirenone, 709*t*
estradiol/norgestimate, 709*t*
estramustine, 559*t*
**estrogen/progestin conjugated
    estrogens, 706*t***

    actions and uses, 706*t*
    administration alerts, 706*t*
    adverse effects, 706*t*, 709*t*
    interactions, 706*t*
    pharmacokinetics, 706*t*
    route and adult dose, 709*t*
ESTROGENS:
    adverse effects, 708*t*
    consequences of loss in menopause, 705*t*
    definition, 787
    drugs classified as
        combination drugs
            conjugated estrogens with medroxy-
            progesterone. *See* **conjugated estro-
            gens with medroxyprogesterone**
            estradiol/drospirenone, 709*t*
            estradiol/norgestimate, 709*t*
            ethinyl estradiol/norethindrone
                acetate, 709*t*
        estradiol, 709*t*, 801
        estradiol cypionate, 709*t*
        estradiol valerate, 709*t*
        estrogen/progestin conjugated
            estrogens. *See* **estrogen/progestin
            conjugated estrogens**
        estropipate, 709*t*
        ethinyl estradiol. *See* ethinyl
            estradiol
    functions, 697–98
    for specific conditions
        dysfunctional uterine bleeding, 709
        hormone replacement therapy. *See*
            HORMONE REPLACEMENT THERAPY
        oral contraception. *See* ORAL
            CONTRACEPTIVES
        overview, 706, 706*t*
estropipate, 709*t*
eszopiclone, 165, 165*t*, 167
etanercept, 465*t*, 746, 767*t*, 768
ethacrynic acid, 428*t*
ethambutol, 507*t*
ethchlorvynol, 165*t*
ethinyl estradiol:
    adverse effects, 709*t*
    for cancer chemotherapy, 568, 568*t*
    in oral contraceptives,
        699, 700*t*, 709*t*
    in transdermal patch, 700
ethinyl estradiol with levonorgestrel, 704*t*
ethinyl estradiol with norethindrone, 702*t*
    actions and uses, 702*t*
    administration alerts, 702*t*
    adverse effects, 702*t*
    interactions, 702*t*
    pharmacokinetics, 702*t*
ethinyl estradiol/norethindrone
    acetate, 709*t*
ethionamide, 507*t*
ethnic, 102, 787
ethnic/racial considerations:
    ACE inhibitor action, 320*t*
    alcoholism, 101*t*
    angina, 348*t*

    communication techniques, 71*t*
    depression treatment, 187*t*
    diarrhea treatment, 630*t*
    dietary habits, 291*t*
    enzyme deficiencies, 62*t*
    healthcare access, 102*t*
    in immunization, 461*t*
    mental illness, 212*t*
    osteoporosis, 743*t*
    pain expression and perception, 225*t*
    pharmacotherapy, 101–3
    tobacco use, 126*t*
ethosuximide, 181*t*
    actions and uses, 181*t*
    administration alerts, 181*t*
    adverse effects, 180*t*, 181*t*
    interactions, 181*t*
    overdose treatment, 181*t*
    pharmacokinetics, 181*t*
    route and adult dose, 180*t*
Ethrane. *See* enflurane
ethyl alcohol. *See* alcohol
etidocaine, 248*t*
etidronate disodium, 741*t*
    actions and uses, 741*t*
    administration alerts, 741*t*
    adverse effects, 741*t*
    interactions, 741*t*
    overdose treatment, 741*t*
    pharmacokinetics, 741*t*
    route and adult dose, 741*t*
etodolac, 233*t*, 473*t*, 802
etomidate, 255*t*
etoposide, 555*f*, 566, 566*t*
etretinate, 767*t*, 768
eugenol, 247*t*
Euglucon. *See* glyburide
Eulexin. *See* flutamide
Eurax. *See* crotamiton
Euthroid. *See* liotrix
evaluation:
    definition, 68, 787
    in drug administration, 72–73
evening primrose, 110*t*, 191*t*
Evista. *See* **raloxifene**
Evoxac. *See* cevimeline HCl
excoriation, 765, 787
excretion, drug:
    definition, 51, 787
    factors affecting, 51–52
    mechanisms, 48*f*, 51
    in older adults, 86
    in pregnancy, 77
Exelderm. *See* sulconazole
Exelon. *See* rivastigmine
exemestane, 568*t*, 569
exenatide, 690*t*, 691
exercise-induced asthma, 596
exfoliative dermatitis, 766*t*
Ex-Lax. *See* phenolphthalein
Exna. *See* benzthiazide
exocrine, 682
Exosurf. *See* colfosceril

EXPECTORANTS:
    definition, 591, 787
    guaifenesin, 589t, 590t, 591
    pharmacotherapy with, 591
extended insulin zinc suspension, 685t, 688
extended-spectrum penicillins, 489t, 490.
        See also PENICILLINS
external otitis, 779, 787
extracellular fluid (ECF) compartment, 438,
        438f, 787
extract, 111f
extrapyramidal side effects (EPS):
    with antipsychotic drugs, 213t, 214
    definition, 214, 787
    in Parkinson's disease, 262
Exubera, 684
eye:
    anatomy, 771–72, 771f
    glaucoma. *See* glaucoma
    natural therapy with bilberry, 779t
    pharmacotherapy. *See* ophthalmic drugs
ezetimibe, 292t, 294f, 298–99, 800, 801

F

Factive. *See* gemifloxacin
Factrel. *See* gonadorelin
famciclovir, 544t
famotidine, 615t, 801
Famvir. *See* famciclovir
Fansidar. *See* sulfadoxine–pyrimethamine
Fareston. *See* toremifene
Faslodex. *See* fulvestrant
fat-soluble vitamins. *See* vitamin(s),
        lipid-soluble
FDA. *See* Food and Drug Administration
FDA Modernization Act, 6, 8
febrile seizure, 171, 172t, 173t, 787
Feco-T. *See* ferrous fumarate
Federal Bureau of Chemistry, 6f
Feen-a-Mint. *See* phenolphthalein
felbamate, 178, 178t
Felbatol. *See* felbamate
Feldene. *See* piroxicam
felodipine, 313t
female infertility:
    causes, 714–15
    definition, 714
    pharmacotherapy for
        bromocriptine, 714t, 715
        cetrorelix, 714t
        clomiphene, 714t, 715
        danazol, 714t, 715
        follitropin alfa, 714t
        follitropin beta, 714t
        ganirelix, 714t
        gonadorelin, 714t, 715
        goserelin, 714t
        human chorionic gonadotropin, 714,
            714t
        human menopausal
            gonadotropin–menotropins,
            714, 714t
        leuprolide, 714t, 715

nafarelin, 714t
        therapeutic approach, 714–15
        urofollitropin, 714t
female reproductive function:
    hypothalamic and pituitary regulation,
        697, 698f
    infertility. *See* female infertility
    ovarian control, 697–98
Femara. *See* letrozole
FemCare. *See* clotrimazole
Femhrt. *See* ethinyl estradiol/norethindrone
        acetate
Feminone. *See* ethinyl estradiol
Femiron. *See* ferrous fumarate
Femizole. *See* clotrimazole
Femogex. *See* estradiol
Femstat. *See* butoconazole
fenfluramine, 635
Fenicol. *See* chloramphenicol
fenofibrate, 292t, 800
fenoprofen, 233t, 473t
fen-phen, 635
fentanyl, 255, 255t, 256t
fentanyl/droperidol, 255, 256t
Feosol. *See* **ferrous sulfate**
Feosol-caps. *See* carbonyl iron
Feostat. *See* ferrous fumarate
Fergon. *See* ferrous gluconate
Fer-Iron. *See* **ferrous sulfate**
ferritin, 403, 787
Ferronyl. *See* carbonyl iron
ferrous fumarate, 402t, 650t
ferrous gluconate, 402t, 650t
ferrous sulfate, 404t
    actions and uses, 404t
    administration alerts, 404t
    adverse effects, 402t, 404t, 650t
    interactions, 404t
    nursing considerations, 404–6
        client teaching, 406
        lifespan considerations, 406
    nursing process focus, 405t
    overdose treatment, 404t
    route and adult dose, 402t, 650t
Fertinex. *See* urofollitropin
fetal–placental barrier, 50, 787
fever:
    drug-induced, 478
    effects, 478
    pharmacotherapy. *See* antipyretics
feverfew:
    drug interactions
        aspirin, 235t
        ibuprofen, 475t
        overview, 113t
        warfarin, 384t
    for migraine, 241t
fexofenadine, 583t
    actions and uses, 583t
    administration alerts, 583t
    adverse effects, 581t, 583t
    interactions, 583t
    pharmacokinetics, 583t

prescription ranking, 800, 801
    route and adult dose, 581t
fexofenadine with pseudoephedrine, 801
Fiberall. *See* calcium polycarbophil
FiberCon. *See* calcium polycarbophil
FIBRIC ACID AGENTS:
    adverse effects, 292t
    drugs classified as
        clofibrate, 292t
        fenofibrate, 292t, 800
        gemfibrozil. *See* **gemfibrozil**
    nursing considerations, 298
        client teaching, 298
    pharmacotherapy with, 298
    route and adult doses, 292t
fibrillation, 362, 787
fibrin, 379, 787
fibrinogen, 379, 787
fibrinolysis, 379, 380f, 787
fight-or-flight response, 131, 787
filgrastim, 399t
    actions and uses, 398, 399t
    administration alerts, 399t
    adverse effects, 395t, 399t
    interactions, 399t
    nursing process focus, 400t
    pharmacokinetics, 399t
    route and adult dose, 395t
filtrate, 424, 787
Finacea. *See* azelaic acid
finasteride, 727t
    actions and uses, 727t
    administration alerts, 727t
    adverse effects, 726t, 727t
    interactions, 727t
    nursing process focus, 728–29t
    pharmacokinetics, 727t
    route and adult dose, 726t
Fioricet. *See* butalbital/acetaminophen/
        caffeine
first trimester, drug therapy during, 77. *See
        also* pregnancy
first-pass effect, 51, 51f, 787
fish oils:
    for chronic obstructive pulmonary
        disease, 606t
    drug interactions, 606t
    for inflammation, 476t
    uses, 114t
five rights of drug administration, 29, 787
Flagyl. *See* **metronidazole**
flaxseed oil, 114t
flecainide, 366t, 367t
Fleet Phospho-Soda. *See* sodium
        biphosphate
Flexeril. *See* **cyclobenzaprine**
Flexon. *See* orphenadrine
flight-or-fight response, 131, 787
Flomax. *See* tamsulosin
Flonase. *See* **fluticasone**
Florone. *See* diflorasone
Flovent. *See* **fluticasone**
Floxin. *See* ofloxacin

floxuridine, 561t

fluconazole, 519t
  actions and uses, 519t
  administration alerts, 519t
  adverse effects, 519t
  interactions, 519t
  pharmacokinetics, 519t
  prescription ranking, 800
  route and adult dose, 519t
flucytosine, 515, 516, 516t, 798
Fludara. *See* fludarabine
fludarabine, 561t
fluid balance:
  body fluid compartments, 438–39, 438f
  intake and output regulation, 439
  movement of fluids, 439, 439f
fluid replacement agents:
  blood products
    fresh frozen plasma, 413t
    packed red blood cells, 413t
    plasma protein fraction, 413t
    whole blood, 413t
  colloids. *See* COLLOIDS
  crystalloids. *See* CRYSTALLOIDS
  nursing considerations, 413–14
    client teaching, 414
  nursing process focus, 416t
  therapeutic approach, 411
flukes, 528
Flumadine. *See* rimantadine
flumazenil, 177, 177t
flunisolide, 585t, 601t
fluocinolone, 765t
fluocinonide, 765t
Fluolar. *See* fluocinolone
fluorine, 653t, 654
5-fluorocytosine. *See* flucytosine
Fluoroplex. *See* fluorouracil
FLUOROQUINOLONES:
  adverse effects, 499, 499t
  drugs classified as
    first-generation
      cinoxacin, 499t
      nalidixic acid, 499, 499t
    fourth-generation
      gemifloxacin, 499t
      moxifloxacin, 499, 499t
      trovafloxacin mesylate, 499, 499t
    second-generation
      ciprofloxacin. *See* **ciprofloxacin**
      enoxacin, 499t
      lomefloxacin, 499t
      norfloxacin, 499t
      ofloxacin, 499t, 507t
    third-generation
      gatifloxacin, 499, 499t
      levofloxacin, 499t, 800
      sparfloxacin, 499t
  nursing considerations, 500
    client teaching, 500
  pharmacotherapy with, 499
  route and adult doses, 499t
fluorouracil, 555, 555f, 561t, 562f

Fluothane. *See* **halothane**
fluoxetine, 160t, 189t, 271, 800
fluoxymesterone, 568t, 569, 720t, 798
fluphenazine, 212t
flurandrenolide, 765t
flurazepam, 162t, 798
flurbiprofen, 233t, 473t
FluShield. *See* influenza vaccine
flutamide, 568t, 569
fluticasone, 586t
  actions and uses, 586t
  administration alerts, 586t
  adverse effects, 585t, 586t
  interactions, 586t
  pharmacokinetics, 586t
  prescription ranking, 800
  for specific conditions
    allergic rhinitis, 585t
    asthma, 601t
    dermatitis, 765t
fluvastatin, 292t
Fluvirin. *See* influenza vaccine
fluvoxamine, 160t, 189t
Fluzone. *See* influenza vaccine
Folacin. *See* **folic acid/folate**
Folex. *See* **methotrexate**
FOLIC ACID ANTAGONISTS.
    See also ANTIMETABOLITES
  methotrexate. *See* **methotrexate**
  pemetrexed, 561t
folic acid inhibitors. *See* SULFONAMIDES
folic acid/folate, 648t
  for anemia, 402–3, 402t
  deficiency, 395t, 402, 643t
  functions, 501, 643t, 787
  mechanisms of action, 412
  nursing considerations, 403
    client teaching, 403
  nursing process focus, 649t
  pharmacotherapy with
    actions and uses, 648t
    administration alerts, 648t
    adverse effects, 647t, 648t
    interactions, 648t
    pharmacokinetics, 648t
    route and adult dose, 402t, 647t
  in pregnancy, 395t, 642t, 648t
  prescription ranking, 800
  recommended dietary allowance, 643t
  sources, 647
  structure, 562f
follicle-stimulating hormone (FSH):
  for female infertility, 714t
  in female reproductive function,
    697, 699f
  in male reproductive function, 718
  secretion, 663f, 787
follicular cells, 666, 787
Follistim. *See* follitropin beta
follitropin alfa, 714t
follitropin beta, 714t
Folvite. *See* **folic acid/folate**
fondaparinux, 382t

Food and Drug Administration (FDA):
  medication error reporting, 93
  MedWatch, 96
  new drug approval process
    recent changes, 8
    stages, 7–8, 7f
    time length, 8
  pregnancy categories, 78, 78t
  roles, 6, 787
Food Directorate, 9
Food, Drug, and Cosmetic Act, 5, 6f
food poisoning, 485t
Foradil. *See* formoterol
Forane. *See* isoflurane
Forest. *See* acamprosate calcium
formoterol, 137t, 597, 597t
formulary, 5, 787
Fortamet. *See* metformin
Fortaz. *See* ceftazidime
Forteo. *See* teriparatide
Fortovase. *See* **saquinavir**
Fosamax. *See* alendronate
fosamprenavir, 537t
foscarnet, 544t
Foscavir. *See* foscarnet
fosfomycin, 503t
fosinopril, 316t, 333t
fosphenytoin, 178t
Fosrenol. *See* lanthanum carbonate
Fostex. *See* benzoyl peroxide
foxglove, 338
Fragmin. *See* dalteparin
Frank–Starling law, 331, 788
frequency distribution curve,
    57–58, 57f, 788
fresh frozen plasma, 413t
Frova. *See* frovatriptan
frovatriptan, 238t
FSH. *See* follicle-stimulating hormone
5-FU. *See* fluorouracil
FUDR. *See* floxuridine
fulvestrant, 568t
Fulvicin. *See* griseofulvin
fungal infections. *See* mycoses
fungi, 514, 515t, 788. *See also* mycoses
Fungi-Nail. *See* undecylenic acid
Fungizone. *See* **amphotericin B**
Furadantin. *See* nitrofurantoin
Furalan. *See* nitrofurantoin
Furanite. *See* nitrofurantoin
furazolidone, 628t
Furomide. *See* **furosemide**
furosemide, 336t
  actions and uses, 336t
  administration alerts, 336t
  adverse effects, 333t, 336t, 428t
  Canadian/U.S. trade names, 798
  interactions, 336t
  overdose treatment, 336t
  pharmacokinetics, 336t
  prescription ranking, 800
  for specific conditions
    heart failure, 333t

hypertension, 310*t*
renal failure, 428, 428*t*
Furoxone. *See* furazolidone
Fuzeon. *See* enfuvirtide

G

G6PD (glucose-6-phosphate dehydrogenase) deficiency, 62*t*, 480*t*, 525*t*
gabapentin:
adverse effects, 175, 175*t*
for bipolar disorder, 200
prescription ranking, 800
for seizures, 175*t*
Gabitril. *See* tiagabine
GAD (generalized anxiety disorder), 154, 788
galantamine hydrobromide, 143*t*, 269*t*
Galvus. *See* vildagliptin
Galzin. *See* zinc acetate
Gamastan. *See* immune globulin
intramuscular
Gamimune N. *See* immune globulin
intravenous
gamma-aminobutyric acid (GABA),
173, 174*f*, 788
Gammagard. *See* immune globulin
Gammar-P. *See* immune globulin intravenous
ganciclovir, 544*t*
ganglion, 133, 788
ganglionic blockers, 135
ganglionic synapse, 132
ganirelix, 714*t*
Gantanol. *See* sulfamethoxazole
Gantrisin. *See* sulfisoxazole
Garamycin. *See* **gentamicin**
garlic:
for cardiovascular health, 380*t*
for dementia, 263*t*
drug interactions
alpha-glucosidase inhibitors, 689
aspirin, 235*t*
ibuprofen, 475*t*
insulin, 686*t*
overview, 113*t*
warfarin, 384*t*
uses, 110*t*
Gastozepine. *See* pirenzepine
gastric ulcer, 613
gastroesophageal reflux disease (GERD),
613, 788
gastrointestinal anthrax, 22*t*
gastrointestinal tract. *See* lower gastrointestinal tract; upper gastrointestinal tract
gastrostomy (G) tube, 33*t*, 34
Gas-X. *See* simethicone
gatifloxacin, 499, 499*t*
gefitinib, 571*t*
gemcitabine, 561*t*
gemfibrozil, 298*t*
actions and uses, 298*t*
administration alerts, 298*t*
adverse effects, 292*t*, 298*t*
interactions, 298*t*
pharmacokinetics, 298*t*

prescription ranking, 801
route and adult dose, 292*t*
gemifloxacin, 499*t*
gemtuzumab ozogamicin, 571*t*
Gemzar. *See* gemcitabine
gender, influences on pharmacotherapy, 104–5
general anesthesia:
characteristics, 245, 245*t*, 249–50, 788
stages, 251*t*
GENERAL ANESTHETICS:
adjuncts
barbiturates
amobarbital. *See* amobarbital
butabarbital, 164*t*, 256*t*
pentobarbital. *See* pentobarbital
sodium
secobarbital. *See* secobarbital
bethanechol chloride, 256*t*, 258
droperidol, 256*t*
nursing considerations, 258
client teaching, 258
opioids
alfentanil hydrochloride, 256*t*
fentanyl, 256*t*
fentanyl/droperidol, 256*t*
remifentanil hydrochloride, 256*t*
sufentanil citrate, 256*t*
pharmacotherapy with, 256–58
promethazine. *See* promethazine
succinylcholine. *See* **succinylcholine**
tubocurarine, 256*t*, 257
follow-up care, 254*t*
gas
adverse effects, 252*t*
characteristics, 251
nitrous oxide. *See* **nitrous oxide**
intravenous
adverse effects, 255*t*
barbiturates
etomidate, 255*t*
methohexital sodium, 255*t*
propofol, 255*t*
benzodiazepines
diazepam. *See* **diazepam**
lorazepam. *See* **lorazepam**
midazolam, 30*t*, 161, 255*t*
ketamine, 124, 255, 255*t*
nursing considerations, 255–56
client teaching, 256
opioids
alfentanil hydrochloride, 255*t*
fentanyl, 255, 255*t*
remifentanil hydrochloride, 255*t*
sufentanil citrate, 255*t*
pharmacotherapy with, 255
thiopental. *See* **thiopental**
nursing process focus, 253*t*
pharmacotherapy with, 250–53
volatile liquid
adverse effects, 252*t*
characteristics, 252, 252*t*
drugs classified as
desflurane, 252*t*

enflurane, 252*t*
halothane. *See* **halothane**
isoflurane, 252*t*, 254
methoxyflurane, 252*t*
sevoflurane, 252*t*
nursing considerations, 254
client teaching, 254
lifespan considerations, 254
generalized anxiety disorder (GAD), 154, 788
generalized seizure, 171, 172*t*, 788
generic drugs, vs. brand-name drugs, 14
generic name, 13, 788
genetic polymorphisms, 104, 104*t*, 788
genetics:
influences on pharmacotherapy, 104, 104*t*
seizure etiologies and, 171*t*
Genotropin. *See* somatropin
Gen-Salbutamol. *See* albuterol
gentamicin, 498*t*
actions and uses, 498*t*
administration alerts, 498*t*
adverse effects, 498*t*
Canadian/U.S. trade names, 798
cream and ointment, 756
interactions, 498*t*
pharmacokinetics, 498*t*
route and adult dose, 498*t*
Gentran 40. *See* **dextran 40**
Gentran 75. *See* dextran 75
Geocillin. *See* carbenicillin
Geodon. *See* ziprasidone
Geopen. *See* carbenicillin
Geopen Oral. *See* carbenicillin
GERD (gastroesophageal reflux disease),
613, 788
gestational age, drug therapy and, 77–78, 77*f*
gestational diabetes mellitus, 688
GFR (glomerular filtration rate), 425–26
GH (growth hormones), 663, 664–65
Giardia lamblia, 526*t*, 528*t*
giardiasis, 526*t*, 528*t*
ginger:
drug interactions
aspirin, 235*t*
ibuprofen, 475*t*
overview, 113*t*
warfarin, 384*t*
for gastrointestinal disorders, 621*t*
with general anesthesia, 251*t*
standardization, 110*t*
uses, 110*t*
ginkgo:
for dementia, 263*t*
drug interactions
alteplase, 388*t*
aspirin, 235*t*
heparin, 383*t*
ibuprofen, 475*t*
imipramine, 191*t*
overview, 113*t*
reteplase, 357*t*
sumatriptan, 239*t*
labeling, 111*f*

ginkgo *(continued)*
    standardization, 110*t*
    uses, 110*t*
Ginkgo biloba. See ginkgo
ginseng:
    drug interactions
        alpha-glucosidase inhibitors, 689
        digoxin, 339*t*
        diuretics, 358*t*
        insulin, 686*t*
        overview, 113*t*
        phenelzine, 196*t*
        sumatriptan, 239*t*
        warfarin, 358*t*
    for myocardial ischemia, 358*t*
    standardization, 110*t*
    uses, 110*t*
glaucoma:
    diagnosis, 772
    incidence, 773*t*
    nursing considerations, 776
        client teaching, 776, 778
    pathophysiology, 772
    pharmacotherapy, 773. *See also*
        ANTIGLAUCOMA DRUGS
    risk factors, 772
    types, 772–73, 772*f*
Gleevec. *See* imatinib mesylate
Gliadel. *See* carmustine
glimepiride, 690*t*, 801
glioma, 553*t*
glipizide, 692*t*
    actions and uses, 692*t*
    administration alerts, 692*t*
    adverse effects, 690*t*, 692*t*
    interactions, 692*t*
    overdose treatment, 692*t*
    pharmacokinetics, 692*t*
    prescription ranking, 801
    route and adult dose, 690*t*
glipizide/metformin, 690*t*, 691
glomerular filtration rate (GFR), 425–26
glucagon, 682–83, 683*f*, 684
Glu-calcium. *See* calcium gluceptate
Glucamide. *See* chlorpropamide
GLUCOCORTICOIDS:
    adverse effects, 476–77, 476*t*, 675, 675*t*
    definition, 788
    drugs classified as
        alclometasone, 765*t*
        amcinonide, 765*t*
        beclomethasone. *See* **beclomethasone**
        betamethasone. *See* betamethasone
        budesonide, 585*t*, 601*t*, 801, 802
        clobetasol, 765*t*
        clocortolone, 765*t*
        cortisone, 476*t*, 675*t*
        desonide, 765*t*
        desoximetasone, 765*t*
        dexamethasone. *See* dexamethasone
        diflorasone, 765*t*
        flunisolide, 585*t*, 601*t*
        fluocinolone, 765*t*

fluocinonide, 765*t*
flurandrenolide, 765*t*
fluticasone. *See* **fluticasone**
halcinonide, 765*t*
hydrocortisone. *See* **hydrocortisone**
methylprednisolone. *See*
    methylprednisolone
mometasone, 585*t*, 765*t*, 800
prednisolone, 476*t*, 675*t*, 799
prednisone. *See* **prednisone**
triamcinolone. *See* triamcinolone
inhaled. *See* INHALED GLUCOCORTICOIDS
intranasal. *See* INTRANASAL
    GLUCOCORTICOIDS
mechanisms of action, 476, 673–74
nursing considerations. *See specific*
    conditions
nursing process focus, 676–77*t*
for specific conditions
    adrenocortical insufficiency, 674–75,
        675*t*
    allergic rhinitis. *See* INTRANASAL
        GLUCOCORTICOIDS
    asthma. *See* INHALED GLUCOCORTICOIDS
    cancer, 568, 568*t*
    dermatitis, 765–66, 765*t*
    gout, 747
    inflammatory disorders, 476–77, 476*t*
    nausea and vomiting, 633, 634*t*
    osteoarthritis, 745
    overview, 674–75
    psoriasis, 768
    rheumatoid arthritis, 746
    topical
        for dermatitis, 765–66, 765*t*
        for psoriasis, 768
Glucophage. *See* metformin
glucosamine, 114*t*, 746*t*
glucose, 355*t*
glucose-6-phosphate dehydrogenase
    (G6PD) deficiency, 62*t*, 480*t*, 525*t*
Glucotrol. *See* **glipizide**
Glucotrol XL. *See* **glipizide**
Glucovance. *See* glyburide/metformin
Glumetza. *See* metformin
glutethimide, 165*t*
glyburide, 690*t*, 798, 800
glyburide/metformin, 690*t*, 801
glycerin anhydrous, 774*t*, 776
GlycoLax. *See* polyethylene glycol
glycoprotein IIb/IIIa, 358, 386, 788
GLYCOPROTEIN IIB/IIIA RECEPTOR ANTAGONISTS:
    adverse effects, 386*t*
    drugs classified as
        abciximab, 358, 386*t*
        eptifibatide, 386*t*
        tirofiban, 386*t*
    mechanisms of action, 386
    route and adult doses, 386*t*
glycopyrrolate, 147*t*
GLYCYLCYCLINES:
    tigecycline, 494*t*, 506
Glynase. *See* glyburide

Glyset. *See* miglitol
G-mycin. *See* **gentamicin**
goals:
    definition, 67, 788
    in medication administration, 70
GOLD SALTS:
    auranofin, 747*t*
    aurothioglucose, 747*t*
    gold sodium thiomalate, 747*t*
gold sodium thiomalate, 747*t*
gold thioglucose. *See* aurothioglucose
goldenseal, 113*t*, 509*t*
gonadocorticoids, 673
gonadorelin, 714*t*, 715
gonadotropin-releasing hormone (GnRH),
    697, 714, 714*t*, 788
Gonal-F. *See* follitropin alfa
gonorrhea, 485*t*
Gordochom. *See* undecylenic acid
goserelin, 568*t*, 714*t*
gotu-kola, 163*t*
gout:
    characteristics, 746, 788
    classification, 746
    nursing considerations, 748, 750
        client teaching, 750
        lifespan considerations, 750
    pathophysiology, 746
    pharmacotherapy, 747–48. *See also* URIC
        ACID INHIBITORS
    prophylaxis, 747–48
graded dose–response relationship, 59, 59*f*,
    788
gram-negative bacteria, 485, 788
gram-positive bacteria, 485, 788
grand mal. *See* tonic–clonic (grand mal)
    seizure
granisetron, 634*t*
granulocyte colony-stimulating factor
    (G-CSF), 398. *See also* COLONY-
    STIMULATING FACTORS
granulocyte/macrophage colony-stimulating
    factor (GM-CSF), 398. *See also*
    COLONY-STIMULATING FACTORS
grape seed, 110*t*, 308*t*
grapefruit juice, drug interactions:
    fexofenadine, 583*t*
    nifedipine, 314*t*
    overview, 30*t*
    statins, 295*t*
Graves' disease, 664*t*, 670, 788
Gravol. *See* dimenhydrinate
green tea, 110*t*, 564*t*
griseofulvin, 520*t*, 521, 798
Grisovin-FP. *See* griseofulvin
growth, 76
growth fraction, 555, 788
growth hormones (GH), 663, 664–65
guaifenesin, 589*t*, 590*t*, 591
guanabenz, 321*t*
guanadrel, 321*t*
guanethidine, 191, 321*t*
guanine, 562*f*

guttate psoriasis, 766*t*
Gyne-Lotrimin. *See* clotrimazole
Gynergen. *See* ergotamine

H

H⁺, K⁺-ATPase, 617, 788

H$_1$-receptor, 473, 581, 788

H$_1$-RECEPTOR ANTAGONISTS:
  adverse effects, 581*t*
  drugs classified as
    first-generation
      azatadine, 581*t*
      azelastine, 581*t*, 582
      brompheniramine, 581*t*, 582, 797
      chlorpheniramine, 581*t*, 582, 797
      clemastine, 581*t*, 582
      cyproheptadine, 581*t*
      dexbrompheniramine, 581*t*, 582
      dexchlorpheniramine, 581*t*
      diphenhydramine. *See*
        diphenhydramine
      promethazine. *See* promethazine
      tripelennamine, 581*t*, 799
      triprolidine, 581*t*
    second-generation
      cetirizine. *See* cetirizine
      desloratadine, 581*t*, 801
      fexofenadine. *See* **fexofenadine**
      loratadine, 581*t*
  nursing considerations, 582
    client teaching, 584
    lifespan considerations, 584
    nursing process focus, 584–85*t*
  for specific conditions
    allergic rhinitis, 581–82, 581*t*
    pretreatment of drug allergies, 420
H$_2$-receptor, 473, 788
H$_2$-RECEPTOR ANTAGONISTS:
  adverse effects, 615*t*
  drugs classified as
    cimetidine, 191, 615*t*, 638, 797
    famotidine, 615*t*, 801
    nizatidine, 615*t*
    ranitidine HCl. *See* **ranitidine HCl**
  mechanisms of action, 614*f*, 788
  nursing considerations, 616–17
    client teaching, 617
    nursing process focus, 616*t*
  pharmacotherapy with, 615
  route and adult doses, 615*t*
  vitamin B$_{12}$ absorption and, 617*t*
HAART (highly active retroviral therapy),
      536, 788. *See also* ANTIRETROVIRALS
Haemophilus, 485*t*
haemophilus type B conjugate vaccine, 460*t*
HAIg (hepatitis A immunoglobulin), 547
halazepam, 161, 162*t*
halcinonide, 765*t*
Halcion. *See* triazolam
Haldol. *See* **haloperidol**
hallucinations, 210, 788
hallucinogens:
  dependency characteristics, 120*t*

LSD, 123–24
  mescaline, 124, 124*f*
  psilocybin, 123, 123*f*
  toxicity signs, 120*t*
  types, 124
  withdrawal symptoms, 120*t*
Halog. *See* halcinonide
haloperidol, 215*t*
  actions and uses, 215*t*, 271
  administration alerts, 215*t*
  adverse effects, 215*t*
  Canadian/U.S. trade names, 798
  genetic polymorphisms affecting
      metabolism, 104*t*
  interactions, 215*t*
  overdose treatment, 215*t*
  pharmacokinetics, 215*t*
  route and adult dose, 215*t*
haloprogin, 520*t*
Halotestin. *See* fluoxymesterone
Halotex. *See* haloprogin
halothane, 252*t*
  actions and uses, 252*t*
  adverse effects, 252*t*
  interactions, 252*t*
  pharmacokinetics, 252*t*
hash oil, 122
hashish, 122
Havrix. *See* hepatitis A vaccine
hawthorn, 342*t*
hay fever. *See* allergic rhinitis
H-BIG. *See* hepatitis B immunoglobulin
HBIg (hepatitis B immunoglobulin), 458*t*,
      548
hBNP (human beta-type natriuretic
      peptide), 342
HCG (human chorionic gonadotropin),
      714, 714*t*, 721
HCTZ. *See* **hydrochlorothiazide**
HDL. *See* high-density lipoprotein
headaches, 237, 237*t*. *See also* migraine
health beliefs, cultural and ethnic
      influences, 103
Health Canada, 9
health history assessment, 68–69, 68*t*
Health Products and Food Branch (HPFB), 9
health status, community influences, 104*t*
healthcare access:
  community influences, 103
  minority status and, 102*t*
hearing impairments, 69*t*
heart attack. *See* myocardial infarction
heart block, 363*t*
heart failure (HF):
  definition, 330, 788
  etiology, 330
  hypertension and, 305
  incidence, 330*t*
  natural therapy with hawthorn, 342*t*
  pathophysiology, 331–32, 331*f*
  pharmacotherapy
    ACE inhibitors. *See* ANGIOTENSIN-
      CONVERTING ENZYME (ACE) INHIBITORS

angiotensin-receptor blockers, 334
  beta-adrenergic agonists, 342
  beta-adrenergic antagonists.
      See BETA-ADRENERGIC ANTAGONISTS
  cardiac glycosides. *See* CARDIAC GLYCOSIDES
  diuretics. *See* DIURETICS
  increasing compliance, 341*t*
  mechanisms of action, 332*f*
  nesiritide, 342
  overview, 333*t*
  phosphodiesterase inhibitors. *See*
      PHOSPHODIESTERASE INHIBITORS
  psychosocial issues in compliance, 341*t*
  therapeutic approach, 330
  vasodilators. *See* VASODILATORS
  symptoms, 331–32
Helicobacter pylori, 613, 614*f*, 620–21, 788
helminthic infection, 514*t*, 528,
      pharmacotherapy, 528
      ANTIHELMINTHICS, 358*t*
      See also ANTIHELMINTHICS
helminths, 514*t*, 527*t*, 528, 528*t*, 788.
      See also ANTIHELMINTHICS
helper T cells, 459, 788
Hemabate. *See* carboprost tromethamine
hematopoiesis, 394–95, 394*f*, 788
HEMATOPOIETIC GROWTH FACTORS:
  drugs classified as
    colony-stimulating factors.
        See COLONY-STIMULATING FACTORS
    darbepoetin alfa, 395*t*, 396
    epoetin alfa. *See* **epoetin alfa**
    platelet enhancers.
        See PLATELET ENHANCERS
  nursing considerations, 395–96
    client teaching, 396, 398
    lifespan considerations, 396
    nursing process focus, 397*t*
  pharmacotherapy with, 395
hemophilia, 378*t*, 380, 788
hemosiderin, 403, 788
hemostasis:
  definition, 378, 788
  diseases of, 380–81
  mechanisms of modification, 381, 381*f*, 381*t*
  process, 378–79, 379*f*
HEMOSTATICS:
  adverse effects, 390*t*
  drugs classified as
    aminocaproic acid. *See* **aminocaproic
        acid**
    aprotinin, 390*t*
    tranexamic acid, 390*t*
  mechanisms of action, 381, 381*t*, 389, 788
  nursing considerations, 390
    client teaching, 390
  pharmacotherapy with, 389–90
  route and adult dose, 390*t*
henbane, 583*t*
Hepalean. *See* **heparin**
heparin, 383*t*
  actions and uses, 383*t*
  administration alerts, 383*t*

heparin *(continued)*
  adverse effects, 382*t*, 383*t*
  Canadian/U.S. trade names, 798
  interactions, 113*t*, 383*t*
  overdose treatment, 383*t*
  pharmacokinetics, 383*t*
  route and adult dose, 382*t*
hepatic microsomal enzyme system, 50, 788
Hepatic-Aid II, 655
hepatitis, 547, 788
hepatitis A, 547
hepatitis A immunoglobulin (HAIg), 547
hepatitis A vaccine, 547
hepatitis B:
  characteristics, 547–48
  pharmacotherapy, 548, 548*t*
hepatitis B immunoglobulin (HBIg),
    458*t*, 548
hepatitis B vaccine, 460*t*
  actions and uses, 460*t*
  administration alerts, 460*t*
  adverse effects, 460*t*
  interactions, 460*t*
  pharmacokinetics, 460*t*
  schedule and age, 460*t*, 548
hepatitis C:
  characteristics, 549
  pharmacotherapy, 548*t*
Heplock. *See* **heparin**
Hepsera. *See* adefovir
herb, 108, 788
herbal therapies. *See also* Natural Therapies;
    specific therapies
  best-selling, primary uses, 110*t*
  drug interactions, 113*t*
  formulations, 109–11
  history, 108–9
  liquid formulations, 111*t*
  medication errors and, 96*t*
  in older adults, 109*t*
  pharmacological actions and safety,
    112, 114
  regulation, 111–12
  standardization, 110*t*
Herceptin. *See* trastuzumab
heroin:
  adverse effects during breast-feeding, 79*t*
  fetal effects, 80*t*
herpes simplex, 756
herpes zoster, 545*t*, 756
herpesviruses:
  classification, 544
  eye infections, 545
  home and community considerations, 545*t*
  incidence, 534*t*
  pharmacotherapy. *See* ANTIVIRALS
Herplex. *See* idoxuridine
Hespan. *See* hetastarch
hetastarch, 413*t*, 414
Hetrazan. *See* diethylcarbamazine
hexaBetalin. *See* vitamin B$_6$
Hexadrol. *See* dexamethasone
Hexalen. *See* altretamine

Hexastate. *See* altretamine
HF. *See* heart failure
HibTITER. *See* haemophilus type
    B conjugate vaccine
high-density lipoprotein (HDL):
  characteristics, 289, 289*f*, 788
  laboratory values, 290*t*
  ratio to LDL, 290
highly active retroviral therapy (HAART),
    536, 788. *See also* ANTIRETROVIRALS
hippocampus, 269, 788
Hiprex. *See* methenamine
Hismanal. *See* astemizole
Hispanic Americans:
  depression treatment considerations,
    187*t*
  hot and cold theory of illness, 488*t*
  mental illness treatment, 212*t*
  pain management, 225*t*
histamine, 472, 472*t*, 581, 788
histamine receptor antagonists. *See* H$_1$-RE-
    CEPTOR ANTAGONISTS; H$_2$-RECEPTOR
    ANTAGONISTS
histamine receptors, 473, 581, 615
Histantil. *See* promethazine
Histerone. *See* **testosterone**
Histoplasma capsulatum, 515*t*
histoplasmosis, 515*t*
histrelin, 568*t*, 569
HIV (human immunodeficiency virus). *See*
    HIV-AIDS; human immunodefi-
    ciency virus
HIV-AIDS:
  in children, 544*t*
  complementary and alternative medicine
    for, 548*t*
  definition, 534, 788
  home and community considerations,
    545*t*
  incidence, 534*t*
  mortality rate, 534*t*
  in older adults, 544*t*
  pathophysiology, 534
  pharmacotherapy
    antiretrovirals. *See* ANTIRETROVIRALS
    classification of drugs, 536
    structured treatment interruptions,
      536
    therapeutic approach, 534–36
  postexposure prophylaxis following
    occupational exposure, 543
  prevention of perinatal transmission, 543
  stages, 535
Hivid. *See* zalcitabine
HMG-CoA reductase, 291, 293*f*, 788
HMG-CoA reductase inhibitors. *See* STATINS
HNKC (hyperosmolar nonketotic
    coma), 691, 789
holistic, 100, 788
homatropine, 779*t*
Home and Community Considerations:
  Alzheimer's disease, 268*t*
  anaphylaxis, recurrent, 421*t*

anticoagulant therapy, 380*t*
aspirin for cardiovascular event risk
    reduction, 479*t*
asthma management
  peak-flow meter for, 605*t*
  in schools, 599*t*
autonomic nervous system agents, safety
    with, 150*t*
bone and joint disorders, accommoda-
    tions for, 738*t*
diabetes impact on community
    resources, 694*t*
diuretic therapy at home, 433*t*
dysrhythmia therapy, 374*t*
erectile dysfunction drugs, 725*t*
heart disease, CPR and other education
    for, 348*t*
heart failure treatment, increasing
    compliance, 341*t*
hematopoietic disorders, 396*t*
hepatotoxicity with long-term drug
    therapies, 529*t*
herpes zoster, 545*t*
HIV-AIDS, 545*t*
hormone therapy, side effects, 702*t*
hypernatremia in athletes, 444*t*
medication errors
  in children, educating parents
    to reduce, 95*t*
  preventing, 93*t*
muscle relaxant therapy, 281*t*
neural tube defects and folic acid levels
    in pregnancy, 648*t*
ophthalmic drugs, 778*t*
over-the-counter drugs
  for bowel disorders, nausea, and
    vomiting, 638*t*
  interactions, 618*t*
  medication errors and, 96*t*
postanesthesia follow-up care, 254*t*
pseudoephedrine and drug abuse, 588*t*
skin disorders and self-esteem, 765*t*
viral infections, 545*t*
homocysteine, 395*t*
Honval. *See* diethylstilbestrol
HORMONE ANTAGONISTS:
  adverse effects, 568*t*
  for cancer chemotherapy
    abarelix, 568*t*, 569
    aminoglutethimide, 568*t*
    anastrozole, 568*t*, 569
    bicalutamide, 568*t*, 569
    exemestane, 568*t*, 569
    fulvestrant, 568*t*
    goserelin, 568*t*, 714*t*
    histrelin, 568*t*, 569
    letrozole, 568*t*, 569
    leuprolide, 568*t*, 569
    mechanisms of action, 555*f*
    nilutamide, 568*t*
    tamoxifen. *See* **tamoxifen**
    toremifene, 568*t*, 569
  route and adult doses, 568*t*

selective estrogen-receptor modifiers. *See* SELECTIVE ESTROGEN-RECEPTOR MODIFIERS

hormone replacement therapy (HRT). *See also* ESTROGENS
  adverse effects, 705–6, 708*t*
  benefits, 705, 706*t*
  definition, 788
  nursing considerations, 708
    client teaching, 708
  nursing process focus, 707–8*t*

HORMONES:
  adverse effects, 702*t*
  androgens. *See* ANDROGENS
  for cancer chemotherapy
    diethylstilbestrol, 568*t*, 569
    ethinyl estradiol, 568, 568*t*
    fluoxymesterone, 568, 568*t*
    mechanisms of action, 555*f*
    medroxyprogesterone. *See* **medroxyprogesterone acetate**
    megestrol, 568*t*, 569
    nursing considerations, 569–70
      client teaching, 570
    pharmacotherapy with, 569–70
    testolactone, 568, 568*t*
    testosterone. *See* **testosterone**
  for contraception. *See* CONTRACEPTIVES
  definition, 788
  estrogens. *See* ESTROGENS
  functions, 661, 788
  pharmacotherapy with, 662
  production, 661–62, 661*f*
host flora, 488, 788
household system of measurement, 31, 31*t*, 788
H.P. Acthar. *See* repository corticotropin
HPFB (Health Products and Food Branch), 9
HRT. *See* hormone replacement therapy
HTN. *See* hypertension
huffing, 120*t*
Humalog. *See* insulin lispro
human beta-type natriuretic peptide (hBNP), 342
human chorionic gonadotropin (HCG), 714, 714*t*, 721
human immunodeficiency virus (HIV). *See also* HIV-AIDS
  postexposure prophylaxis following occupational exposure, 543
  prevention of perinatal transmission, 543
  replication, 534, 535*f*
  structure, 533*f*
  transmission, 534
human integration pyramid care model, 100, 100*f*
human menopausal gonadotropin–menotropins, 714, 714*t*
Humatin. *See* paromomycin
Humatrope. *See* somatropin
Humegon. *See* human menopausal gonadotropin–menotropins

Humira. *See* adalimumab
humoral immunity, 456, 456*f*, 788
Humorsol. *See* demecarium
Humulin 70/30. *See* NPH 70% Regular 30%
Humulin L. *See* insulin zinc suspension
Humulin N. *See* isophane insulin suspension
Humulin R. *See* **regular insulin**
Humulin U. *See* extended insulin zinc suspension
hunger, 635
Huntington's chorea, 261*t*
Hyalgan. *See* sodium hyaluronate
Hybolin. *See* nandrolone phenpropionate
Hycodan. *See* hydrocodone bitartrate
Hycomine Compound, 590*t*
Hycotuss Expectorant, 590*t*
HYDANTOINS:
  adverse effects, 178*t*
  fosphenytoin, 178*t*
  nursing considerations, 178–80
    client teaching, 179–80
    lifespan considerations, 179
  phenytoin. *See* **phenytoin**
  route and adult doses, 178*t*
Hydeltrasol. *See* prednisolone
hydralazine, 325*t*
  actions and uses, 325*t*
  administration alerts, 325*t*
  adverse effects, 324*t*, 325*t*
  Canadian/U.S. trade names, 798
  genetic polymorphisms affecting metabolism, 104*t*
  interactions, 325*t*
  overdose treatment, 325*t*
  pharmacokinetics, 325*t*
  for specific conditions
    heart failure, 333*t*, 338
    hypertension, 324*t*
Hydrastis canadensis. *See* goldenseal
Hydrea. *See* hydroxyurea
Hydrex. *See* benzthiazide
hydrochlorothiazide, 311*t*
  actions and uses, 311*t*
  administration alerts, 311*t*
  adverse effects, 311*t*
  Canadian/U.S. trade names, 798
  in combination drugs for hypertension, 309*t*
  interactions, 311*t*
  overdose treatment, 311*t*
  pharmacokinetics, 311*t*
  prescription ranking, 800
  for specific conditions
    heart failure, 333*t*
    hypertension, 310*t*
    renal failure, 429*t*
hydrocodone bitartrate:
  adverse effects, 227*t*, 589*t*
  as antitussive, 589, 589*t*
  Canadian/U.S. trade names, 798
  in combination cold drugs, 480*t*
  for pain management, 227*t*
  route and adult dose, 227*t*, 589*t*

hydrocodone polistirex and chlorpheniramine polistirex, 590*t*, 802
hydrocodone with APAP, 800
hydrocortisone, 676*t*
  actions and uses, 676*t*
  administration alerts, 676*t*
  adverse effects, 476*t*, 675*t*, 676*t*
  Canadian/U.S. trade names, 798
  interactions, 676*t*
  pharmacokinetics, 676*t*
  for specific conditions
    adrenocortical insufficiency, 675*t*
    dermatitis, 765*t*
    psoriasis, 768
    severe inflammation, 476*t*
HydroDIURIL. *See* **hydrochlorothiazide**
hydroflumethiazide, 429*t*
hydrogen cyanide, 24*t*
hydrolysis, 788
hydromorphone hydrochloride, 227*t*
Hydromox. *See* quinethazone
Hydropres, 309*t*
hydroxyamphetamine, 779*t*
hydroxychloroquine sulfate, 748*t*
  actions and uses, 748*t*
  administration alerts, 748*t*
  adverse effects, 523*t*, 747*t*, 748*t*
  interactions, 748*t*
  overdose treatment, 748*t*
  pharmacokinetics, 748*t*
  route and adult dose, 523*t*, 747*t*
  for specific conditions
    malaria, 523*t*
    rheumatoid arthritis, 746, 747*t*
hydroxyurea, 571*t*, 767*t*, 768
hydroxyzine, 137, 634*t*, 798, 801
Hygroton. *See* chlorthalidone
Hyoscine. *See* scopolamine
Hyperab. *See* rabies immune globulin
hypercalcemia:
  definition, 442*t*
  supportive treatment, 442*t*
  symptoms, 652, 733
hyperchloremia, 442*t*
hypercholesterolemia, 289, 789
hyperemesis gravidarum, 632
hyperemia, 789
hyperglycemia, 691*t*, 789. *See also* diabetes mellitus
HyperHep. *See* hepatitis B immunoglobulin
Hypericum perforatum. *See* St. John's wort
hyperkalemia:
  causes, 445
  definition, 442*t*, 445
  pharmacotherapy, 442*t*, 445
  potassium-sparing diuretics and, 308
  in renal failure, 426*t*
hyperlipidemia:
  in childhood, 289
  definition, 289, 789
  incidence, 287*t*
  laboratory values, 290, 290*t*
  nonpharmacological treatment, 290–91

hyperlipidemia *(continued)*
  pharmacotherapy
    bile acid resins. *See* BILE ACID RESINS
    ezetimibe, 292*t*, 294*f*, 298–99, 800, 801
    niacin. *See* vitamin B₃
    nursing considerations, 292,
      294–95, 297, 298
      client teaching, 292–93, 295, 297, 298
      lifespan considerations, 292, 295
    nursing process focus, 296*t*
    statins. *See* STATINS
hypermagnesemia, 442*t*
hypernatremia:
  in athletes, 444*t*
  causes, 443
  definition, 442*t*, 443, 789
  pharmacotherapy, 442*t*, 443
hyperosmolar nonketotic coma
    (HNKC), 691, 789
hyperphosphatemia, 426*t*, 442*t*
Hyperstat IV. *See* diazoxide
hypertension (HTN):
  classification, 302–3, 303*t*
  definition, 302, 789
  etiology, 305
  incidence, 302*t*
  management recommendations, 303*t*
  natural therapy with chocolate and grape
    seed extract, 308*t*
  nonpharmacological management, 305–6
  pathogenesis, 305–6
  pharmacotherapy
    ACE inhibitors. *See* ANGIOTENSIN-
      CONVERTING ENZYME (ACE) INHIBITORS
    adrenergic agonists. *See*
      ALPHA-ADRENERGIC AGONISTS
    adrenergic antagonists. *See*
      ALPHA-ADRENERGIC ANTAGONISTS;
      BETA-ADRENERGIC ANTAGONISTS
    calcium channel blockers. *See* CALCIUM
      CHANNEL BLOCKERS
    combination drugs, 308, 309*t*
    diuretics. *See* DIURETICS
    mechanisms of action, 307*f*
    therapeutic approach, 306–8
    vasodilators. *See* VASODILATORS
  primary, 305
  secondary, 305
hypertensive emergency, 324
HyperTet. *See* tetanus immune globulin
hyperthyroidism:
  incidence, 666*t*
  natural therapies, 667*t*
  pharmacotherapy, 670, 672. *See also*
    ANTITHYROID AGENTS
hypertonic solutions:
  characteristics, 439, 439*f*
  crystalloid, 440, 440*t*. *See also*
    CRYSTALLOIDS
  saline, 413*t*
hypertriglyceridemia, 298
hyperuricemia, 746, 789
hypervitaminosis, 644, 789

hypervolemia, 426*t*
hypnotics, 159, 789
hypocalcemia:
  causes, 734
  definition, 442*t*
  nonpharmacological therapy, 734
  pharmacotherapy. *See* CALCIUM SALTS
  in renal failure, 426*t*
  supportive treatment, 442*t*
  symptoms, 651, 733, 734
hypochloremia, 442*t*
hypodermis, 753
hypoglycemia, 684, 789
hypoglycemic effect, 682
hypogonadism:
  causes, 718–19
  definition, 718, 789
  incidence, 718*t*
  pharmacotherapy. *See* ANDROGENS
  symptoms, 719
hypokalemia:
  causes, 308, 445
  definition, 442*t*, 445
  nursing considerations, 445
    client teaching, 445–46
  pharmacotherapy, 442*t*, 445, 446*t*
hypomagnesemia, 442*t*, 651–52
hyponatremia, 442*t*, 443, 444, 789
hypophosphatemia, 651
HYPOTHALAMIC AGENTS:
  octreotide, 664*t*, 665
  pegvisomant, 664*t*, 665
  protirelin, 664*t*
hypothalamus:
  in anxiety, 155, 155*f*
  disorders, 662
  hormone production, 662, 663*f*
hypothyroidism:
  amiodarone and, 667
  incidence, 666*t*
  natural therapies, 667*t*
  pharmacotherapy. *See* THYROID AGENTS
  in shift workers, 667*t*
  symptoms, 667
hypotonic solutions:
  characteristics, 439, 439*f*
  colloid, 440*t*. *See also* COLLOIDS
  crystalloid, 440, 440*t*. *See also* CRYSTALLOIDS
hypovolemic shock, 410, 410*t*, 412*t*, 789
Hyskon. *See* **dextran 40**
Hytone. *See* **hydrocortisone**
Hytrin. *See* terazosin
Hyzaar. *See* losartan/hydrochlorothiazide

I

I-131. *See* radioactive iodine
ibandronate, 741*t*
ibritumomab tiuxetan, 571*t*
ibuprofen, 475*t*
  actions and uses, 474, 475*t*
  administration alerts, 475*t*
  adverse effects, 233*t*, 474, 475*t*
  Canadian/U.S. trade names, 798

  interactions, 475*t*
  pharmacokinetics, 475*t*
  prescription ranking, 800
  route and adult dose, 233*t*
ibutilide, 367*t*, 371
ICD (implantable cardioverter
    defibrillator), 364
ICF (intracellular fluid) compartment,
    438, 438*f*, 789
ID (intradermal) drug administration, 38,
    39*f*, 40*t*, 789
Idamycin. *See* idarubicin
idarubicin, 563, 564*t*
idiopathic hypertension, 305. *See also*
    hypertension
idiosyncratic responses, 62, 789
idoxuridine, 544*t*, 545
Ifex. *See* ifosfamide
ifosfamide, 559*t*
IGIV. *See* immune globulin intravenous
Iletin II. *See* protamine zinc insulin
ileum, 624, 625*f*, 789
illusions, 210, 789
IM (intramuscular) drug administration,
    39, 40*t*, 41, 42*f*, 789
imatinib mesylate, 571, 571*t*
Imdur. *See* isosorbide mononitrate
Imfed. *See* iron dextran
Imferon. *See* iron dextran
imipenem-cilastatin, 503*t*, 506
imipramine, 191*t*
  actions and uses, 191*t*
  administration alerts, 191*t*
  adverse effects, 191*t*, 238*t*
  Canadian/U.S. trade names, 798
  genetic polymorphisms affecting
    metabolism, 104*t*
  interactions, 191*t*
  overdose treatment, 191*t*
  pharmacokinetics, 191*t*
  for specific conditions
    ADHD, 204
    depression, 189*t*
    migraine, 238*t*
    panic disorders, 159*t*
Imitrex. *See* **sumatriptan**
immune globulin intramuscular, 458*t*
immune globulin intravenous, 458*t*
IMMUNE GLOBULINS:
  cytomegalovirus immune globulin, 458*t*
  hepatitis A immune globulin, 547
  hepatitis B immune globulin, 458*t*, 548
  immune globulin intramuscular, 458*t*
  immune globulin intravenous, 458*t*
  rabies immune globulin, 458*t*
  Rho(D) immune globulin, 458*t*
  tetanus immune globulin, 458*t*
immune response, 455–56, 456*f*, 789
immunity. *See also* vaccines
  active, 457, 459*f*
  cell-mediated, 459–61
  passive, 457, 459*f*
immunization, 457, 795. *See also* vaccines

immunoglobulins, 456
IMMUNOSTIMULANTS:
  adverse effects, 461*t*
  drugs classified as
    aldesleukin, 461*t*, 462
    Bacillus Calmette-Guérin (BCG)
      vaccine, 461*t*, 462
    interferons. *See* INTERFERONS
    levamisole, 461*t*, 462, 571*t*
  nursing considerations, 462–63
    client teaching, 463
  nursing process focus, 464*t*
  pharmacotherapy with, 461–62, 461*t*
  route and adult doses, 461*t*
IMMUNOSUPPRESSANTS:
  adverse effects, 465*t*, 466
  characteristics, 463, 466
  definition, 789
  drugs classified as
    antibodies. *See* MONOCLONAL ANTIBODIES
    antimetabolites and cytotoxic agents
      anakinra, 465*t*, 746, 747*t*
      azathioprine, 465*t*, 466, 630, 746
      cyclophosphamide. *See*
        cyclophosphamide
      etanercept, 465*t*, 746, 767*t*, 768
      methotrexate. *See* **methotrexate**
      mycophenolate mofetil, 465*t*
      sirolimus, 465*t*, 466
      thalidomide, 465*t*
    calcineurin inhibitors
      cyclosporine. *See* **cyclosporine**
      tacrolimus. *See* tacrolimus
    glucocorticoids. *See* GLUCOCORTICOIDS
  mechanisms of action, 463, 466–67
  nursing considerations, 468
    client teaching, 468
  nursing process focus, 467*t*
  route and adult doses, 465*t*
  for transplant rejection prevention, 463
Imodium. *See* loperamide
Imogam Rabies-HT. *See* rabies
  immune globulin
impetigo, 485*t*, 756
Implanon, 700. *See also* desogestrel
implantable cardioverter defibrillator
  (ICD), 364
impotence, 721, 789. *See also* erectile
  dysfunction
Impril. *See* **imipramine**
Imuran. *See* azathioprine
inamrinone, 333*t*
Inapsine. *See* droperidol
incident report, 93–94
indapamide, 310*t*, 429*t*, 798
Inderal. *See* **propranolol**
Inderal LA. *See* **propranolol**
Inderide, 309*t*
indinavir, 537*t*
Indocin. *See* indomethacin
indomethacin, 233*t*, 473*t*, 747
Infanrix. *See* diphtheria, tetanus, and
  pertussis vaccine

infants:
  definition, 789
  drug administration challenges, 29*t*, 72
  drug administration guidelines, 81–82, 81*f*
Infasurf. *See* calfactant
infectious agents, 20*t*
infectious diseases, 20*t*
Infergen. *See* interferon alfacon-1
infertility:
  definition, 789
  female. *See* female infertility
  male, 721
infiltration anesthesia, 246*f*, 246*t*
Inflamase. *See* prednisolone
inflammation:
  chemical mediators, 472*t*
  classification, 471
  definition, 789
  function, 471
  natural therapy with fish oils, 476*t*
  pharmacotherapy
    glucocorticoids. *See* GLUCOCORTICOIDS
    nonsteroidal anti-inflammatory
      drugs. *See* NONSTEROIDAL
      ANTI-INFLAMMATORY DRUGS
  process, 472, 472*f*
inflammatory bowel disease, 630
inflammatory disorders, 471–72, 471*t*
infliximab:
  adverse effects, 465*t*
  as immunosuppressant, 465*t*, 468
  for inflammatory bowel disease, 630
  for psoriasis, 768
  for rheumatoid arthritis, 746
influenza:
  characteristics, 546, 789
  pharmacotherapy
    prophylaxis, 546
      amantadine, 546, 547*t*
      rimantadine, 546, 547*t*
    treatment
      oseltamivir, 546, 547*t*
      zanamivir, 546, 547*t*
influenza vaccine, 460*t*, 546
infusion, herbal, 111*t*
INH. *See* **isoniazid**
inhalation, for drug administration, 595
inhalation anthrax, 22*t*
inhalations, 34
INHALED GLUCOCORTICOIDS:
  adverse effects, 601*t*
  for asthma, 601, 601*t*
  beclomethasone, 601*t*. *See also*
    beclomethasone
  budesonide, 601*t*, 801, 802
  flunisolide, 601*t*
  fluticasone. *See* **fluticasone**
  nursing considerations, 603
    client teaching, 603
  pharmacotherapy with, 301
  triamcinolone. *See* triamcinolone
Innohep. *See* tinzaparin
Innovar. *See* fentanyl/droperidol

Inocor. *See* inamrinone
INOTROPIC AGENTS:
  drugs classified as
    digoxin. *See* **digoxin**
    dobutamine. *See* dobutamine
    dopamine. *See* **dopamine**
  mechanisms of action, 417, 789
  nursing considerations, 418
    client teaching, 418
inotropic effect, 336, 789
insomnia:
  anxiety and, 156–57
  definition, 156, 789
  incidence, 157*t*
  insulin resistance and, 157*t*
  long-term, 157
  natural therapies, 157*t*
  pharmacotherapy
    barbiturates, 164*t*. *See also*
      BARBITURATES
    benzodiazepines, 162*t*. *See also*
      BENZODIAZEPINES
    nonbenzodiazepine, nonbarbiturate,
      165*t*. *See also* NONBENZODIAZEPINE,
      NONBARBITURATE CNS DEPRESSANTS
    nursing considerations, 161–62
      client teaching, 162–63
      lifespan considerations, 162
      nursing process focus, 166*t*
  rebound, 157
  short-term (behavioral), 157
Inspra. *See* eplerenone
installations, 34
Institute for Safe Medication Practices
  (ISMP), 96
insulin:
  functions, 682, 683*f*
  pancreatic secretion, 682, 682*f*
  pharmacotherapy with. *See* INSULINS
insulin analogs, 684, 789. *See also* INSULINS
insulin aspart, 685*t*
insulin detemir, 685*t*, 688
insulin glargine, 685*t*, 688, 801
insulin lispro, 685*t*, 688, 801
insulin pump, 684, 685*f*
insulin resistance, 157*t*, 689, 789
insulin zinc suspension, 685*t*
insulin-dependent diabetes. *See* diabetes
  mellitus, type 1
INSULINS:
  adverse effects, 684
  herb–drug interactions, 113*t*
  inhaled, 684, 685*f*
  nursing considerations, 686, 688
    client teaching, 688
    lifespan considerations, 688
    nursing process focus, 687*t*
  pharmacotherapy with
    principles, 684
    routes of administration, 684, 685*f*
  preparations
    extended insulin zinc suspension,
      685*t*, 688

INSULINS *(continued)*
    insulin aspart, 685t
    insulin detemir, 685t, 688
    insulin glargine, 685t, 688, 801
    insulin lispro, 685t, 688
    insulin zinc suspension, 685t
    isophane insulin suspension,
        685t, 686
    NPH 50% Regular 50%, 685t
    NPH 70% Regular 30%, 685t
    protamine zinc insulin, 688
    regular insulin. *See* **regular insulin**
Intal. *See* cromolyn
Integrilin. *See* eptifibatide
interferon alfa-2a, 463t
    actions and uses, 463t, 570
    administration alerts, 463t
    adverse effects, 461t, 463t
    interactions, 463t
    pharmacokinetics, 463t
    route and adult dose, 461t, 571t
    for specific conditions
        cancer, 570, 571t
        hepatitis, 548t
interferon alfa-2b, 461t, 548t, 570
interferon alfacon-1, 548t
interferon alfa-n1, 548t
interferon beta-1a, 461t
interferon beta-1b, 461t
INTERFERONS (IFNs):
    adverse effects, 461t, 478
    definition, 461, 789
    drugs classified as
        interferon alfa-2a. *See* **interferon
            alfa-2a**
        interferon alfa-2b, 461t, 548t, 570
        interferon alfacon, 548t
        interferon alfa-n1, 548t
        interferon beta-1a, 461t
        interferon beta-1b, 461t
        peginterferon alfa-2a, 461t, 548t
        peginterferon alfa-2b, 548t
    mechanisms of action, 461–62
    nursing considerations, 462–63
        client teaching, 463
    nursing process focus, 464t
    pharmacotherapy with, 461, 570
    for specific conditions
        cancer, 570, 571t
        hepatitis, 548t, 549
INTERLEUKINS (ILs):
    aldesleukin, 461t, 462, 570
    definition, 462, 789
    mechanisms of action, 462
    oprelvekin, 395t, 399, 462
intermittent claudication, 386, 386t, 789
intermittent infusion, 43, 43f
International Union of Pure and Applied
        Chemistry (IUPAC), 13
interpersonal therapy, 187
interstitial space, 438, 438f
interventions:
    definition, 67–68, 789

in medication administration,
        71–72, 72t
intracellular fluid (ICF) compartment, 438,
        438f, 789
intracellular parasites, 533, 789
intradermal (ID) drug administration, 38,
        39f, 40t, 789
intramuscular (IM) drug administration,
        39, 40t, 41, 42f, 789
intranasal cromolyn, 586
INTRANASAL GLUCOCORTICOIDS:
    for allergic rhinitis, 584–86, 585t
    beclomethasone. *See* **beclomethasone**
    budesonide, 585t, 801, 802
    flunisolide, 585t
    fluticasone. *See* **fluticasone**
    mometasone furoate, 585t, 800
    nursing considerations, 586
        client teaching, 586
    triamcinolone. *See* triamcinolone
intraocular pressure (IOP), 772
intravascular space, 438, 438f
intravenous (IV) drug administration, 42f,
        43, 43f, 789, 845–46
intrinsic factor, 401, 612, 789
Intron-A. *See* interferon alfa-2b
Intropin. *See* **dopamine**
Invanz. *See* ertapenem
Invirase. *See* **saquinavir**
iodine, 653, 653t, 666
iodoquinol, 526t
Iodotope. *See* radioactive iodine
ion trapping, 448
ionization, 49, 49f
ionizing radiation, 23–25, 789
IOP (intraocular pressure), 772.
        See also glaucoma
Iopidine. *See* apraclonidine
IPOL. *See* poliovirus vaccine
ipratropium bromide, 599t
    actions and uses, 147t, 599, 599t
    administration alerts, 599t
    adverse effects, 147, 597t, 599t
    interactions, 599t
    pharmacokinetics, 599t
    prescription ranking, 801
    for specific conditions
        asthma, 597t, 599
        chronic obstructive pulmonary
            disease, 606
        nasal congestion, 587, 587t
ipratropium bromide with albuterol
        sulfate, 801
Iprivask. *See* desirudin
irbesartan, 316t, 801
irbesartan/hydrochlorothiazide, 801
Iressa. *See* gefitinib
irinotecan, 566, 566t
iron, 403–4, 653, 653t. *See also*
        IRON SALTS
iron dextran, 402t, 404, 650t
IRON SALTS:
    adverse effects, 402t

drugs classified as
    ferrous fumarate, 402t, 650t
    ferrous gluconate, 402t, 650t
    ferrous sulfate. *See* **ferrous sulfate**
    iron dextran, 402t, 404, 650t
    iron sucrose injection, 650t
    nursing considerations, 404–6
        client teaching, 406
        lifespan considerations, 406
    pharmacotherapy with, 404
    route and adult dose, 402t
iron sucrose injection, 650t
irrigations, 34
irritable bowel syndrome (IBS):
    incidence, 624t
    nursing considerations, 631–32
        client teaching, 632
        lifespan considerations, 632
    pharmacotherapy, 630, 632t
    symptoms, 630, 789
islets of Langerhans, 682, 682f, 789
Ismelin. *See* guanethidine
ISMO. *See* isosorbide mononitrate
Ismotic. *See* isosorbide
Iso-Bid. *See* **isosorbide dinitrate**
isocarboxazid, 189t
isoetharine, 597, 597t
isoflurane, 252, 252t
isoniazid, 508t
    actions and uses, 508t
    administration alerts, 508t
    adverse effects, 507t, 508t
    Canadian/U.S. trade names, 798
    genetic polymorphisms affecting
        metabolism, 104, 104t
    interactions, 508t
    overdose treatment, 508t
    pharmacokinetics, 508t
    route and adult dose, 507t
isophane insulin suspension,
        685t, 686
isoproterenol:
    actions and uses, 137t
    as bronchodilator, 597, 597t
    for heart failure, 342
    for shock, 414
Isoptin. *See* **verapamil**
Isopto Atropine. *See* **atropine**
Isopto Carbachol. *See* carbachol
Isopto Carpine. *See* pilocarpine
Isopto Homatropine. *See* homatropine
Isopto Hyoscine. *See* scopolamine
Isordil. *See* **isosorbide dinitrate**
isosorbide, 774t, 776
isosorbide dinitrate, 338t
    actions and uses, 338, 338t
    administration alerts, 338t
    adverse effects, 333t, 338t, 350t
    Canadian/U.S. trade names, 798
    interactions, 338t
    overdose treatment, 338t
    pharmacokinetics, 338t
    prescription ranking, 800

for specific conditions
angina, 350, 350t
heart failure, 333t
isosorbide mononitrate, 350t
Isotamine. See **isoniazid**
isotonic crystalloids, 440, 440t. See also
CRYSTALLOIDS
isotretinoin, 762t
actions and uses, 762t
administration alerts, 762t
adverse effects, 761t, 762t
interactions, 762t
nursing considerations, 764
nursing process focus, 763–64t
pharmacokinetics, 762t
for rosacea, 762
route and adult dose, 761t
isradipine, 313t
Isuprel. See isoproterenol
itraconazole, 30t, 518, 519t, 521
IUPAC (International Union of Pure and
Applied Chemistry), 13
IV bolus (push) administration, 43, 43f
IV (intravenous) drug administration, 42f,
43, 43f, 789, 845–46
Iveegam EN. See immune globulin intravenous
ivermectin, 528t

J
Jadelle, 700. See also levonorgestrel
Januvia. See sitagliptin
jejunum, 624, 625f, 789
Jenamicin. See **gentamicin**
jock itch, 515t, 520
See also tinea cruris
Joint Commission on Accreditation of
Healthcare Organization (JCAHO),
disaster planning requirements, 20
joint disorders:
gout. See gout
osteoarthritis. See osteoarthritis
rheumatoid arthritis. See rheumatoid
arthritis
juvenile-onset diabetes. See diabetes
mellitus, type 1

K
K+. See potassium
Kabikinase. See streptokinase
Kalcinate. See calcium gluconate
Kaletra. See lopinavir/ritonavir
kanamycin, 498t, 507t
Kantrex. See kanamycin
Kaposi's sarcoma, 789
kappa receptors, 226, 226f, 226t, 789
Karasil. See **psyllium mucilloid**
kava:
for anxiety and insomnia, 157t
drug interactions
chlorpromazine, 213t
clozapine, 219t
diazepam, 177t
haloperidol, 215t

lorazepam, 163t
morphine sulfate, 228t
overview, 113t
phenobarbital, 176t
thiopental, 255t
parkinsonism and, 265t
standardization, 110t
Kayexalate. See polystyrene sulfate
KCl. See **potassium chloride**
K-Dur. See **potassium chloride**
Keflex. See cephalexin
Kefurox. See cefuroxime
Kefzol. See cefazolin
Kemadrin. See procyclidine hydrochloride
Kenacort. See triamcinolone
Kenalog. See triamcinolone
keratolytic, 761, 789
Ketalar. See ketamine
ketamine, 124, 255, 255t
Ketek. See telithromycin
ketoacids, 683, 789
ketoconazole:
adverse effects, 519t
for Cushing's syndrome, 678
interactions, 30t, 113t
route and adult dose, 518, 519t
ketogenic diet, 173t
KETOLIDES:
telithromycin, 504t, 506
ketoprofen, 233t, 473t, 798
ketorolac tromethamine, 233t
Key-Pred. See prednisolone
KI (potassium iodide), 24–25, 653, 668, 672
kidneys:
disorders. See renal failure
drugs toxic to, 426t
functions, 424–25, 425f, 443f
transplants, 424t
Kidrolase A. See asparaginase
Kineret. See anakinra
Klaron. See sulfacetamide
Klebsiella, 485t
Klonopin. See clonazepam
Klor-Con. See **potassium chloride**
K-Phos MF. See monobasic potassium and
sodium phosphates
K-Phos neutral. See monobasic potassium
and sodium phosphates
K-Phos original. See monobasic potassium
phosphate
Kwell. See **lindane**
Kytril. See granisetron

L
labetalol, 321t
Lacri-lube. See lanolin alcohol
lactase dehydrogenase, 355t
lactated Ringer's, 413t
lactation. See breast-feeding
Lactobacillus acidophilus, 629, 629t
Lamictal. See lamotrigine
Lamisil. See terbinafine
lamivudine, 537t, 543, 548

lamotrigine:
adverse effects, 178t, 200t
for bipolar disorder, 200, 200t
prescription ranking, 801
for seizures, 178, 178t, 181
Laniazid. See **isoniazid**
lanolin alcohol, 779t
Lanoxicaps. See **digoxin**
Lanoxin. See **digoxin**
lansoprazole, 617t, 800
lanthanum carbonate, 426t
Lantus. See insulin glargine
Lanvis. See thioguanine
Largactil. See **chlorpromazine**
large-volume infusion, 42f, 43
Lariam. See mefloquine
Larodopa. See **levodopa**
Lasix. See **furosemide**
latanoprost, 775t
actions and uses, 773, 775t
administration alerts, 775t
adverse effects, 774t, 775t
interactions, 775t
pharmacokinetics, 775t
prescription ranking, 801
route and adult dose, 774t
laughing gas. See **nitrous oxide**
LAXATIVES:
definition, 625, 789
drugs classified as
bulk forming
calcium polycarbophil, 626t
characteristics, 626
methylcellulose, 626t, 779t
psyllium mucilloid. See
psyllium mucilloid
herbal
senna. See senna
lubiprostone, 626t, 627
mineral oil, 626t, 627
saline and osmotic
characteristics, 626
magnesium hydroxide, 626t
polyethylene glycol, 626t, 801
sodium biphosphate, 626t
stimulant
bisacodyl, 626t
castor oil, 626t
characteristics, 626
phenolphthalein, 626t
stool softener/surfactant
characteristics, 626
docusate, 626t
fluid-electrolyte balance and, 445t
nursing considerations, 627–28
client teaching, 628
lifespan considerations, 628
LD50 (median lethal dose), 58,
58f, 790
L-Deprenyl. See selegiline hydrochloride
L-dopa. See **levodopa**
lecithins, 287, 789
leflunomide, 747t

Leishmania, 526*t*
leishmaniasis, 526*t*
lemon balm, 667*t*, 669*t*
Lente Iletin II. *See* insulin zinc suspension
Lente L. *See* insulin zinc suspension
lepirudin, 382, 382*t*
leprosy, 485*t*, 508
Lescol. *See* fluvastatin
letrozole, 568*t*, 569
leucovorin, 562*t*, 567*t*
leukemia, 553*t*, 789
Leukeran. *See* chlorambucil
Leukine. *See* sargramostim
leukopoiesis, 398
LEUKOTRIENE MODIFIERS:
  adverse effects, 601*t*
  drugs classified as
    montelukast, 601*t*, 603, 800
    zafirlukast. *See* **zafirlukast**
    zileuton, 601*t*, 603
  nursing considerations, 604–5
    client teaching, 604–5
    lifespan considerations, 604
  pharmacotherapy with, 603–4
leukotrienes, 472*t*, 603, 789
leuprolide:
  for cancer chemotherapy, 568*t*, 569
  for female infertility, 714*t*, 715
Leustatin. *See* cladribine
levalbuterol, 597, 597*t*
levamisole, 461*t*, 462, 571*t*
Levaquin. *See* levofloxacin
Levarterenol. *See* **norepinephrine**
Levate. *See* amitriptyline
Levemir. *See* insulin detemir
Levitra. *See* vardenafil
levobunolol, 773, 774*t*
levobupivacaine, 248*t*
levodopa, 265*t*
  actions and uses, 265*t*
  administration alerts, 265*t*
  adverse effects, 263*t*, 265*t*
  interactions, 113*t*, 265*t*
  mechanisms of action, 264*f*
  nursing considerations, 264–65
  nursing process focus, 266–67*t*
  overdose treatment, 265*t*
  pharmacokinetics, 265*t*
  route and adult dose, 263*t*
Levo-Dromoran. *See* levorphanol tartrate
levofloxacin, 499*t*, 800
levonorgestrel:
  for emergency contraception, 704, 704*t*
  implants, 700
  in oral contraceptives, 700, 700*t*
Levophed. *See* **norepinephrine**
levorphanol tartrate, 227*t*
Levothroid. *See* **levothyroxine**
levothyroxine, 669*t*
  actions and uses, 669*t*
  administration alerts, 669*t*
  adverse effects, 668*t*, 669*t*
  interactions, 669*t*

overdose treatment, 669*t*
  pharmacokinetics, 669*t*
  prescription ranking, 800, 802
  route and adult dose, 668*t*
Levoxyl. *See* **levothyroxine**
lewisite mixture, 24*t*
Lexapro. *See* **escitalopram oxalate**
Lexiva. *See* fosamprenavir
LH. *See* luteinizing hormone
libido, 719, 789
Librium. *See* chlordiazepoxide
lice:
  characteristics, 756–57, 756*f*
  pharmacotherapy. *See* PEDICULICIDES
  psychosocial and community impact,
    758*t*
licorice, 430*t*, 477*t*
Lidex. *See* fluocinonide
Lidex-E. *See* fluocinonide
lidocaine, 249*t*
  actions and uses, 249*t*
  administration alerts, 249*t*
  adverse effects, 248*t*, 249*t*, 367*t*
  Canadian/U.S. trade names, 798
  chemical structure, 248*f*
  interactions, 249*t*
  overdose treatment, 249*t*
  pharmacokinetics, 249*t*
  for specific conditions
    dysrhythmias, 366*t*, 367*t*
    as local anesthetic, 248*t*, 760
limbic system, 155, 155*f*, 789
Lincocin. *See* lincomycin
lincomycin, 503*t*
lindane, 757*t*
  actions and uses, 757*t*
  administration alerts, 757*t*
  adverse effects, 757*t*
  interactions, 757*t*
  nursing process focus, 757*t*
  overdose treatment, 757*t*
  pharmacokinetics, 757*t*
  pharmacotherapy with, 757
linezolid, 503*t*, 505
Lioresal. *See* baclofen
liothyronine, 668*t*
liotrix, 668*t*
lipid solubility, 49
lipids, 287, 288*f*. *See also* cholesterol
lipid-soluble vitamins. *See* vitamin(s),
  lipid-soluble
Lipitor. *See* **atorvastatin**
lipodystrophy, 537, 789
lipoproteins, 289, 289*f*, 789. *See also*
  cholesterol
liposomes, 564*t*, 789
liquids, administration guidelines,
  32–33, 33*t*
Liquifilm. *See* polyvinyl alcohol
lisinopril, 334*t*
  actions and uses, 334*t*
  administration alerts, 334*t*
  adverse effects, 316*t*, 333*t*, 334*t*

interactions, 334*t*
  overdose treatment, 334*t*
  pharmacokinetics, 334*t*
  prescription ranking, 800
  for specific conditions
    heart failure, 333*t*
    hypertension, 316*t*
    myocardial infarction, 358
literacy, healthcare and, 103–4
lithium, 200*t*
  actions and uses, 200*t*
  administration alerts, 200*t*
  adverse effects, 79*t*, 200*t*
  for bipolar disorder, 200–201, 200*t*
  Canadian/U.S. trade names, 798
  interactions, 200*t*
  nursing considerations, 202
    client teaching, 202
    lifespan considerations, 202
  nursing process focus, 201–2*t*
  overdose treatment, 200*t*
  pharmacokinetics, 200*t*
Lithizine. *See* **lithium**
10% LMD. *See* **dextran 40**
LMWHs. *See* LOW-MOLECULAR-WEIGHT
  HEPARINS
loading dose, 53–54, 53*f*, 789
local anesthesia, 245, 789
LOCAL ANESTHETICS:
  administration techniques, 245,
    246*f*, 246*t*
  adverse effects, 248, 248*t*
  classification, 246–48
  drugs classified as
    amides
      articaine, 248*t*
      bupivacaine, 248*t*
      chemical structure, 246, 248*f*
      dibucaine, 248*t*
      etidocaine, 248*t*
      levobupivacaine, 248*t*
      lidocaine. *See* **lidocaine**
      mepivacaine, 248*t*
      prilocaine, 248*t*
      ropivacaine, 248*t*
    dyclonine, 248*t*
    esters
      benzocaine. *See* **benzocaine**
      chemical structure, 246, 248*f*
      chloroprocaine, 248*t*
      procaine, 247, 248*f*, 248*t*
      tetracaine, 248*t*
    pramoxine, 248*t*
  mechanisms of action, 245–46, 247*f*
  nursing considerations, 248, 249
    client teaching, 249
    nursing process focus, 250*t*
Locoid. *See* **hydrocortisone**
Lodine. *See* etodolac
Loestrin 1.5/30 Fe, 700*t*
lomefloxacin, 499*t*
Lomotil. *See* **diphenoxylate with atropine**
lomustine, 559*t*

long-term insomnia, 157, 790
Loniten. *See* minoxidil
LOOP DIURETICS:
    adverse effects, 308, 310*t*, 333*t*, 428*t*
    drugs classified as
        bumetanide. *See* bumetanide
        ethacrynic acid, 428*t*
        furosemide. *See* **furosemide**
        torsemide. *See* torsemide
    mechanisms of action, 427, 427*f*
    for specific conditions
        heart failure
            nursing considerations, 335–36
            route and adult doses, 333*t*
            therapeutic approach, 335
        hypertension
            nursing considerations, 310
            route and adult doses, 310*t*
            therapeutic approach, 308
        renal failure
            nursing considerations, 428–29
            route and adult dose, 428*t*
            therapeutic approach, 428
Lo/Ovral, 700*t*
loperamide, 628*t*
Lopid. *See* **gemfibrozil**
lopinavir/ritonavir, 537*t*
Lopressor, 309*t*. *See also* **metoprolol**
Loprox. *See* ciclopirox olamine
Lopurin. *See* allopurinol
Lorabid. *See* loracarbef
loracarbef, 492*t*
loratadine, 581*t*
lorazepam, 163*t*
    actions and uses, 163*t*
    administration alerts, 163*t*
    adverse effects, 162*t*, 163*t*
    Canadian/U.S. trade names, 798
    interactions, 163*t*
    overdose treatment, 163*t*
    pharmacokinetics, 163*t*
    prescription ranking, 800
    for specific conditions
        anxiety, 162*t*
        as general anesthesia adjunct, 255*t*
        nausea and vomiting, 634*t*
        seizures, 173*t*, 175*t*, 177
        as skeletal muscle relaxant, 276*t*
losartan, 316*t*, 800
losartan/hydrochlorothiazide, 309*t*, 801
Losec. *See* **omeprazole**
Lotensin, 309*t*. *See also* benazepril
Lotrel. *See* amlodipine/benazepril
Lotrisone. *See* clotrimazole
lovastatin, 30*t*, 292*t*, 800
Lovenox. *See* enoxaparin
low-density lipoprotein (LDL):
    characteristics, 289, 289*f*, 790
    laboratory values, 290*t*
    ratio to HDL, 290
    subclasses, 290
lower gastrointestinal tract:
    anatomy, 612*f*, 625*f*

disorders
    constipation, 625. *See also* LAXATIVES
    diarrhea, 628. *See also* ANTIDIARRHEALS
    incidence, 624*t*
    normal function, 624, 625*f*
lower respiratory tract, 594–95, 594*f*
LOW-MOLECULAR-WEIGHT
    HEPARINS (LMWHs):
    adverse effects, 382*t*
    characteristics, 381–82, 790
    drugs classified as
        ardeparin, 382*t*
        dalteparin, 382*t*
        danaparoid, 382*t*
        enoxaparin, 358, 382*t*, 383
        tinzaparin, 382*t*
    mechanisms of action, 381–82
    nursing considerations, 382–84
        client teaching, 384
        lifespan considerations, 383
    route and adult dose, 382*t*
    for specific conditions
        myocardial infarction, 358
        thromboembolic disease, 381–82, 382*t*
Loxapac. *See* loxapine succinate
loxapine succinate, 215*t*, 798
Loxitane. *See* loxapine succinate
Lozide. *See* indapamide
Lozol. *See* indapamide
LSD, 123–24, 123*f*
L-tryptophan, 193*t*
lubiprostone, 626*t*, 627
LUBRICANTS, OPHTHALMIC:
    lanolin alcohol, 779*t*
    methylcellulose, 779*t*
    polyvinyl alcohol, 779*t*
Ludiomil. *See* maprotiline
Lugol's solution, 653, 668*t*, 672
Lumigan. *See* bimatoprost
Luminal. *See* **phenobarbital**
Lunelle, 700. *See also*
    medroxyprogesterone acetate
Lunesta. *See* eszopiclone
Lupron. *See* leuprolide
Lupron Depot. *See* leuprolide
luteinizing hormone (LH), 69*f*, 663*f*,
    697, 718, 789
Lutrepulse. *See* gonadorelin
Luvox. *See* fluvoxamine
Lyme disease, 485*t*
lymphatic system, 455
lymphocyte, 455
lymphocyte immune globulin, 465*t*
lymphoma, 553*t*, 790
lypressin, 664*t*, 666
Lysodren. *See* mitotane

M

ma huang, drug interactions:
    digoxin, 339*t*
    lorazepam, 163*t*
    oxytocin, 712*t*
    phenelzine, 196*t*

Maalox. *See* magnesium hydroxide and
    aluminum hydroxide
Maalox Plus. *See* magnesium hydroxide
    and aluminum hydroxide with
    simethicone
MAC (*Mycobacterium avium complex*), 508
Macrobid. *See* nitrofurantoin
macrocytic anemia, 401, 401*t*
Macrodantin. *See* nitrofurantoin
Macrodex. *See* dextran 70
MACROLIDES:
    adverse effects, 496, 496*t*
    drugs classified as
        azithromycin, 496, 496*t*, 508, 800, 801
        clarithromycin, 496*t*, 508, 620
        dirithromycin, 496*t*
        erythromycin. *See* **erythromycin**
        troleandomycin, 496*t*
    for *H. pylori*, 620
    nursing considerations, 496–97
        client teaching, 497
    pharmacotherapy with, 496
    route and adult doses, 496*t*
MACROMINERALS:
    calcium. *See* calcium
    characteristics, 651, 790
    chloride, 442*t*, 651*t*
    functions, 651*t*
    magnesium. *See* magnesium
    nursing considerations, 652–53
        client teaching, 653
    pharmacotherapy with, 650*t*, 651–52
    phosphorus. *See* phosphorus/phosphate
    potassium. *See* potassium
    recommended dietary allowances, 651*t*
    sodium. *See* sodium
    sulfur, 651*t*
magaldrate, 619*t*
magnesium:
    for dysrhythmias, 374*t*
    functions, 651, 651*t*
    imbalances, 442*t*, 651. *See also* hypermag-
        nesemia; hypomagnesemia
    pharmacotherapy with
        magnesium chloride, 650*t*
        magnesium hydroxide, 619*t*, 626*t*
        magnesium hydroxide and aluminum
            hydroxide, 619*t*
        magnesium hydroxide and aluminum
            hydroxide with simethicone, 619*t*
        magnesium oxide, 650*t*
        magnesium sulfate. *See* **magnesium**
            sulfate
    recommended dietary allowance, 651*t*
magnesium chloride, 650*t*
magnesium hydroxide, 619*t*, 626*t*
magnesium hydroxide and aluminum
    hydroxide, 619*t*
magnesium hydroxide and aluminum
    hydroxide with simethicone, 619*t*
magnesium oxide, 650*t*
magnesium sulfate, 652*t*
    actions and uses, 652, 652*t*

magnesium sulfate (*continued*)
administration alerts, 652*t*
adverse effects, 650*t*, 652*t*, 711*t*
interactions, 652*t*
nursing considerations, 652–53
client teaching, 653
overdose treatment, 652*t*
pharmacokinetics, 652*t*
route and adult dose, 650*t*, 711*t*
as tocolytic, 711*t*
Mag-Ox. *See* magnesium oxide
maintenance dose, 54, 790
malaria:
characteristics, 790
incidence, 514, 524
pathophysiology, 524, 524*f*
pharmacotherapy. *See* ANTIMALARIALS
prevention, 524
Malarone. *See* atovaquone and proguanil
malathion, 757
male infertility, 721
male reproductive function:
disorders
anticholinergics and, 147*t*
erectile dysfunction. *See* erectile
dysfunction
hypogonadism. *See* hypogonadism
incidence, 718*t*
infertility, 721
hypothalamic and pituitary regulation,
718, 719*f*
malignant, 790
malignant hyperthermia, 478
malignant tumor, 553*t*
Malogen. *See* **testosterone**
Malogex. *See* testosterone enanthate
Mandelamine. *See* methenamine
mandrake, 565
manganese, 653*t*
mania, 199, 790. *See also* bipolar disorder
manic depression. *See* bipolar disorder
mannitol, 433, 433*t*, 774*t*, 776
manual healing, 109*t*
MAO (monoamine oxidase), 134, 790
MAOIs. *See* MONOAMINE OXIDASE
INHIBITORS
Maolate. *See* chlorphenesin
Maox. *See* magnesium oxide
maprotiline, 188, 189*t*
MAR (medication administration record),
93, 790
Marcaine. *See* bupivacaine
Marezine. *See* cyclizine hydrochloride
marijuana:
dependency characteristics, 120*t*
effects, 122–23
fetal effects, 80*t*
toxicity signs, 120*t*
withdrawal symptoms, 120*t*, 123
Marinol. *See* dronabinol
Marplan. *See* isocarboxazid
Marzine. *See* cyclizine hydrochloride
masculinization, 719

MAST CELL STABILIZERS:
adverse effects, 601*t*
drugs classified as
cromolyn, 586, 601*t*, 605
nedocromil sodium, 601*t*, 605
pharmacotherapy with, 605
mast cells, 472, 790
mastoiditis, 779–80, 790
Material Medica, 3
mature acne, 761
maturity-onset diabetes. *See* diabetes
mellitus, type 2
Maxair. *See* pirbuterol acetate
Maxalt. *See* rizatriptan
Maxaquin. *See* lomefloxacin
Maxeran. *See* metoclopramide
Maxidex. *See* dexamethasone
Maxiflor. *See* diflorasone
Maxipime. *See* cefepime
May apple, 565
Mazepine. *See* carbamazepine
MCT Oil, 655
MDA, 124
MDI (metered dose inhaler),
595, 595*f*, 790
MDMA, 124
measles, mumps, and rubella vaccine, 460*t*
measurement systems, 31–32, 31*t*
Mebaral. *See* mephobarbital
mebendazole, 529*t*
actions and uses, 529*t*
administration alerts uses, 529*t*
adverse effects, 528*t*, 529*t*
interactions, 529*t*
pharmacokinetics, 529*t*
route and adult dose, 528*t*
mechanism of action, 12, 790
mechlorethamine, 559*t*
meclizine, 633, 634*t*, 798, 801
median effective dose (ED$_{50}$), 58, 58*f*, 790
median lethal dose (LD$_{50}$), 58, 58*f*, 790
median toxicity dose (TD$_{50}$), 58–59, 790
medication, 4, 790
medication administration record
(MAR), 93, 790
medication error index, 90, 91*f*, 790
medication errors:
categories, 94, 95*f*
in children, 95*t*
definition, 80, 790
factors contributing to, 90–92
in the home, 92, 93*t*
impact, 93
OTC drugs and, 96*t*
reporting and documenting
documenting in client's medical
record, 93
reporting to national databases, 93
writing an incident report, 93–94
strategies for reducing
case studies, 191*t*, 299*t*, 374*t*, 386*t*,
468*t*, 496*t*, 587*t*, 662*t*, 745*t*

client education, 95, 95*t*
in healthcare facilities, 96
nursing process in, 94–95
supplements and, 96*t*
tracking, 96
Medihaler-Iso. *See* isoproterenol
Medilium. *See* chlordiazepoxide
MEDMARX, 96
Medrol. *See* methylprednisolone
medroxyprogesterone acetate, 710*t*.
See also **conjugated estrogens with
medroxyprogesterone**
actions and uses, 710*t*
administration alerts, 710*t*
adverse effects, 568*t*, 709*t*, 710*t*
interactions, 710*t*
pharmacokinetics, 710*t*
for specific conditions
cancer, 568*t*, 709
dysfunctional uterine bleeding, 709, 709*t*
injection for contraception, 700
mefenamic acid, 233*t*
mefloquine, 523*t*
Mefoxin. *See* cefoxitin
Megace. *See* megestrol
Megacillin. *See* **penicillin G potassium**
megaloblastic (pernicious) anemia,
402, 647, 792
megestrol, 568*t*, 569
MEGLITINIDES:
adverse effects, 690*t*
characteristics, 690
drugs classified as
nateglinide, 690*t*
repaglinide, 690*t*
route and adult doses, 690*t*
melanin, 753
melanocytes, 753
melatonin, 157*t*
Melissa officinalis. See lemon balm
Mellaril. *See* thioridazine
meloxicam, 233*t*, 473*t*, 801
melphalan, 559*t*
memantine, 269–70, 270*f*
memory B cells, 456
meningitis, 485*t*
menopause:
definition, 705, 790
estrogen loss in, 705*t*
hormone replacement therapy in. *See*
hormone replacement therapy
natural therapy with black cohosh, 706*t*
menorrhagia, 709, 790
menotropin, 714, 715*t*, 721
Mentax. *See* butenafine
meperidine, 194, 227*t*, 358, 638
mephentermine, 414*t*
mephenytoin hydroxylase, 104, 104*t*
mephobarbital, 164*t*, 174
mepivacaine, 248*t*
meprobamate, 165*t*
mercaptopurine, 555*f*, 561*t*
Meridia. *See* **sibutramine**

meropenem, 503, 506
merozoites, 524, 524f
Merrem IV. *See* meropenem
mesalazine, 630
mesoridazine, 212t, 214
Mestinon. *See* pyridostigmine
metabolic acidosis, 426t, 447t. *See also*
    acidosis
metabolism:
  alcohol, 122
  definition, 790
  drug
    factors affecting, 50
    mechanism, 48f, 50–51
    in older adults, 86
    in pregnancy, 77
Metaglip. *See* glipizide/metformin
Metahydrin. *See* trichlormethiazide
Metamucil. *See* **psyllium mucilloid**
Metandren. *See* methyltestosterone
Metaprel. *See* metaproterenol
metaproterenol, 137t, 597, 597t
metaraminol, 137t
metastasis, 552, 552f, 790
metaxalone, 276t, 801
metered dose inhaler (MDI), 595, 595f, 790
metformin, 689, 690t, 800, 801
methacycline, 494t
methadone:
  for opioid dependence, 121, 232
  for pain management, 227t
methadone maintenance, 232, 790
methamphetamine, 124–25, 203, 204t, 588t
methazolamide, 433t, 774t
methenamine, 503t
Methergine. *See* methylergonovine maleate
methicillin-resistant *S. aureus* (MRSA), 506
methimazole, 668t, 670
methocarbamol, 276t
methohexital sodium, 255t
methotrexate, 562t
  actions and uses, 562t
  administration alerts, 562t
  adverse effects, 562t, 747t
  interactions, 113t, 562t
  mechanisms of action, 555f
  overdose treatment, 562t
  pharmacokinetics, 562t
  prescription ranking, 801
  for specific conditions
    cancer chemotherapy, 561, 562t
    immunosuppression, 465t
    inflammatory bowel disease, 630
    psoriasis, 767t, 768
    rheumatoid arthritis, 746, 747t
  structure, 562f
methotrexate with misoprostol, 704t, 705
methoxyflurane, 252t
methsuximide, 180t
Methulose. *See* methylcellulose
methyclothiazide, 429t
methyl sulfonyl methane (MSM), 114t
methylcellulose, 626t, 779t

methyldopa, 137t, 321t, 798
methylergonovine maleate, 711t
methylparaben, 248
methylphenidate, 205t
  abuse, 125, 203
  actions and uses, 205t
  for ADHD, 203–4
  administration alerts, 205t
  adverse effects, 205t
  interactions, 205t
  mechanisms of action, 125
  nursing considerations, 204
    client teaching, 205
  nursing process focus, 205–6t
  overdose treatment, 205t
  pharmacokinetics, 205t
  prescription ranking, 801
  zero tolerance policies and, 204t
methylprednisolone:
  for adrenocortical insufficiency, 675t
  adverse effects, 476t
  as antiemetic, 633, 634t
  prescription ranking, 800
  for severe inflammation, 476t
methyltestosterone, 720t, 798
METHYLXANTHINES:
  aminophylline, 597t, 600, 797
  characteristics, 600, 790
  nursing considerations, 600–601
    client teaching, 600–601
  pharmacotherapy with, 600
  theophylline, 113t, 597t, 600, 799
methysergide, 238t
Meticorten. *See* **prednisone**
metipranolol, 773, 774t
metoclopramide, 634t, 798, 801
metolazone, 310t, 429t
metoprolol, 337t
  actions and uses, 140t, 337t
  administration alerts, 337t
  adverse effects, 333t, 337t, 350t
  Canadian/U.S. trade names, 798
  genetic polymorphisms affecting
    metabolism, 104t
  interactions, 337t
  overdose treatment, 337t
  pharmacokinetics, 337t
  prescription ranking, 800
  for specific conditions
    angina and myocardial infarction, 350t
    heart failure, 333t
    hypertension, 321t
    migraine, 238t
metric system of measurement, 31, 31t, 790
Metrodin. *See* urofollitropin
metronidazole, 527t
  actions and uses, 527t
  administration alerts, 527t
  adverse effects, 527t
  as antibacterial, 505
  interactions, 527t
  pharmacokinetics, 527t
  prescription ranking, 801

  for specific conditions
    H. pylori, 620
    protozoal infections, 726
    rosacea, 764
metyrapone, 678
Mevacor. *See* lovastatin
Mexate. *See* **methotrexate**
mexiletine, 367t
Mexitil. *See* mexiletine
MI. *See* myocardial infarction
Miacalcin. *See* calcitonin–salmon
mibefradil, 30t
micafungin, 516t
Micardis. *See* telmisartan
Micatin. *See* miconazole
miconazole, 519t, 521, 756
MICRhoGAM. *See* Rho(D) immune
    globulin
microcytic anemia, 401, 401t
Micro-K. *See* **potassium chloride**
Microlipid, 655
MICROMINERALS:
  chromium, 653t
  cobalt, 653t
  copper, 653t
  definition, 790
  fluorine, 653t
  functions, 653t
  iodine, 653, 653t, 666
  iron, 403–4, 653, 653t. *See also* IRON SALTS
  manganese, 653t
  molybdenum, 653t
  recommended dietary allowances, 653t
  selenium, 554t, 653t
  zinc, 653t
    zinc acetate, 650t
    zinc gluconate, 650t
    zinc sulfate, 650t
Micronase. *See* glyburide
Micronor. *See* norethindrone
Microsporum audouini, 515t
Microsulfon. *See* sulfadiazine
microvilli, 611
Midamor. *See* amiloride
midazolam, 30t, 161, 255t
middle adulthood, 84–85, 790
Mifeprex. *See* mifepristone
mifepristone, 704t, 705, 711
miglitol, 690t
migraine:
  definition, 237, 790
  incidence, 237t
  natural therapy with feverfew, 241t
  pharmacotherapy. *See* ANTIMIGRAINE DRUGS
  prophylaxis
    beta-adrenergic blockers, 238t
    calcium channel blockers, 238t
    methysergide, 238t
    riboflavin, 238t
    tricyclic antidepressants, 238t
    valproic acid, 238t
Milk of Magnesia. *See* magnesium
    hydroxide

milk thistle, 110*t*, 122*t*, 251*t*
milrinone, 341*t*
  actions and uses, 341*t*
  administration alerts, 341*t*
  adverse effects, 333*t*, 341*t*
  interactions, 341*t*
  overdose treatment, 341*t*
  pharmacokinetics, 341*t*
  route and adult dose, 333*t*
mind–body interventions, 109*t*
mineral oil, 626*t*, 627
mineralocorticoids, 673
minerals:
  macrominerals. *See* MACROMINERALS
  microminerals. *See* MICROMINERALS
minimum effective concentration,
    53, 53*f*, 790
minipills, 699
Minipress. *See* **prazosin**
Minizide, 309*t*
Minocin. *See* minocycline
minocycline, 494, 494*t*, 801
minoxidil, 324*t*, 325
Miocarpine. *See* pilocarpine
miosis, 779, 790
Miostat. *See* carbachol
MIOTICS:
  carbachol, 774*t*
  demecarium, 774*t*
  physostigmine, 774*t*
  pilocarpine, 774*t*, 775
Miradon. *See* anisindione
MiraLax. *See* polyethylene glycol
Mirapex. *See* pramipexole
Mirena, 700. *See also* levonorgestrel
mirtazapine, 188, 189*t*, 801
misoprostol, 621, 704*t*, 705, 711*t*
Mithracin. *See* plicamycin
Mithramycin. *See* plicamycin
mitomycin, 564*t*
mitotane, 571, 571*t*
mitoxantrone, 564*t*
Mitrolan. *See* calcium polycarbophil
Mivacron. *See* mivacurium
mivacurium, 257
MMR II. *See* measles, mumps, and rubella
    vaccine
Moban. *See* molindone
Mobenol. *See* tolbutamide
Mobic. *See* meloxicam
modular formulas, 655
Moduretic, 309*t*
moexipril, 316*t*
molindone, 215*t*
molybdenum, 653*t*
mometasone, 585*t*, 765*t*, 800
Monistat. *See* miconazole
Monitan. *See* acebutolol
monoamine oxidase (MAO), 134, 790
MONOAMINE OXIDASE INHIBITORS (MAOIs):
  adverse effects, 159*t*, 160, 189*t*, 190, 194
  drugs classified as
    isocarboxazid, 189*t*

phenelzine. *See* **phenelzine**
    tranylcypromine, 159*t*, 189*t*
  interactions, 160, 194, 195*t*
  mechanisms of action, 194, 195*f*, 790
  nursing considerations, 195–96
    client teaching, 196
  nursing process focus, 197–99*t*
  for specific conditions
    depression, 189*t*, 194
    panic disorders, 159*t*
monobasic potassium and sodium
    phosphates, 650*t*
monobasic potassium phosphate, 650*t*
Monocid. *See* cefonicid
MONOCLONAL ANTIBODIES (MABs):
  adverse effects, 465*t*, 478
  for autoimmune disorders, 468
  drugs classified as
    adalimumab, 465*t*, 746
    alemtuzumab, 570, 571*t*
    basiliximab, 465*t*, 468
    bevacizumab, 571, 571*t*
    cetuximab, 571, 571*t*
    daclizumab, 465*t*, 468
    gemtuzumab ozogamicin, 571*t*
    ibritumomab tiuxetan, 571*t*
    infliximab. *See* infliximab
    lymphocyte immune globulin, 465*t*
    muromonab-CD3, 465*t*, 468
    rituximab, 571*t*
    tositumomab, 571*t*
    trastuzumab, 570, 571*t*
  mechanisms of action, 466
  for specific conditions
    cancer chemotherapy, 570, 571*t*
    immunosuppression, 465*t*, 466–68
Monodox. *See* doxycycline
Monoket. *See* isosorbide mononitrate
Monopril. *See* fosinopril
monosodium glutamate (MSG), 237
montelukast, 601*t*, 603, 800
Monurol. *See* fosfomycin
mood disorder, 186, 790. *See also* bipolar
    disorder; depression
mood stabilizers, 199, 790. *See also* **lithium**
morning sickness, 632
morphine sulfate, 228*t*
  actions and uses, 228*t*
  administration alerts, 228*t*
  adverse effects, 227*t*, 228*t*
  Canadian/U.S. trade names, 798
  genetic polymorphisms affecting
    metabolism, 104*t*
  interactions, 228*t*
  in myocardial infarction, 358
  overdose treatment, 228*t*
  pharmacokinetics, 228*t*
  route and adult dose, 227*t*
motion sickness, 624*t*, 633
Motofen. *See* difenoxin with atropine
Motrin. *See* ibuprofen
moxifloxacin, 499, 499*t*
MSG (monosodium glutamate), 237

MSM (methyl sulfonyl methane), 114*t*
mu receptors, 226, 226*f*, 226*t*, 790
MUCOLYTICS:
  acetylcysteine, 589*t*, 591
  characteristics, 591, 790
  dornase alfa, 591
  pharmacotherapy with, 591, 606
Mucomyst. *See* acetylcysteine
Mucorales, 515*t*
mucormycosis, 515*t*
mucosa layer, 611, 790
mucositis, 556, 790
mucous colitis, 630
multiple sclerosis, 261*t*
mupirocin, 756
Murine Plus. *See* tetrahydrozoline
muromonab-CD3, 465*t*, 468
muscarinic antagonists. *See*
    ANTICHOLINERGICS
muscarinic receptors, 135–36, 135*t*, 790
muscle relaxants. *See* SKELETAL MUSCLE
    RELAXANTS
muscle spasms:
  causes, 275
  definition, 275, 790
  home care considerations, 281*t*
  incidence, 275*t*
  natural therapy with cayenne, 277*t*
  nonpharmacological treatment, 275
  pharmacotherapy. *See also* SKELETAL
    MUSCLE RELAXANTS
    nursing process focus, 280*t*
    therapeutic approach, 275–76, 276*t*
Mustargen. *See* mechlorethamine
Mutamycin. *See* mitomycin
mutations, 487, 790
myasthenia gravis:
  characteristics, 143, 790
  cholinergic agents for, 143
  nitrous oxide use in, 251
  nursing considerations, 146
Mycamine. *See* micafungin
Mycelex. *See* clotrimazole
Mycifradin. *See* neomycin
Myciguent. *See* neomycin cream/ointment
Myclo-Gyne. *See* clotrimazole
Mycobacterium avium complex (MAC), 508
Mycobacterium leprae, 485*t*, 508
Mycobacterium tuberculosis, 485*t*, 506. *See*
    also tuberculosis
mycophenolate mofetil, 465*t*
Mycoplasma pneumoniae, 485*t*
mycoses:
  community-acquired, 514
  definition, 515, 790
  incidence, 514*t*
  natural therapy with tea tree oil, 529*t*
  opportunistic, 514
  pathogens, 515*t*
  pharmacotherapy. *See* ANTIFUNGALS
  superficial, 515, 515*t*, 794
  systemic, 515, 515*t*, 794
Mycostatin. *See* **nystatin**

Mydfrin. *See* **phenylephrine**
Mydriacyl. *See* tropicamide
MYDRIATICS:
  characteristics, 778, 790
  hydroxyamphetamine, 779*t*
  phenylephrine, 779, 779*t*
Mykrox. *See* metolazone
Mylanta. *See* magnesium hydroxide and aluminum hydroxide with simethicone
Mylanta AP. *See* famotidine
Mylanta Gas. *See* simethicone
Mylanta Gel-caps. *See* calcium carbonate with magnesium hydroxide
Myleran. *See* busulfan
Mylotarg. *See* gemtuzumab ozogamicin
myocardial infarction (MI):
  definition, 355, 790
  diagnosis, 355, 355*t*
  incidence, 347*t*
  natural therapy with ginseng, 358*t*
  pathophysiology, 355, 356*f*
  pharmacotherapy
    goals, 355
    for symptoms and complications
      ACE inhibitors, 358
      anticoagulants, 358
      antiplatelets, 358
      beta-adrenergic antagonists, 358
      nitrates, 358
    thrombolytics. *See* THROMBOLYTICS
myocardial ischemia, 346, 358*t*, 790
Myochrysine. *See* gold sodium thiomalate
myoclonic seizure, 172*t*, 173*t*, 176, 790
myoglobin, 355*t*
Myolin. *See* orphenadrine
Mysoline. *See* primidone
Mytelase. *See* ambenonium
myxedema, 664*t*, 667, 790

N
Na⁺. *See* sodium
nabilone, 633, 634*t*
nabumetone, 233*t*, 473*t*, 801
N-acetylcysteine, 479*t*, 589*t*
NaCl. *See* **sodium chloride**
nadir, 557
nadolol, 140*t*
Nadostine. *See* **nystatin**
nafarelin, 714*t*
Nafcil. *See* nafcillin
nafcillin, 489*t*
Nafrine. *See* **oxymetazoline**
naftifine, 520*t*
Naftin. *See* naftifine
NaHCO₃. *See* **sodium bicarbonate**
nalbuphine hydrochloride, 227*t*
Nalfon. *See* fenoprofen
nalidixic acid, 499, 499*t*
nalmefene hydrochloride, 227*t*
naloxone hydrochloride, 231*t*
  actions and uses, 226, 231, 231*t*
  administration alerts, 231*t*
  adverse effects, 227*t*, 231*t*

interactions, 231*t*
  overdose treatment, 231*t*
  pharmacokinetics, 231*t*
  route and adult dose, 227*t*
naltrexone hydrochloride, 227*t*, 232
Namenda. *See* memantine
NANDA (North American Nursing Diagnosis Association), 67
nandrolone phenpropionate, 720*t*
Napamide. *See* disopyramide phosphate
naphazoline HCl, 587*t*, 779, 779*t*
Naprelan. *See* naproxen
Naprosyn. *See* naproxen
naproxen, 233*t*, 473*t*, 798, 800
naproxen sodium, 233*t*, 473*t*
Naqua. *See* trichlormethiazide
naratriptan, 238*t*
Narcan. *See* **naloxone hydrochloride**
narcotic, 226, 790
narcotic analgesics. *See* OPIOID (NARCOTIC) ANALGESICS
Nardil. *See* **phenelzine**
Naropin. *See* ropivacaine
narrow-spectrum antibiotics, 487, 790. *See also* ANTIBACTERIALS
narrow-spectrum penicillins, 489*t*. *See also* PENICILLINS
Nasacort AQ. *See* triamcinolone
nasal drug administration, 36*t*, 37, 38*f*
Nasalcrom. *See* intranasal cromolyn
Nasalide. *See* flunisolide
Nasarel. *See* flunisolide
nasogastric (NG) tube, 33*t*, 34
Nasonex. *See* mometasone
nateglinide, 690*t*
National Coordinating Council for Medication Error Reporting and Prevention (NCC MERP), 93, 95*f*
National Formulary (NF), 5, 6*f*
Native Americans:
  mental illness treatment, 212*t*
  pain management, 225*t*
Natrecor. *See* nesiritide
Natulan. *See* procarbazine
Naturacil. *See* **psyllium mucilloid**
Natural Therapies. *See also* herbal therapies; *specific substances*
  acidophilus for diarrhea, 629*t*
  for anxiety, 157*t*
  bilberry for eye health, 779*t*
  black cohosh for menopausal symptoms, 706*t*
  burdock root for acne and eczema, 765*t*
  cayenne for muscular tension, 277*t*
  chocolate for hypertension, 308*t*
  chondroitin for osteoarthritis, 746*t*
  cloves and anise as dental remedies, 247*t*
  coenzyme Q10, 295*t*
  cranberry for urinary tract infections, 433*t*
  echinacea for immune system enhancement, 462*t*
  feverfew for migraine, 241*t*

fish oils
    for chronic obstructive pulmonary disease, 606*t*
    for inflammation, 476*t*
  garlic
    for cardiovascular health, 380*t*
    for dementia, 263*t*
  ginger for gastrointestinal disorders, 621*t*
  ginkgo for dementia, 263*t*
  ginseng for myocardial ischemia, 358*t*
  glucosamine for osteoarthritis, 746*t*
  goldenseal, antibacterial properties, 509*t*
  grape seed extract for hypertension, 308*t*
  hawthorn for heart failure, 342*t*
  for HIV-AIDS, 548*t*
  for insomnia, 157*t*
  kava for anxiety and insomnia, 157*t*
  ketogenic diet for seizures, 173*t*
  magnesium for dysrhythmias, 374*t*
  medication errors and, 96*t*
  melatonin for insomnia, 157*t*
  milk thistle for alcohol liver damage, 122*t*
  saw palmetto for benign prostatic hyperplasia, 728*t*
  sea vegetables for acidosis, 447*t*
  selenium for cancer prevention, 554*t*
  St. John's wort for depression, 193*t*
  stevia for hyperglycemia, 691*t*
  tea tree oil for fungal infections, 529*t*
  thyroid disease treatments, 667*t*
  valerian for anxiety and insomnia, 157*t*
  vitamin C and the common cold, 647*t*
Naturetin. *See* bendroflumethiazide
nausea, 632, 790. *See also* nausea and vomiting
nausea and vomiting:
  pathophysiology, 632–33
  pharmacotherapy. *See* ANTIEMETICS
Navane. *See* thiothixene
Naxen. *See* naproxen
NDA review, 8, 790
NE. *See* **norepinephrine**
Nebcin. *See* tobramycin
nebulizer, 595, 595*f*, 790
Nebupent. *See* pentamidine
nedocromil sodium, 601*t*, 605
nefazodone, 188, 189*t*
negative feedback, 662, 790
negative formulary list, 14
negative inotropic agents, 331
negative symptoms, 211, 790
NegGram. *See* nalidixic acid
Neisseria gonorrhoeae, 485*t*
Neisseria meningitidis, 485*t*
nelarabine, 561*t*
nelfinavir, 537*t*
Nembutal. *See* pentobarbital sodium
Neoloid. *See* castor oil
neomycin, 497, 498*t*
neomycin cream/ointment, 756
neomycin with polymyxin B cream/ointment, 756
neoplasm, 552, 791

Neoral. *See* cyclosporine
Neosar. *See* **cyclophosphamide**
Neosporin. *See* neomycin with polymyxin B cream/ointment
neostigmine, 143, 143*t*
Neo-Synephrine. *See* **oxymetazoline; phenylephrine**
nephron, 424, 425*f*, 791
Nephronex. *See* nitrofurantoin
nephrotoxic drugs, 426*t*
Neptazane. *See* methazolamide
nerve agents, 23, 24*t*, 791
nerve block anesthesia, 246*f*, 246*t*
Nesacaine. *See* chloroprocaine
nesiritide, 342
NesTrex. *See* vitamin B$_6$
netilmicin, 498*t*
Netromycin. *See* netilmicin
Neulasta. *See* pegfilgrastim
Neumega. *See* oprelvekin
Neupogen. *See* **filgrastim**
neural tube defects, 648*t*
neurofibrillary tangles, 267, 270*f*, 791
neurogenic shock, 410*t*, 412*t*, 791
neurohypophysis, 662, 791
NEUROKININ RECEPTOR ANTAGONIST:
    aprepitant, 633, 634*t*
neuroleptanalgesia, 255, 791
neuroleptic malignant syndrome, 213*t*, 214, 478, 791
neuroleptics, 212. *See also* ANTIPSYCHOTICS
NEUROMUSCULAR BLOCKERS:
    definition, 791
    as general anesthesia adjunct, 257
    nursing considerations, 258
        client teaching, 258
    succinylcholine. *See* **succinylcholine**
Neurontin. *See* gabapentin
neuropathic pain, 224, 791
Neutra-Phos. *See* potassium and sodium phosphates
Neutra-Phos-K. *See* potassium phosphate
Neutrexin. *See* trimetrexate
nevirapine, 539*t*
    actions and uses, 539*t*
    administration alerts, 539*t*
    adverse effects, 537*t*, 539*t*
    interactions, 539*t*
    lipid profile effects, 538
    pharmacokinetics, 539*t*
    route and adult dose, 537*t*
New Drug Application (NDA), 8
Nexavar. *See* sorafenib
Nexium. *See* esomeprazole
NF (*National Formulary*), 5, 6*f*
Niac. *See* vitamin B$_3$
niacin. *See* vitamin B$_3$
Niaspan. *See* vitamin B$_3$
Niazide. *See* trichlormethiazide
nicardipine, 313*t*, 324, 350*t*
Nicobid. *See* vitamin B$_3$
Nicolar. *See* vitamin B$_3$

nicotine:
    characteristics, 125
    dependency characteristics, 120*t*, 125
    effects, 125
    toxicity signs, 120*t*
    withdrawal symptoms, 120*t*
nicotinic acid. *See* vitamin B$_3$
nicotinic receptors, 135, 135*t*, 791
nifedipine, 314*t*
    actions and uses, 314*t*
    administration alerts, 314*t*
    adverse effects, 238*t*, 313*t*, 314*t*, 711*t*
    Canadian/U.S. trade names, 798
    interactions, 314*t*
    mechanisms of action, 314
    overdose treatment, 314*t*
    pharmacokinetics, 314*t*
    prescription ranking, 802
    for specific conditions
        angina and myocardial infarction, 350*t*
        hypertension, 313*t*
        migraine, 238*t*
        as tocolytic, 711*t*
NIG. *See* immune globulin
Nilandron. *See* nilutamide
Nilstat. *See* **nystatin**
nilutamide, 568*t*
nimodipine, 238*t*
Nimotop. *See* nimodipine
Nipent. *See* pentostatin
Nisocor. *See* nisoldipine
nisoldipine, 313*t*
Nitro-Bid. *See* **nitroglycerin**
Nitro-Dur. *See* **nitroglycerin**
nitrofurantoin, 503*t*, 798, 801
nitrogen mustard, 24*t*
NITROGEN MUSTARDS. *See also* ALKYLATING AGENTS
    chlorambucil, 559*t*
    cyclophosphamide. *See* **cyclophosphamide**
    estramustine, 559*t*
    ifosfamide, 559*t*
    mechlorethamine, 559*t*
    melphalan, 559*t*
nitroglycerin, 351*t*
    actions and uses, 351*t*
    administration alerts, 351*t*
    adverse effects, 350*t*, 351*t*
    interactions, 351*t*
    nursing process focus, 352*t*
    overdose treatment, 351*t*
    pharmacokinetics, 351*t*
    prescription ranking, 802
    route and adult dose, 350*t*
    in suspected myocardial infarction, 358
Nitropress. *See* nitroprusside
nitroprusside, 324, 324*t*, 325
NitroQuick. *See* **nitroglycerin**
NITROSOUREAS. *See also* ALKYLATING AGENTS
    carmustine, 557, 559*t*
    lomustine, 559*t*
    streptozocin, 559*t*

Nitrostat. *See* **nitroglycerin**
nitrous oxide, 251*t*
    actions and uses, 251*t*
    administration alerts, 251*t*
    adverse effects, 251*t*
    interactions, 251*t*
    overdose treatment, 251*t*
    pharmacokinetics, 251*t*
nits, 756, 791
Nix. *See* permethrin
nizatidine, 615*t*
Nizoral. *See* ketoconazole
NOC (Notice of Compliance), 9
nociceptor, 224, 234*f*, 791
nociceptor pain, 224
Noctec. *See* chloral hydrate
Nolvadex. *See* **tamoxifen**
Nolvadex-D. *See* **tamoxifen**
NONBENZODIAZEPINE, NONBARBITURATE CNS DEPRESSANTS:
    for anxiety and insomnia, 164–65, 164*t*
    drugs classified as
        buspirone, 165, 165*t*, 271, 801
        chloral hydrate, 165*t*
        dexmedetomidine HCL, 165*t*
        eszopiclone, 165, 165*t*, 167
        ethchlorvynol, 165*t*
        glutethimide, 165*t*
        meprobamate, 165*t*
        paraldehyde, 165*t*
        zaleplon, 165*t*, 167
        zolpidem, 164*t*, 165*t*
    mechanisms of action, 164–65
    nursing process focus, 166*t*
non-English-speaking clients:
    communication considerations, 71*t*
    pharmacotherapy considerations, 103–4, 103*f*
nonmaleficence, 90, 791
NONNUCLEOSIDE REVERSE TRANSCRIPTASE INHIBITORS. *See* ANTIRETROVIRALS
NONOPIOID ANALGESICS:
    acetaminophen. *See* **acetaminophen**
    centrally-acting
        clonidine. *See* clonidine
        tramadol, 233*t*, 800, 802
    nonsteroidal anti-inflammatory drugs. *See* NONSTEROIDAL ANTI-INFLAMMATORY DRUGS (NSAIDs)
NONPHENOTHIAZINES:
    adverse effects, 215, 215*t*
    drugs classified as
        chlorprothixene, 215*t*
        haloperidol. *See* **haloperidol**
        loxapine succinate, 215*t*, 798
        molindone, 215*t*
        pimozide, 215*t*
        thiothixene, 215*t*
    nursing considerations, 218
        client teaching, 218
        lifespan considerations, 218
    nursing process focus, 216–17*t*

nonspecific cellular responses, 61, 791
nonspecific defenses, 455, 791
NONSTEROIDAL ANTI-INFLAMMATORY DRUGS
   (NSAIDs):
   drugs classified as
      ibuprofen and ibuprofen-like drugs
         diclofenac, 233t, 473t, 801
         diflunisal, 233t, 473t
         etodolac, 233t, 473t, 802
         fenoprofen, 233t, 473t
         flurbiprofen, 233t, 473t
         ibuprofen. See **ibuprofen**
         indomethacin, 233t, 473t, 747
         ketoprofen, 233t, 473t, 798
         ketorolac tromethamine, 233t
         mefenamic acid, 233t
         meloxicam, 233t, 473t, 801
         nabumetone, 233t, 473t, 801
         naproxen, 233t, 473t, 798, 800
         naproxen sodium, 233t, 473t
         oxaprozin, 233t, 473t
         piroxicam, 233t, 473t
         sulindac, 233t
         tolmetin, 233t, 473t
      salicylates
         aspirin. See **aspirin**
         choline salicylate, 233t
         salsalate, 233t
      selective COX-2 inhibitors
         celecoxib, 233t, 473t, 800
   herb–drug interactions, 113t
   mechanisms of action, 232–33
   nursing considerations, 234–35, 475
      client teaching, 235, 475
      lifespan considerations, 235, 475–76
   nursing process focus, 236–37t
   for specific conditions
      inflammation, 473–75, 745
      pain management, 232–34, 233t, 745
   usage statistics, 471t
norepinephrine (NE), 415t
   actions and uses, 137t, 415t
   administration alerts, 415t
   adverse effects, 414t, 415t
   characteristics, 791
   interactions, 415t
   overdose treatment, 415t
   pharmacokinetics, 415t
   physiology, 134–35
   receptors. See adrenergic receptors
   for specific conditions
      heart failure, 342
      shock, 414, 414t
norethindrone, 699, 700t, 709t
norethindrone acetate, 709t, 798
Norflex. See orphenadrine
norfloxacin, 499t
norgestimate, 700t, 801
norgestrel, 700t
Norlutate. See norethindrone acetate
normal saline, 413t
normal serum albumin, 413t
   actions and uses, 413t

   administration alerts, 413t
   adverse effects, 413t
   interactions, 413t
   pharmacokinetics, 413t
Normiflo. See ardeparin
normochromic anemia, 401, 401t
normocytic anemia, 401, 401t
Normodyne. See labetalol
Norometoprol. See **metoprolol**
Noroxin. See norfloxacin
Norpace. See disopyramide phosphate
Norplant, 700. See also levonorgestrel
Norpramin. See desipramine
Nor-Q.D. See norethindrone
North American Nursing Diagnosis
   Association (NANDA), 67
nortriptyline, 159t, 189t, 802
Norulate. See norethindrone
Norvasc. See amlodipine
Norvir. See ritonavir
nosocomial infections, 791
Notice of Compliance (NOC), 9
Novahistine DH, 590t
Novantrone. See mitoxantrone
Novasen. See **aspirin**
Novastan. See argatroban
Novo-Ampicillin. See ampicillin
Novobutamine. See tolbutamide
Novocain. See procaine
Novochlorhydrate. See chloral hydrate
Novochlorocap. See chloramphenicol
Novochlorpromazine. See **chlorpromazine**
Novocimetine. See cimetidine
Novoclopate. See clorazepate
Novocloxin. See cloxacillin
Novocolchicine. See **colchicine**
Novoflupam. See flurazepam
Novoflurazine. See trifluoperazine
Novofuran. See nitrofurantoin
Novohexidyl. See trihexyphenidyl
Novo-Hylazin. See **hydralazine**
Novolexin. See cephalexin
Novolin 70/30. See NPH 70% Regular 30%
Novolin L. See insulin zinc suspension
Novolin N. See isophane insulin suspension
Novolin R. See **regular insulin**
NovoLog. See insulin aspart
Novonaprox. See naproxen
Novo-Nifedin. See **nifedipine**
Novopentotarb. See pentobarbital sodium
Novopheniram. See chlorpheniramine
Novopoxide. See chlordiazepoxide
Novopramine. See **imipramine**
Novopranol. See **propranolol**
Novopropamide. See chlorpropamide
Novopropoxyn. See propoxyphene
   hydrochloride
Novoquinidin. See quinidine sulfate
Novoquinine. See quinine
Novoridazine. See thioridazine
Novorythro. See **erythromycin**
Novosalmol. See albuterol
Novosecobarb. See secobarbital

Novosorbide. See **isosorbide dinitrate**
Novospiroton. See **spironolactone**
Novotetra. See **tetracycline**
Novothalidone. See chlorthalidone
Novotriptyn. See amitriptyline
Novo-Veramil. See **verapamil**
NPH. See isophane insulin suspension
NPH 50% Regular 50%, 685t
NPH 70% Regular 30%, 685t
NPH Iletin II. See isophane insulin
   suspension
NREM sleep, 158, 158t
NSAIDs. See NONSTEROIDAL ANTI-
   INFLAMMATORY DRUGS
Nubain. See nalbuphine hydrochloride
NUCLEOSIDE REVERSE TRANSCRIPTASE
   INHIBITORS. See ANTIRETROVIRALS
nucleosides, 536
NUCLEOTIDE REVERSE TRANSCRIPTASE
   INHIBITORS. See ANTIRETROVIRALS
Numorphan. See oxymorphone
   hydrochloride
Nupercainal. See dibucaine
Nupercaine. See dibucaine
nurse practice act, 92, 791
nursing considerations:
   ACE inhibitors
      for heart failure, 334–35
      for hypertension, 317–20
   acne-related disorders, 764
   adrenergic agonists (sympathomimetics),
      137–38
   adrenergic antagonists (sympatholytics),
      141, 322
   alkylating agents, 558–60
   alpha-adrenergic agonists, 323
   alpha-adrenergic antagonists, 322, 728
   5-alpha-reductase inhibitors, 728
   aminoglycosides, 497–98
   ammonium chloride for alkalosis, 449–50
   androgens, 720
   anorexiants, 636–37
   antacids, 619–20
   antiadrenal therapy for Cushing's syn-
      drome, 678
   antianemia therapy, 403, 404–6
   anticholinergics
      for asthma, 599–600
      overview, 149–50
      for Parkinson's disease, 267–68
   anticoagulants, 382–84, 385
   antidiarrheals, 629–30
   antidiuretic hormone, 666
   antiemetics, 633–35
   antifungals
      azoles, 520
      superficial, 521–22
      systemic, 515–16
   antiglaucoma drugs, 776, 778
   antigout drugs, 748, 750
   antihelminthics, 529–30
   antimetabolites, 561, 563
   antimigraine drugs, 237–41

nursing considerations (*continued*)
  antineoplastics
    alkylating agents, 558–60
    antimetabolites, 561, 563
    antitumor antibiotics, 563, 565
    hormone and hormone antagonists, 569–70
    natural product extracts, 566–67
  antiplatelets, 386–87
  antiprostatic agents, 728
  antipsychotics
    atypical, 218–19
    nonphenothiazines, 217–18
    phenothiazines, 214
  antipyretics, 478–80
  antiretrovirals, 539–40
  antispasmodics, 279, 281
  antithyroid agents, 672–73
  antituberculosis drugs, 509t
  antitussives, 590–91
  antivirals for non-HIV infections, 545–46
  attention deficit–hyperactivity disorder, 204–5
  atypical antipsychotics, 218–19
  barbiturates, 174–76
  benign prostatic hyperplasia, 728
  benzodiazepines
    for anxiety and insomnia, 161–63
    for seizures, 176–77
  beta-adrenergic agonists, 598
  beta-adrenergic antagonists
    for angina, 352–53
    for dysrhythmias, 371
    for heart failure, 337
    for hypertension, 323–24
  bile acid resins, 294–95
  bisphosphonates, 743
  calcium channel blockers
    for angina, 354–55
    for dysrhythmias, 373–74
    for hypertension, 314–16
  calcium supplements, 735
  cardiac glycosides, 339–41
  cephalosporins, 493–94
  cholinergics (parasympathomimetics)
    for Alzheimer's disease, 271–72
    overview, 144
  colloidal solutions, 413–14, 441–42
  colony-stimulating factors, 398–99
  crystalloids for shock, 413–14
  diuretics
    for heart failure, 335–36
    for hypertension, 309–11
    for renal failure, 428–29, 431–32
  dopaminergics for Parkinson's disease, 264–65
  enteral feeding, 655
  epoetin alfa, 395–96, 398
  ferrous sulfate, 404–6
  fibric acid agents, 298
  filgrastim, 398–99
  fluid replacement for shock, 413–14
  fluoroquinolones, 500

folic acid for anemia, 403
general anesthetics, 254, 255–56
glucocorticoids
  for adrenocortical insufficiency, 675, 678
  inhaled, 603
  intranasal, 586
  systemic, 477–78, 603
H_1-receptor antagonists, 582, 584
H_2-receptor antagonists, 616–17
hemostatics, 390
hormone antagonists for cancer chemotherapy, 569–70
hormone replacement therapy, 708
hormones for cancer chemotherapy, 569–70
hydantoins, 178–80
immunostimulants, 462–63
immunosuppressants, 468
inotropic agents for shock, 418
insulins, 686, 688
iron salts, 404–6
isotretinoin, 764
laxatives, 627–28
leukotriene modifiers, 604–5
lithium, 202
local anesthetics, 248, 249
macrolides, 496–97
macrominerals, 652–53
magnesium sulfate, 652–53
methylphenidate, 204–5
methylxanthines, 600–601
minor skin irritation, 760
monamine oxidase inhibitors, 195–96
nasal decongestants, 588
neuromuscular blockers, 258
niacin (vitamin B_3) for hyperlipidemia, 297
nonphenothiazines, 217–18
nonsteroidal anti-inflammatory drugs, 234–35, 475–76
opioid analgesics, 228, 230
opioid antagonists, 231–32
oral contraceptives, 701–2
oral hypoglycemics, 691–92, 694
organic nitrates, 350–51
otic preparations, 780–81
oxytocics, 712–14
pancreatic enzymes, 638
pediculicides, 757–58
penicillins, 490–92
phenothiazines, 214
phenytoin-like drugs, 178–80
phosphodiesterase inhibitors, 342
potassium channel blockers, 372
potassium replacement therapy, 445–46
potassium-sparing diuretics, 431–32
progestins, 709–10
protease inhibitors, 539–40
proton pump inhibitors, 617–18
reverse transcriptase inhibitors, 539–40
scabicides, 757–58
selective serotonin reuptake inhibitors, 194

sodium bicarbonate for acidosis, 447–49
sodium channel blockers, 369
sodium replacement therapy, 444
statins, 292–93
succinimides, 181
sulfonamides, 501–2
sunburn, 760
taxanes, 566–67
tegaserod, 631–32
tetracyclines, 494–95
thrombolytics, 357, 388–89
thyroid agents, 668
topoisomerase inhibitors, 566–67
tricyclic antidepressants, 190–92
vaccines, 458–59
vasoconstrictors
  for anaphylaxis, 420–21
  for shock, 415
vasodilators
  for heart failure, 338
  for hypertension, 324–25
vinca alkaloids, 566–67
vitamin B_3 (niacin) for hyperlipidemia, 297
vitamin B_{12} for anemia, 403
vitamins
  lipid-soluble, 646
  water-soluble, 648–49
nursing diagnoses:
  for client receiving medications, 69–70, 70t
  definition, 67, 791
nursing process:
  definition, 67, 791
  in medication administration
    assessment, 68–69, 68t
    evaluation, 72–73
    goals and outcomes, 70–71
    interventions, 71–72, 72t
    nursing diagnoses, 69–70, 70t
  in medication error reduction and prevention, 94
  steps, 67–68
Nursing Process Focus:
  ACE inhibitor therapy, 319–20t
  adrenergic blocking therapy, 139–40t, 323–24t
  amphotericin B (Fungizone), 518t
  androgen therapy, 722t
  antibacterial therapy, 504–5t
  anticholinergic therapy, 148–49t
  anticoagulant therapy, 385t
  antidepressant therapy, 197–99t
  antidiarrheal therapy, 631t
  antidysrhythmic therapy, 370t
  antihistamine therapy, 584–85t
  antineoplastic therapy, 572–73t
  antipyretic therapy, 480t
  antiretroviral drugs, 541–42t
  antiseizure therapy, 182–83t
  antispasmodics, 280t
  antithyroid therapy, 671–72t
  antituberculosis therapy, 509–10t

atypical antipsychotic therapy, 220–21t
benzodiazepine and nonbenzodiazepine antianxiety therapy, 166t
beta-adrenergic antagonist therapy, 323–24t
bisphosphonates, 742t
bronchodilator therapy, 602–3t
calcium channel blocker therapy, 315–16t
calcium supplements, 737t
cardiac glycoside therapy, 340t
cholinergic-blocking agents (anticholinergics), 148–49t
cholinergics (parasympathomimetics), 145–46t
colchicine, 749–50t
colony-stimulating factors, 399t
conventional antipsychotic therapy, 216–17t
direct vasodilator therapy, 326t
diuretic therapy (for hypertension), 312–13t
diuretic therapy (for renal failure), 434–35t
drugs for muscle spasms or spasticity, 280–81t
epoetin alfa (Epogen, Procrit), 397t
ferrous sulfate (Feosol, others), 405t
filgrastim (Neupogen), 399t
finasteride (Proscar), 728–29t
folic acid (Folacin, Folvite), 649t
general anesthesia, 253t
H1-receptor antagonists, 584–85t
H2-receptor antagonist therapy, 616t
HMG-CoA reductase inhibitor therapy, 296t
hormone replacement therapy, 707–8t
immunostimulant therapy, 464t
immunosuppressant therapy, 467t
insulin therapy, 687t
iron salts, 405t
isotretinoin (Accutane), 763t
IV fluid therapy for shock, 416t
levodopa (Larodopa), 266–67t
lindane (Kwell), 759t
lithium (Eskalith), 201–2t
local anesthesia, 250t
methylphenidate (Ritalin), 205–6t
nitroglycerin (Nitrostat), 352t
nonsteroidal anti-inflammatory (NSAID) therapy, 236–37t
ophthalmic solutions for glaucoma, 777–78t
opioid therapy, 229–30t
oral contraceptive therapy, 703–4t
oral hypoglycemic therapy, 693t
oxytocin (Pitocin Syntocinon), 713t
parasympathomimetic therapy, 145–46t
pharmacotherapy for superpficial fungal infections, 522–23t
sympathomimetics therapy, 139–40t, 142t, 323–24t
systemic glucocorticold therapy, thrombolytic therapy, 389t
thyroid hormone replacement, 669–70t

total parenteral nutrition, 656–57t
triptan therapy, 240t
uric acid inhibitors, 749–50t
vasodilators, 326t
nutraceuticals, 9
nutritional supplements:
    enteral. See enteral nutrition
    indications, 654
    total parenteral nutrition. See total parenteral nutrition
NuvaRing, 700
Nu-Verap. See **verapamil**
Nyaderm. See **nystatin**
Nydrazid. See **isoniazid**
nystatin, 521t
    actions and uses, 521t
    administration alerts, 521t
    adverse effects, 520t, 521t
    Canadian/U.S. trade names, 798
    pharmacokinetics, 521t
    route and adult dose, 520t
Nystex. See **nystatin**

O

obesity:
    nursing considerations, 636–37
    pharmacological treatment, 635–36, 636t
objective data, 67, 791
obsessive–compulsive disorders (OCD), 154, 791
Octagam. See immune globulin
octreotide, 664t, 665
OcuClear. See **oxymetazoline**
Ocupress. See carteolol
Office of Natural Health Products, 9
ofloxacin, 499t, 507t
Ogen. See estropipate
olanzapine, 218t, 271, 801
older adulthood, 84, 791
older adults:
    adverse drug effects in, 51t
    chemotherapy in, 570t
    dietary supplement use, 109t
    drug administration challenges, 72, 94t
    drug administration guidelines, 85–86
    H2-receptor blockers and vitamin B12 in, 617t
    HIV infection, 544t
    ophthalmic drug administration, 778t
    pain expression and perception, 231t
    pharmacokinetics
        absorption, 86
        distribution, 86
        excretion, 86
        metabolism, 86
    prescription drug costs and, 8t
oligomenorrhea, 709, 791
oligomeric formulas, 654
oligospermia, 721, 791
olmesartan medoxomil, 316t, 801
olopatadine, 801
olsalazine, 630

omapatrilat, 317
omega-3 fatty acids. See fish oils
omeprazole, 618t
    actions and uses, 618t, 638
    administration alerts, 618t
    adverse effects, 617t, 618t
    Canadian/U.S. trade names, 799
    interactions, 618t
    pharmacokinetics, 618t
    prescription ranking, 801
    route and adult dose, 617t
Omnicef. See cefdinir
Omnipen. See ampicillin
Oncaspar. See pegaspargase
oncogenes, 553, 791
oncotic pressure, 411
ondansetron, 634t
open-angle glaucoma, 772, 772f, 773, 791
Ophthalgan. See glycerin anhydrous
ophthalmic drugs:
    administration, 35, 36f, 36t, 37
    antiglaucoma. See ANTIGLAUCOMA DRUGS
    cycloplegics
        atropine, 779t
        characteristics, 777, 778, 779
        cyclopentolate, 779t
        homatropine, 779t
        scopolamine, 779t
        tropicamide, 779t
    home care considerations, 778t
    lubricants
        lanolin alcohol, 779t
        methylcellulose, 779t
        polyvinyl alcohol, 779t
    mydriatics
        characteristics, 778
        hydroxyamphetamine, 779t
        phenylephrine, 779, 779t
    pemirolast, 779
    vasoconstrictors
        naphazoline HCl, 779, 779t
        oxymetazoline. See **oxymetazoline**
        tetrahydrozoline, 779, 779t
opiate, 226, 791
opioid(s). See also OPIOID (NARCOTIC) ANALGESICS
    definition, 226, 791
    dependence/abuse
        characteristics, 120t, 121
        treatment, 232
        withdrawal symptoms, 120t
    endogenous, 225, 225f, 787
    in general anesthesia
        alfentanil hydrochloride, 255t, 256t
        fentanyl citrate, 255, 255t, 256t
        remifentanil hydrochloride, 255t, 256t
        sufentanil citrate, 255t, 256t
    receptors, 226, 226f, 226t
OPIOID (NARCOTIC) ANALGESICS:
    in children and older adults, 231t
    combined with nonnarcotic analgesics, 227–28

OPIOID (NARCOTIC) ANALGESICS (*continued*)
dependence. *See* opioid(s),
  dependence/abuse
drugs classified as
  mixed opioid agonists
    buprenorphine hydrochloride, 226*f*,
      227*t*, 232
    butorphanol tartrate, 226*f*, 227*t*
    characteristics, 226, 226*f*
    dezocine, 227*t*
    nalbuphine hydrochloride, 227*t*
    pentazocine hydrochloride,
      226, 226*f*, 227*t*
  opioid agonists
    characteristics, 226, 226*f*
    codeine. *See* codeine
    hydrocodone bitartrate. *See* hy-
      drocodone bitartrate
    hydromorphone hydrochloride, 227*t*
    levorphanol tartrate, 227*t*
    meperidine hydrochloride. *See*
      meperidine
    methadone. *See* methadone
    morphine sulfate. *See* **morphine sul-
      fate**
    oxycodone hydrochloride, 227*t*, 801
    oxycodone terephthalate, 227*t*
    oxymorphone hydrochloride, 227*t*
    propoxyphene hydrochloride,
      227*t*, 799
    propoxyphene napsylate, 227*t*, 799
herb–drug interactions, 113*t*
nursing considerations, 228, 230
  client teaching, 230
nursing process focus, 229–30*t*
for specific conditions
  myocardial infarction, 358
  pain management, 226–28, 227*t*
toxicity signs, 120*t*
OPIOID ANTAGONISTS:
characteristics, 226, 226*f*
drugs classified as
  nalmefene hydrochloride, 227*t*
  naloxone hydrochloride. *See* **naloxone
    hydrochloride**
  naltrexone hydrochloride, 227*t*, 232
nursing considerations, 231–32
  client teaching, 232
opportunistic infections, fungal, 514
opportunistic organisms, 488
oprelvekin, 395*t*, 399, 462
Optimine. *See* azacitidine
OptiPranolol. *See* metipranolol
Ora Testryl. *See* fluoxymesterone
Oradexon. *See* dexamethasone
ORAL CONTRACEPTIVES:
for acne, 761*t*, 762
administration, 699, 701*f*
adverse effects, 700, 700*t*
benefits, 697*t*
estrogens and progestins as,
  699–700, 700*t*
extended regimen

Seasonal, 700
Seasonique, 700
formulations, 699
  biphasic
    characteristics, 699
    Ortho-Novum 10/11, 700*t*
  monophasic
    Alesse, 700*t*
    characteristics, 699
    Desogen, 700*t*
    Loestrin 1.5/30 Fe, 700*t*
    Lo/Ovral, 700*t*
    Ortho-Cyclen, 700*t*
    Ortho-Novum 1/35. *See* ethinyl
      estradiol with norethindrone
    Yasmin, 700*t*
  progestin only
    characteristics, 699–700
    Micronor, 700*t*
    Nor-Q.D., 700*t*
    Ovrette, 700*t*
  triphasic
    characteristics, 699
    Ortho Tri-Cyclen, 700*t*
    Ortho-Novum 7/7/7, 700*t*
    Tri-Levlen, 700*t*
    Triphasil, 700*t*
interactions, 701
nursing considerations, 701–2
nursing process focus, 703–4*t*
progestin-only, 699, 700*t*
ORAL HYPOGLYCEMICS:
adverse effects, 690*t*
drugs classified as
  alpha-glucosidase inhibitors
    acarbose, 689, 690*t*
    characteristics, 689
    miglitol, 690*t*
  biguanides
    characteristics, 689
    metformin, 689, 690*t*, 800, 801
  combination drugs
    glipizide/metformin, 690*t*, 691
    glyburide/metformin, 690*t*
    pioglitazone/metformin, 690*t*
    rosiglitazone/glimepiride, 690*t*
    rosiglitazone/metformin, 690*t*
  meglitinides
    characteristics, 690
    nateglinide, 690*t*
    repaglinide, 690*t*
  newer agents
    aloglipton, 691
    characteristics, 691
    denaglipton, 691
    exenatide, 690*t*, 691
    pramlintide, 691
    saxaglipton, 691
    sitagliptin, 690*t*, 691
    vildaglipton, 691
  sulfonylureas
    acetohexamide, 690*t*
    characteristics, 689

chlorpropamide, 690*t*
glimepiride, 690*t*
glipizide. *See* **glipizide**
glyburide, 690*t*, 800
tolazamide, 690*t*
tolbutamide, 690*t*
thiazolidinediones
  characteristics, 689–90
  pioglitazone, 690*t*, 800
  rosiglitazone, 690*t*, 800
herb–drug interactions, 113*t*
nursing considerations, 691–92
  client teaching, 692, 694
  lifespan considerations, 692
  nursing process focus, 693*t*
  route and adult doses, 690*t*
Orap. *See* pimozide
Oratrol. *See* dichlorphenamide
Orazinc. *See* zinc sulfate
organ transplants:
frequency, 455*t*
rejection, 463
ORGANIC NITRATES:
drugs classified as
  amyl nitrite, 350*t*
  isosorbide dinitrate. *See* **isosorbide
    dinitrate**
  isosorbide mononitrate, 350*t*
  nitroglycerin. *See* **nitroglycerin**
mechanisms of action, 349–50, 349*f*
nursing considerations, 350–51
  client teaching, 351
  nursing process focus, 352*t*
  route and adult doses, 350*t*
in suspected myocardial infarction, 358
therapeutic approach, 349–50
Organ. *See* danaparoid
Orinase. *See* tolbutamide
orlistat, 636
orphenadrine, 276*t*
Ortho Tri-Cyclen, 700*t*
Ortho Tri-Cyclen Lo, 801
Orthoclone OKT3. *See* muromonab-CD3
Ortho-Cyclen, 700*t*
Ortho-Evra, 700, 800
Ortho-Novum 1/35. *See* **ethinyl estradiol
  with norethindrone**
Ortho-Novum 7/7/7, 700*t*
Ortho-Novum 10/11, 700*t*
Ortho-Prefest. *See* estradiol/norgestimate
orthostatic hypotension, 309, 791
Orudis. *See* ketoprofen
Oruvail. *See* ketoprofen
Os-Cal 500. *See* calcium carbonate
oseltamivir, 546, 547*t*
Osmitrol. *See* mannitol
osmolality, 439, 791
osmosis, 439, 439*f*, 791
OSMOTIC DIURETICS:
adverse effects, 433*t*, 774*t*
drugs classified as
  glycerin anhydrous, 774*t*, 776
  isosorbide, 774*t*, 776

mannitol, 433, 433t, 774t, 776
  urea, 433, 433t
mechanisms of action, 427f, 433
for specific conditions
  glaucoma, 774t, 776
  renal failure, 433, 433t
osteitis deformans. *See* Paget's disease
osteoarthritis:
  characteristics, 745, 745f, 745t, 791
  incidence, 745t
  natural therapy with glucosamine and
      chondroitin, 746t
  pharmacotherapy, 745
osteoclasts, 733
osteomalacia:
  causes, 738
  characteristics, 738, 791
  diagnosis, 738
  nursing considerations, 738
    client teaching, 739
    lifespan considerations, 738
  pharmacotherapy
    calcifediol, 736t
    calcitriol. *See* **calcitriol**
    ergocalciferol, 736t
osteoporosis:
  calcium metabolism in, 740f
  causes, 739
  characteristics, 791
  ethnic/racial considerations, 743t
  incidence, 740t
  lifestyle considerations, 743t
  pharmacotherapy
    bisphosphonates. *See*
        BISPHOSPHONATES
    hormonal agents
      calcitonin, 741t, 743
      estrogen replacement therapy, 743–44
      raloxifene. *See* **raloxifene**
      teriparatide, 740, 741t
  risk factors, 739
Ostoforte. *See* ergocalciferol
otic preparations:
  administration, 36t, 37, 37f
  formulations
    acetic acid and hydrocortisone, 780t
    aluminum sulfate and calcium
        acetate, 780t
    benzocaine and antipyrine, 780t
    carbamide peroxide, 780t
    ciprofloxacin hydrochloride and
        hydrocortisone, 780t
    polymyxin B, neomycin, and
        hydrocortisone, 780t
    triethanolamine polypeptide oleate
        10% condensate, 780t
  nursing considerations, 780–81
    client teaching, 781
    lifespan considerations, 781
  pharmacotherapy with, 778, 780–81
otitis media, 485t, 779, 791
ototoxicity, 791
Otrivin. *See* xylometazoline

outcomes:
  definition, 67, 791
  in medication administration,
      70–71
over-the-counter (OTC) drugs:
  advantages and disadvantages, 5
  client teaching, 638t
  definition, 5
  interactions, 618t
  medication errors and, 96t
Ovide. *See* malathion
Ovrette, 700t
ovulation, 697, 791
oxacillin, 489t, 490
oxaliplatin, 559t
oxaprozin, 233t, 473t
oxazepam, 162t, 799
OXAZOLIDINONES:
  linezolid, 503t, 505
oxcarbazepine, 200
oxiconazole, 519t
Oxistat. *See* oxiconazole
Ox-Pam. *See* oxazepam
oxybutynin, 147t
oxycodone hydrochloride,
      227t, 801
oxycodone terephthalate, 227t
oxycodone/APAP, 800
OxyContin. *See* oxycodone
  hydrochloride
Oxydess II. *See* dextroamphetamine
oxymetazoline, 588t
  actions and uses, 137t, 588t
  administration alerts, 588t
  adverse effects, 587t, 588t
  Canadian/U.S. trade names, 799
  interactions, 588t
  pharmacokinetics, 588t
  for specific conditions
    nasal decongestion, 587t
    ophthalmic irritation, 779t
oxymorphone hydrochloride, 227t
OXYTOCICS:
  definition, 710
  drugs classified as
    carboprost tromethamine, 704t, 705,
        711t
    dinoprostone, 704t, 705, 711t
    ergonovine maleate, 711t
    methylergonovine maleate, 711t
    misoprostol, 621, 704t, 705, 711t
    oxytocin. *See* **oxytocin**
  nursing considerations, 712–13
    client teaching, 713–14
  nursing process focus, 713t
oxytocin, 712t
  actions and uses, 710–11, 712t
  administration alerts, 712t
  adverse effects, 711t
  functions, 711, 712f, 791
  interactions, 712t
  overdose treatment, 712t
  pharmacokinetics, 712t

route and adult dose, 711t
secretion, 663f

P
p53 gene, 553
pacemaker, 363
Pacerone. *See* **amiodarone**
Pacific yew, 565
packed red blood cells, 413t
paclitaxel, 555f, 565, 566t
Paget's disease, 744, 791
pain:
  assessment, 224
  classification, 224
  definition, 224
  expression and perception
    age and, 231t
    ethnic/racial considerations, 225t
  incidence, 224t
  mechanisms
    neural, 225–26, 225f
    nociceptor level, 234f
  nonpharmacologic management, 224–25
  pharmacotherapy
    acetaminophen. *See* **acetaminophen**
    clonidine. *See* clonidine
    nonsteroidal anti-inflammatory drugs.
        See NONSTEROIDAL ANTI-
        INFLAMMATORY DRUGS
    opioid. *See* OPIOID (NARCOTIC)
        ANALGESICS
    salicylates
      aspirin. *See* **aspirin**
      choline salicylate, 233t
      salsalate, 233t
    tramadol, 233t, 800
Paladron. *See* aminophylline
palliation, 554, 791
palonosetron, 634t
Paludrine. *See* proguanil
Pamelor. *See* nortriptyline
pamidronate disodium, 741t
Panax quinquefolius. See ginseng
pancreas, 682–83, 683f
Pancrease. *See* **pancrelipase**
pancreatic enzymes:
  actions and uses, 637, 638
  drugs classified as
    pancreatin, 638
    pancrelipase. *See* **pancrelipase**
  nursing considerations, 638
    client teaching, 638
pancreatin, 638
pancreatitis:
  acute, 637–38
  chronic, 638
  nursing considerations, 638
    client teaching, 638
  pharmacotherapy, 637–38
  psychosocial and community impact,
      638t
pancrelipase, 637t
  actions and uses, 637t

pancrelipase (*continued*)
administration alerts, 637*t*
adverse effects, 637*t*
interactions, 637*t*
overdose treatment, 637*t*
pharmacokinetics, 637*t*
panic disorder:
definition, 154, 791
pharmacotherapy, 159–60, 159*t*
Pankreon. *See* pancreatin
Panmycin. *See* **tetracycline**
pantoprazole, 617, 617*t*, 800
pantothenic acid, 643*t*
papaverine, 723
Paracetaldehyde. *See* paraldehyde
Paraflex. *See* chlorzoxazone
parafollicular cells, 666, 791
Parafon Forte. *See* chlorzoxazone
paraldehyde, 165*t*
paranoia, 210, 791
Paraplatin. *See* cisplatin
parasitic infections:
childhood play areas and, 527*t*
lice. *See* lice
scabies. *See* scabies
parasympathetic nervous system, 132, 132*f*,
133*f*, 791
PARASYMPATHOMIMETICS. *See* CHOLINERGICS
parathyroid gland, 733, 734*f*
parathyroid hormone (PTH), 733, 734*f*
Paredrine. *See* hydroxyamphetamine
Paregoric. *See* camphorated opium tincture
parenteral route, 38, 791. *See also* drug
administration, parenteral
parietal cells, 612, 791
parkinsonism, 213*t*, 214, 261, 791
Parkinson's disease:
characteristics, 261–62, 262*t*, 791
incidence, 261, 262*t*
living with, 262*t*
pharmacotherapy
anticholinergics. *See* ANTICHOLINERGICS
dopaminergics. *See* DOPAMINERGICS
mechanisms of action, 264*f*, 267
nursing considerations, 264–65,
267–68
client teaching, 265, 268
nursing process focus, 266–67*t*
Parlodel. *See* bromocriptine
Parnate. *See* tranylcypromine
paromomycin, 497, 498*t*, 526*t*
paroxetine, 160*t*, 189*t*, 800, 801
partial agonist, 61–62, 791
partial (focal) seizure, 171,
172*t*, 173*t*, 791
passive immunity, 457, 459*f*, 792
passive transport, 47
Patanol. *See* olopatadine
pathogen, 484, 792
pathogenicity, 484, 792
Paveral. *See* codeine
Paxil. *See* paroxetine
Paxipam. *See* halazepam

PBZ-SR. *See* tripelennamine
PCP, 124
Pediapred. *See* prednisolone
pediatric clients. *See* children; infants
PEDICULICIDES:
definition, 757, 792
drugs classified as
lindane. *See* **lindane**
malathion, 757
permethrin, 757
pyrethrin, 757
nursing considerations, 757–58
client teaching, 758
lifespan considerations, 758
nursing process focus, 759*t*
pharmacotherapy with, 757
pediculosis:
characteristics, 756–57, 756*f*
pharmacotherapy. *See* PEDICULICIDES
psychosocial and community impact, 758*t*
Pediculus capitis, 756, 756*f*
Pediculus corpus, 756
PedvaxHIB. *See* haemophilus type
B conjugate vaccine
pegaspargase, 555*f*, 571*t*
Pegasys. *See* peginterferon alfa-2a
pegfilgrastim, 395*t*, 398
peginterferon alfa-2a, 461*t*, 548*t*
peginterferon alfa-2b, 548*t*
PEG-Intron, 548*t*
PEG-L-asparaginase. *See* pegaspargase
pegvisomant, 664*t*, 665
pegylation, 549, 792
Pelamine. *See* tripelennamine
pellagra, 646, 792
pemetrexed, 561*t*
pemirolast, 779
pemoline, 203, 204*t*
Pen Tsao, 3
Penbritin. *See* ampicillin
penciclovir, 544*t*
Penetrex. *See* enoxacin
Penglobes. *See* bacampicillin
penicillamine, 746, 747*t*
penicillin G benzathine, 489*t*
penicillin G potassium, 491*t*
actions and uses, 491*t*
administration alerts, 491*t*
adverse effects, 489*t*, 491*t*
Canadian/U.S. trade names, 799
interactions, 491*t*
pharmacokinetics, 491*t*
route and adult dose, 489*t*
penicillin G procaine, 489*t*
penicillin G sodium, 489*t*
penicillin V, 489*t*, 799
penicillin VK, 800
penicillinase, 490, 490*f*, 784
penicillinase-resistant penicillins, 489*t*, 490.
See also PENICILLINS
penicillin-binding protein, 490
PENICILLINS:
adverse effects, 489*t*, 490

allergy to, 490
drugs classified as
broad-spectrum (aminopenicillins)
amoxicillin. *See* amoxicillin
amoxicillin–clavulanate, 489*t*, 490
ampicillin, 489*t*, 490, 797
bacampicillin, 489*t*, 797
characteristics, 490
extended-spectrum
(antipseudomonal)
carbenicillin, 489*t*, 490, 797
characteristics, 490
piperacillin sodium, 489*t*, 490
piperacillin tazobactam, 489*t*
ticarcillin, 489*t*
narrow-spectrum/penicillinase
sensitive
penicillin G benzathine, 489*t*
penicillin G potassium. *See*
penicillin G potassium
penicillin G procaine, 489*t*
penicillin G sodium, 489*t*
penicillin V, 489*t*, 797
penicillinase-resistant
characteristics, 490
cloxacillin, 489*t*, 490
dicloxacillin, 489*t*
nafcillin, 489*t*
oxacillin, 489*t*, 490
mechanisms of action, 490, 490*f*
nursing considerations, 490–91
client teaching, 491–92
pharmacotherapy with, 490
route and adult doses, 489*t*
Pentacarinat. *See* pentamidine
Pentam 300. *See* pentamidine
pentamidine, 526*t*, 799
Pentamycetin. *See* chloramphenicol
Pentasa. *See* mesalazine
Pentazine. *See* promethazine
pentazocine hydrochloride, 226, 226*f*, 227*t*
Penthrane. *See* methoxyflurane
Pentids. *See* **penicillin G potassium**
pentobarbital sodium:
Canadian/U.S. trade names, 799
as general anesthesia adjunct, 256*t*
for sedation and insomnia, 164*t*
for seizures, 175*t*
Pentolair. *See* cyclopentolate
Pentostam. *See* sodium stibogluconate
pentostatin, 561*t*
Pentothal. *See* **thiopental**
pentoxifylline, 386, 386*t*
Pen-Vee K. *See* penicillin V
Pepcid. *See* famotidine
Peptamen Liquid, 655
peptic ulcer disease:
definition, 612, 792
herbal therapy, 621*t*
nonpharmacological therapy, 613
pathophysiology, 612–13
pharmacotherapy
antacids. *See* ANTACIDS

H$_2$-receptor antagonists. *See*
H$_2$-RECEPTOR ANTAGONISTS
mechanisms of action, 614*f*
misoprostol, 621
pirenzepine, 621
proton pump inhibitors. *See* PROTON
PUMP INHIBITORS
sucralfate, 620
therapeutic approach, 613–14
risk factors, 612–13
symptoms, 613
Pepto-Bismol. *See* bismuth subsalicylate
Peptol. *See* cimetidine
Percocet, 228
Percocet-5. *See* oxycodone terephthalate
Percodan, 228
percutaneous transluminal coronary
angioplasty (PTCA), 348, 792
performance anxiety, 154
perfusion, 594, 594*f*, 792
pergolide, 263, 263*t*
Pergonal. *See* human menopausal
gonadotropin–menotropins
Periactin. *See* cyproheptadine
Peridol. *See* **haloperidol**
perindopril, 316*t*
peripheral edema, 331
peripheral nervous system (PNS),
131, 132*f*, 792
peripheral resistance, 304, 304*f*, 792
peristalsis, 611, 792
periwinkle, 565
Permax. *See* pergolide
permethrin, 757
Permitil. *See* fluphenazine
pernicious (megaloblastic) anemia,
402, 647, 792
perphenazine:
genetic polymorphisms affecting
metabolism, 104*t*
for nausea and vomiting, 634*t*
for psychoses, 212*t*, 213
Persantine. *See* dipyridamole
Pertofrane. *See* desipramine
petit mal. *See* absence (petit mal) seizure
pH:
definition, 446, 792
effect on absorption, 49, 49*f*
plasma, 446
pharmacodynamics:
cellular receptors, 60–61, 61*f*
customization of drug therapy, 62
definition, 57, 792
drug–receptor interactions, 61–62
efficacy, 59–60, 60*f*
graded dose–response relationship,
59, 59*f*
interclient variability, 57–58, 57*f*
potency, 59–60, 60*f*
second messenger events, 61
therapeutic index, 58–59, 58*f*
pharmacogenetics, 62, 104, 792.
See also genetics

pharmacokinetics:
absorption, 48–49, 48*f*, 49*f*
definition, 47, 792
distribution, 48*f*, 49–50, 49*f*
drug plasma concentration, 52–53, 53*f*
excretion, 48*f*, 51–52
loading dose, 53–54, 53*f*
maintenance dose, 54
metabolism, 48*f*, 50–51
in older adults, 86
plasma half-life, 53
in pregnancy, 77
therapeutic range, 53, 53*f*
pharmacologic classification:
definition, 12, 792
example, 13*t*
pharmacology:
definition, 4, 792
history, 3
vs. therapeutics, 4
pharmacopoeia, 5, 792
pharmacotherapy. *See also* drug
administration
community and environmental
influences, 103–4
cultural and ethnic influences, 101–3
definition, 4, 792
gender influences, 104–5
genetic influences, 104, 104*t*
holistic, 100–101
psychosocial influences, 101
Pharmacotherapy Illustrated:
active and passive immunity, 459*f*
Alzheimer's disease drugs, 270*f*
angina drugs, 349*f*
antihypertensive drugs, 307*f*
antiparkinsonism drugs, 264*f*
antispasmodics, 278*f*
antiulcer drugs, 614*f*
benign prostatic hyperplasia, 726*f*
cholesterol-lowering agents, 294*f*
diuretics, 427*f*
GABA receptor–chloride channel
molecule, 174*f*
heart failure drugs, 332*f*
limbic system and reticular activating
system, 155*f*
local anesthetics, 247*f*
PharmFacts:
alternative therapies, attitudes toward,
109*t*
anesthesia and anesthetics, 245*t*
angina, 347*t*
anxiety disorders, 156*t*
arthritis, 745
asthma, 596*t*
attention deficit–hyperactivity disorder,
202*t*
bacterial infections, 484*t*
cancer, 553*t*
clotting disorders, 378*t*
community health statistics in the
U.S., 104*t*

degenerative diseases of the central
nervous system, 262*t*
depression, 187*t*
diabetes mellitus, 684*t*
dysrhythmias, 362*t*
epilepsy, 172*t*
female reproductive conditions, 697*t*
fetal effects of drug use during
pregnancy, 80*t*
fungal infections, 514*t*
gastrointestinal disorders, 624*t*
glaucoma, 773*t*
grapefruit juice and drug
interactions, 30*t*
headaches and migraine, 237*t*
healthcare access among minorities, 102*t*
heart failure, 330*t*
helminthic infections, 514*t*
hematopoietic disorders, 395*t*
high blood cholesterol, 287*t*
hypertension, 302*t*
inflammatory disorders, 471*t*
insomnia and insulin resistance, 157*t*
insomnia incidence, 157*t*
male reproductive disorders, 718*t*
muscle spasms, 275*t*
myocardial infarction, 347*t*
organ transplants, 455*t*
osteoporosis, 740*t*
pain, 224*t*
poisoning, 83*t*
prescription drugs
consumer spending, 5*t*
marketing costs, 14*t*
time length for new drug approvals, 8*t*
protozoal infections, 514*t*
psychoses, 210*t*
renal disorders, 424*t*
shock, 410*t*
skin disorders, 754*t*
Stevens-Johnson syndrome, 28*t*
substance abuse statistics, 15*t*, 119*t*
terrorist attacks, potential chemical and
biologic agents for, 19*t*
thyroid disorders, 666*t*
toxic epidermal necrolysis, 28*t*
upper gastrointestinal tract disorders, 611*t*
vaccines, 455*t*
viral infections, 534*t*
vitamins, minerals, and nutritional
supplements, 642*t*
pharyngitis, 485*t*
Phenazine. *See* perphenazine;
promethazine
phencyclidine, 79*t*
phenelzine, 196*t*
actions and uses, 196*t*
administration alerts, 196*t*
adverse effects, 189*t*, 194, 196*t*
contraindications, 195
interactions, 196*t*
overdose treatment, 196*t*
pharmacokinetics, 196*t*

phenelzine (*continued*)
for specific conditions
depression, 189t
panic disorders, 159t
Phenergan. *See* promethazine
Phenergan with Codeine, 590t
phenindione, 79t
phenobarbital, 176t
actions and uses, 176t
administration alerts, 176t
adverse effects, 79t, 164t, 175t, 176t
interactions, 176t
overdose treatment, 176t
pharmacokinetics, 176t
for specific conditions
sedation and insomnia, 164t
seizures, 173–74, 173t, 175t
phenolphthalein, 626t
PHENOTHIAZINES:
adverse effects, 212t, 213–14, 213t
characteristics, 212–13
drugs classified as
chlorpromazine. *See* **chlorpromazine**
fluphenazine, 212t
mesoridazine, 212t, 214
perphenazine. *See* perphenazine
promazine, 212t
thioridazine, 212t, 214, 799
trifluoperazine, 212t, 214, 799
herb–drug interactions, 113t
mechanisms of action, 211f, 212–13
nursing considerations, 214
client teaching, 214
lifespan considerations, 214
nursing process focus, 216–17t
phensuximide, 180t
phentermine, 635, 636, 802
phentolamine, 140t, 723
phenylephrine, 138t
actions and uses, 137t, 138t
administration alerts, 138t
adverse effects, 138t, 414t
Canadian/U.S. trade names, 799
in cold/allergy combination
drugs, 582t
interactions, 138t
overdose treatment, 138t
pharmacokinetics, 138t
for specific conditions
eye irritation, 779, 779t
nasal congestion/allergic rhinitis, 582,
582t, 587t
shock, 414t
phenylpropanolamine, 635
phenytoin, 179t
actions and uses, 179t
administration alerts, 179t
adverse effects, 178t, 179t, 367t
interactions, 179t, 191
overdose treatment, 179t
pharmacokinetics, 179t
prescription ranking, 802
for specific conditions

dysrhythmias, 367t
seizures, 173t, 178, 178t
PHENYTOIN-LIKE AGENTS:
drugs classified as
carbamazepine. *See* carbamazepine
felbamate, 178, 178t
lamotrigine. *See* lamotrigine
valproic acid. *See* **valproic acid**
zonisamide, 178, 178t, 180
nursing considerations, 178–80
client teaching, 179–80
lifespan considerations, 179
phobias, 154, 792
phosgene, 24t
phosgene oxime, 24t
PhosLo. *See* calcium acetate
phosphodiesterase, 341, 792
PHOSPHODIESTERASE INHIBITORS:
adverse effects, 333t
drugs classified as
inamrinone, 333t
milrinone. *See* **milrinone**
mechanisms of action, 332f, 341
nursing considerations, 342
client teaching, 342
route and adult doses, 333t
therapeutic approach, 341
PHOSPHODIESTERASE-5 INHIBITORS:
adverse effects, 723, 723t
drugs classified as
sildenafil. *See* **sildenafil**
tadalafil, 723, 723t, 801
vardenafil, 723, 723t
nursing considerations, 723–24
client teaching, 724, 725t
Phospholine Iodide. *See* echothiophate
iodide
phospholipids, 287, 288f, 792
phosphorus/phosphate:
functions, 651, 651t
imbalances, 442t. *See also* hyperphosphatemia; hypophosphatemia
for nutritional and electrolyte
disorders
monobasic potassium and sodium
phosphate, 650t
monobasic potassium phosphate, 650t
potassium and sodium phosphates, 650t
potassium phosphate, 650t
recommended dietary allowance, 651t
photosensitivity:
definition, 792
with diuretics, 309
with tetracyclines, 495
Phthirus pubis, 756
physical dependence, 15, 119, 792. *See also*
substance abuse
Physostigma venenosum, 143
physostigmine, 143, 143t, 774t
phytonadione. *See* vitamin D
pilocarpine, 143t, 774t, 775, 799
pimecrolimus, 766
pimozide, 215t

pioglitazone, 690t
pioglitazone/metformin, 690t
Piper methysticum. See kava
piperacillin sodium, 489t, 490
piperacillin tazobactam, 489t
Pipracil. *See* piperacillin sodium
pirbuterol acetate, 597, 597t
pirenzepine, 621
piroxicam, 233t, 473t
Pitocin. *See* **oxytocin**
Pitressin. *See* **vasopressin**
pituitary gland:
anterior. *See* ANTERIOR PITUITARY AGENTS
disorders, 664t
hormone production, 662, 663f
posterior. *See* POSTERIOR PITUITARY AGENTS
Placidyl. *See* ethchlorvynol
Plan B, 704, 704t
planning, 67, 792
plaque, 346, 792
Plaquenil. *See* **hydroxychloroquine sulfate**
plaques, psoriasis, 766, 766f
Plasbumin. *See* **normal serum albumin**
plasma cells, 456, 792
plasma concentration, 52–53
plasma half-life ($t_{1/2}$), 53, 792
plasma membranes, 47–48
plasma protein fraction, 413t, 414
plasma volume expanders. *See* COLLOIDS
Plasmalyte, 413t
Plasmanate. *See* plasma protein fraction
Plasma-Plex. *See* plasma protein fraction
Plasmatein. *See* plasma protein fraction
plasmids, 487, 792
plasmin, 379, 792
plasminogen, 379, 792
Plasmodium, 524, 524f
PLATELET ENHANCERS:
drugs classified as
oprelvekin, 395t, 399, 462
nursing considerations, 399, 401
client teaching, 401
pharmacotherapy with, 399
Platinol. *See* cisplatin
Plavix. *See* **clopidogrel**
Plenaxis. *See* abarelix
Plendil. *See* felodipine
Pletal. *See* cilostazol
plicamycin, 563, 564t
PMS Benztropine. *See* **benztropine**
PMS Isoniazid. *See* **isoniazid**
PMS Sulfasalazine. *See* sulfasalazine
pneumococcal infections, 484t
pneumococcal vaccines, 460t
Pneumococci, 485t
*Pneumocystis carinii (Pneumocystic
jiroveci),* 515t
pneumonia, 485t
Pneumovax 34. *See* pneumococcal vaccines
PNS (peripheral nervous system),
131, 132f, 792
Pnu-Immune 23. *See* pneumococcal
vaccines

Podophyllum peltatum, 566
poisoning:
　incidence, 83*t*
　prevention, 82
Poladex. *See* dexchlorpheniramine
Polaramine. *See* dexchlorpheniramine
Polargen. *See* dexchlorpheniramine
polarized, 364, 792
poliovirus, 22–23
poliovirus vaccine, 460*t*
Polycillin. *See* ampicillin
Polycose, 655
polyenes, 521*t*, 792
polyethylene glycol, 626*t*, 801
Polygam S/D. *See* immune globulin
polymeric formula, 655
polymyxin B, neomycin, and
　hydrocortisone, 780*t*
polypharmacy, 85, 792
polystyrene sulfate, 426*t*
polythiazide, 310*t*, 429*t*
polyvinyl alcohol, 779*t*
Ponstel. *See* mefenamic acid
Pontocaine. *See* tetracaine
Pork Regular Iletin II.
　　　See **regular insulin**
Posicor. *See* mibefradil
positive inotropic agents, 331
positive symptoms, 211, 792
posterior chamber, 771, 771*f*
POSTERIOR PITUITARY AGENTS:
　desmopressin, 664*t*, 665, 666
　lypressin, 664*t*
　vasopressin. *See* **vasopressin**
postganglionic neuron, 133, 792
postmarketing surveillance, 8, 792
postpartum, 792
post-traumatic stress disorder (PTSD),
　　155, 792
postural hypotension, 309
Posture. *See* calcium phosphate tribasic
potassium (K⁺):
　functions, 651*t*
　imbalances. *See* hyperkalemia;
　　hypokalemia
　in kidneys, 431
　in myocardial cells, 364
　pharmacotherapy with. *See* **potassium**
　　chloride
　recommended dietary allowance, 651*t*
　regulation, 443*f*, 444–45
potassium and sodium phosphates, 650*t*
POTASSIUM CHANNEL BLOCKERS:
　drugs classified as
　　amiodarone. *See* **amiodarone**
　　bretylium, 367*t*, 371
　　dofetilide, 367*t*, 371
　　ibutilide, 367*t*, 371
　　sotalol, 367*t*
　nursing considerations, 372
　　client teaching, 372
　　lifespan considerations, 372
　pharmacotherapy with, 371–72

potassium chloride (KCl), 446*t*
　actions and uses, 446*t*
　administration alerts, 446*t*
　adverse effects, 446*t*
　interactions, 446*t*
　ions, 442*t*
　nursing considerations, 445
　　client teaching, 445–46
　overdose treatment, 446*t*
　prescription ranking, 800
potassium iodide (KI), 24–25, 653, 668, 672
potassium ion channels, 364, 366*f*, 792
potassium phosphate, 650*t*
POTASSIUM-SPARING DIURETICS:
　adverse effects, 308, 310*t*, 333*t*
　drugs classified as
　　amiloride, 310*t*, 431*t*
　　eplerenone, 317, 431, 431*t*
　　spironolactone. *See* **spironolactone**
　　triamterene, 310*t*, 431*t*
　mechanisms of action, 427–28, 427*f*, 431
　for specific conditions
　　heart failure
　　　route and adult doses, 333*t*
　　　therapeutic approach, 335
　　hypertension
　　　combination drugs, 309*t*
　　　nursing considerations, 309
　　　route and adult doses, 310*t*
　　　therapeutic approach, 308
　　renal failure
　　　nursing considerations, 431–32
　　　therapeutic approach, 431
potency, 59–60, 60*f*, 792
PPF. *See* plasma protein fraction
pramipexole, 263, 263*t*, 264*f*
pramlintide, 691
pramoxine, 248*t*
Prandin. *See* repaglinide
Pravachol. *See* pravastatin
pravastatin, 292*t*, 800
praziquantel, 528*t*
prazosin, 141*t*
　actions and uses, 140*t*, 141*t*
　administration alerts, 141*t*
　adverse effects, 141*t*, 321*t*
　classification, 140*t*
　interactions, 141*t*
　overdose treatment, 141*t*
　pharmacokinetics, 141*t*
　for specific conditions
　　benign prostatic hypertrophy, 726*t*
　　hypertension, 321*t*
Precedex. *See* dexmedetomidine HCl
preclinical investigation, in drug
　　development, 7, 7*f*, 792
Precose. *See* acarbose
prednisolone, 476*t*, 675*t*, 799
prednisone, 477*t*
　actions and uses, 477*t*
　administration alerts, 477*t*
　adverse effects, 476*t*, 477*t*, 568*t*, 675*t*
　Canadian/U.S. trade names, 799

　interactions, 477*t*
　pharmacokinetics, 477*t*
　prescription ranking, 800
　for specific conditions
　　adrenocortical insufficiency, 675*t*
　　cancer, 568, 568*t*
　　inflammatory disorders, 476*t*
preganglionic neuron, 133, 792
pregnancy:
　anesthesia during, 254
　antiseizure drugs during, 171
　client teaching about drug therapy
　　during, 80–81
　depression after, 186
　drug registries, 79
　FDA drug categories, 78–79, 78*t*
　folic acid supplements in, 395*t*, 648*t*
　gestational age and drug therapy
　　first trimester, 77
　　prenatal stage, 77
　　second trimester, 77
　　third trimester, 78
　pharmacodynamic changes
　　absorption, 77
　　distribution and metabolism, 77
　　excretion, 77
　pharmacological agents for early
　　termination
　　carboprost tromethamine, 704*t*, 705
　　dinoprostone, 704*t*, 705
　　methotrexate with misoprostol,
　　　704*t*, 705
　　mifepristone with misoprostol,
　　　704*t*, 705
Pregnyl. *See* human chorionic gonadotropin
preload, 331, 331*f*, 792
Prelone. *See* prednisolone
Premarin. *See* **estrogen/progestin**
　　conjugated estrogens
premature atrial contractions, 363*t*
premature ventricular contractions
　　(PVCs), 363*t*
Prempro. *See* **conjugated estrogens with**
　　medroxyprogesterone
prenatal stage, 77, 792. *See also* pregnancy
Prepidil. *See* dinoprostone
preschool child, 83, 792. *See also* children
Prescription Drug User Fee Act, 6*f*, 8
prescription drugs:
　abuse, 118
　brand-name vs. generic equivalents, 14
　consumer spending on, 5*t*
　dispensing, 4–5
　effect of costs on older adults, 8*t*
　marketing and promotional
　　spending, 14*t*
Pretz-D. *See* ephedrine
Prevacid. *See* lansoprazole
Preven, 704, 704*t*
Prevnar. *See* pneumococcal vaccines
Prezista. *See* darunavir
priapism, 325
prilocaine, 248*t*

Prilosec. *See* **omeprazole**
Primacor. *See* **milrinone**
primaquine, 523*t*
primary hypertension, 305.
        See also hypertension
Primatene. *See* **epinephrine**
Primaxin. *See* imipenem-cilastatin
primidone, 79*t*, 175*t*, 799
Prinivil. *See* **lisinopril**
Prinzmetal's (vasospastic) angina, 347, 795.
        See also angina pectoris
Privine. *See* naphazoline HCl
PRL (prolactin), 663*f*, 711, 792
PRN order, 31, 792
Probalan. *See* probenecid
Pro-Banthine. *See* propantheline
probenecid, 747, 748*t*, 799
procainamide, 368*t*
    actions and uses, 368*t*
    administration alerts, 368*t*
    adverse effects, 368*t*
    for dysrhythmias, 366*t*, 367*t*
    genetic polymorphisms affecting
        metabolism, 104*t*
    interactions, 368*t*
    overdose treatment, 368*t*
    pharmacokinetics, 368*t*
procaine, 247, 248*f*, 248*t*
Procan. *See* **procainamide**
procarbazine, 559*t*, 799
Procardia. *See* **nifedipine**
prochlorperazine, 635*t*
    actions and uses, 635*t*
    administration alerts, 635*t*
    adverse effects, 634*t*, 635*t*
    Canadian/U.S. trade names, 799
    interactions, 635*t*
    overdose treatment, 635*t*
    pharmacokinetics, 635*t*
    route and adult dose, 634*t*
Procyclid. *See* procyclidine hydrochloride
procyclidine hydrochloride, 267*t*, 799
Procytox. *See* **cyclophosphamide**
prodrugs, 50, 792
Profasi HP. *See* human chorionic
        gonadotropin
progesterone, 698, 708, 792. *See also*
        PROGESTINS
progesterone micronized, 709*t*
PROGESTINS:
    actions and uses, 709
    drugs classified as
        combination drugs
            conjugated estrogens with medroxy-
            progesterone. *See* **conjugated estro-
            gens with medroxyprogesterone**
            estradiol/drospirenone, 709*t*
            estradiol/norgestimate, 709*t*
            ethinyl estradiol/norethindrone
            acetate, 709*t*
            medroxyprogesterone acetate. *See*
                medroxyprogesterone acetate
            norethindrone, 699, 700*t*, 709*t*

norethindrone acetate, 709*t*
progesterone micronized, 709*t*
functions, 698, 708
nursing considerations, 709–10
    client teaching, 710
Prograf. *See* tacrolimus
proguanil, 523*t*, 524
prolactin (PRL), 663*f*, 711, 792
Proleukin. *See* aldesleukin
Prolixin. *See* fluphenazine
promazine, 212*t*
promethazine:
    as adjunct to general anesthesia, 256*t*, 258
    for allergic rhinitis, 581*t*
    Canadian/U.S. trade names, 799
    for nausea and vomiting, 634*t*
    prescription ranking, 801
Prometrium. *See* progesterone micronized
Pronestyl. *See* **procainamide**
propafenone, 367*t*
propantheline, 147*t*
Propine. *See* dipivefrin
Propionibacterium acnes, 761
propofol, 255*t*
propoxyphene hydrochloride, 227*t*, 799
propoxyphene N/APAP, 800
propoxyphene napsylate, 227*t*, 799
propranolol, 369*t*
    actions and uses, 140*t*, 369*t*
    administration alerts, 369*t*
    adverse effects, 165*t*, 238*t*, 321*t*,
        350*t*, 367*t*, 369*t*
    Canadian/U.S. trade names, 799
    ethnic/racial considerations, 371*t*
    genetic polymorphisms affecting
        metabolism, 104*t*, 371*t*
    interactions, 369*t*
    overdose treatment, 369*t*
    pharmacokinetics, 369*t*
    prescription ranking, 801
    for specific conditions
        angina and myocardial infarction, 350*t*
        anxiety, 165*t*
        dysrhythmias, 367*t*
        hypertension, 321*t*
        migraine, 238*t*
proprietary (trade) name, 13. *See also*
        brand-name drugs
propylthiouracil, 671*t*
    actions and uses, 670, 671*t*
    administration alerts, 671*t*
    adverse effects, 668*t*, 671*t*
    Canadian/U.S. trade names, 799
    interactions, 671*t*
    overdose treatment, 671*t*
    pharmacokinetics, 671*t*
    route and adult dose, 668*t*
Propyl-Thyracil. *See* **propylthiouracil**
Prorazin. *See* **prochlorperazine**
Proscar. *See* **finasteride**
Prosom. *See* estazolam
PROSTAGLANDINS:
    characteristics, 711, 792

drugs classified as
    bimatoprost, 773, 774*t*
    carboprost tromethamine, 704*t*,
        705, 711, 711*t*
    dinoprostone, 704*t*, 705, 711, 711*t*
    latanoprost. *See* **latanoprost**
    mifepristone, 704*t*, 705, 711
    misoprostol, 621, 704*t*, 705, 711*t*
    travoprost, 773, 774*t*
    unoprostone, 773, 774*t*
functions, 232–33
mechanisms of action, 472*t*, 474
for specific conditions
    as emergency contraception, 704*t*
    glaucoma, 773, 774*f*
    pharmacological abortion, 704*t*
    as tocolytics, 711, 711*t*
Prostaphlin. *See* oxacillin
prostate. *See* benign prostatic
        hypertrophy
Prostigmin. *See* neostigmine
Prostin E$_2$. *See* dinoprostone
protamine zinc insulin, 688
protease, 534, 792
PROTEASE INHIBITORS:
    adverse effects, 537*t*
    drugs classified as
        amprenavir, 537*t*
        atazanavir, 537*t*
        darunavir, 537*t*, 539
        fosamprenavir, 537*t*
        indinavir, 537*t*
        lopinavir/ritonavir, 537*t*
        nelfinavir, 537*t*
        ritonavir, 537*t*
        saquinavir. *See* **saquinavir**
        tipranavir, 537*t*
    herb–drug interactions, 113*t*
    nursing considerations, 539–40
        client teaching, 540, 543
    nursing process focus, 541–42*t*
    pharmacotherapy with, 538–39
    route and adult dose, 537*t*
Protenate. *See* plasma protein fraction
Proteus mirabilis, 485*t*
prothrombin, 379, 792
prothrombin activator, 378, 792
prothrombin time (PT), 380, 383, 792
protirelin, 664*t*
PROTON PUMP INHIBITORS:
    drugs classified as
        esomeprazole, 617, 617*t*, 800
        lansoprazole, 617*t*, 800
        omeprazole. *See* **omeprazole**
        pantoprazole, 617, 617*t*, 800
        rabeprazole, 617*t*, 801
    mechanisms of action, 614*f*, 793
    nursing considerations, 617–18
        client teaching, 618
    pharmacotherapy with, 617–18
Protonix. *See* pantoprazole
Protopic. *See* tacrolimus
prototype drug, 12–13, 793

protozoal infections:
    incidence, 514*t*
    malaria. *See* malaria
    nonmalarial, 526*t*
protozoans, 522, 793
protriptyline, 189*t*, 799
Protropin. *See* somatrem
Proventil. *See* albuterol
Provera. *See* **medroxyprogesterone acetate**
provitamins, 642, 793
Prozac. *See* fluoxetine
Prozine. *See* promazine
pruritus, 753, 793
pseudoephedrine:
    actions and uses, 137, 137*t*
    in combination cold/allergy drugs, 582*t*
    methamphetamine abuse and, 588*t*
    for nasal decongestion, 587*t*
pseudohermaphrodism, 678
pseudomembranous colitis, antibiotic-associated, 491, 502
Pseudomonas aeruginosa, 485*t*, 487
psilocybin, 123*f*, 124
psoralens, 768, 793
Psorcon. *See* diflorasone
psoriasis:
    characteristics, 766, 766*f*
    drugs triggering, 766
    etiology, 766
    nonpharmacological therapy, 768
    pharmacotherapy
        systemic
            acitretin, 767*t*, 768
            cyclosporine. *See* **cyclosporine**
            etanercept, 767*t*, 768
            etretinate, 767*t*, 768
            hydroxyurea, 767*t*, 768
            infliximab, 768
            methotrexate. *See* **methotrexate**
        topical, 768
            calcipotriene, 767*t*, 768
            tacrolimus, 767*t*, 768
            tazarotene, 767*t*, 768
        types, 766*t*
psoriasis vulgaris, 766*t*
psoriatic arthritis, 766*t*
psoriatic erythroderma, 766*t*
psychedelics, 123, 793. *See also* hallucinogens
psychodynamic therapy, for depression, 187
psychological dependence, 15, 119, 793. *See also* substance abuse
psychology, 101, 793
psychoses. *See also* schizophrenia
    characteristics, 210, 210*t*
    incidence, 210*t*
    pharmacotherapy. *See* ANTIPSYCHOTICS
psyllium mucilloid, 627*t*
    actions and uses, 627*t*
    administration alerts, 627*t*
    adverse effects, 627*t*
    Canadian/U.S. trade names, 799

interactions, 627*t*
    pharmacokinetics, 627*t*
PT (prothrombin time), 380, 383, 792
PTCA (percutaneous transluminal coronary angioplasty), 348, 792
PTH (parathyroid hormone), 733, 734*f*
PTSD (post-traumatic stress disorder), 155, 792
PTU. *See* **propylthiouracil**
pubic lice, 756–57
Public Health Service Act, 6*f*
Pulmicort Turbuhaler. *See* budesonide
Pulmocare, 655
Pulmophylline. *See* theophylline
Pulmozyme. *See* dornase alfa
Pure Food and Drug Act, 5, 6*f*
Purge. *See* castor oil
purine, 561, 793
PURINE ANALOGS. *See also* ANTIMETABOLITES
    cladribine, 561*t*
    clofarabine, 561
    fludarabine, 561*t*
    mercaptopurine, 555*f*, 561*t*
    nelarabine, 561*t*
    pentostatin, 561*t*
    thioguanine, 561*t*, 562*f*
Purinethol. *See* mercaptopurine
Purkinje fibers, 364, 793
push (IV bolus) administration, 43, 43*f*
push package, 21
pustular psoriasis, 766*t*
pyrantel, 528*t*
pyrazinamide, 507*t*, 799
pyrethrin, 757
Pyribenzamine. *See* tripelennamine
pyridostigmine, 143, 143*t*
pyridoxine. *See* vitamin B$_6$
pyrimethamine, 523*t*
pyrimidine, 561, 793
PYRIMIDINE ANALOGS. *See also* ANTIMETABOLITES
    azacitidine, 561, 561*t*
    capecitabine, 561*t*
    cytarabine, 555*f*, 561, 561*t*
    floxuridine, 561*t*
    fluorouracil, 555, 555*f*, 561*t*, 562*f*
    gemcitabine, 561*t*
PZA. *See* pyrazinamide
PZI. *See* protamine zinc insulin

Q

quazepam, 162*t*
Questran. *See* **cholestyramine**
quetiapine fumarate, 218*t*, 800
Quinaglute. *See* quinidine gluconate
Quinamm. *See* quinine
quinapril, 333*t*, 801
quinethazone, 429*t*
Quinidex. *See* quinidine sulfate
quinidine gluconate, 367*t*
quinidine polygalacturonate, 367*t*
quinidine sulfate, 367*t*, 799
quinine, 279*t*, 523*t*, 799, 801

quinupristin–dalfopristin, 503*t*, 506
Quiphile. *See* quinine

R

rabeprazole, 617*t*, 801
rabies immune globulin, 458*t*
racial considerations. *See* ethnic/racial considerations
radiation sickness, 24
radiation therapy, 554
radioactive iodine, 80, 653, 668*t*, 670
Radiostol. *See* ergocalciferol
raloxifene, 744*t*
    actions and uses, 569, 744*t*
    administration alerts, 744*t*
    adverse effects, 741*t*, 744*t*
    interactions, 744*t*
    pharmacokinetics, 744*t*
    prescription ranking, 801
    route and adult dose, 741*t*
ramipril, 316*t*, 333*t*, 800
ranitidine bismuth citrate, 620
ranitidine HCl, 615*t*
    actions and uses, 615*t*
    administration alerts, 615*t*
    adverse effects, 615*t*
    Canadian/U.S. trade names, 799
    interactions, 615*t*
    pharmacokinetics, 615*t*
    prescription ranking, 800
    route and adult dose, 615*t*
Rapamune. *See* sirolimus
rapid eye movement (REM) sleep, 158, 158*t*, 793
RAS (reticular activating system), 155, 793
RDS (respiratory distress syndrome), 606*t*
reabsorption, tubular, 425, 793
Reactine. *See* cetirizine
reasonable and prudent action, 92, 793
Rebif. *See* interferon beta-1a
rebound congestion, 587
rebound insomnia, 157, 793
receptors, 60–61, 61*f*, 793
Recombivax HB. *See* **hepatitis B vaccine**
Recommended Dietary Allowances (RDAs):
    definition, 643, 793
    macrominerals, 651*t*
    microminerals, 653*t*
    vitamins, 643*t*
Recommended Nutrient Intake (RNI), 643
rectal drug administration, 36*t*, 37–38
Rectocort. *See* **hydrocortisone**
rectum, 625*f*
red-man syndrome, 506, 793
Redona. *See* denagliptin
reflex tachycardia, 314, 324, 793
Refludan. *See* lepirudin
refractory period, 365, 793
regional anesthesia, 245
Regitine. *See* phentolamine
Reglan. *See* metoclopramide
Regular Iletin II. *See* **regular insulin**

regular insulin, 686t
actions and uses, 686t
administration alerts, 686t
adverse effects, 685t, 686t
interactions, 686t
overdose treatment, 686t
pharmacokinetics, 686t
route and adult dose, 685t
Regular Purified Pork Insulin. *See* **regular insulin**
Regulax. *See* docusate
Relafen. *See* nabumetone
releasing hormones, 662, 793
Relenza. *See* zanamivir
religious affiliation, disease incidence and, 102t
Relpax. *See* eletriptan
REM (rapid eye movement) sleep, 158, 158t, 793
Remeron. *See* mirtazapine
Remicade. *See* infliximab
remifentanil hydrochloride, 255t, 256t
Reminyl. *See* galantamine hydrobromide
Renagel. *See* sevelamer
renal failure:
causes, 424t
classification, 426
definition, 425
diagnosis, 425–26
drugs causing, 426, 426t
incidence, 424t
pathophysiology, 424t, 425
pharmacotherapy
carbonic anhydrase inhibitors
acetazolamide, 433, 433t
dichlorphenamide, 433t
methazolamide, 433t
loop diuretics. *See* LOOP DIURETICS
osmotic diuretics
mannitol, 433, 433t
urea, 433, 433t
therapeutic approach, 426, 426t
thiazide diuretics. *See* THIAZIDE DIURETICS
Renese. *See* polythiazide
renin–angiotensin system:
characteristics, 316–17, 317f, 793
drugs affecting. *See* ANGIOTENSIN II RECEPTOR BLOCKERS; ANGIOTENSIN-CONVERTING ENZYME (ACE) INHIBITORS
in fluid balance, 439
in hypertension, 305, 305f, 317, 317f
ReoPro. *See* abciximab
repaglinide, 690t
repetitive transcranial magnetic stimulation (rTMS), 187
repository corticotropin, 674
Repronex. *See* human menopausal gonadotropin–menotropins
Requip. *See* ropinirole
Rescriptor. *See* delavirdine
Rescula. *See* unoprostone
reserpine, 321t

resistance, 487, 487f
respiration, 594, 793
respiratory acidosis, 447t. *See also* acidosis
respiratory distress syndrome (RDS), 606t
rest-and-digest response, 132, 793
Restoril. *See* temazepam
Resyl. *See* guaifenesin
Retavase. *See* **reteplase**
reteplase, 357t
actions and uses, 357t
administration alerts, 357t
adverse effects, 357t, 388t
interactions, 357t
pharmacokinetics, 357t
route and adult dose, 388t
reticular activating system (RAS), 155, 793
reticular formation, 124, 155, 155f, 793
Retin-A. *See* tretinoin
RETINOIDS:
characteristics, 762, 793
drugs classified as
adapalene, 761t, 762
isotretinoin. *See* **isotretinoin**
tretinoin, 761t, 762
retinol. *See* **vitamin A**
Retrovir. *See* **zidovudine**
reverse cholesterol transport, 289, 793
reverse transcriptase, 534, 793
REVERSE TRANSCRIPTASE INHIBITORS. *See* ANTIRETROVIRALS
Revex. *See* nalmefene hydrochloride
ReVia. *See* naltrexone hydrochloride
Revimine. *See* **dopamine**
Reyataz. *See* atazanavir
Reye's syndrome, 233, 475, 479, 793
Rezulin. *See* troglitazone
rhabdomyolysis, 291, 793
Rheomacrodex. *See* **dextran 40**
rheumatoid arthritis:
characteristics, 745–46, 746f, 793
incidence, 746t
pharmacotherapy. *See* DISEASE-MODIFYING ANTIRHEUMATIC DRUGS
rheumatoid factors, 746
Rheumatrex. *See* **methotrexate**
Rhinocort. *See* budesonide
rhinophyma, 761, 793
Rhodis. *See* ketoprofen
RhoGAM. *See* Rho(D) immune globulin
Rho(D) immune globulin, 458t
ribavirin/interferon alpha-2b, 548t
riboflavin. *See* vitamin B$_2$
rickets. *See* osteomalacia
Rickettsia rickettsii, 485t
RID. *See* pyrethrin
Ridaura. *See* auranofin
Rifadin. *See* rifampin
rifampin, 191, 507t, 508, 799
rifapentine, 507t
Rifater, 507t
Rimactane. *See* rifampin

rimantadine, 546, 547t
ringworm, 515t
Riopan. *See* magaldrate
risedronate sodium, 741t, 800
risk management, 96, 793
Risperdal. *See* risperidone
risperidone, 218, 218t, 271, 801
Ritalin. *See* **methylphenidate**
ritodrine, 137t, 711, 711t
ritonavir, 537t
Rituxan. *See* rituximab
rituximab, 571t
rivastigmine, 143t, 269, 269t
Rivotril. *See* clonazepam
rizatriptan, 238t
RNI (Recommended Nutrient Intake), 643
Robaxin. *See* methocarbamol
Robidone. *See* hydrocodone bitartrate
Robinul. *See* glycopyrrolate
Robitussin. *See* guaifenesin
Robitussin A-C, 590t
Rocaltrol. *See* **calcitriol**
Rocephin. *See* ceftriaxone
Rocky Mountain spotted fever, 485t
Rofact. *See* rifampin
rofecoxib, 233, 474
Roferon-A. *See* **interferon alfa-2a**
Rolaids. *See* calcium carbonate with magnesium hydroxide
Romazicon. *See* flumazenil
Rondomycin. *See* methacycline
ropinirole, 263, 263t, 264f
ropivacaine, 248t
rosacea:
characteristics, 761, 761f, 793
pharmacotherapy, 762, 764
rosiglitazone, 690t, 800
rosiglitazone/glimepiride, 690t
rosiglitazone/metformin, 690t
rosuvastatin, 292t, 801
roundworms, 528
routine orders, 31, 793
Roxicet. *See* oxycodone terephthalate
rTMS (repetitive transcranial magnetic stimulation), 187
rubella, 756
rubeola, 756
Rubex. *See* **doxorubicin**
Rythmodan. *See* disopyramide phosphate
Rythmol. *See* propafenone

S

SA (sinoatrial) node, 363, 794
SAD (seasonal affective disorder), 187
Safe Medicine, 96
Salagen. *See* pilocarpine
Salbutamol. *See* albuterol
SALICYLATES:
aspirin. *See* **aspirin**
choline salicylate, 233t
salsalate, 233t
salicylism, 474, 793

salmeterol, 598*t*

actions and uses, 137*t*, 597, 598*t*

administration alerts, 598*t*

adverse effects, 597*t*, 598*t*

interactions, 598*t*

overdose treatment, 598*t*

pharmacokinetics, 598*t*

route and adult dose, 597*t*

salmeterol/fluticasone, 800

Salmonella enteritidis, 485*t*

Salmonella typhi, 485*t*

salsalate, 233*t*

Saluron. *See* hydroflumethiazide

Sandimmune. *See* cyclosporine

Sandoglobulin. *See* immune globulin
    intravenous

Sandostatin. *See* octreotide

Sansert. *See* methysergide

saquinavir, 540*t*

actions and uses, 540*t*

administration alerts, 540*t*

adverse effects, 537*t*, 540*t*

interactions, 540*t*

pharmacokinetics, 540*t*

route and adult dose, 537*t*

sarcoma, 553*t*, 793

Sarcoptes scabiei, 756

sargramostim, 395*t*, 398

Sarin, 24*t*

saw palmetto, 110*t*, 727*t*, 728*t*

saxagliptin, 691

Scabene. *See* **lindane**

SCABICIDES:

characteristics, 757, 793

drugs classified as

crotamiton, 757

lindane. *See* **lindane**

permethrin, 757

nursing considerations, 757–58

client teaching, 758

lifespan considerations, 758

nursing process focus, 759*t*

pharmacotherapy with, 757

scabies:

characteristics, 756, 756*f*, 793

pharmacotherapy. *See* SCABICIDES

psychosocial and community impact, 758*t*

scheduled drugs:

Canada, 16*t*

definition, 15, 793

U.S., 15, 15*t*

schizoaffective disorder, 211, 793

schizophrenia:

definition, 210, 793

pathophysiology, 211, 211*f*

pharmacotherapy, 212. *See also*
    ANTIPSYCHOTICS

atypical antipsychotics. *See* ATYPICAL
    ANTIPSYCHOTICS

dopamine system stabilizers, 221

mechanisms of action, 211*f*

nonphenothiazines. *See*
    NONPHENOTHIAZINES

nursing considerations, 214, 217–18,
    218–19

client teaching, 214, 218, 219

lifespan considerations, 214, 218, 219

nursing process focus, 216–17*t*, 220–21*t*

phenothiazines. *See* PHENOTHIAZINES

signs and symptoms, 210–11

school-age child, 83, 793. *See also* children

scopolamine:

actions and uses, 147, 147*t*

as antiemetic, 633, 634*t*

Canadian/U.S. trade names, 799

as cycloplegic, 779*t*

scurvy, 647, 793

seasonal affective disorder (SAD), 187

Seasonale, 700

Seasonique, 700

seborrhea, 761, 793

seborrheic dermatitis, 765

secobarbital:

Canadian/U.S. trade names, 799

as general anesthesia adjunct, 256*t*

for sedation and insomnia, 164*t*

for seizures, 175*t*

Seconal. *See* secobarbital

second messenger events, 61, 793

second trimester, drug therapy during, 77.
    See also pregnancy

secondary hypertension, 305

secretion, tubular, 425, 793

Sectral. *See* acebutolol

sedative–hypnotics, 121, 159, 793

sedatives, 121, 159, 793

seizures:

age-related factors, 171*t*

causes, 170–71, 171*t*

definition, 170, 793

EEG recordings, 170*f*

genetic factors, 171*t*

incidence, 172*t*

natural therapy with ketogenic diet, 173*t*

pharmacotherapy. *See also* ANTISEIZURE DRUGS

nursing considerations, 178–80, 181

nursing process focus, 182–83*t*

by seizure type, 173*t*

therapeutic approach, 171–73

types, 170*f*, 171, 172*t*

SELECTIVE ESTROGEN-RECEPTOR MODIFIERS
    (SERMS):

characteristics, 569, 743, 793

drugs classified as

raloxifene. *See* **raloxifene**

tamoxifen. *See* **tamoxifen**

toremifene, 568*t*, 569

for osteoporosis, 743

SELECTIVE SEROTONIN REUPTAKE INHIBITORS
    (SSRIs):

adverse effects, 160, 160*t*, 189*t*, 193, 478

drugs classified as

citalopram, 160*t*, 189*t*, 271, 800

dolasetron, 634*t*

escitalopram oxalate. *See* **escitalopram
    oxalate**

fluoxetine, 160*t*, 189*t*, 271, 800

fluvoxamine, 160*t*, 189*t*

granisetron, 634*t*

ondansetron, 634*t*

palonosetron, 634*t*

paroxetine, 160*t*, 189*t*, 800, 801

sertraline. *See* **sertraline**

sibutramine. *See* **sibutramine**

herb–drug interactions, 113*t*

mechanisms of action, 192, 192*f*, 793

nursing considerations, 194

client teaching, 194

nursing process focus, 197–99*t*

for specific conditions

anxiety, 160*t*

depression, 189*t*, 193

nausea and vomiting, 633, 634*t*

selegiline hydrochloride, 263, 263*t*

selenium, 554*t*, 653*t*

senior citizens. *See* older adults

senna:

adverse effects, 626*t*

drug interactions, 179*t*, 477*t*, 676*t*

mechanisms of action, 627

route and adult dose, 626*t*

Septa. *See* **trimethoprim–sulfamethoxazole**

septic shock, 410, 410*t*, 412*t*, 793

septicemia, 485*t*

Septodont. *See* articaine

Septra. *See* **trimethoprim– sulfamethoxazole**

Serax. *See* oxazepam

Serentil. *See* mesoridazine

Serevent. *See* **salmeterol**

SERMS. *See* SELECTIVE ESTROGEN-RECEPTOR
    MODIFIERS

Serophene. *See* clomiphene

Seroquel. *See* quetiapine fumarate

serotonin syndrome (SES), 193, 478, 794

serotonin–norepinephrine reuptake
    inhibitors (SNRIs), 188, 189*t*. *See
    also* ATYPICAL ANTIDEPRESSANTS

Serpasil. *See* reserpine

sertaconazole, 519*t*

sertraline, 193*t*

actions and uses, 193*t*, 271

administration alerts, 193*t*

adverse effects, 160*t*, 189*t*, 193*t*

interactions, 193*t*

overdose treatment, 193*t*

pharmacokinetics, 193*t*

prescription ranking, 800

for specific conditions

anxiety, 160*t*

depression, 189*t*

Serzone. *See* nefazodone

sevelamer, 426*t*

sevoflurane, 252*t*

Sherley Amendment, 5, 6*f*

shingles, 545*t*

shock:

definition, 410, 794

mortality rates, 410*t*

pathophysiology, 412*f*

shock (*continued*)
  pharmacotherapy
    effects, 412*f*
    fluid replacement agents. *See* FLUID
        REPLACEMENT AGENTS
    inotropic agents. *See* INOTROPIC AGENTS
    vasoconstrictors. *See*
        VASOCONSTRICTORS
  signs and symptoms, 410, 411*f*
  treatment priorities, 411
  types, 410, 412*t*
short stature, 664, 664*t*
short-term (behavioral) insomnia,
    157, 794
sibutramine, 636*t*
  actions and uses, 636*t*
  administration alerts, 636*t*
  adverse effects, 636*t*
  interactions, 636*t*
  overdose treatment, 636*t*
  pharmacokinetics, 636*t*
sildenafil, 724*t*
  actions and uses, 724*t*
  administration alerts, 724*t*
  adverse effects, 723*t*, 724*t*
  interactions, 724*t*
  pharmacokinetics, 724*t*
  prescription ranking, 800
  route and adult dose, 723*t*
silent angina, 347. *See also* angina pectoris
simethicone, 619
simple partial seizure, 172*t*
Simron. *See* ferrous gluconate
Simulect. *See* basiliximab
simvastatin, 30*t*, 292*t*, 800
Sinemet. *See* carbidopa-levodopa
Sinequan. *See* doxepin
single order, 31, 794
Singulair. *See* montelukast
sinoatrial (SA) node, 363, 794
sinus bradycardia, 363*t*
sinus rhythm, 363, 794
sinusitis, 485*t*
Sinutab Sinus Allergy tablets, 582*t*
sirolimus, 465*t*, 466
sitagliptin, 690*t*, 691
situational anxiety, 154, 794
Skelaxin. *See* metaxalone
SKELETAL MUSCLE RELAXANTS:
  drugs classified as
    baclofen, 276, 276*t*
    carisoprodol, 276*t*, 800
    chlorphenesin, 276*t*
    chlorzoxazone, 276*t*
    clonazepam. *See* clonazepam
    cyclobenzaprine. *See* **cyclobenzaprine**
    diazepam. *See* **diazepam**
    lorazepam. *See* **lorazepam**
    metaxalone, 276*t*, 801
    methocarbamol, 276*t*
    orphenadrine, 276*t*
    tizanidine, 276, 276*t*, 802
  home care considerations, 281*t*

  mechanisms of action, 276
  nursing process focus, 280*t*
Skelid. *See* tiludronate disodium
skin:
  disorders
    acne. *See* acne vulgaris
    causes, 753–54
    classification, 754, 754*t*
    dermatitis. *See* dermatitis
    incidence, 754*t*
    infections, 754, 754*t*, 756
    inflammatory, 754, 754*t*
    neoplastic, 754, 754*t*
    parasites. *See* lice; scabies
    psoriasis. *See* psoriasis
    rosacea, 761, 761*f*, 762, 764
    self-esteem and, 765*t*
    sunburn and minor irritations,
        758–60
  interrelationships with other
      body systems, 755*f*
  layers, 753
  symptoms associated with changing
      health, age, or weakened immune
      system, 755*t*
sleep:
  functions, 156
  stages, 158, 158*t*
sleep debt, 158, 794
sleeping sickness, 526*t*
Slo-Mag. *See* magnesium chloride
smallpox, 23
smoking. *See* nicotine; tobacco use
SNRIs (serotonin–norepinephrine reuptake
    inhibitors), 188, 189*t*. *See also*
    ATYPICAL ANTIDEPRESSANTS
SNS (Strategic National Stockpile), 20, 794
social anxiety, 154, 794
sociology, 101, 794
sodium (Na$^+$):
  functions, 651*t*
  imbalances. *See* hypernatremia;
      hyponatremia
  in kidneys, 431
  in myocardial cells, 364
  pharmacotherapy with. *See* **sodium**
      bicarbonate
  recommended dietary allowance, 651*t*
  regulation, 443, 443*f*
sodium bicarbonate (NaHCO$_3$), 448*t*
  actions and uses, 448*t*
  administration alerts, 448*t*
  adverse effects, 448*t*, 650*t*
  interactions, 448*t*
  ions, 442*t*
  nursing considerations, 447–48
    client teaching, 449
  overdose treatment, 448*t*
  pharmacokinetics, 448*t*
  for specific conditions
    acidosis, 447, 448*t*
    as antacid, 619*t*
    nutritional and electrolyte disorders, 650*t*

sodium biphosphate, 626*t*
SODIUM CHANNEL BLOCKERS:
  drugs classified as
    disopyramide phosphate, 367*t*
    flecainide, 367*t*
    lidocaine. *See* **lidocaine**
    mexiletine, 367*t*
    phenytoin. *See* **phenytoin**
    procainamide. *See* **procainamide**
    propafenone, 367*t*
    quinidine gluconate, 367*t*
    quinidine polygalacturonate, 367*t*
    quinidine sulfate, 367*t*
    tocainide, 367*t*
  for dysrhythmias, 367*t*, 368
  as local anesthetics. *See* LOCAL
      ANESTHETICS
  nursing considerations, 369
    client teaching, 369
  nursing process focus, 370*t*
sodium chloride (NaCl), 444*t*
  actions and uses, 444*t*
  administration alerts, 444*t*
  adverse effects, 444*t*
  interactions, 444*t*
  ions, 442*t*
  nursing considerations, 444
    client teaching, 444
  pharmacokinetics, 444*t*
sodium hyaluronate, 745
sodium hydroxide, 246
sodium ion channels, 364, 366*f*, 794
sodium stibogluconate, 526*t*
sodium sulfate, 442*t*
Solarcaine. *See* **benzocaine**
Solazine. *See* trifluoperazine
Solganal. *See* aurothioglucose
Solium. *See* chlordiazepoxide
Solucalcine. *See* calcium chloride
Solu-Cortef. *See* **hydrocortisone**
Soma. *See* carisoprodol
Soman, 24*t*
somatic nervous system, 131, 794
somatic pain, 224
somatostatin, 665, 794
somatotropin, 664, 794
somatrem, 664, 664*t*
somatropin, 664*t*, 665
Somavert. *See* pegvisomant
Somogyi phenomenon, 684, 794
Somophyllin. *See* aminophylline
Somophyllin-12. *See* theophylline
Sonata. *See* zaleplon
sorafenib, 571, 571*t*
Sorbitrate. *See* **isosorbide**
    dinitrate
Soriatane. *See* acitretin
sotalol, 140*t*, 367*t*, 371
soy, 110*t*
soy isoflavone, 114*t*
sparfloxacin, 499*t*
Sparine. *See* promazine
spastic colon, 630

spasticity:
causes, 277
definition, 276–77, 794
home care considerations, 281t
nonpharmacological treatment, 277
pharmacotherapy. *See also*
ANTISPASMODICS
mechanisms of action, 278f
nursing considerations, 279
client teaching, 281
lifespan considerations, 281
nursing process focus, 280t
therapeutic approach, 278–79, 279t
Special Considerations:
ACE inhibitors and ethnicity, 320t
acetaminophen metabolism, ethnic/racial
considerations, 480t
adverse drug effects in older adults, 51t
age-related issues in drug
administration, 94t
alcoholism, cultural and environmental
influences, 101t
alcohol-related pancreatitis, 638t
Alzheimer's disease, 262t
androgen abuse by athletes, 720t
angina, influence of gender and
ethnicity, 348t
antibacterials, Hispanic cultural
beliefs, 488t
anticholinergics and male sexual
function, 147t
antimalarials and G6PD deficiency, 525t
antiretroviral drug compliance, psychosocial issues, 538t
Asians clients' sensitivity to
propranolol, 371t
botulinum toxin type A, 281t
chemotherapy in older adults, 570t
clients with speaking, visual, or hearing
impairments, 69t
cultural dietary habits, 291t
cultural remedies for diarrhea, 630t
depression, cultural influences, 187t
diabetes in children, psychosocial and
cultural impact, 688t
dietary supplements and the older
adult, 109t
enzyme deficiency in certain ethnic populations, 62t
estrogen use and psychosocial issues, 708t
ethnic groups and smoking, 126t
G6PD deficiency
acetaminophen and, 480t
antimalarials and, 525t
incidence, 62t
Giardia infections in children, 528t
H$_2$-receptor blockers and vitamin B$_{12}$ in
older adults, 617t
heart failure, psychosocial issues and
treatment compliance, 341t
helminthic infections in children, 527t
HIV in the pediatric and geriatric populations, 544t

hypothyroidism in shift workers, 667t
immunizations, cultural effects, 461t
laxatives' effect on fluid-electrolyte balance, 445t
mental illness, cultural views, 212t
non-English-speaking and culturally
diverse clients, 71t
osteoporosis, impacts of ethnicity and
lifestyle, 743t
pain expression and perception
age and, 231t
cultural influences, 225t
parasitic infections in children, 528t
Parkinson's disease, 262t
pediatric drug administration, 29t
pediatric drug research and labeling, 83t
pediatric dyslipidemias, 290t
pediculosis, psychosocial and community impact, 758t
prescription drug costs, effects on senior
citizens, 8t
religious affiliation and disease
incidence, 102t
respiratory distress syndrome, 606t
scabies, psychosocial and community impact, 758t
seizure etiologies based on genetics and
age-related factors, 171t
vitamin supplements and client communication, 645t
volatile inhalants abuse in children and
adolescents, 120t
zero tolerance in schools,
methylphenidate therapy and, 204t
specialty supplement, 114, 114t, 794
Spectazole. *See* econazole
Spectracef. *See* cefditoren pivoxil
Spectrobid. *See* bacampicillin
spinal anesthesia, 246f, 246t
spirilla, 485
spiritual therapies, 109t
spirituality, 101, 794
Spiriva. *See* tiotropium
spironolactone, 432t
actions and uses, 335, 432t
administration alerts, 432t
adverse effects, 310t, 333t, 431t, 432t
Canadian/U.S. trade names, 799
interactions, 432t
overdose treatment, 432t
pharmacokinetics, 432t
prescription ranking, 801
for specific conditions
heart failure, 333t, 335
hypertension, 309t, 310t
renal failure, 431t
Sporanox. *See* itraconazole
Sporothrix schenckii, 515t
sporotrichosis, 515t
SSRIs. *See* SELECTIVE SEROTONIN REUPTAKE
INHIBITORS
St. John's wort:
for depression, 193t

drug interactions
anesthetics, 245t
chlorpromazine, 213t
escitalopram, 161t
ethinyl estradiol with norethindrone,
702t
imipramine, 191t
medroxyprogesterone acetate, 710t
morphine sulfate, 228t
nevirapine, 539t
phenelzine, 196t
saquinavir, 540t
sertraline, 193t
sumatriptan, 239t
zidovudine, 538t
standardization, 110t
uses, 110t
stable angina, 347, 794. *See also* angina
pectoris
Stadol. *See* butorphanol tartrate
standards of care, 92, 794
standing orders, 31, 794
Staphylococcus aureus:
diseases caused by, 485t, 506
methicillin-resistant, 506
resistance to penicillin, 484t, 487
skin infections, 754
Starlix. *See* nateglinide
stasis dermatitis, 765
STAT order, 30, 794
Statex. *See* **morphine sulfate**
STATINS:
administration, 292
adverse effects, 291, 292t
coenzyme Q10 and, 295t
drugs classified as
atorvastatin. *See* **atorvastatin**
fluvastatin, 292t
lovastatin, 30t, 292t, 800
pravastatin, 292t, 800
rosuvastatin, 292t, 801
simvastatin, 30t, 292t, 800
mechanisms of action, 291, 294f
nursing considerations, 292
client teaching, 292–93
lifespan considerations, 292
nursing process focus, 296t
pharmacotherapy with, 291–92
status asthmaticus, 596
status epilepticus, 172t, 173t, 174, 794
stavudine, 537t, 543
steatorrhea, 638
Stelazine. *See* trifluoperazine
stem cell, 394–95, 394f, 794
Stemetil. *See* **prochlorperazine**
steroids, 287, 288f, 794
sterol nucleus, 287, 794
Stevens-Johnson syndrome, 28t
stevia, 691t
Stilbestrol. *See* diethylstilbestrol
Stimate. *See* desmopressin
stimulants, central nervous system:
amphetamines. *See* amphetamines

stimulants, central nervous system (*continued*)
caffeine, 104*t*, 125
cocaine. *See* cocaine
methylphenidate. *See* **methylphenidate**
pemoline, 203, 204*t*
STIs (structured treatment interruptions), 536
stomach, 611–12, 613*f*. *See also* upper gastrointestinal tract
Strategic National Stockpile (SNS), 20, 794
Strattera. *See* atomoxetine
stratum basale, 753
stratum corneum, 753
stratum granulosum, 753
stratum lucidum, 753
stratum spinosum, 753
Streptococcus, 485*t*, 754
Streptococcus pneumoniae, 484*t*, 506
streptogramins, 505
streptokinase, 388*t*
streptomycin, 498*t*, 507*t*
streptozocin, 559*t*
Striant, 719. *See also* **testosterone**
stroke volume, 303, 304*f*, 794
Stromectol. *See* ivermectin
structured treatment interruptions (STIs), 536
subcutaneous drug administration, 38–39, 40*t*, 41*f*, 794
subjective data, 67, 794
Sublimaze. *See* fentanyl
sublingual route, 33, 33*t*, 34*f*, 794
Suboxone, 232
substance abuse:
androgens, 719, 720*t*
definition, 118, 794
incidence and extent, 15*t*
neurobiological and psychosocial components, 118–19
nurse's role, 126
opioids
characteristics, 120*t*, 121
treatment, 232
withdrawal symptoms, 120*t*
overview, 118
physical dependence, 119
psychological dependence, 119
statistics, 119*t*
terminology, 14–15
tolerance, 120
volatile inhalants, 120*t*
withdrawal syndromes, 119, 120*t*
substance dependence, 119
substance P, 225, 225*f*, 794
substantia nigra, 262, 794
SUCCINIMIDES:
drugs classified as
ethosuximide. *See* **ethosuximide**
methsuximide, 180*t*
phensuximide, 180*t*
mechanisms of action, 180
nursing considerations
client teaching, 181
lifespan considerations, 181

succinylcholine, 257*t*
actions and uses, 257*t*
administration alerts, 257*t*
adverse effects, 256*t*, 257*t*
interactions, 257*t*
nursing considerations, 258
overdose treatment, 257*t*
pharmacokinetics, 257*t*
sucralfate, 620
Sudafed. *See* pseudoephedrine
Sudafed PE Nighttime, 582*t*
Sufenta. *See* sufentanil citrate
sufentanil citrate, 255*t*, 256*t*
sulbactam, 490
sulconazole, 519*t*
sulfacetamide, 501*t*, 761, 764
sulfadiazine, 501, 501*t*
sulfadoxine–pyrimethamine, 501, 501*t*
sulfamethizole, 501*t*
sulfamethoxazole, 501, 501*t*
sulfasalazine:
actions and uses, 501
adverse effects, 79*t*, 747*t*
Canadian/U.S. trade names, 799
for inflammatory bowel disease, 630
for rheumatoid arthritis, 746, 747*t*
sulfinpyrazone, 747, 748*t*, 799
sulfisoxazole, 501, 501*t*
sulfites, 247
SULFONAMIDES:
adverse effects, 501*t*
drugs classified as
sulfacetamide, 501*t*, 761, 764
sulfadiazine, 501, 501*t*
sulfadoxine–pyrimethamine, 501, 501*t*
sulfamethizole, 501*t*
sulfamethoxazole, 501, 501*t*
sulfasalazine. *See* sulfasalazine
sulfisoxazole, 501, 501*t*
trimethoprim–sulfamethoxazole. *See* **trimethoprim–sulfamethoxazole**
mechanisms of action, 501
nursing considerations, 501–2
client teaching, 502
pharmacotherapy with, 501
route and adult doses, 501*t*
SULFONYLUREAS:
adverse effects, 690*t*
characteristics, 689
drugs classified as
acetohexamide, 690*t*, 797
chlorpropamide, 690*t*, 797
glimepiride, 690*t*, 801
glipizide. *See* **glipizide**
glyburide, 690*t*, 798, 800
tolazamide, 690*t*
tolbutamide, 690*t*, 799
route and adult doses, 690*t*
sulfur, 651*t*
sulindac, 233*t*
sumatriptan, 239*t*
actions and uses, 239*t*
administration alerts, 239*t*

adverse effects, 238*t*, 239*t*
interactions, 239*t*
overdose treatment, 239*t*
pharmacokinetics, 239*t*
prescription ranking, 801
route and adult dose, 238*t*
Sumycin. *See* **tetracycline**
sunburn:
nursing considerations, 760
client teaching, 760
lifespan considerations, 760
pharmacotherapy, 758, 760*t*
prevention, 758
symptoms, 758–60
superficial mycosis, 515, 515*t*, 794
superinfections, 488, 794
supplements. *See also* Natural Therapies
dietary. *See* dietary supplements
herbal. *See* herbal therapies
specialty, 114, 114*t*, 794
Suprane. *See* desflurane
supraventricular, 362
Suprax. *See* cefixime
surface anesthesia, 245
surfactants, 606*t*
Surfak. *See* docusate
surgical anesthesia, 250, 794
Surmontil. *See* trimipramine
Survanta. *See* beractant
SusPhrine. *See* **epinephrine**
Sustacal Powder, 655
sustained-release tablets, 32, 794
Sustiva. *See* efavirenz
Symlin. *See* pramlintide
Symmetrel. *See* amantadine
sympathetic nervous system, 131, 132*f*, 133*f*, 794
SYMPATHOLYTICS. *See* ADRENERGIC ANTAGONISTS
SYMPATHOMIMETICS. *See* ADRENERGIC AGONISTS
Synalar. *See* fluocinolone
synapse, 132, 794
synaptic transmission, 133, 794
Synarel. *See* nafarelin
Synercid. *See* quinupristin–dalfopristin
Synthroid. *See* **levothyroxine**
Syntocinon. *See* **oxytocin**
systemic mycosis, 515, 515*t*, 794
systolic pressure, 302–3, 303*t*, 794. *See also* blood pressure

T

T cells, 459, 794
tablets:
administration guidelines, 32–33, 33*t*
crushing, 32
types, 32
Tabun, 24*t*
tacrine, 143*t*, 269, 269*t*
tacrolimus:
adverse effects, 465*t*, 767*t*
for dermatitis, 766
as immunosuppressant, 465*t*, 466
for psoriasis, 767*t*, 768

tadalafil, 723, 723t, 801
Tagamet. *See* cimetidine
Takeda. *See* aloglipton
Talwin. *See* pentazocine hydrochloride
Tambocor. *See* flecainide
Tamiflu. *See* oseltamivir
Tamofen. *See* **tamoxifen**
tamoxifen, 569t
   actions and uses, 569t
   administration alerts, 569t
   adverse effects, 568t, 569t
   Canadian/U.S. trade names, 799
   interactions, 569t
   pharmacokinetics, 569t
   for specific conditions
      breast cancer, 568t, 569
      male infertility, 721
tamsulosin, 726t, 727, 801
Tanacetum parthenium. See feverfew
Tao. *See* troleandomycin
Tapazole. *See* methimazole
tapeworms, 528
Tarabine. *See* cytarabine
Taractan. *See* chlorprothixene
Tarceva. *See* erlotinib
tardive dyskinesia, 213t, 214, 794
target tissue, 52
Targretin. *See* bexarotene
Tarka, 309t
Tasmar. *See* tolcapone
Tavist. *See* clemastine
Tavist Allergy 12-hour tablets, 582t
TAXANES:
   characteristics, 565, 794
   drugs classified as
      docetaxel, 565, 566t
      paclitaxel, 555f, 565, 566t
   nursing considerations, 566–67
      client teaching, 567
   pharmacotherapy with, 565
Taxus baccata, 565
tazarotene, 767t, 768
tazobactam, 490
Tazorac. *See* tazarotene
3TC. *See* lamivudine
TCAs. *See* TRICYCLIC ANTIDEPRESSANTS
TD$_{50}$ (median toxicity dose), 58–59, 790
tea, 111t
tea tree oil, 529t
Tebrazid. *See* pyrazinamide
Teebaconin. *See* **isoniazid**
tegaserod, 632t
   actions and uses, 630, 632t
   administration alerts, 632t
   adverse effects, 632t
   interactions, 632t
   nursing considerations, 631–32
   pharmacokinetics, 632t
Tega-Tussin Syrup, 590t
Tegison. *See* etretinate
Tegopen. *See* cloxacillin
Tegretol. *See* carbamazepine
telithromycin, 504t, 506

telmisartan, 316t
temazepam, 162t, 801
Temodar. *See* temozolomide
Temovate. *See* clobetasol
temozolomide, 559t
tenecteplase, 388, 388t
teniposide, 566, 566t
tenofovir, 536, 537t
Tenoretic. *See* atenolol/chlorthalidone
Tenormin. *See* **atenolol**
Tensilon. *See* edrophonium
tension headache, 237, 794
Tequin. *See* gatifloxacin
teratogen, 77, 795
Terazol. *See* terconazole
terazosin, 140t, 321t, 726t, 727, 801
terbinafine, 520t, 521
terbutaline:
   actions and uses, 137t
   adverse effects, 597t, 711t
   for asthma, 597, 597t
   as tocolytic, 711t, 712–13
terconazole, 519t
Terfluzine. *See* trifluoperazine
teriparatide, 740, 741t
Teslac. *See* testolactone
Tessalon. *See* benzonatate
Testim, 719. *See also* **testosterone**
Testoderm, 719. *See also* **testosterone**
Testoderm TTS, 719. *See also* **testosterone**
testolactone, 568t, 569, 720t, 721
Testone LA. *See* testosterone enanthate
Testopel, 719. *See also* **testosterone**
testosterone, 721t
   actions and uses, 721t
   administration alerts, 721t
   adverse effects, 568t, 720t, 721t
   Canadian/U.S. trade names, 799
   formulations, 719, 720t
   functions, 718, 719f, 795
   interactions, 721t
   pharmacokinetics, 721t
   secretion, 718
   for specific conditions
      cancer chemotherapy, 568t
      hypogonadism, 719, 720t
testosterone cypionate, 719, 720t
testosterone enanthate, 719, 720t, 799
Testred. *See* methyltestosterone
tetanus immune globulin, 458t
tetracaine, 248t, 760
tetracycline, 495t
   actions and uses, 495t
   administration alerts, 495t
   adverse effects, 494t, 495t
   Canadian/U.S. trade names, 799
   interactions, 495t
   pharmacokinetics, 495t
   route and adult doses, 494t
   for specific conditions
      acne, 761t
      H. pylori, 620
      skin infections (topical), 756

TETRACYCLINES:
   adverse effects, 494, 494t
   drugs classified as
      demeclocycline, 494t
      doxycycline. *See* doxycycline
      methacycline, 494t
      minocycline, 494, 494t, 801
      tetracycline. *See* **tetracycline**
      tigecycline, 494t, 506
   factors affecting absorption, 49
   nursing considerations, 494–95
      client teaching, 495–96
      lifespan considerations, 495
   pharmacotherapy with, 494
tetrahydrocannabinol (THC), 122, 123, 795
tetrahydrozoline, 587t, 779, 779t
Teveten. *See* eprosartan
TG. *See* thioguanine
thalidomide, 465t
Thalomid. *See* thalidomide
THC (tetrahydrocannabinol), 122, 123, 795
Theo-Dur. *See* theophylline
theophylline, 113t, 597t, 600, 799
TheraCys. *See* Bacillus Calmette-Guérin
      (BCG) vaccine
therapeutic classification, 12, 12t, 795
therapeutic index, 58–59, 58f, 795
Therapeutic Products Programme
      (TPP), 9
therapeutic range, 53, 53f, 795
therapeutics, 4, 795
thiamine. *See* vitamin B$_1$
THIAZIDE DIURETICS:
   adverse effects, 310t, 333t
   drugs classified as
      bendroflumethiazide, 429t
      benzthiazide, 310t, 429t
      chlorothiazide. *See* **chlorothiazide**
      chlorthalidone, 310t, 429t, 797
      hydrochlorothiazide. *See* **hy-
         drochlorothiazide**
      hydroflumethiazide, 429t
      indapamide, 310t, 429t, 798
      methyclothiazide, 429t
      metolazone, 310t, 429t
      polythiazide, 310t, 429t
      quinethazone, 429t
      trichlormethiazide, 310t, 429t
   mechanisms of action, 427, 427f
   for specific conditions
      heart failure
         nursing considerations, 335–36
         route and adult doses, 333t
         therapeutic approach, 335
      hypertension
         combination drugs, 309t
         nursing considerations, 309–11
         route and adult doses, 310t
         therapeutic approach, 308
      renal failure
         nursing considerations, 430–31
         route and adult dose, 429t
         therapeutic approach, 429–30

THIAZOLINEDIONES:
adverse effects, 690*t*
characteristics, 689–90
drugs classified as
pioglitazone, 690*t*, 800
rosiglitazone, 690*t*, 800
route and adult doses, 690*t*
thioguanine, 561*t*, 562*f*, 799
thiopental, 255*t*
actions and uses, 255*t*
administration alerts, 255*t*
adverse effects, 255*t*
interactions, 255*t*
overdose treatment, 255*t*
pharmacokinetics, 255*t*
Thioplex. *See* thiotepa
thioridazine, 212*t*, 214, 799
thiotepa, 559*t*
thiothixene, 215*t*
third trimester, drug therapy during, 78. *See also* pregnancy
Thorazine. *See* **chlorpromazine**
three checks of drug administration, 29, 795
thrombin, 379, 795
thrombocytopenia, 380, 795
thrombocytopoiesis, 399
thromboembolic disorders, 380, 795
THROMBOLYTICS:
drugs classified as
alteplase. *See* **alteplase**
anistreplase, 388*t*
reteplase. *See* **reteplase**
streptokinase, 388*t*
tenecteplase, 388, 388*t*
mechanisms of action, 381, 381*t*, 387, 795
nursing considerations, 357, 388–89
client teaching, 357, 389
nursing process focus, 389*t*
pharmacotherapy with, 355–56, 387–88
thrombopoietin, 399, 795
thrombus, 380, 795
Thypinone. *See* protirelin
Thyrar. *See* thyroid
Thyro-Block, 668*t*
Thyrogen. *See* thyrotropin
thyroid, 668*t*
THYROID AGENTS:
adverse effects, 668*t*
drugs classified as
levothyroxine. *See* **levothyroxine**
liothyronine, 668*t*
liotrix, 668*t*
thyroid, 668*t*
nursing considerations, 668
client teaching, 668, 670
lifespan considerations, 668
nursing process focus, 669–70*t*
pharmacotherapy with, 667–68
thyroid gland:
in calcium metabolism, 733, 734*f*
disorders, 664*t*, 666*t*. *See also* THYROID AGENTS
functions, 666–67, 667*f*

thyroid storm, 672, 795
Thyroid USP. *See* thyroid
thyroid-stimulating hormone (TSH), 663*f*, 664*t*
Thyrolar. *See* liotrix
thyrotoxic crisis, 672, 795
thyrotropin, 664*t*
thyroxine, 666
tiagabine, 175, 175*t*
Tiamate. *See* **diltiazem**
Tiazac. *See* **diltiazem**
Ticar. *See* ticarcillin
ticarcillin, 489*t*
Tice. *See* Bacillus Calmette-Guérin (BCG) vaccine
Ticlid. *See* ticlopidine
ticlopidine, 358, 386, 386*t*
tigecycline, 494*t*, 506
Tikosyn. *See* dofetilide
Tilade. *See* nedocromil sodium
tiludronate disodium, 741*t*
Timentin, 490
Timolide, 309*t*
timolol, 776*t*
actions and uses, 140*t*, 776*t*
administration alerts, 776*t*
adverse effects, 321*t*, 350*t*, 776*t*
interactions, 776*t*
pharmacokinetics, 776*t*
for specific conditions
angina and myocardial infarction, 350*t*
glaucoma, 773, 774*t*
hypertension, 321*t*
migraine, 238*t*
Timoptic. *See* **timolol**
Timoptic XE. *See* **timolol**
Tinactin. *See* tolnaftate
tincture, 111*f*
Tindamax. *See* tinidazole
tinea capitis, 515*t*, 756
tinea cruris, 515*t*, 520, 756
See also jock itch
tinea pedis, 515*t*, 520, 756
tinea unguium, 756
tinidazole, 526*t*, 527
tinzaparin, 382*t*
tioconazole, 519*t*
tiotropium, 597*t*, 599
tipranavir, 537*t*
tirofiban, 386*t*
tissue plasminogen activator (TPA), 379, 795
titer, 457, 795
Titralac. *See* calcium carbonate
tizanidine, 276, 276*t*, 802
TNKase. *See* tenecteplase
tobacco use. *See also* nicotine
ethnic considerations, 126*t*
fetal effects, 80*t*
tobramycin, 498*t*
tocainide, 367*t*
TOCOLYTICS:
characteristics, 710, 711, 795
drugs classified as

magnesium sulfate. *See* **magnesium sulfate**
nifedipine. *See* **nifedipine**
ritodrine, 137*t*, 711, 711*t*
terbutaline sulfate. *See* terbutaline
pharmacotherapy with, 711–12
tocopherols, 645, 795. *See also* vitamin E
toddlerhood, 82, 795. *See also* children
Tofranil. *See* **imipramine**
Tolamide. *See* tolazamide
tolazamide, 690*t*
tolbutamide, 690*t*, 799
tolcapone, 263, 263*t*
Tolectin. *See* tolmetin
tolerance, 120, 795
Tolinase. *See* tolazamide
tolmetin, 233*t*, 473*t*
tolnaftate, 520*t*, 521
tolterodine tartrate, 801
tonic spasm, 275, 795
tonic–clonic (grand mal) seizure, 172*t*, 173*t*, 795
tonicity, 439, 439*f*, 795
Tonocard. *See* tocainide
tonometry, 772, 795
Topamax. *See* topiramate
topical anesthesia, 246*f*, 246*t*. *See also* **benzocaine**
topical antibiotics, 756
topical drug administration. *See* drug administration, topical
topical glucocorticoids:
for dermatitis, 765–66, 765*t*
for psoriasis, 768
Topicort. *See* desoximetasone
Topicort LP. *See* desoximetasone
Topicycline. *See* **tetracycline**
topiramate, 175*t*, 200, 801
topoisomerase I, 566, 795
TOPOISOMERASE INHIBITORS:
drugs classified as
etoposide, 555*f*, 566, 566*t*
irinotecan, 566, 566*t*
teniposide, 566, 566*t*
topotecan, 555*f*, 566, 566*t*
nursing considerations, 566–67
client teaching, 567
pharmacotherapy with, 566
topotecan, 555*f*, 566, 566*t*
Toprol. *See* **metoprolol**
Toprol-XL. *See* **metoprolol**
Toradol. *See* ketorolac tromethamine
toremifene, 568*t*, 569
Tornalate. *See* bitolterol mesylate
torsades de pointes, 372
torsemide:
adverse effects, 310*t*, 333*t*
for heart failure, 333*t*
for hypertension, 310*t*
for renal failure, 428, 428*t*
tositumomab, 571*t*
total parenteral nutrition (TPN):
definition, 655, 795

indications, 655
  nursing considerations, 655
    client teaching, 655
    nursing process focus, 656–57*t*
toxic concentration, 53, 53*f*, 795
toxic epidermal necrolysis, 28*t*
toxic shock syndrome, 485*t*
toxins, 21, 795
toxoids, 456, 795
Toxoplasma gondii, 526*t*
toxoplasmosis, 526*t*
TPA. *See* **alteplase**
TPA (tissue plasminogen activator), 379, 795
TPN. *See* total parenteral nutrition
TPP (Therapeutic Products Programme), 9
trabecular meshwork, 772
trace minerals. *See* MICROMINERALS
trade (proprietary) name, 13, 795. *See also*
    brand-name drugs
tramadol, 233*t*, 800, 802
tramadol/acetaminophen, 802
Trandate. *See* labetalol
trandolapril, 316*t*
tranexamic acid, 390*t*
tranquilizer, 159, 795. *See also* sedatives
transdermal drug administration, 35, 35*f*, 36*t*
Transderm-Scop. *See* scopolamine
Transderm-V. *See* scopolamine
transferrin, 403, 795
transplant rejection, 463, 795
Tranxene. *See* clorazepate
tranylcypromine, 159*t*, 189*t*
trastuzumab, 570, 571*t*
Trasylol. *See* aprotinin
Travatan. *See* travoprost
traveler's diarrhea, 485*t*
travoprost, 773, 774*t*
trazodone, 160*t*, 188, 189*t*, 800
Trental. *See* pentoxifylline
tretinoin, 761*t*, 762
Trexan. *See* naltrexone hydrochloride
Triacin-C Cough Syrup, 590*t*
Triadapin. *See* doxepin
triamcinolone:
  adverse effects, 476*t*, 601*t*, 675*t*
  prescription ranking, 801
  for specific conditions
    adrenocortical insufficiency, 585*t*, 675*t*
    asthma, 601*t*
    severe inflammation, 476*t*
    topical, 765*t*
Triaminic Cold/Allergy, 582*t*
triamterene, 310*t*, 431*t*
triamterene/HCTZ, 800
Triassic. *See* **diltiazem**
triazolam, 162*t*
trichlormethiazide, 310*t*, 429*t*
Trichomonas vaginalis, 526*t*
trichomoniasis, 526*t*
Trichophyton, 515*t*
Tricor. *See* fenofibrate
TRICYCLIC ANTIDEPRESSANTS (TCAs):
  adverse effects, 159*t*, 160, 189*t*

contraindications, 160
definition, 795
drugs classified as
  amitriptyline. *See* amitriptyline
  amoxapine, 189*t*
  clomipramine, 159*t*, 188
  desipramine, 159*t*, 189*t*, 204
  doxepin, 159*t*, 189*t*, 798
  imipramine. *See* **imipramine**
  maprotiline, 188, 189*t*
  nortriptyline, 159*t*, 189*t*, 802
  protriptyline, 189*t*, 799
  trimipramine, 189*t*
herb–drug interactions, 113*t*
mechanisms of action, 188, 190*f*
nursing considerations, 190–91
  client teaching, 191–92
  nursing process focus, 197–99*t*
for specific conditions
  ADHD, 204
  depression, 188, 189*t*, 190
  enuresis, 188
  migraine, 238*t*
  obsessive-compulsive disorder, 188
  panic disorders, 159*t*
Tridesilon. *See* desonide
triethanolamine polypeptide oleate 10%
    condensate, 780*t*
trifluoperazine, 212*t*, 214, 799
trifluridine, 544*t*, 545
triglycerides:
  characteristics, 287, 288*f*, 795
  laboratory values, 290*f*
trihexyphenidyl, 147*t*, 267*t*, 799
Tri-Immunol. *See* diphtheria, tetanus, and
    pertussis vaccine
triiodothyronine, 666
Trilafon. *See* perphenazine
Trileptal. *See* oxcarbazepine
Tri-Levlen, 700*t*
trimethoprim–sulfamethoxazole, 502*t*
  actions and uses, 502*t*
  administration alerts, 502*t*
  adverse effects, 502*t*
  interactions, 502*t*
  overdose treatment, 502*t*
  pharmacokinetics, 502*t*
  prescription ranking, 800
  route and adult dose, 502*t*
trimetrexate, 526*t*
trimipramine, 189*t*
Trimox. *See* amoxicillin
Trinalin, 581*t*
Trinessa, 801
Triostat. *See* liothyronine
Tripedia. *See* diphtheria, tetanus, and
    pertussis vaccine
tripelennamine, 581*t*, 799
Triphasil, 700*t*
triprolidine, 581*t*
TRIPTANS:
  drugs classified as
    almotriptan, 238*t*

    eletriptan, 238*t*
    frovatriptan, 238*t*
    naratriptan, 238*t*
    rizatriptan, 238*t*
    sumatriptan. *See* **sumatriptan**
    zolmitriptan, 238*t*
  nursing considerations, 237–41
    client teaching, 241
    nursing process focus, 240*t*
Triptil. *See* protriptyline
Trisenox. *See* arsenic trioxide
Tritec. *See* ranitidine bismuth citrate
troglitazone, 8, 689
troleandomycin, 496*t*
Tronothane. *See* pramoxine
Tropicacyl. *See* tropicamide
tropicamide, 779*t*
troponin I, 355*t*
troponin T, 355*t*
trovafloxacin mesylate, 499, 499*t*
Trovan. *See* trovafloxacin mesylate
Truphylline. *See* aminophylline
Trypanosoma brucei, 526*t*
trypanosomiasis, 526*t*
TSH (thyroid-stimulating hormone),
    663*f*, 664*t*
TSPA. *See* thiotepa
tube feeding. *See* enteral nutrition
tubercles, 506, 795
tuberculosis:
  incidence, 506
  pathophysiology, 506
  pharmacotherapy. *See* ANTITUBERCULOSIS
    DRUGS
  prevention, 508
  transmission, 506
tubocurarine, 256*t*, 257
tumor, 552, 553*t*, 795
tumor suppressor genes, 553
Tums. *See* calcium carbonate
Tussionex. *See* hydrocodone polistirex and
    chlorpheniramine polistirex
Twinrix, 548
Tygacil. *See* tigecycline
Tylenol. *See* **acetaminophen**
Tylenol Allergy Sinus caplets, 582*t*
type 1 diabetes mellitus, 683, 786.
    See also diabetes mellitus
type 2 diabetes mellitus, 689, 786.
    See also diabetes mellitus
typhoid fever, 485*t*
typical antipsychotics. *See*
    NONPHENOTHIAZINES; PHENOTHIAZINES
tyramine:
  definition, 194, 795
  foods containing, 195*t*
  MAOIs and, 160, 194
Tyzine. *See* tetrahydrozoline

U

ulcer, 612
ulcerative colitis, 624*t*, 630, 795
Ultane. *See* sevoflurane

Ultiva. *See* remifentanil hydrochloride
Ultracet. *See* tramadol/acetaminophen
Ultralente. *See* extended insulin zinc suspension
Ultram. *See* tramadol
ultraviolet light therapy, 768
Unasyn, 490
undecylenic acid, 520*t*, 521, 756
undernutrition, 654, 795
Unipen. *See* nafcillin
Uniretic, 309*t*
unoprostone, 773, 774*t*
unstable angina, 347, 795. *See also* angina pectoris
upper gastrointestinal tract:
  acid production, 611–12
  anatomy, 612*f*
  digestive process, 611
  disorders
    gastroesophageal reflux disease. *See* gastroesophageal reflux disease
    incidence, 611*t*
    peptic ulcer disease. *See* peptic ulcer disease
upper respiratory tract, 579–80, 579*f*
Urabeth. *See* **bethanechol**
uracil, 562*f*
urea, 433, 433*t*
Ureaphil. *See* urea
Urecholine. *See* bethanechol
Urex. *See* methenamine
URIC ACID INHIBITORS:
  drugs classified as
    allopurinol. *See* allopurinol
    colchicine. *See* **colchicine**
    probenecid, 747, 748*t*, 799
    sulfinpyrazone, 747, 748*t*, 799
  nursing considerations, 748, 750
    client teaching, 750
    lifespan considerations, 750
    nursing process focus, 749–50*t*
  pharmacotherapy with, 747
Uridon. *See* chlorthalidone
urinalysis, 425, 795
urinary tract infection (UTI):
  bacteria causing, 485*t*
  incidence, 484*t*
  natural therapy with cranberry, 433*t*
urine, 424
Urocide. *See* **hydrochlorothiazide**
urofollitropin, 714*t*
Uro-KP neutral. *See* potassium and sodium phosphates
U.S. Adopted Name Council, 13
U.S. Department of Health and Human Services, 6*f*
U.S. drug schedules, 15
U.S. Pharmacopoeia (USP):
  history, 5, 6*f*
  medication error reporting system, 96
U.S. Pharmacopoeia-National Formulary (USP-NF), 5, 6*f*
USP label, 5, 5*f*

uterus:
  dysfunctional bleeding. *See* dysfunctional uterine bleeding
  relaxants. *See* TOCOLYTICS
  stimulants. *See* OXYTOCICS

V

vaccination, 457, 795. *See also* vaccines
vaccines:
  administration, 457–58
  adverse effects, 458
  anthrax, 33
  definition, 456
  diphtheria, tetanus, and pertussis, 460*t*
  ethnic/racial considerations, 461*t*
  haemophilus type B conjugate, 460*t*
  hepatitis B. *See* **hepatitis B vaccine**
  influenza, 460*t*, 546
  measles, mumps, and rubella, 460*t*
  nursing considerations, 458
    client teaching, 458–59
  pneumococcal, 460*t*
  poliovirus, 460*t*
  public health effects, 455*t*
  schedules and ages, 460*t*
  smallpox, 23
  types, 456
  varicella zoster/chicken pox, 460*t*
Vaccinum myrtillus. *See* bilberry
vaginal drug administration, 36*t*, 37, 38*f*
Vagistat. *See* tioconazole
valacyclovir, 544*t*, 801
valdecoxib, 475
Valergen. *See* estradiol valerate
valerian:
  drug interactions
    lorazepam, 163*t*
    morphine sulfate, 228*t*
    overview, 113*t*
    phenobarbital, 176*t*
    thiopental, 255*t*
  uses, 110*t*, 157*t*
Valeriana officinalis. *See* valerian
Valisone. *See* betamethasone
Valium. *See* **diazepam**
valproic acid (divalproex sodium), **180***t*
  actions and uses, 180*t*
  administration alerts, 180*t*
  adverse effects, 165*t*, 178*t*, 179, 180*t*, 200*t*
  Canadian/U.S. trade names, 799
  interactions, 180*t*
  overdose treatment, 180*t*
  pharmacokinetics, 180*t*
  prescription ranking, 801
  for specific conditions
    anxiety, 165*t*
    bipolar disorder, 200, 200*t*
    migraine, 238*t*
    seizures, 173*t*, 178*t*
valrubicin, 563, 564*t*
valsartan, 316*t*, 334, 800
Valstar. *See* valrubicin
Vancenase. *See* **beclomethasone**

Vanceril. *See* **beclomethasone**
Vancocin. *See* vancomycin
vancomycin, 504*t*, 506
Vanlev. *See* omapatrilat
Vantas. *See* histrelin
Vantin. *See* cefpodoxime
VAQTA. *See* hepatitis A vaccine
vardenafil, 723, 723*t*
varicella, 756
varicella zoster/chicken pox vaccine, 460*t*, 545*t*
Varivax. *See* varicella zoster/chicken pox vaccine
Vascor. *See* bepridil
Vaseretic, 309*t*
VASOCONSTRICTORS:
  adverse effects, 414*t*, 587*t*
  drugs classified as
    mephentermine, 414*t*
    naphazoline HCl, 587*t*, 779, 779*t*
    norepinephrine. *See* **norepinephrine**
    oxymetazoline. *See* **oxymetazoline**
    phenylephrine. *See* **phenylephrine**
    tetrahydrozoline, 587*t*, 779, 779*t*
  nursing considerations, 415
    client teaching, 415
  for specific conditions
    ophthalmic irritation, 779, 779*t*
    shock, 414–15, 414*t*
VASODILATORS:
  adverse effects, 324*t*, 333*t*
  drugs classified as
    diazoxide, 324, 324*t*, 325
    hydralazine. *See* **hydralazine**
    isosorbide dinitrate. *See* **isosorbide dinitrate**
    minoxidil, 324*t*, 325
    nitroprusside, 324, 324*t*, 325
  mechanisms of action, 332*f*, 338
  for specific conditions
    heart failure
      nursing considerations, 338
      route and adult doses, 333*t*
      therapeutic approach, 338
    hypertension
      nursing considerations, 324–25
      nursing process focus, 326*t*
      route and adult doses, 324*t*
      therapeutic approach, 324
vasomotor center, 304, 795
vasopeptidase inhibitors, 317
vasopressin, 665*t*
  actions and uses, 665*t*
  administration alerts, 665*t*
  adverse effects, 664*t*, 665*t*
  interactions, 665*t*
  overdose treatment, 665*t*
  pharmacokinetics, 665*t*
  route and adult dose, 664*t*
vasopressors. *See* VASOCONSTRICTORS
vasospastic (Prinzmetal's) angina, 347, 795. *See also* angina pectoris
Vasotec. *See* **enalapril**

vastus lateralis site, 41, 82
Veetids. *See* penicillin V
Velban. *See* vinblastine
Velbe. *See* vinblastine
Velcade. *See* bortezomib
Velosef. *See* cephradine
vendor-managed inventory (VMI)
    package, 21, 795
venlafaxine, 160*t*, 188, 189*t*, 800
Venofer. *See* iron sucrose injection
Venoglobulin-S. *See* immune globulin
    intravenous
ventilation, 594–95
Ventolin. *See* albuterol
ventricular fibrillation, 363*t*
ventricular flutter, 363*t*
ventricular tachycardia, 363*t*
ventrogluteal site, 39, 41
verapamil, 373*t*
    actions and uses, 373*t*
    administration alerts, 373*t*
    adverse effects, 238*t*, 350*t*, 367*t*, 373*t*
    Canadian/U.S. trade names, 799
    interactions, 373*t*
    mechanisms of action, 314
    overdose treatment, 373*t*
    pharmacokinetics, 373*t*
    prescription ranking, 800
    for specific conditions
        angina and myocardial infarction, 350*t*
        dysrhythmias, 367*t*
        migraine, 238*t*
Verelan. *See* **verapamil**
Vermox. *See* **mebendazole**
Versed. *See* midazolam
very low-density lipoprotein (VLDL),
    289, 289*f*
vesicants, 557, 795
vestibular apparatus, 795
Vfend. *See* voriconazole
Viagra. *See* **sildenafil**
Vibra Tabs. *See* doxycycline
Vibramycin. *See* doxycycline
Vibrio cholerae, 485*t*
Vicodin, 228
vidarabine, 544*t*, 545
Vidaza. *See* azacitidine
Videx. *See* didanosine
vildaglipton, 691
villi, 611
Vimicon. *See* cyproheptadine
vinblastine, 555*f*, 565, 566*t*, 799
VINCA ALKALOIDS:
    adverse effects, 566*t*
    characteristics, 565, 795
    drugs classified as
        vinblastine, 555*f*, 565, 566*t*, 799
        vincristine. *See* **vincristine**
        vinorelbine, 565, 566*t*
    nursing considerations, 566–67
        client teaching, 567
    pharmacotherapy with, 565
    route and adult doses, 566*t*

Vinca rosea, 565
vincristine, 567*t*
    actions and uses, 555, 555*f*, 565, 567*t*
    administration alerts, 567*t*
    adverse effects, 566*t*, 567*t*
    interactions, 567*t*
    overdose treatment, 567*t*
    pharmacokinetics, 567*t*
    route and adult dose, 566*t*
vinorelbine, 565, 566*t*
Vioxx. *See* rofecoxib
Vira-A. *See* vidarabine
Viracept. *See* nelfinavir
viral infections, 534*t*. *See also* specific
    viruses
Viramune. *See* nevirapine
Viread. *See* tenofovir
virilization, 719, 796
virion, 533, 795
Viroptic. *See* trifluridine
virulence, 484, 795
viruses, 533–34, 533*f*, 796
visceral pain, 224
Visculose. *See* methylcellulose
Visine. *See* tetrahydrozoline
Visine LR. *See* **oxymetazoline**
Vistaril. *See* hydroxyzine
Vistide. *See* cidofovir
visual impairments, 69*t*
Vita-C. *See* vitamin C
vitamin(s):
    characteristics, 642, 796
    classification, 642–43
    deficiencies, 643*t*, 644
    excess, 644
    functions, 643*t*
    lipid-soluble
        characteristics, 643
        nursing considerations, 646
            client teaching, 646
        vitamin A. *See* **vitamin A**
        vitamin D. *See* vitamin D
        vitamin E. *See* vitamin E
        vitamin K. *See* vitamin K
    recommended dietary allowances,
        643, 643*t*
    supplements, 642*t*, 645*t*
    water-soluble
        characteristics, 643
        nursing considerations, 648–49
            client teaching, 648–49
        vitamin B_1. *See* vitamin B_1
        vitamin B_2. *See* vitamin B_2
        vitamin B_3. *See* vitamin B_3
        vitamin B_6. *See* vitamin B_6
        vitamin B_9. *See* **folic acid/folate**
        vitamin B_{12}. *See* **vitamin B_{12}**
        vitamin C. *See* vitamin C
vitamin A, 645*t*
    characteristics, 644
    deficiency, 643*t*
    functions, 643*t*
    pharmacotherapy with

actions and uses, 644, 645*t*
    administration alerts, 644*t*
    adverse effects, 644*t*, 645*t*
    interactions, 645*t*
    route and adult dose, 644*t*
    recommended dietary allowance, 643*t*
    sources, 644
vitamin B complex, 643*t*
vitamin B_1:
    deficiency, 643*t*, 646
    functions, 643*t*
    pharmacotherapy with, 646, 647*t*
    recommended dietary allowance, 643*t*
    sources, 646
vitamin B_2:
    deficiency, 643*t*, 646
    functions, 643*t*
    for migraine prophylaxis, 238*t*
    pharmacotherapy with, 646, 647*t*
    recommended dietary allowance, 643*t*
    sources, 646
vitamin B_3 (niacin):
    deficiency, 643*t*, 646
    functions, 643*t*
    for hyperlipidemia
        adverse effects, 292*t*, 296–97
        mechanisms of action, 294*f*
        nursing considerations, 297
            client teaching, 297
        pharmacotherapy with, 296–97
        route and adult dose, 292*t*
    pharmacotherapy with, 646, 647*t*
    prescription ranking, 801
    recommended dietary allowance, 643*t*
    sources, 646
vitamin B_6:
    deficiency, 395*t*, 643*t*, 647
    drug interactions, 265
    functions, 643*t*, 647
    pharmacotherapy with, 647, 647*t*
    recommended dietary allowance, 643*t*
vitamin B_9. *See* **folic acid/folate**
vitamin B_{12} (cyanocobalamin), 403*t*
    deficiency, 395*t*, 402, 643*t*, 644
    functions, 643*t*, 647
    H_2-receptor blockers and, 617*t*
    metabolism, 401–2, 402*f*
    pharmacotherapy with
        actions and uses, 403*t*
        administration alerts, 403*t*
        adverse effects, 402*t*, 403*t*, 647*t*
        interactions, 403*t*
        nursing considerations, 403
            client teaching, 403
        route and adult dose, 402*t*, 647*t*
    recommended dietary allowance, 643*t*
    sources, 647
vitamin C:
    common cold and, 647*t*
    deficiency, 643*t*, 647
    functions, 643*t*, 647
    pharmacotherapy with, 647, 647*t*
    recommended dietary allowance, 643*t*

vitamin D:
deficiency, 643t
functions, 643t
pharmacotherapy with, 644, 644t
calcifediol, 736t
calcitriol. See **calcitriol**
ergocalciferol, 736t
nursing considerations, 738
client teaching, 738–39
lifespan considerations, 738
recommended dietary allowance, 643t
sources, 644
synthesis, 733, 735f
vitamin E:
deficiency, 643t, 645
functions, 643t
nursing considerations, 646
client teaching, 646
pharmacotherapy with, 644t, 645
recommended dietary allowance, 643t
sources, 645
vitamin K:
deficiency, 643t, 645
functions, 643t
nursing considerations, 646
client teaching, 646
pharmacotherapy with, 644t, 645
recommended dietary allowance, 643t
sources, 645
Vita-Plus E. See vitamin E
vitiligo, 753, 796
Vivactil. See protriptyline
Vivonex T.E.N, 655
VLDL (very low-density lipoprotein), 289, 289f
volatile inhalants, abuse, 120t
Voltaren. See diclofenac
vomiting, 632–33. See also nausea and vomiting, emesis
vomiting center, 632, 796
von Willebrand's disease, 378t, 380–81, 796
voriconazole, 519t
VoSol. See acetic acid and hydrocortisone
VX, 24t
Vytorin, 299. See also ezetimibe; simvastatin

W

warfarin, 384t
actions and uses, 384t
administration alerts, 384t
adverse effects, 382t, 384t
Canadian/U.S. trade names, 799
genetic polymorphisms affecting metabolism, 104t
interactions
drug, 50
herbal therapies, 113t, 384t
oral contraceptives, 701
nursing considerations, 382–84
client teaching, 384
lifespan considerations, 383

overdose treatment, 384t
pharmacokinetics, 384t
prescription ranking, 800, 801
for specific conditions
after myocardial infarction, 358
thromboembolic disease, 381, 382t
Warfilone. See **warfarin**
WBC (white blood cell count), 355t
Welchol. See colesevelam
Wellbutrin. See bupropion
Wellbutrin XL. See bupropion
Wellferon. See interferon alfa-n1
Westcort. See **hydrocortisone**
white blood cell count (WBC), 355t
whole blood, 413t
Winpred. See **prednisone**
WinRho SDF. See Rho(D) immune globulin
withdrawal, 15, 119, 796
withdrawal syndromes, 119, 120t, 796
Wyamine. See mephentermine
Wycillin. See penicillin G procaine
Wymox. See amoxicillin
Wytensin. See guanabenz

X

Xalatan. See **latanoprost**
Xanax. See alprazolam
Xeloda. See capecitabine
Xenical. See orlistat
Xopenex. See levalbuterol
Xylocaine. See **lidocaine**
Xylocard. See **lidocaine**
xylometazoline, 587t

Y

Yasmin, 700t
yeasts, 514, 796
Yodoxin. See iodoquinol
yohimbe, 228t
young adulthood, 84, 796
Yutopar. See ritodrine

Z

zafirlukast, 605t
actions and uses, 603, 605t
administration alerts, 605t
adverse effects, 601t, 605t
interactions, 605t
pharmacokinetics, 605t
route and adult dose, 601t
Zagam. See sparfloxacin
zalcitabine, 537t
zaleplon, 165t, 167
Zanaflex. See tizanidine
zanamivir, 546, 547t
Zanosar. See streptozocin
Zantac. See **ranitidine HCl**
Zapex. See oxazepam
Zarontin. See **ethosuximide**
Zaroxolyn. See metolazone
Zebeta. See bisoprolol
Zefazone. See cefmetazole

Zenapax. See daclizumab
Zerit. See stavudine
Zestoretic, 309t. See also **lisinopril**
Zestril. See **lisinopril**
Zetia. See ezetimibe
Zevalin. See ibritumomab tiuxetan
Ziac, 309t
Ziagen. See abacavir
zidovudine, 538t
actions and uses, 538t
administration alerts, 538t
adverse effects, 537t, 538t
interactions, 538t
pharmacokinetics, 538t
resistance, 537
for specific conditions
HIV prophylaxis after occupational exposure, 543
HIV-AIDS, 536, 537t
prevention of perinatal HIV transmission, 543
zileuton, 601t, 603
Zinacef. See cefuroxime
zinc, 653t, 654
zinc acetate, 650t
zinc gluconate, 650t
zinc sulfate, 650t
Zincate. See zinc sulfate
Zingiber officinalis. See ginger
ziprasidone, 218t
Zithromax. See azithromycin
Zocor. See simvastatin
Zofran. See ondansetron
Zoladex. See goserelin
zoledronic acid, 571t
Zollinger-Ellison syndrome, 618t, 796
zolmitriptan, 238t
Zoloft. See **sertraline**
zolpidem, 164t
actions and uses, 164t, 165
administration alerts, 164t
adverse effects, 164t, 165, 165t
contraindications, 165
interactions, 164t
overdose treatment, 164t
pharmacokinetics, 164t
prescription ranking, 800
route and adult dose, 165t
Zometa. See zoledronic acid
Zomig. See zolmitriptan
Zonegran. See zonisamide
zonisamide, 178, 178t, 180
Zosyn. See piperacillin tazobactam
Zovirax. See **acyclovir**
Zyban. See bupropion
Zyflo. See zileuton
Zyloprim. See allopurinol
Zyprexa. See olanzapine
Zyrtec. See cetirizine
Zyrtec-D. See cetirizine/pseudoephedrine
Zyvox. See linezolid

Pearson Education, Inc.

YOU SHOULD CAREFULLY READ THE TERMS AND CONDITIONS BEFORE USING THIS DVD-ROM PACKAGE. USING THIS DVD-ROM PACKAGE INDICATES YOUR ACCEPTANCE OF THESE TERMS AND CONDITIONS.

Pearson Education, Inc. provides this program and licenses its use. You assume responsibility for the selection of the program to achieve your intended results, and for the installation, use, and results obtained from the program. This license extends only to use of the program in the United States or countries in which the program is marketed by authorized distributors.

LICENSE GRANT

You hereby accept a nonexclusive, nontransferable, permanent license to install and use the program ON A SINGLE COMPUTER at any given time. You may copy the program solely for backup or archival purposes in support of your use of the program on the single computer. You may not modify, translate, disassemble, decompile, or reverse engineer the program, in whole or in part.

TERM

The License is effective until terminated. Pearson Education, Inc. reserves the right to terminate this License automatically if any provision of the License is violated. You may terminate the License at any time. To terminate this License, you must return the program, including documentation, along with a written warranty stating that all copies in your possession have been returned or destroyed.

LIMITED WARRANTY

THE PROGRAM IS PROVIDED "AS IS" WITHOUT WARRANTY OF ANY KIND, EITHER EXPRESSED OR IMPLIED, INCLUDING, BUT NOT LIMITED TO, THE IMPLIED WARRANTIES OR MERCHANTABILITY AND FITNESS FOR A PARTICULAR PURPOSE. THE ENTIRE RISK AS TO THE QUALITY AND PERFORMANCE OF THE PROGRAM IS WITH YOU. SHOULD THE PROGRAM PROVE DEFECTIVE, YOU (AND NOT PRENTICE-HALL, INC. OR ANY AUTHORIZED DEALER) ASSUME THE ENTIRE COST OF ALL NECESSARY SERVICING, REPAIR, OR CORRECTION. NO ORAL OR WRITTEN INFORMATION OR ADVICE GIVEN BY PRENTICE-HALL, INC., ITS DEALERS, DISTRIBUTORS, OR AGENTS SHALL CREATE A WARRANTY OR INCREASE THE SCOPE OF THIS WARRANTY.

SOME STATES DO NOT ALLOW THE EXCLUSION OF IMPLIED WARRANTIES, SO THE ABOVE EXCLUSION MAY NOT APPLY TO YOU. THIS WARRANTY GIVES YOU SPECIFIC LEGAL RIGHTS AND YOU MAY ALSO HAVE OTHER LEGAL RIGHTS THAT VARY FROM STATE TO STATE.

Pearson Education, Inc. does not warrant that the functions contained in the program will meet your requirements or that the operation of the program will be uninterrupted or error-free.

However, Pearson Education, Inc. warrants the DVD-ROM on which the program is furnished to be free from defects in material and workmanship under normal use for a period of ninety (90) days from the date of delivery to you as evidenced by a copy of your receipt.

The program should not be relied on as the sole basis to solve a problem whose incorrect solution could result in injury to person or property. If the program is employed in such a manner, it is at the user's own risk and Pearson Education, Inc. explicitly disclaims all liability for such misuse.

LIMITATION OF REMEDIES

Pearson Education, Inc.'s entire liability and your exclusive remedy shall be:
1. the replacement of any DVD-ROM not meeting Pearson Education, Inc.'s "LIMITED WARRANTY" and that is returned to Pearson Education, or
2. if Pearson Education is unable to deliver a replacement DVD-ROM that is free of defects in materials or workmanship, you may terminate this agreement by returning the program.

IN NO EVENT WILL PRENTICE-HALL, INC. BE LIABLE TO YOU FOR ANY DAMAGES, INCLUDING ANY LOST PROFITS, LOST SAVINGS, OR OTHER INCIDENTAL OR CONSEQUENTIAL DAMAGES ARISING OUT OF THE USE OR INABILITY TO USE SUCH PROGRAM EVEN IF PRENTICE-HALL, INC. OR AN AUTHORIZED DISTRIBUTOR HAS BEEN ADVISED OF THE POSSIBILITY OF SUCH DAMAGES, OR FOR ANY CLAIM BY ANY OTHER PARTY.

SOME STATES DO NOT ALLOW FOR THE LIMITATION OR EXCLUSION OF LIABILITY FOR INCIDENTAL OR CONSEQUENTIAL DAMAGES, SO THE ABOVE LIMITATION OR EXCLUSION MAY NOT APPLY TO YOU.

GENERAL

You may not sublicense, assign, or transfer the license of the program. Any attempt to sublicense, assign or transfer any of the rights, duties, or obligations hereunder is void.

This Agreement will be governed by the laws of the State of New York.

Should you have any questions concerning this Agreement, you may contact Pearson Education, Inc. by writing to:

Director of New Media
Higher Education Division
Pearson Education, Inc.
One Lake Street
Upper Saddle River, NJ 07458

Should you have any questions concerning technical support, you may contact:

Product Support Department: Monday–Friday 8:00 A.M. –8:00 P.M. and Sunday 5:00 P.M.-12:00 A.M. (All times listed are Eastern). 1-800-677-6337

You can also get support by filling out the web form located at http://247.prenhall.com

YOU ACKNOWLEDGE THAT YOU HAVE READ THIS AGREEMENT, UNDERSTAND IT, AND AGREE TO BE BOUND BY ITS TERMS AND CONDITIONS. YOU FURTHER AGREE THAT IT IS THE COMPLETE AND EXCLUSIVE STATEMENT OF THE AGREEMENT BETWEEN US THAT SUPERSEDES ANY PROPOSAL OR PRIOR AGREEMENT, ORAL OR WRITTEN, AND ANY OTHER COMMUNICATIONS BETWEEN US RELATING TO THE SUBJECT MATTER OF THIS AGREEMENT.

NURSING EXCELLENCE

Success in Skills, Review, & Test Preparation

Excellence in Nursing Skills

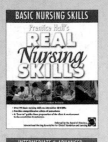
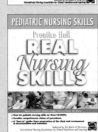
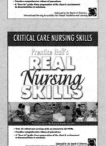
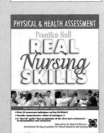
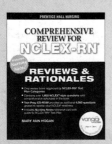

Prentice Hall's Real Nursing Skills on CD-ROMs

Prentice Hall Real Nursing Skills series offers you the complete foundation for competency in performing clinical skills. The CD-ROMS provide comprehensive procedures demonstrated in hundreds of videos, animations, illustrations, and photographs. These skills CD-ROMs are designed to help you visualize how to perform each skill and understand the concepts and rationales for each skill.

Basic Nursing Skills:
94 skills on 5 CD-ROMs. 2005, ISBN: 0-13-191526-6
Intermediate & Advanced Nursing Skills:
84 skills on 5 CD-ROMs. 2005, ISBN: 0-13-119344-9
Physical & Health Assessment Nursing Skills:
25 skills on 5 CD-ROMs. 2006, ISBN: 0-13-191525-8
Maternal-Newborn & Women's Health Nursing Skills:
24 skills on 2 CD-ROMs. 2005, ISBN: 0-13-191527-4
Pediatric Nursing Skills:
65 skills on 3 CD-ROMs. 2006, ISBN: 0-13-191524-X
Critical Care Nursing Skills:
35 skills on 2 CD-ROMs. 2005, ISBN: 0-13-119264-7

Excellence in NCLEX-RN® Review

Prentice Hall's Comprehensive Review for NCLEX-RN® is designed specifically to help you achieve nursing excellence by simplifying your review and making the most of your valuable study time. This review book is uniquely organized according to the April 2007 NCLEX-RN® Test Plan, providing you with both a comprehensive content review and practice questions in sections covering * Safe, Effective Care Environment * Health Promotion * Physiological Integrity, and * Psychosocial Integrity. Throughout this book, you will find:

- **Memory Aids** that help you remember key concepts.
- **NCLEX® Alerts** that identify critical concepts you are likely to see on the NCLEX-RN®.
- **Check Your NCLEX® IQ** boxes that help you to assess your readiness for the NCLEX-RN® on the topics covered in the chapter.
- **Practice Tests** at the end of the chapter that review the concepts from that chapter and provide comprehensive rationales and test-taking strategies to help you find the right answers.

2008, ISBN 0-13-119599-9

The **NCLEX-RN® Test Prep CD-ROM** that comes with your book simulates the test-taking environment by allowing you to practice questions on the computer. It contains all the questions in the book PLUS thousands of additional questions. You can choose to practice in Study, Quiz, or Exam modes, and you will receive detailed reports that will help you focus your preparation for NCLEX-RN®.

For additional information and resources